Clinical Practice in Small Incision Cataract Surgery (Phaco Manual)

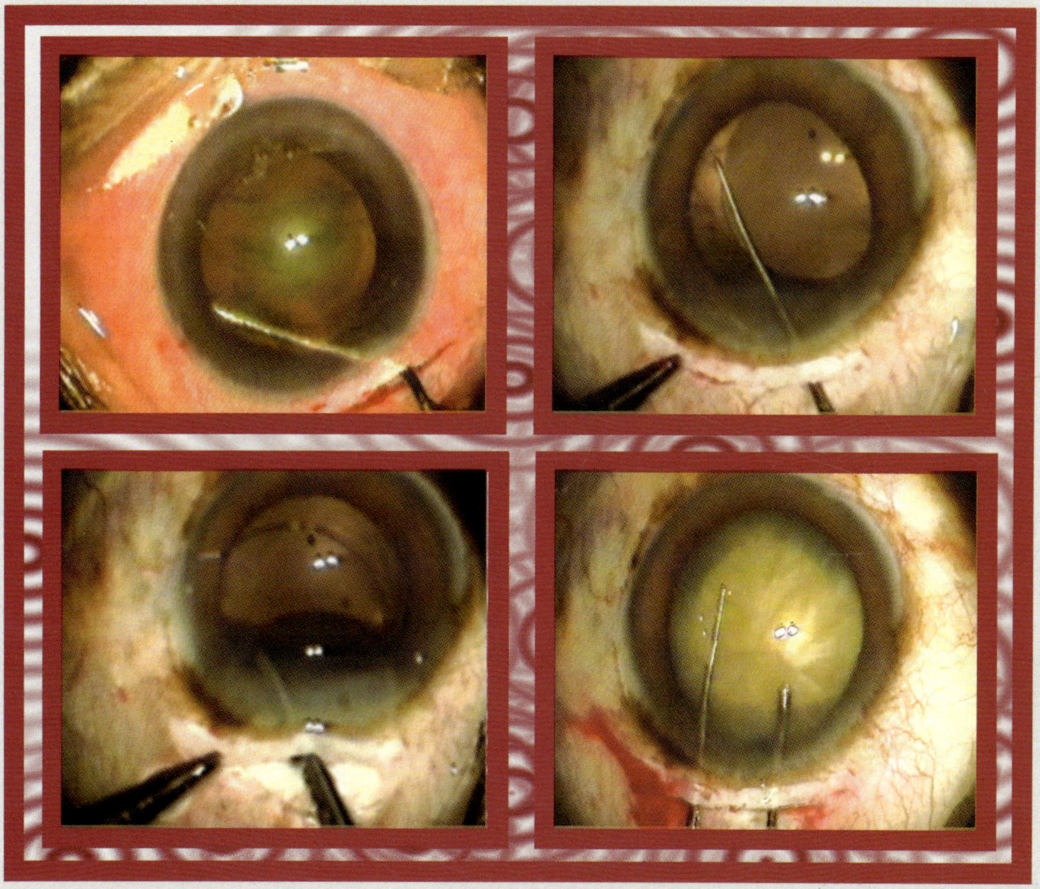

Clinical Practice in Small Incision Cataract Surgery Phaco Manual

Editors

Ashok Garg MS, PhD, FIAO(Bel), FRSM, ADM, FICA, FAIMS, FICS
National and International Gold Medalist
Medical Director
Garg Eye Institute & Research Centre
235-Model Town, Dabra Chowk
Hisar, India

Luther L Fry MD
Fry Eye Associates
PA/Ophthalmology
Garden City
Kansas, USA

Geoffery Tabin MD
Associate Professor of Ophthalmology
University of Vermont
College of Medicine
Burlington, Vermont, USA

Francisco J Gutiérrez-Carmona MD, PhD
Associate Professor
Ophthalmologic Research Institute
Ramon Castroviejo
Hoyo de Manzanares
Madrid, Spain

Suresh K Pandey MD
Instructor, John A Moran Eye Center
Department of Ophthalmology
and Visual Sciences
University of Utah
Salt Lake City, Utah, USA

Foreword
Pandelis A Papadopoulos

Taylor & Francis
Taylor & Francis Group
LONDON AND NEW YORK
A MARTIN DUNITZ BOOK

First published in India in 2004 by
Jaypee Brothers Medical Publishers (P) Ltd, New Delhi, India.
EMCA House, 23/23B Ansari Road, Daryaganj, New Delhi 110 002, India
Phones: 23272143, 23272703, 23282021, 23245672 m\, Fax: +91-011-23276490
e-mail: jpmedpub@del2.vsnl.net.in, Visit our website: www.jaypeebrothers.com

First published in the United Kingdom by Taylor & Francis, a member of the Taylor & Francis Group in 2004. Exclusively distributed worldwide (excluding the Indian Subcontinent) by Martin Dunitz, a member of the Taylor & Francis Group.

Tel.: +44 (0) 20 7583 9855
Fax.: +44 (0) 20 7842 2298
E-mail: info@dunitz.co.uk
Website: http://www.dunitz.co.uk

A CIP record for this book is available from the British Library.

ISBN 1 84184 467 5

Distributed in North and South America by

Taylor & Francis
2000 NW Corporate Blvd
Boca Raton, FL 33431, USA

Within Continental USA
Tel.: 800 272 7737; Fax.: 800 374 3401
Outside Continental USA
Tel.: 561 994 0555; Fax.: 561 361 6018
E-mail: orders@crcpress.com

Distributed in the rest of the world (excluding the Indian Subcontinent) by
Thomson Publishing Services
Cheriton House
North Way
Andover, Hampshire SP10 5BE, UK
Tel.: +44 (0)1264 332424
E-mail: salesorder.tandf@thomsonpublishingservices.co.uk

Dedicated to

My Respected Param Pujya Guru Sant Gurmeet Ram Rahim Singh Ji
for his blessings and guidance.

My Respected Parents, my wife Dr. Aruna Garg, son Abhishek and daughter Anshul
for their endless support and constant encouragement.

My dear friend Dr. Amar Agarwal
for his expert advice and whole hearted support in this endeavour.

ASHOK GARG

My wife, Ardis and my sons, Eric and David
whose sacrifices have made my career in Ophthalmology possible.

LUTHER L FRY

My wife, Jean, son Danny and daughters Sara, Ali, Emilia, and Livia
for their love and support.

To my partner in Himalayan Cataract Project, Dr. Sanduk Ruit.

To Dr Ashok Garg
for making this book come to life.

GEOFFERY TABIN

My wife, Carmen and my daughters Marta, Laura
for their love and support.

All my teachers and particularly Prof. Ramon Castroviejo
who taught me the elegance and excellence in ocular surgery.

Dr Amar Agarwal for his friendship

FRANCISCO J GUTIÉRREZ-CARMONA

Param Pujya Gurudev, Pt. Shri Ram Sharma Acharya and
Mata Bhagawati Devi Sharma, Shantikunj, Haridwar, India
for their blessings.

My respected parents (Shri Kameshwar Prasad Pandey, and Smt. Maya Devi Pandey)
for helping me set higher goals.

My loving spouse, Dr. Vidushi
for her constant support.

My teacher and colleagues (particularly Dr Liliana Werner, Prof. David J Apple)
for transmitting their skills and expertise with passion and enthusiasm.

SURESH K PANDEY

Contributors

Albrecht Hennig
Lahan Eye Hospital
C/o UMN
PO Box 126
Kathmandu
Nepal

Amar Agarwal
Director
Dr Agarwal's Eye Hospital Pvt Ltd
19, Cathedral Road
Chennai-600086
India

Andrea M Izak
Department of Ophthalmology
Storm Eye Institute
Charleston SC
USA

Arif Adenwala
Consultant
Aditya Jyot Eye Hospital
Aashirwad, Vikaswadi, Dadar TT
Mumbai-400014
India

Arun Kshetrapal
Kshetrapal Eye Hospital and Research Centre
Kutchery Road
Ajmer-305001
India

Ashok Garg
Medical Director
Garg Eye Institute and Research Centre
235, Model Town, Dabra Chowk
Hisar-125005
India

Athiya Agarwal
Dr Agarwal's Eye Hospital Pvt Ltd
19, Cathedral Road
Chennai-600086
India

Azimuddin Azim Siraj
Dr Agarwal's Eye Hospital Pvt Ltd
19, Cathedral Road
Chennai-600086
India

Clement K Chan
Southern California Desert
Retina Consultant
PO Box 2467
Palm Springs CA 92263
USA

Cyres Mehta
Consultant
Mehta International Eye Institute
Colaba Eye Hospital
Sea side, 147-Colaba Road
Mumbai-400005
India

David J Apple
Director
John A Moran Eye Centre
Department of Ophthalmology and
Visual Sciences
5th Floor, University of Utah
50, North Medical Drive
Salt Lake City
Utah-84132
USA

David Meyer
Professor and Chairman
Department of Ophthalmology
Faculty of Health Sciences
University of Stellenbosch and
Tygerberg, Academic Hospital
South Africa

Edward Wilson
Professor and Chairman
Storm Eye Institute
Charleston SC
USA

Francisco J Gutiérrez-Carmona
Zarracin, 25-Urb
La Berzosa
28240, Hoyo de Manzanares
Madrid
Spain

Gaurav Shah
Consultant
Gaurav Laser Academy and
Varsha Nursing Home
105-A, Patel Shopping Centre
Chandavarkar Road
Borivili (W)
Mumbai-400092
India

Geoffery Tabin
Associate Professor of Ophthalmology
University of Vermont
College of Medicine
Burlington, Vermont
USA

Gerald R Schultz
Assistant Clinical Professor
Department of Ophthalmology
Loma Linda University
Loma Linda
California
USA

Haripriya Aravind
Aravind Eye Hospital
Madurai
India

Jagannath Boramani
Surya Netralaya
51, 4th Floor, Shanti Centre
Sector 17, Vashi
Navi Mumbai-400703
India

Jean-Marc Legeais
Hospital Hotel Dieu
Service d'ophtalmologie
1, Place due Parvis Notre Dame
75181, Paris Cedex 04,
France

KPS Malik
Department of Ophthalmology
Vardhman Mahavir Medical College
and Safdarjung Hospital
New Delhi, India

K Thiruvenkata Krishnan
Aravind Eye Hospital
Abhishekapakkam
Pondicherry-605007
India

Kamal Nagpal
Consultant
Retina Foundation
Shahibaug, Near Underbridge
Ahmedabad 380004
India

Kamaljeet Singh
Associate Professor, Ophthalmology
410, MLN Medical College
Allahabad
India

Keiki Mehta
Medical Director
Mehta International Eye Institute
Colaba Eye Hospital
Sea side, 147, Colaba Road
Mumbai-400005
India

Liliana Werner
Assistant Professor
John A Moran Eye Centre
Department of Ophthalmology and Visual Sciences
5th Floor, University of Utah
50, North Medical Drive
Salt Lake City
Utah-84132
USA

Luther L Fry
Fry Eye Associates
PA/Ophthalmology
310, East Walnut
Garden City
Kansas-67846-2562
USA

MS Ravindra
Director
Karthik Netralaya
Ashok Nagar, 89, 7th Cross, NR Colony
Bangalore-560050
India

Manish Nagpal
Consultant
Retina Foundation, Shahibaug
Near Underbridge, Ahmedabad 380004
India

Minu Mathen
Arvind Eye Hospital
Madurai
India

Nikhilesh Trivedi
Bhatera Road
Balaghat-481001
India

Nilesh Kanjani
Dr Agarwal's Eye Hospital Pvt Ltd
19, Cathedral Road
Chennai-600086
India

PN Nagpal
Medical Director
Retina Foundation
Shahibaug, Near Underbridge
Ahmedabad-380004
India

Pandelis A Papadopoulos
Director
Ophthalmology Department
Athens Metropolitan Hospital
Medical Director
Diagnostic, Therapeutic and Research Centre
Ophthalmo-check, 42, Poseidon Ave
Paleo Faliro, 17561, Athens, Hellas
Greece

Paul Liebenberg
Faculty of Medicine
Department of Ophthalmology
Cape Town
South Africa

RD Ravindran
Aravind Eye Hospital
Abhishekapakkam
Pondicherry-605007
India

Ramesh Kshetrapal
Kshetrapal Eye Hospital and Research Centre
Kutchery Road, Ajmer-305001
India

Ranjit S Dhaliwal
Eye Infirmary
Hira Mahal, Radha Soami Marg
Nabha-147201
India

Ruchi Goel
Consultant
Hindu Rao Hospital
New Delhi
India

RM Shanbhag
Hon Prof of Ophthalmology
Grant Medical College, Mumbai
Hon Ophthalmic Surgeon
PD Hinduja Hospital
Mumbai
India

Sasikanth
Dr Agarwal's Eye Hospital Pvt Ltd
19, Cathedral Road
Chennai -600086
India

Rupal H Trivedi
Storm Eye Institute
Department of Ophthalmology
Medical University of South Carolina
167, Ashley Avenue
Charleston SC
USA

Samuel L Pallin
Medical Director
The Lear Eye Clinic
10615 W, Thunderbird A100
Sun City, AZ 85351-3018
USA

Sanduk Ruit
Consultant
Tilganga Eye Centre
Gaushala, Kathmandu
Nepal

Shushmita
Consultant
Gaurav Laser Academy and
Varsha Nursing Home
105-A, Patel Shopping Centre
Chandavarkar Road
Borivili(W)
Mumbai-400092
India

S Natarajan
Medical Director
Aditya Jyot Eye Hospital
Aashirwad, Vikaswadi
Dadar TT, Mumbai-400014
India

Steve Charles
Charles Retina Institute
6401, Poplar Avenue, Suite 190
Memphis, Tennessee
USA

Steven G Lin
Southern California Desert Retina
Consultant, Palm Springs
USA

Sunita Agarwal
15, Eagle Street
Langford Town
Bangalore (India)
Villa No.2, Roundhouse 3
Al Wasl Road
Dubai PB 9168
Dubai

Suresh K Pandey
John A Moran Eye Centre
Department of Ophthalmology and
Visual Sciences
5th Floor, University of Utah
50, North Medical Drive, Salt Lake City
Utah-84132
USA

Tamer A Macky
Assistant Professor
Department of Ophthalmology
Cario University, Cario
Egypt

Tobias H Neuhann
Founder and Medical Director
Aam Augenklinik
AM Marienplatz
Marienplatz 18, Munich
Germany

Venkatesh Rengaraj
Aravind Eye Hospital
Abishekapakkam
Pondicherry-605007
India

Vidushi Sharma
RP Centre for Ophthalmic Sciences
AIIMS
New Delhi-110029
India

Yogesh Shah
Medical Director
Gaurav Laser Academy and
Varsha Nursing Home
105-A, Patel Shopping Centre
Chandavarkar Road
Borivili (W) Mumbai-400092
India

Foreword

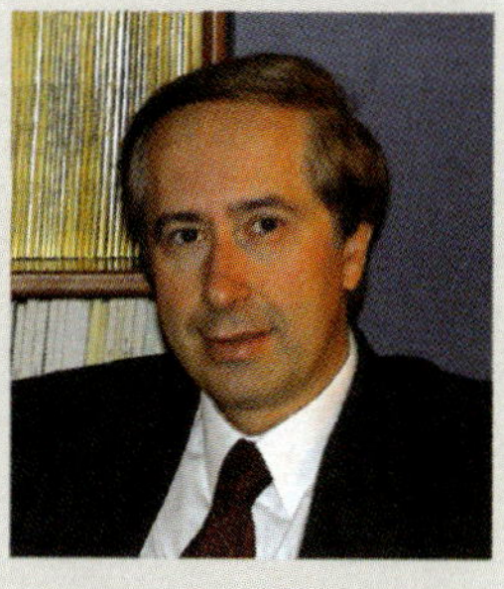

Since the invention of phacoemulsification by Dr. Charles Kelman, the incision size has been a challenge for the modern cataract surgeon. The incision size has continuously been reduced in the past thirty years. The importance of incision size is related to the safety provided by the smallest incision that can be left without suturing, the neutrality in astigmatism, one of the important steps in the realization of refractive cataract surgery and the ability to implant or inject an IOL through a very small, sealed incision.

Intraocular lens technology, kept the pace in this race against time, making significant steps in the recent years. The dream of the pioneers of this field, to operate through the smallest incision possible, with an IOL that can be inserted or injected through it, has finally come true at the dawn of the new millennium.

The *Clinical Practice in Small Incision Cataract Surgery (SICS)* is the first book on this new exciting era of cataract surgery. The editors, Drs. Ashok Garg, Luther L Fry, Geoffery Tabin, Francisco J Gutiérrez-Carmona, Suresh K Pandey and an international team of expert ophthalmic surgeons have contributed in the realization of this manual, that will become a very valuable source for the colleagues that are interested to adapt these techniques.

The "Clinical Practice in Small Incision Cataract Surgery" consists of 57 chapters divided in four sections that analyze every detail on small incision cataract surgery. The first chapter describes the anatomy and the biochemistry of the human crystalline lens. The etiology of cataract, its classification and various treatment modalities are beautifully illustrated. Drs. Sunita and Amar Agarwal wrote the next chapters on two very important issues in modern cataract surgery, the optical and acoustical biometry and the sterilization. Anesthesia, topical or non-topical, and also modern anesthetic viscoelastics compose the next chapters. The fluidics and the various viscosurgical devices play a significant role in the safety of cataract surgery, as described in the following chapters. Several pages are devoted to the preoperative preparation of the patient, the dynamics of SICS and surgical techniques utilized during the various operative steps.

Modern IOL materials and IOL implantation techniques through very small incision are some of the important issues that are covered in the "Clinical Practice in Small Incision Cataract Surgery". A significant amount of information on manual phacofragmentation through small incision, combined SICS and glaucoma surgery, and pediatric cataract surgery are also included. The management of complications from the anterior or posterior segment is extensively described. The etiology, the clinical manifestations and the pharmacological prevention of the posterior capsule opacification, a problem still to be solved, are presented in detail. The final chapter is an update on twenty-first century cataract-intraocular lens surgery, that describes the shape of things to come.

The "Clinical Practice in Small Incision Cataract Surgery" presents an overview of SICS with a look towards the future. I am very honored by the request of **Dr. Ashok Garg and his internationally known coauthors to write a foreword to this new manual. I would like to congratulate all the contributors of this excellent book, that will become a very important reference for the modern ophthalmic surgeon.**

Pandelis A. Papadopoulos MD, PhD, FEBO
Director, Ophthalmology Department Athens Metropolitan Hospital
Director Ophthalmo-Check Eye Center of Athens
General Secretary, Hellenic Society of Cataract and Refractive Surgery
42, Poseidon Avenue, Paleo Faliro, 17561 Athens, Hellas
tel: +30 210 9881800
fax:+30 210 9848505
e-mail: eyedoc@hol.gr

Preface

Cataract is currently the main cause of avoidable blindness specially in the developing world accounting for about three quarters of blindness. In developed world Phacoemulsification is the primary method of performing cataract surgery. However, in many developing countries involving the majority of cataract blindness in the world today, phacoemulsification is not viable due to density of cataract involved and high cost of the equipments. Significant efforts are being undertaken to increase the output of cataract surgical services in such countries. Manual small incision cataract surgery (MSICS) has emerged as first choice alternative to phacoemulsification to achieve a best unaided visual acuity with rapid postsurgical recovery and minimal surgery related complications. Incision size has been a challange for ophthalmologist and it has continuously been reduced in past two decades. Clinical significance of small incision has increased manifold related to safety provided by self sealing smallest incision and neutrality in astigmatism a vital factor in realization of best postoperative visual acuity and ability to implant modern foldable or Hydrogel and Artisan IOLs and faster rehabilitation.

This book on SICS has been written through a team effort with the sole aim of providing latest knowledge on Modern Techniques in SICS to ophthalmologists who are interested in manual small incision cataract surgery clinical practice. Fifty seven chapters of this book cover all aspects of SICS from Anatomy of Lens to various operative techniques, complications, management and recent advances.

We are highly thankful to all contributors who are masters of SICS techniques at an international level to share their knowledge and surgical skills in this book. We are thankful to our family members and friends who have extended every cooperation and stood by us to prepare this useful book.

Our special gratitude to Mr. JP Vij, Chairman and Managing Director and staff of Jaypee Brothers Medical Publishers (P) Ltd, a leading name in Medical Publication at an international level who extended full cooperation and never ruffled to prepare this high quality international book on small incision cataract surgery. Each author in this book has already left footprints on the sands of time and made every effort to shape this book as a worthwhile companion to our readers. Along with this book a complimentary CD Rom is also being provided showing various operative techniques of manual SICS by masters of this field.

We hope our book shall provide a comprehensive and complete up to date information on SICS to every ophthalmologist.

Editors

Contents

SECTION TWO
Manual Small Incision Cataract Surgery (MSICS) Techniques

SECTION THREE
Complications and Their Management

SECTION FOUR
Recent Advances and Future Considerations

CD Contents

CD 1

CD 2

Introduction

Thoughts on Small Incision Manual Extracapsular Surgery

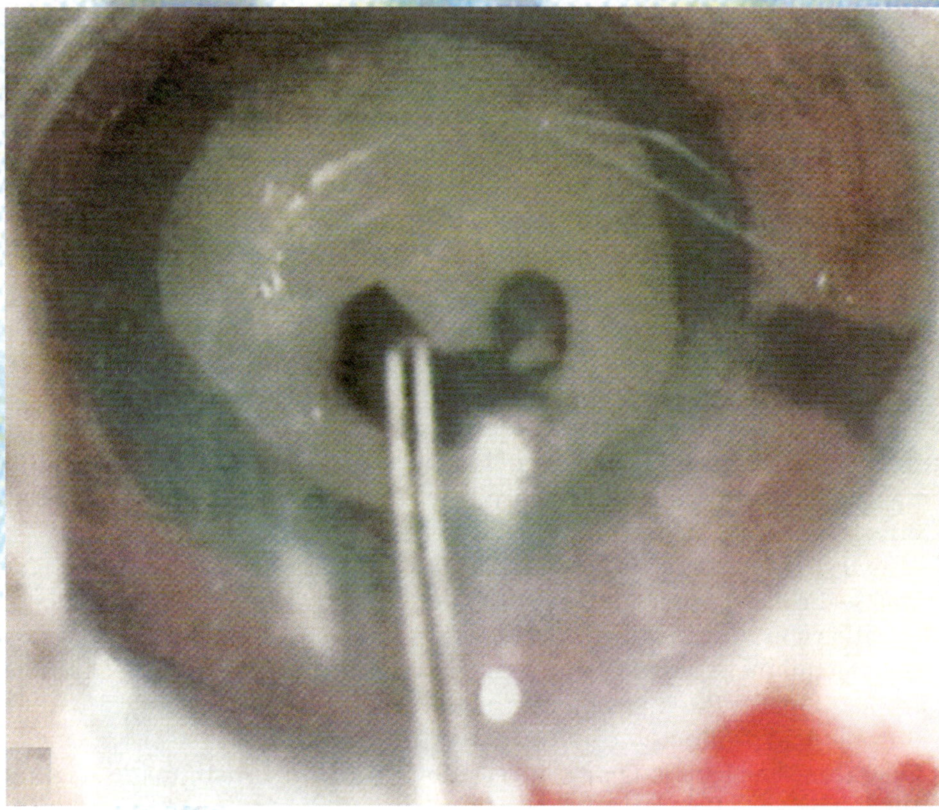

Thoughts on Small Incision Manual Extracapsular Surgery

Luther L Fry (USA)

In more affluent areas of the world, Phakoemulsification has become the primary method of performing extracapsular cataract surgery. There are, however, many areas, possibly involving the majority of cataract blindness in the world today, where phakoemulsification is not appropriate. This is because of the density of cataracts involved, and the cost and maintenance demands of the equipment.

I believe small incision manual extracapsular techniques, such as outlined in this book, give visual results equivalent to Phako, based on many years of doing both techniques in parallel on my personal patients. From my experience on the dense cataracts encountered in mission work, I believe small incision manual is superior to phako in these cases.

I would like to mention a few things which might be helpful to those starting with my small incision manual technique.

Start with an 8 mm incision, particularly for mature black cataracts.

This procedure works well under topical anesthesia. The patient may feel slight sensation with scleral cautery. This is not enough to bother them, but warn them before cauterizing, so they aren't startled. The procedure is otherwise painless under topical anesthesia. I like lidocaine 2% jelly for topical anesthesia and feel 0.2cc of 1% non-preserved lidocaine intracamerally through the side port before starting surgery makes it more comfortable. I have also used preserved lidocaine intracamerally. This did not cause any apparent endothelial problem in the small volume used, and might be an alternative if non-preserved is not available.

Povidone Iodide is equal to, or better than, even the newest generation of antibiotics, and much less expensive. I like the 5% (1/2 strength) on a saturated 4x4 gauze over the lids for 10 minutes pre-op, plus 2.5% (1/4 strength) in the cul-de-sac placed 15 minutes pre-op and not irrigated out. This2.5% can be re-applied post-op, particularly if antibiotics are not available. 5% causes mild punctuate keratitis if placed in the cul-de-sac; 2.5% does not, and is probably just as bacteriacidal.

Although the 7mm incision self-seals in nearly all cases, you might want to start with a 10-0 nylon "X" suture with buried knot. The 10-0 nylon can be placed on a 4x4 gauze pad and re-autoclaved without damage, allowing one suture to be used for multiple cases. (Dexon and Vicryl disintegrate if you attempt to autoclave them.)

This technique works just as well with can-opener capsulotomy as with capsulorhexis. In mature cataracts, the can-opener may be safer and easier, particularly if capsular dye is not available. (When using either the can-opener or capsulorhexis, make the opening as large as possible.)

This technique is viscoelastic dependent. Using the "sandwich" technique under air will result in striate keratopathy. Methylcellulose, however, works well and may be a more cost effective alternative to hyaluronic acid products.

Operating on steep axis of K gives about a 1 diopter astigmatic flattening on that axis (depending somewhat on age). Presently, it is easier for me to do everyone from a temporal approach, and add limbal relaxing incisions for cylinder.

In closing, I believe that one of the small incision manual techniques, such as outlined in this book, should be in the armamentarium of every cataract surgeon. Even those doing virtually all phako (such as myself) will encounter the occasional rock hard cataract which is probably better managed by manual technique. Anyone doing small incision manual techniques can be assured they are performing state-of-the art surgery for their patients, with results just as good as with phakoemulsification.

Section One

Preoperative Evaluation and Preliminary Considerations

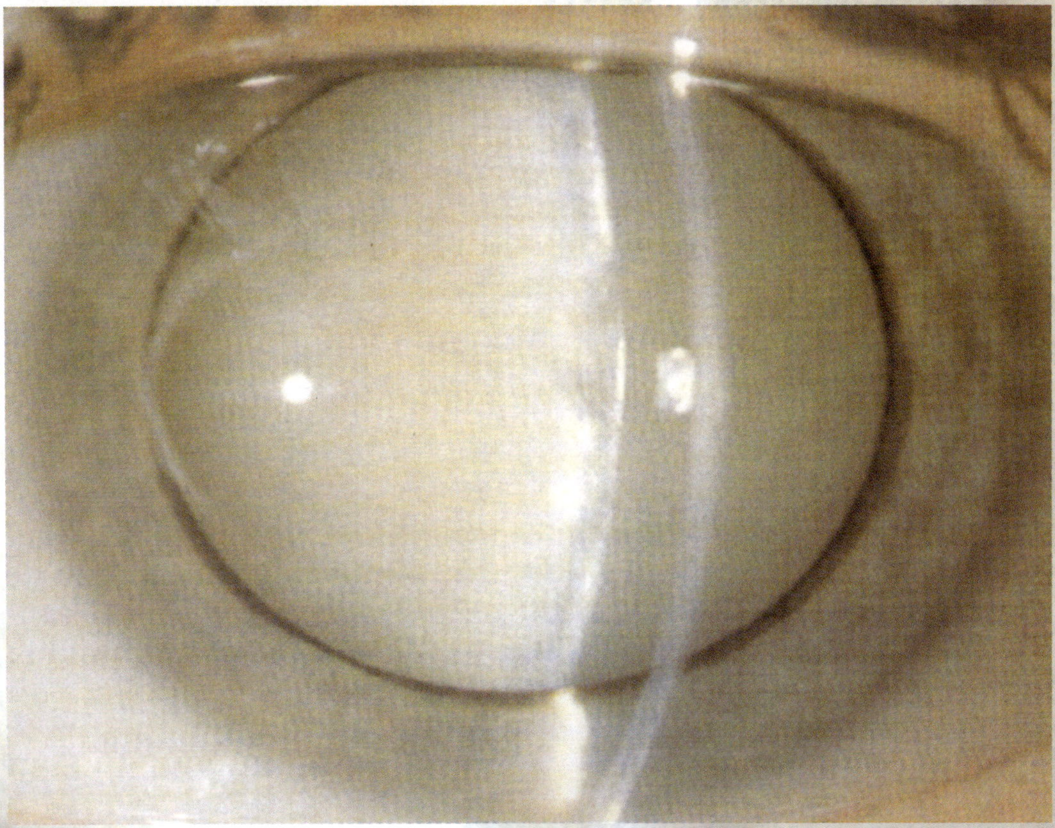

- Anatomy of Human Crystalline Lens, Capsular Bag, Zonules and its Relevance to Cataract Surgery
- Biochemistry of the Lens
- Cataract Etiology: A Comprehensive Review
- Cataract Classification and Various Treatment Modalities
- Ocular Biometry
- Sterilization
- Anesthesia in Cataract Surgery
- Viscoanesthetic Solutions for Small Incision Cataract Surgery: Experimental Studies and Clinical Applications
- Dynamics of Ocular Surgical Adjuncts in Cataract Surgery
- Update on Ophthalmic Viscosurgical Devices
- Corneal Topography in Cataract Surgery
- Capsular Dye Enhanced Cataract Surgery
- Relevance and Clinical Significance of SICS (Manual Phaco) in Modern Cataract Surgery
- Learning Curve in Small Incision Cataract Surgery
- Preoperative Preparation of the Patient in Small Incision Cataract Surgery

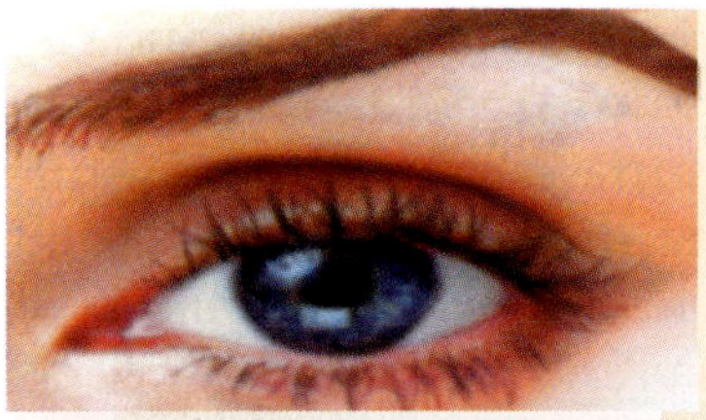

One

Anatomy of Human Crystalline Lens, Capsular Bag, Zonules and its Relevance to Cataract Surgery

Suresh K Pandey
Liliana Werner
David J Apple (USA)
Vidushi Sharma (India)

ANATOMY-HISTOLOGY OFTHE HUMAN CRYSTALLINE LENS
GROWTH OFTHE HUMAN CRYSTALLINE LENS
LENS CAPSULE
LENS EPITHELIAL CELLS
LENS SUBSTANCE (CORTEX AND NUCLEUS)

ANATOMY- HISTOLOGY OFTHE HUMAN CRYSTALLINE LENS

The adult crystalline lens measures approximately 9.6 $\pm$ 0.4 mm in diameter with an approximate anterior-posterior diameter of 4.2 $\pm$ 0.5 mm. [1,3,11] Figure 1.1 shows the empty capsular bag after removal of the crystalline lens. The diameter of ciliary sulcus 11.1 $\pm$ 0.5-mm, according to studies performed at the Center for Research on Ocular Therapeutics and Biodevices, Storm Eye Institute, Charleston, SC, USA (now renamed as David Apple, MD, Laboratory for Ophthalmic Devices Research, John A Moran Eye Center, Salt Lake City, Utah, USA).[3] The anterior and posterior poles form the optical and geometrical axis of the lens. Although the normal lens is transparent and clear in vivo, it is seldom completely colorless; even in childhood a slight yellowish tint is present that tends to intensify with age.

The crystalline lens is a unique transparent, biconvex intraocular structure, which lies in the anterior segment of the eye suspended radially at its equator by the zonular fibers and the ciliary body, between the iris and the vitreous body. Enclosed in an elastic capsule, the lens has no innervation or blood supply after fetal development. Its

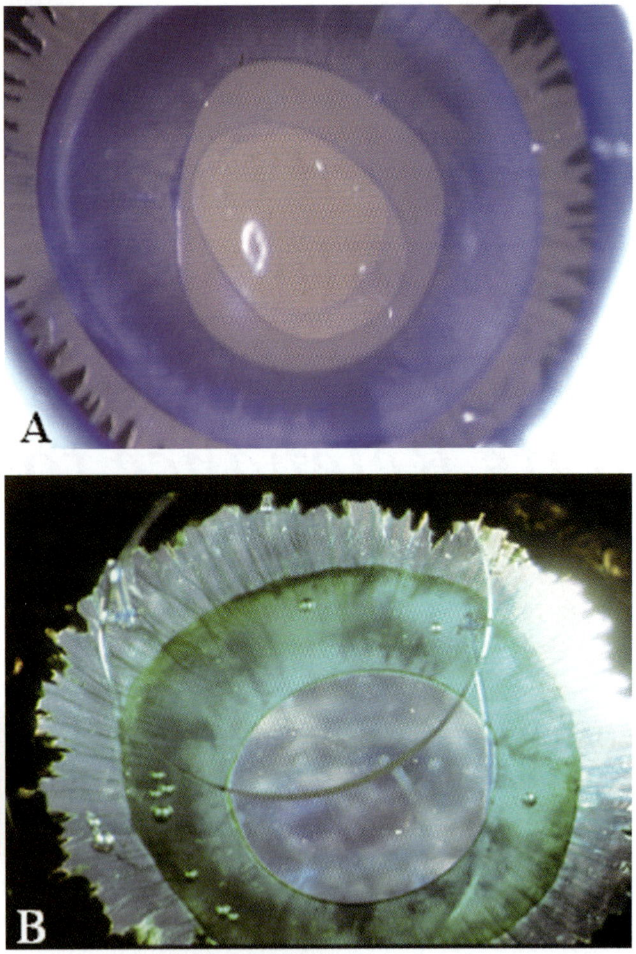

Figs 1.1A and B: Gross photographs of the pediatric and adult human eyes obtained postmortem showing the capsular bag, zonules shape, status after phacoaspiration/phacoemulsification of the lens substance. Both pictures were taken from an anterior (surgeon's) view; cornea and iris were excised to allow better visualization. (A) Empty capsular bag of a pediatric (aged 24 months) human eye obtained postmortem stained with 0.1% trypan blue.The diameter of the crystalline lens and empty capsular bag were 9.2 mm and 9.6 mm, respectively. The anterior and posterior capsulorhexis are also visible. (B) Empty capsular bag of an adult (aged 44 years) human eye obtained postmortem stained with 0.5% indocyanine green dye. The diameter of human crystalline lens and empty capsular bag were 9.9mm and 10.4 mm, respectively. Note the zonules are stained green and clearly visible.

nourishment must be obtained from the surrounding aqueous and vitreous, and the same media must also remove metabolic waste products. Therefore, disturbances in circulation of these fluids, or inflammatory processes in these chambers, play a large role in the pathogenesis of lens abnormalities. The aqueous humor continuously flows from the ciliary body to the anterior chamber, bathing the anterior surface of the lens. Disturbances in permeability of the lens capsule and epithelium can occur, leading to the formation of cataracts. Posteriorly, the crystalline lens is supported by the vitreous (hyaloid) face and lies in a small depression called the "patellar fossa." In younger eyes, the vitreous comes in contact with the posterior capsule in a circular area of thickened vitreous, the ligamentum hyaloidocapsular. The potential space between the capsule and the circle of condensed vitreous is called Berger's space. The lateral border of the lens is the equator, formed from the joining of the anterior and posterior capsules, and is the site of insertion of the zonules.

The lens consists of three components : capsule, epithelium, and lens substance. The lens substance is a product of the continuous growth of the epithelium and consists of the cortex and nucleus. The transition between the cortex and nucleus is gradual. It does not reveal a concise line of demarcation when observed in histological sections. The lines of demarcation are often better visualized by slitlamp microscopy.

GROWTH OFTHE HUMAN CRYSTALLINE LENS

The pediatric ocular structures, including the crystalline lens, are significantly smaller than in the adult, especially in the first 1-3 years of life.[9,10,11-13,17] the mean axial length of a newborn's eye is 17.0 mm compared to 23-24 mm in an adult. The human crystalline lens grows throughout life by the deposition of new fibers. Figure 1.2 shows the growth of the human crystalline lens. The most rapid lens-growth occurs from birth to 2 years-of-age. The mean diameter of the capsular bag is about 7.0-7.5 mm at birth, which increases to about 9.0-9.5 mm by the age of 2-years.[9,10,11-13,17] Human crystalline lens growth is slower after the second decade. The lens does not increase much in size thereafter because of a relative loss of hydration and shrinkage of the lens nucleus, which offsets some of the increase from new fiber deposition. Nuclear opacities (nuclear sclerosis) is the physiologic change that occur as the result of the above changes in hydration and nuclear size. The lens

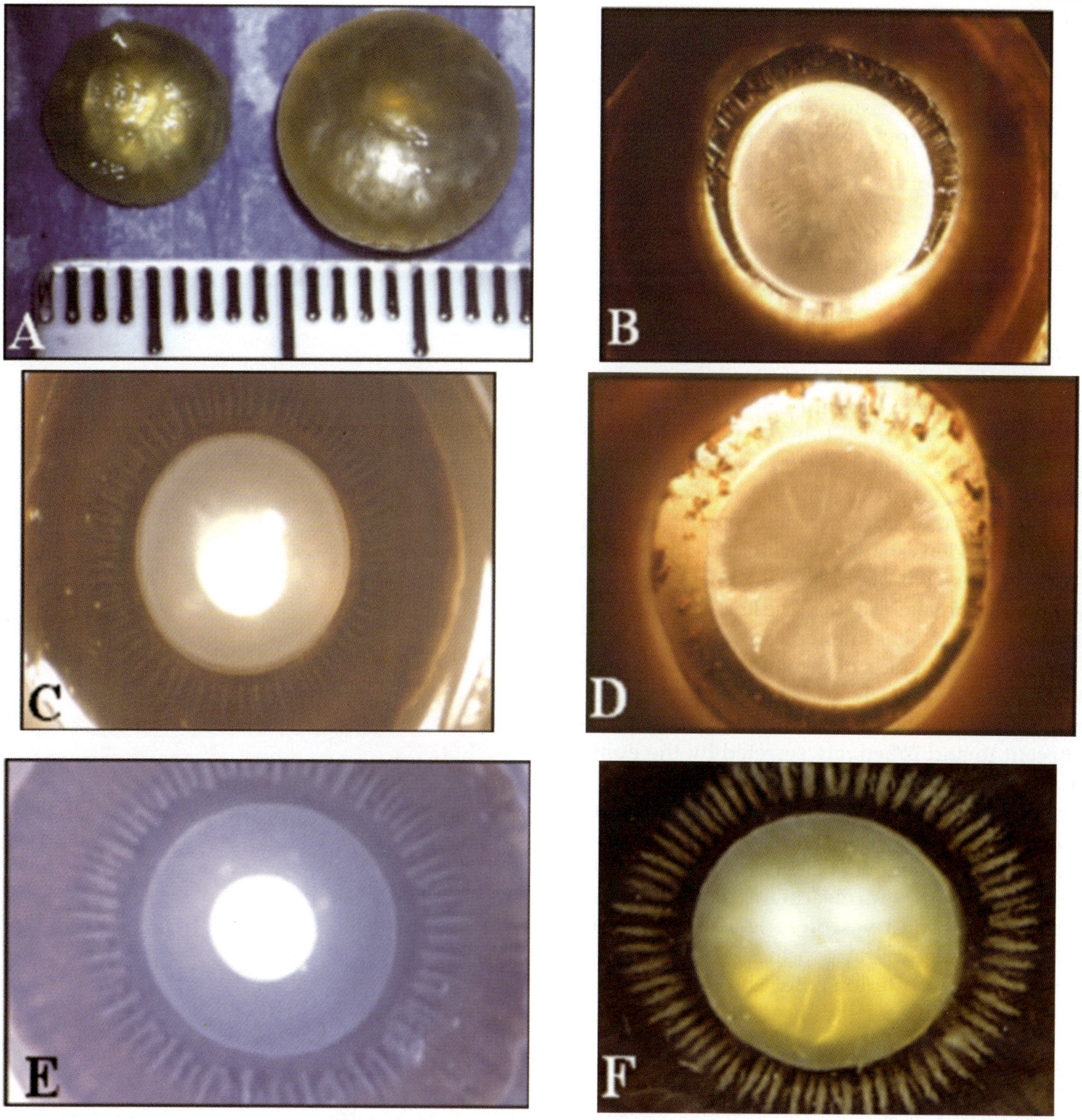

Figs 1.2A to F: Growth of the human crystalline lens. (A) Gross photographs of human crystalline lens taken from a child aged 4 months (left side). On the right side photographs human crystalline lens from the adult aged 70 years. (B) Gross pictures of a pediatric human lens obtained postmortem, 20 months, showing human crystalline, zonules and ciliary body (anterior or surgeon's view). The diameter of human crystalline lens was 8.5 mm. (C) Gross pictures of a pediatric human lens obtained postmortem, 20 months, showing human crystalline, zonules and ciliary body (Miyake-Apple posterior view). (D) Gross photographs of pediatric human eyes obtained postmortem aged 3 years showing crystalline lens zonules and ciliary body. Anterior (surgeon's view): The diameter of human crystalline lens was 9.3 mm. (E) Gross photographs of pediatric human eyes obtained postmortem aged 3 years showing crystalline lens zonules and ciliary body (Miyake-Apple posterior view). (F) Gross photographs of an adult human eye obtained postmortem (aged 60 years) showing crystalline lens, zonules and ciliary body (Miyake-Apple posterior view). The diameter of human crystalline lens was 9.8 mm.

nucleus may become sufficiently opaque to cause visual difficulties. Also, the lens capsule thickens with age and loses some of the inherent elasticity, which further decreasing the capacity for accommodation and helping to lead to presbyopia.[5,6]

LENS CAPSULE

The lens capsule is a basement membrane elaborated by the lens epithelium anteriorly and by superficial fibers posteriorly. By light microscopy the lens capsule appears as a structureless, elastic membrane, which completely surrounds the lens. It is a true Periodic acid-Schiff (PAS) positive basement membrane, a secretory product of the lens epithelium.[1,15] Figure 1.3 demonstrates histology of the anterior, equatorial, and posterior lens capsule using 2 different staining techniques. The capsule functions as a metabolic barrier and may play a role in lens shaping during accommodation. The lens capsule is of variable thickness in various zones. At its thickest regions the lens capsule represents the thickest basement membrane in the body. The relative thickness of the anterior capsule compared with the much thinner posterior capsule, may result from the fact that the former lies directly adjacent to and is actively secreted by the epithelium, whereas the lens epithelium is not present on the posterior surface. Local differences in capsular thickness are important surgically, particularly because of the danger of tears or rupture of the thin posterior capsule during cataract surgery. Remnants of the tunica vasculosa lentis are common and appear as light-gray opacities (Mittendorf dots) at or near the posterior pole. These opacities are rarely responsible for significant visual loss.

LENS EPITHELIAL CELLS

It is pertinent to discuss some details about the lens epithelial cells and their behavior after cataract surgery. Postoperative proliferation of these cells may lead to opacification of the posterior lens capsule, which in-turn may contribute to decrease vision after the cataract surgery and implantation of the intraocular lenses.[12-15] The lens epithelium is confined to the anterior surface and the equatorial lens bow (Fig. 1.4). It consists of a single row of

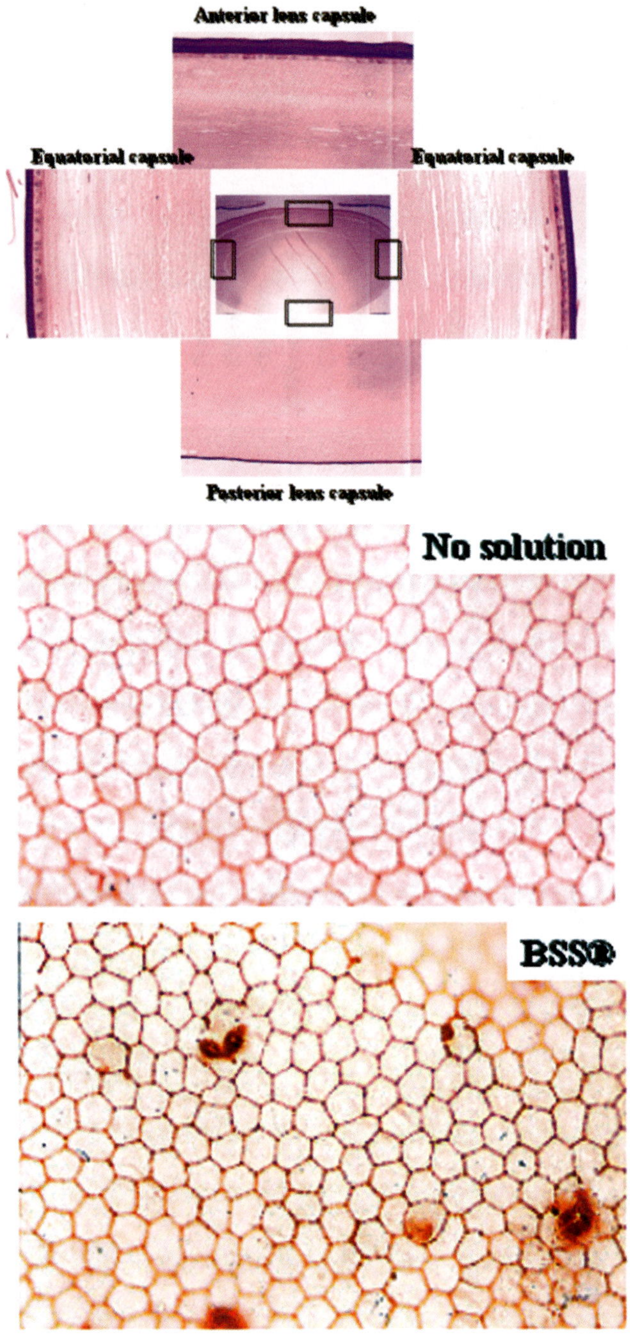

Figs 1.3A and B: Histological section of human crystalline lens showing anterior, equatorial and posterior lens capsules. (A) Anterior lens surface stained by the PAS stain, which imparts a brilliant red hue to the basement membranes. The anterior lens epithelium lays down a basement membrane, which is thick anteriorly; it is the thickest basement membrane in the body. (Original magnification X 100). (B) Masson's Trichome stain. (Original magnification X 100).

Section 1

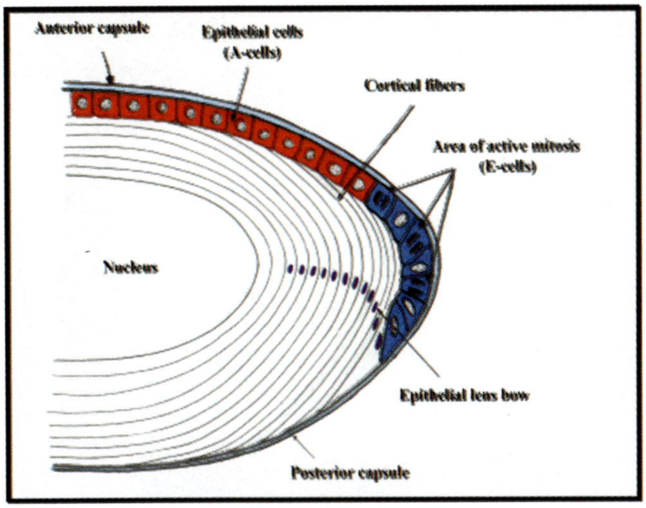

Fig. 1.4: Schematic illustration of the microscopic anatomy of the lens, showing the "A" cells of the anterior epithelium and the "E" cells, the important germinal epithelial cells of the equatorial lens bow. These lens epithelial cells plays predominant role in the pathogenesis of various complication as postoperative opacification of anterior and posterior capsule.

cuboidal-cylindrical cells, which can biologically be divided into two different zones with two different types of cells:

1. **A-cells** are located in the anterior–central zone (corresponding to the central zone of the anterior lens capsule). They consist of relatively quiescent epithelial cells with minimal mitotic activity. When disturbed, they tend to remain in place and not migrate. However, in a variety of disorders (e.g. inflammation, trauma), an anterior subcapsular epithelial plaque may form. The primary type of response of the anterior epithelial cells is to proliferate and form fibrous tissue by undergoing fibrous metaplasia.
   Recently, a new potential complication of A-cell proliferation has emerged in the field of refractive surgery. The anterior subcapsular opacities that have been described with various phakic posterior chamber (PC) IOLs are based on A-cell proliferation. The fibrotic response of the anterior lens epithelium is what determines the degree of anterior capsular thickening following implantation of a phakic PC IOL in close proximity (or on) the anterior surface of the crystalline lens.
2. **E-cells** are located in the second zone, as a continuation of the anterior lens epithelial cells around the equator, forming the equatorial lens bow, with the germinal cells. These cells normally show mitotic capability, and new lens fibers are continuously produced at this site. Because cell production in this region is relatively active, the cells are rich in enzymes and have extensive protein metabolism. E-cells are responsible for the continuous formation of all cortical fibers, and they account for the continuous growth in size and weight of the lens throughout life. During lens enlargement the location of older fibers becomes more central as new fibers are formed at the periphery.

In pathologic states, the E-cells tend to migrate posteriorly along the posterior capsule; instead of undergoing a fibrotic transformation, they tend to form large, balloon-like bladder cells (i.e. Wedl cells). These are the cells that are clinically visible as "pearls." These equatorial cells are the primary source of classic secondary cataract, especially the pearl-form of posterior capsule opacification (PCO). E-cells are responsible for the formation of a Soemmering's ring, which is a donut-shaped lesion, composed of retained/regenerated lens cortex and cells that may form following any type of disruption of the anterior lens capsule. This lesion was initially described in connection with ocular trauma. It is the basic precursor of classic PCO. The E-cells have also been implicated in the pathogenesis of opacification between piggyback IOLs, also termed interlenticular opacification.[14]

LENS SUBSTANCE (CORTEX AND NUCLEUS)

The lens substance consists of the lens fibers themselves, which are derived from the equatorial lens epithelium. On cross-section these cells are hexagonal, and are bound together by ground substance. After formation, the cellular nuclei of the lens fibers are present only temporarily. Subsequently they disappear, leaving the lens center devoid of cell nuclei except in certain pathologic situations (e.g., the maternal rubella syndrome).

The original lens vesicle represents the primary embryonic nucleus; in later stages of gestation the fetal nucleus encircles the embryonic nucleus. The

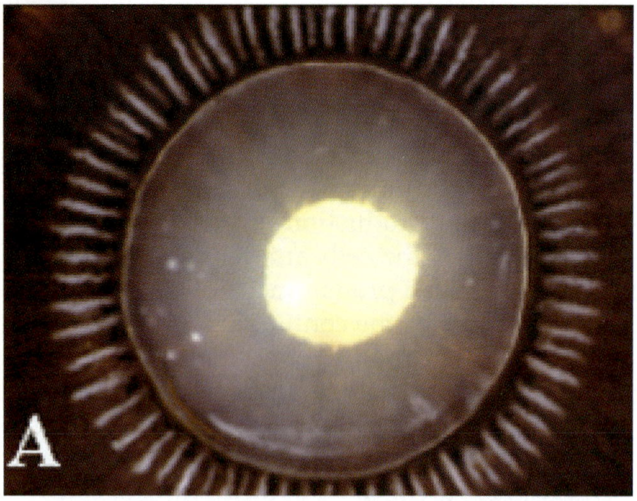

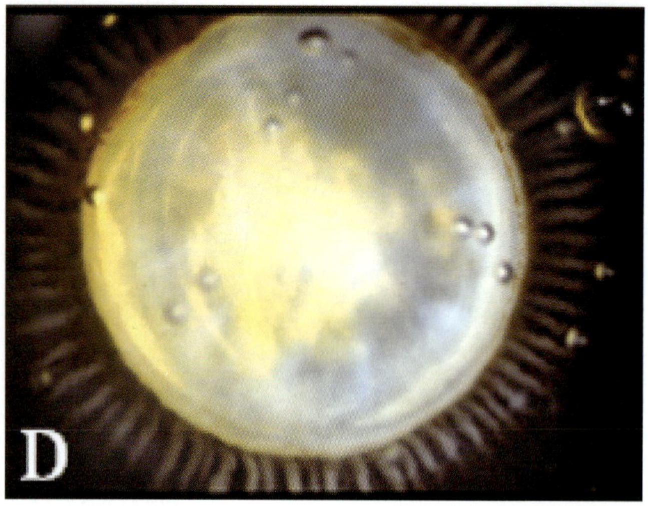

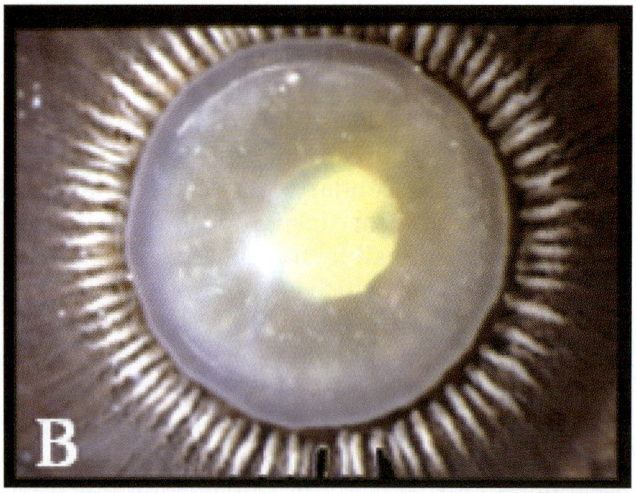

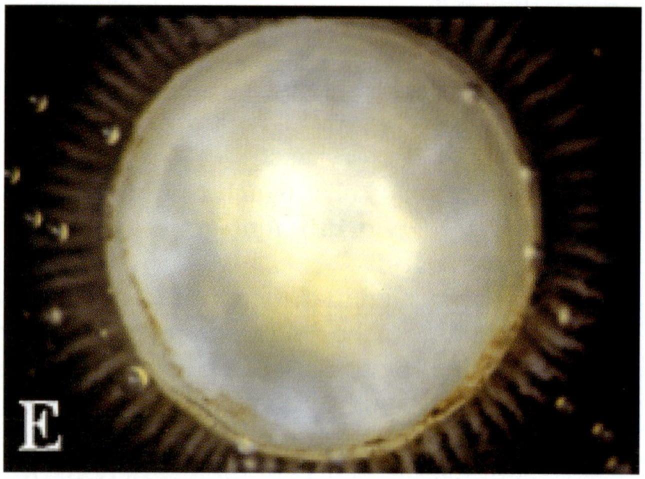

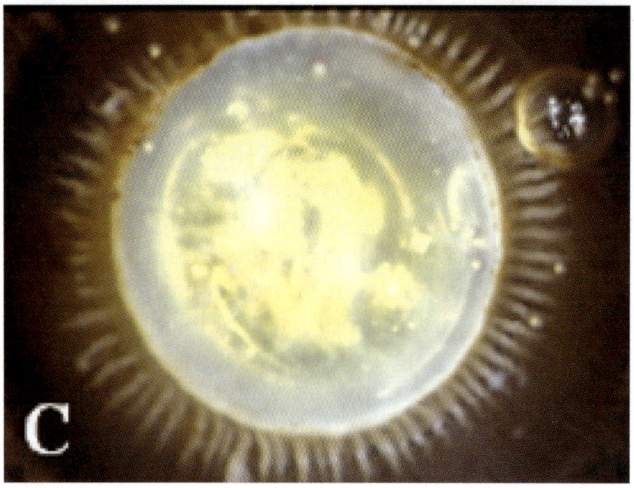

Figs 1.5A to E: Aging of the lens substance (nuclear sclerosis). Emery-Little's classification was proposed for the hardness of nuclear cataract (varying from soft, semi-soft, medium hard, hard and rock-hard), in clinical setting. We have presented posterior view of the postmortem phakic human eye showing an experimental example of induction of different degrees of nuclear sclerotic cataract after injection of Karnovsky's solution in the lens substance.[8] (A) Miyake-Apple posterior view of a human eye obtained post-mortem from a 79-year-old male, showing the crystalline lens. There is a grade 1 of nuclear hardness (soft cataract, according to the Emery-Little classification). (B, C, D and E) Same eye 5, 15, 20 and 30 minutes after the injection of Karnovsky's solution within the nucleus, with the creation of grades 2, 3, 4 and 5 of nuclear hardness, respectively.

various layers surrounding the fetal nucleus are designated according to stages of growth. The most peripherally located fibers, which underlie the lens capsule, form the lens cortex. The designation of cortex is actually an arbitrary term signifying a peripheral location within the lens, rather than specific fibers.

The relationship between sclerosis and hardness is uncertain. Traditionally the word "sclerosis" has been associated with decreased water content of the crystalline lens. Although there is no consensus in the past literature about the extent to which the lens hardens, recent evidence has demonstrated more consistently that increased hardness of the crystalline lens occurs with age. Emery-Little proposed a classification of lens nuclei depending on varying degree of hardness.[4] Using postmortem human eyes, we have developed a model of inducing cataract of varying degree of hardness in a laboratory setting using the Miyake-Apple posterior video technique and this is shown in Figure 1.5.[2,7,8] Figure 1.6 summarizes the anatomical relationship of the human crystalline lens, ciliary body and zonules.

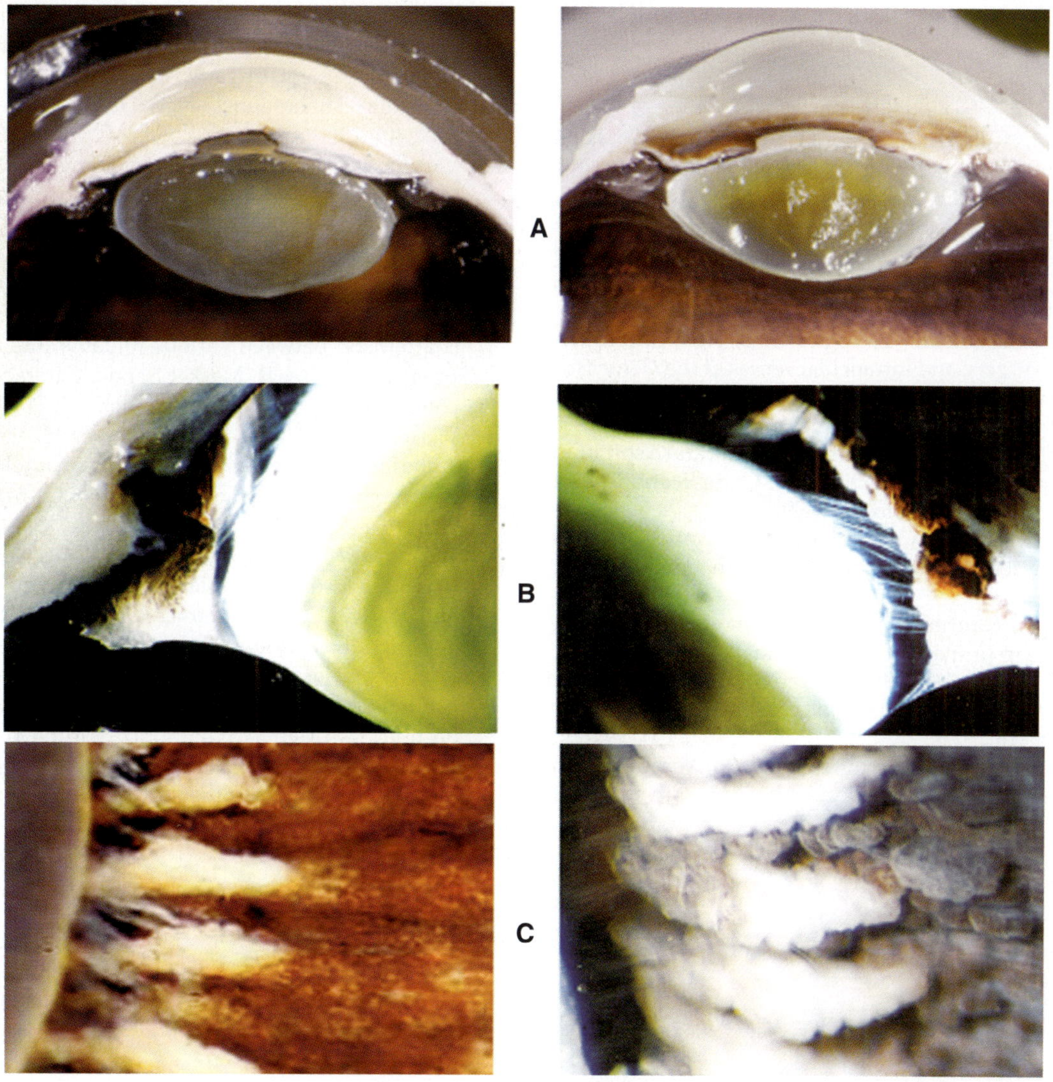

Figs 1.6A to C: Parasagittal section of the phakic human eye obtained postmortem. Note the crystalline lens suspended by the ciliary zonule. (A) Crystalline lens and zonules. (B) Higher magnification of crystalline lens, ciliary body and zonules from another case. (C) Higher magnification of ciliary body and zonules from another case. Miyake-Apple posterior view.

In summary, the crystalline lens is a unique transparent, biconvex intraocular structure, which lies in the anterior segment of the eye suspended radially at its equator by the zonular fibers and the ciliary body, between the iris and the vitreous body. The lens consists of three components : capsule, epithelium, and lens substance. The lens substance is a product of the continuous growth of the epithelium and consists of the cortex and nucleus.

Acknowledgement

The authors gratefully acknowledge the partial support of an unrestricted grant from Research to Prevent Blindness, Inc, New York, NY, USA.

REFERENCES

1. Apple DJ, Auffarth GU, Peng Q, Visessook N. Foldable Intraocular Lenses. Evolution, Clinicopathologic Correlations, Complications. Thorofare, NJ:Slack, Inc., 2000.
2. Apple DJ, Lim E, Morgan R, et al. Preparation and study of human eyes obtained postmortem with the Miyake posterior photographic technique. Ophthalmology 1990; 97:810-16.
3. Assia EI, Castaneda VE, Legler UFC, et al. Studies on cataract surgery and intraocular lenses at the Center for Intraocular Lens Research. Ophthal Clin North Am 1991; 4:251-266.
4. Emery JM, Little JH. Phacoemulsification and Aspiration of Cataracts; Surgical Techniques, Complications, and Results. St Louis: CV Mosby, 1979;45-8.
5. Glasser A, Croft MA, Kaufman P Aging of the human crystalline lens and presbyopia. Int Ophthalmol Clin 2001; 41:1-15.
6. Glasser A, Kaufman PL. The mechanism of accommodation in primates. Ophthalmology. 1999;106:863-72.
7. Miyake K, Miyake C. Intraoperative posterior chamber lens haptic fixation in the human cadaver eye. Ophthalmic Surg 1985;16:230-6.
8. Pandey SK, Werner L, Escobar-Gomez M, Apple DJ, et al. Creating cataracts of varying hardness to practice extracapsular cataract extraction and phacoemulsification. J Cataract Refract Surg 2000;26:322-29.
9. Pandey SK, Wilson ME, Trivedi RH, Werner L, Apple DJ, et al. Pediatric cataract surgery and intraocular lens implantation: Current techniques, complications and management. Int Ophthalmol Clin 2001;41:175-96.
10. Pandey SK, Wilson ME, Apple DJ, Werner L, Ram J. Childhood cataract surgical technique, complications and management. In: Garg A, Pandey SK, Eds., Textbook of Ocular Therapeutics. Jaypee Brothers, New Delhi, India.
11. Pandey SK, Thakur J, Werner L, Wilson ME, Werner LP, Izak AM, Apple DJ. The Human Crystalline Lens, Ciliary Body and Zonules: Their Relevance to Presbyopia. In: Agarwal A, ed., Presbyopia: A Surgical Text. Slack Inc., Thorofare, NJ, USA 2002: Chapter 2, 15-25.
12. Pandey SK, Werner L, Apple DJ. Posterior capsule opacification: Etiopathogenesis, clinical manifestations, and management. In: Garg A, Pandey SK, Eds., Textbook of Ocular Therapeutics. New Delhi, Jaypee Brothers, 2002;408-25.
13. Vargas LG, Peng Q, Escobar-Gomez M, Apple DJ. Overview of modern foldable intraocular lenses and clinically relevant anatomy and histology of the crystalline lens. Int Ophthalmol Clin 2001;41(3):1-15.
14. Werner L, Apple DJ, Pandey SK. Postoperative proliferation of anterior and equatorial lens epithelial cells: A comparison between various foldable IOL designs. In: Buratto L, Osher R, Masket S, Eds, Cataract surgery in complicated cases. Thorofare, NJ: Slack. 2000;399-17.
15. Werner L, Pandey SK, Escobar-Gomez M, Apple DJ, et al. Anterior capsule opacification: A histopathological study comparing different IOL styles. Ophthalmology 2000;107:463-71.
16. Wilson ME, Apple DJ, Bluestein EC, Wang XH. Intraocular lenses for pediatric implantation: biomaterials, designs and sizing. J Cataract Refract Surg 1994;20:584-91.
17. Wilson ME, Pandey SK, Werner L, Ram J, Apple DJ. Pediatric Cataract Surgery: Current Techniques, Complications and Management. In: Agarwal S, Agarwal A, Sachdev MS, Mehta KR, Fine IH, Agarwal A, eds., Phacoemulsification, Laser Cataract Surgery and Foldable IOLs. New Delhi, Jaypee Brothers, 2000;369-88.

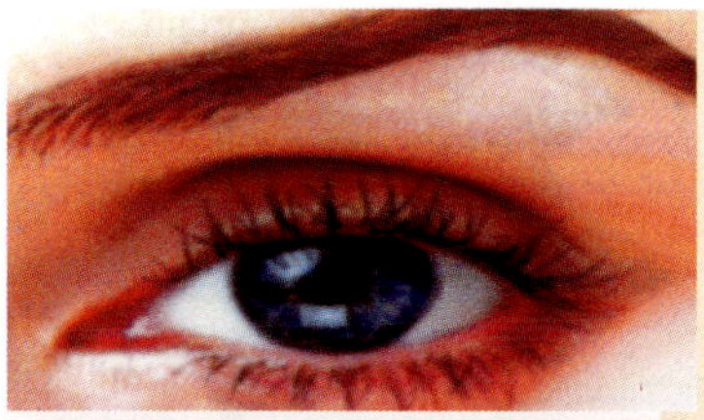

Two

Biochemistry of the Lens

Ashok Garg (India)

INTRODUCTION

Crystalline lens which is positioned behind the iris is the chief refractive medium of the eye having the maximum refractory power. It is a transparent, elastic and biconvex lens enclosed in a capsule. It refracts the light entering the eye through the pupil and focuses it on the retina. The transparency of lens depends on maintenance of structural and functional integrity (physiologic).

BIOCHEMISTRY OF THE LENS

The human lens is the least hydrated organ of the body. It contains 66 percent water, and the 33 percent remaining bulk is composed mainly of protein. The lens cortex is more hydrated than the lens nucleus. **Lens dehydration is maintained by an active Na^+ ion water pump that resides within the membranes of cells in the lens epithelium and each lens fiber.**

The inside of lens is electronegative. Proteins of –64 to 78 mV are recorded across the intact lens capsule and of –23 mV in the lens fibers. There is a –23 mV difference between anterior and posterior surfaces of the lens. Thus, the flow of electrolytes into the lens is directed by an electrical gradient.

LENS PROTEINS 100%

- Soluble crystallins 85%
  - α-crystallin 15%
    - M.W. = 1,000,000
    - Fast electrophoretic mobility toward anode
    - has separable subunits (M.W. 21,000-23,000)
  - β-crystallin 55%
    - M.W. = 50,000-100,000
    - Intermediate electrophoretic mobility
    - Marked molecular heterogeneity
  - γ-crystallin 15%
    - M.W. = 20,000
    - Slow electrophoretic mobility
    - No subunits
    - Precipitates reversibly in the cold
- Insoluble (albuminoid) 15%
  - Membrane protein fraction
  - ? Aggregated crystallins

Fig. 2.1: Human lens protein composition

CRYSTALLINE LENS AS AN OSMOMETER

The capsule of the lens acts as an intact cell and induces properties like swelling in hypotonic media and dehydration in the hypertonic media. The osmolarity of the human lens is 302 mOsm and equals the osmolarity of aqueous. The cations like sodium and potassium with concentration of 145 mEq/L and anions (chloride, bicarbonate, sulfate, ascorbate and glutathione) with concentration of 50 to 60 mEq/L contribute to lens osmolarity. An anionic deficit of 90 mEq/L is probably made by acidic groups of lens protein and glycoproteins.

Water increase in the lens breaks the lens fibers membranes and results in microscopic vacuoles. The water equilibrium between the lens and the surrounding fluids is disrupted if the concentration of osmotically active compounds (Na^+,K^+, etc.) increases inside the lens. Increase in Na^+ and K^+ levels also follows lens exposure to surface active detergents or antibiotics. When retained inside the cell, abnormal products of sugar metabolism such as sorbitol can exert osmotic effects and result in water influx and lens swelling.

LENS PROTEINS

The human lens contains the highest concentration of protein (33%) of any tissue in the body. Proteins are synthesized in the anterior epithelium and at equatorial region. The perfect physiochemical arrangement of the lens protein living in an optimum environment of water, electrolytes and sulfhydryl gives transparency to the lens. Amino acids which are actively transported by the anterior lens epithelium are used by the lens to synthesize lens proteins. Since the lens protein is sequestered from the body immune system during embryonic life, later exposure of the lens protein can result in an autoimmune reaction. The separation of lens proteins is based initially on their solubility of water. Fifteen percent of the lens proteins are insoluble in water, these form the albuminoid fraction which is thought to include membrane bound protein and aggregated crystallins. The remaining 85 percent are soluble in water and are classified as alpha, beta and gamma crystallins on the basis of molecular weight, electrophoretic mobility and presence or absence of subunits as shown in Figure 2.1. The soluble alpha and gamma crystallins leak into the aqueous humor during cataract formation causing a reduction in total lens protein.

The water soluble lens proteins are grouped as: (i) α-crystallins (15%), (ii) β-crystallins (55%), and (iii) γ-cystallins (15%). On the basis of their electrophoretic mobility towards the anode, α-crystallin is fastest, β-crystallin is intermediate and γ-crystallins is slowest. The molecular weight of crystallins in daltons is α-crystallin 1,000,000, β-crystallin 50000-200000 and γ-crystallin 20000. α and β-crystallins are made of subunits and aggregation or separation of these subunits determines the physiochemical characteristics of each crystallin.

The protein subunits are assembled by the alignment of amino acids through ribonucleic acid (RNA) as specified by the genetic code (Fig. 2.2). Lens proteins are degraded by proteases and amino peptidases. In the normal lens, the membrane of lens fibers and lens capsule do not allow the passage of protein molecules from the lens to the aqueous humor. **When a mature cataract develops, the membranes of the lens fibers are lysed, the capsule becomes more permeable and protein can leak out of the lens. Lens proteins in the anterior chamber can act as an antigen which lead to inflammation of the uveal tissues known as lens induced or phacogenic uveitis.**

Sometimes degraded lens proteins leak through the capsule into the aqueous humor and are engulfed by macrophages which plug up the trabecular meshwork thus blocking aqueous humor outflow and producing increased intraocular pressure (IOP)—phacolytic glaucoma.

ACTIVE TRANSPORT PROCESSES

Water and Electrolyte Transport

The electrolyte and water content of the lens resembles that of an intact cell as shown in Figure 2.3. Whereas the Na^+, Cl^- and K^+ ion and water content of aqueous and vitreous is similar to that in plasma or extracellular fluids. To maintain electrolyte and water gradients against the surrounding fluids, the lens generates chemical and electrical energy. Chemical energy extrudes Na^+ ions and water is provided by ATP through glucose metabolism.

Cation Transport

The energy dependent cation pump in the lens accumulates K^+ intracellularly and extrudes sodium (Na^+). The influx of K^+ and efflux of Na^+ are thought to be linked and mediated by the membrane bound enzyme, Na^+-K^+-ATPase which degrades ATP to adenosine diphosphate (ADP) inorganic phosphate and energy with which to power this cation pump. The action of Na^+-K^+-ATPase of lens can be inhibited by cardiac glycoside such as digitalis thereby stopping the cation pump.

It is generally believed that the cation pump of the lens functions at the anterior epithelial surface because the concentration of Na^+-K^+-ATPase is greater in this area than elsewhere. When K^+ is pumped into the lens and Na^+ is pumped out at the anterior surface, a chemical gradient is gene-

Section 1

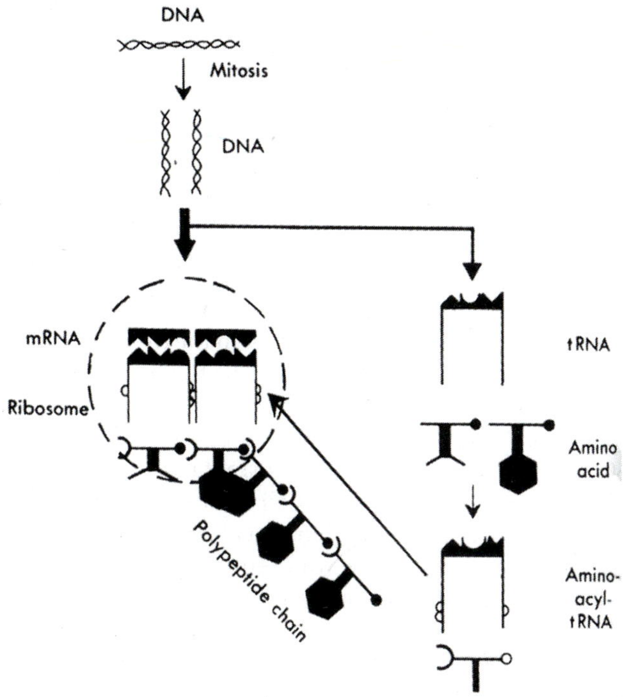

Fig. 2.2: Biochemistry of lens protein synthesis

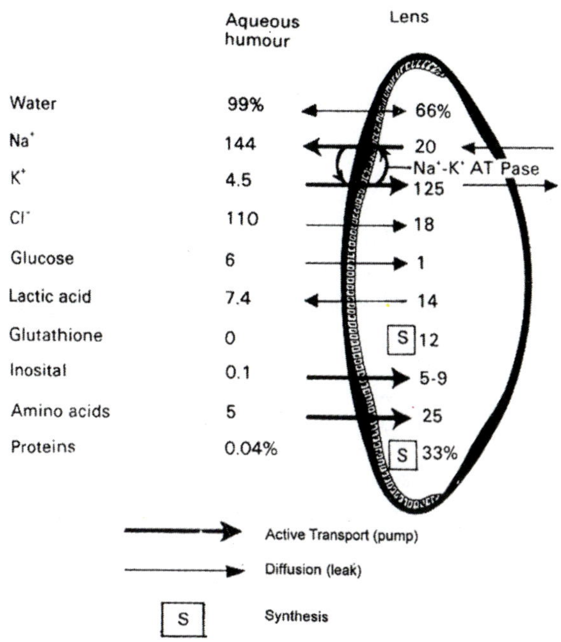

Fig. 2.3: Chemical composition of human lens.
(All values in mmol/kg of lens water), unless otherwise stated

rated that stimulates a diffusion of Na^+ into the lens and K^+ out of the primarily through the posterior surface. This process of active transport (pump) stimulating passive diffusion (leak) has been termed as "pump and leak" theory of cation transport (Fig. 2.4). This cation transport system performs three important functions.

- It regulates the water content of the lens, thereby allowing the lens to act as a perfect osmometer. This prevents colloid osmotic swelling.
- It produces and maintains an electrical potential difference (approximately–70 mV) between the lens and the medium surrounding it.
- It promotes the proper physiochemical environment within the lens to maintain transparency and optimal enzymatic activity.

Surface active agents (antibiotics, detergents, lysophospholipids and fatty acids) disrupt the physiochemical integrity of the membrane and Na^+ extrusion pump with subsequent gain of Na^+ ions and water by the lens, lens swelling and eventually complete loss of lens transparency follow.

AMINO ACIDS

Amino acids and inositol are actively transported into the lens at the anterior epithelial surface (Fig. 2.5). Once in the lens, free amino acids are incorporated into RNA to form lens protein, can be metabolized with formation of CO_2, or can efflux from the lens. The turnover of free amino acids in the lens is very rapid, the renewal rate for lysine being 16 percent of the total in the lens per hour. There are three separate pumps for acidic, basic and neutral amino acids. Once in the lens these amino acids are metabolized and used for energy.

Glutathione-Sulfhydryl Proteins

Glutathione, a polypeptide is actively synthesized in the lens. It is a tripeptide containing glycine, cysteine and glutamic acid. The levels of glutathione in the lens are high and most of lens glutathione is in the reduced form (GSH). Only 6.8 percent of all lens Glutathione is in the oxidized form (GSSG). GSH and GSSG are in equilibrium.

$$2GSH + \frac{1}{2} O_2 \rightleftharpoons = GSSG + H_2O$$

GSH concentrations are 12.0 micromoles/gm in human lens. GSH levels are much higher in the cortex than in the nucleus of the lens. A reducing agent by virtue of its free sulfhydryl group, glutathione maintains membrane stability in the lens by supporting the protein complexes of the membrane.

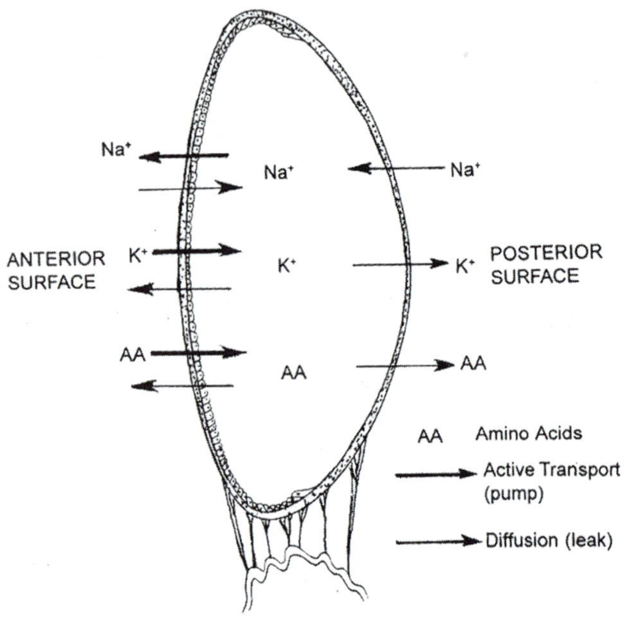

Fig. 2.4: Active transport process of lens (pump-leak) mechanism

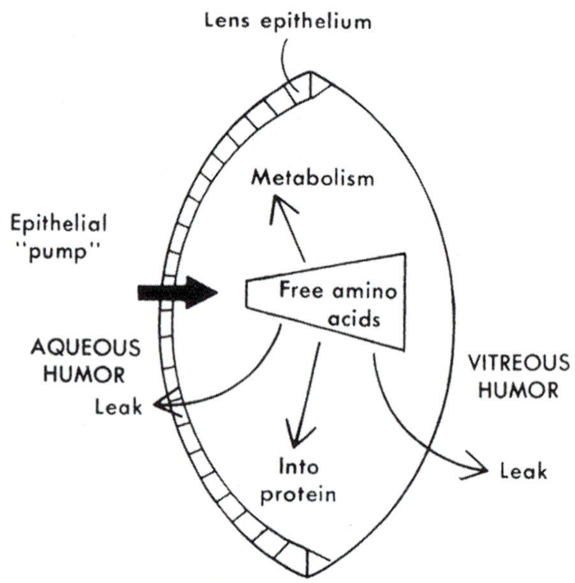

Fig. 2.5: Schematic diagram showing amino acid active transport into the lens (epithelial pump)

GSH levels decrease slightly with age. One of the earliest changes noted in the lens in different types of cataracts is the loss of glutathione. This allows the cross-linkage of proteins by the formation of disulfide bonds through sulfhydryl oxidation.

Another polypeptide ophthalmic acid is also found in the lens in concentrations of 1/10 to 1/100 those of GSH.

The pentose shunt of glucose metabolism active in the lens generates NADPH (reduced nicotinamide-adenine dinucleotide phosphate) that maintains glutathione in the reduced state by the following reductase:

$$GSSH + NADPH + H^+ \rightleftharpoons 2GSH + NADP$$

Lens proteins contain reduced sulfhydryl groups (PSH) and oxidized disulfide groups (PSSP) maintaining high levels of GSH as shown in the following reaction

$$2PSH + GSSG — 2GSH + PSSP$$

Thus, decreased GSH or increased GSSG will result in PSH oxidation and alterations in protein linkages, their solubility and their transparency.

The main functions of lens GSH are:

- To preserve the physiochemical equilibrium of lens proteins by maintaining high levels of reduced sulfhydryl (SH^-) groups.
- To maintain transport pumps and the molecular integrity of lens fiber membranes.

Synthesis of lens glutathione proceeds via α-glutamyl cysetine synthetase which is markedly decreased in human senile cataracts. The enzyme glutathione peroxidase removes H_2O_2 or toxic lipid peroxides but decreases rapidly with age and in senile cataracts. Thus, the ability of lens to remove toxic oxygen appears impaired in early senile cataracts.

LIPIDS

The lipids of human lens are unique and differ markedly from those of other species. Lipids represent about 3 to 5 percent of the dry weight of lens. In human lens cholesterol is about 50 percent of lipids followed by phospholipids (45%) and glycosphingolipids and ceramides (5%). The lipids are major components of the lens fiber membranes and either decrease in their synthesis or impaired degradation brings about lens membrane damage and lens opacities. Cataracts develop in humans if treated with anticholesterolemic agents such as triparanol. Esterification of cholesterol takes place in human lens where 25 percent of total cholesterol is in the ester form. Among phospholipids, the human lens is specially rich in sphingomyelin and its precursor ceramides may increase in senile cataracts. Ceramide synthesis proceeds via fatty acids and sphingosine. Its degradative enzyme ceramidase is present in the human lens. Sphingomyelin is degraded by sphingomyelinase which is somewhat decreased in senile cataract.

The cholesterol-phospholipid ratio of human lens fiber membranes is the highest among cell or organelle membranes, thus conferring the lens resistance to deformation. Lipids as structural components of lens fiber membranes are associated with the insoluble lens proteins. The increased insolubility of the proteins with age or during cataract formation may be due to derangements in the stereochemical arrangement between lipids and proteins in the membrane and soluble proteins inside the fibers.

ASCORBIC ACID

In human lens ascorbic acid values are higher in the lens than in the aqueous. The role of ascorbic acid in the lens is not clear; but it could participate in oxidation-reduction reactions alone or coupled to glutathione.

GLUCOSE METABOLISM

Lens is avascular and surrounded by aqueous and vitreous humors. Both of which are rich in glucose and poor in oxygen. Glucose used by the lens is metabolized through following four main pathways.

- The glycolytic pathway
- The Krebs (oxidative) cycle
- The hexose monophosphate (pentose) shunt
- The sorbitol pathway.

End products of glucose metabolism are lactic acid, carbon dioxide and water. Lactic acid from the lens diffuses to the aqueous and is eliminated via this circulating fluid.

About 80 percent of glucose used by the lens is metabolized anaerobically by the glycolytic pathway to produce lactic acid and adenosine triphosphate (ATP). A small proportion of lens glucose may be metabolized via oxidative Krebs' citric acid cycle which is 18 times more efficient in producing ATP than glycolysis (Fig. 2.6). About 15 percent of the glucose consumed by the lens is metabolized by the pentose or hexose monophosphate shunt. Although this pathway produces no energy in the form of ATP it does provide five carbon sugars (pentoses) for the synthesis of RNA and NADPH to maintain glutathione in a reduced state.

The sorbitol pathway in which glucose is converted to sorbitol by aldose reductase in the normal lens is relatively insignificant, but it is extremely important in the production of cataracts in diabetic and galactosemic patients (Fig. 2.7).

The lens uses the energy of metabolism for two principle processes, reproduction and growth and active transport processes.

The synthesis of RNA, DNA, lens fiber membrane constituents, enzymes and other lens proteins occurs mainly at the anterior surface and equatorial region of the lens.

Glucose metabolism generates adenosine triphosphate. ATP breakdown is required for active transport of ions and amino acids, maintenance of lens dehydration, lens transparency and for conti-

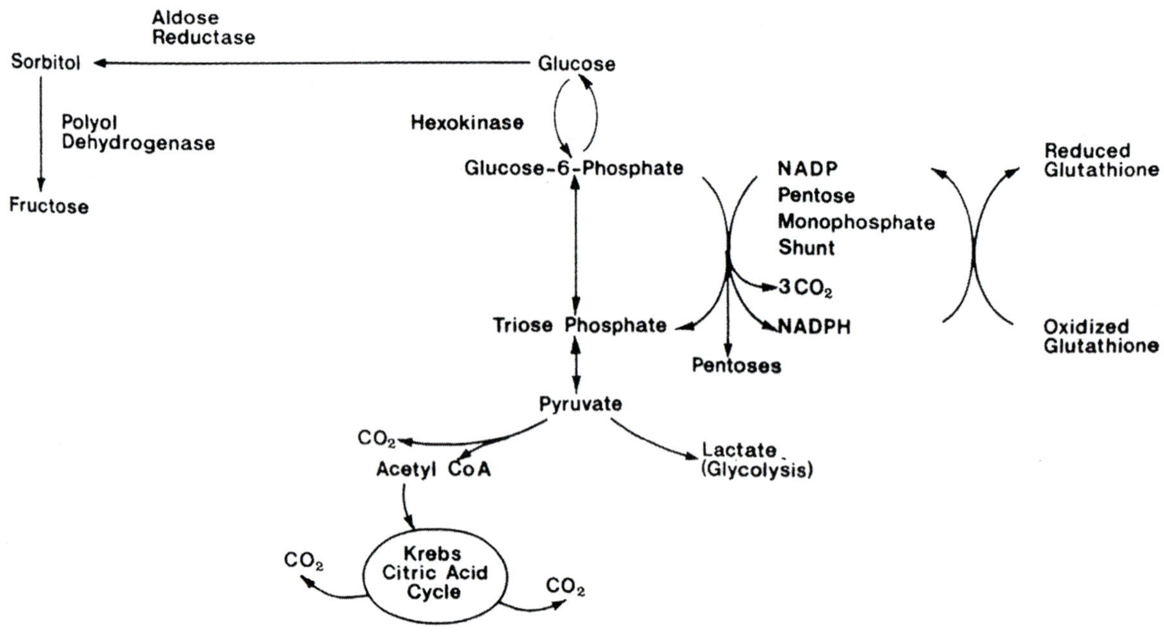

Fig. 2.6: Lens glucose metabolism pathway (Krebs' cycle)

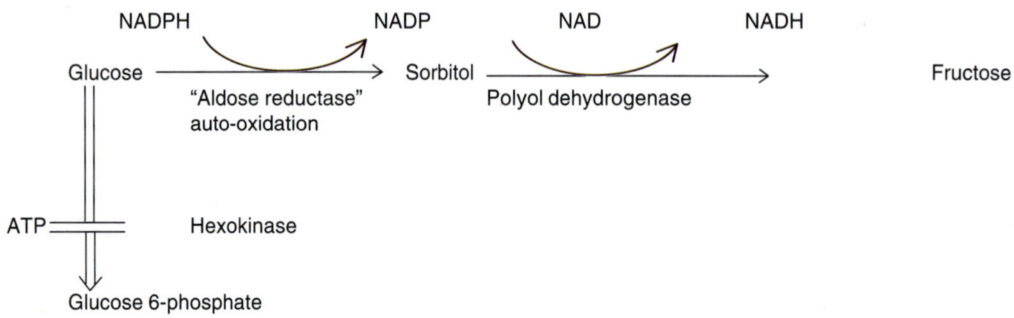

Fig. 2.7: Lens glucose metabolism (sorbitol pathway)

nuous protein and GSH synthesis. The pentose shunt does not generate ATP, but it forms pentoses required for RNA synthesis. NADPH generated from the shunt is needed to maintain lens glutathione in the reduced state. The pentose shunt is extremely active in the lens. In addition, an active mechanism for pyruvate decarboxylation exists in the lens which results in formation of carbon dioxide and acetaldehyde. The latter is metabolized through lens aldehyde dehydrogenase. The carbon dioxide combination with water to form bicarbonate (HCO_3^-) may be partially active in the lens nucleus where the levels of carbonic anhydrase exceed those in lens cortex. However, carbonic anhydrase inhibitors do not produce cataracts.

The enzymes hexokinase and phosphofructokinase regulate the rate of glucose metabolism by the lens, whereas oxygen is not essential for glucose metabolism. Conversion of glucose to amino acids such as glutamic acid, aspartic acid, glycine and others may account for 6 to 8 percent of glucose metabolism. Oxygen consumption by the lens is minimal 0.5 mmol/glens/hour. The Krebs' cycle requires oxygen and it is very inactive in the lens as there is paucity of mitochondria and oxidative enzymes. If the lens is deprived of glucose, it will utilize its own endogenous energy reserves.

When deprived of glucose the lens will gain water and lose transparency. In infantile hypoglycemia, cataract develops because of the low plasma glucose level are present.

The levels of glucose are higher in the aqueous (5.5 mmol/ml) than in the lens (1 mmol/ml) and glucose diffuses readily into the lens. Transport of glucose into the lens is not affected by the absence of sodium or calcium ions. However, other sugars or phloretin can inhibit lens glucose transport.

Studies of Intact lens metabolism or protein structure can be done by noninvasive techniques. The ^{31}P nuclear magnetic resonance (NMR) spectra of intact lens sugar phosphates and dinucleoside phosphate are among the best resolved in biological tissues. For lens protein analysis, laser spectroscopy techniques are available. The Raman laser signals allow determination of the axial distribution of protein subgroups such as tryptophan, sulfhydryl and disulfide which suffer modifications during cataract formation.

APPLIED PHYSIOLOGY

Chemical Changes in Lens Proteins in Senile Cataractogenesis

Lens proteins glycosylation happens on exposure to high glucose levels. These high glucose levels lead to protein conformational changes, near similar to those that occurs in glycosylated hemoglobin. The amino acid terminals of lens α- and β-crystallins are acetylated. Thus sugar attachment in lens proteins occurs primarily by binding to amino groups of lysine and formation of covalent sugar-lysine bonds. Glucosyl-lysine combination results in conformational protein changes, protein formation of S-S bonds through oxidation of adjacent sulfhydryl groups, protein aggregation and opacification. These findings explain in part the protein aggregation in human cataracts. Levels of Σ-amino acids in diabetic senile cataracts are substantially reduced as compared to age-related cataract. Another chemical modification of lens protein includes carbamylation, i.e. addition of cyanate which occurs secondary to accumulation of urea cycle metabolites in uremia or secondary to dehydration. Urea cycle enzymes are active in human lens and cataracts.

Research studies have now clearly shown that formation of protein S-S bonds is the major primary or secondary event associated in senile cataracts. Oxidation of lens protein SH groups with H_2O_2 induces protein conformation changes leading to opacification.

Protection against oxidation of protein SH groups is vital. Cysteine and glutathione have proven effective to prevent formation of S-S protein bonds. Protein unfolding due to primary modification of exposed lysine amine groups can be prevented by lysine acetylation. Lysine acetylation of protein prevents attachment of glycosyl, cyanate or other reactive groups like keto groups of steroids.

BIOCHEMISTRY OF CORTICAL CATARACTS

Cortical cataract is characterized by abnormalities in fiber permeability that causes vacuoles or clefts in the lens cortex. Damage to the membranes of lens fibers represents the initial insult due to X-rays, diabetes, galactosemia, arachidonic acid or other surface active agents. The various chemical changes some of which develop prior to clinical cortical changes include :

- Loss of glutathione with compensatory increase in NADPH synthesis
- Increase K^+ ion efflux
- Loss of K^+ ions, inositol and amino acids from lens
- Gain in Na^+ ions
- Decrease lens protein synthesis with decrease in the proportion of soluble protein and increase in insoluble protein
- Increase in protein S-S groups and in Ca^{++} ions.
- Decreased activity of most enzymes and increased activities of hydrolytic enzymes
- Decreased ATP content.

The majority of cataractogenic agents damage the ability of the lens to maintain GSH synthesis or increase its efflux through more permeable membranes. Thus a cycle of increased exudation of K^+ ions, amino acids and inositol is initiated. The lens epithelium tries to maintain the concentration of these compounds by increased pumping. Depending upon the magnitude of cataractogenic stimuli, the GSH leak out may continue or stop. To maintain normal levels, of NADPH is required which in turn stimulate the glucose metabolism through the pentose shunt. If the epithelium or lens fibers are structurally damaged and are unable to extrude Na^+ ions water gain will occur. This is followed by a decrease in protein synthesis which manifest itself by decreased levels of soluble lens proteins. This is compounded by the retention of cations and formation of disulfide S-S bonds with increased turbidity and protein insolubility. At this stage of cataractogenesis, the increased activity of glycolysis and other engymes is detected. The generalized disarray of lens metabolism is accompanied by ATP loss. The end result is a total opaque or cataractous lens.

NUCLEAR SCLEROSIS

The human lens normally undergoes changes with age. It slowly increases in size as new lens fibers develop throughout life. Older lens fibers in the center of the lens become dehydrated and compacted. The cross-linking of proteins in the nucleus increases its optical density and decreases its transparency. Clinically this condition is known as nuclear sclerosis which may cause refractive changes. Simultaneously splits in sutures or clefts in the cortical fibers are visible causing damage to the permeability of the lens. The nucleus of the lens becomes more compact and resists mechanical disruption with aging. There is extensive cross-linkage of the lens protein. The cataract protein cross-linkage is accompanied by increased pigmentation in certain cases. In senile cataracts, changes in lens color to dark yellow, yellow brown or brown and hardening of the nucleus parallel lead to decreased transparency. Three major types of cross-links are identified in senile cataracts.

- Disulfide cross-links (S-S)
- Lysine modification
- Dityrosine cross-links.

Protein SH groups are oxidized and noncovalent S-S protein cross-links are formed in senile cataracts.

These S-S bonds are susceptible to dissociation by a variety of reducing agents. The origin of oxidative insult is attributed to either the loss of lens glutathione, excessive H_2O_2 or lipid peroxidase in aqueous humor, increased permeability to oxygen into the aqueous or lack of oxygen detoxiflying enzymes. S-S cross-links may explain the conformational changes in protein causing opacity, the presence of covalent bonds is a feature of senile cataracts.

Superoxide anion-free radicals (O_2^-) or its derivative peroxide (H_2O_2), singlet, oxygen ($^1O_2$) and OH^- induce oxidative damage to a variety of cells. The lens is highly susceptible to these radicals. Peroxide (H_2O_2) is catalyzed through catalase and peroxidase and synthesized through superoxide dismutase. This oxidative damage as a result of free radicals to human lens leads to cataract formation (Fig. 2.8).

Diabetic Cataract

Snow flake cortical lens opacities also known as metabolic cataract is found in diabetic patients.

Increased levels of glucose in the aqueous and lens are found in patients with diabetes mellitus. In general glucose concentration in the aqueous is similar to concentrations in the plasma. From the

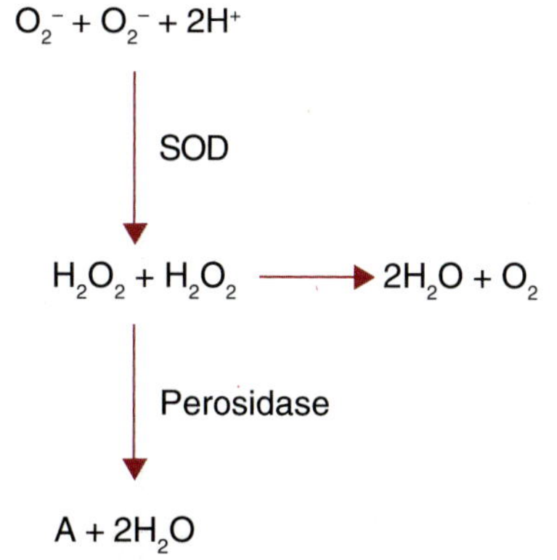

Fig. 2.8: Oxidative damage of lens (by free radicals)

aqueous glucose diffuses rapidly into the lens. The lens metabolizes glucose through the four main pathways as already mentioned in this chamber. In diabetes excessive glucose in the lens (more than 200 mg/100 ml) saturates hexokinase. Excessive glycosylation of lens proteins takes place and glucose is converted to sorbitol by auto-oxidation and protein binding (aldose reductase). These chemical changes are present in human diabetic cataract. However, glucose oxidation to sorbitol plays a more important role in the rapidly developing diabetic cataract. Whereas, abnormal protein glycosylation is of greater significance in the slowly developing senile cataracts in patients with diabetes.

REFERENCES

1. Garg Ashok. In: Text Book of Ophthalmology, New Delhi, Jaypee Brothers, 2002;1: 117-26.
2. Langston Pavan. Manual of Ocular Diagnosis & Therapy, Lippincot Williams & Wilkins, Philadelphia; 2002;140-63.
3. Pirie A, Van Heyningen R : Biochemistry of the Eye, Charles C. Thomas Publisher; 1956;32-44.
4. Cotlier F : Active Transport by the Crystalline Lens, Invest Ophthalmol; 1970;9:681.
5. Frohman CE, Kinsey VE : Studies on the Crystalline Lens, Arch. Ophthalmol; 1976;62: 8.
6. Gabby KH : The Sorbitol Pathway and the Complications of the Diabetes, N Eng J Med 1973;288: 831.

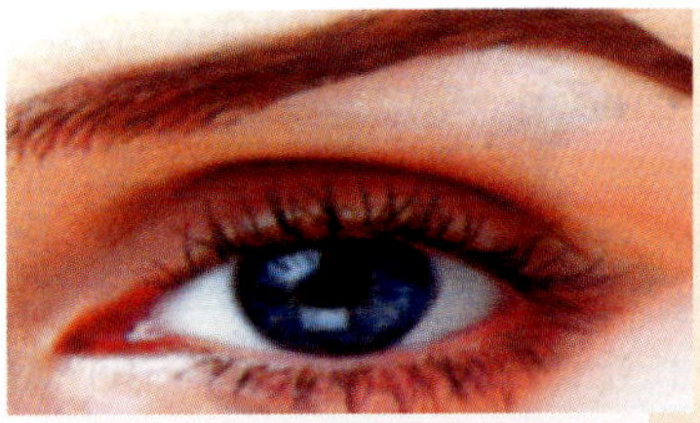

Three

Cataract Etiology: A Comprehensive Review

David Meyer
Paul Liebenberg
(South Africa)

INTRODUCTION

The term cataract is derived from the Latin *cataracta* and from the Greek *katarraktes* which denotes a waterfall or a portcullis. Analogously a cataract is a complete or partial opacification of sufficient severity, on or in the human lens or capsule, to impair vision.

Vision is one of the most valued senses. Proper vision is achieved by a series of eye tissues working harmoniously in concert. Most eye debilities involve dysfunction in the lens or retina, and hence this chapter will focus on and elucidate etiological factors which may affect the proper function of the lens as target organ.

The lens is an elegantly simple tissue. It is made up of only two types of cells.

- *Epithelial cells*, which have not yet completely differentiated and not yet elaborated the major gene products, and
- *Fiber cells*, in which these processes have been initiated or even completed.

Cataract is one of the major causes of visual impairment leading eventually to blindness. In the USA alone 1,35 million cataract extractions are performed annually. In developing countries the magnitude of the problem is overwhelming.

Management of this age-old impairment of vision requires one of the three following approaches, or a combination of these approaches.

1. Surgical, i.e. extracapsular lens extraction (either manually or by phacoemulsification) and intraocular lens (IOL) implantation;
2. Development and application of drug-related strategies to counteract the development of cataract;
3. Identification and elimination of risk factors.

It is now well-established that cataract formation is a multifactorial disease. Several of the etiological factors are constitutional and hence difficult to manipulate. Others are environmental in nature and a little easier to control whilst a significant number are behavioral in nature and fall well within the individuals' own ability to control or modify.

- This review will briefly touch on congenital and infantile cataract but will focus on etiological factors in adults (Fig. 3.1) and especially those implicated as risk factors in age-related cataract.

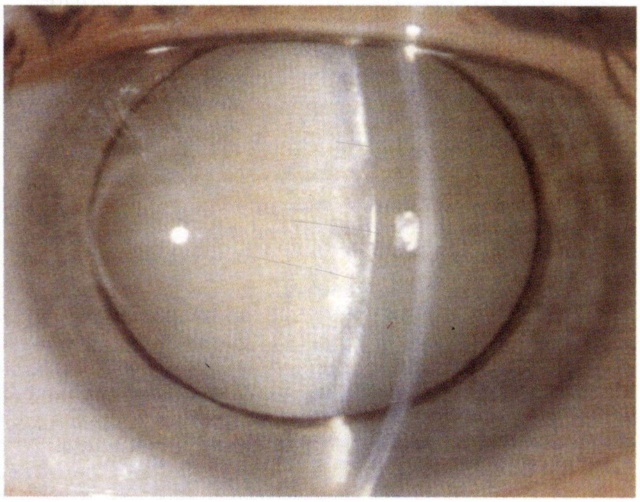

Fig. 3.1 : Mature senile cataract

CONGENITAL AND INFANTILE CATARACT

Congenital cataract is numerically the most important cause of remediable blindness in children, being far more common than, for example, retinoblastoma or congenital glaucoma.

The prevalence of infantile cataract has been reported to be between 1.2 and 6 cases per 10,000 births. Furthermore, it has been estimated that between 10 percent and 38.8 percent of all blindness in children is caused by congenital cataract (Figs 3.2 to 3.4) and that one out of every 250 newborns (0.4%) has some form of congenital cataract.

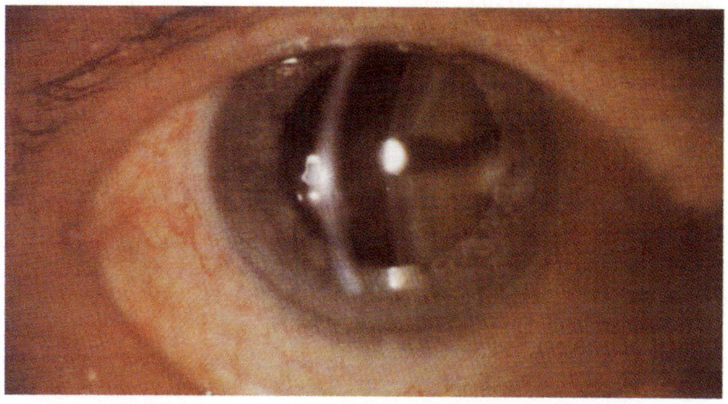

Fig. 3.2: Anterior polar congenital cataract

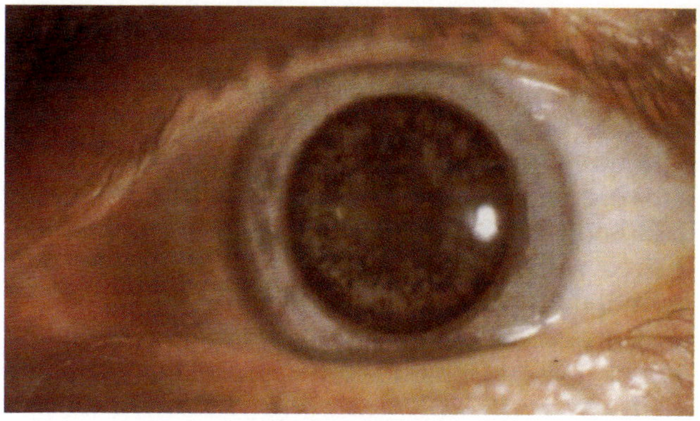

Fig. 3.3: Congenital cortical cataract

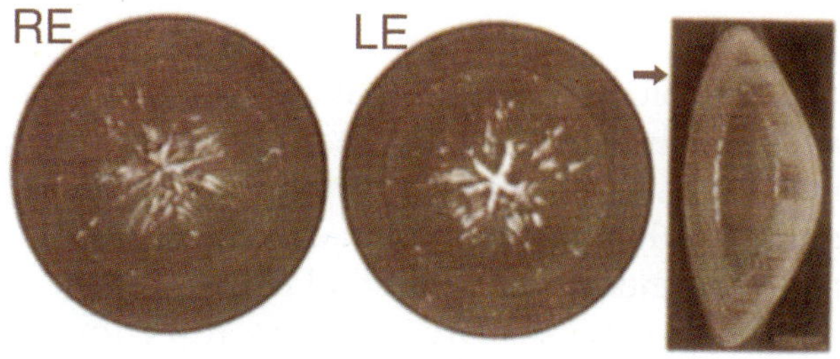

Fig. 3.4: Congenital coronary cataract

Table 3.1: Etiology of infantile cataract

A. Idiopathic

B. Intrauterine infection
1. Rubella
2. Varicella
3. Toxoplasmosis
4. Herpes simplex

C. Drug induced
Corticosteroids

D. Metabolic disorders
1. Galactosemia
2. Galactokinase deficiency
3. Hypocalcemia
4. Hypoglycemia
5. Mannosidosis

E. Trauma
1. Accidental
2. Non-accidental

F. Miscellaneous
1. Radiation
2. Laser photocoagulation

G. Other ocular diseases
1. Microphthalmia
2. Aniridia
3. Persistent hyperplastic primary vitreous (PHPV)
4. Prematurity
5. Peters' anomaly
6. Corneal guttata
7. Endophthalmitis

H. Dental anomalies
1. Nance-Roran syndrome

I. Cardiac disease
Hypertrophic cardiomyopathy

J. Renal disease
1. Lowe syndrome
2. Hallermann-Streiff-Francois syndrome

K. Inherited with systemic abnormalities
Chromosomal abnormalities
1. Trisomy 21
2. Turner syndrome
3. Trisomy 13
4. Trisomy 18
5. Translocation 3;4
6. Cri-du-chat syndrome
7. Translocation 2;14

Craniofacial syndromes
Cerebro-oculo-facio- skeletal syndrome (COFS)

Mitochondrial abnormalities
Complex I deficiency

L. Skeletal disease
1. Smith-Lemli-Opitz syndrome
2. Conradi syndrome
3. Weill-Marchesani syndrome

M. Syndactyly, polydactyly or digital abnormalities
1. Bardet-Biedl syndrome
2. Rubenstein-Taybi syndrome

N. Central nervous system abnormalities
1. Zellweger syndrome
2. Meckel-Gruber syndrome
3. Marinesco-Sjögren syndrome
4. Infantile neuronal ceroid-lipofuscinosis (Batten's disease)

O. Dermatological
1. Crystalline cataract and uncombable hair
2. Cockayne syndrome
3. Rothmund-Thomson syndrome
4. Atopic dermatitis
5. Incontinentia pigmenti
6. Progeria
7. Ichthyosis
8. Ectodermal dysplasia

The etiology of infantile cataract (Table 3.1) can be established in up to one-half of children with bilateral cataract, but in a smaller proportion of infants with unilateral cataract.Infantile cataract most commonly occur secondary to genetic or metabolic diseases, intrauterine infections or trauma. Less commonly they may occur as a side effect of treatment with certain medications or radiation therapy.

Genetic

Infantile cataract may be inherited as autosomal dominant, autosomal recessive or X-linked recessive traits. Autosomal dominant cataract are most commonly bilateral nuclear opacities, but marked variability can be present even within the same pedigree. In an extended pedigree of 28 patients with autosomal dominant nuclear cataract,

Scott *et al* reported that 19 of the affected family members had unilateral cataract while 9 had bilateral cataract. Less commonly, anterior polar, posterior polar, and posterior lentiglobus cataract can be autosomal dominantly inherited. In the United States, infantile cataract are most commonly inherited as autosomal dominant traits, however, in countries where there is a high prevalence of parental consanguinity, infantile cataract are more commonly inherited as autosomal recessive traits. In Egypt where one-third of all marriages are consanguineous, Mostafa *et al* reported autosomal recessive inheritance for six of seven pedigrees with inherited infantile cataract. Linkage analysis has been used to determine the genetic loci of certain autosomal dominant cataract. Coppock-like cataract has been linked to the gamma E-crystalline gene on chromosome 2, Coppock cataract to chromosome 1q21-q25, Marner cataract to 16q22, and cerulean cataract to 17q24. The Cerulean cataract links closely to the galactokinase gene, but galactokinase levels in these patients are normal.

Metabolic

The most common metabolic disturbance causing cataract during infancy is galactosemia. Galactosemia may be caused by a transferase, galactokinase or epimerase deficiency. Galactose-1-phosphate uridyl transferase (GALT) deficiency occurs in 1:40,000 newborns in the United States and 1:23,000 newborns in Ireland. A homozygous mutation of Q188R on exon 6 of the GALT gene on chromosome 9 is found in two-third of children with the transferase deficiency. This results in the accumulation of galactose 4-phosphate in the blood. Galactose is then converted to galactitol in the crystalline lens, resulting in an influx of water into the lens by osmosis. The hydration of the lens then disrupts the normal structure of the lens fibers, resulting in a loss of transparency. Early on, these lens changes have the appearance of an oil-droplet in the center of the lens. These changes are initially reversible with the elimination of galactose from the diet. If left untreated, a lamellar cataract develops which may then progress to a total cataract. In addition to cataract, these children have failure to thrive as infants, which may lead to death, if milk and milk products are not eliminated from their diet. Later in childhood, these children may have delayed development, abnormal speech, growth delay, ovarian failure and ataxia. While eliminating galactose from the diet can prevent the life-threatening problems which occur during infancy, dietary compliance does not always correlate closely with the formation of cataract in later childhood or with the associated abnormalities of late childhood. The N314D mutation of the GALT gene causes the milder Duarte form of galactosemia. Combinations of Q188R, N314D and unknown mutations may result in phenotypically different forms of galactosemia.

Galactokinase deficiency may cause cataract with few or no systemic abnormalities. The galactokinase gene is on chromosome 17 and has recently been cloned and found to harbor homozygous mutations in some patients with cataract. Heterozygotes for galactokinase deficiency have half normal values on blood tests. Conflicting results have been reported in the literature as to whether partial loss of enzyme activity leads to presenile cataract. Alpha mannosidosis can also be associated with early onset cataract.

Lamellar cataract may also develop in children with neonatal hypoglycemia or hypocalcemia. Neonatal hypoglycemia is more common in low birth weight infants.

Infectious

The congenital rubella syndrome was one of the most common causes of congenital cataract in the United States until the widespread employment of the rubella vaccine. During the rubella epidemic in the United States during 1963-64, 16 percent of all children with the congenital rubella syndrome developed cataract. Infantile cataract also occur occasionally in children after intrauterine varicella, toxoplasmosis and herpes simplex infections, or after bacterial or fungal endophthalmitis. Cataract may also develop after a varicella infection during early childhood.

Prematurity

Transient cataract occur occasionally in premature infants. They are usually bilateral and begin as clear vacuoles along the apices of the posterior lens suture. They may progress to posterior subcapsular vacuoles. In most cases, they clear completely over the course of several months. All of the premature infants with transient cataract reported by Alden *et al* were septic and had been treated with Kanamycin, 80 percent of these infants also had an unexplained metabolic acidosis. These authors suggested that osmotic changes in the lens of these infants might have caused these cataract.

Trauma

While trauma is not a common cause of cataract during infancy it should be considered, particularly when a cataract is associated with other ocular signs suggestive of a traumatic injury. The trauma can be either blunt or penetrating. Nonaccidental causes for the trauma must always be considered. Eyes with suspected traumatic cataract should also be examined carefully for both retinal and optic nerve injuries.

Laser Photocoagulation

Laser photocoagulation has been used in recent years to ablate the avascular retina of infants with threshold retinopathy of prematurity (ROP). Laser-induced cataract are transient in some instances, but progress in some cases to total opacification of the lens. Drack *et al* reported cataract in six eyes following argon laser photoablation of the avascular retina in four infants with threshold retinopathy of prematurity.

Radiation Induced

Radiation used to treat ocular and periocular tumors may induce cataract in children. A radiation dose of 15 Gy has been shown to be associated with a 50 percent risk of cataract formation. Radiation usually causes posterior subcapsular cataract, which typically have their onset 1 to 2 years after the completion of radiation therapy.

Medications

Systemic corticosteroids cause cataract in up to 15 percent of children once a cumulative dose of 1000 mg of prednisone or the equivalent has been reached. This cataract usually begin as central posterior subcapsular opacities, but may progress to involve the entire lens.

Idiopathic

In most series, at least 50 percent of bilateral infantile cataract are idiopathic. The percentage of idiopathic unilateral infantile cataract is even higher.

AGE RELATED CATARACT

Personal Factors

Gender

It has often been observed that more females than males have cataract and undergo cataract surgery. This is partly explicable by the longer life span of women and therefore, their over-representation in the age groups where cataract is most common. It does appear however, that there is an additional effect—a true excess risk of cataract in females. In Nepal the prevalence of cataract was greater in females than in males at all ages. The overall risk ratio was 1.4, which would be detectable only in larger studies. In most case-control studies the two groups were age- and sex-matched so that the effect of sex could not be explored. Hiller *et al* had to combine the results from three earlier studies in the United States and India to find a significant excess relative risk of 1.13 in females. This follow-up study of data from the National Health and Nutrition Examination Survey (NHANES) also suggested that such an excess risk for women is specific to cortical cataract. In a population-based prevalence survey in Beaver Dam, Wisconsin, women had more cortical opacities compared to men within similar age groups. The Beaver Dam Study reported a protective effect for nuclear opacities with current use of postmenopausal estrogens. Older age at menopause was associated with decreased risk of cortical opacities, suggesting hormonal influences in cataractogenesis. It was also suggested that hormone replacement therapy (HRT) may protect against cortical cataract. The

Epidemiology of Cataract in Australia, study found that a protective relationship of HRT and cortical cataract exists at the univariate level, but that this relationship was not significant in multivariate analysis. Nuclear cataract cases were more likely to be female in the above study, even after age adjustment. They were however unable to support the hypothesis that HRT is protective against nuclear cataract.

Tavani *et al* studied 287 Italian women who had undergone cataract extraction and 1277 control subjects who were in the hospital for acute, nonneoplastic, nonophthalmologic, nonmetabolic, nongastroenterologic diseases in a case-control study in Northern Italy. The results of this study support the association in women between cataract extraction and diabetes, (OR 4.6 for those younger than 60 years and 1.7 for those age 60 and over) current overweight, (OR 2.2) history of clinically relevant obesity, (OR 1.5) hypertension(OR 1.5) and hyperlipidemia (OR 1.8). They suggest that these factors may have some biologically independent impact on the risk of cataract in women and therefore supports the association in women between cataract extraction on the other hand and diabetes, current overweight, history of clinically relevant obesity, hypertension and hyperlipidemia on the other.

Body Mass Index

Body mass index (BMI) is computed as weight in kilograms divided by the square of the height in meters (kg/m^2) and is frequently identified as a risk factor for cataract, but the nature of the association is unclear. Several mechanisms may play a role:

- BMI affects glucose levels, which are associated with increased risk of cataract
- Higher BMI also increases uric acid concentrations and the risk of gout, which were associated with cataract in some studies
- BMI is also an important determinant of hypertension which has a controversial relationship with cataract.

Experimental evidence also supports a possible protective effect of restriction of energy intake on the risk of cataract by protection against oxidative stress to the lens.

In developing countries some studies have associated low BMI with cataract. A recent case control study in India , however failed to confirm this association.

Hankinson *et al* in a prospective study examined the association of BMI with cataract extraction in a large cohort of women and found elevated rates of cataract in those with higher BMI. Women with BMI of 23 or above had significantly elevated rates of extraction, between 46 percent and 65 percent higher than those with BMI of less than 21. Glynn *et al* in a prospective cohort study of a total of 17,764 apparently healthy US male physicians aged 40 to 84 years who were free of cataract at baseline were followed for 5 years. In this group higher BMI was especially strongly related to risk of posterior subcapsular and nuclear sclerotic cataract and was also significantly related to risk of cataract extraction. Furthermore BMI below 22 appeared especially protective against posterior subcapsular cataract, with reductions in risk of 50 percent or more relative to each of the groups with a higher BMI. They concluded that BMI appears to be a strong and independent risk factor for cataract in this well-nourished and socioeconomically homogenous study population. Even modest elevations in weight were associated with increased risk.

In so far as BMI index is modifiable, cataract caused by overweight is therefore, potentially preventable.

Social Economic Status

Less education and lower income are related to increased morbidity and mortality from a number of diseases, even after controlling the known risk factors. These relations have been attributed to underuse of health care resources, high-risk behaviors, exposure to noxious work or adverse home environment, and poor nutrition. In population studies, less education and lower income consistently have been associated with impaired vision and cataract. The relationship of education, income, marital status, employment status to age-related cataract and impaired vision was addressed in the population-based Beaver Dam Eye Study.

A private census of the population of Beaver Dam, Wisconsin, was performed from September 15, 1987 to May 4, 1988. Eligibility requirements for entry into the study included living in the city or township of Beaver Dam and being 43 to 84 years of age at the time of the census. A total of 5924 eligible people were identified. Of these, 4926 (83.1%) participated in the examination.

While controlling for age and sex in this study, less education was significantly ($P< 0.05$) related to higher frequency of nuclear sclerotic and cortical cataract. Lower reported total household income was significantly associated with higher frequencies of cortical and posterior subcapsular cataract. These relations between total household income and cataract were observed in both men and women.

Less education has been associated with higher frequencies of history of heavy drinking, cigarette smoking and less vitamin supplement intake, all of which have been found to be related to specific types of cataract. However, the association of education and income with cataract persisted, despite controlling these exposures in their population. It is possible that poorer nutrition occurring earlier in life, may be related to the development of age-related cataract. A second possible reason explaining the relation of education and income to cataract is that people with less education or lower income are less likely to see an ophthalmologist or have cataract surgery.

Marital status is a measure of social support which is postulated to be an important factor in developing and managing complications associated with disease. While controlling for age and sex, people who were never married had a higher frequency of impaired vision than those currently married. This may be due to the fact that married people may have more social pressure to seek health care and to maintain familial responsibilities, and they may have more transportation assistance than their unmarried/widowed counterparts.

In summary, less education and income are related to cataract and visual impairment, but not to age-related maculopathy. These data suggest that access to medical, surgical, and low vision care may be of benefit to people with low socioeconomic status.

Social Factors

Smoking

Tobacco is the leading preventable cause of disease, disability and premature death.

Tobacco smoking is considered a major risk factor for 6 of the 15 leading causes of death. An individual who smokes has about twice the risk of premature death as a non-smoker, and the heavier the cigarette consumption, the higher the risk.

Of the 4 000 active substances in tobacco smoke, most are hazardous to human health. More than 40 of these chemicals are carcinogens and many others are deleterious to the cardiovascular and the pulmonary systems. They include nicotine, tars, nitrosamines, polycyclic aromatic hydrocarbons, hydrogen cyanide, formaldehyde, and carbon monoxide. Cigarette smoking is also a substantial source of intake of heavy metals and toxic mineral elements, such as cadmium, aluminum, lead, and mercury, all known to be poisonous in high concentrations.

Tobacco smoke also contains numerous compounds with oxidative properties; their existence is linked to the pathogenesis of several of the most common eye disorders, such as cataract and age-related macular degeneration.

Epidemiological data link cigarette smoking to several ophthalmologic disorders like ocular irritation, ocular ischemia, age-related macular degeneration (AMD), cataract, thyroid ophthalmopathy, tobacco-alcohol amblyopia, primary open-angle glaucoma, conjunctival intraepithelial neoplasia, uveal melanoma, Leber hereditary optic neuropathy, type II diabetes, ocular sarcoidosis and strabismus in the offspring of smoking mothers. The effects of smoking on ocular disorders show significant dose dependence; higher levels of smoking increase the risk of developing cataract. It is important to note, however that the interpretation

Table 3.2: Smoking and the risk of cataract

Study	*Relative risk (RR)*	*95% CI*	*Comments*
Leske *et al*, 1991[90]	1.68	0.96-1.94	Association was found to nuclear cataract
Hankinson *et al*, 1992[91]	1.63	1.8-2.26	Conducted on 50,828 women; RR for developing posterior subcapsular cataract is 2.59
Christen *et al*, 1992[92]	2.16	1.46-3.20	N = 22,071 males; RR for nuclear cataract is 2.24 and for posterior subcapsular, 3.17
Klein *et al*,1993[93]	1.09	1.04-1.16	Beaver Dam Eye Study; same RR for women and men
West *et al*,1995[94]	2.40	1.00-6.00	Conducted on 442 watermen of the Chesapeake Bay

of results of different studies may be inherently biased, as smokers in these studies use cigarettes of different types, containing different concentrations of toxic substances. Moreover, some of the cigarettes have filters and others do not. Smoking habits may also be associated with other potentially noxious habits, such as excessive alcohol consumption, which may contribute a further bias to the results.

Table 3.2 summarizes five very thought-provoking studies all supporting the view that smoking is associated with the development of cataract.

Several authors have reported a significant link between tobacco smoking and an increased risk of cataract development. Nuclear sclerosis appears to be the type of cataract most commonly associated with smoking.

In the Beaver Dam Eye Study, the relationship between cigarette smoking and lens opacities was examined in 4926 adult subjects. A significant correlation was found between severe levels of nuclear sclerosis and the number of pack-years smoked. For both sexes, the odds ratio associated with 10 years was 1.09 (confidence interval, 1.04–1.16). The frequency of posterior subcapsular opacities was also increased (odds ratios, 1.05 [confidence interval, 1.00–1.11] for men and 1.06 [confidence interval, 0.98–1.14] for woman). Cortical opacities were not found to be linked to smoking. Leske *et al* studied, 1380 patients with cataract, aged 40 to 79 years, in an attempt to identify possible risk factors for the development of cataract, current smoking was correlated with the risk of developing nuclear cataract (odds ratio, 1.68; confidence interval, 0.96–1.94), but not other forms of cataract. The City Eye Study reported epidemiological data concerning 1029 volunteers, aged 54 to 65 years, from London, UK. The findings showed a significant relationship between nuclear lens opacities and moderate to heavy cigarette smoking. The relative risk for nuclear-type cataract ranged from 1.0 for past light smokers to 2.6 for past heavy smokers, and 2.9 for current heavy smokers.

Klein *et al* presented evidence that smoking has a detrimental effect on the development of cataract in the type II diabetic population.

Several prospective studies have investigated the relationship between cataract formation and cigarette smoking. In an 8-year prospective study, Hankinson *et al* examined the association between cigarette smoking and the risk of cataract extraction in 50,828 female nurses aged 45 to 67 years. The age-adjusted relative risk among female smokers of at least 65 pack-years was 1.63 (confidence interval, 1.18–2.26).

Smoking was also strongly associated with posterior subcapsular opacities for smokers of 65 or more pack-years (relative risk 2.59). In a 5-year prospective study of 22,071 men aged 40 to 84 years, current smokers of at least 20 cigarettes a day showed a significantly increased risk of developing cataract (relative risk 2.16; confidence interval, 1.46–3.20). When calculated for the different types, the relative risk was 2.24 for developing nuclear sclerosis and 3.17 for posterior subcapsular cataract. Past smokers were also at increased risk of developing posterior subcapsular opacities (relative risk 1.44), whereas, current light smokers had the same chance of developing any type of cataract as subjects who had never smoked. In a study of 838 watermen from Chesapeake Bay, Maryland, West *et al* found a significantly increased risk of development of nuclear opacities associated with cigarette smoking (relative risk 2.40; confidence interval, 1.00–6.00).

A 5-year prospective study of this cohort of subjects reported an increase in the incidence and degree of nuclear opacities with increasing age. The risk of progression of nuclear opacities from less than grade 3 at baseline to grade 3 or worse was 2.4-fold higher among current smokers than among ex-smokers or non-smokers.

A significant increase (18%) in the risk of cataract progression was associated with each pack-year that a subject had smoked during the 5-year study period.

Mechanism The way in which smoking induces cataract formation is probably through its effect on the oxidant-antioxidant status of the lens. Oxidative damage plays a major role in cataractogenesis. Animal, laboratory, clinical, and epidemiological data support the relationship between cataract prevention and diets rich in nutritional factors with antioxidant properties, such as riboflavin, vitamins C and E, and the carotenoids.

Smoking appears to further impair lenticular function by imposing an additional oxidative challenge as well as by contributing to the depletion of endogenous anti-oxidant pools. Tobacco smoke also contains large amounts of heavy metals, such as cadmium, lead and copper, which appear to accumulate in the lens and exert further toxicity.

The above data strongly support an association between tobacco smoking and cataract formation. Given the magnitude and seriousness of the cataract problem, an important preventive measure in fighting this disorder is to quit smoking. It is important to note that smoking is on the increase in the developing world, where cataract surgery is not always readily available.

Alcohol

Excessive alcohol use is associated with numerous chronic health problems, such as liver disease, varicosities, blood dyscrasias, and elevated blood pressure. Some studies have reported a relationship between alcohol consumption and cataract, while other studies have found no relationship. One study reported that both abstainers and heavy drinkers were more likely to have cataract than moderate users, while another found that total abstainers were more likely to have cataract than alcohol users.

As far back as 1973 Sabiston clinically observed in 40 patients over a 5-year period a definite correlation between alcohol intake, Dupuytren's contracture, and cataract. He stated that the mechanism of cataract formation was uncertain, but that an element of chronic dehydration was possible. In New Zealand, where he did his observations, heavy drinking often commenced with the ingestion of large quantities of beer. The national average consumption of beer there is 100 liters per head annually, with manual labourers ingesting a daily total of 4 liters of beer per person per day on average. These persons were almost invariably heavy cigarette smokers as well. He further noted that the cataract commenced in a posterior subcapsular position, and could progress to almost full maturity in six months. There was almost universally a history of heavy cigarette smoking as well. Malnutrition was only sometimes seen.

Drews in 1970 also drew attention to the association of ethanol and cataract. Two decades later he writes: "A patient in his or her 40s or 50s who appears with a posterior subcapsular cataract should be investigated for alcoholism. In the author's practice, about 25 percent of patients younger than age 65 years who present with cataract are found to be alcoholic on careful investigation. It has been his experience that if the opacities are incipient and if the consumption of alcohol is stopped completely, the posterior subcapsular changes may reverse and even disappear."

Two decades later attention is once again drawn to the possible link between alcohol and cataract in the Archives of Ophthalmology by two different sets of authors. Munoz *et al* from the Wilmer Eye Institute, Baltimore, MD, USA conducted a follow-up study of surgical cases of posterior subcapsular cataract(PSC) and their controls to evaluate the possible association of alcohol intake and posterior subcapsular opacities. Two hundred thirty-eight cases and controls were interviewed. Current alcohol intake and usual and maximum weekly consumption ever were assessed. In this population, 57 percent of the cases and 56 percent of the controls were nondrinkers, 22 percent of the cases and 36 percent of the controls had an average of seven or fewer drinks per week, and 17 percent of the cases and 8 percent of the controls had more than seven drinks per week. Heavy drinkers were more likely to be cases than were nondrinkers (odds ratio, 4.6;$P<0.05$), and light drinkers were not at an increased risk. Light drinkers, defined as those who drink less than 91g/wk (i.e., one drink or less per day), were at a lower risk than were nondrinkers, although this difference did not reach statistical significance. Moderate to heavy drinkers, that is, those drinking an average of more than one drink per day (more than 91g/wk) were 2.7 times more likely to have PSC. This U-shaped relationship between alcohol and the risk of PSC was more pronounced in the logistic regression model when controlling for all the factors found to be related to PSC. Some studies have suggested that heavy drinking patterns are associated with lower socioeconomic status. In this study after adjustment for education level, the risk of PSC was still higher among drinkers. Smoking was also not related to PSC. Heavy alcohol use has been linked to poor nutritional status, so the presence of PSC may be related to poor nutrition rather than alcohol consumption *per se*. Dietary assessment however, was not performed in this study. In summary, this study concluded that moderate to heavy alcohol consumption is associated with a four-fold increase of PSC cataract whereas light drinkers, those consuming one drink per day or less, were not at an increased risk.

The second study reported on in the same journal was on alcohol use and lens opacities in the Beaver Dam Eye Study group of patients. The relationship between alcohol use and lens opacities was examined in a large (N=4926) population-based study of adults. Alcohol history was determined by a standardized questionnaire and the cataract severity was determined by masked grading of photographs obtained using a slit lamp camera and retroillumination. Several significant findings were made and conclusions drawn:

- In both sexes and every age group, a higher percentage of current heavy drinkers had late nuclear sclerotic changes. Similar results were seen for cortical and PSC changes.
- Past heavy drinkers were found to have increased odds of nuclear sclerosis (OR, 1.34; 95% confidence interval[CI], 1.12 to 1.59). There was an additional significant effect of past heavy drinking on the severity of cortical opacity(OR, 1.36; 95%CI, 1.04 to 1.77). The presence of posterior subcapsular opacity was also significantly associated with past heavy drinking(OR, 1.57; 95%CI, 1.10 to 2.25).
- Wine was associated with less severe nuclear sclerosis (OR, 0,84; 95%CI, 0.74 to 0.94) in general. Participants who drank liquor were less likely to have severe nuclear sclerosis than those who did not (OR, 0,81; 95%CI, 0,72 to 0.95). Liquor use was also associated with lower frequencies of any cataract (OR, 0.83; 95%CI, 0.72 to 0.94) and fewer past cataract surgeries (OR, 0.75; 95%CI, 0.57 to 0.98).
- A significant relationship was found between beer consumption and cortical cataract. Those who drank larger amounts of beer were more likely to have cortical cataract than those who drank smaller quantity of beer. An increased risk of cortical cataract was associated with increased beer consumption. An increased risk of cortical cataract was not associated with consumption of wine, hard liquor, or a combination of alcohol types when considered as continuous variables. These different relationships for the different types of alcohol (wine and hard-liquor consumption was generally associated with OR's or less than 1, while beer consumption was associated with OR's of more than 1) raises the possibility that other components of wine or hard liquor confer protective effects on cataract development. However, no such theoretical links have yet been established.

Alcohol has many metabolic effects, and modifies the absorption of drugs and dietary components. These effects may be important in the alcohol-cataract relationship. However, one cannot exclude the possibility that alcohol itself, especially when consumed in high volume, may be a direct toxin to the human phacos.

Metabolic Factors

Diabetes Mellitus

Juvenile diabetic cataract classically known as the "snow flake cataract" is now uncommon with the advent of effective hypoglycemic therapy. It occurs in insulin-dependent diabetics whose onset was before the age of 30. The limited period over which snowflake cataract may occur (chiefly in the first two decades of life) contrasts with the extended period over which lenticular change occurs (from youth into the eighth decade). It is of interest that snow flake cataract occurs at a period of life when the lens is undergoing a major physiological shape change, with negligible sagittal and major equatorial expansion. It may very well be that the mechanisms for refractive change and cataract are the same but age-related factors such as the decreasing ability of the lens to swell may protect the older lens from this type of cataract formation. Other typical features of this type of cataract are subcapsular and cortical "snow flakes", and polychromatic opacities and vacuoles (Fig. 3.5). These may proceed to mature cataract within weeks or months and rarely, may be reversible after normalization of blood glucose over some weeks or even as rapidly as 24 hours.

The rat sugar cataract model is an attractive model for juvenile diabetic cataract in terms of its acute development and other features. It is also relevant to human galactosemic cataract, in which the lens is exposed to high levels of aqueous galactose. The first visible indication of galactosemic cataract is the "oil-droplet" change on retroillumination, due to a change in refractive index between the inner and outer parts of the lens.

It has been noted that there are difficulties in accepting a role of aldose reductase in human cataract. Even though sorbitol is found in increased amount in the human diabetic lens, the amounts detected have been quite low, and insufficient on a lens mass basis to account for osmotic damage.

Data on a cell-to-cell basis, which would be appropriate, are not available.

Although Vadot and Guibal considered that there was sufficient sorbitol in young diabetic lenses to induce cataract, Lerman and Moran could not demonstrate the accumulation of significant amounts in sugar-incubated lenses over the age of 20 years. There is no information about levels in juvenile diabetic cataract itself. Jedziniak *et al* found a higher aldose reductase activity in the young lens than in the adult lens and calculated that it was sufficient to generate a significant osmotic stress. However, these calculations referred to the lens epithelium and assumed that sorbitol was not removed. Since, polyol dehydrogenase is more active than aldose reductase in the human lens, the calculated levels would be expected to be lower. Lin *et al* demonstrated accumulation of dulcitol and loss of myoinositol in 72- hour cultures of infantile human lens epithelium in a 30 mlQI galactose medium, associated with vacuolar changes at ultrastructural level. Sorbinil and AL1576 reversed these changes. Similar changes have been produced in dog epithelial culture within 6 hours. Lin *et al* suggest that damage in the human lens

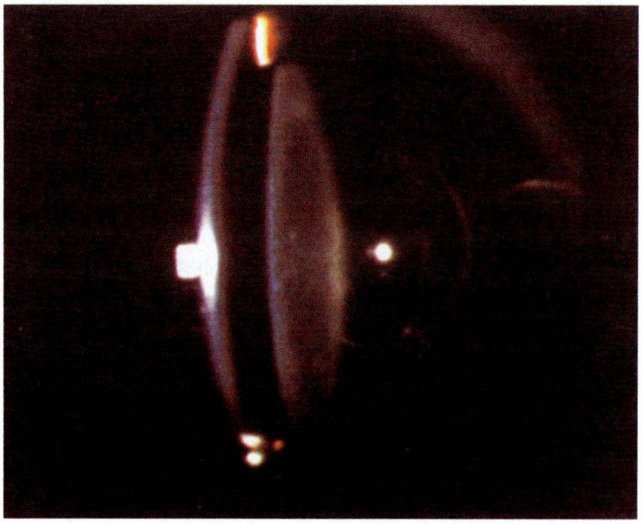

Fig. 3.5: Diabetic cataract

may reflect compartmentalization of aldose reductase activity, for instance in the epithelium. If sorbitol accumulation in the epithelium (and not the fibers) were the basis of juvenile cataract, then a failure of epithelial permeability or pumping functions would be a more likely cause of lens swelling and cataract than an osmotic mechanism. There is no information available as to whether an oxidative mechanism, dependent on the polyol pathway or not, is operative in juvenile diabetic cataract.

Cataract in diabetic adults Cataract has a greater prevalence in diabetics with a greater risk for women, and is dependent on the duration of diabetics. The morphology is no different from that of age-related cataract, although the frequency of some subtypes is increased.

Klein *et al* in a population study found cataract to be more prevalent in early and late onset diabetes with significant association with age, severity of retinopathy and diuretic usage. Diabetes duration and the level of glycosylated hemoglobin were also associations in early onset diabetics. In a second report, cataract was found to be the second most common cause of severe visual loss in adult onset diabetics. Various other reports have shown an association between cataract, and diabetes duration or retinopathy.

The frequency of cataract extraction is greater in diabetics than non-diabetics. The Framingham study showed a significant excess risk in the 50 to 64 year age group (relative risk 4.02), while the HANES study showed a relative risk of 2.97 in this age group and 1.63 in the 65 to 74 year age group. Both studies reported an excess prevalence of cataract in diabetics in 50 to 64 year age groups, which disappeared at an older age. This has been attributed to the higher mortality in diabetics with cataract. However, a case-control study in Oxford, found an increased risk for cataract extraction in diabetics in the age group of 50 to 79 years, and a small increase in risk for women relative to men.

As has been noted the morphology of cataract in the adult diabetic resembles that seen in age-related cataract in the absence of diabetes. Thus the major features are nuclear cataract (increased nuclear scattering and brunescence) and cortical spoke and posterior subcapsular cataract. In the Lens Opacity Case Control study, diabetes increased the risk of posterior subcapsular, cortical and mixed forms of cataract. Individual features may not have an identical etiology, but it is likely that those metabolic changes identified in experimental cataract are relevant for the human are in varying degrees. There is no relation between cataract type, and the level of either sorbitol or myoinositol in lens epithelium from patients with cataract and diabetes.

It has been suggested that the increased nuclear scattering and brunescence in diabetic lenses is likely to be the result of increased glycation and the formation of advanced glycation end products.

There is evidence for a fall in free lysine amino groups in the human diabetic lens. It is also possible to induce a change in tertiary structure in alpha-crystalline (bovine) incubated with glucose and glucose-6-phosphate.

A three-fold increase in glycation was measured in diabetics and controls by Vidal *et al* but there was no correlation with the degree of browning of the lenses measured spectrophotometrically, and they concluded that other chromophores were responsible for the browning at the relevant wavelengths.

Certainly a number of other factors have been proposed to contribute to nuclear brunescence of the non-diabetic lens, but since the diabetic state is not anticipated to increase their concentration, glycation products are still the most likely candidates responsible for diabetic cataract.

Cortical cataract can be caused experimentally by agents which interfere with membrane permeability, ion and water control. Oxidation of membrane thiols causes lens clouding and incubation of the lens with ouabain causes lens swelling and cataract. The non-diabetic, aging human lens, free of cataract, has an increased membrane permeability which parallels the increase in optical density which occurs from about the fifth decade. There is evidence of degradation of the lens protein MIP26 with age in non-diabetics, which could be responsible for a functional abnormality. This channel protein has until recently been regarded as the gap junctional protein, but may in fact serve as a volume regulating channel. Disturbance of either function could increase the risk of cataract. It would be of interest to examine these events in the diabetic lens. The greater thickness of the diabetic compared to the non-diabetic lens could be relevant to this point. The disturbance in Na' K'-ATPase kinetics reported by Garner and Spector during exposure to glucose-6-phosphate is similar to the change noted in diabetic human lenses. Hydrogen peroxide is present in normal human aqueous, and present at raised levels in the aqueous of patients with cataract. Higher levels are found in the aqueous of diabetic patients with cataract. Simonelli *et al* have also shown an increase in malondialdehyde in cataractous compared with non-cataractous lenses which is greater in the cataract of diabetic patients. Malondialdehyde is a product of lipid peroxidation of cell membranes, and is regarded as an indicator of oxidative membrane damage. These are important findings, although the methods of measurement are not entirely specific.

The potential role of the sorbitol (polyol) pathway in juvenile cataract was discussed earlier. Recent studies of cultured lens epithelium from cataract patients have shown negligible or absent levels of sorbitol in the epithelium of non-diabetics. In diabetic epithelium sorbitol levels are higher than blood glucose levels, while there is an inverse relationship between blood glucose and myo-inositol.

It has been noted that oxidative stress may cause lens membrane damage experimentally. It may also cause damage to DNA. Subcapsular cataract may be regarded as due to an aberration of lens mitosis and lens fiber differentiation, and could be the result of oxidative damage. There are no data, which link this to human subcapsular cataract.

Other cataract-related events A higher rate of capsular rupture reported in diabetics undergoing intracapsular or extracapsular extraction could be related to structural and chemical changes which are known to occur in the capsule. Thickening of the capsule has been reported in diabetic humans and animals, including the genetically determined diabetic kk mouse. There is an increased risk for death in patients with cataract and diabetes. Cohen *et al* found lens opacities to be a powerful predictor of death, independent of other factors and with an odds ratio of 2.4 (95% confidence interval 1.5-3.9).

Dyslipidemia

Lens opacification and cardiovascular disease are two of the main causes of morbidity worldwide. Lens opacity, manifesting as cataract, is responsible for an estimated 40 percent of the 42 million cases of blindness in the world. On the other hand, heart disease is the single greatest cause of death in developed countries. The relationship between cholesterol and cardiovascular heart disease is well documented. The relationship between cholesterol and lens opacity is, however, far less well appreciated.

Issues relating to drug safety and inherited defects in enzymes mediating cholesterol metabolism have brought renewed attention to a possible interrelationship between lipid metabolism and cataract induction in humans. The lens is unique in that it contains a relative abundance of cholesterol in the fiber cell plasma membrane (the highest of any cell group in the body), and furnishes its needs for cholesterol by onsite biosynthesis. It has been shown that inhibition of cholesterol synthesis in the lens leads to cataract formation in man.

Smith-Limli-Opitz syndrome, mevalonic aciduria and cerebrotendinous xanthomatosis are inherited disorders of cholesterol metabolism and affected patients may present with lens opacities. Triparanol, a hypolipidemic agent that inhibits cholesterol biosynthesis was withdrawn from clinical use because of its propensity to induce cataract formation in humans. The very widely used vastatin class of hypolipidemic medicines is potent inhibitors of cholesterol biosynthesis and is able to lower serum lipid concentration effectively. Although high ocular safety in older patients over periods of up to 5 years, has been reported, it is still not clear whether these agents have the potential to be cataractogenic, particularly in younger patients and over longer periods.

In order to assess the prevalence of lenticular opacities in patients with dyslipidemia (raised serum cholesterol and triglycerides) a group of 80 dyslipidemic patients were subjected to a general physical examination and an ophthalmic examination of the fully dilated eye at the Tygerberg Academic Hospital, University of Stellenbosch, South Africa (unpublished data).

Patients (n = 80) of both genders and irrespective of age were enrolled in the trial if they met the inclusion criteria for dyslipidemia. Patients were included if their fasting serum cholesterol and triglyceride concentrations were > 5.2 mmol/l and > 2.3 mmol/l, respectively when measured on three separate occasions over a one-month period (Fig. 3.6). Patients were excluded if they suffered from any condition known to cause or predispose them to elevated lipid levels or lenticular opacification.

Results The study group was predominantly male Caucasian and smokers. Most patients—68.8 percent admitted regular alcohol consumption. The mean systolic and diastolic blood pressure data, 134 ± 18 and 84 ± 9 mm Hg, respectively, fell within the normal range for age. The BMI of the group was significantly greater than the norm (i.e. 28.89 ± 4.82 kg/m).

The prevalence of lenticular opacities divided the study group into two cohorts, i.e. those with normal lenses (62%) and those with opacities (39%) (Fig. 3.7).

The prevalence of lenticular opacity in dyslipidemic patients in the age group of 30 to 40 years was 33 percent. This age group was not studied in the Barbados Eye Study (BES) or in The Beaver Dam Eye Study (BDES) and consequently data for comparison are not available (Table 3.3). In the 40 to 50 year age group, the prevalence of lenticular opacity in our patients was 50 percent compared to 4.7 percent in the BES and 8.3 percent in BDES. Differences in the older age groups were not prominent (Fig. 3.8).

Modern medicine today aspires to early detection of disease processes with the aim of early intervention in an attempt either to halt the progression or to reverse the process.

Although the classic systemic signs of dyslipidemia are well appreciated, i.e. xanthomata, xanthelasma, thickening of the Achilles tendon and corneal arcus, in our study the prevalence of one or more of the ocular signs was far greater than that of the systemic signs, 23.8 percent for the former as opposed to 47.3 percent for the latter.

The distribution of dyslipidemia-related signs in this study was:

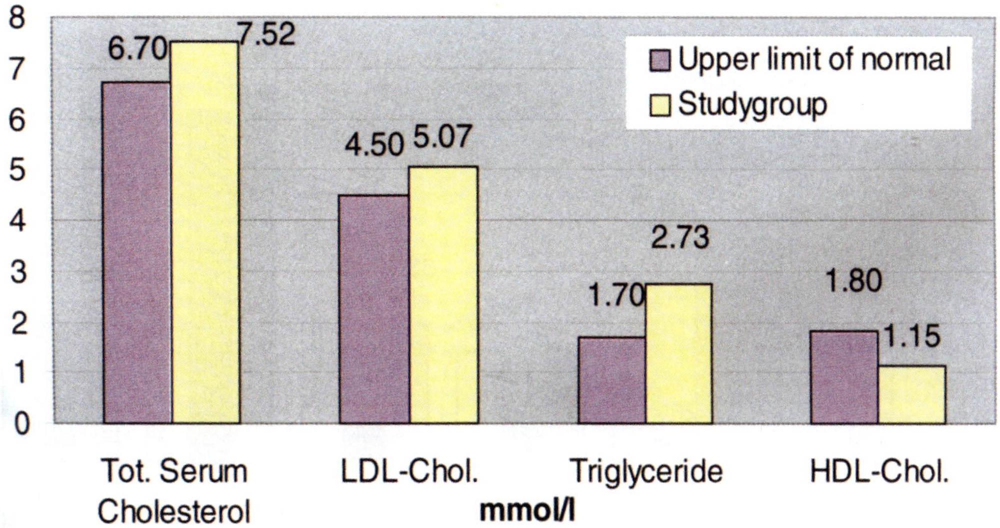

Fig. 3.6: The lipid profile of the study group

Table 3.3: Age distribution of patients with lenticular opacities compared to other population based studies

Age group (years)	*Percentage of opacities Study group*	*BES*[201]	*BDES*[202]
30-40	33.33	N/A	N/A
40-50	50.00	4.7	8.3
50-60	18.51	24.5	26.5
60-70	33.33	57.5	56.7
70-80	66.67	85.9	70.5
80+	33.33	98.3	N/A

BES: Barbados Eye Study
BDES: Beaver Dam Eye Study
N/A: Not available.

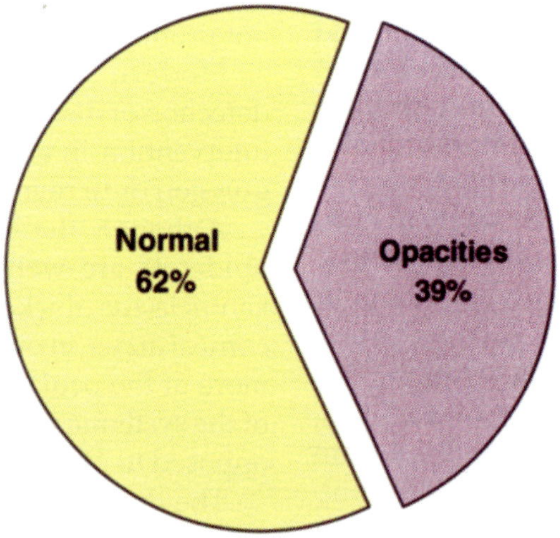

Fig. 3.7: The prevalence of lens opacities in the study group

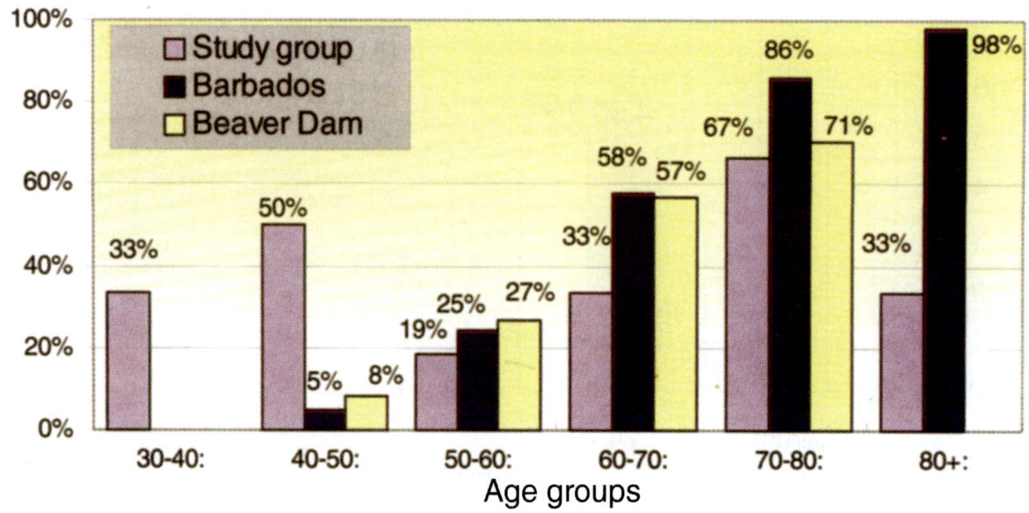

Fig. 3.8: Prevalence of lenticular opacities in two population-based studies compared to the dyslipidemic study group

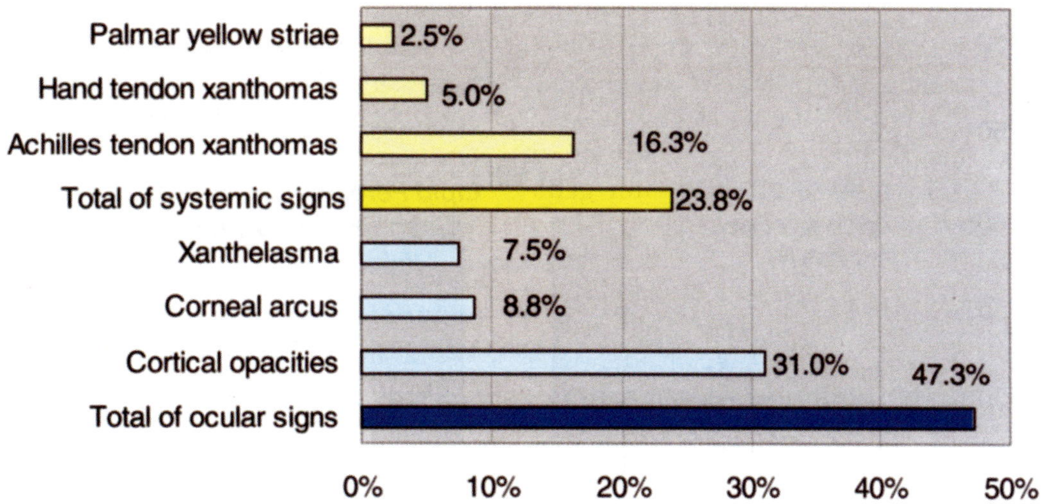

Fig. 3.9: Physical signs associated with dyslipidemia

- Xanthelasma—7.5 percent
- Corneal arcus—8.8 percent
- Achilles tendon involvement—16.3 percent
- Cortical lenticular opacity—31.0 percent.

It is noteworthy that the most frequent ocular sign—cortical lenticular opacity—occurred twice as frequently as the most frequent systemic sign—Achilles tendon thickening (Fig. 3.9).

This work leads the investigators to conclude that:

- Dyslipidemic patients are more likely to develop cortical opacification than the normal population.
- Cortical lens opacification in dyslipidemics manifests at a younger age than does nuclear opacification.
- Cortical lens opacification in the patient younger than 50 years of age should alert the ophthalmologist to arrange for diagnostic serum lipid assessment.
- Cortical lenticular opacification should be regarded as one of the most common, and hence reliable, clinical signs of dyslipidemia.

Jahn *et al* attempted to determine the role of glucose and lipid metabolism in the formation of cataract in elderly people undergoing cataract extraction. They found that patients with posterior subcapsular cataract had higher concentrations of fasting serum triglycerides and were significantly younger than patients with nuclear or cortical cataract. Their results furthermore suggest that the association of hypertriglyceridemia, hyperglycemia and obesity favors the formation of a specific morphologic type of lens opacity, posterior subcapsular cataract, occurring at an early age. Because these factors are potentially modifiable by lifestyle changes, these observations may prove important as the modification of these parameters could constitute an effective mode of prevention or retardation in a subgroup of patients developing cataract at an early age.

Acetylator Status

The human acetylation polymorphism has been known for more than three decades since its discovery during the metabolic investigation of the antituberculous hydrazine drug, isoniazid. The trait was originally known as the "isoniazid acetylation polymorphism" but is now usually abbreviated as "acetylation polymorphism" because acetylation of numerous hydrazine and arylamine drugs and other chemicals are subject to this trait. Individuals phenotype as "slow" acetylators when homozygous for the slow acetylator gene, "rapid" when homozygous for the rapid acetylator gene or "intermediate" when heterozygous. The acetylator phenotype is a lifelong, relatively stable characteristic of the individual that can phenotypically be determined by procedures using any of several test agents (e.g. caffeine, isoniazid, sulfamethazine, sulfapyridine). Certain disease states such as AIDS can change the phenotype expression in an individual. On the other hand, acetylator genotype can be determined by specialized polymerase chain reaction (PCR) methods.

Several diseases have been linked to acetylator pheno- and/or genotype. The best documented are bladder cancer (slow), colorectal adenomas (frapid), Gilbert's syndrome (slow), allergic diseases Type I diabetes mellitus (fast), Type II diabetes mellitus (slow) and familial Parkinson's disease (slow).

Recent work (PhD level, unpublished) at the departments of Ophthalmology and Pharmacology at the University of Stellenbosch, South Africa have also established an association between age-related cataract and acetylation status as determined both phenotypically and genotypically. Sixty adult patients of both sexes with classic age-related lens opacities presenting for cataract surgery were enrolled in a prospective controlled study. Patients were included in the trial if they perceived themselves to be colored and if this was verified by at least one independent observer. The South African population of mixed ancestry (including Malay, Khoisan, Negroid and Caucasoid stock) is referred to as "colored" and all patients were selected from this well studied subgroup of the population. Care was taken to exclude all patients with well known etiological factors for cataract formation such as diabetes mellitus, previous ocular trauma, other metabolic and/or inherited diseases. One hundred and twenty patients of the same race group served as controls.

Figure 3.10 demonstrates that in the control group (representing the population at large) the distribution of the phenotypic acetylation status was 20 percent "rapid", 50 percent "intermediate" and 30 percent "slow". In the cataract group the distribution was 5 percent "rapid", 42 percent "intermediate" and 53 percent "slow". This clearly seems to suggest that cataract possibly occur more frequently in slow acetylators than in the rest of the population. Could this finding perhaps suggest a possible etiologic role for chemical substances possessing a primary aromatic amine or hydrazine group in human lenticular opacification?

Lipid Peroxidation, Free Radicals and Nutritional Influences on Cataract Formation

Oxygen and oxygen-derived free radicals and a failure of intracellular calcium homeostatic mechanisms are recurring themes in a wide variety of cell injuries.

The addition of electrons to molecular oxygen leads to the formation of toxic free oxygen radicals or reactive oxygen species (ROS), e.g.

O_2^- = superoxide (one electron)
H_2O_2 = hydrogen peroxide (two electrons)
OH^- = hydroxyl radical (three electrons)

Iron is very important in this process according to the Haber-Weiss reaction:

$$H_2O_2 + O_2^{-Fe2+}. OH + OH^- + O_2$$

These free radical species cause lipid peroxidation and other deleterious effects on cell structure. Recent studies have shown that lipid peroxidation, an event caused by imbalance between free radical production and antioxidant defense, may play a role in the genesis of cataract. Higher levels of malondialdehyde (MDA), a final product of the lipid peroxidation process, have been observed in diabetic and myopic cataract compared with senile cataract. Protection of the cell against damage by these free radicals takes place indirectly (enzymatically) by antioxidant enzymes—superoxide dismutase (SOD), glutathione peroxidase (GPX) and catalase (CAT). Direct protection is offered by mainly dietary antioxidants—ascorbate (Vit C), tocopherol (Vit E), carotenoids(Vit A) and glutathione (GSH).

Light and oxygen as risk factors for cataract Various epidemiological studies demonstrate associations between elevated risk of various forms of cataract and exposure to higher intensities of incident and/or reflected ultraviolet light (Table 3.4).

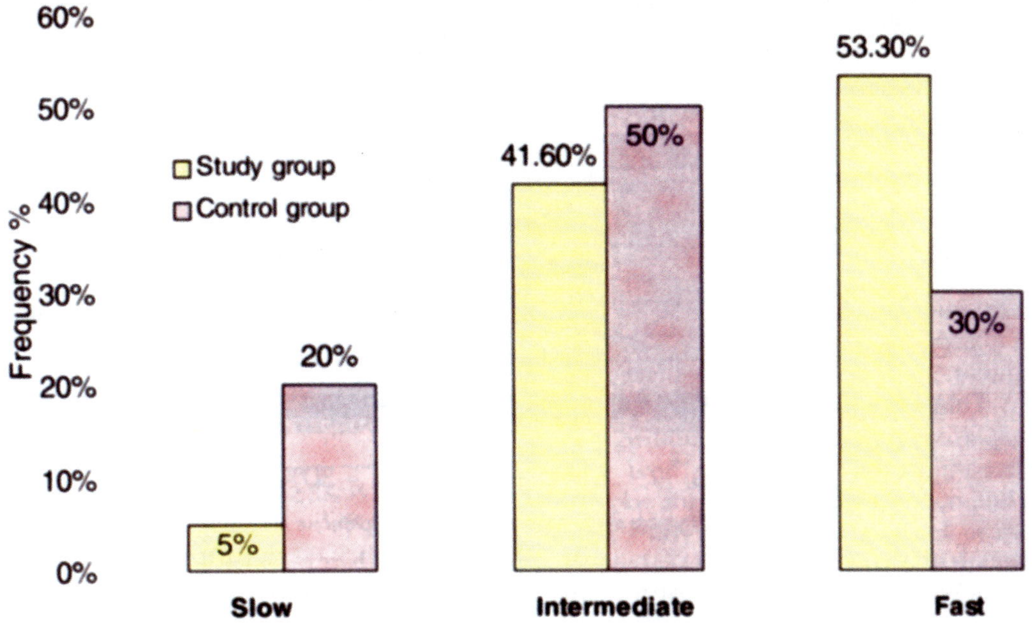

Fig. 3.10: Acetylator status of cataract vs normal patients

Elevated levels of oxygen exposure perhaps show the clearest causal relationship between oxidative stress and cataract. Nuclear cataract was observed in patients treated with hyperbaric oxygen therapy, and markedly elevated levels of mature cataract were observed in mice that survived exposure to 100 percent oxygen twice weekly for 3 hours. A higher incidence of cataract was noted in lenses exposed to hyperbaric oxygen *in vitro*. Very early stages of cataract in guinea pigs exposed to hyperbaric oxygen was noted by Giblin.

Role of cellular antioxidants against lens damage

Protection of the organism against photooxidative insult can be viewed as two interrelated processes. Primary defenses offer protection of proteins and other lens constituents by lens antioxidants and antioxidant enzymes whereas, secondary defenses include proteolytic and repair processes. The primary defenses shall form the focus of our attention.

The major aqueous antioxidants in the lens are ascorbate and GSH.

Ascorbate is probably the most effective, least toxic antioxidant identified in mammalian systems. The following has been observed

- The lens and aqueous concentrate ascorbate >10 times the level found in human plasma.
- The concentration of ascorbate in the lens nucleus is only 25 percent that of the surrounding cortex.
- Ascorbate levels in normal lenses are higher than in cataractous lenses.
- Ascorbate levels are higher in the older guinea pig lens than in younger animals despite the same dietary intake of ascorbate.
- Increasing lens ascorbate concentrations by two-fold is associated with protection against cataract-like damage.

With this basic science knowledge several epidemiological, clinical and even interventional studies have been undertaken. Vitamin C was considered in approximately 9 published studies and observed to be inversely associated with at least one type of cataract in eight of these studies.

In the Nutrition and Vision Project, age-adjusted analyzes based on 165 women with high vitamin C intake (mean = 294 mg/day) and 136 women with low vitamin C intake (mean = 77mg/day) indicated that the women who took vitamin C supplements

Table 3.4: Extent of light exposure and the risk of cataract

Study	Exposure		PR	95% CI
USA: NHANES survey[222]	Daily hours of sunlight in area; ages 65 -74	< 6.6 h	1.0	
		7.1 – 7.7 h	1.7	1.2 – 2.7
		>8.2 h	2.7	1.6 – 4.6
Australia[223]	Daily hours of sunlight in area	<8 h	1.0	
		8.5 – 9 h	2.9	0.6 – 13.2
		>9.5 h	4.2	0.9 – 18.9
	Average mean erythemal dose of area	2000	1.0	
		2500	1.3	0.8 – 2.3
		3000	1.8	1.0 – 3.4
Nepal[224]	Average hours of sunlight	7 – 9 h	1.0	
		10 – 11 h	1.2	0.9 – 1.4
		>12 h	2.5	2.1 – 3.0

PR = prevalence ratio
CI = confidence interval

for ≥ 10 years had > 70 percent lower prevalence of early opacities (RR: 0.23; CI: 0.09-0.60) and > 80 percent lower risk of moderate opacities (RR: 0.17; CI: 0.03-0.87) at any site compared with women who did not use vitamin C supplements.

In comparison to the above data, Mares-Perlman and *et al* report that past use of supplements containing vitamin C was associated with a reduced prevalence of nuclear cataract, but an increased prevalence of cortical cataract after controlling for age, sex, smoking, and history of heavy alcohol consumption.

Glutathione (GSH) levels in the lens are several fold the levels found in whole blood and plasma. GSH levels also diminish in the older and cataractous lenses. Pharmacological opportunities could be suggested by observations that incorporating the industrial 0.4 percent butylated hydroxytoluene in diets of galactose-fed (50% of diet) rats diminished prevalence of cataract. Clinical studies however, have not yet been forthcoming.

Vitamin E, a natural lipid-soluble antioxidant, can inhibit lipid peroxidation and appears to stabilize lens cell membranes. Consumption of Vit E supplements was inversely correlated with cataract risk in two studies. Robertson *et al* found among age- and sex-matched cases and controls that the prevalence of advanced cataract was 56 percent lower (RR: 0.44: CI: 0.24-0.77) in persons who consumed vitamin E supplements (>400 I.U./day) than in persons not consuming supplements. Jacques and Chylack (unpublished) observed a 67 percent (RR: 0.33; CI:0.12-0.96) reduction in prevalence of cataract for vitamin E supplement users after adjusting for age, sex, race and diabetes.

Two prospective studies demonstrated a reduced cataract progress among individuals with higher plasma vitamin E. Rouhianen *et al* found a 73 percent reduction in risk for cortical cataract progression (RR:027; CI: 0.08-0.83), whereas Leske *et al* reported a 42 percent reduction in risk for nuclear cataract progression (RR: 0.58; CI 0.36-0.94). Vitamin E supplementation was related to a lower risk for progress of nuclear opacity (RR:0.43; CI 0.19-0.99).

The carotenoids, like vitamine E, are also natural lipid-soluble antioxidants. Beta-carotene is the best known carotenoid because of its importance as a vitamin A precursor. However, it is only one of the 400 naturally occurring carotenoids, and other carotenoids may have similar or greater antioxidant potential. In addition to β-carotene, α-carotene, lutein and lycopene are important carotenoid components of the human diet. Jacques and Chylack were the first to observe that persons with carotene intakes above 18,700 IU/day had the same prevalence of cataract as those with intakes below 5,677 IU/day (RR:0.91; CI:0.23-3.78). Hankinson *et al* followed this report with a study that reported that the multivariate-adjusted rate of cataract surgery was about 30 percent lower (RR: 0.73; CI 0.55-0.97) for women with high carotene intakes (median = 14,558 IU/day) compared with women with low intakes of this nutrient (median = 2,935 IU/day). However, while cataract surgery was inversely associated with total carotene intake, it was not strongly associated with consumption of carotene-rich foods, such as carrots. Rather, cataract surgery was associated with lower intakes of foods such as spinach that are rich in lutein and xanthin carotenoids, rather than β-carotene. This would appear to be consistent with the observation that the human lens contains lutein and zeaxanthin but no β-carotene.

This observation would appear to be consistent with the observation that lutein and zeaxanthin are the most prevalent carotenoids in lens. However, Mares-Perlman did not detect a significantly altered risk for cataract among consumers of these nutrients.

Intervention studies To date only one intervention trial designed to assess the effect of vitamin supplements on cataract risk has been completed. Sperduto *et al* took advantage of two ongoing, randomized, double-blinded vitamin and cancer trials to assess the impact of vitamin supplements on cataract prevalence. The trials were conducted among almost 4,000 participants aged 45 to 74 years from rural communities in Linxian, China. Participants in one trial received either a multisupplement or placebo. In the second trial, a more complex factorial design was used to evaluate the effects of four different vitamin/mineral combinations:

- Retinol (5000 IU) and zinc (22 mg)
- Riboflavin (3 mg) and niacin (40 mg)
- Vitamin C (120 mg) and molybdenum (30 mg)
- Vitamin E (30 mg), β-carotene (15 mg), and selenium (50 mg).

At the end of the five to six year follow-up, the investigators conducted eye examinations to determine the prevalence of cataract. In the first trial there was a significant 43 percent reduction in the prevalence of nuclear cataract for persons aged 65 to 74 years receiving the multisupplement (RR: 0.57; CI: 0.36-0.90). The second trial demonstrated a significantly reduced prevalence of nuclear cataract in persons receiving the riboflavin/niacin supplement relative to those persons not receiving the supplement (RR: 0.59; CI 0.45-0.79). The effect was strongest in those aged 65 to 74 years (RR: 0.45; CI 0.31-0.64). However, the riboflavin/niacin supplement appeared to increase the risk of posterior subcapsular cataract (RR:2.64; CI: 1.31-5.35). The results further suggested a protective effect of the retinol/zinc supplement (RR: 0.77; CI: 0.58-1.02) and the vitamin C/molybdenum supplement (RR:0.78; CI: 0.50-1.04) on prevalence of nuclear cataract.

Conclusion Although light and oxygen are necessary for physiological function, when present in excess they seem to be causally related to cataractogenesis. Aging might diminish the bodies primary antioxidant reserves, antioxidant enzyme abilities, and diminished secondary defenses such as proteases.

The literature creates the strong impression that antioxidant intake might diminish the risk for cataract formation.

Longitudinal studies and more intervention studies are essential in order to establish the value of dietary antioxidants and to determine the extent to which cataract progress is affected by nutritional supplements. This fact becomes significant when one appreciates that poor education and lower socioeconomic status are directly related to poor nutrition. It is, therefore, not irrational to contemplate the value of intervention for populations at risk. The work available, albeit preliminary, indicates that nutrition may provide the least costly and most practicable means to attempt the objectives of delaying cataract. Ocular Disease

Many ocular diseases have been associated with cataract formation either as direct cause and effect relationships or as common associations.

Myopia

Weale suggested that lenses of myopes are subject to excessive mechanical stress which could lead to cataract. This hypothesis was tested by several investigators and Harding *et al* during their Oxford case-control studies found that the risk of cataract after the age of 50 was doubled in myopes. Weale

(1980) also suggested that there is a graded risk for increasing degrees of myopia. This was eloquently confirmed two decades later by Lim *et al* in the Blue Mountains Eye Study. Eyes with onset of myopia before age 20 had the greatest posterior subcapsular (PSC) cataract risk(odds ratio[OR] 3.9; confidence interval [CI] 2.0-7.9) Refraction-related increasing odds were found between PSC cataract and myopia: low myopia (OR 2.1; CI 1.4-3.5), moderate myopia (OR3.1; CI 1.6-5.7), and high myopia (OR 5.5; CI 2.8-10.9). High myopia was associated with PSC, cortical, and late nuclear cataract. Conversely PSC cataract was inversely associated with hyperopia (OR 0.6; CI 0.4-0.9). They finally concluded that early-onset myopia(before 20 years of age) may be a strong and independent risk factor for PSC cataract, that nuclear cataract was associated with presumed acquired myopia, whereas high myopia was associated with all three types of cataract.

Wensor *et al* demostrated that a myopic shift is associated with nuclear cataract. In the population based study of 3,271 Australians an association between myopia of 1 diopter or more and both nuclear and cortical cataract was observed. Between posterior subcapsular cataract and myopia such a relationship did not exist. It is not sure that a causal relationship exists between cortical cataract and myopia or rather that a myopic shift occurs after people develop cortical cataract. The temporality of this relationship should still be explored in future prospective analyses.

Glaucoma

Glaucoma has been shown to be strongly associated with the pathogenesis of cataract in many studies undertaken in many countries. The relative risk (odds ratio [OR]) of cataract developing in a glaucoma patient can be as high as six times normal. This risk more than doubles to an OR of 14.3 after glaucoma filtration surgery. This rise in risk is most probably due to the trauma of surgery for glaucoma. Vesti in Helsinki, Finland investigated cataract progression after trabeculectomy in a study of 47 eyes with exfoliative glaucoma (EXG) and in 20 eyes with primary open-angle glaucoma (POAG). EXG, age, hypotony (IOP < or = 5 mm Hg) lasting > or = 5 days and early postoperative IOP rise > 30 mm Hg were observed to be risk factors for cataract progression.

Besides formal filtering procedures like full thickness procedures, laser procedures for the management of different types of glaucomas are frequently performed such as argon laser trabeculoplasty, argon laser iridoplasty and Nd-YAG peripheral iridotomy. Each of these procedures carries the risk of inducing a cataract especially of the focal type. Zadok *et al* has described a previously unreported complication of a posterior chamber intraocular lens (IOL) implanted in a phakic eye. The left eye of a 25-year old patient with high myopia was treated prophylactically with Nd: YAG laser iridotomy prior to phakic IOL implantation. Slit lamp examination of the same eye disclosed an opacity of the anterior capsule of the crystalline lens under the iridotomy site.

Miotics, particularly long-acting cholinesterase inhibitors, if used for long-term, may cause tiny anterior subcapsular vacuoles and, occasionally, more advanced opacities. Cessation of medication may stop, retard or occasionally reverse their progression.

Acute congestive angle-closure glaucoma is associated with the subsequent formation of glaukomflecken consisting of small, gray-white, anterior, subcapsular or capsular opacities in the pupillary zone (Fig. 3.11).

Ophthalmic Surgical Procedures

Many different ophthalmic procedures carry the risk of inducing cataract. Among others are surgical iridectomy, filtration surgery, corneal transplants, retinal detachment surgery with and without intraocular silicone oil as well as pars plana vitrectomy especially in diabetics. Assessing the surgical outcome in a series of 63 consecutive patients treated for rhegmatogenous retinal detachment by primary vitrectomy Oshima reported the reattachment rate by final examination as 100 percent, but there was a high incidence (53.8 percent) of cataract progression in phakic eyes.

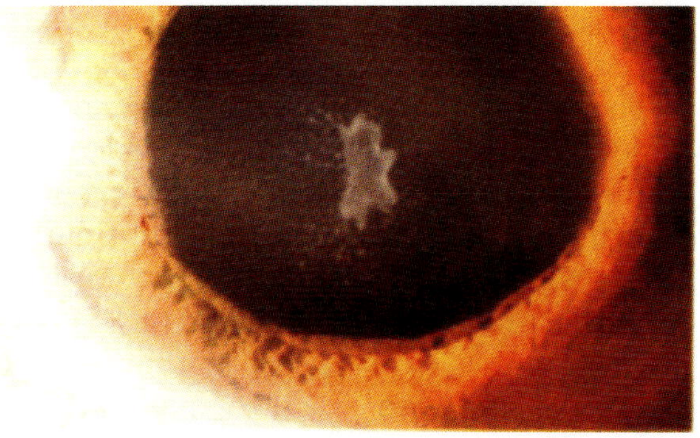

Fig. 3.11 : Anterior subcapsular flecks after acute closed angle glaucoma

More recently with the advent of minus power phakic IOL implantation surgery, several reports have appeared of cataract induction secondary to the implantation of these lenses into the ciliary sulcus. These cataract have occurred both with silicone and collamer materials. Some have taken as short a time as 6 months, whilst others took 7 years to form. In another series of 38 consecutive eyes with high myopia implanted with a silicone posterior chamber plate-style intraocular lens (Chiron, Adatomed) over a period of 21 months and followed for between 3 and 24 months not a single cataract occurred. The lens style and design may play a significant role in the cataract pathogenesis, because in a recent study Brauweiler *et al* attempted to assess the effectiveness and safety of implantation of a silicone, posterior chamber IOL in the ciliary sulcus of phakic, highly myopic eyes in a noncomparative consecutive interventional series. Eighteen eyes of 10 patients underwent implantation of a Fyodorov 094M-1 IOL by the same surgeon and were evaluated for a 2-year postoperative period. Cataract formation of the anterior subcapsular (8 eyes) or nuclear (only 1 eye) type was observed in overall 9 (52.9%) of 17 eyes. When considering only the patients with a follow-up of 2 years, the incidence of cataract formation was 81.9 percent (9 of 11 eyes). Obviously this very high incidence of cataract formation should discourage the implantation of the type of IOL used in this study.

Ocular Trauma

The development of cataract is a known complication following blunt or penetrating ocular trauma. However, traumatic cataract and zonular dehiscence is only one complication of the injured ocular tissues. Other complications include glaucoma, retinal detachment, optic nerve damage, extraocular muscle imbalance and injury to the bony orbit.

Ocular trauma is a major cause of monocular blindness in both the developed and developing world, but this is not seen as a significant cause of bilateral blindness. Trauma can therefore be considered as a major cause of blind eyes but not of blind people.

Crystalline lens subluxation, total dislocation, or localized cortical or diffuse opacities are often observed secondary to blunt ocular trauma. An unusual complication of blunt trauma is rupture of the posterior capsule with subsequent lens fiber hydration leading to rapidly progressive lens opacification (Fig. 3.12). Posterior capsular breaks have been reported to develop thick, fibrous, opaque margins approximately 6 weeks after blunt trauma.

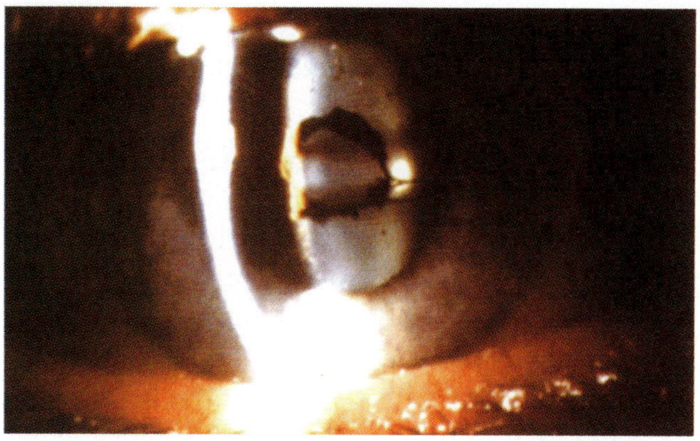

Fig. 3.12: Vossius' ring after blunt ocular trauma

Secondary Cataract

Uveitis A secondary cataract develops as a result of some other primary ocular disease. The most common cause of secondary cataract is chronic anterior uveitis. The earliest finding is a polychromatic luster at the posterior pole of the lens. If the uveitis is controlled, the progression of cataract may be arrested. If the inflammation cannot be controlled, anterior and posterior subcapsular opacities develop and the lens may become completely opaque. The lens opacification seems to progress more rapidly in the presence of posterior synechiae.

Hereditary posterior segment disease Hereditary fundus dystrophies such as retinitis pigmentosa, Leber's congenital amaurosis, gyrate atrophy, Wagner's and Stickler's syndromes may be associated with posterior subcapsular lens opacities. In a study of 384 eyes of 192 patients with a mean age of 39.1 years who presented with typical retinitis pigmentosa, cataract was found in 46.4 percent of the eyes. Among these, 93,6 percent showed posterior subcapsular opacification. The incidence of cataract increased with age.

Wagner's vitreoretinal degeneration is characteristically associated with high myopia, glaucoma, choroidal atrophy, retinal detachment and presenile cataract.

Persistent hyperplastic primary vitreous (PHPV) is a congenital disorder that manifests a range of ocular anomalies including leukoria, microphthalmia, a retrolental fibrovascular membrane and cataract. In general the prognosis for visual acuity with PHPV is poor.

Iris color McCarty *et al* in their Australian population study of 3,271 adults aged 40 years and older found an association between cortical cataract and brown or dark brown irides for all ages that was not explained by country of birth or language spoken. In all age categories, brown iris color was also associated with nuclear cataract. No such association was found for posterior subcapsular cataract however.

In the Italian-American Cataract Study, there was an increased, although not significant, risk of cortical cataract in people with brown irides. Dark iris color was not associated with cortical cataract in the Lens Opacities Case-Control Study. In the National Health and Nutrition Examination Survey, blacks, who have dark brown irides, were found to have significantly increased risk of cortical cataract. In both the above mentioned studies, dark iris color was also found to be a significant risk factor for nuclear cataract.

The relationship of nuclear cataract and iris color could result from genetic susceptibility associated with iris color or other factors not yet determined. This finding may partially explain the variation in the prevalence of nuclear cataract observed in different countries with different racial groups.

Systemic Diseases

Hypertension

The association between hypertension and cataract was first noted in the Framingham study where earlier detection of elevated blood pressure was more common in those later found to have cataract. It was also noted in the same study that consumption of diuretics which restores normal blood pressure in many patients does not protect against this risk. There may however be a variety of interactions in these patients in that hypertension may be associated with high blood glucose, diabetes and other conditions as well as with use of diuretics. Diuretics have different effects on plasma urea levels, with frusemide and acetazolamide associated with the highest levels, and parallel effects on cataract. Overall diuretic use was associated with an odds ratio of 1:6 but cyclopenthiazide (Navidrex), which had least effect on plasma urea, was reported by a greater proportion of controls than cases. Loop diuretics were reported by more than twice the proportion of cases than of controls. Hypertension and diuretic consumption did not appear as risk factors in Oxford but the graded properties of different diuretics did emerge and with a similar sequence to that found in Edinburgh. The only significant association of individual diuretics was an apparent protective effect by cyclopenthiazide and a risk associated with spironolactone which itself is a steroid. There was no significant association of particular sites of opacity with diuretic use.

Dehydrational Crisis

Harding has proposed that frequent episodes of diarrhea may be related to cataractogenesis and may account for the excess prevalence in some developing countries. Four intermediate events have been suggested to explain the role of diarrhea in the development of cataract:

- Malnutrition secondary to malabsorption of nutrients
- Relative alkalosis from administration of rehydrating fluids with bicarbonate
- Dehydration induced osmotic disturbance between the lens and the aqueous humor and
- Increased levels of urea and ammonium cyanate which may denature lens proteins by the process of carbamylation.

Six case-control studies have examined the relationship of severe diarrhea and increased risk of cataract, with discordant results. Two case-control, clinic-based studies done in Madhya Pradesh and Orissa, India have suggested a three- to four-fold increase in the risk for cataract for those with remembered episodes of life-threatening dehydration crises, severe enough to render the patient bedridden for at least three days. However, these findings were not replicated in two other epidemiologic investigations done in India. Using a less stringent definition of diarrhea (confinement to bed for one day), the India-US Case-Control Study found no associations with cataract. Also, a village-based case-control study in Southern India showed no association between severe diarrhea and risk of cataract. Furthermore, an observational study done in Matlab, Bangladesh, revealed that diarrhea from all causes was not significantly associated with cataract, although it was difficult to determine how cataract was defined in the study. The case-control study in Oxford found a marginally significant excess risk of cataract with reported severe diarrhea, but a significant risk in the subgroup aged 70 and older. Adjustments for the other possible confounding factors also found in the study were not done. Considering the potential public health importance of diarrhea as a risk factor, as well as the biologically plausible role of dehydration in cataractogenesis, further research to clarify this association is needed. Prospective studies involving closer follow-up of groups of patients who suffered from acute life-threatening diarrhea may provide more convincing evidence. Moreover, studies that examine the cumulative effect of milder, chronic dehydration episodes in cataractogenesis may also add to the current understanding of this issue.

Renal Failure

Cataract has been reported in many cases of renal failure. Sometimes cataract, often transient, was associated with hemodialysis and thought to be caused by the osmotic shock that dialysis causes, but Laqua (1972) noted lens opacities before dialysis and suggested they were caused by uremia. Increased blood urea could lead to cataract in a similar way to that postulated in severe diarrhea. After renal transplantation patients are treated with immunosuppressants usually including corticosteroids that may cause cataract. Posterior subcapsular lens opacities were observed in 19 out of 22 renal transplant recipients, aged 21 to 54 years in Hiroshima. Half of the patients suffered visual loss, attributed to steroid-induced cataract. In a study of diabetic patients receiving renal transplants in the USA, only one patient developed a visually-impairing cataract but lesser degrees of lens opacification were seen in 26 percent of eyes. Fourteen of 55 non-diabetic renal transplant patients were found to have cataract. The case-control study in Edinburgh did not report on renal failure as such but did find that the mean urea level was significantly higher in the plasma of cataract patients compared with controls. The level was not high enough to indicate renal failure. The raised urea levels are still present when subjects are subdivided by age and sex. Diuretics may raise urea levels and thus contribute to these differences but when all diabetics and individuals receiving diuretics were excluded, a relationship between high plasma urea and cataract remained.

Environmental Factors: Ultraviolet Radiation

There is considerable international interest in the association between solar ultraviolet B (UVB) radiation and cataract. Much of this interest has resulted from concern about the health effects of the increasing levels of UVB reaching the earth's surface as a consequence of depletion of the stratospheric ozone layer.

Young suggests that sunlight is the primary causal factor in cataractogenesis, and strongly advocates the widespread distribution of sunglasses to prevent cataract. Harding on the other hand suggests that sunlight is not a major etiological factor in human cataract formation.

The lens is known to absorb UVB and UVA, and change in lens clarity has been linked in animal experiments with short-term, high intensity exposure and chronic exposure to UVB.

Epidemiologic studies have demonstrated cataract to be more prevalent in sunny countries, such as Israel, than in cloudy countries, such as England. Moreover, in Romania and the United States, cataract are more prevalent in dry hot areas with more sun exposure within each country than in areas with prolonged cloud cover. The Beaver Dam Eye Study, found an association between ultraviolet B radiation exposure and cortical cataract in men only.

The Lens Opacity Case-Control Study did not find an association between sun exposure and any type of cataract development. However, this study investigated only urban populations, and this may explain why no association was found. In both the Italian-American Cataract Study and India-US Case-Control Study, sunlight exposure was associated with cataract formation. Taylor studied 797 watermen and went to great lengths to calculate an ultraviolet radiation exposure index on the basis of field variables such as outdoor hours worked, work location, and attenuation due to spectacle use and hat cover. He found a significant association between ultraviolet B radiation index and cortical cataract but found no association with other morphological cataract types.

Bochow *et al* studied the relationship between ultraviolet radiation exposure and posterior subcapsular cataract. He not only discovered a significant association but also a dose-response relationship.

Two unique studies, one prospective and one case-control, provide indirect evidence that ultraviolet light plays a role in cataract formation. Schein *et al* studied the distribution of cortical opacities by lens quadrant in a prospective study of Chesapeake Bay watermen. The prevalence of cortical lens opacities increased with age, with a high degree of concordance between eyes. The inferonasal lens quadrant was the most common location involved both for new cataract development and for progression of pre-existing cataract. Cataract formation in this quadrant was presumed to be the most consistent with ultraviolet radiation damage on the basis of greater exposure in this area of the lens. Resnikoff *et al* studied the association of lens opacities with two other presumed ultraviolet radiation-associated ocular diseases, climatic droplet keratopathy and exfoliation syndrome. There was a strong correlation between the diseases in this case-control study.

Based on the available epidemiological evidence, the following conclusions can be drawn:

- There is sufficient experimental evidence that exposure to artificial sources of UVB can cause lens opacities in laboratory animals.
- There is limited evidence suggesting that exposure to solar UVB causes cortical opacities in humans.
- There is also limited evidence suggesting that exposure to solar UVB causes posterior subcapsular cataract in humans.
- The epidemiological evidence is consistent in suggesting that nuclear cataract are not causally associated with exposure to solar UVB.

Drug Related Factors

A number of well-known and widely used drugs have been implicated in cataract etiology with oral corticosteroids probably the widest recognized of all.

Corticosteroids

In 1930, Hench postulated that a naturally occurring substance might be responsible for the clinical improvement seen in women with rheumatoid arthritis when they became pregnant. He called this substance "compound E", but it was not until 1948 that this substance (soon to be called cortisone) was synthesized and became available for clinical use. In the 50 years since then, corticosteroids have had an enormous impact in medicine, however it soon became clear that hydrocortisone has significant mineral corticoid as well as antiinflammatory activity and that this could produce dose-related toxicity. It is now known that the principal naturally occurring corticosteroids secreted by the adrenal cortex are hydrocortisone (cortisol), a glucocorticoid involved in the regulation of carbohydrate, protein and lipid metabolism and aldosterone, a mineralocorticoid affecting fluid and electrolyte balance. Because hydrocortisone also exerts some mineralocorticoid (salt-retaining) effects, several structurally modified glucocorticoids with relatively greater antiinflammatory and lower salt-retaining properties were synthesized once the therapeutic potential of their anti-inflammatory and immunosuppressive properties became apparent. Anti-inflammatory and immunosuppressive effects occur at doses above the normal physiological levels of daily glucocorticoid production, i.e. at pharmacological doses. However since many physiological and pharmacological actions are mediated by the same receptor, it is not surprising that prolonged use of pharmacological doses can lead to adverse physiological effects.

It is estimated that between 10 to 60 percent of patients using systemic corticosteroids develop cataract, especially of the posterior subcapsular (PSC) type. Glucocorticosteroids are lipophilic and therefore diffuse easily across the cell membrane after which they bind and activate a cytoplasmic glucocorticoid receptor. The resulting receptor steroid complex enters the cell nucleus, binds to the glucocorticoid response elements on the DNA and up- or down-regulates the expression of corticosteroid-responsive genes with resultant effects on protein synthesis in target tissues.

Several ways have been identified in which corticosteroids may induce cataract formation (Fig. 3.13) including:

- Elevation of glucose level
- Inhibition of Na, K-ATPase
- Increased cation permeability
- Inhibition of glucose-6-dehydrogenase
- Inhibition of RNA-synthesis
- Loss of ATP
- Covalent bonding of steroids to lens proteins.

Posterior subcapsular cataract is the hallmark of steroid cataract (Fig. 3.14). It starts as fine granular and vacuolated opacities at the posterior aspect of the lens. PSC opacities occur frequently with high doses (more than 15 mg prednisone or equivalent per day) and prolonged use (more than one year) of corticosteroids. Clinical trials have shown that PSC opacities secondary to oral corticosteroids may develop within as short a time as 4 months.

Recent studies have suggested that the use of inhaled corticosteroids may be a significant risk factor for the development of cataract, may be even more so than the use of oral corticosteroids. These studies have again pointed out the importance of the "first-order effect". A drug absorbed through the nasal mucosa or conjunctiva "drains" to the right atrium and ventricle. The drug is then pumped in part, to the head (i.e. the eye as a target organ)

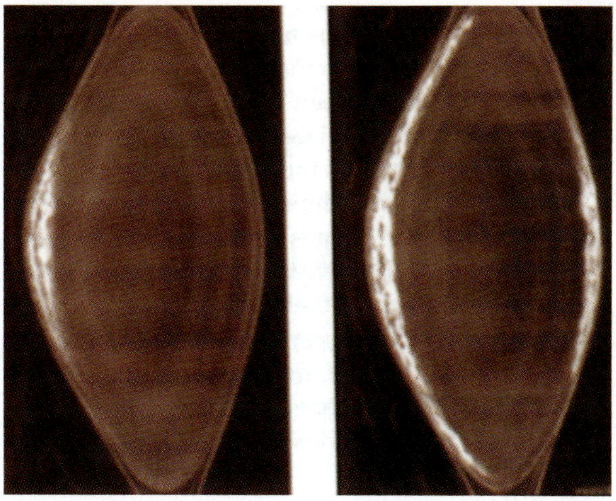

Fig. 3.13: Progession of steroid-induced cataract

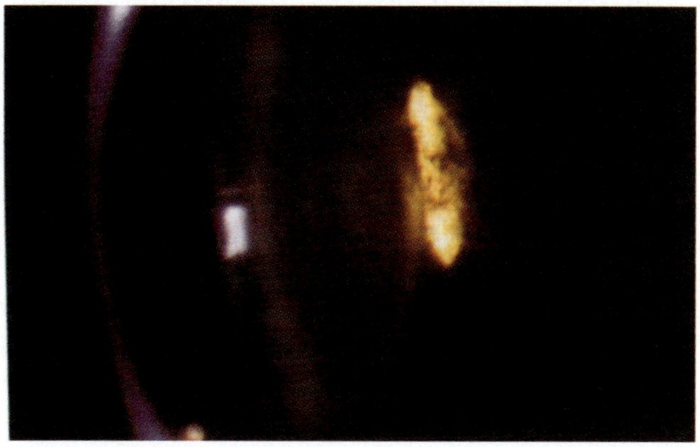

Fig. 3.14: Posterior subcapsular cataract

before returning to the left atrium and ventricle. The second passage is then to the liver and kidneys, where the drug is metabolized and detoxified. With oral medication—the first pass includes absorption from the gut via the liver where, depending on the drug, more than 90 percent of the drug is detoxified before going to the right atrium. Therefore, oral medications are metabolized even before the first pass, while ocular or nasally administered drugs are not metabolized until the second pass. This, in part, may be a reason why more potent steroid inhalants have greater ocular exposure and some ocular medications cause significant systemic adverse effects.

Considering the widespread use of corticosteroids and their association with PSC cataract, clinicians should be aware of a patient's medication history and recognize the distinguishing features of PSC cataract.

Allopurinol

Allopurinol is an antihyperuricemic drug widely used for the treatment of hyperuricemia and chronic gout. It inhibits the terminal step in uric acid synthesis, which results in a reduction of uric acid concentrations in both serum and urine. In about 85 percent of patients with gout, serum urate concentrations can be normalized by an allopurinol dose of 300 mg/d, and in some patients a dose of 100 to 200 mg/d is sufficient. Treatment with allopurinol is usually well tolerated, with hypersensitivity reactions constituting the most common adverse effects.

In 1982, Fraunfelder *et al* reported 30 cases of cortical and subcapsular cataract associated with long-term use of allopurinol reported to the National Registry of Drug-Induced Ocular Side Effects (Oregon Health Sciences University, Portland). The observed lens changes appeared to have the characteristics of early age-related cataract. At about the same time, Lerman *et al* used phosphorescence spectroscopy to demonstrate *in vitro* the probable presence of allopurinol in cataractous lenses that had been extracted from patients treated with allopurinol. The phosphorescence peaks characteristic of allopurinol could not be demonstrated in lenses from patients who had not ingested allopurinol. Evidence from epidemiologic studies on the possible cataractogenic effects of allopurinol is, however, inconclusive. Two separate epidemiologic studies did not show an increased risk. Another study reported an unusual morphologic thinning of the anterior clear zone of the lens in patients receiving long-term treatment with allopurinol. In the Lens Opacities Case Control Study, wherein gout medications were found to be associated with a 2.5-fold increased risk of mixed cataract, no distinction was made between allopurinol and other medications for gout. In a case control study conducted by Garbe *et al* using data from the Quebec universal health program for all elderly patients they established that a clear relationship exists between the long-term administration of allopurinol and an increased risk for cataract extraction.

Phenothiazines

In 1965, the occurrence of ocular pigmentation and lens opacity in patients on high dose phenothiazine drugs, particularly chlorpromazine, was reported in several papers. Phenothiazine has been thought to cause pigmentation by virtue of its ability to combine with melanin and form a photosensitive product. It is also postulated that this process might accelerate any predisposition to lens opacification from environmental insults such as solar radiation. A study involving schizophrenic patients showed an association between severity or grade of lenticular pigmentation and equivalent dose of phenothiazine intake. Epidemiologic research on the role of phenothiazines in cataractogenesis is limited. A case-control study done in North Carolina found a two-fold increased risk of cataract in those with history of tranquilizer use, although the types of tranquilizers and cataract were not characterized. A health maintenance organization based, non-concurrent prospective study that controlled for steroid use and diabetes documented at least three-fold increased risk for cataract extraction among current and past (two to five years prior to extraction) users of two groups of tranquilizers: "anti-psychotic phenothiazine drugs" (chlorpromazine, thioridazine, trifluoperazine, perphenazine, fluphenazine) and "other phenothiazine drugs" (chlorperazine, prochlorperazine, promethazine, trimeprazine).

Given the paucity and limitations of available epidemiologic data, more studies, such as those characterizing the specific types of senile cataract and phenothiazines, are needed to verify any association.

Diuretics and Antihypertensives

Harding and van Heyningen reported that thiazide diuretics were used less frequently by patients who underwent cataract surgery than control subjects. More recently, the Beaver Dam Eye Study found that use of thiazides was associated with lower prevalence of nuclear cataract and increased prevalence of posterior subcapsular cataract. Several other studies have found that use of diuretics was associated with increased risk of cataract. The Beaver Dam Eye Study also found a raised overall risk (OR, 1.3) for potassium-sparing diuretics, but this was not statistically significant. A cataractogenic effect of potassium-sparing diuretics is biologically plausible, as these diuretics disturb sodium transport across the lens fiber membrane.

The calcium channel blocker nifedipine has been associated with increased risk of cataract extraction and angiotensin-converting enzyme inhibitors with decreased risk of nuclear cataract. Hypertension and other cardiovascular conditions is a potential confounding problem in studies of cataract and antihypertensive medications, including diuretics.

Antimalarial Drugs

Most drugs used in the treatment of malaria produce phototoxic side effects in both the skin and the eye. Cutaneous and ocular effects that may be caused by light include: cataract formation, changes in skin pigmentation, corneal opacity and other visual disturbances including irreversible retinal damage (retinopathy) leading to blindness. The mechanism for these reactions in humans is unknown. A number of studies have been published that suggest a strong relationship between chloroquine use and cataract formation. The basis of the relationship seems to lie in the phototoxicity of chloroquine and related drugs.

Because malaria is a disease most prevalent in regions of high light intensity, protective measures (clothing, sunblock, sunglasses or eye wraps) should be recommended whilst taking antimalarial drugs.

Amiodarone

Amiodarone hydrochloride is a benzofurane derivative used for cardiac abnormalities. Its use is commonly associated with an asymptomatic keratopathy. The antiarrhythmic drug also produces anterior subcapsular lens opacities that are usually asymptomatic. Anterior subcapsular lens opacities were observed in 7 of 14 patients treated with moderate to high doses of amiodarone at the Veterans Administration Medical Center in San Francisco in 1982. In 1993, a report was published that summarized the status of these same 14 patients 10 years later. Anterior subcapsular lens opacities developed or progressed in all patients continuing treatment with this antiarrhythmic agent during the ensuing 10-year interval. Although Snellen visual acuities were not decreased, subtle visual impairment was present as measured by contrast sensitivity measurements with and without glare. The authors of the report concluded that decrease in visual acuity should not be a contraindication for therapy with this potentially life saving drug.

Hypocholesterolemic Drugs

Cataract in animals and men are in some instances associated with genetic defects in enzymes that regulate cholesterol metabolism and the use of drugs which inhibit lens cholesterol biosynthesis. The basis of this relationship apparently lies in the need of the lens to satisfy its sustained requirement for cholesterol by on-site synthesis, and impairing this synthesis can lead to alteration of lens membrane structure. The lens membrane contains the highest cholesterol content of any known membrane. The genetic defects Smith-Lemli-Opitz syndrome, mevalonic aciduria, and cerebrotendinous xanthomatosis all involve mutations in enzymes of cholesterol metabolism, and affected patients can develop cataract. Questions about the ocular safety of drugs, which can inhibit lens cholesterol biosynthesis, persist. Concern over potential damage to the lens from the use of hypocholesterolemic drugs stems from the reports in 1962 by Kirby *et al* and Laughlin *et al* that treatment of patients with Triparanol (Mer 29, Wm. S. Merrel Co.) to lower blood cholesterol was associated with development of cataract. Drugs used to lower blood cholesterol are among the most widely prescribed medicines. One drug in the group, lovostatin (Mevacor, Merck), is alone the third most prescribed drug in the United States. This drug can inhibit cholesterol synthesis in lens and produce cataract in dogs. Whether these drugs inhibit cholesterol biosynthesis in human lenses at therapeutic doses is unknown.

The clinical safety trials indicate that treatment with lovastatin for up to five years does not significantly increase the development of cataract or grossly alter visual function. The ocular safety in an older patient population (>50 years) appears high. This seems also to apply to simvastin, except that one clinical trial showed a significant increase in cortical opacities with the use of this drug (Fig. 3.15).

An unpublished study conducted at the University of Stellenbosch Medical School found that the rate at which opacification occurs in dyslipidemic patients on Cerivastatin was 4.5 percent per year (Fig. 3.15). Although this rate of opacification is not statistically noteworthy it would seem that if this data is projected over a period of 20 years and compared the normal rate of opacification reported by Boccuzzi and Leino *et al*, an alarming amount of opacities would be present in the group of patients on cerivistatin.

Hypolipidemic drugs are intended for life-long use and patients as young as 18 years can receive these drugs. Although the human lens grows throughout life, the rate of growth is slow after 10 years of age. About 40 years are required for the lens cortex to double in width. The size of the nucleus remains essentially constant after 10 years of age. Thus, the consequences of inhibiting lens growth due to block of cholesterol biosynthesis may be difficult to assess in only a 1 to 5 year period. A considerable body of evidence indicates that sustained alteration of lens sterol content and composition due to genetic mutations or exposure to drugs can lead to altered lens clarity. Long-term ocular safety of the vastatin drugs should perhaps

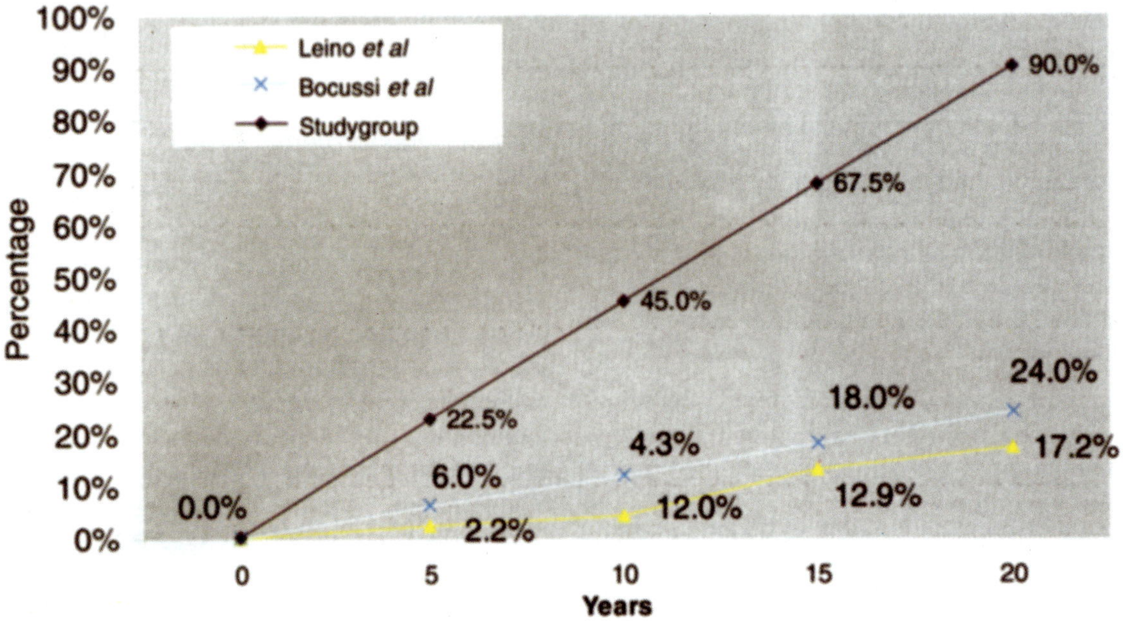

Fig. 3.15: Tempo of lens opacification with Vastatin therapy

be viewed in units of 10 to 20 years. Certainly a 20-year-old person required to have cataract surgery at age 40 because of some chronic treatment would constitute a medical crisis for this individual, particularly if a less toxic treatment had been available. The question of whether the vastatin drugs inhibit lens cholesterol biosynthesis in humans treated with standard therapeutic doses is unanswered. Since very low concentrations of lovastatin and simvastatin are required to inhibit cholesterol synthesis in animal lenses (3–22 nM), and only five times the therapeutic dose of lovostatin decreased cholesterol accumulation by the rat lens, it at least appears possible that therapeutic doses could inhibit lens cholesterol biosynthesis in humans.

CONCLUSION

Human lenticular opacification leading to the clinical challenge of cataract formation is etiologically multifactorial. It does seem however that evidence is slowly mounting to encourage clinicians to consider cataract as belonging to the growing list of preventable ocular diseases.

BIBLIOGRAPHY

1. Adler NE, Boyce T, Chesney MA et al. Socioeconomic inequalities in health. No easy solution. JAMA 1993;269:3140-45.
2. Alden ER, Ralina RE, Hodson WA: Transient cataract in low-birth-weight infants. J Pediatr 1973;82:318-31.
3. Amaya LG, Speedwell L, Taylor D. Contact lenses for infant aphakia. Br J Ophthalmo1 1990;74:154-56.
4. Ames GM, Janes CR. Heavy and problem drinking in an American blue-collar population: implications for prevention. Soc Sci Med 1987;8:949-60.
5. Ansari NH, Awasthi YG, Srivastava SK. Role of glycosylation in protein disulphide formation and cataractogenesis. Exp Eye Res 31: 9-19, 1980.
6. Armitage MM, Kivun JD, Farrell RE. A progressive early onset cataract gene maps to human chromosome 17q24. Nature Facet 1995;937-40.
7. Assmann et al. Lipid Metabolism Disorders and Coronary Heart Disease. MMV-Medizin-Verl (2nd ed), 1993.
8. Baghdassarian SA, Tabbara KF: Childhood blindness in Lebanon. Am J Ophthalmol 1975;79:827-30.
9. Bandmann O, Vaughan J, Holmans P et al. Association of slow acetylator genotype for N-Acetyltransferase 2 with familial Parkinson's disease. Lancet 1997;350:1136-39.
10. Barnes PJ. Anti-inflammatory mechanisms of glucocorticoids. Biochem Soc Trans 1995;23:940-45.
11. Behrens-Baumann W, Thiery J, Wieland E et al. 3-Hydroxy-3-methylglutaryl coenzyme—a reductase inhibitor simvastatin and the human lens: clinical results of 3-year follow-up. Arzneim-Forsch 1992;42(11):1023-24.
12. Beigi B, O'Keefe M, Bowell R et al. Ophthalmic findings in classical galactosaemia—prospective study. Br J Ophthalmol 1993;77:1624-64.
13. Belpoliti M, Maraini G. Sugar alcohols in the lens epithelium of age-related cataract. Exp Eye Res 1993;56:3-6.
14. Benos DJ. Amiloride. a molecular probe of sodium transport in tissues and cells. Am J Physiol 1982;242:C131-45.
15. Benson WH, Farber ME, Caplan RJ. Increased mortality rates after cataract surgery: A statistical analysis. Ophthalmology 1988;95:1288-92.
16. Berger J, Shepard D, Morrow F et al. Relationship between dietary intake and tissue levels of reduced and total vitamin C in the guinea pig. J Nutr 1989;119:1-7.
17. Bernstein HN. Chloroquine ocular toxicity. Surv Ophthalmol 1967;12(5):415-47.
18. Bhatnagar R, West KP (Jr), Vitale S et al. Risk of cataract and history of severe diarrheal disease in Southern India. Arch Ophthalmol 1991;109:696-99.
19. Bhuyan KC, Bhuyan DK, Podos SM. Free radical enhancer xenobiotic is an inducer of cataract in rabbit. Free Radical Res Comm 1991;12-13:609-20.
20. Bhuyan KC, Bhuyan DK, Podos SM. Lipid peroxidation in cataract of the human. Life Sci 1986;38:1463-71.
21. Bialas MC, Routledge PA. Adverse effects of corticosteroids. Adverse Drug React Toxicol Rev 1998;17(4):227-35.
22. Björkhem, I Boberg KM. Inborn errors in bile biosynthesis and storage of sterols other than cholesterol. Metabolic Basis of Inherited Disease; New York, McGraw-Hill 1995;7: 2073-99.
23. Blondin J, Baragi VJ, Schwartz E et al. Delay of UV-induced eye lens protein damage in guinea pigs by dietary ascorbate. Free Radic Biol Med 1986;2:275-81.
24. Boccuzzi SJ, Bocanegra TS, Walker JF et al. Long-term safety and efficiency profile of simvastatin. Am J Cardiol 1991;86:1127-31.
25. Bochow TW, West SK, Axar A et al. Ultraviolet light exposure and risk of posterior subcapsular cataract. Arch Ophthalmol 1989;107:369-72.
26. Bonting SJ. Na'K' activated adenosine triphosphatase and active cation transport in the lens. Invest Ophthalmol 1965;4:723.
27. Brauweiler PH, Wehler T, Busin M. High incidence of cataract formation after implantation of a silicone posterior chamber lens in phakic, highly myopic eyes. Ophthalmology 1999;106(9):1651-55.

28. Brilliant LB, Grasset NC, Pokrel RP et al. Associations among cataract prevalence, sunlight hours and altitude in the Himalayas. Am J Epidemiol 1983;118:250-64.
29. Brown CA, Burman D: Transient cataract in a diabetic child with hyperosmolar coma. Br J Ophthalmol 57: 429-33, 1973.
30. Burke JP, O'Keefe M, Bowell R et al. Ophthalmic findings in classical galactosemia: a screened population. Pediatr Ophthal Strabismus 1989;26:165-68.
31. Caird Fl, Pirie A, Ramsell TG. Diabetes and the Eye. Blackwell Scientific: Oxford 1969.
32. Caird Rl, Hutchinson M, Pirie A. Cataract and diabetes. BMJ 1964;2:665-68.
33. Cenedella RJ. Cholesterol and cataract. Surv Ophthalmol 1996;40:320-37.
34. Chatterjee A, Milton RC, Thyle S. Prevalence and aetiology of cataract in Punjab. Br J Ophthalmol 1982;66:35-42.
35. Chiba M, Masironi R. Toxic and trace elements in tobacco and tobacco smoke. Bull World Health Organ 1992;70:270-76.
36. Christen WG, Manson JE, Seddon JM et al. A prospective study of cigaret smoking and risk of cataract in men. JAMA 1992;268:989-93.
37. Chylack LT Jr, Henriques H, Tung W. Inhibition of sorbitol production in human lenses by an aldose reductase inhibitor. Invest Ophthalmol Vis Sci 1978;17:ARVO (Suppl): 300.
38. Cigala O, Pancallo MT, Della Valle M et al. La simvastatina nel trattamento delle piercolesterolemie. La Clinica Terapeu 1991;137:333-37.
39. Clair WK, Chylack LTJ, Cook EF et al. Allopurinol use and the risk of cataract formation. Br J Ophthalmol 1989;73:173-76.
40. Clayton RM, Cuthbert J, Duffy J et al. Some risk factors associated with cataract in SE Scotland: a pilot study. Trans Ophthalmol Soc UK 1982;102:331-36.
41. Clayton RM, Cuthbert J, Philips CJ et al. Analysis of individual cataract patients and the lenses: a progress report. Exp Eye Res 31:553-66.
42. Clayton RM, Cuthbert J, Philips CJ et al. Epidemiological and other studies in the assessment of factors contributing to cataractogenesis. Ciba Fdn Symp 1984;106:25-47.
43. Clayton RM, Cuthbert J, Philips CJ et al. Some risk factors associated with cataract in SE Scotland: A pilot study. Trans Ophthalmol Soc UK, 1982;102:331-36.
44. Clayton RM, CuthbertJ, Phillios CI et al. Analysis of individual cataract patients and their lenses: a progress report. Exp Eye Res 1980;31:553-56.
45. Cohen DL, Neil HA, Sparrow J et al. Lens opacity and mortality in diabetes. Diabetic Med 1990;7:615-17.
46. Collman GW, Shore DL, Shy CH et al. Sunlight and other risk factors for cataract: an epidemiological study. Am J Public Health 1988;78:1459-62.
47. Cooperative Study of Lipoproteins and Atherosclerosis. Evaluation of serum lipoprotein and cholesterol measurements as predictors of clinical complications of atherosclerosis. Circulation 1956;14.2:691-741.
48. Cotlier E, Kwan B, Beatty C. The lens as an osmometer. Bioctfm Biophys Acta 1968;150:705.
49. Cotlier E, Rice P. Cataract in the Smith-Lemli-Opitz syndrome. Am J Ophthalmol 1971;72:955-59.
50. Cotlier E. Congenital rubella cataract. In Cotlier E, Lambert SR, Taylor D (Eds): Congenital Cataract. RG Landes/ CRC: Boca Raton, 1994;65-76.
51. Cotlier E. Congenital varicella cataract. Am Ophihalmol 1978;86:627-29.
52. Cruickshanks KI, Klein BEK, Klein R. Ultraviolet light exposure and lens opacities: the Beaver Dam Eye Study. Am J Public Health 1992;82:1658-62.
53. Cuthbert J, Clayton RM, Philips: Cuneiform cataract: a special case? Colloq D'INSERM, 147:387-96.
54. Dawber TR: The Framingham Study: The Eipidemiology of Atherosclerotic Disease. Cambridge Harvard University Press: London 1980.
55. de Vries ACJ, Cohen LH: Different effects of the hypolipidemic drugs pravastatin and lovastatin on the cholesterol biosynthesis of the human ocular lens in organ culture and on the cholesterol content of the rat lens in viva. Biochim Biophys Acta 1993;1167:63-69.
56. Dohi K, Fukuda K et al. Cataract in kidney transplant patients. Horishima J Med Sci 1984;33:275-78.
57. Dolan BJ, Flach AJ, Peterson JS: Amiodarone keratopathy and lens opacities. J Am Optom Assoc 1985;56(6):468-70.
58. Donahue RP, Bias WB, Renwickj H et al. Probable assignment of the Duffy blood group locus to chromosome I in man. Proc Natl Acad Sci USA 1968;61:949-55.
59. Dorland's Illustrated Medical Dictionary (28th edn) WB Saunders: Philadelphia 276.
60. Drack AV, Burke JP, Pulido JS et al. Transient punctate lenticular opacities as a complication of argon laser photoablation in an infant with retinopathy of prematurity. Am J Ophthalmol 1992;113:583-84.
61. Drews RC. Alcohol and cataract. Arch Ophthalmol 1993;111:1312.
62. Drews RC. Ethanol cataract. In Solanes M (Ed): XXI Concilium Ophthalmologicum Mexico 1970. Amsterdam: the Netherlands Exerpta Medica 1970;753-58.
63. Duncan G, Hightower KR, Gandolfi SA, Tomlinson J, Maraini G. Human lens membrane cation permeability increases with age. Invest Ophthalmol Vis Sci 1989;30:1855-59.
64. Dunn JP, Jabs DA, Wingard JC et al. Bone marrow transplantation and cataract development. Arch Ophthalmol 1993;11:1367-73.
65. Duthie GG, Arthur JR, James WP. Effects of smoking and vitamin E on blood antioxidant status. Am J Clin Nutr 1991;53(Suppl):1061S-64S.
66. Ederer F, Hiller R, Taylor HR: Senile lens changes and diabetes in two population studies. Am J Ophthalmol 1981;91: 381-95.

67. Eiberg H, Marner E, Rosenberg T et al. Marner's cataract (AM) assigned to chromosome 16: linkage to haptoglobin. Clin Cenet 1988;34:272-75.
68. Elsas U II, Fridovich-Keil JL, Leslie ND: Galactosemia: a molecular approach to the enigma. Pediatr 8: 101-09, 1993.
69. Elsas U, Dembure PP, Langley S et al. A common mutation associated with the Duarte galactosemia allele. Am J Hum Cenet 1994;54:1030-36.
79. El-Yazigi A, Johansen K, Raines DA et al. N-Acetylation Polymorphism and diabetes mellitus among Saudi-Arabians. J Clin Pharmacol 1992;32(10):905-10.
71. Emmelot P. The organization of the plasma membrane of mammalian cells: structure in relation to function. In Jamieson GA, Robinson DM (Eds): Mammalian Cell Membranes, Butterworths: Boston, 1977;2:1-54.
72. Emmerson BT. The management of gout. N Engl J Med 1996;446:445-51.
73. Epstein FH. Cardiovascular Disease Epidemiology; A Journey from the Past Into the Future. Circulation 1996;93:1755-64.
74. Erdman J. The physiologic chemistry of carotenes in man. Am J Clin Nutr 1988;7:101-106.
75. Fechner PU. Cataract formation with a phakic IOL. J Cataract Refract Surg 1999;25(4):461-62.
76. Fink AM, Gore C, Rosen E. Cataract development after implantation of the Staar Collamer posterior chamber phakic lens. J Cataract Refract Surg 1999;25(2):278-82.
77. Finley SC, Finley WH, Monsky DM: Cataract in girl with features of Smith-Lemli-Opitz syndrome. J Pediatr 1969'75:706-07.
78. Flach AJ, Dolan BJ, Sudduth B et al. Amiodarone-induced lens opacities. Arch-Ophthalmol 1983;101(10):1554-56.
79. Flach AJ, Dolan BJ. Progression of amiodarone induced cataract. Doc Ophthalmol 1993;83(4):323-29.
80. Flaye DE, Sullivan KN, Cullinan TR et al. Cataract and cigaret smoking: the City Eye Study. Eye 1989;3:379-84.
81. Francois J: Congenital Cataract, Charles C Thomas (Ed): Springfield, 1963.
82. Francois J: Late results of congenital cataract surgery. Ophthalmol 1979;86:1586-98.
83. Franfelder FT: Do inhaled corticosteroids significantly increase cataract surgery in elderly patients? Arch Ophthalmol 1998;116:1369.
84. Fraunfelder FT, Hanna C, Dreis MW et al. Cataract associated with allopurinol therapy. Am J Ophthalmol 1982;94:137-40.
85. Friend J, Chylack LT, Khu P et al. The MSDRL Study Group: Lack of human cataractogenic potential of lovastatin: results of three year study. Invest Ophthalmol Vis Sci 1992;33:1301.
86. Garbe E, Suissa S, LeLorier J. Exposure to allopurinol and the risk of cataract extraction in elderly patients. Arch Ophthalmol 1998;116:1652-56.
87. Garner MH, Spector A: ATP hydrolysis kinetics by Na, K-ATPase in cataract. Exp Eye Res 1986;42:339-48.
88. Gibbs ML, Jacobs M, Wilkie AOM et al. Posterior lens. Surv Ophthalmol 1996;40(6).
89. Giblin FJ, Padgaonkar VA, Leverenz VR et al. Nuclear light scattering, disulfide formation and membrane damage in lenses of older guinea pigs treated with hyperbaric oxygen. Exp Eye Res 1995;60:219-35.
90. Giblin FJ, Schrimscher L, Chakrapani B et al. Exposure of rabbit lens to hyperbaric oxygen in vitro: regional effects on GSH level. Invest Ophthalmol Vis Sci 1988;29:1312-19.
91. Glynn RJ, Christen WG, Manson JE et al. Body Mass Index—an independent predictor of cataract. Arch Ophthalmol 1995;113:1131-37.
92. Gofman et al. The role of lipids and lipoproteins in atherosclerosis. Science 111: 166-71, 1950.
93. Gretton C: Like falling off a cliff. Med Ad News 3-25, 1994.
94. Grundy SM: HMG-KoA reductase inhibitors for treatment of hypercholesterolemia. N Engl J Med 319: 24:33, 1988.
95. Gumming RG, Mitchell P, Leeder SR. Use of inhaled corticosteroids and the risk of cataract. N Engl J Med 1997;337:8-14.
96. Hankinson SE, Seddon JM, Colditz et al. A prospective study of aspirin use and cataract extraction in women. Arch Ophthalmol 1989;111:503-08.
97. Hankinson SE, Stampfer MJ, Seddon JM et al. Intake and cataract extraction in women: a prospective study. Br Med J 1992;305:335-39.
98. Hankinson SE, Willet WC, Colditz GA et al. A prospective study of cigaret smoking and risk of cataract surgery in woman. JAMA 1992;268:994-98.
99. Harding J: Cataract: Biochemistry, Epidemiology and Pharmacology. Chapman and Hall: London, 1991;122-23.
100. Harding JJ, Crabe MJC: The lens: development, proteins, metabolism and cataract. In Davidson H (Ed): The Eye, Academic Press: London, 207-492.
101. Harding JJ, Egerton M, Harding RS: Protection against cataract by aspirin, paracetamol and ibuprofen. Acta Ophthalmol 1989;67:518-24.
102. Harding JJ, Harding RS, Egerton M: Risk factors for cataract in Oxfordshire: diabetes, peripheral neuropathy, myopia, glaucoma and diarrhoea. Acta Ophthalmol 1989;67:510-17.
103. Harding JJ, van Heyningen R: Beer, cigarets and military work as risk factors for cataract. Dev Ophthalmol 1989;17:13-16.
104. Harding JJ, van Heyningen R: Drugs including alcohol that act as risk factors for cataract and possible protection against cataract by aspirin like drugs. Br J Ophthalmol 1989;73:579-80.
105. Harding JJ, van Heyningen R: Drugs including alcohol, that act as risk factors for cataract, and possible protection against cataract by aspirin-like analgesics and

cyclopenthiazide. Br J Ophthalmol 1988;72:809-14.
106. Harding JJ: Cataract Biochemistry, Epidemiology and Pharmacology. Chapman and Hall 1991;116-18
107. Harding JJ: Physiology, biochemistry, pathogenesis, and epidemiology of cataract. Curr Opinion Ophthalmol 1992;3:3-12.
108. Harding JJ: Possible causes of the unfolding of proteins in cataract and a new hypothesis to explain the high prevalence of cataract in some countries. In Regnault F, Hockwin O, Courtois Y (Eds): Ageing of the lens. Proceedings of the symposium on the aging of the lens held in Paris, September 1979. Biomedical Press: Amsterdam, 1980;71-80.
109. Havel et al. Lovastatin (Mevolin) in the treatment of heterozygous familial hypercholesterolemia. Ann Intern Med 1987;107:609-15.
110. Hayes RB, Bi W, Rothman N et al. N-Acetylation phenotype and genotype and risk of bladder cancer in benzidine-exposed workers. Carcinogenesis (United States); 1993;14(4): 675-78.
111. Henkj M, Whitelocke RAF, Warrington AlP et al. Radiation dose to the lens and cataract formation. Radiat Oncol Biol Phys 1993;25:815-20.
112. Hesker H: Antioxidative vitamins and cataract in the elderly. Z Ernahrungswiss 1995;34:167-76.
113. Hiller R, Giacometti L, Yuen K: Sunlight and cataract—an epidemiologic investigation. Am J Epidemiol 1977;105.
114. Hiller R, Sperduto RD, Ederer F: Epidemiologic associations with cataract in the 1971-1972 National Health and Nutrition Examination Survey. Am J Epidemiol 1983;118:239-49.
115. Hiller R, Sperduto RD, Ederer F: Epidemiologic associations with nuclear, cortical, and posterior subcapsular cataract. Am J Epidemiol 1986;124:916-25.
116. Hiller R, Yuen K: Sunlight and cataract: an epidemiological investigation. Am J Epidemiol 1977;105:450-59.
117. Hing S, Speedwell L, Taylor D: Lens surgery in infancy and childhood. Br J Ophthalmol 1990;74:73-77.
118. Hockwin O, Koch H: Cataract of toxic etiology. In Bellows (Ed): Cataract and Abnormalities of the Lens. Grune and Stratton 1975;234-45.
119. Hoffmann G, Gibson KM, Brandt IK et al. Mevalonic aciduria: an inborn error of cholesterol and nonsterol isoprene biosynthesis. N Engl J Med 1986;314:1610-14.
120. Holowich F, Boateng A, Kolck B: Toxic Cataract. In Bellows JG (Ed): Cataract and Abnormalities of the Lens. Grune and Stratton: New York 1975;230-43.
121. Hunninghake et al. Lovastatin—follow up ophthalmological data. JAMA 1988;259:354-55.
122. Hyman L: Epidemiology of eye disease in the elderly. Eye 1987;1:330-41.
123. Jaafar MS, Robb RM: Congenital anterior polar cataract. Ophthalmology 1984;91:249-54.
124. Jackson RC: Temporary cataract in diabetes mellitus. Br J Ophthalmol 1955;39:629-31.
125. Jacques PF, Chylack LT (Jr): Epidemiologic evidence of a role for the antioxidant vitamins and carotenoids in cataract prevention. Am J Clin Nutr 1991;53:352S-55S.
126. Jacques PF, Taylar A, Hankinson SE et al. Long-term vitamin C supplement use and prevalence of early age-related lens opacities. Am J Clin Nutr 1997;66:911-16.
127. Jahn CE, Janke M, Winowski H et al. Identification of metabolic risk factors for posterior subcapsular cataract. Ophthalmic Res 1986;18:112-16.
128. Jay B, Black RE, Wells RS: Ocular manifestations of ichthyosis. Br J Ophthalmol 1968;52:217-26.
129. Jedziniak JA, Chylack LT Jr, Cheng HM et al. The sorbitol pathway in the human lens: aldose reductase and polyol dehydrogenase. Invest Ophthalmol Vis Sci 1981;20:314-26.
130. Jick H, Brandt DE: Allopurinol and cataract. Am J Ophthalmol 1984;98:355-58.
131. Kahn HA, Leibowitz HM, Ganley JP et al. The Framingham Eye Study. II—Association of ophthalmic pathology with single variables previously measured in the Framingham Heart Study. Am J Epidemiolo 1997;106:33-41.
132. Kahn MU, Kahn MR, Sheikh AK: Dehydrating diarrhoea and cataract in rural Bungladesh. Ind J Med Res 1987;85:311-15.
133. Kallner AB, Hartmann D, Horning DH: on the requirements of ascorbic acid in men: steady-state turnover and blood pool in smokers. Am J Clin Nutr 1981;34:1347-55.
134. Kanski JJ: Clinical Ophthalmology (3rd edn). Butterworth-Heineman: Oxford. 1994;289.
135. Kasai K, Nakamura T, Kase N et al. Increased glycosylation of proteins from cataractous lenses in diabetes. Diabetologia 1983;25:36-38.
136. Kench PS, Kendall EC, Slocumb CH, Polley HF. The effect of a hormone of the adrenal cortex (17-hydroxy-11-dehydrocorticosterone; compound E) and of pituitary and adrenocorticotrophic hormone on rheumatoid arthritis. Mayo Clin Prvc 1949;4:181-97.
137. Keys A. Atherosclerosis: a problem in newer public health. J Mt Sinai Hosp 1953;20:118-39.
138. Kirby TJ, Achor RWP, Perry HO et al. Cataract formation after triparanol therapy. Arch Ophthalmol 68: 486-89, 1962.
139. Klein BEK, Klein R, Jensen SC et al. Hypertension and lens opacities from the Beaver Dam Eye Study. Am J Ophthalmol 1995;119:640-46.
140. Klein BEK, Klein R, Lee KE: The incidence of age-related cataract, the Beaver Dam Eye Study. Arch Ophthalmol 1998;116:219.
141. Klein BEK, Klein R, Linton KL et al. Cigaret smoking and lens opacities: the Beaver Dam Eye Study. Am J Prev Med 1993;9:27-30.
142. Klein BEK, Klein R, Linton KL et al. The Beaver Dam Eye Study: the relation of age-related maculopathy to smoking. Am J Epidemiol 1993;137:190-200.
143. Klein BEK, Klein R, Moss SE. Prevalence of cataract in a population-based study of persons with diabetes mellitus. Ophthalmology 1985;92:1191-96.

144. Klein BEK, Klein R, Ritter LL: Is there evidence of an estrogen effect on age-related lens opacities? The Beaver Dam Eye Study. Arch Ophthalmol 1994;112:85-91.
145. Klein R, Klein BEK, Jenses SC et al. The relation of socioeconomic factors to age-related cataract, maculopathy, and impaired vision. Ophthalmology 101(21):1969-79.
146. Klein R, Klein BEK, Moss SE: Visual impairment in diabetes. Ophthalmology 1984;91:1-8.
147. Klein R, Moss SE, Klein BE et al. Relation of ocular and systemic factors to survival in diabetes. Arch Intern Med 1989;149:266-72.
148. Kleinman NJ, Spector A: The relationship between oxidative stress, lens epithelial cell DNA and cataractogenesis. Exp Eye Res 1992;55(Suppl):1 (abstract 807).
149. Koga T, Shimada Y, Kuroda M et al. Tissue-selective inhibition of cholesterol synthesis in viva by pravastatin sodium, a 3-hydroxy-3-methylglutaryl coenzyme: a reductase inhibitor. Biochim Biophys Acta 1990;1045:115-20.
150. Köhler L, Stigmar G. Vision screening of four-year-old children. Acta Paediatr Scand 1973;62:17-27.
151. Kreines K, Rowe KW. Cataract and adult diabetes. Ohio Med J 1979;75:782-86.
152. Kretzer FL, Hittner HM, Mehta RS. Ocular manifestations of the Smith-Lemli-Opitz syndrome. Arch Ophthalmol 1981;99:2000-06.
153. Kuchle M, Schonherr U, Dieckmann U. Risk factors for capsular rupture and vitreous loss in extracapsular cataract extraction. The Erlangen Ophthalmology Group. Fortschr Ophthalmol 1989;86:417-21.
154. Kuriyama M, Fujiyama J, Yoshidome H et al. Cerebrotendinous xanthomatosis: clinical and biochemical evaluation of eight patients and review of the literature. J Neurol Sci 1991;102:225-32.
155. Kuzma JW, Kissinger DG: Patterns of alcohol and cigarette use in pregnancy. Neurobehav Toxicol Teratol 1981;3:211-21.
156. Lambert SR, Taylor D, Kriss A et al. Ocular manifestations of the congenital varicella syndrome. Arch Ophthalmol 1989;107:52-56.
157. Laqua H: Kataract bei chronisher Nierensuffinzeinz und Dialysebehanlung. Klin MBl Augenheilk 1972;160:346-49.
158. Laties AM, Shear CL, Lippa EA et al. Expanded clinical evaluation of lovastatin (EXCEL) study results II. Assessment of the human lens after 48 weeks of treatment with lovastatin. Am J Cardiol 1991;67:447-53.
159. Laughlin RC, Carey TF: Cataract in patients treated with triparanol. JAMA 1962;181:339-40.
160. Laurent M, Kern P, Regnault F: Thickness and collagen metabolism of lens capsule from genetically prediabetic mice. Ophthalmic Res 1981;13:93.
161. Law MR, Wald NJ: An ecological study of serum cholesterol and ischeamic heart disease between 1950 and 1990. Eur J Clin Nutr 1994;48:305-25.
162. Leino M, Pyorala K, Lehto S et al. Lens opacities in patients with hypercholesterolemia and ischemic heart disease. Doc Ophthalmol 1992;80:309-15.
163. Lerman S, Megaw JM, Fraunfelder FT: Further studies on allopurinol therapy and human cataractogenesis. Am J Ophthalmol 1984;97:205-09.
164. Lerman S, Megaw JM, Gardner K: Allopurinol therapy and cataractogenesis in humans. Am J Ophthalmol. 1982;94:141-46.
165. Lerman S, Moran M: Sorbitol generation and its inhibition by Sorbinil in the aging normal human and rabbit lens and human diabetic cataract. Ophthalmic Res 1988;20:348-52.
166. Leske MC, Chylack LT (Jr), He Q et al. The LSC Group: Antioxidant vitamins and nuclear opacities—The longitudial study of cataract. Ophthalmology 1998;105:831-36.
167. Leske MC, Chylack Lt (Jr), Wu S: The lens opacities case-control study: Risk factors for cataract. Arch Ophthalmol 1991;109:244-51.
168. Leske MC, Connel AMS, Schadat A: Prevalence of lens opacities in the Barbados Eye Study. Arch Ophthalmol 1997;115:105.
169. Lessel S, Forbes AP: Eye signs in Turner's syndrome. Arch Ophthalmol 1966;76:211-13.
170. Letson RD, Desnick RJ: Punctate lenticular opacities in Type II mannosidosis. Am J Ophthalmol 1978;85:218-24.
171. Leveille PJ, Weidruch R, Walford RL et al. Dietary restriction retards age-related loss of gamma crystalline in the mouse lens. Science 1998;224:1247-49.
172. Liang J, Chakrabarti B: Sugar-induced change in near ultraviolet circular dichroism of alpha-crystallin. Biochem Biophys Res Commun 1981;102:180.
173. Libondi T, Menzione M, Auricchio G: In vitro effect of alpha-tocopherol on lysophosatiphatidylcholine-induced lens damage. Exp Aye Res 1985;40:661-66.
174. Lim R, Mitchell P, Cumming RG: Refractive associations with cataract: the Blue Mountains Eye Study. Invest Ophthalmol Vis Sci 1999;40(12):3021-26.
175. Lin LR, Reddy VN, Giblin FJ et al. Polyol accumulation in cultured human lens epithelial cells. Exp Eye Res 1991;52:93-100.
176. Liu CS, Brown NA, Leanard TJ et al. The prevalence and morphology of cataract in patients on allopurinol treatment. Eye 1988;2:600-06.
177. Lovastatin Study Group II: Therapeutic response to lovastatin (mevolin) in non-familial hypercholesterolemia. JAMA 1988;260:359-66.
178. Lovastatin Study Group III: A multicenter comparison of lovastatin and cholestyramine therapy for severe primary hypercholesterolemia. JAMA 1988;260:359-66.
179. Lovastatin Study group IV: A multicenter comparison of lovastatin and probucol for treatment of severe primary hypercholesterolemia. Am J Cardiol 1990;66:22B-30B.

180. Lubkin VL: Steroid cataract—a review and conclusion. J Asthma Res 1977;14:55-59.
181. Lubsen NH, Renwickjfl, Tsui LC et al. A locus for a human hereditary cataract is closely linked to the gamma-crystallin gene family. Proc NatI Acad Sri USA 1987;84:489-92.
182. Machlin LJ, Bendich A: Free radical tissue damage: protective role of antioxidants. FASEB J 1987;1:441-45.
183. Marais JS: The Cape Coloured People 1652 to 1932 (1st edn) 1-31. Witwatersrand University Press: Johannesburg, 1957.
184. Mares-Perlman JA, Brady WE, Klein BEK et al. Diet and nuclear lens opacities. Am J Epidemiol 1995b;141:322-34.
185. Mares-Perlman JA, Klein BEK, Klein R et al. Relation between lens opacities and vitamin and mineral supplement use. Ophthalmology 1994;101:315-25.
186. Marinho A, Neves MC, Pinto MC et al. Posterior chamber silicone phakic intraocular lens. J Refract Surg 1997;13(3):219-22.
187. Marmot MG, Kogevinas M, Elston MA: Social/economic status and disease. Ann Rev Public Health 1987;8:111-35.
188. Marmot MG, Smith GD, Stansfeld S et al. Health inequalities among British civil servants: the Whitehall II study. Lancet 1991;337:1387-93.
189. Matthews KA, Kelsy SF, Meilahn EN et al. Educational attainment and behavioral and biologic risk factors for coronary heart disease in middle-aged women. Am J Epidemiol 1989;129:1132-44.
190. McCarty CA, Mukesh BN, Fu CL et al. The epidemiology of cataract in Australia. Am J of Ophthal 1999;128(4):446-65.
191. McCornsick AQ: Transient cataract in prensature infants:a new clinical entity. Can J Ophthalmol 1968;3:302-08.
192. Meltzer EO: Prevalence, economic, and medical impact of tobacco smoking. Ann Allergy 1994;73:381-91.
193. Merin S, Crawbird S: The etiology of congenital cataract. Can J Ophthalmol 1971;6:1782-84.
194. Merits S, Craw S: Hypoglycemia and infantile cataract. Arch Ophthalmol 1993;86:495-98.
195. Micozzi MS, Beecher GR, Taylor HR et al. Carotenoid analyses of selected raw and cooked foods associated with a lower risk for cancer. J Natl Cancer Inst 1990;82:282-85.
196. Minassian DC, Mehra V, Jones BR: Dehidrational crisis from severe diarrhoea or heatstroke and risk factor for cataract. Lancet 1984;1:751-53.
197. Minassian DC, Mehra V, Jones BR: Dehidrational crisis: a major risk factor in the risk of blinding cataract. Br J Ophthalmol 1989;73:100-105.
198. Minchin RF, Kadlubar FF, Ilett KF: Role of acetylation in colorectal cancer. Mutat Res 2901993;(1):35-42.
199. Mitchell RN, Cotran RS: In Kumar V, Cotran RS, Robinson SL (Eds): Basic Pathology (6th edn): WB Saunders Company.
200. Mohan M, Sperduto RD, Angra SK et al. India US case control study of age-related cataract. Arch Ophthalmol 1989;107:670-76.
201. Molgaard J, Lundh B, van Schenck H et al. Long- term efficacy and safety of simvastatin alone and in combination therapy in treatment of hypercholesterolemia. Atherosclerosis 1991;91:S21-24.
202. Mosley ST, Kalinowski SS, Schafer BL et al. Tissue-selective acute effects of inhibitors of 3-hydroxy-3-methyl- glutaryl coenzyme: a reductase on cholesterol biosynthesis in lens. J Lipid Res 1989;50:1411-20.
203. Mostafa MSE, Teintamy S, EI-Gammal MY et al. Genetic studies of congenital cataract. Metah Pediatr Ophthalmol 1981;5:233-42.
204. Motten AG, Martinez LJ, Holt N et al. Photophysical studies on antimalarial drugs. Photochem Photobiol 1999;69(3):282.
205. Mune M, Meydani M, Jahngen-Hodge J et al. Effect of calorie restriction on liver and kidney glutathione in aging emory mice. AGE 1995;18:49.
206. Munoz B, Tajchman U, Bochow T et al. Alcohol use and risk of posterior subcapsular opacities. Arch Ophthalmol 1993;111:110-12
207. Nagata M, Hohmann TC, Nisihimura C et al. Polyol and vacuole formation in cultured canine kens epithelial cells. Exp Eye Res 1989;48:667-77.
208. Nakamura B, Nakamura O, Ufer das vitamin C in der linse und dem Kammerwasser der menschlichen katarakte. Graefes Arch Clin Exp Ophthalmol 1935;134:197-200.
209. Neilson NV, Vinding T: The prevalence of cataract in insulin-dependent and non-insulin-dependent diabetes mellitus: an epidemiological study of diabetics treated with insulin and oral hypoglycaemic agents (OHA). Acta Ophthalmol 1984;62:591-602.
210. O'Neil WM, Gilfix BM, DiGirolamo A et al. N-acetylation among HIV-positive patients and patients with AIDS: when is fast, fast and slow, slow? Clin Pharmacol Ther 1997;62(3):261-71.
211. Orzechowska-Juzwenko K, Milejski P, Patkowski J et al. Acetylator phenotype in patients with allergic diseases and its clinical significance. Int J Clin Pharmacol Ther Toxicol 1990;28(10):420-25.
212. Oshima Y, Emi K, Motokura M et al. Survey of surgical indications and results of primary pars plana vitrectomy for rhegmatogenous retinal detachments. Jpn J Ophthalmol 1999;43(2):120-26.
213. Oxman TE, Berkman LF, Kasl S et al. Social support and depressive symptoms in the elderly. Am J Epidemiol 1992;135: 356-68.
214. Pacurariu I, Marin C: Changes in the incidence of ocular disease in children and old people. Ofthalmologia (Buchuresti). 1973;17:289-308.

215. Palmquist BM, Phillipson B, Barr PO: Nuclear cataract and myopia during hyperbaric oxygen therapy. Br J Ophthalmol 1984;60:113-17.
216. Pande A, Gamer WH, Spector A: Glucosylation of human lens protein and cataractogenesis. Biochem Biophys Res Commun 1979;89:1260-66.
217. Petrohelos MA: Chloroquine-induced ocular toxicity. Ann Ophthalmol 1974;6(6):615.
218. Pirie A, van Heyningen R: The effect of diabetes on the content of sorbitol, glucose, fructose and inositol in the human lens. Exp Eye Res 1964;3:124-31.
219. Probst-Hensch NM, Haile RW, Ingles SA et al. Acetylation polymorphism and prevalence of colorectal adenomas. Cancer Res (US) 1995;55(10):2017-20.
220. Pruett RC: Ritinitis pigmentosa: clinical observations and correlations. Trans Am Ophthalmol Soc 1983;81:693-35.
221. Racz P, Erdohelyi A: Cadmium, lead and copper concentrations in normal and senile cataractous human lenses. Ophthalmic Res 1988;20:10-13.
222. Rafferty iVS: Lens morphology. In Maisel H (Ed): The Ocular Lens: Structure, Function and Pathology. Marcel Dekker: New York 1985;1-60.
223. Ramsay RC, Barbosa JJ: The visual status of diabetic patients after renal transplantation. Am J Ophthalmol 1979;87:305-10.
224. Reddy VN: Glutathione and its function in the lens—an overview. Exp Eye Res 1990;150:771-78.
225. Renwick JH, Lawler SD: Probably linkage between a congenital cataract locus and the Duffy blood group locus. Ann Ham Genet 1963;27:67-84.
226. Resnikoff S, Filliard G, Dell'Aquila B: Climatic droplet kera-topathy, exfoliation syndrome, and cataract. Br J Ophthalmol 1991;75:734-36.
227. Risch A, Wallace DM, Bathers S et al. Slow N-Acetylation genotype is a susceptibility factor in occupational and smoking related bladder cancer. Hum Mol Genet 1995;4(2):231-36.
228. Ritter LL, Klein EK, Klein R et al. Alcohol use and lens opacities in the Beaver Dam Eye Study. Arch Ophthalmol 1993;111:113-17.
229. Robertson J McD, Donner AP, Trevithick JR. Vitamin E intake and risk for cataract in humans. Ann NY Acad Sci 1989;570:372-82.
230. Rouhianen P, Rouhiainen H, Salonen TJ: Association between low plasma vitamin E concentration and progression of early cortical lens opacities. Am J Epidemiol 1996;144:496-500.
231. Rubb RM: Cataract acquired following varicella infectims. Ault Ophthalmol 1972;873-2254.
232. Sabiston DW: Cataract, Dupuytren's contracture, and Alcohol Addiction. Am J Ophthalmol 1973;76:1005-07.
233. Sacanove A: Pigmentation due to phenothiazines in high and prolonged dosage. JAMA 1965;19I:263-68.
234. Salive ME, Guralnik J, Christen W et al. Functional blindness and viusal impairment in older adults from three communities. Ophthalmology 1992;99:1840-47.
235. Salmon JF, Wallis CE, Murray ADN: Variable expressivity of autosomal dominant microcornea with cataract. Arch Ophthalmol 1988;106:505-10.
236. Scales DK: Immunomodulatory agents. In Mauger TF, Craig EL (Eds): Haveners Ocular Pharmacology (Mosby-Yearbook: St Louis 402-14, 1994).
237. Schein OD, West S, Mlnoz B et al. Cortical lenticular opacification: distribution and location in a longitudinal study. Invest Ophthalmol Vis Sci 1994;35:363-66.
238. Schocket SS, Esterson J, Bradford B et al. Induction of cataract in mice by exposure to oxygen. Israel J Med 1972;8: 1596-1601.
239. Scott MR, Hejtmaucik F, Wozencraft LA et al. Autosomal dominant congenital cataract; interocular phenotypic variability. Ophthalmol 1994;101:866-71.
240. Shun Shin GA, Ratcliffe P, Bron AJ et al. The lens after renal transplantation. Br J Ophthalmol 1990;73:522-27.
241. Siddall JR: The ocular toxic findings with prolonged and high dosage chlorpromazine intake. Arch Ophthalmol 1965;74:460-64.
242. Siegmund W, Fengler JD, Frane G et al. N-Acetylation and debrisoquine hydroxylation polymorphisms in patients with Gilbert's syndrome. Br J Clin Pharmacol 1991;32(4):467-72.
243. Simonelli F, Nesti A, Pensa M et al. Lipid peroxidation and human cataractogenesis in diabetes and severe myopia. Exp Eye Res 1989;49:181-87.
244. Simons LA. Interrelations of lipids and lipoproteins with coronary artery disease mortality in 19 countries. Am J Cardiol 57: 5G-10G, 1985.
245. Sirtori CR. Tissue selectivity of hydroxymethylglutaryl co-enzyme A (HMG CoA) reductase inhibitors. Pharmacol Ther 1993;60:431-59.
246. Solberg Y, Rosner M, Belkin M. The association between cigaret smoking and ocular diseases. Surv Ophthalmol 1998;42:535-57.
247. Spector A, Garner WH. Hydrogen peroxide and human cataract. Exp Eye Res 1981;33:673-81.
248. Sperduto RD, Hu T-S, Milton RC et al. The Linxian Cataract Studies: two nutrition intervention trials. Arch Ophthalmol 1993;111:1246-53.
249. Srivastava S, Ansari NH: Prevention of sugar induced cataractogenesis in rats by mutilated hydroxytoluene. Diabetes 1988;37:1505-08.
250. Stambolian D: Galactose and cataract. Surv Ophthalmol 1988;32:333-49.
251. Stayte M, Reeves B, Wortham C: Ocular and vision defects in preschool children. Br J Ophthalmol 1993;77:228-32.
252. Steele G, Peters R: Persistent hyperplastic primary vitreous with myopia: a case study. J Am Optom Assoc 1999;70(9):593-97.

253. Stewart Brown SL, Raslum MN: Partial sight and blindness in children of the 1970 birth cohort at 10 years of age. J Epidemiol Community Health 1988;42:17-23.
254. Stoll C, Alembik Y, Dott B, Roth MP: Epidemiology of congenital eye malformations in 131,760 consecutive births. Ophthalmic Pediatr Genet 1993;39:433-35.
255. Stryker WS, Kaplan LA, Stein EA et al. The relation of diet, cigaret smoking, and alcohol consumption to plasma beta-carotene and alpha-tocopherol levels. Am J Epidemiol 1988;127:283-96.
256. Subar AF, Block G. Use of vitamin and mineral supplements: demographics and amounts of nutrients consumed—the 1987 Health Interview Survey. Am J Epidemiol 1990;132:1091-1101.
257. Summers CG, Letson RD: Is the phakic eye normal in monocular pediatric aphakia? J Pediatr Ophthalmol Strabismus 1992;29:324-27.
258. Szmyd L Jr, Schwartz B: Association of systemic hypertension and diabetes mellitus with cataract extraction: A case-control study. Ophthalmology 1989; 96:1248-52.
259. Takemoto L, Takehana M, Horwitz J: Covalent changes in MIP 26K during aging of the human lens membrane. Invest Ophthalmol Vis Sci 1986;27:443-46.
260. Tavani A, Negri E, La Vecchia C: Selected diseases and risk of cataract in Women. A case-control study from northern Italy. Ann Epidemiol 1995;5(3):234-38.
261. Taylor A, Jacques P, Nadler D et al. Relationship in humans between ascorbic acid consumption and levels of total and reduced ascorbic acid in lens, aqueous humor , and plasma. Curr Eye Res 1997;16:857-64.
262. Taylor A, Jacques PF, Nadler D et al. Relationship in humans between ascorbic acid consumption and levels of total and reduced ascorbic acid in lens, aqueous humor, and plasma. Curr Eye Res 1991;10:751-59.
263. Taylor A, Jaques PF, Epstein EM: Relations among aging, antioxidant status, and cataract. Am J Clin Nutr 1995;62(Suppl):1439S-47S.
264. Taylor A: Nutritional and Environmental Influences on the Eye. CRC Press, London; 1999;1-5.
265. Taylor A: Nutritional and Environmental Influences on the Eye. CRC Press: London. 1999;56-81.
266. Taylor D, Rice NSC: Congenital cataract, a cause of preventable child blindness. Arch Dis Child 1982;57:165-67.
267. Taylor HR, West S, Munoz B et al. The long-term effects of visible light on the eye. Arch Ophthalmol 1992;110:99-104.
268. Taylor HR: The environment and the lens. Br J Ophthalmol 1980;64:303-10.
269. Taylor HR: Ultraviolet radiation and the eye: an epidemiologic study. Trans Am Ophthalmol Soc 1989;87:802-53.
270. Teramoto S, Fukuchi Y, Uejima Y: Influences of chronic tobacco smoke inhalation on ageing and oxidant-antioxidant balance in the senescence-accelerated mouse (SAM)-P/2. Exp Gerontol 1993;28:87-95.
271. Thaler JS, Curinga R, Kiracofe G: Relation of graded ocular anterior chamber pigmentation to phenothiazine intake in schizophrenics: quantification procedures. Am J Optom Physiol Optics 1985;62:600-04.
272. The Italian-American Cataract Study Group: Risk factors for age-related cortical, nuclear, and posterior subcapsular cataract. Am J Epidemiol 1991;133:541-53.
273. Tielsch JM, Sommer A, Katz J et al. Socioeconomic status and visual impairment among urban Americans. Arch Ophthalmol 1991;109:637-41.
274. Tint et al. Defective cholesterol biosynthesis associated with the Smith-Lemli-Opitz syndrome. N Engl J Ed 1994;330:107-13.
275. Tobert JA. New developtments in lipid-lowering therapy: the role of inhibitors of hydroxymethylglutaryl-coenzyme A reductase. Circulation 1987;76:534-38.
276. Traboulsi El, Weinberg RJ. Familial congenital cornea guttata with anterior polar cataract. Am J Ophthalmol 1989;108:123-25.
277. Trindade F, Pereira F. Cataract formation after posterior chamber phakic intraocular lens implantation. J Cataract Refract Surg 1998;24(12):1661-63.
278. Tsutomu Y, Mihori K, Yoshito H. Traumatic cataract with ruptured posterior capsule from a nonpenetrating ocular injury.
279. Tuormaa TE. The adverse effects of tobacco smoking on reproductive and health: A review from the literature. Nutr Health 1995;10:105-120.
280. Ughade SN, Zodpey SP, Khanolkar VA. Risk factors for cataract: a case control study.
281. Urban RC (Jr), Cotlier E: Corticosteroid-induced cataract. Surv Ophthalmol 1986;31:102-110.
282. Vadot E, Guibal JP: Pathogenic de la cataracte diabetique. Bull Soc Ophthalmol Fr 1982;82:1513-14.
283. Vajpayee RB, Angra SK, Honavar SG et al. Pre-existing posterior capsular breaks from penetrating ocular injuries. J Cataract Refract Surg 1994;20:991-94.
284. Van Heyningen R, Harding JJ: A case-control study of cataract in Oxford: some risk factors. Br J Ophthalmol 1988;72:804-08.
285. van Heyningen R, Harding JJ: Do aspirin-like analgesics protect against cataract? Lancet 1986;i:1111-13.
286. van Heyningen R: The human lens. I—a comparison of cataracts extracted in Oxford (England) and Shikarpur (W Pakistan). Exp Eye Res 1972;13:136-47.
287. Varma S, Schocket SS, Richards RD: Implications of aldose reductase in cataract in human diabetes. Invest Ophthalmol Vis Sci 1979;18:237-41.
288. Vesti E. Development of cataract after trabeculectomy. Acta Ophthalmol 1993;71(6):777-81.
289. Vidal P, Fernandez-Vigo J, Cabezas-Cerrato J: Low glycation level and browning in human cataract. Acta Ophthalmol 1988;66:220–22.

290. Vitale S, West S, Hallfrisch J et al. Plasma antioxidants and risk of cortical and nuclear cataract. Epidemiol 1994;4:195-203.
291. Waxman SL, Bergen RL: Wagner's vitreoretinal degeneration. Ann Ophthalmol 1980;12(10):1150-51.
292. Weale R: A note on a possible relation between refraction and a disposition for senile nuclear cataract. Br J Ophthalmol 1980;64:311-14.
293. Weber WW: Acetylation. Birth Defects Orig Artic Ser 1990;26(1):43-65.
294. Wensor MD, McCarty CA, Taylor HR. The prevalence and risk factors of myopia in Victoria, Australia. Arch Ophthalmol 1999;117:658-63.
295. West S, Munoz B, Emmett EA et al. Cigaret smoking and risk of nuclear cataract. Arch Ophthalmol 1989;107:1166-69.
296. West S, Munoz B, Schein OD et al. Cigaret smoking and risk for progression nuclear opacities. Arch Ophthalmol 1995;113:1377-80.
297. Wiechens B, Winter M, Haigis W et al. Bilateral cataract after phakic posterior chamber top hat-style silicone intraocular lens. J Refract Surg 1997;13(4):392-97.
298. Wilczek M, Zygulska-Machowa H: Zawartosc witaminy C W.roznych typackzaem. J Klin Oczna 1968;38:477-80.
299. Winkleby MA, Fortmann SP, Barret DC. Social class disparities in risk factors for disease: eight-year prevalence patterns by level of education. Prev Med 1990;19:1-12.
300. Wolff SM. The ocular manifestations of congenital rubella. Sri Am Ophthalmol Soc 1972;70:577-14.
301. World Health Organization: Management of Cataract in Primary Health Care Services. WHO: Geneva 1990.
302. Ye JJ, Zadunaisky JA: A Na^+/H^+ exchanger and its relation to oxidative effects in plasma membrane vesicles from lens fibers. Exp Eye Res 1992;55:251-60.
303. Young RW. Optometry and the preservation of visual health. Optom Vis Sd 1993;70:255-62.
304. Zadok D, Chayet A: Lens opacity after neodymium: YAG iridectomy for phakic intraocular lens implantation. J Cataract Refract Surg 1999;25(4):592-93.
305. Zelenka PS: Lens lipids. Curr Eye Res 1984;3:1337-59.

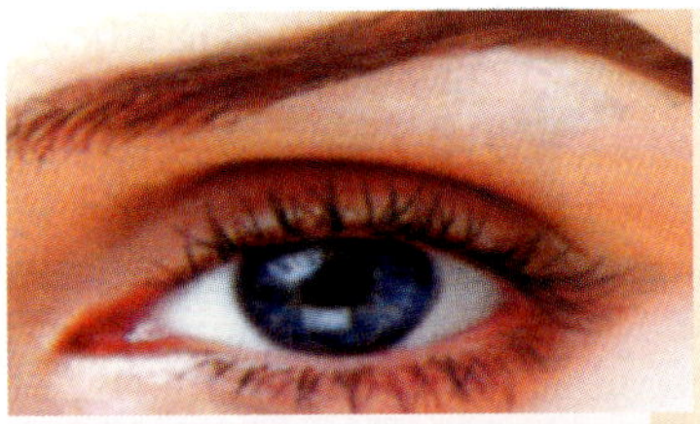

Four

Cataract Classification and Various Treatment Modalities

Ashok Garg (India)

INTRODUCTION

The word cataract is used to define the condition of opacification of the crystalline lens of the eye. In other words any opacity in the lens or its capsule whether congenital or acquired is known as cataract. When the transparency of the crystalline lens decrease enough to disturb vision, a clinically significant cataract exists. The lens being an avascular structure, inflammatory disease cannot develop in it. The most common disease of lens is development of opacity of lens fibers leading to cataract formation. The decrease in lens transparency and subsequent cataract formation is usually the result of foci of light scattering or absorption in the axial part of the lens (Figs 4.1 and 4.2). The term cataract is often used to refer to change in color of the lens as well as a decrease in its transparency.

Before going into the details of classification of cataract let me first discuss in brief about the general

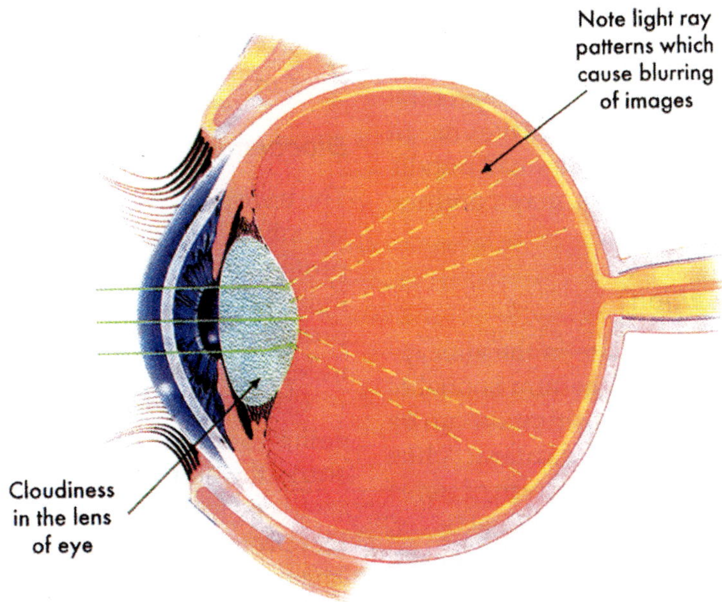

Fig. 4.1: Early cataractous lens with light rays scattered (*Courtesy:* Allergan India Ltd)

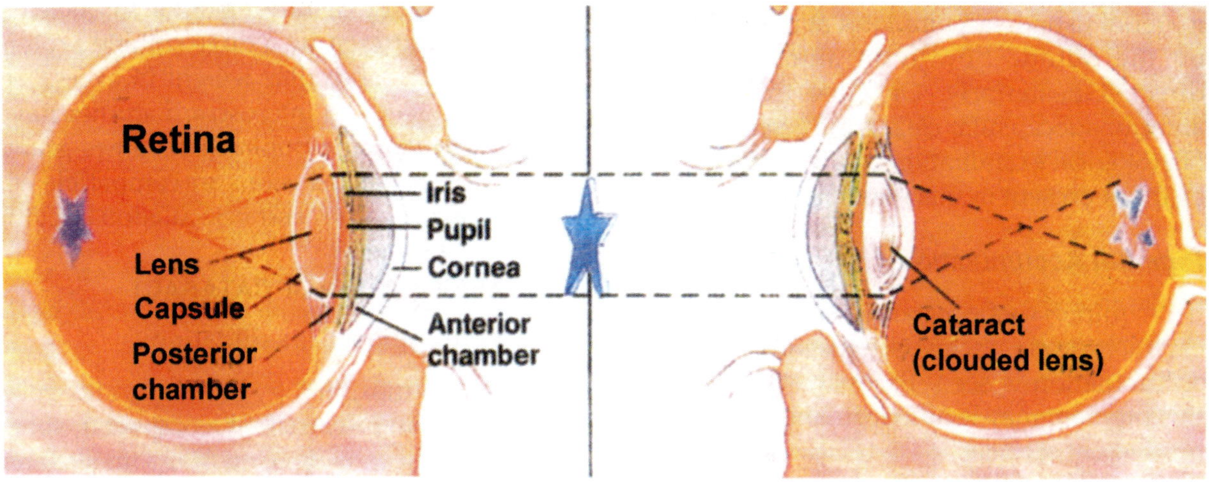

Fig. 4.2: Image formation in normal and cataract lens

mechanism of cataract formation which is common to cataracts of diverse etiology.

The various steps in general mechanism of cataract formations are as follows.

Lens Fibers Opacification

Previously clear, superficially situated youngest lens fibers present in subcapsular clear zone area, are more prone to physical injuries like concussion, trauma and to metabolic disturbances like diabetes. Due to this change many acquired cataracts associated with trauma, diabetes and hypoparathyroidism are present clinically as subcapsular type. In senile cortical cataracts deeper lens fibers are affected most.

Thus opacification of the deeper cortical fibers is the most common mechanism of cataract formation. Biochemically the lens fibers protein get irreversibly denatured and coagulated.

New Opaque Fibers Development

Newly developed lens fibers that are opaque at the time of formation are seen specially in congenital and developmental cataracts. However in developmental cataracts, all fibers or a small bundle of fibers may be opaque and lens may continue normal growth.

Granular Material Deposition

Granular material may accumulate in the subcapsular region of lens in which epithelium is unable to produce new lens fibers. Such a situation can be seen in developmental and acquired cataracts like toxic cataract, radiation cataract, some form of senile cataract, metabolic and complication cataracts.

It has been shown that mitotic activity of the epithelium gives rise to cellular debris and proliferation of epithelial cells. These debris or cells shift in the subcapsular clear zone in the direction normally taken by the growing lens fibers. This material usually accumulates at the posterior pole by the mitotic flow from anterior epithelium directed posteriorly. On close examination the anterior subcapsular clear zone is seen obliterated. Histological examination confirms the cataractous changes present in this region as well.

Pigment Accumulation

In acquired senile cataract specially in nuclear cataract (senile nuclear sclerosis) typical pigment accumulation is seen. Excessive accumulation of this pigment may lead to formation of deep amber brunescent cataract.

Lens Epithelium Opacification

Primary opacification of lens epithelium is seen typically with punctate traumatic cataract, toxic cataract, anterior subcapsular cataract and in glaucoma flecks. These changes lead to fluctuation in refractive index, light scattering and loss of lens transparency.

Deposition of Extraneous Material in Lens

Such type of cataract is seen typically in the patients suffering from Wilson disease in which copper is deposited in lens capsule and lens fibers. In drug-induced cataract like chlorpromazine cataract, the drug or its derivative is precipitated in lens fibers.

Biochemical Alterations in Lens

The transparency of normal crystalline lens is based on small spatial fluctuations in the number of protein molecules over dimensions comparable to light wavelength due to high concentration of these protein molecules in the lens, none scattering light independently of another.

Cataract is explained by large molecular aggregation or by separation of molecules due to the entry of water.

In cortical, supranuclear and subcapsular cataract protein deficient fluid collects between fibers. The refractive index of this fluid is much less than that of fiber cytoplasm and light scattering occurs at this interface. Light scattering may also occur from large protein aggregates linked to the cell membrane by disulfide bonds. In nuclear cataract light is scattered by a huge soluble protein aggregates with molecular weight in excess of 5×10^6 daltons. Electron microscopic studies have shown that in cataract cytoplasm becomes granular and electron dense inclusions are compatible with molecular aggregation and vesiculation of cytoplasm.

CLASSIFICATION OF CATARACT

Morphological Classification

Based on morphology (size, site and appearance) cataract can be classified as capsular, subcapsular, cortical, supranuclear, nuclear, lamellar and sutural cataract. The individual location and configuration of each type of morphological cataract is described here.

CAPSULAR CATARACT

Congenital capsular thickening may involve both anterior and posterior polar opacities and also pyramidal cataracts in which opacity projects into the anterior chamber. Acquired capsular opacities may occur in Lowe and Miller syndromes, thermal cataract, pseudoexfoliation syndrome, gold toxicity and Vossious ring.

Common form of capsular opacity is polar cataract which develops in anterior, posterior and bipolar forms. The anterior polar cataract is more frequent. The opacity is generally disc-shaped and most commonly lies in the anterior subcapsular clear zone.

Posterior polar cataract reduces visual acuity more frequently than anterior polar cataract. Polar opacities are usually congenital but can also develop due to trauma.

Capsular opacities usually remain static but underlying cortical opacities may develop.

SUBCAPSULAR CATARACT

Granular opacities develop in subcapsular clear zone and are more commonly posterior subcapsular type in comparison to anterior one.

- Posterior subcapsular opacities are seen typically in secondary cataract, complicated, toxic and radiation cataract, traumatic cataract, dermatogenic cataract, nutritional cataract, and some forms of senile and presenile cataract (Fig. 4.3).

  These granular opacities form a sheath beneath the capsule and tend to collect towards the poles specially the posterior pole.

  The concave disc-shaped opacities at the posterior pole are typically seen in the senile cataract (cupuliform cataract). The complicated cataract with granular opacities involves the cortex in front of the posterior pole.
- Anterior subcapsular opacities are less common and in early stage are difficult to be recognized on slit-lamp examination. Such opacities occur in glaukomflecken, Wilson's disease, miotic therapy and chlorpromazine and amiodarone administration.

Subcapsular cataracts frequently develop as a result of damage to subcapsular epithelium.

In posterior subcapsular cataract development, first change that occurs in the posterior migration of epithelial cells. Subcapsular cataracts tend to deteriorate during the period of months if the initial trauma was severe or if the stimulating cause is not removed.

CORTICAL CATARACT

Congenital cortical opacities are common and do not usually interfere with vision. These opacities may be white or of deep blue hue. Coronary cataract, a subtype of a congenital cataract surrounds the lens nucleus like a crown. Developmental punctate opacities in the cortex are common and are found in most of the lenses. They increase in number with age but rarely interfere with vision.

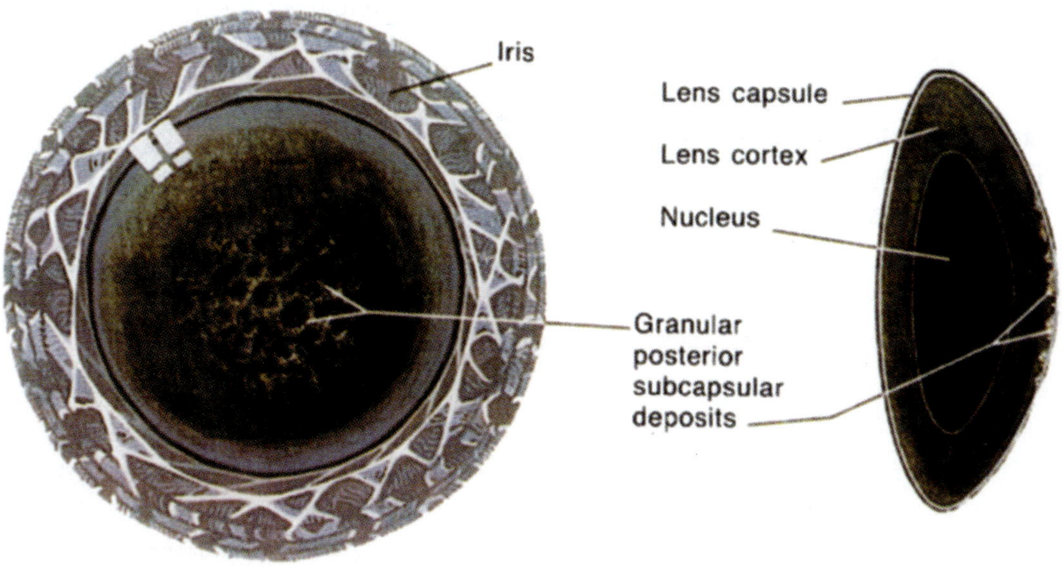

Fig. 4.3: Posterior subcapsular cataract (*Courtesy:* Ciba Geigy *Clinical Symposia*)

Senile cortical cataract (cuneiform cataract) is the most common cataract in acquired type. It becomes manifest in the deep layers of the cortex, although its site or origin is adjacent to the subcapsular epithelium. Cuneiform cataract starts as vacuoles and clefts between the lens fibers. Opacification of the clefts leads to the formation of the typical radial spoke-like pattern which is best seen by fundal retroillumination. Cortical opacities specially in the complicated cataract may also originate from subcapsular opacities which appear within the cortex as the lens grows and lays down new fibers superficial to them.

SUPRANUCLEAR CATARACT

Deep cortical cataracts like coronary in congenital type may be separately classified as supranuclear cataract. The coronary cataract surrounds the nucleus like a crown. As it originates during embryonic development stage, it lies in the deeper layer of the cortex. These opacities are of rounded contour and are associated with contour changes which may be white or cerulean. The number of opacities increases gradually with time and interferes with the vision.

NUCLEAR CATARACT

Congenital opacities are invariably of nuclear type because there is no cortex in the lens at the time of birth. Congenital nuclear opacities occur in rubella, galactosemia and cataracta centralis pulverulenta in which the entire embryonic nucleus is opaque. Nuclear cataract may consist of only punctate opacities or may extend to involve the embryonic nucleus. Usually nuclear cataract is associated with a lamellar opacity and is rarely total.

The nucleus tends to remain free from acquired cataract until the onset of senile nuclear sclerotic cataract in which brown pigment, deposits within the nucleus. The pigment is confined to the nucleus and does not spread into the cortex. Histologically there is sharp demarcation between the homogeneous nucleus and the liquefied or fragmented cortex. Nuclear sclerosis may be secondary to trauma or uveitis.

In nuclear sclerosis the refractive index of nucleus increases which causes a myopic shift in the refractive error. This myopia is known as second sight, as it allows the patient to discard his presbyopic glasses (Fig. 4.4). If refractive index increase is extreme and limited to the central nucleus then peripheral lens shall be relatively hypermetropic resulting in monocular diplopia.

LAMELLAR (ZONULAR) CATARACT

Lamellar cataract is invariably congenital as it involves one lamella of the fetal or nuclear zones so that it encircles the lens both anteriorly and posteriorly forming an apparent hollow disc. It

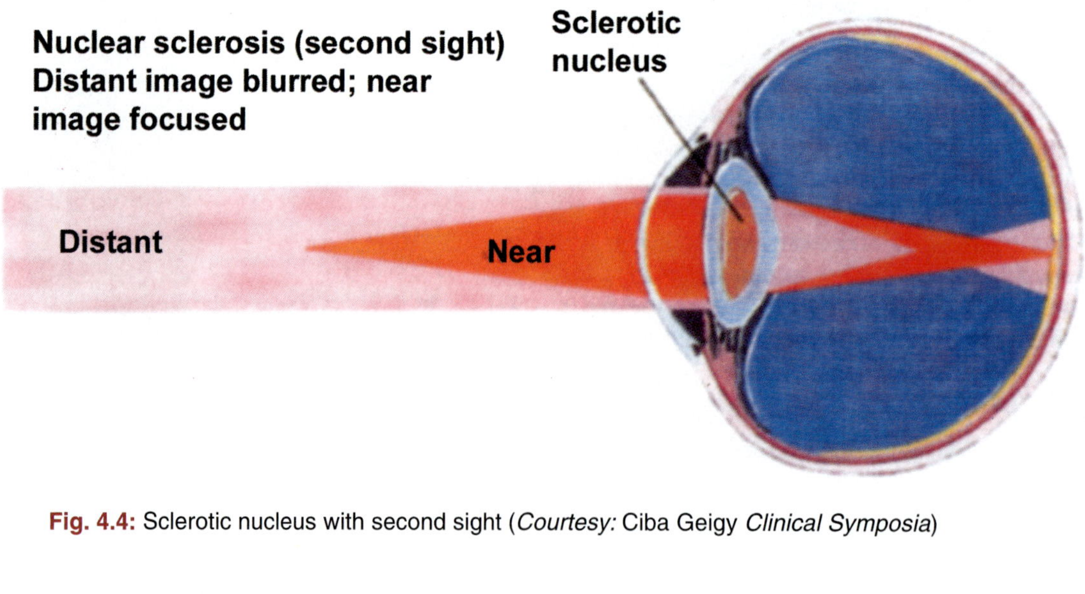

Fig. 4.4: Sclerotic nucleus with second sight (*Courtesy:* Ciba Geigy *Clinical Symposia*)

usually consists of many white dots. This opacity develops as a result of insult that affects the developing lens fibers for a specific period of time. Preexisting and newly developed lens fibers are clear. Radial spoke-like opacities (riders) frequently surround the cataract.

SUTURAL CATARACT

These are very frequent, congenital Y-shaped opacities within the lens nucleus as the Y-sutures are formed earlier than any others. They depict the line of intersection of primary lens fibers and form the anterior and posterior borders of the embryonic nucleus. Most of sutural cataracts develops at this level and thus are usually congenital static and bilateral and have no clinical significance in relation to the vision.

More superficial sutural cataracts are developmental in origin and have peculiar patterns. Floriform and coralliform cataracts represents extended form of sutural cataracts.

Classification According to Maturity

Cataracts have also been classified according to developmental stage (mature, immature, etc.) These are:

IMMATURE CATARACT

Immature cataract is defined as that in which scattered opacities are separated by clear zones. Lens appears gray in color.

INTUMESCENT CATARACT

In this type of cataract lens becomes swollen by imbibed water. It can be immature or mature. The anterior chamber becomes shallow.

MATURE CATARACT

In this type of cataract, the entire cortex becomes opaque white (Fig. 4.5). The outlines of the opaque lens fibers are visible. The vision is sharply reduced to perception of hand movement only. The swelling of lens usually subsides but the intumescent stage may persist. On fundal retroillumination no fundal glow is visible.

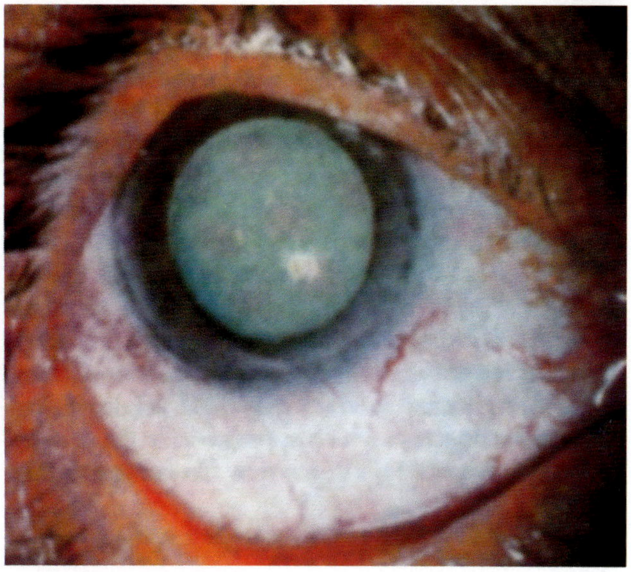

Fig. 4.5: Mature cataract when entire lens becomes opaque (*Courtesy:* Lim and Constable *Color Atlas of Ophthalmology*)

HYPERMATURE CATARACT

Hypermature cataract is mature cataract which has become smaller and has a wrinkled capsule due to leakage of water out of the lens. There may be two types of hypermature cataract.

Hypermature Morgagnian Cataract

In this type of cataract the total liquefaction of the cortex allow the nucleus to sink inferiorly. The whole of the cortical matter liquefies to form milky fluid so that the lens is now converted into a bag of milky fluid with the nucleus settled at the bottom of the bag. The cataract appears milky white uniformly without any visible (Figs 4.6 and 4.7) outlines of the lens fibers. There may be deposits of calcium on the lens capsule. The anterior chamber may be shallow or normal. Vision is reduced to perception of hand movement.

Hypermature Sclerotic Cataract

Due to alterations in the permeability of lens capsule, some of the cortical matter goes out and is absorbed. The lens becomes flatter, the capsule becomes thick and cataract appears brownish. Vision remains reduced to perception of hand movement only.

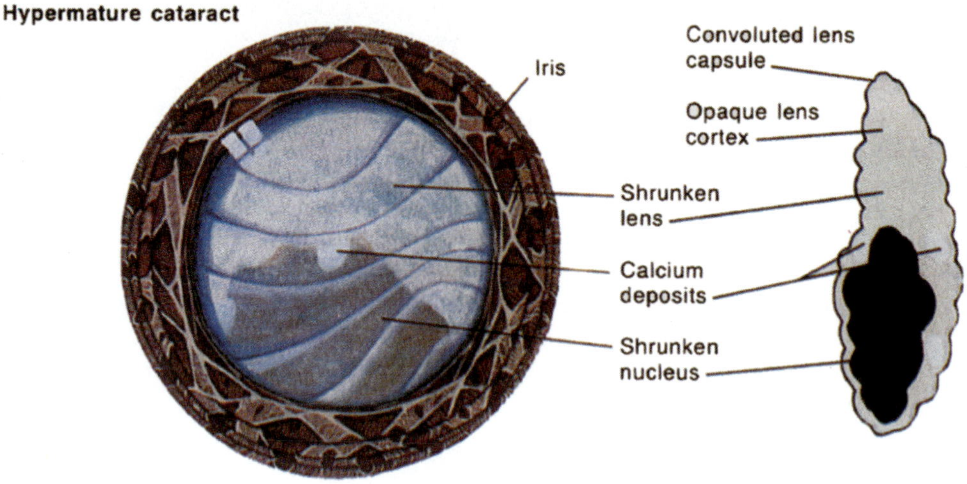

Fig. 4.6: Hypermature senile cataract (*Courtesy:* Ciba Geigy *Clinical Symposia)*

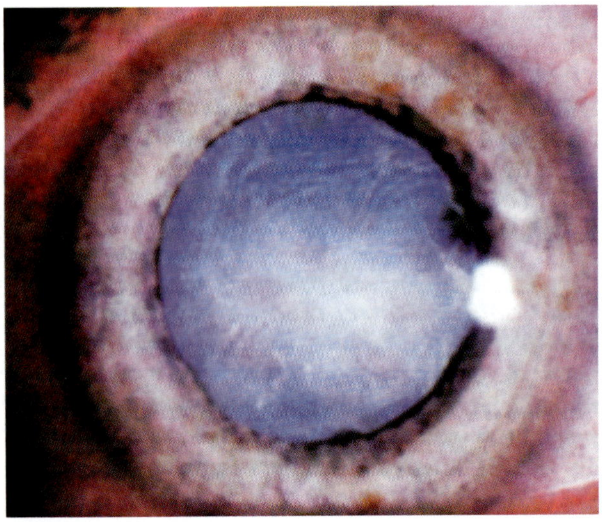

Fig. 4.7: Hypermature cataract with wrinkled anterior lens capsule (*Courtesy:* Kanski Clinical Ophthalmology, Butterworth International Edition)

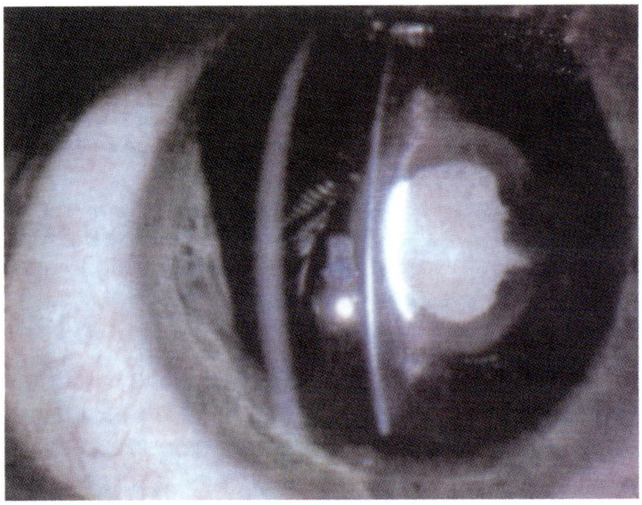

Fig. 4.8: Congenital cataract (*Courtesy:* Kanski *Clinical Ophthalmology,* Butterworth International Edition)

Etiological Classification

Etiological classification is ideally considered as the most widely accepted classification of cataract. Various types of cataracts under this classification are as follows.

CONGENITAL CATARACT

Congenital cataract is present at birth. These cataracts develop due to some disturbances in the normal growth of the lens (Fig. 4.8). When the disturbances occur before birth and child is born with congenital cataract. Therefore in congenital cataract the opacity is limited to either embryonic or fetal nucleus (Fig. 4.9). Lens fibers developed either previous to or later than the period of disturbance remain normal. These types of cataract are usually stationary. Fifteen percent of all cases of childhood blindness are due to congenital cataracts. These cataracts occur about 30 percent as

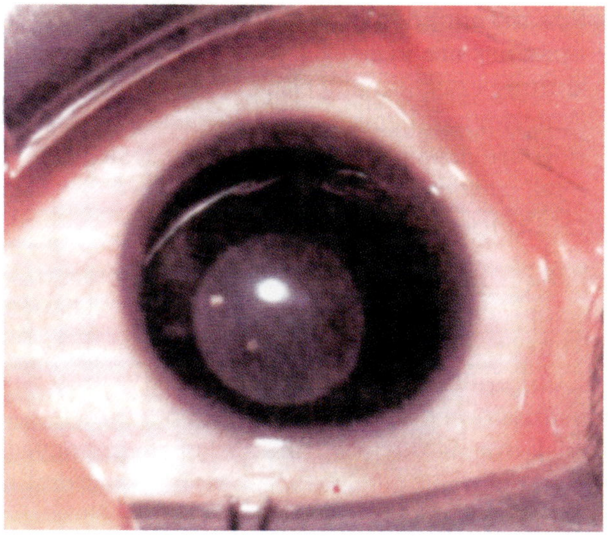

Fig. 4.9: Congenital cataract affecting the nucleus of lens

hereditary factors and are commonly dominant. About 8 percent of congenital cataracts are associated with other ocular anomalies like coloboma, persistent hyperplastic primary vitreous, aniridia, anterior chamber cleavage syndrome or ectopia lentis. Certain factors are associated with congenital cataracts. These are:

Heredity

Genetically determined cataract (in about 30% cases as already mentioned) is due to an anomaly in the chromosomal pattern of the individual. Common familial cataracts include zonular cataract, coronary cataract, all soft cataracts and cataracta pulverulenta.

Maternal Factors

- Maternal malnutrition during pregnancy is associated with non-familial zonular cataract.
- Maternal infections like rubella are usually associated with congenital cataracts in 50 percent of cases. Other maternal infections like toxoplasmosis and cytomegalovirus inclusion disease are also associated with congenital cataract.
- Maternal drug ingestion like thalidomide and corticosteroids during pregnancy are associated with congenital cataracts in newborn babies.
- Maternal exposure to radiation during pregnancy may also cause congenital cataract.

Fetal Factors

These are
- Deficient oxygenation (anoxia) due to placental hemorrhage.
- Metabolic disorders of fetus like galactosemia, galactokinase deficiency and neonatal hypoglycemia.
- Cataract abnormalities like Lowe's syndrome, myotonia dystrophia and congenital ichthyosis.
- Malnutrition of early infancy.

Idiopathic

In about 50 percent cases etiology of congenital cataract is unknown. Various types of clinical congenital cataracts are.

Capsular Cataract

Anterior polar capsular cataract may be associated with persistent pupillary membrane and corneal opacity. Corneal opacification with anterior polar cataract may be caused by one of the anterior chamber cleavage syndromes.

Posterior polar capsular cataract is caused by persistent hyaloid artery remnant.

Polar capsular cataracts are usually of dominant inheritance and bilateral.

Embryonic Nuclear Cataract

Embryonic nuclear cataract is also known as cataracta centralis pulverulenta. It has dominant genetic trait and occurs due to inhibition of the lens development at a very early stage and this involves the embryonal nucleus. This type of cataract is usually bilateral and is characterized by a small rounded opacity lying exactly in the center of the lens. This opacity has a powdery appearance (pulverulenta) and usually does not affect the vision.

Lamellar Cataract

Lamellar cataract is the most common type of congenital cataract developing in about 50 percent of total congenital cataracts. Hereditary lamellar cataracts are often of a prenatal size and are commonly associated with riders (Fig. 4.10). Bilateral

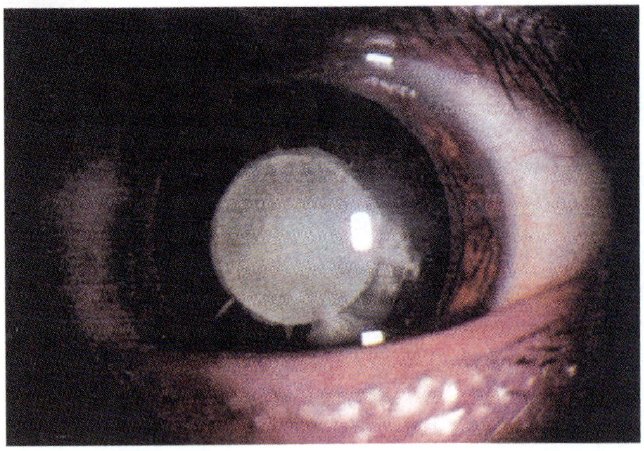

Fig. 4.10: Congenital cataract with riders (*Courtesy :* Kanski *Clinical Ophthalmology*, Butterworth International Edition)

hereditary lamellar cataracts are usually transmitted in an autosomal dominant fashion. Typically this cataract occurs in a zone of fetal nucleus surrounding the embryonic nucleus. The main mass of the lens fibers internal or external to zone of cataract is clear except for small liner opacities like spokes of a wheel (riders) which may be seen towards the equator. Maternal rubella infection during 7 to 8th week of gestation, and maternal metabolic disease during pregnancy such as parathyroid deficiency may cause lamellar cataract.

Lamellar cataracts frequently have a powdery appearance and the effect on vision varies according to the diameter and density of the affected lamella. It is usually bilateral and condition is stationary.

Sutural Cataract

These cataracts are often familial and when inherited transmission is usually autosomal dominant. An X-linked inheritance in which young male patients are severely affected and female carrier show minor symptoms.

Sutural cataract is one of the common form of congenital cataract present and it consists of a series of punctate opacities scattered around the anterior and posterior Y-sutures. Such cataracts are usually static, bilateral and have least effect on the vision. Various forms of sutural cataract present are

- Floriform cataract in which opacities are arranged in flower petal pattern.
- Coralliform cataract where the opacities are present in coral form.
- Spear-shaped cataract where the lenticular opacities are in the form of scattered heaps of shining crystalline needles.
- Anterior axial embryonic cataract in which fine dots are present near the anterior Y-suture.

Total Congenital Cataract

Rubella is the most important causative factor for development of total congenital cataract. About 20 percent of all congenital cataracts are of total type.

Congenital rubella is caused by maternal transmission of the virus to the fetus which is at the risk during the first trimester of pregnancy.

Total congenital cataract may be unilateral or bilateral and has hereditary character.

Typically the child is born with a dense white nuclear cataract and with intumescence, a spherophakic total cataract may develop. It is progressive type of cataract. The lens matter may remain soft or liquefy (congenital Morgagnian cataract).

Congenital rubella cataract may occur alone or as a part of classic triad of congenital rubella syndrome. It consists of

- Ocular abnormalities (congenital cataract, salt and pepper retinopathy (in 40% of cases) and microphthalmos, strabismus (in 35% of cases), nystagmus, optic atrophy, corneal haze, glaucoma and iris atrophy.
- Ear defects include deafness due to destruction of organ of Corti.
- Heart defects include patent ductus arteriosis, (PDA) pulmonary stenosis and ventricular septal defects (VSD). This classic rubella syndrome may also include hepatosplenomegaly, jaundice, purpura and pneumonitis.

Congenital Morgagnian cataract and ring form cataract in which lens nucleus is absent leaves only a doughnut-shaped lens remnant. Maternal infections and metabolic disorders are other causes of congenital total cataract.

Congenital Membranous Cataract

There may occur total or partial absorption of congenital cataract leaving behind thin membranous cataract. Sometimes there is complete disappearance of all lens fibers and only a fine transparent lens capsule remains behind. Such a patient can be misdiagnosed as having congenital aphakia.

DEVELOPMENTAL CATARACT

Developmental cataract may occur from infancy to adolescence. Therefore, such cataract may involve infantile or adult nucleus, deeper parts of cortex or capsule. These small opacities develop after birth at the time of deposition of newly formed but opaque lens fibers. The opacities tend to have a round outline that is not related to the course of the fibers. Developmental cataract typically affects the particular zone which is being formed when this process is disturbed. The lens fibers developed previous and subsequently are often normal and remain clear. The quantity of developmental cataract increases with age but normally they do not interfere with vision.

Developmental cataract assumes the most variegated forms and is common in its minor manifestations various types of developmental cataract are as follows.

Punctate Cataract

Punctate cataract is one of the most common type of developmental cataract present and in minute form it is almost universal in occurrence. It is also called blue dot cataract or cataract a punctata cerulea. It usually develops in first two decades of life. These are small round discrete opacities that appear blue, white or brown situated in the peripheral part of adolescent nucleus and deeper layers of cortex. Punctate opacities are usually stationary and do not affect the vision. However large punctate opacities which are associated with coronary cataract may marginally reduce the vision. Dominant inheritance may be found.

Coronary Cataract

Coronary cataract is another extremely common form of developmental cataract occurring about puberty thus involving either the adolescent nucleus or deeper layers of the cortex.

Coronary cataract appears as corona of club-shaped opacities near the periphery of the lens usually hidden by the iris while the axial region and extreme periphery of the lens remain free.

Each opacity is a flattened disc with a white to brown or bluish hue. These cataracts are known to be transmitted by dominant inheritance. Since these opacities are located peripherally, the vision is unaffected except when they are extensive or present with subcapsular cataract.

Anterior Polar Cataract

Anterior capsular (polar) cataract may be developmental due to delayed formation of anterior chamber. Usually this condition is acquired and follows contact of the capsule with the cornea usually after ulcer perforation in ophthalmia neonatorum, or any other cause. Anterior polar cataract may develop as any of the following morphological patterns.

- Thickened white plaque in the center of anterior lens capsule in the pupillary area.
- Anterior pyramidal cataract where thickened capsular opacity is cone shaped with its apex towards the cornea.

  This opacity may project into the anterior chamber in form of a pyramid.
- Reduplicated cataract (double cataract) Sometimes along with thickening of central point of anterior capsule, lens fibers lying immediately beneath it also becomes opaque and are subsequently separated from the capsule by laying of transparent fibers in between. The buried opacity is called "imprint" and two together constitute "reduplicated cataract." Such opacities are not progressive and rarely affects the vision.

Posterior Polar Cataract

Posterior polar cataract is due to persistence of the posterior part of the vascular sheath of the lens. It is very common lens anomaly and consists of small circular circumscribed opacity involving the posterior pole. In minimum degree it is quite common and rarely affects the vision.

Zonular Cataract

In this type of cataract, development has been interfered with at a later stage and an area around embryonic nucleus becomes opacified, its extent depending on the duration of the inhibiting factor.

The opacity is usually sharply demarcated and area of the lens zone is clear.

Such zonular cataracts have a genetic origin with a strong hereditary tendency of the dominant type.

Lack of vitamin D is apparently a potent factor and evidence of rickets may be found in the affected children. This deficiency may also inhibit the development of other epithelial structures, specially the enamel of permanent teeth which is being formed at the time. It is usually bilateral and frequently causes severe visual defect.

ACQUIRED CATARACT

In acquired cataract opacification occurs due to degeneration of already formed normal lens fibers. The exact mechanism and reasons for degeneration of lens fibers are not yet fully clear. However, in general any factor physical, chemical or biological which affects the critical intra and extracellular equilibrium of water and electrolytes or deranges the colloid system within the lens fibers tends to develop opacification. The common varieties of acquired cataract are as follows:

Senile Cataract

Senile cataract is the most common variety of cataract. It is an affection of advanced life and is essentially an ageing process. Sometimes there appears to be a familial tendency to cataract in which case the condition may develop at an earlier age in successive generations and phenomenon is known as anticipation and as a rule is usually bilateral but develops earlier in one eye than the other. Usually some degree of cataract is present after the age of 50 years and it equally affects both the sexes. Although the precise etiopathogenesis is not clear, yet the various factors involved in senile cataractogenesis are as follows.

Factors Affecting Onset Type and Maturation of Senile Cataracts

- Hereditary factor plays a significant role in the incidence, age of onset and maturation of senile cataracts in different generations.
- *Ultraviolet irradiation* More frequent exposure to UV irradiation from sunlight and artificial sources may stimulate the early onset and maturation of senile cataract.
- *Dietary factors* Anomalous diet in relation to certain proteins, amino acids, vitamins (vitamin E, C and riboflavin) and essential elements also contribute to early onset and maturation of senile cataract.
- Severe dehydrational crisis due to diarrhea, cholera, etc. can predispose to early onset and maturation of cataract.

Mechanism of Loss of Lens Transparency

It is essentially different in nuclear and cortical senile cataracts.

- In senile cortical cataract main biochemical changes are decreased levels of total protein, amino acids and potassium alongwith increased concentration of sodium and marked hydration of the lens followed by coagulation of proteins.

The detailed mechanism of senile opacification of cortex is discussed in separate chapter of this textbook.

Senile Nuclear Cataract

In this cataract usually degenerative change is intensification of the age related nuclear sclerosis (Fig. 4.11) associated with dehydration and compaction of the nucleus resulting in hard nucleus. It is associated with significant increase in water insoluble protein. However total protein content and distribution of cations remain normal. There may be associated deposition of urochrome or melanin derived from the amino acids in the lens.

Senile cataract is of various types and occur in subcapsular, cortical and nuclear regions of the lens. The locations of the predominant senile cataract have been shown to be cortical (70%), nuclear (25%) and subcapsular (5%).

Subcapsular Senile Cataract (Cupuliform Cataract)

These cataracts may be anterior or posterior. These opacities are seen as brown granules and cysts in the shape of a shallow cup in the subcapsular

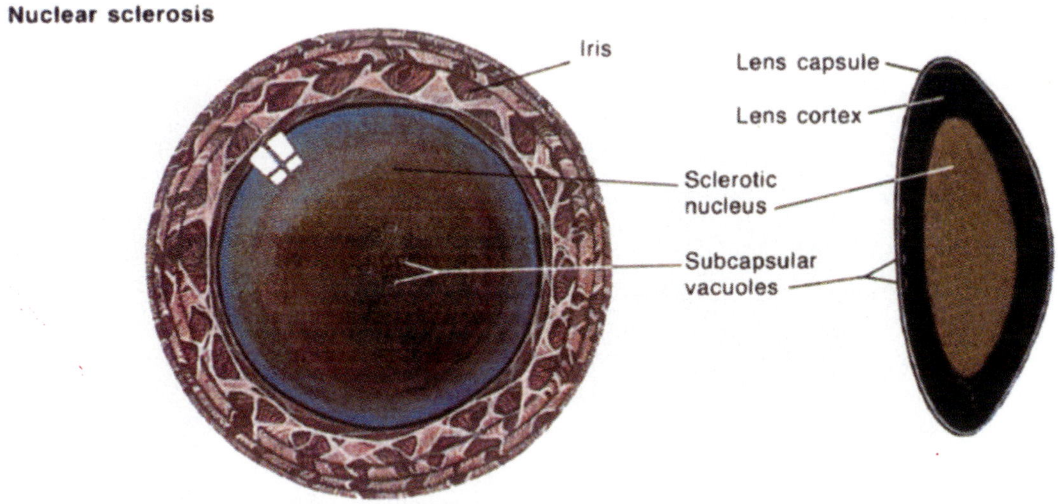

Fig. 4.11: Nuclear sclerosis (*Courtesy* : Ciba Geigy *Clinical Symposia)*

region. The anterior subcapsular cataract lies directly under the lens capsule and is associated with fibrous metaplasia of the anterior epithelium of the lens. The posterior subcapsular cataract lies just in front of the posterior capsule and is associated with posterior migration of epithelial cells of the lens.

These cataracts usually develop in 60 to 80-year-old age group patients but may be present in an inherited form at an earlier age. Patients of posterior subcapsular senile cataract specifically get troubled by bright sun light and head lights of incoming vehicles.

Cortical Senile Cataract (Cuneiform or Soft Cataract)

Cortical senile cataract is the most common form of senile cataract prevalent in the aging population.

In this type of cataract the opacities develop in the cortical fibers and appear to be due to an accumulation of globules and vacuoles between adjacent fibers (Fig. 4.12). Lens fibers of the cortex are mainly affected. There is hydration due to accumulation of water droplets in between the fibers followed by changes in the colloid system within the fibers. The proteins are first denatured and then are coagulated forming an opacity. Ultimately the whole of lens becomes opaque and assumes a pearly white appearance.

The appearance of cuneiform cataract with its vacuoles, radial spoke-like separation of lens fibers and wedge-shaped water clefts and shield-like configuration is salient feature of this senile cataract. Cuneiform opacities represent areas in which lens fiber membranes get damaged allowing a sodium influx and osmotic imbibition of water. Increased membrane permeability and inactivation of active transport process in these areas leads to loss of potassium, glutathione, soluble protein and inositol. These biochemical changes eventually lead to precipitation, opacification and aggregation of lens protein.

Stages of maturation of senile cortical cataract are important to understand. These are as follows:

Stage of lamellar separation Here the earlier senile change is demarcation of cortical fibers probably to excessive shear stress developed between the fibers at the onset of presbyopia. These initial changes are known as lamellar separation and are reversible and are best seen on slit lamp examination.

Incipient cataract stage In this stage in cuneiform senile cataract typical wedge-shaped opacities with clear areas in between are seen (Fig. 4.13). These opacities extend from equator towards the center. On distant direct ophthalmoscopy these opacities appear as dark lines against the red fundal glow. Since cuneiform cataract starts at periphery and

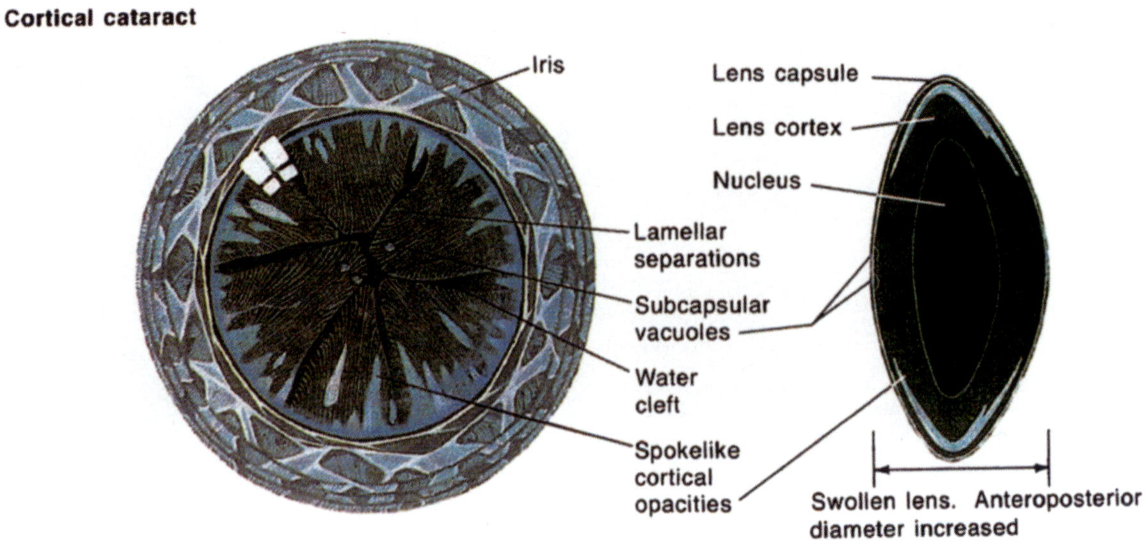

Fig. 4.12: Senile cortical cataract (*Courtesy :* Ciba Geigy *Clinical Symposia*)

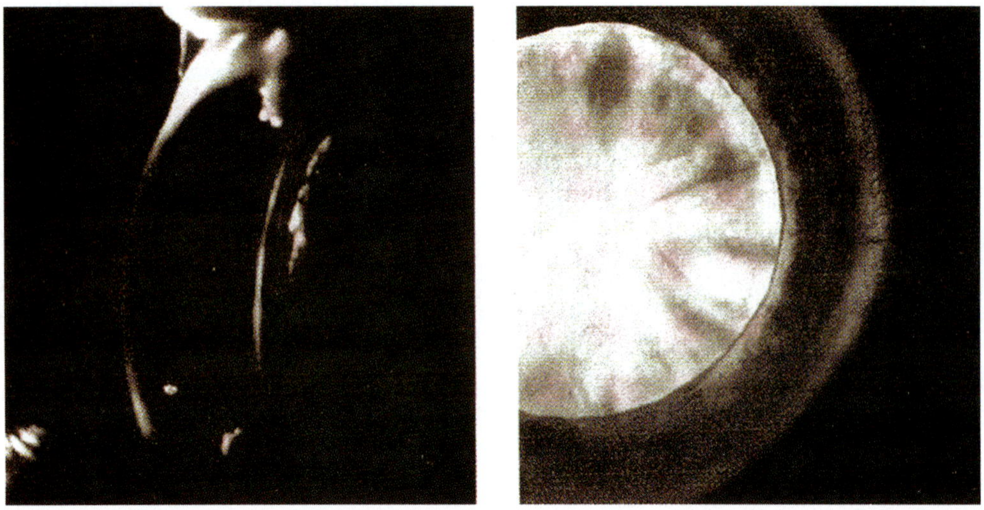

Fig. 4.13: Slit lamp appearance of early senile cortical cataract: (a) oblique illumination, and (b) reflex illumination

extends centrally, the visual disturbances are noticed at a comparatively later stage.

Progressive stage In this stage further wedge-shaped opacities develop, with clear area in between becoming lesser and lesser (Figs 4.14 and 4.15).

Immature senile cataract stage In this stage opacification progresses further. The cuneiform or cupuliform patterns can be recognized till the advanced stage of ISC develops when opacification becomes more diffuse and irregular, the lens appears greyish white. But clear cortex is still present and iris shadow is visible. Very little fundal flow can be seen because the pupillary area is almost fully occupied by the cataract. In certain patients when the cataract is still in immature stage the lens becomes swollen due to imbibition of fluid. The anterior chamber becomes shallow. This condition is known as "intumescent cataract." This stage may persist even in the next stage of maturation.

Mature senile cataract (MSC) In this stage opacification is complete (Fig. 4.16). The whole of

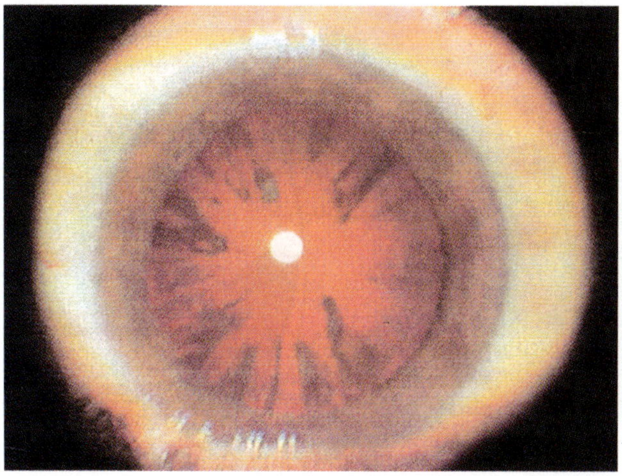

Fig. 4.14: Peripheral cortical cataract (*Courtesy :* Lim and Constable *Color Atlas of Ophthalmology)*

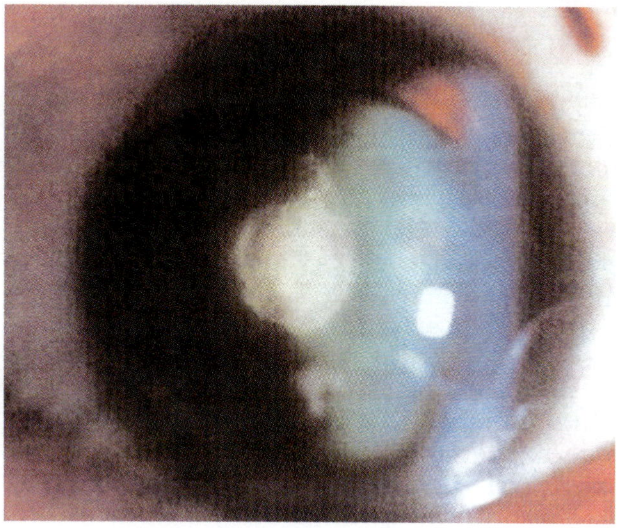

Fig. 4.15: Central cortical cataract (*Courtesy :* Lim and Constable *Color Atlas of Ophthalmology)*

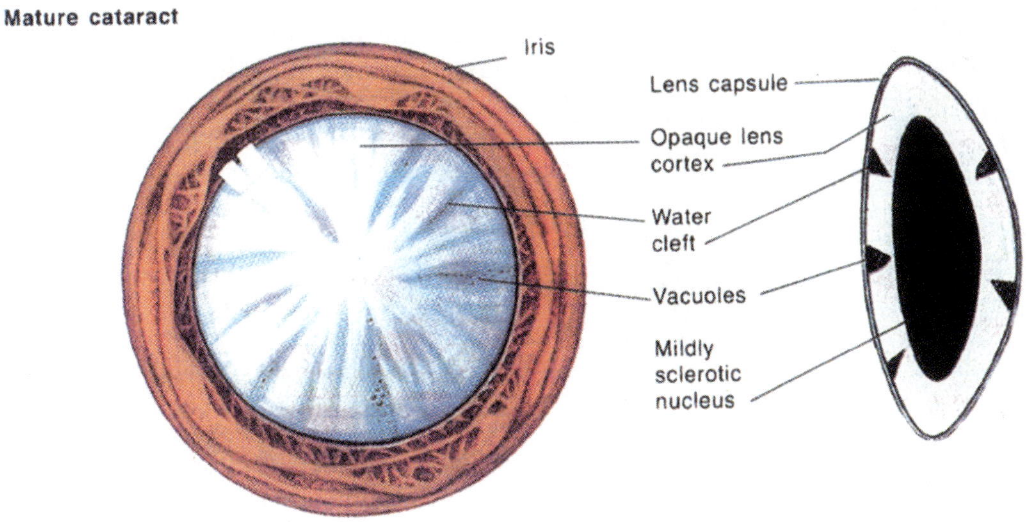

Fig. 4.16: Senile mature cataract (*Courtesy :* Ciba Geigy *Clinical Symposia)*

cortex is opacified. The outlines of opaque lens fibers are visible. The lens becomes pearly white in color. Such a cataract is known as mature senile cataract. The vision becomes reduced to perception of hand movements only. The original cuneiform clefts may still be recognizable on the surface of this opaque lens.

Hypermature senile cataract (HMSC) When the mature cataract is left *in situ* the stage of hypermature sets in. The hypermature cataract may occur in any of two following forms

- Morgagnian hypermature senile cataract: In this type of cataract after maturity liquefaction of cortical fibers may occur and with maceration of these fibers a pultaceous fluid is retained within the lens capsule and lens is converted into a bag of milky fluid (Figs 4.17 and 4.18).

The small brownish nucleus falls to the bottom of the capsule. Sometimes in this stage calcium deposits may also be seen on the lens capsule. Such a cataract is known as morgagnian cataract.

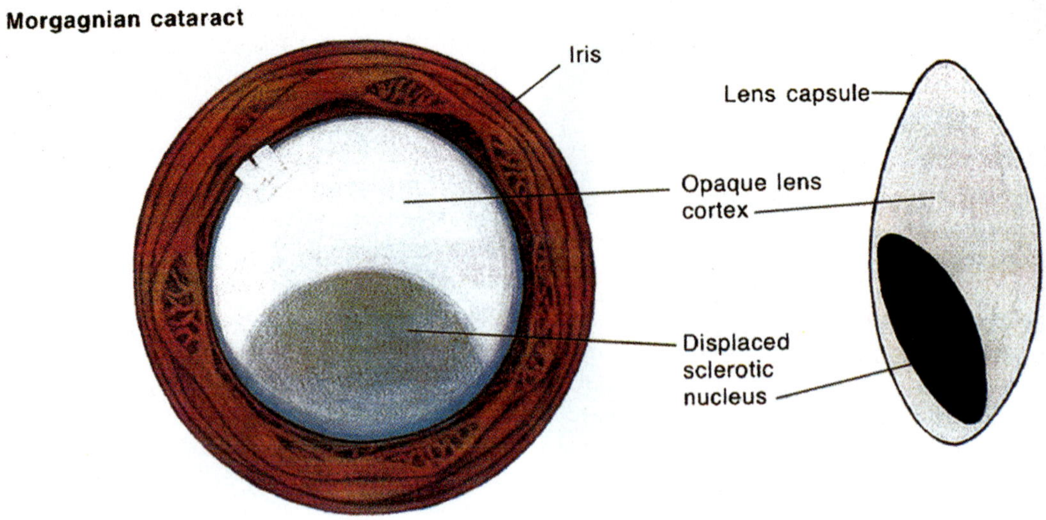

Fig. 4.17: Morgagnian cataract (hypermature type) (*Courtesy :* Ciba Geigy *Clinical Symposia)*

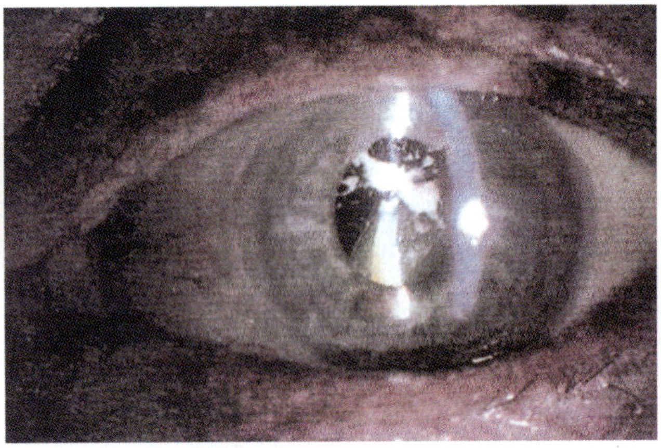

Fig. 4.18: Hypermature morgagnian cataract, (*Courtesy :* Kanski *Clinical Ophthalmology,* Butterworth International Edition)

- Sclerotic hypermature senile cataract: Sometimes after the stage of maturity, the cortex becomes disintegrated and the lens becomes shrunken due to water leakage. The anterior capsule is wrinkled and thickened due to proliferation of anterior cells and a dense white capsular cataract may be formed in the pupillary area. Due to shrinkage of lens, anterior chamber becomes deep and iris becomes tremulous (iridodonesis).

Nuclear Senile Cataract (Hard Cataract)

In this type of cataract, the nucleus gradually becomes opaque and cortex being clear (Fig. 4.19).

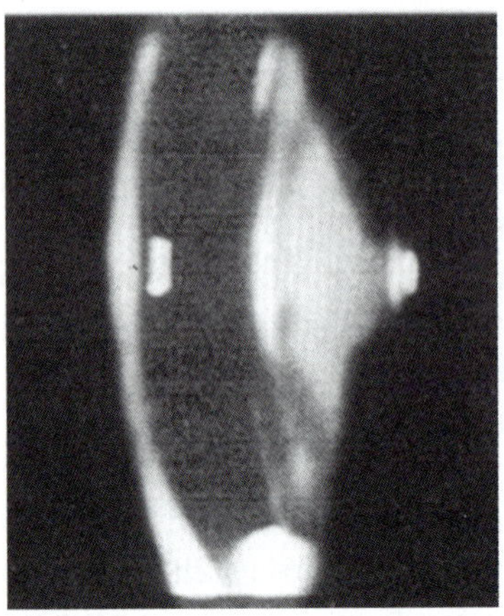

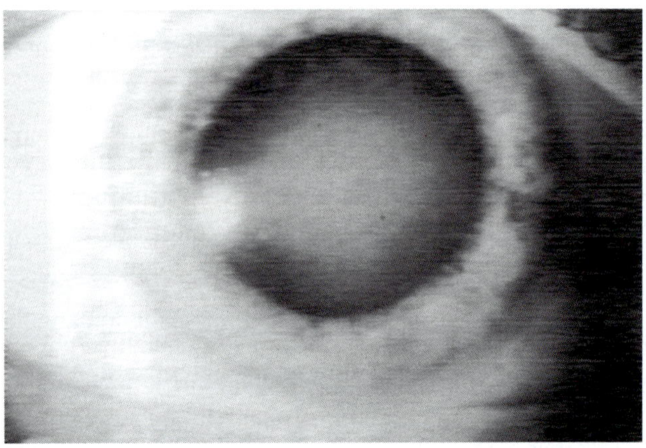

Fig. 4.19: Slit lamp appearance of early senile nuclear cataract: (a) oblique illumination, and (b) reflex illumination

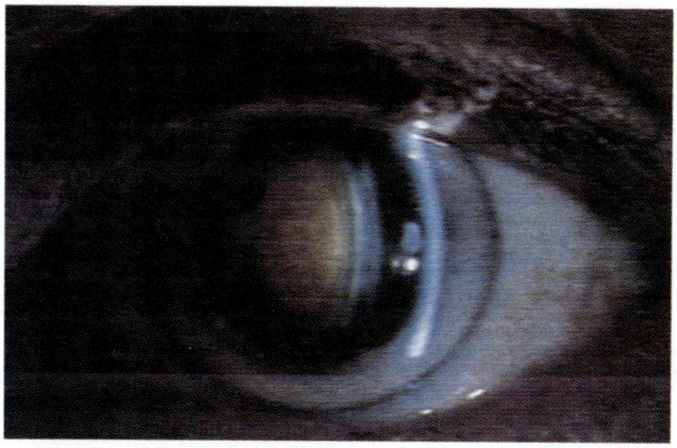

Fig. 4.20: Dense nuclear cataract (*Courtesy* : Kanski *Clinical Ophthalmology*, Butterworth International Edition)

Increased optical density of nucleus occurs normally with aging but it may be stimulated to excess with the formation of brown nucleus (cataracta brunescens) or even a black nucleus (cataracta nigra) and is usually bilateral (Fig. 4.20).

Dehydration and compaction of nucleus are associated with the process of nuclear sclerosis. The sclerotic process renders the lens inelastic and hard and decreases its ability to accommodate. At first a certain degree of myopia is induced. These changes start centrally and spread towards periphery.

This type of cataract do not develop into hypermature stage. The progress of cataract is slow and myopic eyes are more prone to develop this type of cataract.

Biochemical changes in nuclear senile cataract include an increase in the concentrations of protein, corresponding decrease in the degree of hydration, marked increase in sodium level along with decrease in potassium concentration. These changes are associated with accumulation of yellow brown pigment urochrome which may represent an oxidation product of amino acids or lipids.

Nuclear sclerosis begins between 50 to 60 years of age and progresses very slowly unless accelerated by the superimposition of subcapsular cataract.

METABOLIC CATARACT

Diabetic Cataract

Two types of cataracts are associated with diabetes.

- Senile cataract in diabetic patients tends to develop at an earlier age and progresses more rapidly than the usual cataract.
- True diabetic cataract or osmotic cataract is also known as "snow flake" or "snow-storm" cataract. It is although rare condition but usually develops in young adults due to osmotic overhydration of the lens. Initially a large number of fluid vacuoles appear under the anterior and posterior capsules which soon takes the appearance of snow flake-like white opacities in the lens. A rapid influx of water leads to acute swelling and opacification of the lens.

Galactosemic Cataract

Galactosemic cataract is associated with autosomal recessive inborn error of galactose metabolism, a deficiency of galactose-1-phosphate uridyl transferase. It occurs in two forms.

- Classical galactosemia It occurs due to deficiency of galactose-1 phosphate uridyl transferase (GPUT).
- Related disorder which occurs due to deficiency of galactokinase (GK).

Galactosemia is frequently associated with the development of bilateral cataract (oil droplet central nuclear lens opacity) within first few days or weeks of life. The lens changes may be reversible and occurrence of cataract may be prevented if milk and milk products are excluded from the diet when diagnosed at an early stage. Classic galactosemia patients also suffer from systemic disease like renal disease, hepatosplenomegaly, mental retardation and growth retardation if the disease goes untreated.

Galactokinase Deficiency Cataract

In this autosomal recessive disorder lack of enzyme galactokinase leads to accumulation of galactose which is then converted to galactitol. The same osmotic events as in galactosemia occur and lead to cataract formation.

Systemic manifestations of galactosemia are absent. Here children are healthy although they are at increased risk of developing cataract in the first few years of life. Dulcitol accumulation within the metabolizing lens cells leads to an increase in intralenticular osmotic pressure with disruption of lens fibers and opacification.

Hypocalcemic Cataract (Tetanic Cataract)

Hypocalcemic cataract occurs in association with infantile tetany or with hypoparathyroidism or rickets in other age groups. In the infants depression of serum calcium produces a zonular cataract with a thin opacified lamella deep in the infantile cortex.

In adults acquired or surgical hypoparathyroidism is associated with punctate red, green and highly refractile opacities occurring in the subcapsular area. In pseudohypoparathyrodism lamellar opacities are found in the lens nucleus. It is believed that calcium is necessary to maintain membrane integrity and this calcium deficiency leads to membrane disruption and increased permeability.

Nutritional Cataract

Subcapsular cataracts have been shown to develop in patients with anorexia nervosa. An earlier onset of subcapsular cataract specially in peoples who have alcohol abuse developed Dupuytren's contracture has been observed. It may be associated with poor nutrition characteristic of such people.

Cataract in Wilson's Disease

Inborn error of copper metabolism results in Wilson disease (hepatolenticular degeneration).

A characteristic opacity may develop in the anterior capsular region. It has a bright colored sunflower pattern usually red. It represents the deposition of metallic copper in the lens capsule. Ocular features include the characteristic Kayser-Fleischer ring which is present nearly in all cases.

Hypoglycemic Cataract

Neonatal hypoglycemia occurs in about 20 percent of newborns. Repeated hypoglycemia episode may lead to a characteristic lamellar cataract in which layers of cortical opacity are separated from a deeper zonular cataract by clear cortex. Cataract usually develops when child is 2 to 3 years old and in many patients no visual disturbances are encountered.

Cataract in Lowe's Syndrome

Lowe's syndrome (oculo-cerebral-renal) syndrome is inborn error of amino acid metabolism which predominantly affects boys. Ocular features include congenital cataract along with congenital glaucoma. Bilateral nuclear cataract and microphakia are always present in this X-linked recessive disorder. The lens is small, thin and disc like. The lens opacities may be capsular, lamellar, nuclear or total. Most striking feature is blue sclera (scleral thinning). Mothers of the affected children may also show multiple punctate lens opacities. Frequently in Lowe's syndrome patients, there is associated mental retardation, glycosuria, renal calculi and convulsions.

Cataract in Fabry's Disease

Fabry's disease is due to deficiency in the enzyme α-galactosidase A. Ocular features include spoke-like lens opacities and cornea verticillata. The ocular lesions however do not affect the vision. Systemic features include cardiovascular and renal impairment, angiokeratomas and severe pain in fingers and toes.

Cataract in Mannosidosis

This disorder is due to deficiency of enzyme α-mannosidase leading to accumulation of mannose rich oligosaccharide in the tissues. Ocular features consist of spoke-like or wheel-like posterior capsular opacities. Systemic features include mental retardation, short stature, skeletal changes and hepatosplenomegaly.

Cataract in Myotonic Dystrophy

It is inherited as an autosomal dominant trait and is the result of a defect in the gene encoding myotonin protein kinase. Early cataracts are characteristic and consist of fine, scattered dust-like opacities in the cortex and in subcapsular region. Multicolor (red and green) refractile bodies are scattered among these finer dust-like opacities. This is commonly referred as a "Chrismas tree cataract." Later on in the disease, a granular posterior subcapsular cataract develops. The cataract may remain stationary, if it progresses the operative prognosis is good.

Mongolian Idiocy and Hypothyroidism

Cretinism and mongolian idiocy are associated with punctate subcapsular cataracts.

Other Metabolic Conditions

A number of other metabolic conditions including congenital abnormalities are associated with development of cataract. These are aminoaciduria, homocystinuria, Hurler's disease, Fanconi's syndrome, Miller's syndrome, chronic renal failure, hypophosphatasia, phenylketonuria, Werner's syndrome, congenital ichthyosis, Refsum's disease, neurofibromatosis type II, Niemann-Pick disease (type A), mucolipidosis and Thomson syndrome.

TRAUMATIC CATARACT

Both penetrating and non-penetrating physical injuries can cause cataract. Trauma is the most common cause of unilateral cataract in young individuals.

- Penetrating injuries (mechanical trauma) may lead to direct injury to the lens and subsequent development of lens opacities (Fig. 4.21).
- Concussion cataract Concussion injuries may lead to development of concussion cataract which may take many varied forms. It is due partly to the mechanical effects of the injury on the lens fibers and largely to the entrance of aqueous due to damage to the capsule as a result of actual tear. Concussion of lens without rupture of the capsule may result in cataract that is initially subcapsular and commonly has a star-shaped appearance. The lens fibers are usually affected in both the anterior and posterior subcapsular clear zones and initially the loss may show, only as a loss of this zone which accounts for delayed traumatic cataract which becomes evident months or years after the injury. Most typical appearance of concussion cataract is rosette-shaped cataract. This develops usually in the posterior cortex in a star-shaped manner. The posterior capsule is thin so it is easily damaged and the opacity develops. It may remain stationary or may progress until the entire lens becomes opaque.

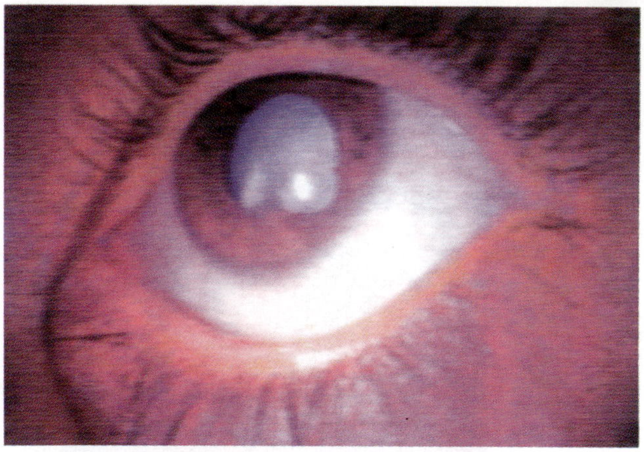

Fig. 4.21: Traumatic cataract

Sometimes concussion may result in subcapsular punctate opacities that are indistinguishable from glaucomatous flecks.

Concussion injury may also cause the imprinting of circle of iris pigment, known as Vossious ring on to the anterior lens capsule just behind pupillary margin.

Perforation of capsule usually results in a rapidly maturing cataract (total cataract).

TOXIC CATARACT

Toxic cataract has been reported in human being following the local and systemic use of certain drugs, exposure to irradiation and electric current shock. Various cataracts under this group are as follows.

Corticosteroids (Steroid-induced Cataract)

Prolonged use of systemic, topical and inhaled corticosteroids is associated with the development of axial posterior subcapsular cataract (Fig. 4.22). These cataracts frequently assume a diskoid morphology and due to their axial position near the nodal point of the eye produces significant visual loss. The higher the dose of corticosteroid and longer the course of treatment, there are more chances to develop cataract. The exact relationship

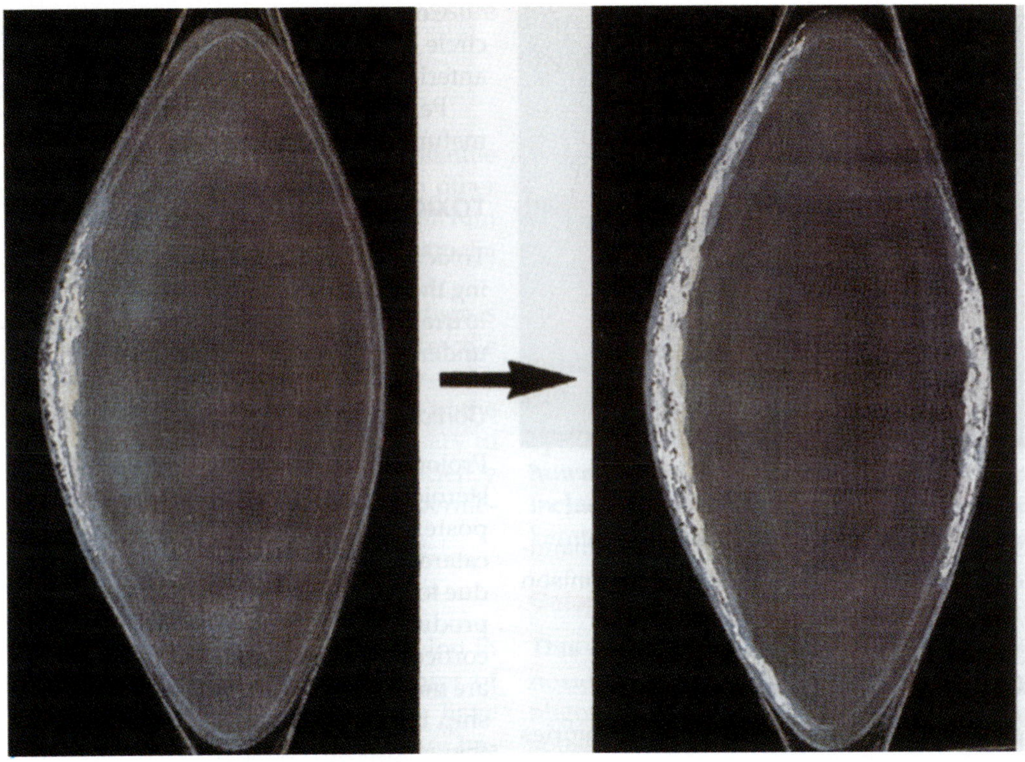

Fig. 4.22: Progression of steroid-induced cataract
(*Courtesy*: Kanski *Clinical Ophthalmology*, Butterworth International Edition)

between the dose and duration of corticosteroid therapy with the development of cataract is still not clear. Patients in whom lens changes develop should have their steroid therapy reduced to minimum consistent with the control of the disease and if possible alternate day therapy should be given because patients develop less lens changes who receive intermittent therapy. Regression of early opacities may occur when the drug is stopped or reduced although progression may occur despite withdrawal. So, all patients with disease requiring prolonged corticosteroid therapy should be periodically evaluated by an ophthalmologist.

Miotics-induced Cataract

Long-term use of miotics specially long acting cholinesterase inhibitors such as echothiophate, demecarium bromide, di-isopropyl fluorophosphate (DFP) may cause formation of tiny anterior subcapsular vacuoles and sometimes more advanced opacities. Stoppage of drug reduces the risk of progression and may even be associated with reversal of cataract.

Chlorpromazine-induced Cataract

Prolonged administration of chlorpromazine may lead to the deposition of fine yellowish brown granules under the anterior lens capsule. These deposits are initially situated within the pupillary area but are rarely dense enough to interfere with vision. If the drug is used in high dosage it may cause retinal damage.

Busulphan

Patients who are put on Busulphan for the treatment of chronic myeloid leukemia may develop lens opacities.

Amiodarone

Patients put on amiodarone for the treatment of cardiac arrhythmias may produce anterior subcapsular lens opacities which do not interfere with the vision.

Gold Treatment

Patients who are receiving gold treatment for rheumatoid arthritis for a prolonged time (3 years or more) may develop anterior capsular lens opacities.

Other Drugs

Toxic cataracts develop in patients who are put on nitro compounds such as dinitrophenol, trinitrotoluene, napthalene, thallium, carbromal, triparanol and tetracaine for a long time.

Radiational Cataract

Exposure to almost all types of radiant energy is known to produce cataract by causing damage to lens epithelium. Various types of radiational cataract are as follows.

Infrared radiation cataract (Glass blower's and Glass worker's cataract) Prolonged exposure (over several years) to infrared radiation may lead to exfoliation of the anterior lens capsule. In true exfoliation large pieces of lens capsule flake off and may curl back on themselves in the pupillary area of the lens. Prolonged exposure may also lead to the formation of diskoid posterior subcapsular opacity with many high refractile spots.

X-ray radiation cataract Ionizing radiation (X-rays, gamma rays or neutrons) may lead to characteristic posterior subcapsular opacity. The degree of cataract formation is related to radiation dose. A little single dose of 300 to 400 rad may lead to cataract formation. There is usually a latent period of 6 months to few years between exposure and cataract development. Neutron and alpha beam produce greater ionization and pose the greatest risk of cataract formation. As gamma and X-rays are most frequently used forms of radiation in medicine, so these forms are more linked to cataract formation. Proper shielding of technician working on X-ray plant, patients being treated for malignant tumors and workers of atomic energy plants is required.

Microwave-induced cataract Exposure to microwave radiation at radar installations in to army personnel for a long time may lead to cataract formation. Therefore microwave radiation is a potential cataractogenic factor.

Ultraviolet (UV) radiation cataract Exposure to UV radiation has been shown to develop senile cataract in many studies. Ultraviolet radiation B (UV-B) (320-290 nm) is more dangerous in relation to lens in formation of cortical and nuclear cataracts. Ocular exposure to UV-B may be reduced sharply by wearing goggles or UV screener fitted into the spectacle lenses.

Laser radiation It has been shown recently to induce localized capsular opacity in human being.

Electrical Cataract

Electrocution injury (passage of powerful electric current through the body) may lead to cataract formation. The cataract may involve both anterior and posterior subcapsular and cortical areas and are usually more extensive on the side with the greater electrical burn. The morphology of these cataracts may include punctate dust-like vacuoles as well as linear and cortical spokes.

Copper (Chalcosis) and Iron (Siderosis) Cataracts

Intraocular foreign bodies containing copper and iron may lead to cataract formation.

- Copper is extremely toxic to the eye and may produce sunflower cataract with small yellowish brown dots in the subcapsular cortex with in the pupillary zone. There is significant visual loss.
- Intraocular iron induction may produce a brownish subcapsular opacity. Intralentricular iron may produce a mature cataract.

Syndermatotic Cataract (Dermatogenic Cataract)

Lens opacities associated with cutaneous diseases are termed syndermatotic cataract. They are bilateral and develop at younger age. Atopic dermatitis is the most common skin disease associated with cataract. A posterior subcapsular cataract usually develop in the third decade of life.

- Rothmund syndrome is a recessive inherited disorder and occurs mainly in females. Such patients develop zonular cataract at 3 to 4 year of age.
- Werner's syndrome is associated with the formation of posterior subcapsular cataract. Other skin diseases associated with cataract formation are ectodermal dysplasia, vascular atrophicus scleroderma, keratitis follicularis, congenital ichthyosis and psoriasis.

Infectious Diseases Associated with Cataract

Congenital rubella is already discussed in this chapter. Other congenital diseases like toxoplasmosis, syphilis, cytomegalovirus disease, variola and herpes simplex are associated with cataract formation.

Co-cataractogenic Factors

Cataractogenesis has been shown to develop as the result of multiple subthreshold cataractogenic stresses. The superimposition of toxic stresses on an aging lens may accelerate the rate of cataract formation. Elimination of one or more subcataractogenic stresses may delay or prevent cataract formation.

CATARACTS ASSOCIATED WITH SYSTEMIC DISEASES

Certain systemic diseases are related to cataract formation. These diseases are as follows.

Down's Syndrome

Cataract develops in about 75 percent of trisomy-21 (Down's syndrome) cases. In small percentage of cases congenital cataract is present in the fetal nucleus. More commonly scattered punctate and flake-like opacities develop in cortex early in life. Brushfield's spots which are iris thickening (gray in color) in the midperiphery are seen in about 85 percent of the patients.

Dystrophia Myotonica

Adult form of this disease usually starts in third decade of life. Besides systemic features a characteristic punctate form of cataract is the most common ocular feature of this condition. The multicolored particles are present in the subcapsular region specially posteriorly in star-shaped pattern. The cataract is present in about 90 percent of the cases. The inheritance is dominant. Cataract and other systemic manifestations occur at an earlier age in successive generations.

Skeletal Abnormalities

Cataract may also be associated with skeletal abnormalities like Conradi's syndrome, van der Hoeve's syndrome and Hallermann syndrome.

Neuroectodermal Syndromes

Cataract may also develop in neuroectodermal syndromes like oligophrenia and Sjögren-Larsson syndrome. Other chromosomal disorders associated with cataract formation are Patau's syndrome, Edward's syndrome and Turner's syndrome.

Other Systemic Disorders

Other systemic disorders associated with middle age cataract formation (posterior subcapsular type) include Alström syndrome, Cockayne's syndrome, Leber congenital amaurosis, Usher's syndrome, Refsum's syndrome, Alport syndrome, Miller syndrome, etc.

COMPLICATED (SECONDARY) CATARACT

Complicated (secondary) cataract refers to the lens opacification secondary to some other primary ocular disease. As we know that lens depends for its nutrition on intraocular fluids. Therefore any condition in which ocular circulation is disturbed or in which inflammatory toxins are formed shall disturb nutrition of crystalline lens resulting in development of complicated cataract. Some important ocular conditions giving rise to complicated cataract are given.

Cataract Secondary to Ocular Inflammation

Chronic iridocyclitis (Fig. 4.23) keratitis, posterior uveitis, pars planitis, corneal ulcer, Fuch's heterochromic cyclitis and endophthalmitis may all lead

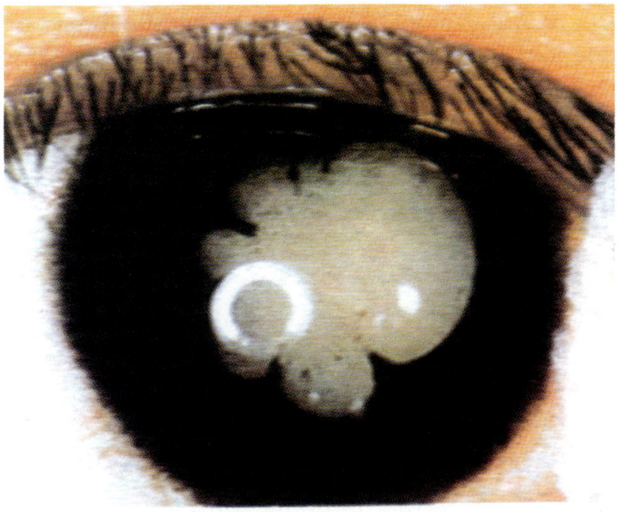

Fig. 4.23: Secondary cataract due to chronic iridocyclitis

to cataract formation. Anterior uveitis is the most common cause of secondary cataract. The earliest finding is a polychromatic luster at the posterior pole of the lens. The exact mechanism of lens opacification is poorly understood but treatment of such cataract is primarily to control the ocular inflammation while minimizing the dose of steroid used to treat the inflammation. If the inflammation cannot be controlled then anterior and posterior subcapsular opacities develop and the lens may become completely opaque. The lens opacification progresses more rapidly in the presence of posterior synechiae.

Hereditary Retinal

Degenerative conditions such as long standing retinal detachment, retinitis pigmentosa, Leber's congenital amaurosis, gyrate atrophy, vitreoretinal disorder and Myopic chorioretinal degeneration may be associated with posterior subcapsular lens opacities. The removal of cataract may rarely be indicated as vision improves even in the presence of severe retinal changes.

Primary or Secondary Glaucoma

Primary or secondary glaucoma may result in complicated cataract. The underlying cause here is probably the embarrassment to the intraocular circulation consequent to the raised IOP.

High Myopia

High myopia is frequently associated with secondary posterior lens opacities as well as early development of nuclear sclerosis.

Intraocular Tumors

Tumors such as ocular melanoma and retinoblastoma may lead to cataract formation. Metastatic tumors involving the choroid or anterior segment may also cause cataract.

Other Ocular Conditions

In other ocular conditions like ocular ischemia, Raynaud's disease, Berger's disease and after ocular surgery, specially glaucoma filtering surgery may lead to cataract formation.

Glaukomflecken

These are small, gray white anterior subcapsular or capsular opacities in the pupillary zone and are typically diagnostic of a previous attack of congestive angle-closure glaucoma.

Typically complicated cataracts occur in two forms.

Posterior cortical complicated cataract This type of secondary cataract usually occurs due to affections of the posterior segment. Such cataract is located in a posterior subcapsular site where they consist of granules and vacuoles that often appear to extend into the cortex anterior to the main opacity. The opacity is irregular in outline and variable in density. On slit lamp examination these opacities have "bread-crumb" appearance. A characteristic sign is presence of polychromatic luster of red, green and blues. A diffuse yellow haze is seen in the adjoining cortex. Slowly the opacity spreads to whole of cortex and ultimately the whole of lens becomes opaque giving chalky white appearance. Deposition of calcium also takes place in the later stage.

Anterior cortical complicated cataract This type of cataract occurs primarily in anterior segment lesions such as glaucoma, acute iritis, etc. Earliest changes are appearance of vacuoles below the anterior capsule followed by opacities in the nearby cortical fibers and thickening of the anterior capsule.

AFTERCATARACT

Aftercataract is a membrane formed by the remnants of the anterior and the posterior capsule following, extracapsular cataract extraction (ECCE) or discission operation.

Membrane may be thick due to various reasons. These are:

- Abortive attempts by the cubical cells underneath the anterior capsule to form lens fibers.
- Deposition of fibrin on the membrane following postoperative hemorrhage in the anterior chamber.
- Formation of inflammatory exudates on the membrane following postoperative iridocyclitis.

The cubical cells underneath the lens capsule instead of developing normal lens fibers may form large balloon like cells known as "Elschnig's pearls." Sometimes the lens fibers grow between the anterior and posterior lens capsules in the periphery behind the iris to form a ring known as ring of sommering.

CLINICAL FEATURES OF CATARACT

Symptoms of Cataract Formation

Any opacity of lens may be present without producing any symptoms and may be discovered on routine ocular examination. Common cataract symptoms are:

Glare One of the earliest visual disturbances with the cataract is glare or bright light intolerance. Glare is symptomatic manifestation of light scattering. When a patient looks on the direct sunlight or head lights of coming vehicles or looks at a point source of light, the diffusion of bright white and colored light around it drastically reduce visual acuity. The amount of glare or dazzle will vary with the location and size of opacity, usually posterior subcapsular opacities are responsible for much of glare.

Uniocular polyopia Doubling or trebling of object is also one of the early symptoms. It occurs mainly due to irregular refraction by lens owing to variable refractive index as a result of cataractogenesis.

Image blur Image blur occurs when the lens is not able to differentiate (resolve) and separate distinct objects. When this happens the near visual functions like reading, sewing, etc. becomes very difficult. Patients are unable to tolerate image blur as it interferes with their day to day activities.

Distortion In cataract patients the straight edges appear wavy or curved. This may even lead to image duplication. Such a patient should be examined to determine if the diplopia is monocular or binocular. Monocular diplopia is usually associated with corneal, lenticular or macular diseases.

Colored Halos and altered color perception Sometimes cataract patients complain of colored halos due to breaking of white light into colored spectrum due to the presence of water droplets in the lens.

The yellowing of the lens nucleus gradually increases with age. Patients with significant nuclear sclerosis may see object browner or yellower than they actually are.

Blackspots Some cataract patients complain of perceiving black spots in front of the eye in their visual field. These spots are stationary.

Loss of vision Visual deterioration in senile cataracts is usually painless and gradually progressive process. Patients with central type of opacities (i.e. cupuliform cataract) may complain of early loss of vision. Such patients see better in the evening (when pupil is dilated due to dim light) as compared to in the morning and afternoon (day blindness), while in patients with peripheral opacities (cuneiform cataract) visual loss is delayed and vision is improved in bright light when pupil is contracted. Patients suffering from nuclear sclerosis complain of distant vision deterioration due to the progressive index myopia. Such patients may be able to read without presbyopic glasses. This near vision improvement is also known as "second sight." As opacification progresses the vision goes on diminishing until only perception and projection of light remains in the stage of mature cataract.

Behavioral changes

- Children suffering from congenital, traumatic or metabolic cataracts may not be able to express their visual disturbances. In such patients behavioral changes are indicative of a loss of visual acuity or binocular vision may alert the intelligent parents and teachers to the presence of a visual problem. Inability to see the blackboard or read with one eye and sitting very close to television may be such symptoms. Loss of accurate depth perception like inability to catch or hit a ball, pour water from the pitcher into the glass, sitting on chair or bed are seen in such children.

- Young adults suffering from cataract may frequently face the difficulty with night driving.

Signs of Cataract Formation

Visual acuity testing Thorough visual acuity testing (both binocular and monocular) should be performed in every cataract patient. The level of visual acuity is directly related to cataract maturation.

Leukokoria Typical white pupil is seen in mature senile cataracts while is certain immature cataracts whitish gray or yellow patches are seen in the pupillary area. These patches are as a result of light scattering from opacities situated in anterior subcapsular or cortical zones.

Iris shadow test When an oblique beam of light is thrown on the pupil a crescentric shadow of pupillary margin of the iris will be formed on the grayish lens opacity as long as clear cortex is present between the opacity and the pupillary margin. When the lens is completely transparent or opaque, no iris shadow is formed. Presence of iris shadow is sign of immature cataract.

Oblique illumination examination It shows color of the lens in the pupillary area which varies in different type of cataracts.

Subtle signs Examination of red reflex with distant direct ophthalmoscopy frequently reveals a black lens opacity against the reddish-yellow hue to fundal reflex. This is a sensitive method of detecting cataractous changes in the lens. In the complete cataractous lens no red fundal glow is seen.

On distant direct ophthalmoscopy if on upgaze the opacity appears to move down, then opacity is in the posterior half of the lens and if opacity moves up with upgaze, then it is in the anterior half of the lens.

Slit lamp examination It should be performed with a fully dilated pupil. This examination reveals complete morphology of lens opacity (site, size, shape, color and pattern).

DIAGNOSTIC TESTS FOR CATARACT

Snellen visual acuity for distant and near vision with appropriate glasses should be tested.

Non-Snellen visual acuity Certain patients come with complaints of poor visual function despite good Snellen visual acuity. Cataracts may lead to decreased contrast perception leading to visual dysfunction. Cataracts specially posterior subcapsular and cortical may cause debilitating glare. Several readily available commercial instruments can be used to show the effect of glare on visual acuity in cataract patients (Mentor BAT).

Lens and pupil examination When a bright flashlight is used the direct and consensual pupillary responses are not affected by lens opacities. But in dim light test the response may be less marked when illuminating the eye with dens cataract. On flash light examination, anterior lens opacities are visible to the examiner if pupil size is adequate.

Direct ophthalmoscopy On direct ophthalmoscopy nuclear cataracts are visible as lens within a lens when viewed against red fundal glow.

Slit lamp biomicroscopy as already described allows the detailed examination of the anterior segment of the eye.

Refraction and retinoscopy Nuclear cataract patient shows index myopia in the early stages. It can be detected by routine refractive examination. Patients can be corrected for years with a stronger myopic distance glasses and standard reading glasses for near vision.

Retinoscopy shall reveal the abnormal reflexes associated with lenticular opacities and lenticonus.

Ultrasonography A-scan and B-scan ultrasonographies are standard methods for accurately measuring the thickness and location of the lens opacities. B-scan ultrasonography is specially helpful in evaluating abnormalities of posterior segment of the eye with a very dense cataract. Secondary cataract formation in response to posterior segment tumors or inflammation thereby necessitates the use of ultrasonography to ascertain the anatomical state of the eye behind the lens.

MANAGEMENT OF CATARACT IN ADULTS

Treatment of cataract essentially consists of its surgical removal. However, certain non-surgical (medical) measures may be of help in some specific conditions till surgery is taken up.

Medical Treatment (Non-surgical measures) of Cataract

Measures to Improve Vision in the Presence of Early Cataract

Mydriatics In initial stages of senile cataract specially the small axial cataract patients are advised to put mydriatics for pupillary dilatation. Purpose of this therapy is to allow the clear, paraxial lens to participate in light transmission, image formation and focussing and try to eliminate the glare and blurring, caused by these initial small central cataracts. Mydriatics such as 5 percent phenylephrine (1 drop twice a day) or 1 percent tropicamide (1 drop bid) are given to put in the affected eye to temporarily clarify vision so that patient may be able to carry day to day activities.

Refraction In cataract patients refraction often changes with considerable rapidity. So, refractive corrections should be done at frequent intervals.

Illumination instructions Patients suffering from peripheral opacities (free pupillary area) may be advised to use bright illumination so that they may be able to see. Similarly in patients suffering from central opacities should be advised to use dull light placed besides and slightly behind the patient's head shall give the best result. It is important to remember that these remedial measures are for short duration just to delay the cataract surgery.

Wearing dark goggles Patients with central opacities should be advised to wear dark goggles which are of great value and comfort when worn outdoors.

Measures to Delay Cataract Progression

Following therapeutic measures can be given to cataract patients to delay cataract progression. These are:

- Patients can be given topical solutions of
  1. Pyridophenoxazine (catalin eyedrops) (conc. of 0.75 mg/15 ml of solvent)
  2. Cineraria Maritima (homeopathic topical preparation)
  3. Anticataract topical solution containing potassium iodide (3.3%), sodium chloride (0.83%) and calcium chloride (1.0%).

  These topical solutions are given to put in the early stages of senile cataract with dose of 1 drop 2 to 3 times a day in the affected eye. These solutions are found to be effective in slowing down the process of cataractogenesis.
- Oral vitamin E therapy (dosage of 200 mg twice a day for 6 months to 1 year)
- Oral antioxidant therapy when given in early stages of cataractogenesis definitely arrest the progress of senile cataract. Oral antioxidants given are:
  1. Oral mixcarotin softgel capsules containing alpha-and beta-carotene, cryptoxanthin, lutein and zeaxanthin 1 cap daily for a year.
  2. Antioxidant capsule containing zinc, copper, selenium, manganese, vitamin A, vitamin B_{12}, vitamin C and vitamin E) 1 cap daily for 6 months to 1 year.

  These antioxidants are potent free radical scavenger to prevent oxidative stress and premature onset of senile degeneration of lens tissues caused by free radical damage.
- Certain other topical compounds have been tested and holds promise in the arrest of process of cataractogenesis. These are:
  - Topical aspirin (1%) solution
  - Sulindac (topical) 1 percent solution
  - Glutathione (topical) 1 percent solution
  - Benzyl alcohol (0.07%) solution.

Treatment/Removal of Cataractogenic Factors

Toxic cataracts produced by X-rays and infrared radiation and due to certain drugs like steroids, cholinesterase inhibitors, phenothiazine and others can be delayed or further progress can be arrested by the removal of these agents.

Any drug of known cataractogenic agent should be used as briefly and in low dose as possible.

Senile cataracts occur more frequently and mature more rapidly in diabetic patients. So careful control of blood sugar levels can minimize the progress of cataract. However advanced cataracts are not benefited by diabetic control.

Blocking the conversion of glucose to sorbitol by aldose reductase might delay or prevent the adverse osmotic stress and helps in arresting the progress of diabetic cataract. Similarly early and adequate treatment of ocular diseases like uveitis may prevent complicated cataract. The above mentioned medical measures and therapeutics are only to delay the inevitable cataract surgery.

Surgical Treatment of Cataract

Indications of Surgical Treatment

Cataract extraction is essentially indicated for the following reasons.

Visual improvement This is one of the most common indication. When surgery should be advised for visual improvement varies from person to person depending upon the visual needs, it is important to establish the patient-specific visual needs before undertaking cataract surgery. If uniocular cataract is present and patient does not need stereoscopic vision then surgery may be delayed until the cataract is mature as long as visual acuity in the follow eye is sufficient for patient needs. If bilateral cataract is present then cataract extraction from the eye with the worse visual acuity should be done first when the patient considers the visual handicap as a significant deterrent to the maintenance of his usual lifestyle. Usually second eye in bilateral cataracts should be operated only after the first eye is fully rehabilitated. However, opinion differs as to when surgery should be performed in the second eye.

Medical indications Sometimes patient may be comfortable from the visual point (due to good visual acuity of the other eye or otherwise), but such patients may be advised cataract surgery due to medical ground such as lens-induced glaucoma, phacoanaphylactic endophthalmitis, angle-closure glaucoma by an intumescent lens and retinal diseases like diabetic retinopathy or retinal detachment, treatment of these conditions being hampered by the presence of lens opacities.

Cosmetic indication Sometimes cataract extraction is done on patient's insistence in order to obtain a black pupil even when prognosis for obtaining good postoperative vision is not good.

Preoperative Evaluation/Considerations

Preoperative generalized evaluation of patient is necessary to exclude the presence of serious systemic diseases like hypertension, diabetes mellitus, cardiac problems, obstructive lung disorders and any potential source of infection in the body like urinary tract infection (UTI) or septic gums, etc. The necessary testing depends on the patient's age and prior medical history.

Preoperative ophthalmological evaluation Complete and thorough ocular examination is necessary to rule out conditions such as long standing amblyopia, pseudoexfoliation, retinal tears or holes, macular lesions or optic nerve abnormalities that may affect the visual or surgical outcome. The following useful information is required before the patient is declared fit for cataract surgery.

- Retinal functional tests: The retinal functions should be thoroughly evaluated as if it is faulty even a good quality operation shall be useless from vision angle and patient must be warned of the prognosis to avoid unnecessary disappointment and medicolegal problems. A few important retinal functions are described here.
- Perception of light (PL) must be present for potential useful postoperative vision.
- Marcus-Gunn pupillary response test should be done routinely because in its presence visual prognosis is poor.
- Projection of light (PR) is an important test for functions of peripheral retina and should be done routinely. A poor PR inference shall indicate towards the poor visual prognosis.
- Two-light discrimination test should be done to know about macular function. If the patient

perceive two normal lights in this test it indicates normal macular function.

- *Maddox rod test* An accurate perception of red line indicates normal function.
- Color perception indicates macular function is present and optic nerve is relatively normal.
- Entopic visualization is done to know about retinal function.
- Laser interferometry is a good test for measuring the macular potential for visual acuity in the presence of opaque media.
- Objectives tests for evaluating retina are essential when some retinal pathology is suspected. These tests include B-scan ultrasonography of the posterior segment of the eye, electroretinogram (ERG), electro-oculogram (EOG), visually evoked response (VER), indirect ophthalmoscopy and color Doppler ultrasonography.
- Potential local source of infection should be checked by ruling out any conjunctival infections, meibomitis, blepharitis, lacrimal sac infection and chronic dacryocystitis.

  Thorough lacrimal sac examination including syringing should be done. In case of presence of chronic dacryocystitis DCR (dacryocystorhinostomy) or DCT (dacryocystectomy) should be performed before the cataract surgery.
- Complete anterior segment examination by slit lamp biomicroscopy should be done in each case routinely to rule out any keratic precipitate present at the back of cornea, subtle uveitis and state of corneal endothelium, specially when intraocular lens (IOL) implantation is planned.
- An accurate refraction of both eyes, keratometry and A-scan ultrasonography to calculate the appropriate IOL power should be done.
- Preoperative IOP measurement should be done in each case.

  The presence of raised IOP shall require a prior management before cataract surgery.

Preoperative Medications and Preparations

- Topical antibiotics such as ciprofloxacilin or tobramycin three to four times a day 72 hours before surgery should be started as prophylaxis against infections.
- Systemic antibiotics such as gentamicin 80 mg intramuscular (IM) injections are advised by some ophthalmic surgeon at previous night and in the morning before surgery. However opinion differs on the use of IM antibiotic injections.
- Preparation of the eye to be operated includes trimming of eyelashes of upper eyelid at previous night and eye to be operated should be properly marked.
- Each patient should be advised to take scrub bath including face and hair wash with soap and water before surgery. Male patients should get their beard cleaned and hair trimmed.
- Preoperative lowering of IOP is done by giving oral acetazolamide tablets 500 mg stat 2 hours before the surgery.
- To sustain dilated pupil (specially in extracapsular cataract extraction with IOL implantation) the NSAID drops like topical flurbiprofen should be instilled three times a day one day before surgery and half hourly for 2 hours immediately before surgery.
- Adequate dilatation of pupil is achieved by 1 percent tropicamide and 5 to 10 percent phenylephrine every 10 minutes one hour before surgery.
- Sometimes highly anxious and nervous patients are also given oral diazepam in small dose (2.5-5.0 mg) one hour before surgery to alleviate the anxiety.
- Mental preparation of the patient for the surgery should include a full explanation of the potential risks and benefits of the proposed surgery and anesthesia. A written consent should be taken from the patient or from his near relative regarding full explanations of pros and cons of surgery to the patient by the operating doctor.
- Both outpatient and inpatient (indoor) surgical facilities are used for cataract surgery with the latter reserved for medical complications. Well-equipped and certified outpatient surgical facilities offer the patient minimum possible surgical trauma and minimum disruption of patient's normal living routine.
- Preoperative prepping/antibiosis is used to prevent postoperative endophthalmitis. Most surgeons prepare the lids and facial skin with

10 percent providone-iodine and placing drop of 5 percent povidone-iodine into the conjunctival cul-de-sac.

Anesthesia for Cataract Surgery

Cataract extraction may be performed under general anesthesia, local anesthesia or topical anesthesia, depending upon condition of patient's cataract status, and surgeon choice.

General Anesthesia

Usually for cataract surgery general anesthesia is not given. It is advisable only in highly anxious/ nervous patient or when cataract surgery requires a long time for completion. Patients who are extremely apprehensive, deaf, mentally retarded, unstable or cannot communicate well with the surgeon are more suitable for general anesthesia. For general anesthesia, complete anesthetic facilities with expert anesthetist are mandatory.

Local Anesthesia

Local ocular anesthesia is the mainstay of cataract surgery. Local anesthesia minimizes the risk of wound rupture, a complication frequently associated with coughing during extubation and postoperative nausea and vomiting (in general anesthesia). Generally the use of 1:1 mixture of 2 percent Xylocaine and 0.50 percent bupivacaine alongwith adrenaline and hyaluronidase in facial, retrobulbar and peribulbar blocks achieve rapid anesthesia, akinesia and postoperative analgesia for several hours.

Care should be taken to avoid intravascular injections of anesthetic agents because refractory cardiopulmonary arrest may result from an inadvertent intravenous or intra-arterial injections.

Many patients express pain of facial and retrobulbar injections so proper preoperative sedation and good rapport with the surgeon make them quite comfortable.

Following techniques are used for giving local anesthesia.

Orbicularis oculi akinesia Temporary paralysis of the orbicularis oculi muscle is essential before making section for the cataract surgery to prevent potential damage from squeezing of the lids. Two methods are used, for getting orbicularis oculi akinesia.

O'Brien's technique: Usually 10 ml of mixture of 2 percent lidocaine solution (5 ml) and 0.5 percent bupivacaine solution (5 ml) with 1:100,000 epinephrine and 150 units of hyaluronidase are infiltrated for local anesthesia.

O'Brien's method is the injection of above mentioned local anesthetic solution down to the periosteum covering the neck of the mandible where the temporofacial division of facial nerve passes forwards and upwards (Figs 4.24 and 4.25). A 10 ml syringe with preferably No. 17 or 18 needle and 2.5 cm in length is used. The patient is asked to open his mouth and the position of the condyle and temporomandibular joint is located by the forefinger of the operators's left hand. After closing the jaw, the injection is given on a horizontal line through the junction of the upper and middle third of the distance between the zygoma and angle of the mandible. The needle should pass straight down the periosteum. Two to three ml of local anesthetic solution is injected and after withdrawing the needle firm pressure and massage are applied. Paralysis of orbicularis oculi should occur normally within 7 minutes. The injection is unlikely to injure the external carotid artery which lies posterior and

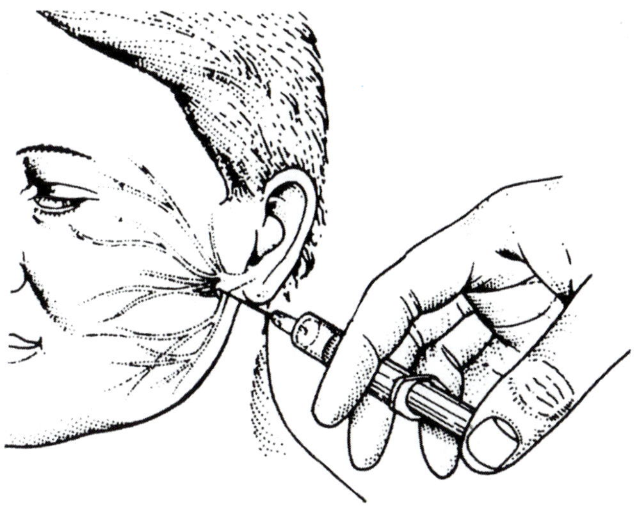

Fig. 4.24: Diagrammatic presentation of O'Brien technique of local anesthesia

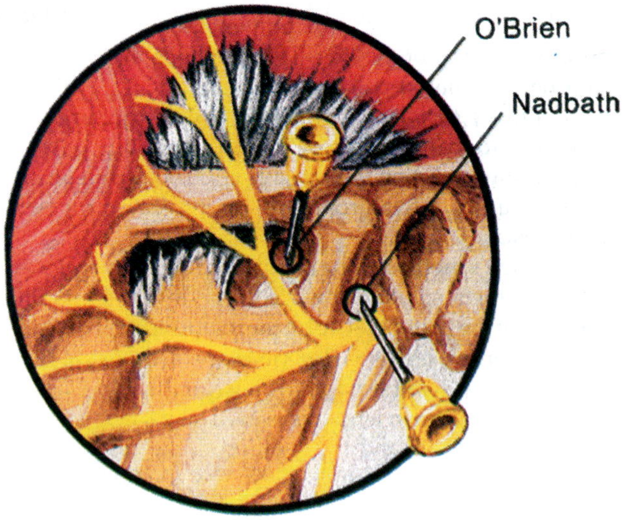

Fig. 4.25: Needle position for O'Brien and Nadbath ocular akinesia (*Courtesy* : Ciba Geigy *Clinical Symposia*)

at a deeper level. However damage may be done to posterior facial vein and the transverse facial artery.

Movement of jaws is sometime painful for few days after this injection.

Van Lint's akinesia: Van Lint's method is a better alternative. The injection of local anesthetic solution is made across the course of branches of the seventh nerve as they pass over the zygomatic bone (Figs 4.26 and 4.27).

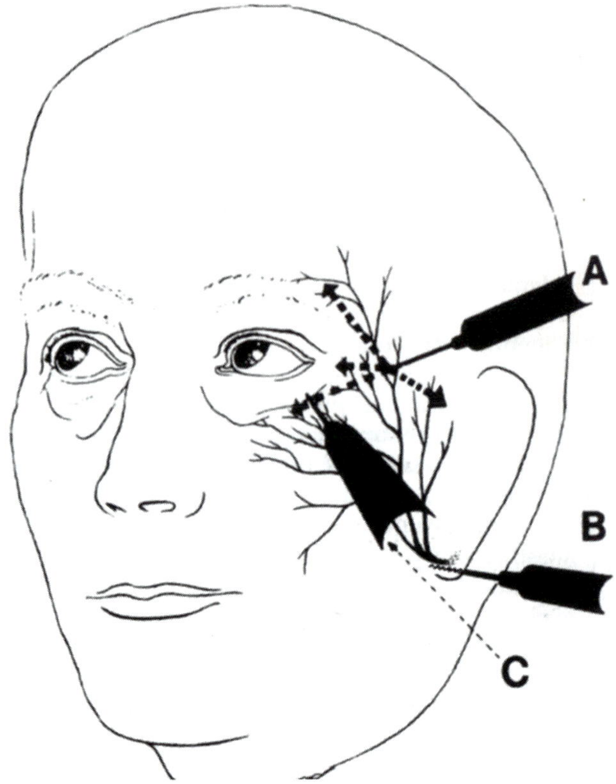

Fig. 4.26: Local anesthesia techniques: (A) Van Lint akinesia (dotted arrows), (B) Nadbath facial nerve block, and (C) Retrobulbar injection position

In this technique a 5 cm in length and 25 gauge needle is passed through the weal down to the periosteum of the zygomatic bone. The needle is than passed upward towards the temporal fossa without touching the periosteum (as it may be painful) and 4 ml of solution is injected and then forwards medially and downwards towards the infraorbital foramen to inject 2 ml and downwards and backwards along the lower margin of the zygoma for 2.5 cm where 3 ml of solution is injected. It is essential to massage the infiltrated area with a gauze swab for motor nerves are less susceptible than sensory nerves to a block with local anesthetic agents.

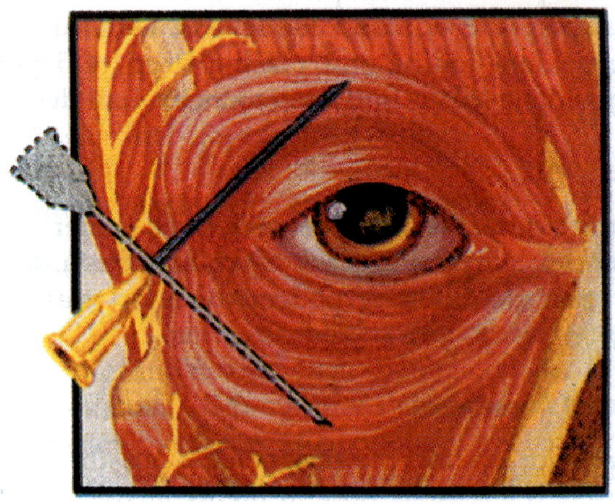

Fig. 4.27: Needle position for Van Lint anesthesia (*Courtesy* : Ciba Geigy *Clinical Symposia*)

The advantage of Van Lint's method is that it provides regional anesthesia as well as paralysis of the orbicularis muscle. After waiting for 5 to 7 minutes akinesia is tested by holding the eyelids open with a small swab on to a holder and asking the patient to close his or her eyelids. If slightest action is observed then injection may be repeated to obtain adequate akinesia.

Retro-ocular (retrobulbar) injection Anesthesia and akinesia of the eye are achieved by injecting a local anesthetic solution into the retrobulbar space within the muscle cone (Fig. 4.28).

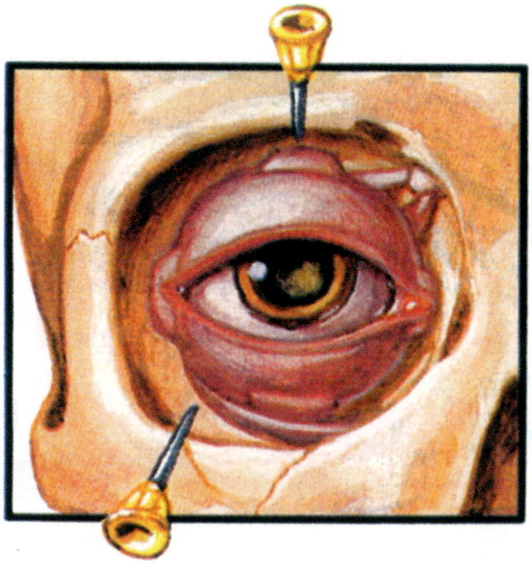

Fig. 4.28: Needle positions for retrobulbar and peribulbar anesthesia

In this method patient is asked to look upwards and to the opposite side. A 3.5 cm length 23 gauge sharp-edged round-tipped needle is inserted in the quadrant between the inferior and the lateral rectus muscles and directed posteriorly until the resistance of orbital septum is encountered. After it has penetrated the orbit the needle is directed towards the apex of the orbit and advanced until it meets the resistance of intermuscular septum. When this structure is penetrated, the needle tip is in the retrobulbar space. About 3 to 4 ml of local anesthetic mixture solution is injected taking care to minimize the needle movement to prevent possible vessels lacerations. Following the injection the globe should be intermittently compressed for several minutes for distributing the anesthetic solution and to ensure hemostasis. A properly placed retrobulbar injection is effective within seconds. It blocks all extraocular muscles except superior oblique muscle, affects the ciliary ganglion and anesthetize the entire globe.

The major complication of retrobulbar injection is orbital hemorrhage. It can be detected by proptosis, subconjunctival hemorrhage, eyelid ecchymosis and elevated IOP. In such situation cataract surgery should be postponed for at least one week. Optic atrophy and blindness have also been reported following retrobulbar blocks but they are fortunately rare. Due to these potential complications retro-ocular injection is out of favor with many eye surgeon worldwide.

Peribulbar (Periocular) technique Since the exit of retrobulbar akinesia, peribulbar akinesia is considered a safe and effective technique of local anesthesia for cataract surgery. It is method of choice with eye surgeons for giving local anesthesia to cataract patients (Fig. 4.29).

Periocular anesthesia is administered at two sites—lower temporal quadrant and nasal to caruncle. This first injection is given in the lower lid at the junction of medial two-third and temporal one-third just above the inferior orbital rim using one inch long 23 gauge disposable needle. The needle is advanced perpendicular to the iris plane to its full depth and after aspirating to rule out intravascular placement, 5 ml of anesthetic mixture is deposited in this location. The second injection is given by introducing needle through the small depression immediately nasal to caruncle and then advanced posteriorly in the transverse plane making an about 5° angulation toward the medial orbital wall. This technique avoids damage to medial rectus muscle and its sheath 5 ml of anesthetic mixture is injected.

A gentle lid massage is given and complete akinesia is achieved within 10 minutes. If complete akinesia is not achieved within 10 minutes after the injection, an additional 3 to 5 ml of anesthetic mixture is injected in the quadrant in which extraocular movement persists.

Adequacy of akinesia is determined by the absence of ocular movements in all directions.

This technique is certainly better than retro-ocular technique and has least complications.

Superior rectus injection The induction of temporary paralysis of the superior rectus muscle is essential for any intraocular operation where the surgical field is upper half of the eye. This injection also affects the action of levator palpebrae superioris.

In this patient is asked to look down. The upper lid is retracted and 2.5 cm long needle is passed

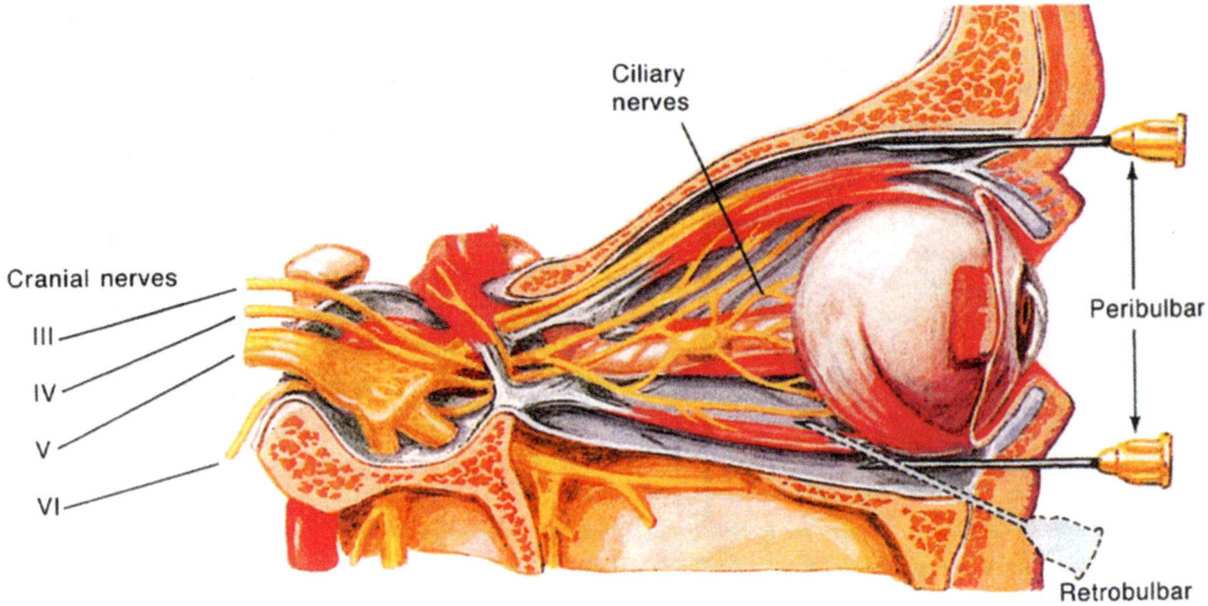

Fig. 4.29: Needle positions for peribulbar and retrobulbar akinesia (*Courtesy*: Ciba Geigy *Clinical Symposia)*

into Tenon's capsule at the temporal edge of the superior rectus muscle. The needle is directed posteromedially and about 1 ml of anesthetic mixture of 2 percent Xylocaine is injected around the muscle belly behind the equator. This injection can also be made through the skin of the upper orbital sulcus.

Tenon's capsule injection The injection of anesthetic mixture can be given into Tenon's capsule around the upper half of the eyeball and into the belly of superior rectus muscle is considered safer than the retroocular injection across the postganglionic fibers of the ciliary body and may be effective in inducing extraocular muscle akinesia.

Topical Anesthesia

In present day high-tech intraocular surgery topical anesthesia is the anesthesia of choice with the eye surgeons.

Topical anesthesia is achieved by instilling 3 applications of 4 percent Xylocaine or 0.4 percent benoxinate HCl or 0.5 to 0.75 percent proparacaine solution 10 minutes apart starting 30 minutes before surgery. A drop is thereafter instilled prior to the incision. 1 cc of 4 percent Xylocaine/0.4 percent benoxinate/0.5-7.5 percent proparacaine is drawn into sterile disposable syringe and OT staff person is asked to instil a few drops of the same prior to caurterization and if required during conjunctival anesthesia is used (pinpoint and mini pinpoint surface anesthesia).

The advantage of topical anesthesia is that it prevents well known complications of retrobulbar and peribulbar injections. There is no immediate postoperative ptosis as seen in retrobulbar, peribulbar and Van lint and O'Brien's infiltrations which lasts for 6 to 8 hours due to temporary akinesia of lids.

However only a highly experienced surgeon can operate with topical anesthesia.

Topical anesthesia cannot be given in all patients specially in anxious stressed patients, deaf, children and very young patients.

No Anesthesia Cataract Surgery

This is the latest technique of cataract surgery in which no anesthesia is required (whether local or topical). Neither the topical or intracameral anesthetic agents are used. This technique is devised by Dr Amar Agarwal (India).

Surgical Techniques for Cataract Surgery

Surgical techniques and their details are a very vast subject. However various techniques are briefly described here. Evolution of various techniques for cataract surgery is shown in Table 4.1.

Table 4.1: Evolution of Techniques for Cataract Surgery

Technique	*Year*	*Author/Surgeon*
Couching	800	Susutra
ECCE' (inferior incision)	1745	Daviel
ECCEE (superior incision)	1860	von Graefe
ICCE** (tumbling)	1880	Smith
ECCE with PC-IOL***	1949	Ridley
ECCE with AC-IOL****	1951	Strampelli
Phacoemulsification	1967	Kelman
Foldable IOLs	1984	Mazzocco
Capsular Surgery	1992	Apple/Assia
Accommodating IOLs	1997	Cummings/Kamman
Phaconit	1998	Agarwal
Dye-enhanced cataract surgery	2000	Pandey/Werner/Apple

* ECCE: extracapsular cataract extraction
** ICCE: intracapsular cataract extraction
***PC-IOL: posterior chamber intraocular lens
****AC-IOL: anterior chamber intraocular lens

Intracapsular Cataract Extraction

Intracapsular cataract extraction (ICCE) is age old traditional method of cataract removal in senile cataract cases.

In ICCE the entire lens is removed with cryoprobe or capsule forceps or by Indian Smith tumbling technique (Figs 4.30 to 4.32).

This procedure has been almost replaced by extracapsular cataract extraction (ECCE).

The main advantages of ICCE over ECCE are

- The technique of ICCE is simple, cheap and does not need sophisticated microinstruments.
- No problem of postoperative opacification of posterior capsule as encountered in ECCE is seen here due to total removal of lens.
- ICCE is less time consuming hence more useful for large scale operations in eye camps.

Disadvantages of ICCE as compared to ECCE

- Posterior chamber IOL implantation is impossible as the posterior capsule is absent due to total removal of lens in ICCE technique.
- ICCE cannot be performed specially in young patients below 35 years of age as the risk of vitreous loss is very high in young patients.
- The incidence of vitreous related anterior segment problems like pupil block, vitreous touch syndrome, vitreous wick syndrome is higher in ICCE cases.
- The incidence of postoperative retinal break formation and aphakic retinal detachment is higher in ICCE cases.
- The incidence of postoperative cystoid macular edema (CME) is higher in ICCE patients.

Extracapsular Cataract Extraction

Extracapsular cataract extraction (ECCE) is the technique of choice for modern cataract surgery. In this technique opaque portions of lens are removed without disturbing the integrity of posterior capsule and anterior vitreous face. So ECCE involves excision of a portion of anterior capsule and nucleus expression through incision and aspiration residual equatorial cortex using either automated irrigation-aspiration machines or manual hand-held devices (Figs 4.33 and 4.34). The posterior capsule is left undisturbed which serves as resting site for posterior chamber IOL implants.

Disadvantages of ECCE technique

- ECCE is more difficult to master and is more dependent on instrumentation.
- Postoperative opacification of posterior capsule occurs in significant number of cases (Fig. 4.35).
- ECCE cannot be performed if zonules are not intact.

Posterior capsule opacification can be easily dealt with man outpatient basis using the neodymium-yttrium-aluminum-garnet (Nd:YAG) laser mounted on slit lamp delivery system (Fig. 4.36).

ECCE is usually done with IOL implantation (Fig. 4.37). IOL implantation is usually not done in patients suffering from proliferative diabetic retinopathy, anterior uveitis and high myopia.

Two main types of IOLs are in current use: (i) anterior chamber lenses (Fig. 4.38), (ii) posterior chamber lenses (Figs 4.39 and 4.40). Each IOL consists of two parts: optical (refractive) portion and haptics (support) which give the lens stability.

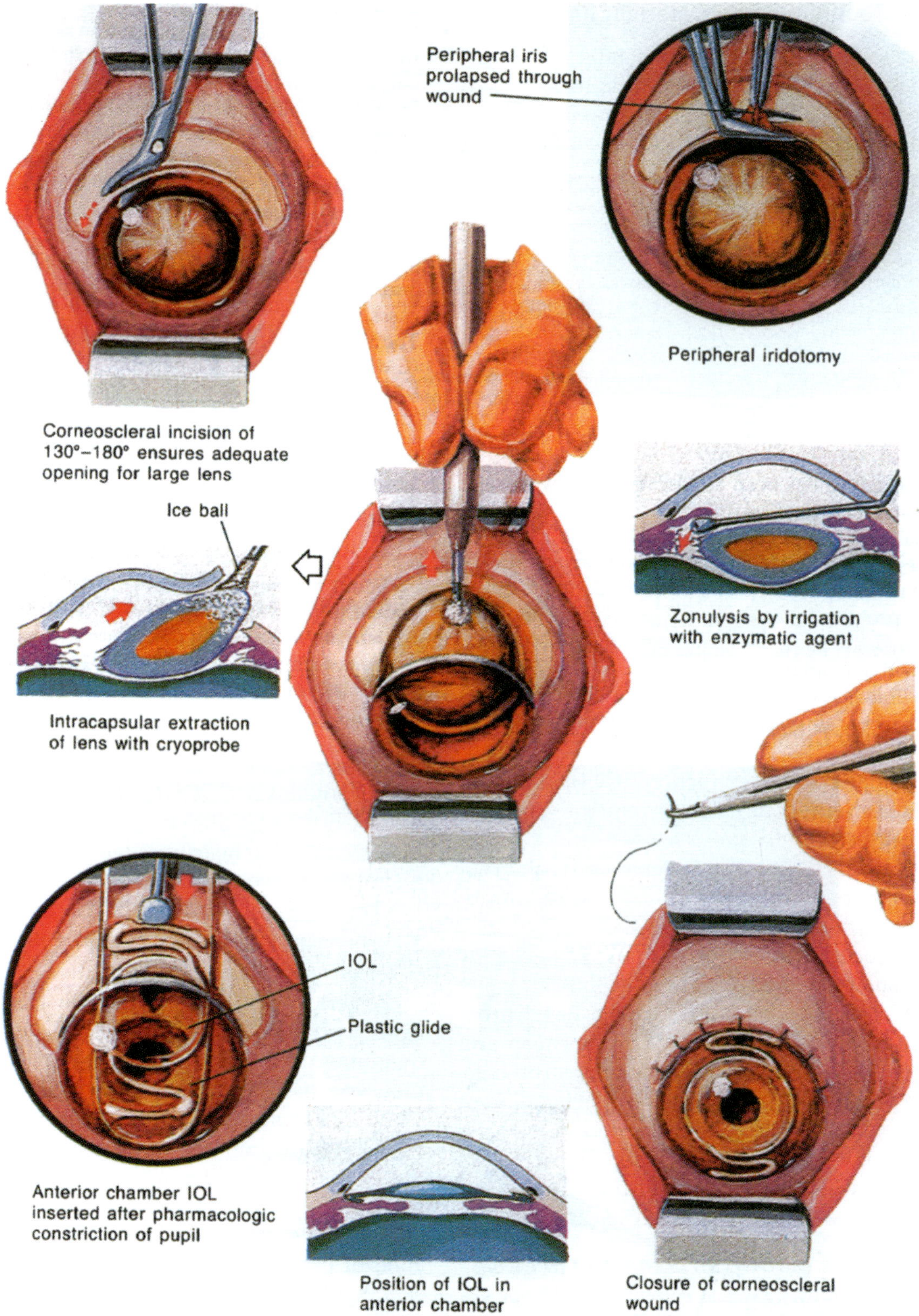

Fig. 4.30: Intracapsular cataract extraction (ICCE) and AC IOL implantation (*Courtesy* : Ciba Geigy *Clinical Symposia*)

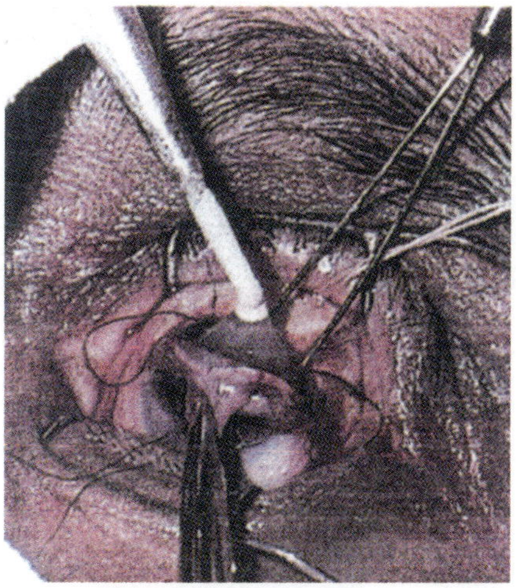

Fig. 4.31: Intracapsular cryoextraction

Usually optics and haptics are made from polymethylmethacrylate (PMMA) (Fig. 4.41). However in some models of IOLs optics are made from PMMA and haptics from polypropylene (prolene). The manufacturing techniques of IOLs are lathe cut, injection molded, compression molded and spin cast.

- Anterior chamber IOLs are implanted in front of the iris and have flexible or semiflexible angle-supported haptics. Anterior chamber IOL implantation is possible with both ICCE and ECCE techniques. They are usually used as standby when the posterior capsule is ruptured accidentally during ECCE making PCIOL implantation impossible.

  Anterior chamber IOLs are also used for secondary implantation in eyes that had previously undergone ICCE.
- Posterior chamber IOLs are fitted behind the iris and have flexible haptics which are inserted either into the capsular bag or into the ciliary sulcus.

Before implanting IOLs the suitable power of IOL is calculated by using special SRK formula which incorporates keratometry readings and length of the globe determined by A-scan ultrasonography (Figs 4.42 and 4.43). K-constant is also used in the formula which is different according to type of IOL to be implanted.

Phacoemulsification

Kelman devised this technique about 25 years ago. It is presently very popular technique of ECCE cataract extraction along with PC IOL implantation. If differs from conventional ECCE in following way:

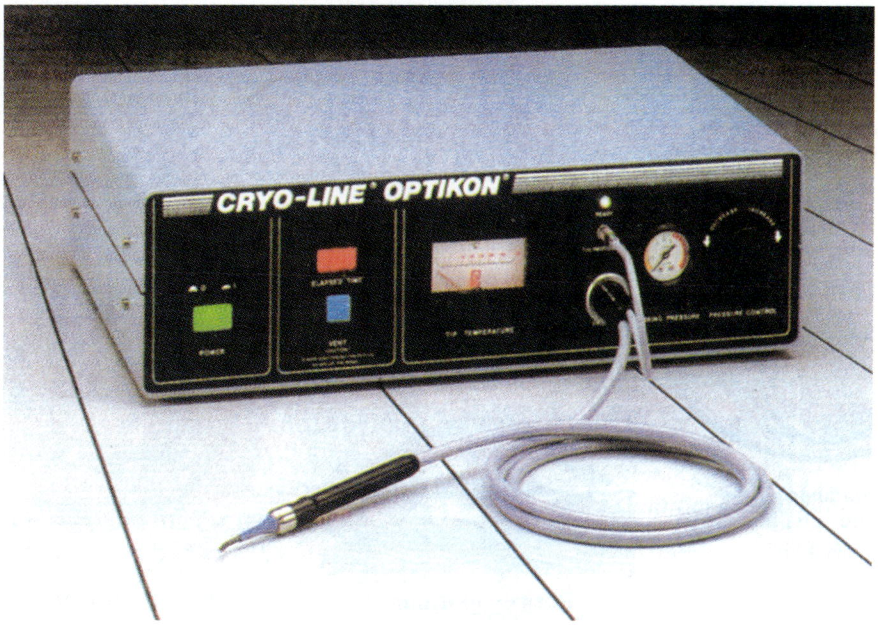

Fig. 4.32: Cryounit for ICCE (*Courtesy :* Towa Optics (India) Pvt Ltd)

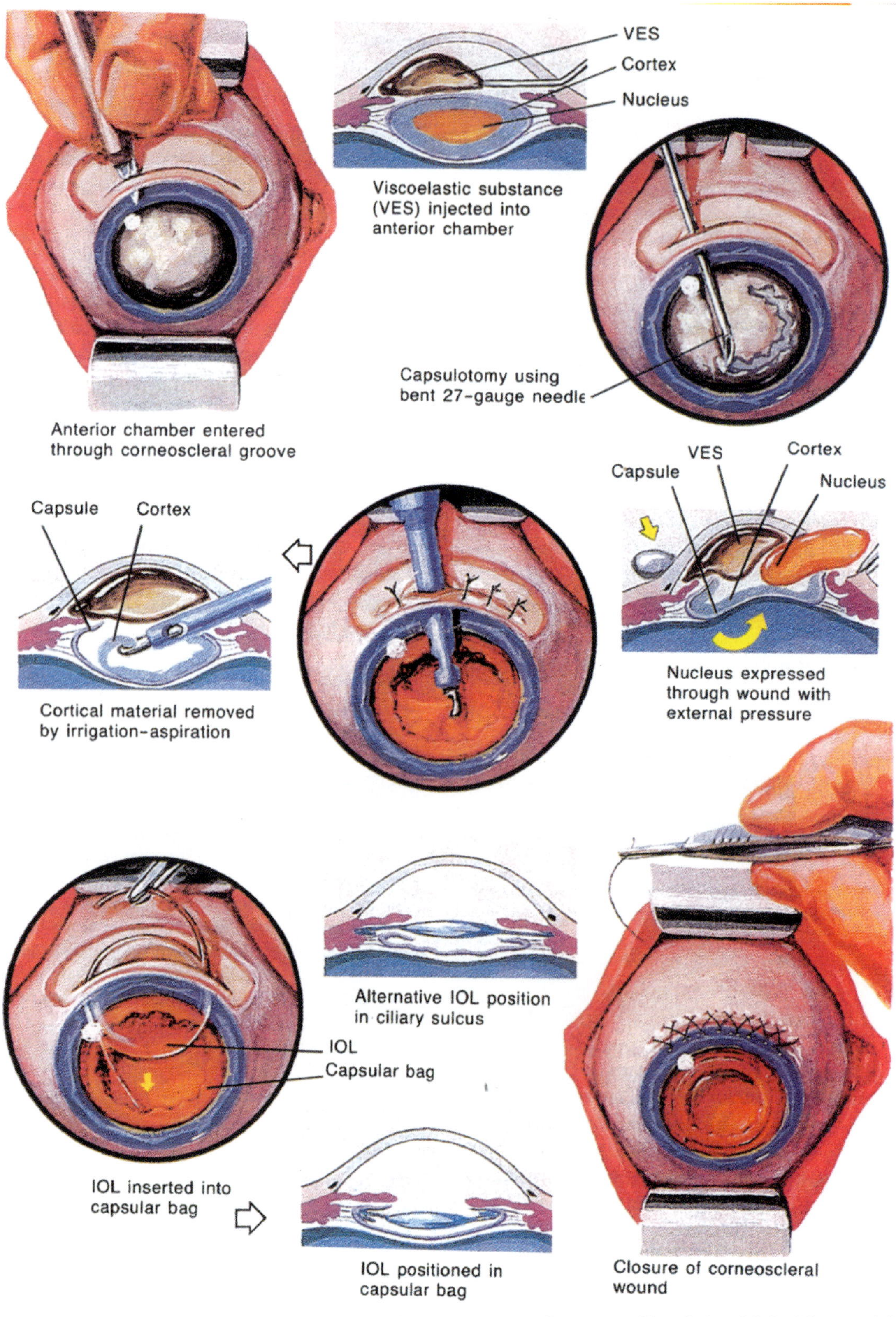

Fig. 4.33: Extracapsular cataract extraction and IOL implantation (*Courtesy* : Ciba Geigy *Clinical Symposia*)

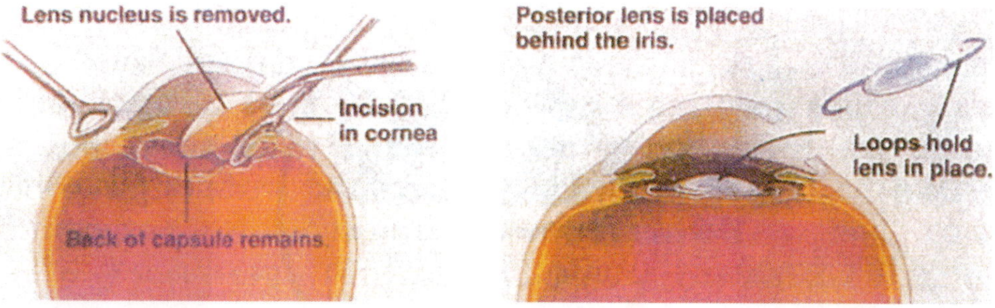

Fig. 4.34: Steps in ECCE with PC IOL implantation

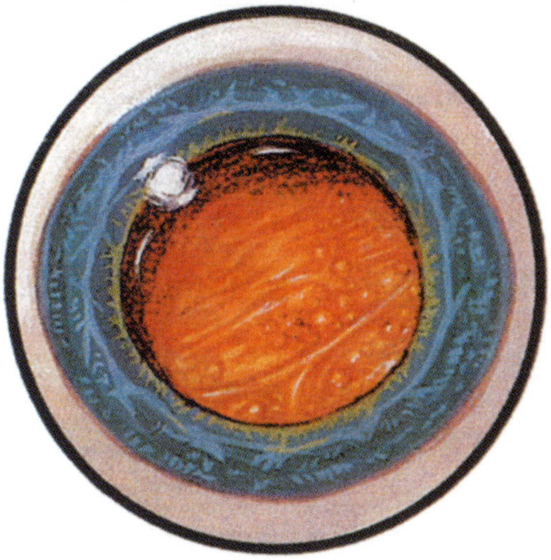
Overgrowth of Proliferative epithelium causes capsule opacification after cataract removal

Fig. 4.35: Posterior capsule opacification after ECCE extraction (*Courtesy* : Ciba Geigy *Clinical Symposia)*

- Corneoscleral incision required is very small (3.0 mm) as compared to conventional ECCE (Fig. 4.44)
- Central capsulorhexis of about 4 mm is preferred over other methods of anterior capsulotomy (Fig. 4.45)
- Nucleus is emulsified and aspirated by phacoemulsifier which acts basically through a hollow 1 mm titanium needle which vibrates in its longitudinal axis at an ultrasonic speed of 40,000 times a second (Figs 4.46 to 4.49).
- The nucleus can be emulsified in the posterior chamber or it can be first brought into the anterior chamber, emulsified and then aspirated (Figs 4.50 and 4.51).
- The remaining cortical lens matter is aspirated with the help of irrigation-aspiration cannula and process of ECCE is completed.

Advantages of phacoemulsification Smaller incision, more rapid wound healing, short convalescence and early stabilization of refractive error with less astigmatism.

Phacoemulsification is now a preferred choice of surgery for all types of cataracts, even the ones previously considered to be pure ECCE. A number of techniques are available for phacoemulsification.

However, "Divide and conquer" is the most favored technique for most of phaco surgeon as it is quite comfortable to perform. However new techniques like phaco flip and supracapsular phacoemulsification have entered into new era.

However there are certain disadvantages of phacoemulsifications. There are higher incidence of complications by novice phaco surgeon as the technique is difficult and needs to be mastered, lens matter is more likely to become mixed with vitreous, iris may prolapse and posterior capsular tear may take place. There is also difficulty in phacoemulsifying hard brunescent cataracts.

Phakonit

Phakonit is the latest technique of phacoemulsification first devised by Dr Amar Agarwal (India). The advantage of Phakonit over conventional phacoemulsification is that here the size of incision is below 1 mm. In other words, the size of incision through which cataract is removed is 0.9 mm. Dr Amar Agarwal performed this technique under no anesthesia first in India in 1998 and then by live

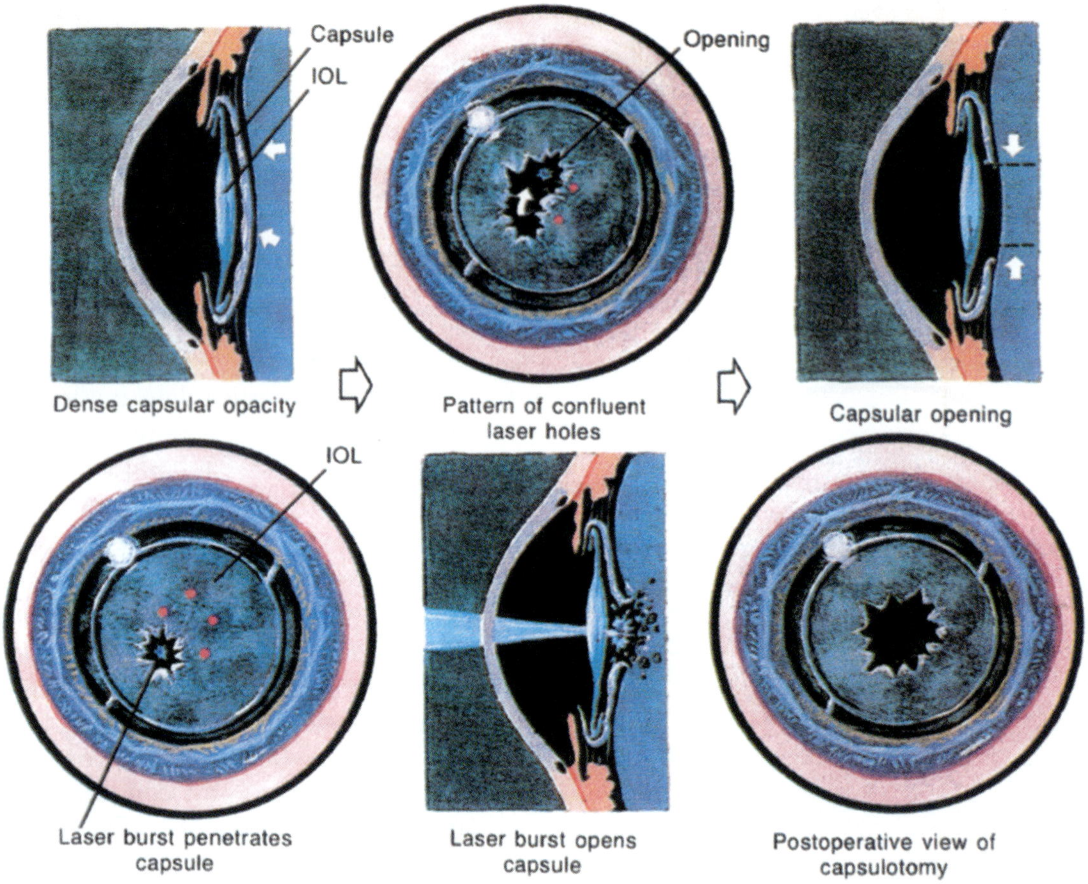

Fig. 4.36: Posterior capsulotomy with Nd:YAG laser (*Courtesy* : Ciba Geigy *Clinical Symposia)*

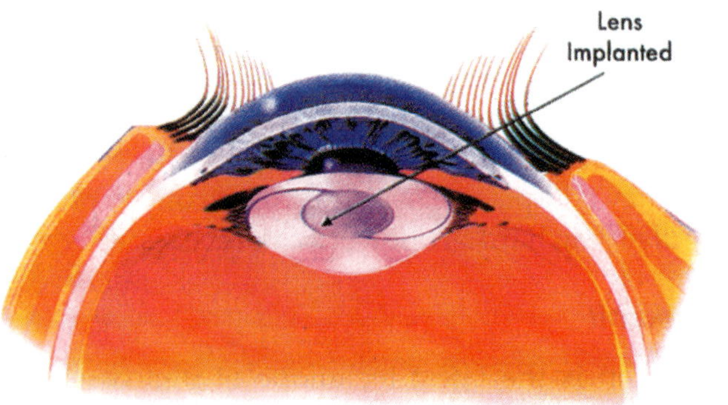

Fig. 4.37: Extracapsular cataract extraction (ECCE) with PC IOL implantation (*Courtesy* : Allergan India Ltd)

surgical telecast from Bangalore to Seattle for ASCRS Conference in 1999.

Phakonit shall revolutionize the cataract surgery because now the foldable lens which usually passes through an incision size of below 2 mm shall have to pass through a below 1 mm incision (Fig. 4.52).

The term Phakonit has been given as it shows Phaco (Phako) being done with a needle (N) opening via an incision (l) and with the phaco tip (T). Dr Amar Agarwal separated the phaco tip from infusion sleeve (which cannot go below an incision of 1.9 mm) (Fig. 4.53). The phako tip is passed inside the eye without infusion sleeve through 0.9 mm incision. In the left hand irrigating chopper is held in side port incision. The assistant injects the BSS fluid continuously at the site of incision to cool the phaco tip. Thus the cataract is removed through a 0.9 mm opening.

Laser Cataract Surgery

Laser cataract surgery is a technique similar as in phacoemulsification procedure. The main

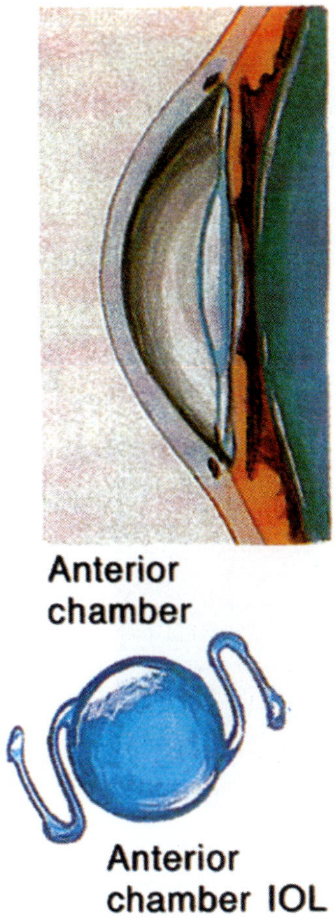

Fig. 4.38: Anterior chamber IOL implantation (*Courtesy* :Ciba Geigy *Clinical Symposia)*

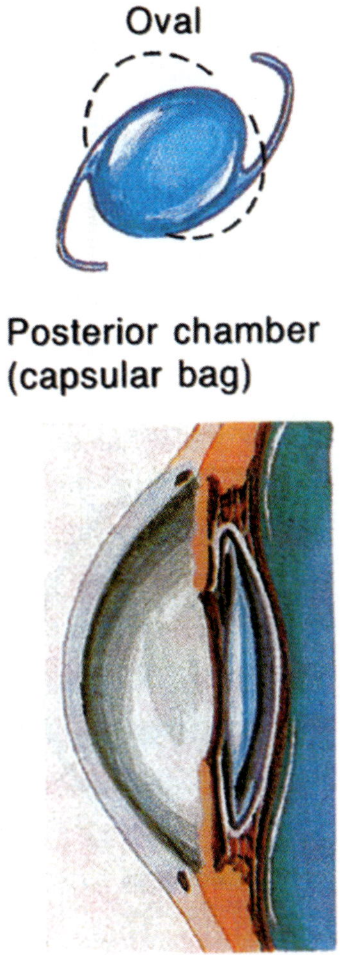

Fig. 4.39: Posterior chamber (capsular bag IOL implantation) (*Courtesy* : Ciba Geigy *Clinical Symposia)*

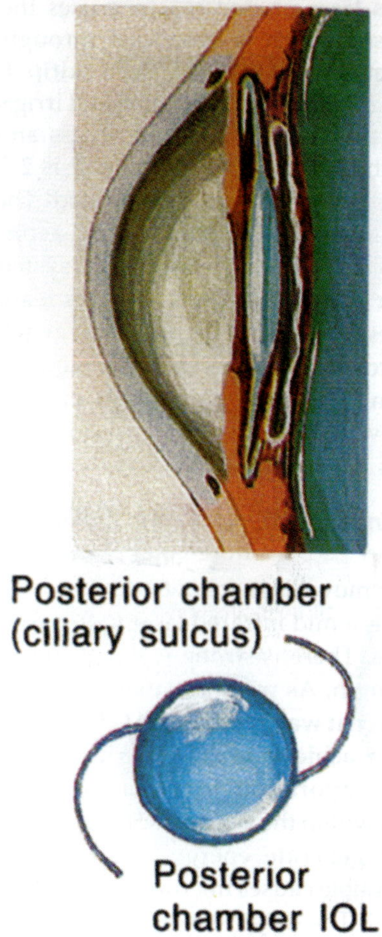

Fig. 4.40: Posterior chamber (ciliary sulcus IOL implantation) (*Courtesy* : Ciba Geigy *Clinical Symposia)*

difference however between the two techniques is that in laser cataract surgery instead of ultrasound power laser energy is used. The rhexis can be done with laser also. After hydrodissection, the laser probe is passed through the incision with the phaco chopper in other hand through the side port opening. The nucleus is split into small pie-shaped pieces and gradually aspirated out followed in the end with foldable PC IOL implantation. Two types of laser systems are being used for laser cataract surgery Nd:YAG and Er:YAG.

Nd:YAG laser system for cataract removal In this system laser photon machine (Paradigm, LISA) which has an inbuilt Nd:YAG laser, phacoemulsification system, vitrectomy system and diathermy unit (Figs 4.54 and 4.55). This laser photon machine uses the 1064 mm Nd:YAG laser which is broadcast through a unique 1.8 mm diameter tip designed like a skitip. It has three functions: fragmentation, aspiration and irrigation. Laser energy travels along a fiber and across an open area called the photofragmentation zone. It is 2.5 mm zone into which nuclear material is aspirated. The resulting nuclear fragments are removed by aspiration and irrigation. Nd:YAG laser-based phaco system have the potential for deep penetration. For this reason,

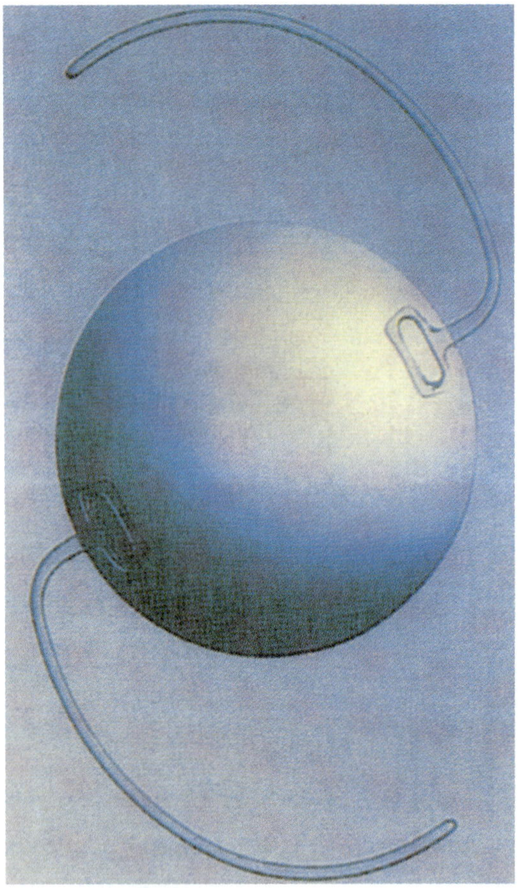

Fig. 4.41: IOL design (Optic refractive element and haptic support element) (*Courtesy* : Ciba Geigy *Clinical Symposia*)

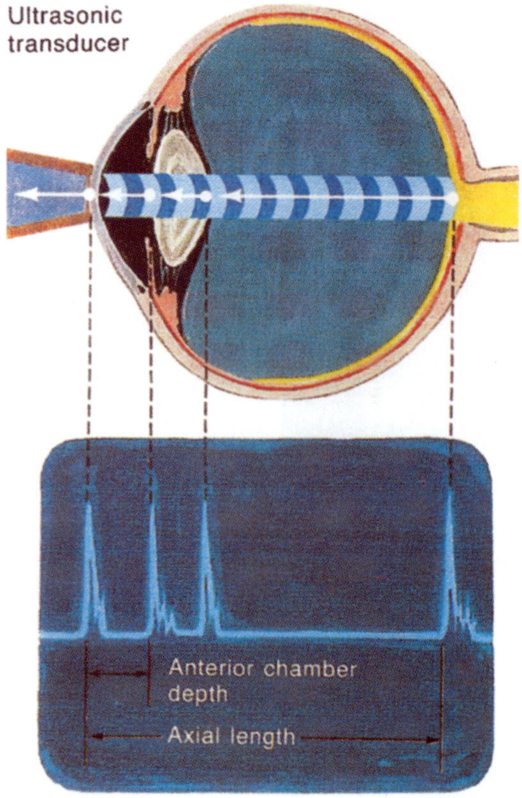

Fig. 4.43: A-scan ultrasonography for IOL power calculation and axial length measurement of globe (*Courtesy* : Ciba Geigy *Clinical Symposia*)

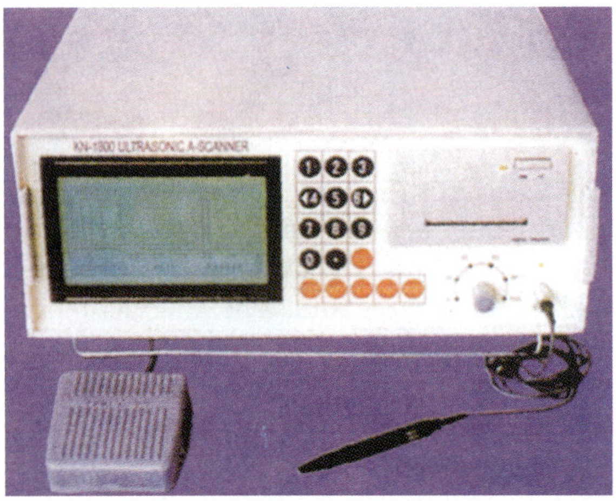

Fig. 4.42: A-scan ultrasound for IOL power calculation and axial length measuring of globe

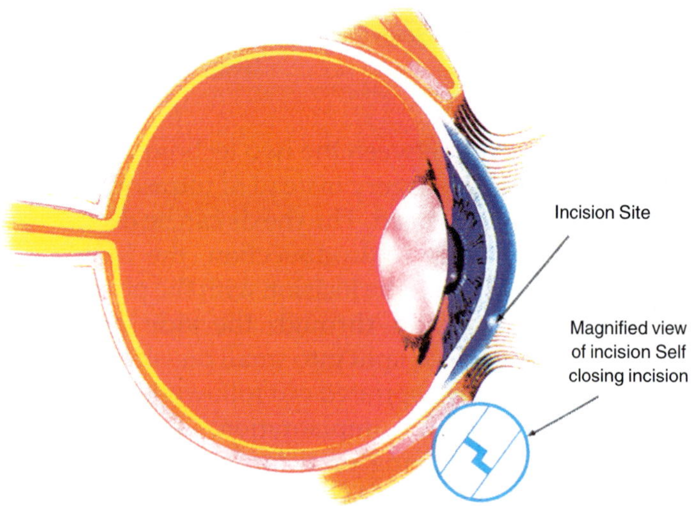

Fig. 4.44: Cataract surgery (phacoemulsification) (*Courtesy* : Allergan India Ltd)

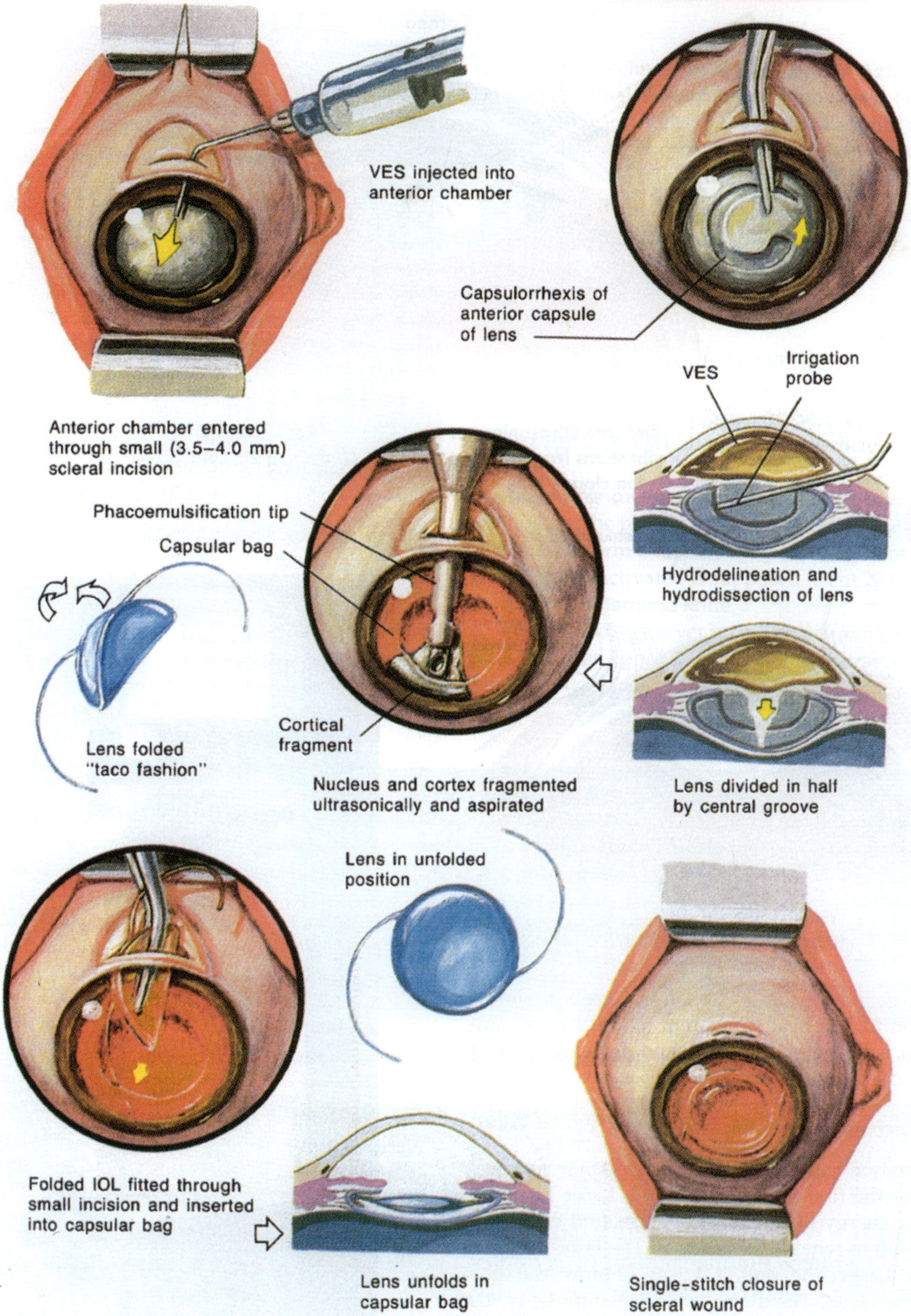

Fig. 4.45: Phacoemulsification and foldable IOL implantation (*Courtesy :* Ciba Geigy *Clinical Symposia)*

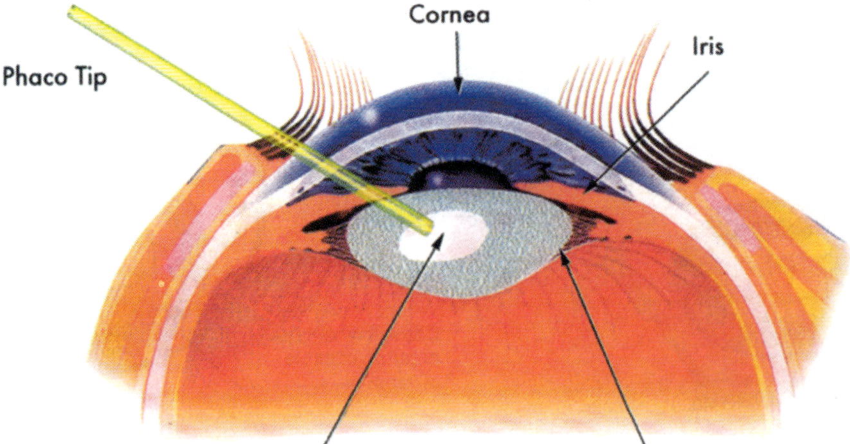

Fig. 4.46: Phacoemulsification surgery for cataract (*Courtesy :* Allergan India Ltd)

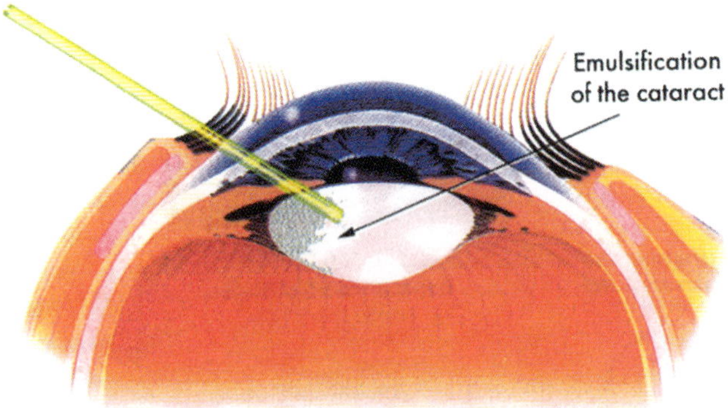

Fig. 4.47: Phacoemulsification surgery in progress (*Courtesy :* Allergan India Ltd)

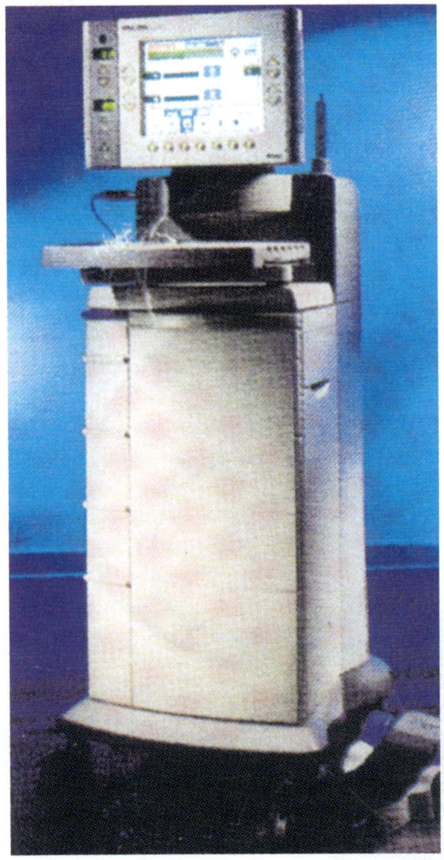

Fig. 4.48: State-of-art phacoemulsifier aspirator system (Alcon Legacy) (*Courtesy :* Alcon International, India)

photon system is designed to deliver laser energy which has an absorption coefficient lower than that required for phaco vaporization. The back stop design of the tip of this machine prevents the beam from damaging the non target tissues (Figs 4.56 and 4.57).

System using Er:YAG laser for cataract removal In Er:YAG laser system the mechanism of action of laser in lens tissue removal is as follows.

Er:YAG is a mid infrared laser with a wavelength of 2.94 microns. There is strong water absorption peak at this wavelength. As we know that lens is

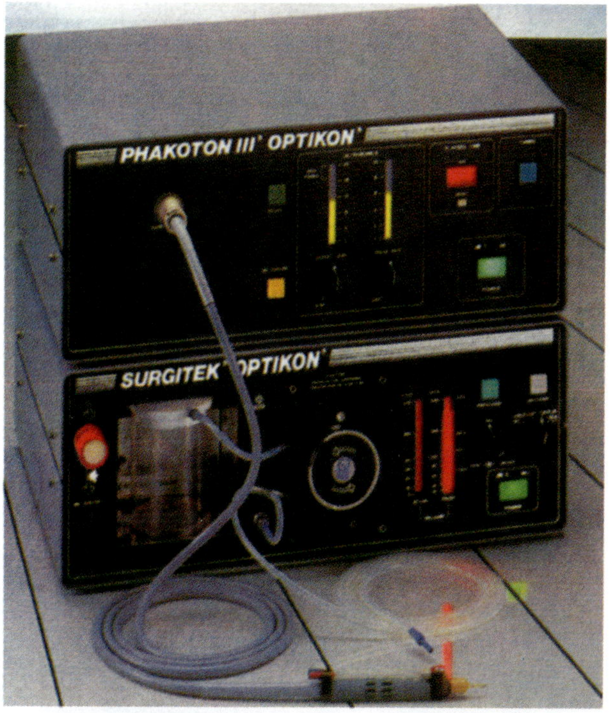

Fig. 4.49: Complete phacoemulsification unit (*Courtesy*: Towa Optics (India) Pvt Ltd)

composed of about 63 percent water, the Er:YAG laser is supposed to be suited to achieve phaco-vaporization of the lens. Explosive evaporation forms a cavitation bubble. Microspikes within the laser pulse traverse this cavitation bubble and generate energy a little beyond it. The cavitation bubble causes microfractures and break up of lens material. The loose lens material is then aspirated out. Laser-based phacoemulsification systems are considered better over conventional ultrasonic phacoemulsification.

The major advantages of laser phaco have been shown in relation to less heat generation (corneal burns uncommon), safer for endothelium and decreased risk of posterior capsule rupture.

Laser Phakonit

This technique has been devised by Dr Amar Agarwal (India) for the first time in the world. Laser Phakonit uses laser energy (coupled with ultrasound energy in hard nuclei) to remove the nucleus. The laser machine used for Laser Phakonit is Laser Photon Machine (Paradigm, USA). The

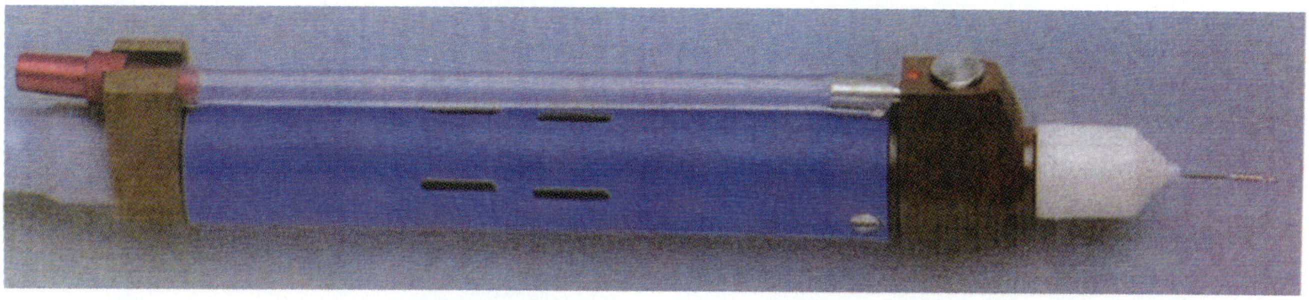

Fig. 4.50: Handpiece or U/S cystotome with cystotome and special sleeve (for phacoemulsification)

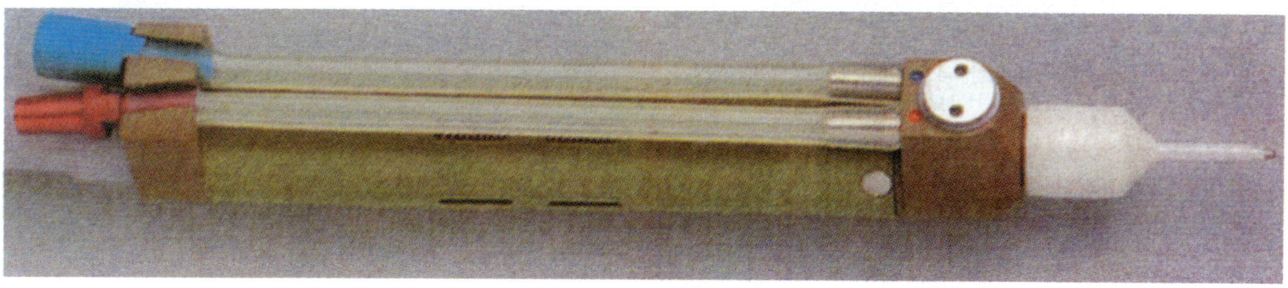

Fig. 4.51: Handpiece for cortical removal and special I/A tip (for phacoemulsification)

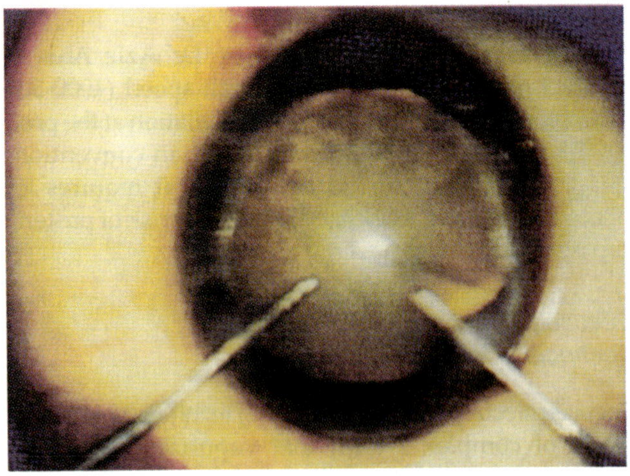

Fig. 4.52: Phakonit surgery [clear corneal incision (0.9 mm)]. Note the left hand has straight rod to stabilize the eye as surgery is being performed under no anesthesia (*Courtesy:* Dr Agarwal's Eye Hospital Ltd, Chennai, India)

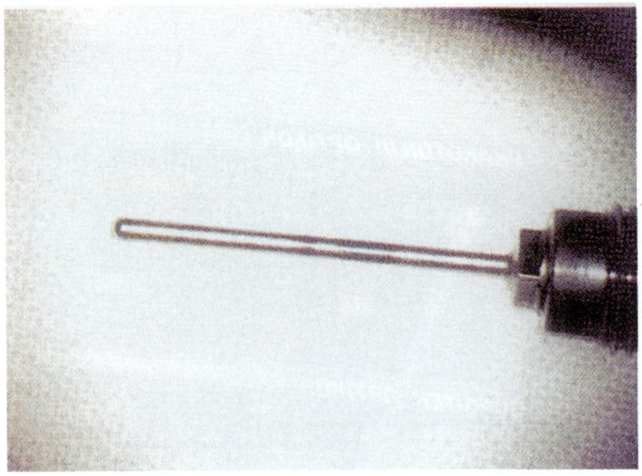

Fig. 4.53: Phakonit surgery—phaco probe without an infusion sleeve (*Courtesy :* Dr Agarwal's Eye Hospital Ltd, Chennai, India)

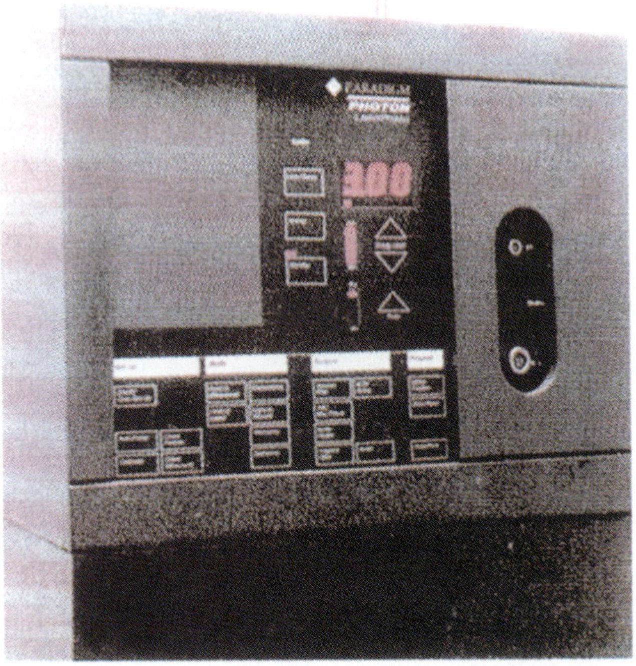

Fig. 4.54: Laser photon machine for laser cataract surgery [*Courtesy* : Dr Agarwal's Eye Hospital Ltd, Chennai (India)]

diameter of phaco probe is 900 microns while the laser probe reduces the orifice opening to 550 microns. Thus the nucleus can be removed through a very small 0.9 mm opening.

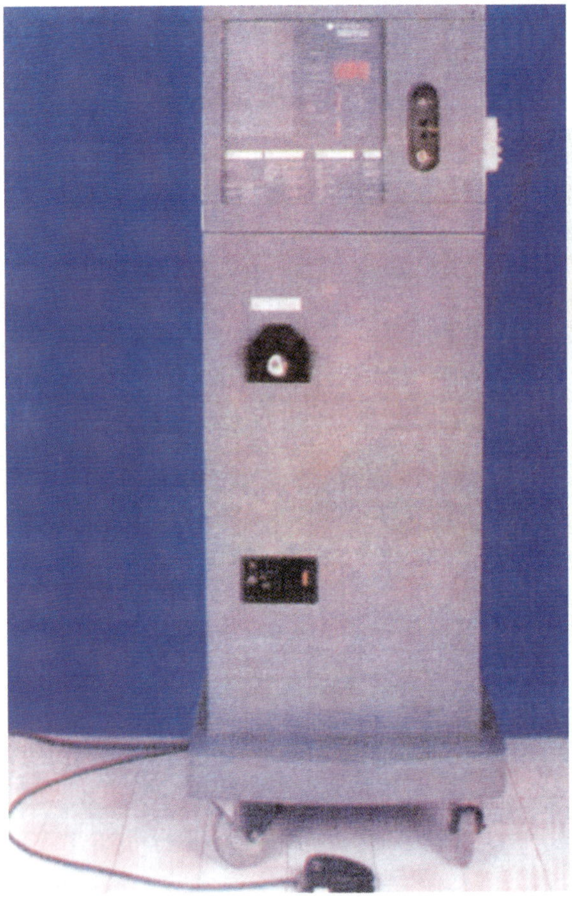

Fig. 4.55: Laser photon machine for laser cataract surgery (*Courtesy :* Dr Agarwal's Eye Hospital Ltd, Chennai, India)

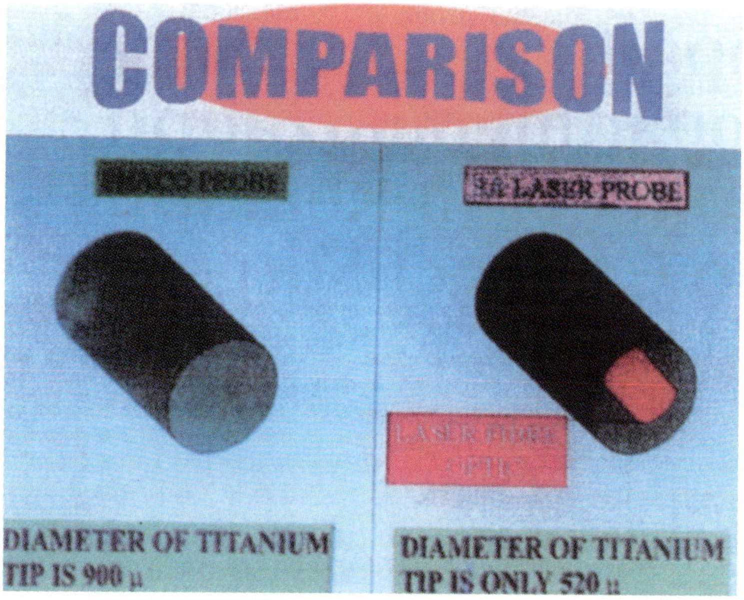

Fig. 4.56: Laser cataract surgery. Comparison of phaco probe and laser phaco probe (*Courtesy* : Dr Agarwal's Eye Hospital Ltd, Chennai, India)

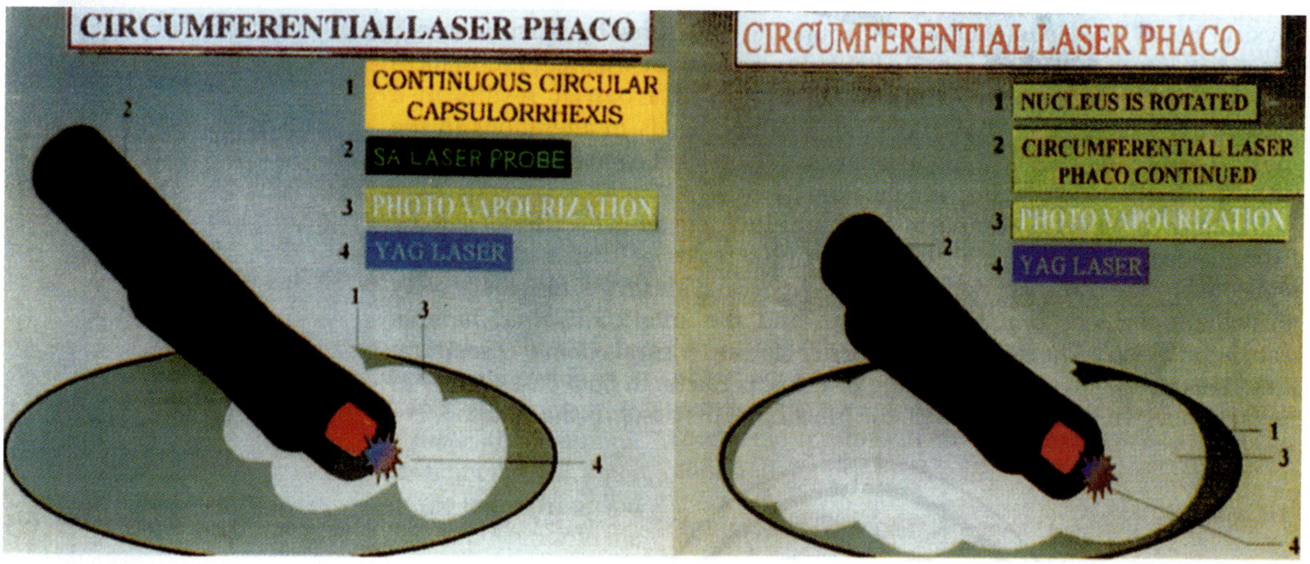

Fig. 4.57: Laser phaco technique for laser cataract surgery (*Courtesy* : Dr Agarwal's Eye Hospital Ltd, Chennai, India)

Phacotmesis

Phacotmesis technology started by Dr Aziz Anis for cataract removal that combines high speed (4000-5000 rpm) rotation and ultrasonic linear oscillation at the probe tip. Phacotmesis is considered safer than conventional ultrasonic phacoemulsification in that it requires less phaco power and is associated with lower risk of posterior capsular dehiscence (PCD).

Focused Electromagnetic Field (FEF) Technology for Cataract Removal

Focused electromagnetic field (FEF) technology is plasma blade of complex system that vaporizes the surface molecules of a hair thin plasma probe, thereby forming a microscopic cloud of cutting plasma particles around the probe.

According to Dr Richard Fugo who devised this technology, the plasma blade has the ability to create an incision, perform a capsulotomy and fragment the lens. The tip when activated is supposed to cut 20 to 30 times sharper than diamond knife.

This technology is yet in the infancy and it shall hold great future as a possible alternative to ultrasonic phacoemulsification.

REFERENCES

1. Garg Ashok. In Textbook of Ophthalmology, New Delhi, Jaypee Brothers, 2002;3;1620-59.
2. Kuck JFR. Cataract Formation, In Biochemistry of the Eye. CN Graymore Ed, New York, 1970.
3. Kinashita JH. Mechanisms initiating Cataract Formation, Proctor Lecture, Invest Ophthalmol 1974;13:713.
4. Merin S. Congenital Cataracts, In Genetic and Metabolic Eye disease, MF Goldberg, Ed. Boston, Little Brown & Co, 1974.
5. Langston Pavan. Manual of Ocular Diagnosis and Therapy, Lippincot Williams & Wilkins, Philadelphia; 2002;140-63.
6. Kanski JJ. Clinical Ophthalmology; Butterworth Heinemann, 3rd Ed, Oxford, 1994.
7. Taylor A : Nutritional and Environmental influences on the eye, CRC Press, London; 1999;1-5.
8. Stambolian D: Glactose & Cataract, Surv Ophthalmol 1988;32:333-49.
9. Drews RC: Alcohol and Cataract, Arch. Ophthalmol 1993;111:110-12.
10. Hesker H : Antioxidative Vitamins & Cataract in the elderly, Z.Ernahrungswiss 1995;34:167-76.
11. Krines K: Cataract and Diabetes, BMJ 1964;2:665-68.
12. Leske MC, Chylack LT : The Lens Opacities Case – Control Study: Risk factors for Cataract, Arch. Ophthalmol 1998;109:244-51.

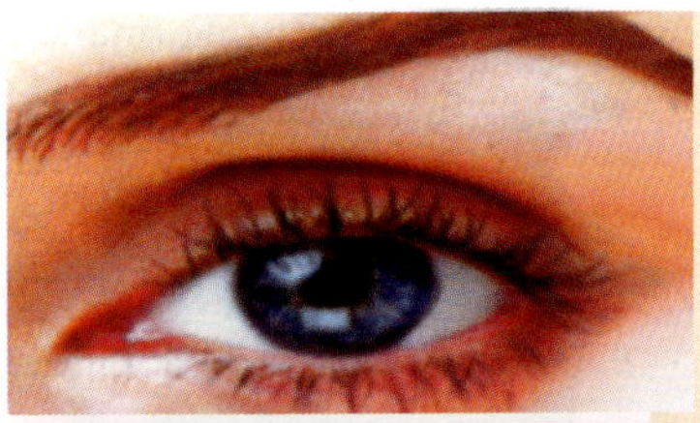

Five

Ocular Biometry

Sunita Agarwal (India)

INTRODUCTION

It is necessary for every ophthalmologist who is working with intraocular lenses to know how to calculate the power of the IOL.

AXIAL LENGTH MEASUREMENT

For IOL implantation, the ultrasonic method affords the best way to calculate the axial length and achieves the desired postoperative refraction. The instruments available to make these measurements are of two basic types:

i. instruments with rigid probe tips, and
ii. instruments with distensible tips or with water baths.

Those instruments with distensible membranes on the front of the probe are approximately 5 percent more accurate in making measurements than those with the rigid tip. The reasons why the distensible tip are better are as follows.

1. The distensible tip prevents indenting the cornea when the measurement is made, and does not cause the eye to appear artificially shortened. A rigid tip can cause corneal indentation between 0.1 and 0.3 mm, resulting in error from 0.3 to 1.0 diopters (Fig. 5.1). In other words if one is buying

an A-scan, one should get one with a distensible tip.

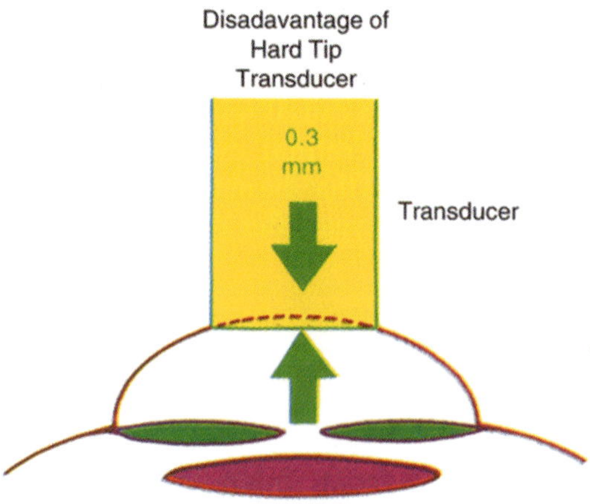

Fig. 5.1: Disadvantage of hard tip transducer—note indentation on the cornea

2. The distensible tip helps to separate the corneal reflection from the signal sent out from the front surface of the transducer, i.e. it makes it more accurate to determine exactly where the front surface of the cornea is, and when it is not in direct contact with the transducer.

KERATOMETRIC MEASUREMENTS

The keratometric measurements can be done through a keratometer or through an autokeratometer. Many biometers (Fig. 5.2) have provision for connecting the autokeratometer to their computer so that once the keratometer reading is taken automatically, the value is entered into the biometer, and one does not have to feed it in again.

IOL FORMULA

There are two major categories of IOL formulae.

Theoretical Formula

Introduction

This formula is based on an optical model of the eye. An optics equation is solved to determine the IOL power needed to focus light from a distant object onto the retina. In the different formulae, different assumptions are made about the refractive index of the cornea, the distance of the cornea to

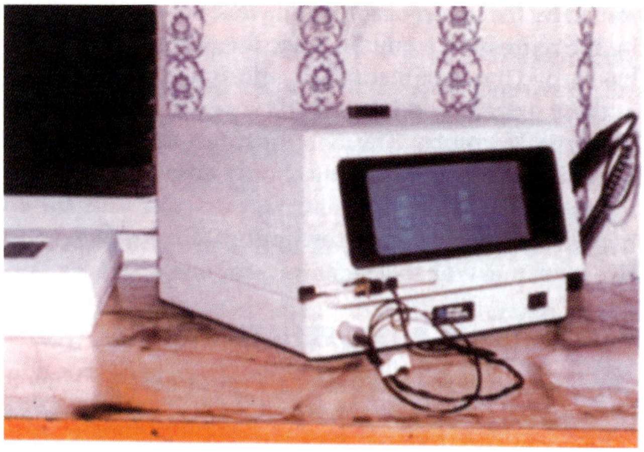

Fig. 5.2: Biometer

the IOL, the distance of the IOL to the retina as well as other factors. These are called theoretical formulae because they are based on a theoretical optical model of the eye. All of these theoretical equations make simplifying assumptions about the optics of the eye, and hence, provide a good (but not perfect) prediction of IOL power.

The most popular formula in this group is the Binkhorst formula. This is based on sound theory. All the theoretical formulae can be algebrically transformed into the following

$$P = [N/(L-C)] - [NK/(N-KC)]$$

where,

P = Dioptric power of the lens for emmetropia,
N = Aqueous and vitreous refractive index,
L = Axial length (mm),
C = Estimated postoperative anterior chamber depth (mm), and
K = Corneal curvature [D].

Binkhorst Formula

Binkhorst has made a correction in his formula for surgically induced flattening of the cornea, using a corneal index of refraction of 1.333. Binkhorst also corrects for the thickness of the lens implant by subtracting approximately 0.05 mm from the measured axial length. Thus with the Binkhorst formula, 0.25 mm is added to the measured axial length to account for the distance between the vitreoretinal interface and the photoreceptor layer, and 0.05 mm is subtracted for lens thickness, resulting in a net addition of 0.20 mm to the measured axial length. The Binkhorst's formula is:

$$D = 1336\ (4r-a)/(a-d)\ (4r-d)$$

where,

D = Dioptric power of IOL in aqueous humor,
1336 = Index of refraction of vitreous and aqueous,
r = Radius of curvature of the anterior surface of the cornea,
a = Axial length of the globe (mm), and
d = Distance between the anterior cornea and the IOL.

Disadvantages

The problem in the theoretical formula is in the axial length measurement. The reason why it is difficult to measure the axial length accurately is that one must know the exact velocities of the ultrasound as it travels through the various structures of the eye. Because of the variation of the acoustic density of a cataract, these velocities cannot be known exactly. As a result, when cataractous lenses are much more acoustically dense than the average lens, the sound wave will move more rapidly through the lens and return to the transducer much more quickly than would have been expected for a given axial length. As a result of the velocity error, the eyes appear to be shorter. The formula consequently calculates an IOL power for an axial length which is too short. The patient then becomes overminused (too myopic). **Theoretical formulae help the surgeon to anticipate what should result, not what will result from implantation.**

Regression Formula (Empirical Formula)

Introduction

The regression formulae or empirical formulae are derived from empirical data and are based on retrospective analysis of postoperative refraction after IOL implantation. The results of a large number of IOL implantations are plotted with respect to the corneal power, axial length of the eye, and emmetropic IOL power. The best-fit equation is then determined by the statistical procedure of regression analysis of the data. Unlike the theoretical formulae, no assumptions are made about the optics of the eye. These regression equations are only as good as the accuracy of the data used to derive them.

Advantages

Implant power calculations can be made much more accurately through the use of regression formulae that are based on the analysis of the actual results of many uncomplicated IOL implantations in previous cataract surgeries. Since regression analysis is based on the results of actual operations, it includes the vagaries of the eye and measuring devices, vagaries that theoretical formulae attempt to address with correction factors.

Sanders-Retzlaff-Kraff (SRK) Formula

The most popular regression formula is the SRK formula which was developed by Sanders, Retzlaff and Kraff in 1980. This is

$$P = A - 2.5\,L - 0.9K$$

where,

P = Implant power to produce emmetropia,
L = Axial length (mm),
K = Average keratometer reading, and
A = Specific constant for each lens type and manufacture.

The SRK formula calculates the IOL power by linearly regressing the results of previous implants. As this is a linear formula, it will underestimate the power of high-powered lenses and it will overestimate the power of the low-powered lenses compared to the theoretical calculation. For example, if the Binkhorst formula predicts that a 28-diopter lens should be used, the SRK formula will predict that a 26-diopter lens should be used. In lenses with low power, if the Binkhorst formula predicts that a 10-diopter lens is necessary, the SRK will predict that a 12-diopter lens should be used.

RELATION OF EQUIPMENT TO SPECIFIC FORMULAE

Most of the instruments calculate the desired power for the IOL at least by three different methods including a regression formula and a theoretical formula. It is the responsibility of the doctor to select which of the formulae he or she wants to use. Rarely, between 18 and 22 diopters, there is a significant difference between the calculated lens powers. But outside this range, there will be a progressive increase in difference between that determined by the theoretical formula and the one calculated by the regression formula. Since the regression formula has turned out to be statistically more accurate, 5 percent at these extremes, it is presently more reliable than the theoretical formulae. The manufacturers vary as to which programs they provide. One should anyway make sure that both the regression and theoretical formulae are included so that one has the opportunity to personally select the most reliable technique for one's surgery.

TARGETING IOL POSTOPERATIVE REFRACTION

The question that comes to one's mind next is "How to predetermine what postoperative refraction the patient should have?" This is the one parameter which the doctor has to decide upon and feed into the computer. The other parameters like axial length, etc. we have no control over. The answer depends on whether we are doing a monocular or binocular correction.

Monocular Correction

If we are considering only one eye (i.e. if the other eye has cataract or is amblyopic), targeting the postoperative refraction for approximately –1.00 diopter is probably the best choice. This is usually best because most people have visual needs for both distance and near. This means that the patient wants to be able to drive and to read without wearing glasses. If we target the postoperative refraction to –1.00 D, it will allow the patient to perform most tasks with no glasses. At times, when they need finer acuity, they can wear regular bifocals, which will correct them for distance and near.

The second reason for targeting the postoperative refraction to –1.00 D is that statistically, between 70 percent and 90 percent of the patients will fall within +1.00 D error of the desired postoperative refraction. The errors, as mentioned earlier are due to our inexact measurements. Therefore, the patient will fall between plano and –2.00 D 90 percent of the time. This will assure most patients of useful vision without glasses. Hence, the error of the ultrasound is best handled by choosing the postoperative refraction to –1.00 D. If we would target for plano, then 90 percent of the patients will be between –1.00 and +1.00 D. When the patient's refraction is on the +1 side he or she has no useful vision at any distance because he or she is hyperopic and does not have the ability to accommodate. Consequently, because it is very undesirable to have a hyperopic correction, targeting for –1.00 D not only optimizes the best vision at all distances, but also minimizes the chance for hyperopia that can result from inaccurate ultrasonic measurements.

Binocular Correction

When the vision in the other eye is good, its refraction must be considered for binocular vision. One overriding rule when prescribing glasses is that one should never prescribe spectacles which gives the patient a difference in the power between the right and left lens greater than 3 D. The reason for this is that even though the patient may have 6/6 vision in primary gaze, when the patient looks up or down, the induced vertical prism difference in the two eyes is so great that it will create double vision. **In a patient who has good vision in the nonoperative eye, one must target the IOL power for a refraction within 2 D of his or her present prescription in the nonoperative eye.** Two diopters, not three, due to our 1 D A-scan variability. For example, if we have a patient who is hyperopic and has +5 D correction in each eye, we cannot target the IOL for a postoperative refraction of –1.00 D because this would produce a 6 D difference between the two lenses resulting in double vision. We must therefore select the IOL power to obtain a refraction which is approximately 2 D less than the nonoperative eye. Consequently, on our patient who is +5 D in both eyes, we should target the postoperative refraction in the eye with the cataract for +3 D, so that there is a 90 percent probability that there will be less than a 3 D difference.

In contrast, if the patient was highly myopic in each eye, for example, –10 D in both eyes, we should target the IOL power to produce refraction of approximately –8 D. Again, we have limited the difference in the spectacles lenses to a 2 D difference in the final prescription. Again, target, for a 2 D difference not a 3 D, because there is approximately a 1 D tolerance in the accuracy of the ultrasonic measurement.

If the operation on the second eye is to be done shortly after the first, the preoperative spectacles refraction can be ignored, and the patient is treated as if he or she were monocular.

FACTORS AFFECTING ACCURACY OF IOL POWER CALCULATION

Many factors can affect the accuracy of the power of the IOL calculated.

Keratometry

Keratometers only measure the radius of curvature of the anterior corneal surface. This measurement must be converted to an estimate of the refracting power of the cornea in diopters, using a fictitious index (the true corneal refractive index of 1.376 could be used only if both the anterior and posterior corneal radii of curvature were known). The variability can alter calculated corneal dioptric power by 0.7 D.

Axial Length Measurement

As explained earlier, indentation of the cornea by the A-scan instrument tip can alter the axial length affecting the accuracy of the power of the IOL.

Axial Length Correction Factor

The distance from the vitreoretinal interface to the photoreceptor layer has been estimated to be about 0.15 to 0.5 mm. This distance can affect the accuracy of the IOL power calculated.

Site of Loop Implantation

Posterior chamber IOLs may be implanted with both loops in the ciliary sulcus or in the capsular bag, or with one loop in the sulcus and one loop in the capsular bag. Positioning the implants within the capsular bag places the implant further back in the eye and decreases the effective power of the lens. There is usually a 0.5 to 1.5 D loss of effectivity by placing the implant in the capsular bag as opposed to the ciliary sulcus. A higher power lens should therefore be used when the implant is placed in the capsular bag.

Orientation of Planoconvex Implants

Some surgeons implant planoconvex posterior chamber lenses with the plano surface forward. Such flipping of the implant decreases the effective power of the lens by 0.75 D even if the position of the lens is unchanged. An additional 0.5 D loss of effectivity occurs because the principal plane of the lens is usually displaced further back into the eye. Thus, a total loss in effectivity of 1.25 D is expected by turning the lens around.

Postoperative Change in Corneal Curvature

Suturing of a cataract incision has a tendency to steepen the vertical meridian. These changes affect the postoperative refraction of the patient.

Density of the Cataract

The density of the cataract also makes a difference. In a dense cataract (Fig. 5.3), the ultrasonic waves travel faster whereas in an early cataract (Fig. 5.4) the ultrasonic waves travel slower.

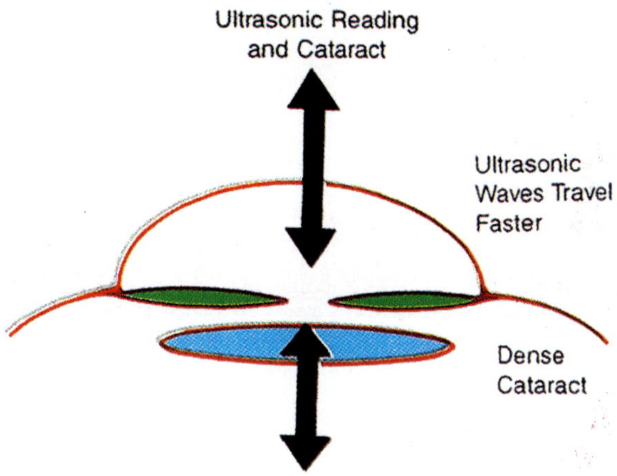

Fig. 5.3: Ultrasonic reading in dense cataract

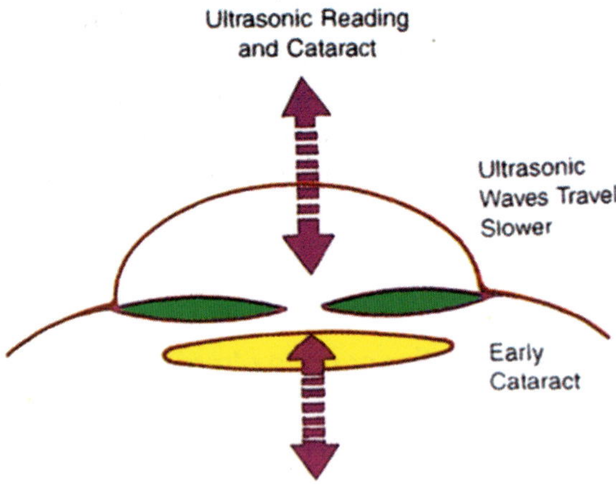

Fig. 5.4: Ultrasonic reading in early cataract

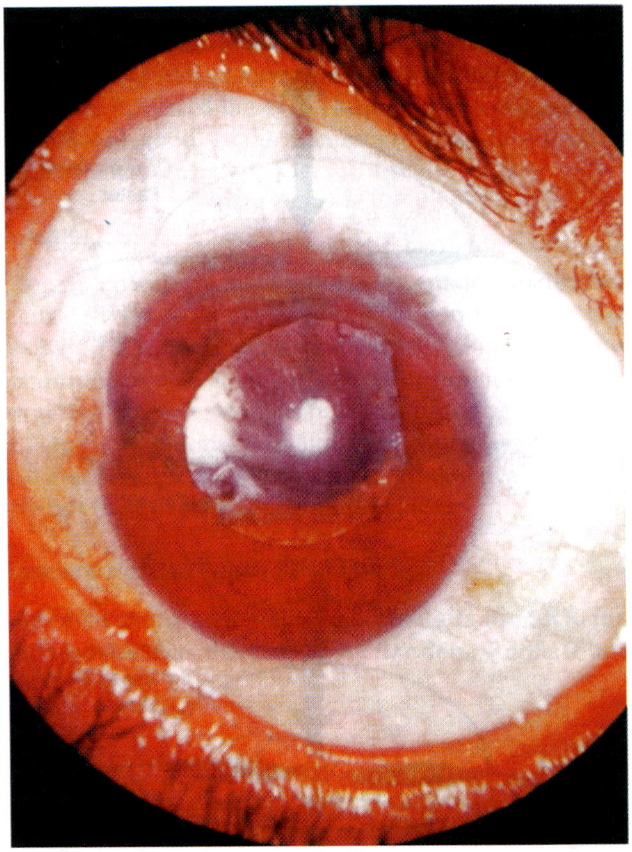

Fig. 5.5: Captive iris syndrome

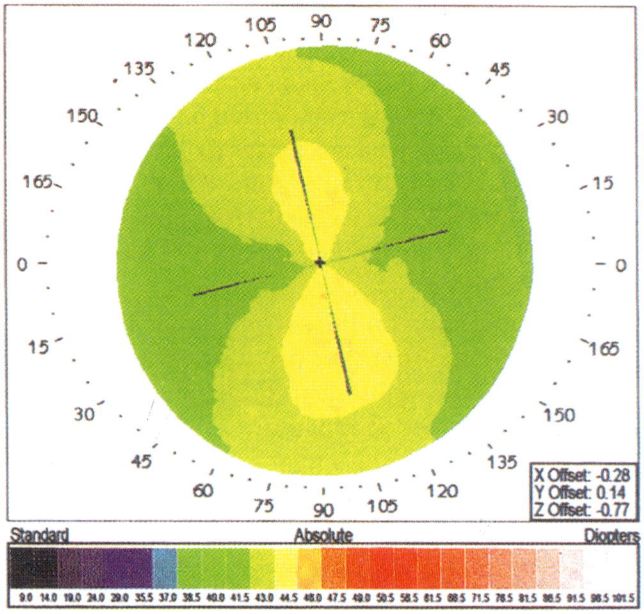

Fig. 5.6: Topograph of a patient in whom a wrong power IOL was implanted

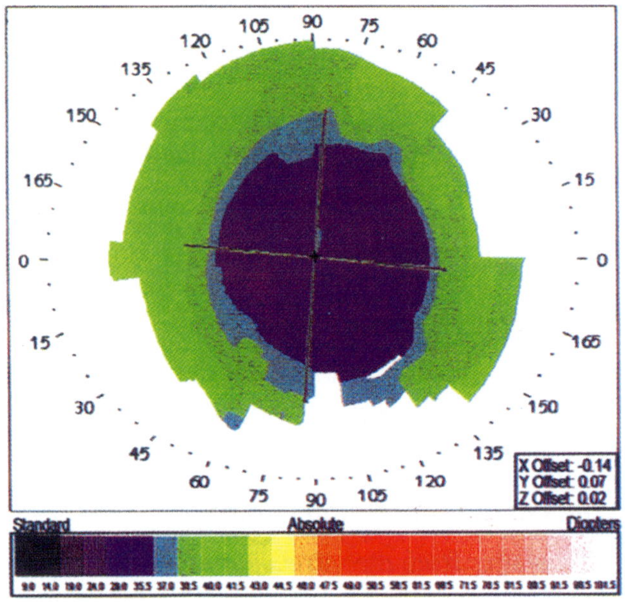

Fig. 5.7: Topograph of the same patient as in Figure 5.6 after LASIK

IOL Tilt and Decentration

When a lens is tilted, its effective power increases and plus cylinder astigmatism is induced about the axis of the lens tilt. The tilting of the lens occurs if one loop is in the capsular bag and the other in the sulcus (Fig. 5.5). Alternatively, residual cortex being left behind can cause an inflammatory response which causes contraction and pulling unequally on parts of the loops and the optic.

PSEUDOPHAKIC LASIK

If a patient has had a wrong biometry then the solution can be to remove the IOL and replace it with a correct powered IOL. Another alternative is to perform LASIK and correct the problem. Figure 5.6 is the topograph before LASIK of a patient who had a power of –10.0 dioptres after IOL implantation. The patient was referred to us and we did a LASIK as the patient was operated a year back. We felt that the IOL might be fixed firmly in the bag. Figure 5.7 is the topograph after LASIK.

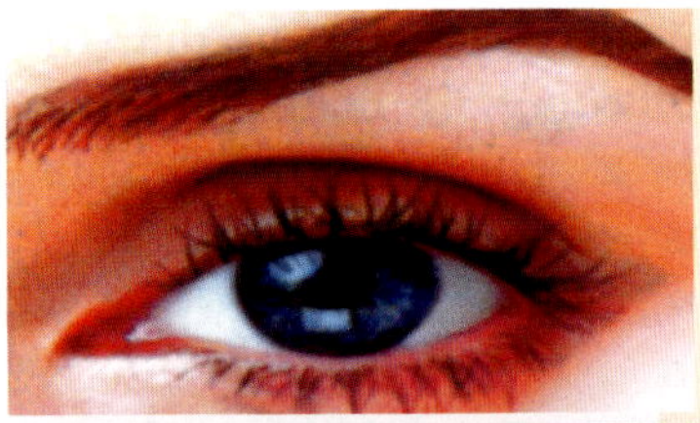

Six

Sunita Agarwal
Amar Agarwal
Ashok Garg (India)

Sterilization

INTRODUCTION

When viewed upon from the broader angle, however good a surgery may have been performed, should it be complicated with infection, the result is fraught with peril. The patient suffers ultimately and the surgeon goes through hell. We have all had our share of infection and its disastrous effects.

Should a surgeon say they have never had infection spoiling their case, either they have never done surgery or the truth lies hidden elsewhere.

Be that as it may we need to understand microorganisms in a much better manner. We need to give this topic full attention in our hospitals and continue to give it the importance, it requires by continuing quality checks at every interval regularly everyday and in every case.

Some basic facts of postsurgical infection in human eyes whether cataract surgery or any intraocular surgery is concerned, are that we need to regard all infections to arise from the operation theatre unless proved otherwise. The operating room is certainly the most guilty in providing the microorganism for postsurgical infection.

It may be very easy to complain about patient compliance and dirtiness to be the cause of infection, and sometimes that may be true, however in our hearts it is safer and better for us to accept that this infection has come from the operating room and then work ourselves backwards in removing the source of the disease.

We may be able to shift blame to a tooth infection or septic foci in the sinus, however, should we be able to first accept the operating room to be at fault, our energies would be directed in improving our facilities, thus averting further mishaps from occurring.

The first rule in sterilization at least where developing countries are concerned is not to believe any manufacturer when they claim to have sterilized their wares. To be taken as guilty of infection unless proved otherwise. This is true of not only suture material, disposable needles and syringes but also of intravenous and intraocular fluids. Many cases have been reported in India where bacteria have grown from the Ringer lactate used. A startling study was carried out in the early 90s where several eyes were lost due to balanced salt solution (BSS) not being of pH 7.4, because the last rinse did not wash of the remnant soap from the glass bottle.

What we all need to remember is that when everything is going fine nobody complains, but as soon as there is a complication the surgeon is the first and often the last person to be held totally responsible for all misdemeanors on anybody's part. Thus as captain of the ship the surgeon has to sink with his or her ship. However, all this can be avoided by taking precautions before entering the operating room.

HISTORY

Dating back to the time that Sushruta from 500 BC explained the importance of washing hands and draping wounds with clean cloth, as well as having a clean environment for surgical procedures, Indian medicine has always kept this part of medical practice in good stead. Practicing principles of Dhanvantri medicine a *Hindu* physician-oculist wrote that surgeons should clean their nails prior to operating, wear fresh clothing, and spray sweet smelling vapors around the operating room. Little did he know the importance of these instructions. However, these were carried down through the ages by the *Vaids* (*Hindu* physicians), now with better knowledge there is more understanding of the topic on infection and sterilization control.

The middle ages saw European medicine catching ground however, sterilization tactics were still very rudimentary. Most surgeons thought it to be fashionable not to wash hands, mayhap due to the cold climate of the temperate zones. Thus centuries of unknown prevailed with thousands being lost to infection and disease even inside the operating room. It was considered hazardous to lay a surgeons hand in the fear of losing the patient to "fever" as it was called then.

However, Hieronymus Fracastorus in 1546 published a landmark book that may have led to the discovery of bacteria. His theory of contagious diseases and their treatment sparked off the original microbe hunter, to identify bacteria with his own saliva in 1675, using his microscope screwed together with some lenses, Anton van Leeuwenhoek had set about 2 centuries of hot debate amongst the European scientists.

In 1840 Jakob Henle postulated the theory of the contagion. This was further specified by Robert Koch in 1876, where he showed that by isolating the anthrax bacillus and was able to infect a normal animal with the same that the theory of contagion was true. This work won him the Nobel Prize for medicine and physiology in 1905.

It took Louis Pasteur to bring out the emphasis of the "little beings" as those responsible for disease. His paper on the importance of washing hands before starting a obstetrical delivery shows the utmost significance of this one act towards a sterile atmosphere.

Throughout the 1800s pioneering technologies of Pasteur, Nizer, Klebs, Escherich, Cohn and Ehrlich played major roles in the evolution of discovery of pathological germs. Today the science of microbiology and medicine are occupied by their names forming important landmarks in the discovery of the importance of sterilization techniques.

Where hospital wards are concerned, making surgery safe and banishing sepsis from hospital wards, an era of pre-Lister and post-Lister can be demarcated. This was the importance of Joseph Lister on surgical outcome. He based a lot of his studies however on Ignaz Semmelweiss (1818-1865)—who was cruelly maligned for his theory of the origins of child-bed fever that led him to be institutionalized and die an unhappy man. The irony of the situation was his studies brought about a revolution in hospital wards and the prevention of infection by antiseptics and cleanliness reiterated by Joseph Lister.

By the time Daimler brought out his first motor cycle in 1884, scientists round the globe had devised the autoclave deriving from the fact that boiling did away with microbes. This revolutionized hospital wards and operation theatre sepsis to a great extent. So much so that till date some contraption of the autoclave is still used in every operation theatre in existence in the modem world.

By 1899 a century was going by and scientists believed this was the ultimate and that internal sepsis was not going to be much more advanced beyond theory and that the field was not likely to advance further. Today with much more information and knowledge we think contrary, that we still know only a drop in this ocean of knowledge against disease and infection.

Change is the spice of life and just as today changes to another day, of more discovery and more scientific achievements so to these pioneers were to discover much more. Sulfanilamide first discovered by Paul Gelmo in 1908 was found to be effective on surgical wounds, by Gerhard Domagk, who first used the drug on humans in 1935. This won Domagk the Nobel Prize for Medicine and Physiology in 1939.

Paul Ehrlich and Toju Hata discovered Salvarsan, the arsenic derivative for the treatment of syphilis, it heralded yet another era, that of the antibiotic.

In 1929, Alexander Fleming published his classical work on Penicillin from London and history followed his every achievement. Through the World Wars his medicine was of immense use in the control of infection and weeding out of disease. He showed first through *in-vitro* studies that a contaminant of *Staphylococcus* medium, *Penicillium notatum* had a destructive effect on the *Staphylococcus* bacteria that was growing on the agar plate. In further experiments he showed that this mould also had strong antibacterial activity against other pathogenic gram-positive bacteria as well as gram-negative cocci and bacilli but was not effective against organisms such as *Escherichia coli.*

While the world raged with war, yet another kind of war was being fought for mankind inside the laboratories of HW FIorey at Oxford University. By 1940 Ernst Chain showed the curative effects of penicillin *in vivo*. In 1945 by the end of the World War II, these three men were awarded the Nobel Prize for Medicine and Physiology. Selman Waksman discovered spates of antibiotics in succession with streptomycin in 1944 for tuberculosis and neomycin in 1949.

Much of today's discoveries have been dependent on the way we see these small "animalcules" of Leeuwenhoek, in 1933. Our eyes could see the destruction of the world with Hitler as the Chancellor of Germany, and could see even greater destruction by microbes since the invention of the first transmission electron microscope by Ruska. Further developed to a phase contrast microscope by 1953, by which time the World War had ended and humanity was once again allowed to prosper. So much so that the scanning tunneling microscope could be developed by 1980 and its fast developing clones that are in use today.

However, very soon the side effects of antibiotics were noted with the classic example of chloramphenicol, the first broad-spectrum antibiotic, discovered in 1949, effective against rickettsial infection, typhoid. A link was established between severe bone marrow depression and aplastic anemia with its use. This curtailed the use of these eyedrops and oral regime in USA.

We owe a lot to these forefathers of modern medicine and surgery, and today's technological advancements have made us more wary of the microbe. It seems to be the more we advance, the more microbes we find the cause of disease. Stress and other dietary factors were believed to be the cause for peptic ulcers, though now we know bacteria to be the root. In a similar manner, there are many more diseases that still retain their shroud of mystery.

Let us not rest on previous laurels and with the close of this century believe that we have reached the ultimate. In reality, we have only skimmed the surface there is much more to be unraveled in this body beautiful of the *Homo sapiens.*

Tempting to say in the words of Louis Pasteur, "Science knows no country, because knowledge belongs to humanity, and is a torch which illuminates the world."

AREAS OF STERILIZATION

Once we enter the operating room, we expect that everything must be in order, and somebody else is in charge, *not me*. However much to our utter astonishment seldom does anything go wrong, though, when it does, the blame is once again pushed on to somebody else, *not me*. This is where the first principle of surgery has to be changed and restructured. **The first and only person responsible for the whole team at work inside an operating room is the main surgeon.** This is the person who everybody in the operation theatre must report to. This is the person who before entering the theatre has to ensure that everything inside this pious area is under strict control of the surgeon. This is the person who must take responsibility if an infection should arise in the patient's eye within one week of surgery.

After carrying out so many tests and sterilization techniques I would rather believe for the benefit of all future patients that infection in a postsurgical eye arises from the operation theatre facilities. It is very difficult to put infection inside a closed eyeball, though it is easy enough while the eye coats are still open. More often than not infection is carried into the eye by instruments themselves.

There is however a small possibility that this may not be the case and there may be a septic foci residing in some corner of the human body like a tooth abscess or such. Still these occurrences are very rare and far between. Moreover, it is far more beneficial to all concerned to garner our resources and give a thorough job of the operating room than to be witch hunting on the patients habits and dirtiness. It is my belief that even a dirty patient cannot infect the inside of his or her eye, if he or she has a postsurgical infection for sure it has been carried in through the workings of the operation theatre.

Going in a methodical manner from without to within anything entering the theatre has to be sterile. First the operating room itself has to be sterile.

The Operating Room Air

The air we breathe can be filled with pollutants, viruses, bacteria and irritants such as pollen, chemical gases, odors and smog. In critical situations—military command centers and public arenas—there is also a threat of chemical and biological agents being released into the air. All these air-borne pollutants can be treated by using various technologies.

We forget about the air coming into the operating room, though, however we should understand that if this itself is clean, it is much easier to retain the cleanliness within. There are many ways of filtering clean air into the operating room. One of the easiest and best is to first make sure the rooms pertaining to the operation theatre complex are sealed shut, with only one entry into the complex. Now we need to bring in clean air into the operating rooms.

Air-Conditioning

Ideally the whole operating area complex must be air-conditioned with the units stationed well outside the complex and only ducts bringing in fresh temperature-controlled air into the complex. The air-conditioning units could be in the form of towers or split units stationed on the terrace or window firmaments outside.

Filtration of air The ducts bringing in the clean oxygenated air need to have the air passing through filters that can ward off bacteria which means they should be 0.2 micron filters. More often these filters need to be changed and or cleansed on a daily pattern.

Ultraviolet radiation Ultraviolet light bulbs could be placed in the path of the filtered air to make sure the air is disinfected as it enters the operating rooms. Alternately these bulbs could be left in the operating area and kept on throughout the night, this would also ensure clean areas the next morning after 12 hours of exposure to the ultraviolet light.

Ozone treatment Another technology gaining ground for clean air is the ozone treatment plants that generate ozone into the air. This breaks up the microorganisms and clean, disinfected air is ensured. One unit for 5000 cubic feet of air space is recommended.

Ozone is a reactive molecule comprising three atoms of oxygen. Because ozone is a reactive molecule it acts as a powerful oxidizing agent against all microbial contaminants, organic toxins and most volatile organic compounds (VOC's) and because of its short half-life it rapidly reverts to water and oxygen.

When a combination of UV, moisture and ozone are used a synergistic effect is seen. The absorption of UV by the ozone-producing highly reactive substances that effectively kill microorganisms including hard to kill spore forming bacteria.

Positive pressure A positive pressure pump is maintained to make sure the air entering the operating rooms are kept at a pressure above the rest of the area. These pumps can be installed in the ducting and positive pressure inside the operating areas would ensure that the air comes only from this area and not through leaks from windows or doors. The main door of the operating room must function for only air escaping the operating area and not for entering it.

Air curtain Entry points in the operating area would do well to have automatic door closers so that the door does not remain open unnecessarily. Also the door can be fitted with an air curtain so that the outside air is curtailed off from entering.

Quality Check

Quality check is ensured by everyday/regularly carrying out the PLATE TEST. This means leaving a bowl of clean sterile water in the room to be tested for 20 minutes. Microorganisms present in the air would settle down on the surface of the water, a small sample is taken from this and grown on a culture plate. If the sterilization techniques have been effective, the culture should be sterile in 24 to 48 hours. If the culture grows positive growth remedial means have to be taken to ensure sterile cultures.

The Operating Room Water

The water coming into the operating room needs to be free of microorganisms. After all the water with which we are cleaning the most important area of the hospital needs to be totally clean. If microorganisms are present in water then they would remain on the items cleansed and the cleaning would be bad. The water coming into the operating room must also contain adequate amounts of minerals.

Filtration

This still finds the safest use in bringing in clean water into the operating area. It could be done by many methods, ceramic is one of them. However today membrane filters seem to have replaced all else as here they bring out the fluid bereft of bacteria. Sometimes a suction pump is attached to the water jet so that the filtration can take place at a faster pace.

Reverse Osmosis

A high pressure is set about in the clean water and a system of reverse osmosis sends back the mineral content of the water while a filtration process blocks out the microbial content. In this way water is able to reach the operating room withless minerals and is absolutely sterile with no bacteria. This is also one of the techniques used in the manufacture of bottled mineral water and can be used very effectively in operating area complexes. This water is now used for cleaning the operating rooms, machines, and for surgeons while scrubbing. The water coming from such a plant is placed in a storage drum, preferably made of stainless steel.

Electronic Control

Water can be made to contain low mineral counts and no bacteria through another technique of manufacturing mineral water. This is by producing cathode and anode electrodes on two ends of the water channel. The anions and cations would respectively move to their corresponding electrodes and this would clear the fluid of mineral content. A filter present below would clear the water of microorganisms. This is another method of producing sterile bottled mineral water.

The Operating Room Walls, Floor, Ceiling and Fixtures

All elements of the operating room need to be first cleansed, then disinfected and last but not the least totally sterile. The three steps in this process can be done by three different fluids and chemicals.

Cleansing

This is best done with a soap and water wash. Every surface, every table, every chair and every fixture needs to be cleansed with a direct application of soap and water on the surface. After cleaning with this it needs to be cleaned with plain water.

Disinfection

Benzalkonium chloride solution 4.5 percent could be used as a disinfectant and as a general cleaning agent for floors.

One of the best solutions used worldwide towards the disinfection of operation theatres and consultation suites is the Bacillocid made by Bode from Germany. This contains 1,6 dihydroxy 2,5 dioxyhexane (chemically bound formaldehyde) with glutaraldehyde, benzalkonium chloride and alkyl urea derivative. A 2 percent solution is used for the operation theatre and a 0.5 percent solution for the consultation areas. With this solution all areas mopped and cleansed of vegetative organisms, fungus and viruses (Figs 6.1 to 6.3).

Formaldehyde in the form of liquid, tablets or gas has been used extensively in the past, however, today its use is put to question since culture tests have proved positive with growth even after formaldehyde sterilization.

The Operating Room Macroinstruments

All fixtures including fans, lights, air-conditioning have to be first cleansed carefully with a dry cloth and then mopped with Bacillocid so that they can be disinfected.

Chairs, stools, operating tables, trays have to be first cleansed with soap water and then mopped with Bacillocid (Fig. 6.1) and left alone for over four hours to ensure disinfection.

Care needs to be taken on operating theatre instruments like Boyles apparatus, microscopes, phaco machines, diathermy machines, suction machines, laser machines. Though delicate, these instruments need to be thoroughly cleansed

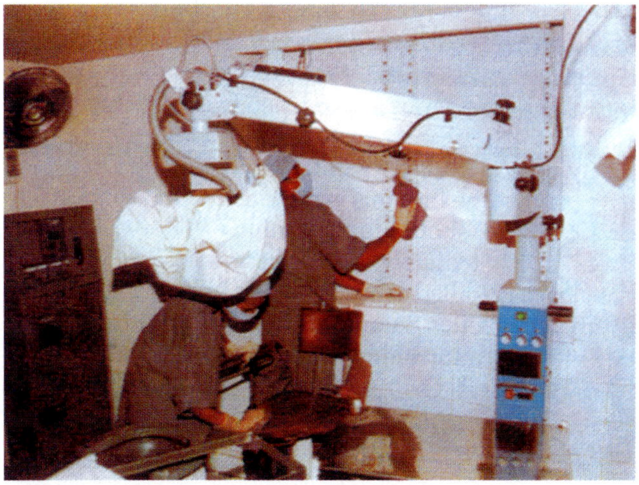

Fig. 6.1: Cleaning of the operation table and chair, external surfaces of the microscope, instrument table, IV poles with Bacillocid

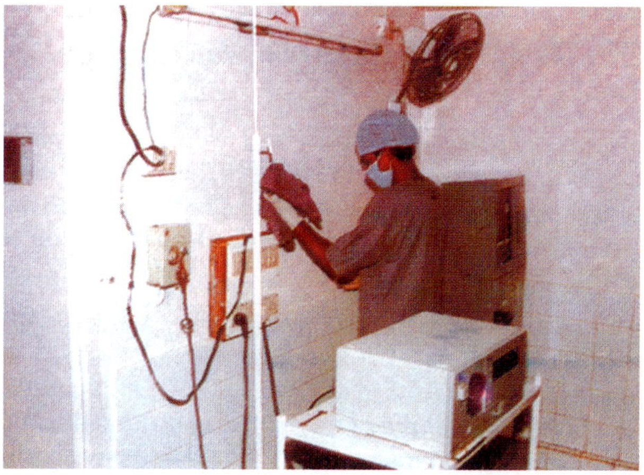

Fig. 6.2: Cleaning of the operation theatre walls with Bacillocid

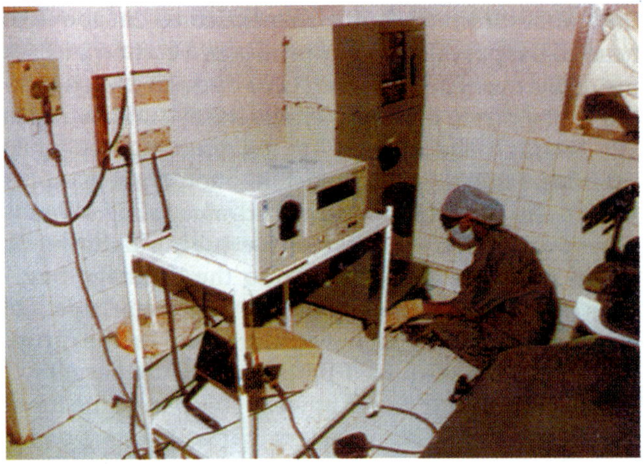

Fig. 6.3: Cleaning of the operation theatre floor with Bacillocid

everyday. Many a time infection is found to be harboring in these areas and they are difficult to clean. More sophisticated the machine more care need to be taken in its cleanliness. This task cannot be given to an untrained personnel and even then ideally there should be a doctor supervising their cleaning.

Microscope

The rest of the microscope can be cleansed with soap water as well as Bacillocid, however the optics need special care and need to cleaned only with a clean cloth preferrably silicon paper. Antifog chemical coating could be given to the optics. After cleaning and before closing for the day the optics should be ideally wrapped in its original cloth or plastic casing and drying agents placed inside like silicon oxide. This allows the moisture inside to be absorbed by the chemical and with less moisture, formation of fungus and other microorganisms on the optics is rare.

Phaco Machines

As eye surgeons we need to be well aware of the pressure maintained inside the eye during phacoemulsification procedures for cataract surgery, but little do we realize the importance of the machinery involved in giving us this information. When the phaco probe is inside the eye of the patient there is a continuous flow of fluid. The fluid arises from the bottle suspended 65 cm above the head of the patient and this produces a certain pressure inside the eye. The fluid then goes through the irrigation line to the phaco tip which enters the eye and leaves the eye through the suction tubing entering the phaco machine. From the phaco machine another set of tubings takes the excess fluid away into a drainage bag. **What we have overlooked is between the tubing entering the phaco machine and exiting into the drainage bag, it goes through a channel inside the phaco machine. This part of the tubing is never sterilized in the proper manner that is required before a cataract surgery.** In fact it cannot be sterilized as well. This part of the tubing is attached to two manometers that gauge the pressure in the tubing and give us a reading on the panel in front. A vent exists that can release the pressure in the tubing to atmospheric levels as soon as our footswitch transfers from position 3 to 2 to 1. In so doing the air from the operating room directly enters the tubings, thus if there should be bacteria in the air they would now have an easy access to the most sterile line that we have been trying to maintain.

These facts were not known to us for a long time, and we had a spate of infections as *Pseudomonas* had managed entry into the tubings present inside the phaco machine. None of the companies' representatives ever let us know of this tubing and its existence and we never racked our brains hard enough to trace the tubings, until this major catastrophy occurred. Over a spate of 12 months we had taken out 4 intraocular lenses (IOL's) from eyes with infection. We were able to save the eyes from blindness, however rendering them aphakic.

We first accepted that the infection came from the operating room and now with a technology of omission went about in a scientific manner trying to decipher where the infection came from.

First the microsurgical instruments and tubings were taken through the 10-step procedure as you will read later on. Now they were tested for sterility by flowing fluids through them and taking this fluid on a culture plate. They were sterile, after fixing the tubings and probe onto the phaco machine the fluids were collected from the drainage bag and sent for culture. The second one was positive. This told us that our sterilization techniques were good, however something was amiss.

We opened the phaco machine and found this tubing running through it and found the vent as well. This vent ideally should have an air filter attached to it. We sent the tubing for culture and replaced it with a fresh sterile piece. The culture proved to us where the culprit lay, the *Pseudomonas* was grown from this tubing.

The internal tubing cannot be changed with every case, though this would be ideal. So we have devised a better structure for its disinfection. That is to keep the air totally sterile and make sure no infection goes into the tubing through the vent. This is ensured with the ozone generator for the total operating room areas.

What we did realize through this study was that not all cases turned up with infection even though the bacteria must have been residing in the tubing for many a day. The cases turned up with infection had something to do with being the last few of the day. The cases which turned up with infection had low immune status, either diabetes or hypertension or such. The cases which turned up with infection had a complication most often a posterior capsular rupture on table thus resorting to vitrectomy. This shows us some characters of infection that we may already have known but not given them their due acknowledgement.

However, what we have realized is that the phaco machine has to be cleansed very well and air filters placed on the vent. The tubing changed every week. And culture tests done for every case before and after surgery (Figs 6.4 and 6.5). What this means is when the tubings and probe are attached to the machine before starting the case first few drops of fluid entering the drainage bag is taken for culture (Fig. 6.6). Once again at the end of the case this is repeated. If and when at any time a culture should turn positive we would know the problem immediately. After these stringent measures have been installed at our hospitals we have neither had

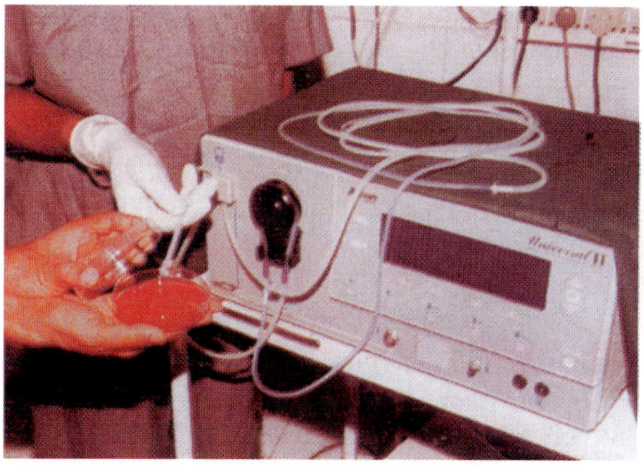

Fig. 6.5: Collection of Ringer lactate solution from the aspiration tube after the operation

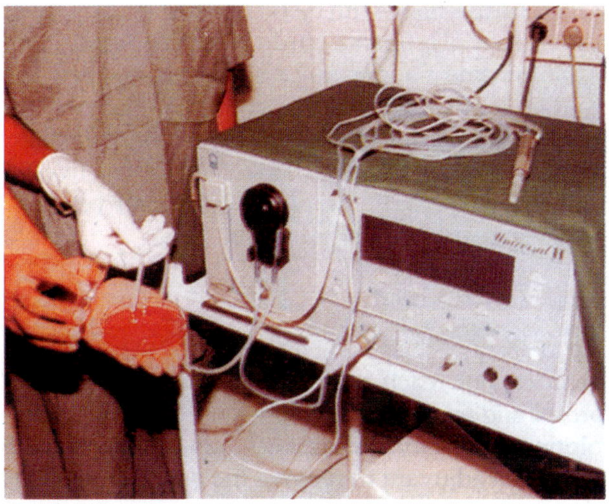

Fig. 6.4: Collection of Ringer lactate solution from the aspiration tube before the operation

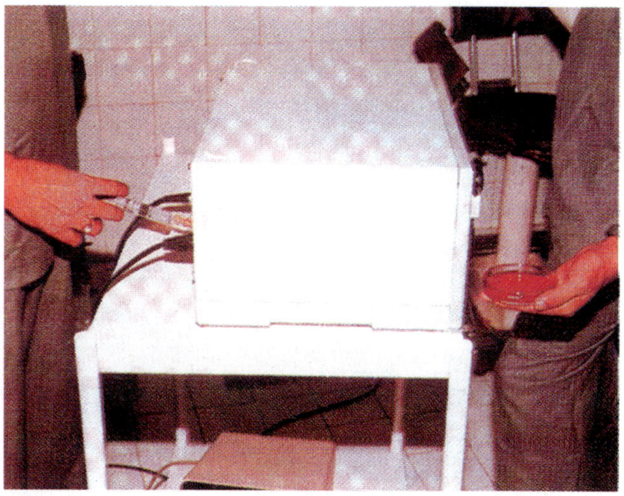

Fig. 6.6: Collection of Ringer lactate solution from the front end of the internal tubing

even one infection coming from the operating room nor had to remove any more intraocular lenses from infected eyes.

Boyles Apparatus

Regular cleaning of all parts of the machine is necessary with spirit as this evaporates and does not leave a residue on it. However the parts of the tubings that enter the human system or are connected to them need to be thoroughly cleansed, disinfected and then sterilized. The method of choice for sterilization, here is the ethylene oxide gas chambers (Fig. 6.7). As most of the tubings are plastic, temperature of below 60°C are comfortably taken by them. Needless to say that oxygen, nitrogen dioxide, halogen levels should be monitored on a daily basis with every case in particular.

The Operating Room Microinstruments

Every case must be treated separately and all instruments must be cleansed thoroughly before the next case. Once a day a 10-step cleansing routine must be established. This 10-step routine includes

1. Soap water wash with toothbrush
2. Ultrasonic cleansing with Lysol
3. Cidex cleansing and soaking for half an hour
4. Isopropyl alcohol cleansing
5. Plain sterile water cleansing
6. Plain sterile water cleansing
7. Plain sterile water cleansing
8. Boiling in sterile water
9. Ethylene oxide sterilization overnight
10. Flash autoclave sterilization three times.

Four trays are kept aside on a long side table (Fig. 6.8). Water used in this sterilization must be mineral sterile water, as this water is totally sterile, prove it by growing the water on a culture plate and making sure it is sterile. The trays are filled with the respective fluids. Each tray is numbered and labeled so that mixing does not occur.

In each tray a toothbrush and 50 ml syringe with a yellow tubing taken off from an IV set is kept. All microsurgical instruments are dipped in each tray periodically. Every instrument is cleansed delicately with gloved hands and toothbrush. When and where required every lumen of every instrument is injected with 50 ml of the liquid that it is dipped in. Thus the cleansing action is from the outside as well as from the inside of every instrument. This is specially true of probes and tubings.

Tray I with Liquid Soap and Sterile Water

The first step in sterilization of instruments is its proper cleansing as whenever the microbial load will be less on the sterilization technique used the better would be the results that can be achieved.

This is best done with the old soap and water wash (Fig. 6.9). Liquid soap is used in a tray with clean sterile mineral water. First a plain cleansing with gloved hands is completed and then using a

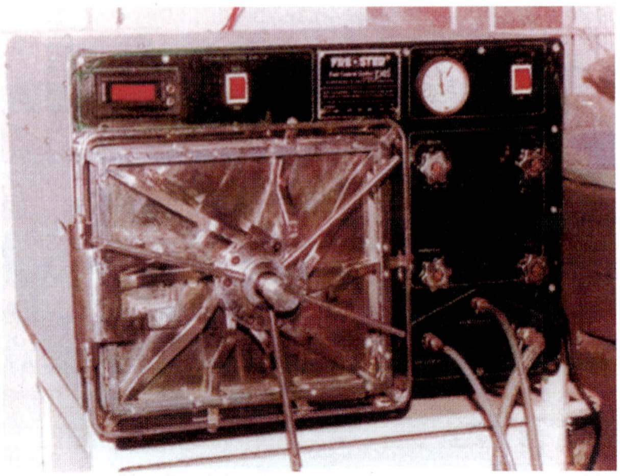

Fig. 6.7: Ethylene oxide sterilizer

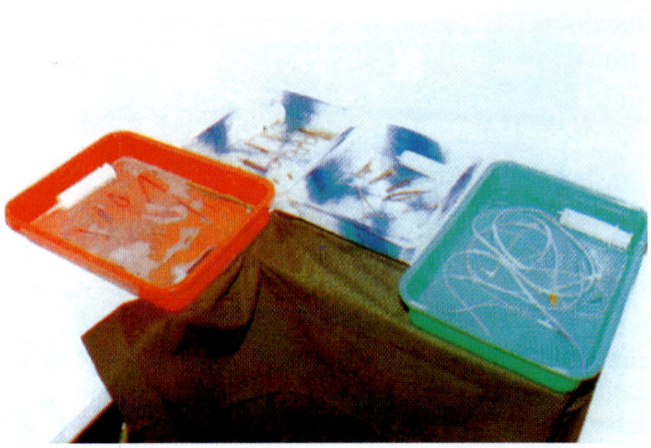

Fig. 6.8: Four trays arranged in sequence containing carbonic soap with mineral water, 2 percent glutaraldehyde, 70 percent isopropyl alcohol and mineral water

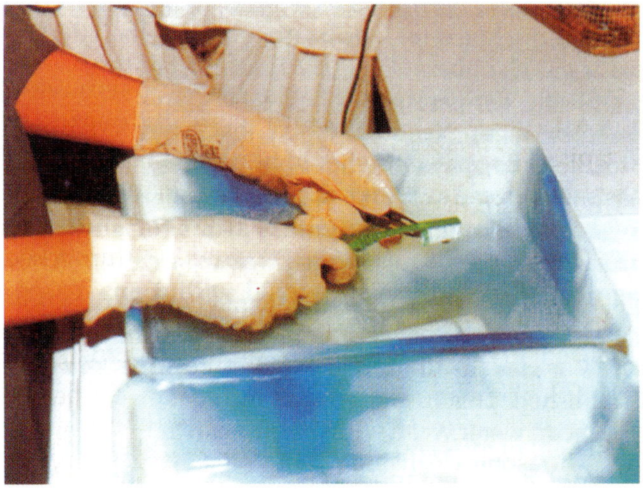

Fig. 6.9: Wash all instruments in a tray of carbonic soap and water with toothbrush

toothbrush into the small crevices of instruments. This is of special importance to instruments filled with blood and tissue. In ophthalmic matters special reference has to be given to machines like the automated flapper in LASIK (laser-assisted *in-situ* keratomileusis) cases, as it is known that corneal tissue gets clogged into the tracks and other areas of the flapper. This can be removed much better using palmolive liquid soap as it contains some of the safest and yet cleanest ways to get grid out of the system.

Ultrasonic Cleansing

The mainstay of cleansing into crevices where the toothbrush cannot reach and this gets into the fulcrum of forceps and scissors to clean the instruments. A chemical solution like Lysol (Cresol and soap solution) could be used as an adjuvant to remove the debris from clogged surfaces. This breaks up the protein and organic matter so that it can come clean from instrument surfaces. Most of the fluids used in the ultrasonic cleanser need to be antiseptics as well so they can be used as disinfectants on the instruments cleaned.

Cidex or Glutaraldehyde 2%

Once activated Cidex solution manufactured by Johnsons & Johnsons must be used within 14 days. Some facts like these go unnoticed in hospital environments and the use of substandard procedures and drugs come into play. Reiterating the fact that the doctor has to be on top of all these activities.

Instruments are left immersed in this solution (Fig. 6.10) for 30 minutes, which is sufficient time for disinfection however for sterilization 10 hours would be needed. Within 10 minutes at room temperature most vegetative organisms would be destroyed, including *Pseudomonas*, fungi, and viruses. The solution is very toxic to the eye and great care has to be taken to get the solution out of the instruments before using on humans.

Isopropyl Alcohol 70%

This is still one of the best ways of killing the microorganisms (Fig. 6.11). Instruments are soaked in the solution for over 15 minutes and then cleansed using a toothbrush and syringe to wash the internal elements of probes and tubings.

Sterile Water

Care must be taken to wash off the deleterious effects of the above mentioned solutions. This is done effectively by first soaking and then washing all the instruments through three trays of sterile water (Fig. 6.12). The lumen of the tubings must be cleansed with sterile water each time 50 ml of the fluid passing through the probes and tubings.

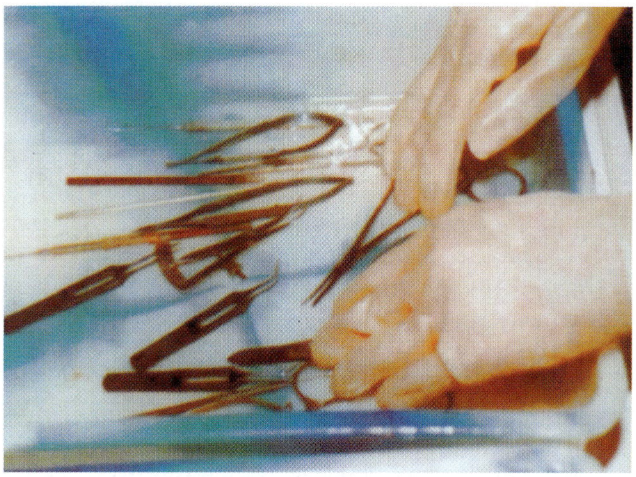

Fig. 6.10: Wash all instruments in a tray of 2 percent glutaraldehyde

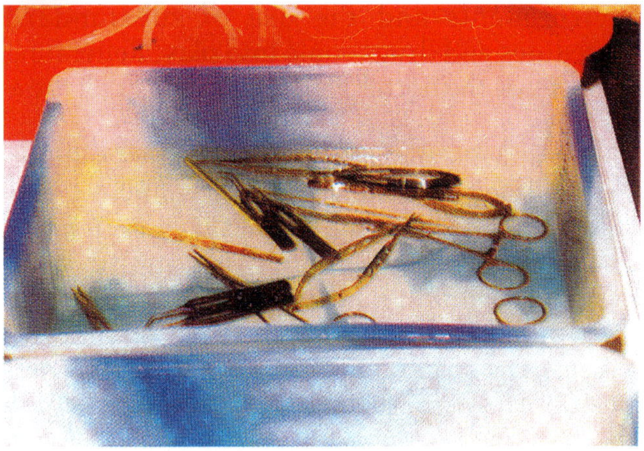

Fig. 6.11: Wash all instruments in a tray of 70 percent isopropyl alcohol

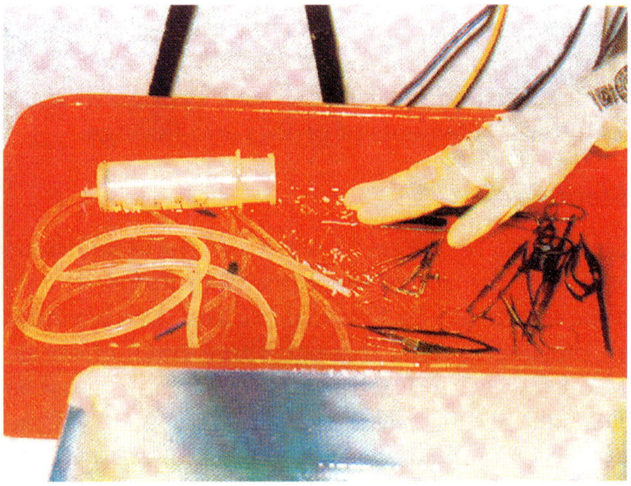

Fig. 6.12: Wash all instruments in a tray of mineral water

Sterile Water

Once again cleansed with sterile water

Sterile Water

Once again cleansed with sterile water

Boiling

After going through a number of tests and methods of sterilization we still find one of the best methods remains the age-old custom of boiling. This brings about total death of the microorganisms. Most rudimentary of operation theatres would still contain means and methods of performing this essential act of sterilization. However, what needs to be detailed is whether the particular article can withstand temperatures of over 100°C.

After having a spate of infections and removing IOLs from infected eyes to save the eyes, my hospital and staff got spurned to find the cause of the infection. Towards this a whole new regimen was set up on cleansing, disinfection and sterilization of microsurgical instruments. After each methodology culture tests would be taken to prove its efficacy. We did understand that the silicon tubings had gram-positive cocci growing in them. In a process of eliminating them we found that the cocci inside the silicon tubing withstood many sterilization techniques like ethylene oxide and autoclave. However, when subjected to boiling for 20 minutes the tubings would be sterile. This once again reiterated our belief in this age-old custom of boiling (Figs 6.13 to 6.15).

Ethylene Oxide Sterilization

This is not a preferred technology of sterilization for microsurgical instruments because of the time duration taken is over 16 hours. However, we have started using this as one more step toward the end of the day. By the time we finish all the cases of the day we take our instruments through this 10-step procedure ending it with a bout of ethylene oxide where the instruments rest for the night. However, the only aspect of this technology is that the

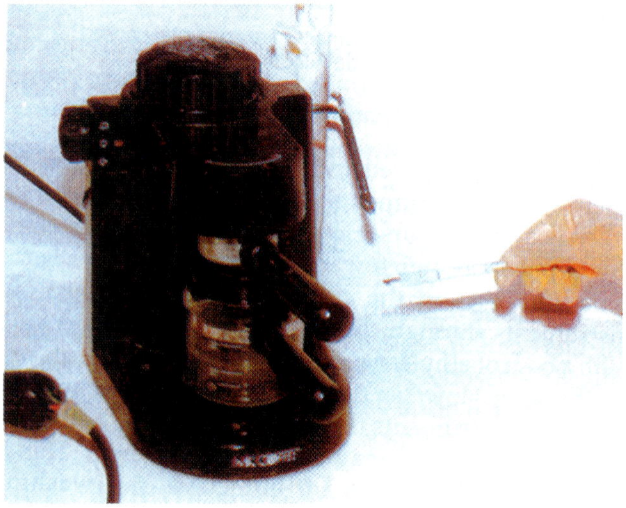

Fig. 6.13: Diamond blades are cleaned using steam

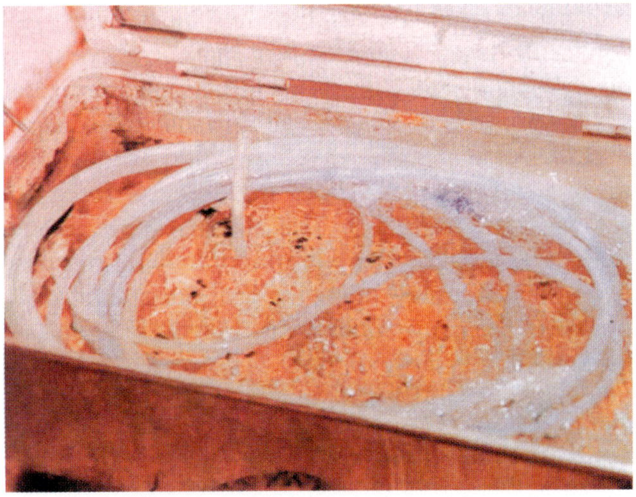

Fig. 6.14: The external tubings, internal tubings, I/A probe and metal knobs are boiled for 30 minutes

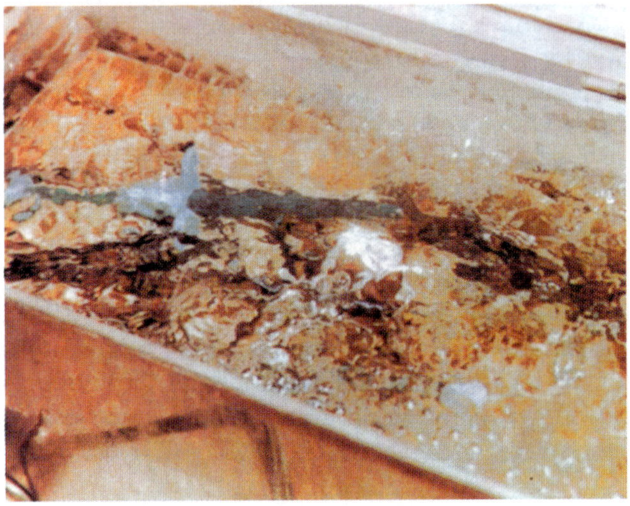

Fig. 6.15. The instruments are separately boiled for 30 minutes

instruments must be cleansed of the ethylene glycol residues that may be found over them. This is effectively done by steam autoclave and washing intraocular instruments with Ringer lactate meant for intravenous use.

Autoclave

As the last step in the sterilization cycle of instruments, they are passed through the flash autoclave for 134°C for 5 minutes and this cycle is repeated three times in the Statim autoclave from Canada (Fig. 6.16). It has a built-in computer that

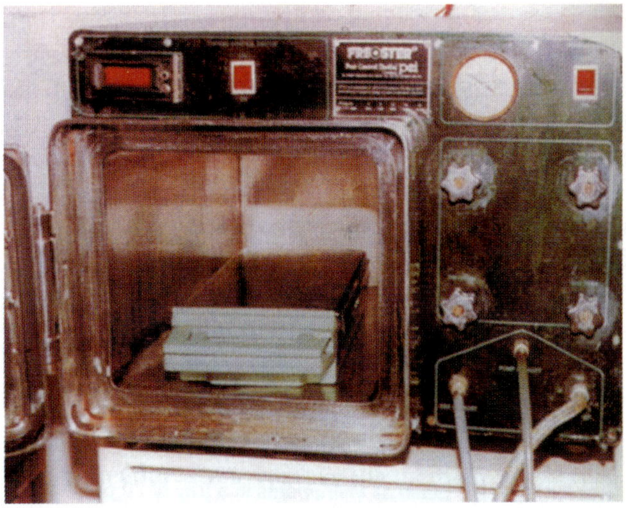

Fig. 6.16: Statim autoclave cassette containing the tubings and instruments is kept in the ethylene oxide sterilizer for a period of six hours

tells us of the efficiency of the cycle. However color indicators would also tell us of the physical measurements reaching the desired levels.

After doing this the instruments are laid on the operating table and each instrument that enters the eye is dipped in Ringer lactate before entering the eye.

The Operating Room Linen and Accessories

All operation theatre linen and accessories must be cleansed before entering the complex. Particular slots should be kept ready and clean for them everyday. Otherwise the operation theatre should be totally bereft of any other article. Anything that is not used everyday need not be found in the operating room. This is not the place to keep stocks and inventory of medicines. They could be kept in the prefunction area of the operating room but not in the operating room itself.

Linen

Sterile operation theatre gowns, towels, gloves could be of disposable variety, this is internationally accepted to be the best. However it is not practical in all kinds of atmospheres. In India we still recycle our operating clothes which are usually made of cloth. The methodology approached toward their care is explained in the same 3-step procedure.

Cleaning This is done by taking all the sullied clothes and first taking away all clothes coming from an infected patient being operated or from the septic operation theatre are treated separately than that coming from a clean operating room. These clothes are preferably disposed off in an incinerator. If they cannot then they are soaked in Dettol solution, before the cleaning process begins.

The clothes are cleansed preferably in a washing machine with adequate soap being used. Then the clothes are passed into a drying machine. Try not to leave these clothes on the drying rope for nature to dry, because with this outside bacteria and fungus can settle on these clothes. Inadvertently they may fly off the clothes line and this would also create much increase of the microbial load for sterilization.

However if machinery is not available these clothes are first soaked for half an hour in hot water with soap solution inside a large tub. A rod is taken and rotated round and round for five minutes. This will shake off the dirt and grind from the clothes.

After this each cloth is taken separately and washed with hand and the clothes thrown into another tub of hot water with a few drops of Dettol solution in it. The clothes are left for another half an hour in this solution and then rinsed off with plain water.

A separate enclosure should be made for the drying of these clothes. When the clothes are placed on the clothesline they should be pinned there as they may fly and hit the floor picking up germs. This could be avoided. Once dry they are picked up, folded and sealed for sterilization.

Sterilization Clothes could be sterilized by two methods, whichever method is used what is important is that they be folded away keeping each procedure in mind. That is to say if for one cataract procedure we need three operating gowns, ten towels and six shoulder bags, then they should be folded in such a way that these are all kept together. One does not have to search for the small items by opening up every item sterilized.

Autoclave: This still finds the pride of place in being the most accepted form of sterilization. However one needs to be aware that the clothes must not come out damp. The steam in the autoclave must be saturated but dry. This means all the water vapor present in the air should be gas and no droplets of water in the steam. **If an autoclave is giving out damp clothes that means it is not working efficiently.** The drums kept in the autoclave must be closed immediately on removal from the autoclave, ensuring that outside air does not enter the drum. Once autoclaved the items can be considered sterile for only 24 hours which means to say they need to be reautoclaved to improve efficiency in sterilization techniques.

Ethylene oxide sterilization: With todays emphasis on better sterilization techniques and total dependence on them, a move has come into using the gas industrial sterilization for hospital purposes. As there is more surety on its efficacy this is even a preferred technology over the autoclave. However it does have its drawbacks which are that the hospital needs to keep a bigger inventory. This is due to the fact that these clothing need to be aired out for over 48 hours before they can come into contact with human skin. Easily achieved by having four times the number of gowns and towels one would ordinarily keep.

The advantage of ethylene oxide sterilization for linen over autoclave is that we never get damp clothing which should be regarded as not sterile. Moreover, the personnel are always sure of ready stocks for operating at any time. We do not have to start the autoclave and wait for sterilization, we always have sterile clothing ready.

Sealing and packing **In ethylene oxide sterilization the methodology employed toward its packaging is very important.** High-grade thick plastic bags could be used, alternately custom-designed bags are available for ethylene oxide sterilization. However, these custom-designed bags are more expensive than plain plastic bags used commercially.

Sealing of these bags has to be immaculate as any porthole left gaping will now allow the atmospheric air containing microbes into the bag and once the seal is broken the contents are not any more registered as sterile. Sealing machines are available in the market and their use is much better than burning the bags with a candle and sealing them.

Ethylene oxide chamber The ethylene oxide (ETO) gas comes compressed in gas cylinders that are attached to the machine. These machines which use the gas cylinder have a vacuum pump attached which first empties the air in the ETO chamber, then we let in the compressed ethylene oxide gas and leave it at about 50°C for over 6 to 12 hours. Now when the chamber has to be opened, once again the vacuum pump empties the gas out. The outlet from the machine needs to be placed 6 ft above and outside into the atmosphere. This gas is toxic and its inadvertent entry inside the hospital premises is a health hazard for personnel. Care must be taken that the outlet tubing is placed well outside the hospital premises, onto the terrace if possible.

Once the ETO has escaped out the atmospheric air is let in and the chamber pressure maintained at atmospheric pressure before it is opened. The materials can now be kept on a shelf for airing. The shelf should be just racks with ample room on either side for the gas to escape from its whereabouts. The linen can be now used as sterile after 48 hours of airing.

Alternately gas ampoules are present which can be placed inside the chamber, these ETO gas ampoules need neither the vacuum pump nor the temperature maintenance and can be easily placed inside a big plastic bag also prescribed by the company that manufactures the ETO gas ampoules. All the clothing is stacked after sealing inside the big plastic bag that occupies the whole of the gas chamber. The ampoule is broken and this allows the ETO gas to permeate through the whole closed plastic bag inside the chamber. This is left so for 12 hours and for another 14 hours when the gas escapes the chamber. After which the contents can be taken out and placed on airing shelves.

Medication

Parenteral

IV fluids and intraocular fluids: Fluids used inside the eye should be regarded as not sterile unless proved otherwise. Toward this exercise we sterilize all our fluids, like Ringer lactate, saline and even 2 percent methylcellulose. Many a surgeon in developing countries has suffered immense loss by placing Ringer lactate into the eye without prior sterilization. *E. coli* has been known to be grown from these fluids. At the moment of an infection occurring not just one eye will be lost, but the whole batch of Ringer lactate would and will be used on several eyes at a time and many losses have been reported. From the Ringer lactate one surgeon lost over 12 eyes to infection from the fluid. This cannot be really taken as a mistake as we understand that fluids meant for IV therapy must be totally sterile, however this is not always the case.

So to protect our patients from such a malady occurring we resterilize these bottles in the autoclave. It is preferrable to use glass bottles. Studies have shown the plastic polymers react with the fluids and can have drastic effects on the cornea of patients. Thus, world over glass is a preferred carrier for use of fluids inside the eye. Moreover, plastic bottles cannot be autoclaved as they would melt with the over 100°C needed for autoclave sterilization.

Even when we are sterilizing these glass bottles care has to be taken in their placement in the autoclave bins. Autoclave indicator stickers are used on every bottle. The bottles are placed head up, and kept in the bin with space all around. Preferrably wrapped in some cloth towel so that should they inadvertently break and blow up, they would do so inside the wrapping. Care has to be taken to let the fluids reach a level of below 80°C temperature before opening the autoclave chamber as they may blow up on exposure to room temperature.

All fluids used inside the eye are kept at 4°C for better trauma control on the eye. As we know cold itself is an anesthetic and controls blood vessels by constricting them, we prefer to use cold fluids inside the eye. This would also ensure better control on the delicate tissues of the eye and less trauma as well.

Methylcellulose 2% (VISCON): Much the same technology is used in autoclaving methylcellulose. Glass containers are once again preferred as plastic would react with the fluids inside. The vials are kept wrapped in cloth and placed inside the autoclave bins. Once sterile these are shifted into a refrigerator to keep them at 4°C, the preferred temperature for methylcellulose as we know at this temperature the viscosity is the greatest and best for intraocular use.

All other medication: These too need our undivided attention as to their expiry. Most drugs are not re-sterilized since the methodologies used might just denature the medication. However, place has to be kept in the operating area complex for essential medication necessary during the course of a surgery. These medicines should not be stocked inside the main operating room but in prefunction area.

Care needs to be taken regularly to keep dusting and keeping the area where medicines are kept to be clean and free from germs. Thus to do so everyday this area must be cleaned, drawers, shelves all cleaned with plain cloth and at least once a week with soap water and/or Bacillocid.

Probes and Tubings

All probes and tubings are usually of disposable variety, and they could be kept in clean shelves or drawers with names written on the outside.

Alternately today we could recycle probes and tubings by first cleaning them well and then passing them through ethylene oxide sterilization. However these tubings and probes are usually made of plastic and for the gas sterilization to be totally safe and non-toxic they need to be kept on the shelf for airing for over 15 days. So the date and time of ETO sterilization needs to be marked on the color indicators when sterilizing these items.

A preferred methodology for sharp instruments to be sterilized is also the ETO chamber, some of these sharp instruments like disposable knives are also made of plastic handles, which can withstand ETO temperatures but not the autoclave. These too need to be kept on a shelf for 15 days before use on human tissues.

The I/A probes, the internal tubing, external tubing, rectal knibs are all cleaned with various disinfectants (Figs 6.17 to 6.26).

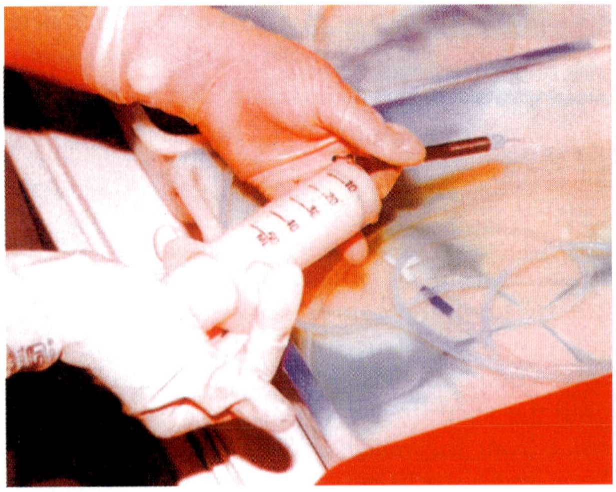

Fig. 6.17: Flushing of I/A probe with 70 percent isopropyl alcohol passing 200 ml of alcohol into every lumen

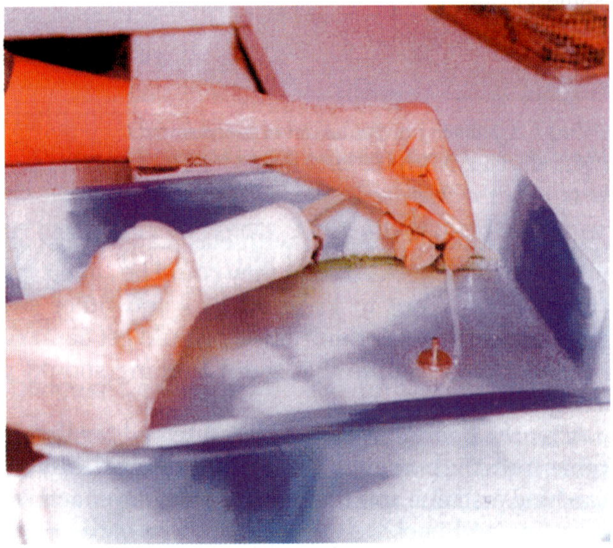

Fig. 6.18: Flushing of the lumen of the internal tubing and the metal knobs with carbonic soap and mineral water passing 200 ml of the same into the lumen

The Operating Room Personnel

Most often surgeons like to operate in the morning, sometimes they need to operate through the whole day, however, it is a good exercise to see that all operating area personnel have a regular bath first thing in the morning before entering the operating area. All street clothing and footwear should be removed before entering the operating area. Thus most hospitals would keep the changing rooms as the first area of the operating area complex.

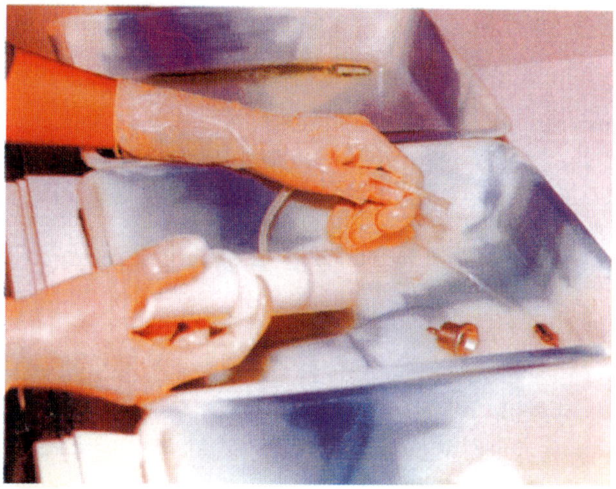

Fig. 6.19: Flushing of the lumen of the internal tubing and the metal knobs with 2 percent glutaraldehyde passing 200 ml of the same into the lumen

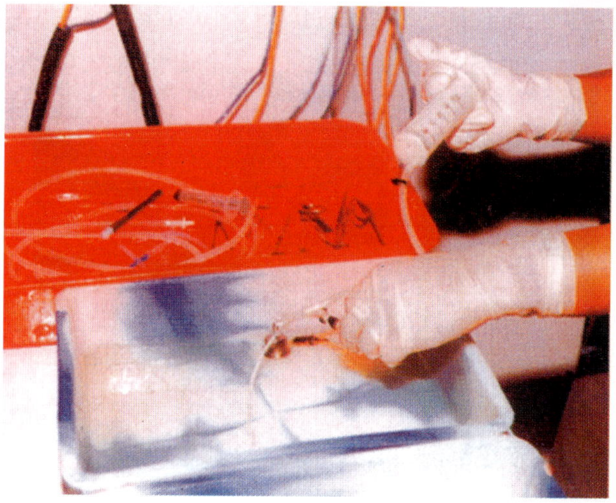

Fig. 6.20: Flushing of the lumen of the internal tubing and the metal knobs with 70 percent isopropyl alcohol passing 200 ml of alcohol into the lumen

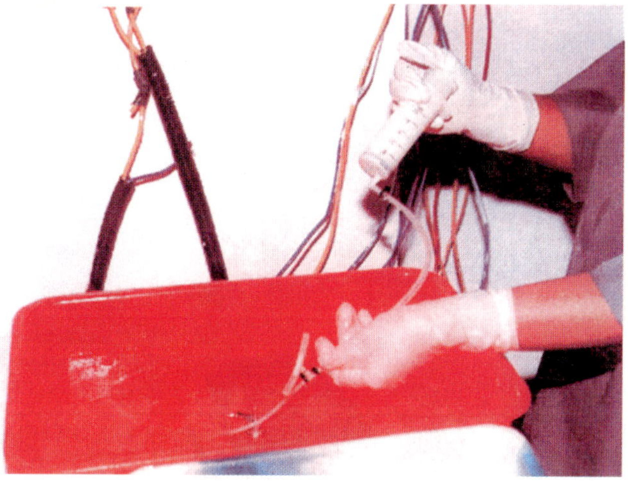

Fig. 6.21: Flushing of the lumen of the internal tubing and the metal knobs with mineral water passing 200 ml of the same into the lumen

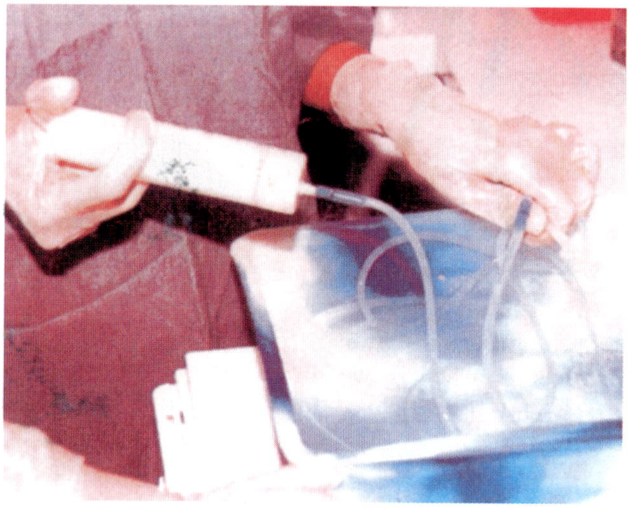

Fig. 6.22: Flushing of the lumen of the external tubing with carbonic soap and mineral water passing 200 ml of the same into the lumen

Footwear

Separate areas should be demarcated to keep footwear. This should be kept outside the operating area complex. However, sometimes they could be kept just inside the door as we have seen many a surgeon goes in taking out his or her shoes and when he or she comes back his or her shoes are gone. This is specially true if he or she wears lovely expensive new shoes.

The personnel take off their shoes and are given alternate operating area clogs, slippers or sandals. The operating area footwear should also undergo vigorous cleaning procedures everyday. At the end of the day, all the footwear is taken in and washed with soap water and cleansed with plain water and left for drying.

Clothing

After changing the footwear all clothing needs to be changed. A changing room has to be kept clean and with lockers so that operating room personnel can keep their clothes and valuables safely. The

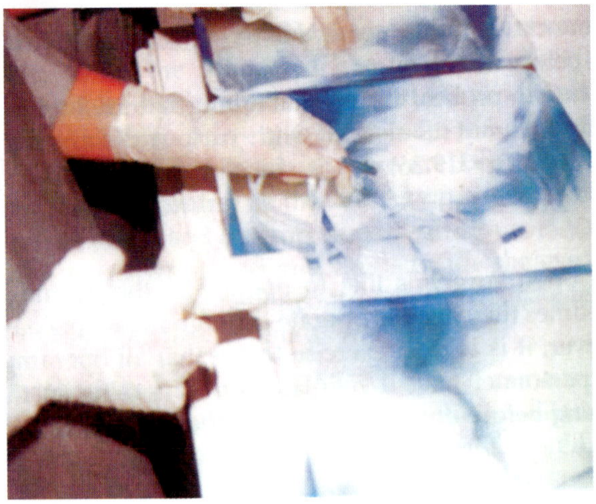

Fig. 6.23: Flushing of the lumen of the external tubing with 2 percent glutaraldehyde passing 200 ml of the same into the lumen

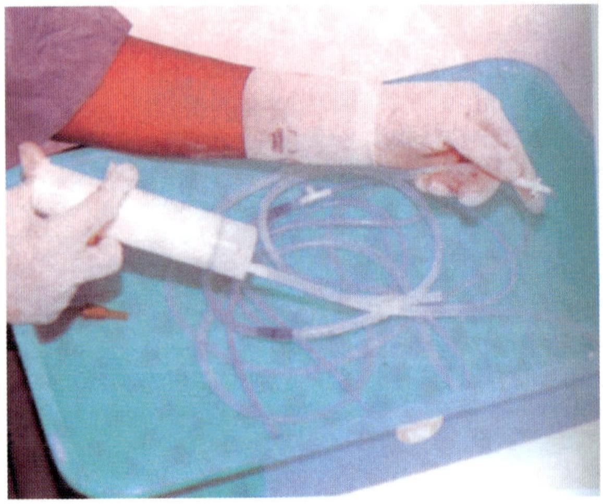

Fig. 6.24: Flushing of the lumen of the external tubings with 70 percent isopropyl alcohol passing 200 ml of alcohol into the lumen

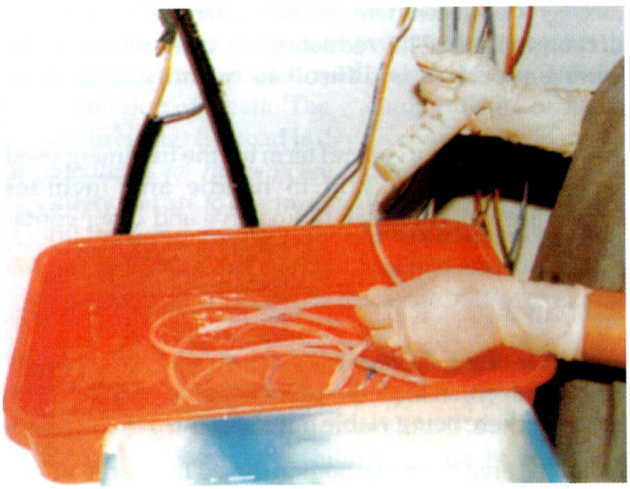

Fig. 6.25: Flushing of the lumen of the external tubings with mineral water passing 200 ml of same into the lumen

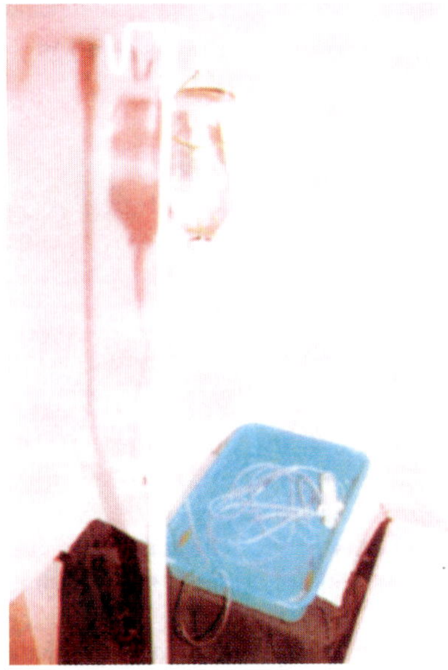

Fig. 6.26: 100 ml of Ringer lactate solution is passed through the lumen of the internal tubings, external tubings, I/A probe and metal knobs

most often used personnel clothing are pant with elasticated waist and shirts with loose necks so that they could be slided into. It is preferrable not to keep buttons and other such accessories on these clothing as they would get damaged in the vigorous routine that these clothing should go through.

After the operation theatre has finished for the day clothes from the personnel lockers are taken ideally into a washing machine and then through the dryer and sent for sealing and packing through ethylene oxide sterilization ready for use four days from the day of sterilization. Toward this rigmarole the hospital would need to keep six times the number of clothes actually required.

However, if this is not possible the clothes could be washed by hand dried and then sent into the autoclave for sterilization. In these clothes one is not really looking for sterility but for disinfection and thus it is better to go a step further and make them sterile before use.

Cap and Mask

The cap and mask need not be sterile, however they should be clean and disinfected. Ideally the cap and mask used can be of disposable variety since their cleaning will then not become necessary. However, if they are not and the hospital needs to use cloth cap and mask, they can go through the same cycle of events like the other clothing.

The Patient

The patient should also be made to go through a process to make him or her clean and disinfected. Ideally all patients should be told to have a bath before they go in for elective planned surgery. This simple process does give large benefits. Shaving, where men are concerned is essential and removal of make-up is necessary, where women are concerned.

Change of Clothes

The patient should change into operating room clothes and take out all street clothes. Footwear has to be removed before entering the operating room. Ideally patients are requested to remove all their clothing including undergarments and a patient gown given to them. This is done in the benefit of the patient so that at any particular time should an emergency procedure be called for it can be applied without interference from essential clothing. Moreover, all patients need to be monitored for their heart and blood oxygen, these electrodes are usually placed close to the heart.

However, in ophthalmic practice it is customary in a day care surgical center that the clothes need not come off the patient. Simple removal of shoes and shirt or dress is sufficient. Patients are then given sterile disposable gowns that can be worn over their undergarments. This process is found to be satisfactory for ophthalmic patients.

All patients are also given a disposable cap so that all hair can be placed inside the cap and not interfere in surgical procedures.

Skin and Incision Site Disinfection

Many solutions are available for wound disinfection some of the best used worldwide are povidone-iodine and chlorhexidine gluconate 1.5 percent with cetrimide 7.5 percent. All these antiseptics will be put to better use if they are used in conjunction with simple cleaning procedures first.

The patient's face could be washed with soap and water and all jewellery and accessories removed. Once the patient lies down on the operating table and is ready for surgery, a scrubbed nurse paints povidone-iodine or any other antiseptic on the skin. This is removed with plain gauze.

If anesthesia is necessary it can be given now after preliminary cleaning of the site. After injections are given the site to be operated is once again cleansed by a scrubbed personnel with antiseptic solution.

Sterile Disposable Surgical Drape

Where the eye is concerned, in todays world the lashes do not have to be cut for intraocular surgery. However, whenever this is not done, then a plastic surgical disposable sterile drape is used over the eyes. This has a gummy on the undersurface, keeping the eyes open the surgeon places the gummy directly on the cornea and keeps the lashes turned out so that they could stick to the gummy surface and keep out of the surgical field.

The drape used in the ophthalmic field manufactured by Dr. Agarwal's Pharma is also equipped with a drainage bag. So, once the drape is stuck to the patient's eye, the central plastic over the palpebral fissure is cut open with sterile scissors after the surgeon has scrubbed and changed.

A whole 20 cc of sterile refrigerated 4°C Ringer lactate fluid is squirted over the eye, to carry out a thorough cleaning procedure as well as to produce cryoanalgesia. The surgery can now be started. This cleaning process is found to be very necessary for a clean fornix and conjunctival sac.

STERILIZERS

Methods of Sterilization

For a very long time we had no idea that sterilization is the basis of surgical correction, after all performing the best of surgery though introducing harmful microbes could mar the effects of surgery irreparably. With the advent of the autoclave in 1884 we got to know a lot of details. However, most surgical ward history can be detailed as that before Lister and the era after Lister as this one person was responsible in explaining antiseptic surgery as we understand it today.

Terminology

To better understand this vast and varied aspect of surgery, first let us understand the terms and conditions often used.

Sterilization is a process used to achieve sterility—an absolute term meaning the absence of all viable micro-organisms.

Disinfection is a process which reduces the number of contaminating microorganisms, particularly those liable to cause infection, to a level which is deemed no longer harmful to health.

Antisepsis is used to describe disinfection applied to living tissue such as a wound.

Cleaning is a soil-removing process which removes many microorganisms. The reduction in contamination by cleaning processes is difficult to quantify other than visually.

Decontamination is a general term for the treatment used to make equipment safe to handle and includes microbiological, chemical, radioactive and other contamination.

Sterilization

An article may be regarded as sterile if it can be demonstrated that there is a probability of less than 1 in a million of there being viable micro-organisms on it.

Methods Five main methods are used for sterilization.

Head: A widely used method needs to reach temperatures above 100°C to ensure bacterial spores are killed.

Moist heat is more effective than dry as it coagulates and denatures the protein, where water participates in the reaction. This requires 121°C for 15 min with moist heat.

Temperatures above that of boiling water can be attained more easily by raising the pressure in a vessel, this is the principle of the autoclave. At sea level water would boil and produce steam at 100°C, increasing the pressure to 2.4 bar would produce steam at 125°C and increasing to 3 bar at 134°C. However at subatmospheric pressures this temperature would fall, thus at higher altitudes water will boil at lower temperatures.

1. *Quality of steam for sterilization* Steam is non-toxic and non-corrosive, though for sterilization it should also be saturated, which means it should hold all the water it can hold. It must also be dry, so it should not contain water droplets. This has a greater lethal action and is quicker in heating up the article to be sterilized.

When dry saturated steam meets a cooler surface it condenses into a small amount of water and liberates latent heat of vaporization. The energy available from this latent heat is considerable. For example, 6 liters of steam at a temperature of 134°C will condense into 10 ml of water and liberate 2162 J of heat energy. By comparison less than 100 J of heat energy is released by the sensible heat from air at 134°C to an article in contact with dry heat.

Steam at a higher temperature than the corresponding pressure would allow is referred to as superheated steam and behaves like hot air. Steam with water droplets is called wet steam and is less efficient.

2. *Types of steam sterilizers*

A. *Sterilizers for porous loads:* For linen, and wrapped instruments, so air could get trapped in the textiles used. Thus, this type of sterilizer should have a vacuum-assisted air removal stage to ensure that adequate air is removed from the load before admission of steam. The vacuum pulsing of air also ensures that the load is dry on completion of cycle.

B. *Sterilizers for fluids in sealed containers:* Must have a safety feature to ensure that the door cannot be opened till the temperature in the glass containers has fallen below 80°C. Otherwise the thermal stress of cold air on opening the door may cause the bottles to explode under pressure.

C. *Sterilizers for unwrapped instruments and utensils:* These should not be used for wrapped articles, recommended for dental clinics and LASIK stations.

D. *Laboratory sterilizers:* Culture media in containers, laboratory glassware and equipment may be contaminated, thus proper cleansing is necessary before sterilization.

3. *Monitoring of steam sterilizers:* Every load everyday every time needs monitoring of some important physical measurements.

- Temperature
- Pressure
- Time with thermometers.

Detailed tests are undertaken with temperature-sensitive probes (thermocouples) inserted into standard test packs. Though most indicators show color change on reaching particular temperatures.

Biological indicators comprising dried spore suspensions of a reference heat-resistant bacterium *Bacillus stearothermopiles,* are not used for routine testing. Although spore indicators are essential for low-temperature gaseous processes in which the physical measurements are very little to kill spores or not reliable. Most often used for ethylene oxide sterilization.

Bowie-Dick test monitors penetration of steam into wrapped pack and detects uneven steam penetration by a bubble of residual air in the pack.

Dry heat causes a destructive oxidation of the essential cell constituents. Thus killing spores here requires 160°C for 2 hours. This may also cause charring of paper, cotton, organic material.

4. *Types of sterilization by dry heat*

A. *Incineration:* Most cities around the world have made it mandatory for most hospitals to have incinerators in their campus for efficient waste disposal where contaminated materials like dressings, sharp needles and other clinical wastes. The high temperatures reached kills all organisms and disposes by charring and burning the material.

B. *Red heat:* Diathermy in ophthalmic hospitals would be done by burning a loop over a flame, this would sterilize as well as cauterize the bleeding vessel. However, this is still used to sterile loops, wires, points of forceps. It is a still very much used in emergency situations.

C. *Flaming:* Inoculating loops and needles are sometimes treated by immersing them in methylated spirit and burning off the alcohol, though this does not produce a sufficiently high temperature for sterilization. This is also done for sterilizing drums and trays over which sterile linen is placed. Once again this is not totally sterile as spores may persist over the short-term flame that is produced with alcohol.

D. *Hot and sterilizer:* Oil, powders, carbon steel instruments, and empty glassware laboratory dishes are sterilized with hot air sterilizers, though the over-all heating up and cooling may take several hours.

E. *Microwave sterilizer:* This is the latest in roads into sterilizers and can offer better results than hot air sterilizers with shorter time spans. Within 10 minutes the material can be sterilized. However, because of the high temperatures reached, it is not very good for organic material or plastics. Very good for microwave transparent material like glass.

5. *Factors influencing sterilization by heat would include*:

A. *Temperature and time:* They are inversely related, i.e. shorter time higher temperatures, holding time is important loading and cooling time would make the total time much longer (Table 6.1).

Table 6.1: Relationship between temperature and time

Process	*Temp (in°C)*	*Hold time (min)*
Dry heat	160	120
	170	60
	180	30
Moist heat	121	15
	126	10
	134	3

B. *Microbial load:* The number of organisms and spores affects the rapidity of sterilization. Thus, it is better to go through vigorous cleaning procedures before sterilization of products.

Ionizing radiation: Both beta (electrons) and gamma (photons) irradiation are employed industrially for the sterilization of single use disposables.

All accelerated electrons are lethal to living cells, that includes, γ-rays, β-rays, X-rays. Bacterial spores are the most resistant. Sterilization is achieved by the use of high-speed electrons from a machine such as a linear accelerator or by an isotope source such as cobalt-60, a dose of 255 kGy is generally adequate, making this an industrial process. It is used for single use prepackaged items like plastic syringes and catheters.

Filtration: Filters are used to remove bacteria and other larger organisms from liquids that are liable to be spoiled by heating. Though virus can crossover they are felt to be unimportant.

Filters using pore size of less than 0.45 microns can render fluids free of bacteria. It is used in the preparation of toxins and thermolabile parenteral fluids such as antibiotic solutions, radiopharmaceuticals, and blood products. Viruses and some bacteria-like mycoplasmas can pass through pore size of less than 0.22 microns.

Filter materials could be unglazed ceramic Chamberland filters, asbestos Seitz filters and sintered glass filters. Though now membrane filters are usually used made of cellulose esters or other polymers.

Sterilant gases: Ethylene oxide is used for sterilization of plastics and other thermolabile material. Formaldehyde in combination with subatmospheric steam is more commonly used in hospitals for reprocessing thermolabile equipment. Both processes are toxic and carry hazards to user and patient.

1. *Ethylene oxide:* Highly penetrative, non-corrosive and microcidal gas which is used to in industry for single use, heat-sensitive medical devices such as prosthetic heart valves and plastic catheters. Ethylene oxide sterilization is usually carried out at temperatures below 60°C in conditions of high relative humidity. To ensure sterility, material should be exposed to a gas concentration of 700 to 1000 mg/l at 45 to 60°C and a relative humidity above 70 percent for about 2 hours. Care must be taken because of toxicity to personnel, flammability and explosion risk. The sterilized product must be aerated to remove residual ethylene oxide before it can be safely used on the patient, and turn round time is consequently slow.

Some recommendations for boosting infection control as well as cut costs on EO sterilization :

- Cleaning is a necessary and important activity before sterilization. I feel that you need to adopt standardized and effective cleaning method.
- Further the items cleaned have to be dried as any wet item will react with ethylene oxide and the efficacy may be reduced.
- The items have to be packed in one of the three materials: linen, paper or plastic. Each has its advantage but the limitation is the period that you can store these sterilized items. You can use plastic bags which are of a proper grade and store the product up to one year after sterilization.
- The sealer used for sealing packs is inappropriate if the heating is too weak for the packaging material used. This results in small holes in pack after sealing. An impulse heat sealer capable of sealing at higher temperatures.
- A safe EO machine which can complete the process of aeration within all items can be used directly without any further handling.
- Aeration is a natural process which can be hastened by installing an aerator.

2. *Low temperature steam and formaldehyde:* A combination process of steam generated at subatmospheric pressure 70 to 80°C and formaldehyde gives an effective sporicidal process. It is appropriate for heat-sensitive articles that can resist temperatures of 80°C.

3. *Propylene oxide:* One of the latest and new techniques is the use of propylene oxide which is a microcidal gas. It has a similar use and toxic effect like propylene oxide.

Sterilant liquids: Glutaraldehyde is generally the least effective and most unreliable method.

Disinfection

Disinfection is applied in circumstances where sterility is unnecessary or impractical, like bedpans, eating utensils, bed linen and other such items. Similarly the skin around the site for an invasive procedure should be cleansed to reduce chances of wound infection.

Cleaning

Thorough cleaning is a prerequisite for successful disinfection and is a process of disinfection by itself. This can be enhanced by ultrasonic baths given to the instruments to remove dried debris.

Methods

Heat: Steam or water could be used

1. Moist heat is the first method of choice, can be precisely controlled, leaves no toxic residues and does not promote the development of resistant strains. Washing or rinsing laundry or eating utensils in water at 70 to 80°C for a few minutes will kill most non-sporing microorganisms present. Similarly, steam maintained at subatmospheric pressure at 73°C is used in low temperature steam disinfectors in hospitals to disinfect thermolabile reusable equipment.
2. Boiling: Exposure to boiling water for 20 min achieves highly effective disinfection, although this is not a sterilization process, it can be useful in emergencies if no sterilizer is available.

Ultraviolet radiation: It has limited application for disinfection of surfaces, some piped water supplies but lacks penetrative power, however newer modifications in use with ozone treatment plants is very effective in disinfection.

This is a low-energy, non-iodising radiation with poor penetrating power that is lethal to microorganisms under optimum conditions. The shorter UV rays that reach the earth's surface in quantity have a wavelength of about 290 nm, but even more effective radiation of 240 to 280 nm is produced by mercury lamps. It is used in the treatment of water, air, thin films and surfaces such as laboratory safety cabinets.

Gases: Formaldehyde is used as a fumigant though it does not have an all pervasive effect. Traditionally formaldehyde gas was used to disinfect rooms previously occupied by patients with contagious diseases such as smallpox. It is still used for disinfection of heat-sensitive equipment, however its efficacy is questionable with better products like Bacillocid available.

Filtration: Air and water supplied to operation theatres and other critical environments are filtered to remove hazardous microorganisms, though viruses cannot remain out altogether. However, they are considered harmless in these environments.

A properly installed high efficiency particulate air (HEPA) filter achieves 99.9 percent or better resistance to particles of 0.5 microns and can produce sterile air at the filter face.

Chemical: Several chemicals with antimicrobial properties are used as disinfectants.

Antiseptic can be regarded as a special kind of disinfectant which is sufficiently free from injurious effects to be applied on the surface of the body, though not suitable for systemic or oral administration.

Some would restrict the use of antiseptic preparations applied to open wounds or abraded tissue and would use the word skin disinfection for removal of organisms from hands and intact skin surfaces.

1. Factors influencing the performance of chemical disinfectants

A. *The concentration of the disinfectant:* The optimum concentration required to produce a standardized microbial effect in practice is described as the in-use concentration. Care must be taken in preparing accurate in-use concentrations while diluting product. Accidental or arbitrary over dilution may result in failure of disinfection.

B. *The number, type and location of microorganism:* The velocity of the reaction depends upon the number and type of organisms present. In general gram-positive bacteria are more sensitive to disinfection than gram-negative bacteria. Mycobacteria and fungus are resistant while spores are highly resistant, while viruses are susceptible.

Glutaraldehyde is highly active against bacteria, viruses and spores. Other disinfectants such as hexachlorophene have a relatively narrow range of activity, predominantly against gram-positive cocci.

C. *The temperature and pH:* Some disinfectants are more active or stable at a particular pH. Though glutaraldehyde is more stable under acidic conditions its microbial effect is seen better when the pH is 8.0

D. *The presence of organic or other interfering substances:* Disinfectants can be inactivated by hard tapwater, cork, plastics, blood, urine, soaps and detergents, or other disinfectants. Information should be sought from the manufacturer or from reference authorities to confirm that the disinfectant will remain active in these circumstances.

2. Common chemicals in use

A. *Alcohols:* Isopropranol, ethanol, and industrial methylated spirit have optimal bactericidal activity in aqueous solution at concentrations of 70 to 90 percent and have little bactericidal effect outside this range. They have limited activity against mycobacteria and are not sporicidal. Action against viruses is generally good. Because they are volatile, alchohols are recommended as rapidly drying disinfectants for skin and surfaces. However, they may not achieve adequate penetration and kill, particularly, if organic matter such as blood or other protein-based contamination is present. Alcohols are suitable for physically clean surfaces such as washed thermometers or trolley tops but not for dirty surfaces. Care must be taken when used on the skin in conjunction with diathermy and other instances of flammable risk. Alcohols with chlorhexidine or povidone-iodine are good choices for hand disinfection, they are applied to the dry skin often with added emollient to counteract the drying effect.

B. *Aldehydes:* Most aldehyde disinfectants are based on glutaraldehyde or formaldehyde formulations, alone or in combination. Glutaraldehyde has a broad spectrum action against vegetative bacteria, fungi, viruses, but acts more slowly against spores. It is often for equipment such as endoscopes that cannot be sterilized or disinfected by heat. It is an irritant to the eyes, skin and respiratory mucosa, and must be used with adequate protection of staff and ventilation of the working environment. It must be thoroughly rinsed after treated equipment with sterile water to avoid carry-over of toxic residues and recontamination. The alkaline buffered solution is claimed to remain active for several days, but this will vary depending on the in-use situation, including the amount of organic material.

C. *Biguanides (chlorhexidine):* This is commonly used for disinfection of skin and mucous membranes. It is less active against gram-negative bacteria such as *Pseudomonas* and *Proteus sp* and in aqueous solution has limited virucidal, tuberculocidal and negligible sporicidal activity. It is often combined with a compatible detergent for handwashing or with alcohol as a handrub. Chlorhexidine has low irritancy and toxicity and is effective even on exposed healing surfaces. It is inactivated by organic matter, soap, anionic detergents, hard water and some natural materials such as cork liners or bottle closures.

D. *Halogens (hypochlorites)*: These broad-spectrum inexpensive chlorine-releasing disinfectants are that of choice against viruses. For heavy spillage such as blood, a concentration of 10,000 ppm of available chlorine is recommended.

These are inactivated by organic matter and corrode metals, so that contact with metallic instruments and equipment should be avoided. The bleaching action of hypochlorites may have a detrimental effect on fabrics and should not be used on carpets.

Chlorine-releasing disinfectants are relatively stable in concentrated form as liquid bleach of as tablets (sodium dichloroisocyanurates) but should be stored in well-sealed containers in a cool dark place. On dilution to the required concentration for use, activity is rapidly lost.

Hypochlorites have widespread application as laboratory disinfectants on bench surfaces and in discard pots. Care should be taken to remove all chlorine-releasing agents from laboratory areas before the use of formaldehyde fumigation to avoid the production of carcinogenic reaction products.

Iodine: Like chlorine, iodine is inactivated by organic matter and has the additional disadvantage of staining and hypersensitivity. The iodophors which contain iodine complexed with an anionic detergent of povidone-iodine a water-soluble complex of iodine and polyvinyl pyrrolidone are less irritant and cause less staining. Aqueous and alcohol-based povidone-iodine preparations are used widely for skin and ocular disinfection as well as other mucous membrane disinfection.

E. *Phenolics:* These have been widely used as general purpose environmental disinfectants in hospital and laboratory practice. They exhibit broad-spectrum activity and are relatively cheap. Clear soluble phenolics have been used to disinfect environmental surfaces and spillages if organic soil and transmissible pathogens may have been present. As hospital disinfection policies are rationalized, phenolics are being replaced by detergents for cleaning and by hypochlorites for disinfection. Most phenolics are stable and not readily inactivated by organic matter, with the exception of the chloroxylenos (Dettol), which are also inactivated by hard water and not recommended for hospital use. Phenolics are incompatible with cationic detergents. Contact should be avoided with rubber and plastics, such as mattress covers, since they are absorbed and may increase the permeability of the material to body fluids. The slow release of phenol fumes in closed environments and the need to avoid skin contact are other reasons for care in use of phenolics.

The bis-phenol hexachlorophane has particular activity against gram-positive cocci, and has been used in powder or emulsion formulations as a skin disinfectant, notably for prophylaxis against staphylococcal infection in nurseries. There has been some concern about the possible toxic effect of absorption across the neonatal skin barrier on repeated exposure. An alternative, which has been used in the control of methicillin-resistant *Staph. aureus* outbreaks is triclosan.

F. *Oxidizing agents and hydrogen peroxide:* Various agents, including chlorine dioxide, peracetic acid and hydrogen peroxide, have good antimicrobial properties but are corrosive to skin and metals. Hydrogen peroxide is highly reactive and has limited application for the treatment of wounds.

G. *Surface active agents:* Anionic, cationic, non-ionic and amphoteric detergents are generally used as cleaning agents. The cationic (quaternary ammonium compounds) and amphoteric agents have limited antimicrobial activity against vegetative bacteria and some viruses but not mycobacteria or bacterial spores. Quaternary ammonium compounds disrupt the membrane of microorganisms, leading to cell lysis. Care must be taken to avoid overgrowth by gram-negative contaminants and inactivation by mixing cationic and anionic agents. Disinfection may be enhanced by appropriate combination of a surface active agent with disinfectant to improve contact spread and cleansing properties.

Quality Control

Every method used must be validated to demonstrate microbial kill. With heat and irradiation a biological test may not be required if the physical conditions can be proved to have reached their ultimate design.

D value The D value or the decimal reduction value is the dose that is required to inactivate 90 percent of the initial population. When the time required or the dose required to reduce the population from 1 000 000 to 1 00 000 is the same as the time or dose required to reduce the population from 1 00 000 to 10 000, the D value remains constant over the full range of the survivor curve. Extending treatment beyond the point where there is one surviving cell does not give rise to fractions of a surviving cell but rather to a statement of the probability of finding one survivor. Thus, by extrapolation from the experimental date it is possible to determine the lethal dose required to give a probability of less than 1 in 1 000 000 which is required to meet the pharmaco-poeial definition of sterile.

Factors Influencing Resistance

Many factors affect the ability of the microorganism to withstand lethal procedures of sterilization. This in fact is the reason why we need to keep updating ourselves as to the methods of sterilization and their efficacies. This also happens to be the reason why living creatures are able to withstand high amounts of torture only to make sure their breed lives on. Bacteria are not that much different from us in this intrinsic need to propagate, grow and leave their legacy behind. Still we need to be on top of them to allow them to grow, where we need them and the operating room is definitely not a place we need any of them at all. Here are some of the reasons why these bacteria do withstand our torture.

Species or strain of microorganism As usual the spores are more resistant than vegetative bacteria or viruses. Though some strains of species have wide variations. *Enterobacteriaceae* D values at 60°C range from a few minutes (*E. coli*) to 1 hour (*Salmonella senftenberg*). The typical D value for *Staphylococcus aureus* at 70°C is less than 1 min compared with 3 min for *Staph. epidermidis*. However, an unusual strain of *Staph. aureus* has been isolated with a D value of 14 min at 70°C. Such variable could be attributed to the morphological and physiological changes such as alterations in cell proteins or specific targets in the cell envelope affecting permeability.

Thus we should not understand the inactivation data for one disease forming organism would withstand by another. Creutzfeldt-Jakob disease is a highly resistant agent requiring six times the normal heat sterilization cycle (134°C for 18 min).

Physiological stage Organisms grown under nutrient-limiting conditions are typically more resistant than those grown under nutrient-rich conditions. Resistance usually increases through the late logarithmic phase of growth of vegetative cells and declines erratically during the stationary phase.

Ability to form spores Bacterial endospores are more resistant than fungal spores, some of them are used as bacterial indicators especially for ethylene oxide sterilizers to monitor their efficacy. Disinfection has no efficacy where spores are concerned.

Suspending menstrum Microorganisms occluded in salt have greatly enhanced resistance to ethylene oxide, the presence of blood or other organic material will reduce the effectiveness of hypochlorite solution. Thus suspended particles will alter efficacy of various techniques.

Number of microorganisms Quite obviously the initial "bio-burden" the more extensive must the process of sterilization be to achieve the same assurance of sterility.

Sterilization and Disinfection Policy

All hospitals should go through a rigmarole of infection control and agree on a particular policy to be followed uniformly by all concerned in this infection control team. This should be headed by the chief surgeon and each one must report to the leader of the team everyday.

It has been noticed over centuries of medical practice when a surgical team gets to do routine surgeries every day for many days and years, a kind of apathy sets into the system and somewhere someone lapses. These instances have been the most common cause for infection. To avoid such lapses the infection control team should meet each week to update themselves on the latest happenings in their hospital and to bring to the notice such lapses so that a tightening of procedures can be applied. At each lapse the chief surgeon must be held responsible for the actions of his or her team.

All members of the team must familiarize themselves with the items to be sterilized and the chemicals necessary to do so. A microbiologist should be included in this team as they alone can monitor the efficacy of the said processes. Along with, should also be a pharmaceutical person who has full knowledge of the various chemicals used, their action and the efficiency in said matters. It is very instrumental to include these persons on the infection control team of a hospital.

The hospital policy should be common and should include

- The sources to be sterilized (equipment, skin, environment, air, water, personnel) for which a choice of process is required to be commonly accepted by the team for infection control.
- The processes and products available for sterilization and disinfection must be made available for all to see and inspect. An effective policy may include a limited number of process options, restrictions on the range of chemical disinfectants eliminate unnecessary costs, confusion and chemical hazards.

- The category of process required for each item, sterilization for surgical instruments and needles, heat disinfection for laundry, crockery, bed-pans, cleaning of floors, walls, furniture and fixtures.
- The specific products and method to be used for each item of equipment, the site of use and the staff responsible for the procedure. These should all be earmarked in a record so that one can get back to the lapse when it happens.

Effective implementation of the policy requires liaison and training of staff and updating the policy. Safety considerations for staff and patients require a careful assessment of specific procedures to minimize risks.

The staff for implementation of these processes must wear protective gear where necessary. Gloves, aprons, caps and masks must be included in the policy. Where dangerous gases are used eye goggles similar to swim goggles can be used to protect the eyes from the noxious gases.

For proper sterilization control, it is important to go back into every case that gets infected to try and pry and find out what was the reason for the infection. This can effectively be done by the weekly meeting of the infection control team where every one tries to pitch in their inputs.

Staff should not be penalized for accepting their wrong-doings, because if they are penalized they will not accept the cause of the infection next time it occurs. The staff should be goaded into performing better by putting the patients best interests in view and not for witch hunting and blaming.

CULTURE RATE

The most important mechanism for the proper functioning of an operation theatre is the fact that no organism should grow from this area. To find out whether an organism is growing or not we need to make sure it is present or not, that can effectively be done by growing it on a culture media. Some of the most common culture media used in hospitals is discussed here.

MacConkey's Agar

To make this culture plate (Fig. 6.27) is simple enough. According to directions 51.5 gm of the

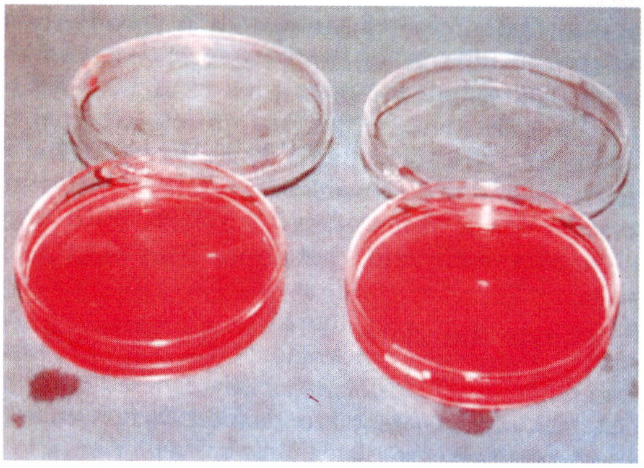

Fig. 6.27: MacConkey's blood agar culture plates

powder made available through Himedia Laboratories is dissolved in 1000 ml of distilled water. This is allowed to boil till the powder is completely dissolved and the fluid has boiled for over 15 minutes, thus sterilizing the fluid further. It could be still sterilized by autoclaving though most hospitals find 15 minutes of boiling to suffice in its sterilization.

This culture medium contains

Peptic digest of animal tissue	17 gm / lit
Peptone	3
Lactose	10
Bile salts	1.5
Sodium chloride	5
Neutral red	0.03
Agar	15
At a final pH of 7.1 at 25°C	

Alternately if the ready-made powder is not available then the following procedure can be applied to the above-mentioned ingredients.

Base solution Dissolve agar in 500 ml of distilled water by autoclaving at 121°C for 20 minutes. Dissolve the peptone, bile salts and sodium chloride in the remaining 500 ml of distilled water, and bring the solution to boil. Combine the two solutions mixing thoroughly. Dissolve the lactose and adjust the pH to 7.2. Distribute in screw-capped bottles and sterilize with autoclaving at 121°C for 15 minutes.

Dissolve 1 gm of neutral red in distilled water and make up the volume to 100 ml. Heat the solution in steam at 100°C for 30 minutes.

Dissolve 0.1 gm of crystal violet in distilled water and make up the volume to 100 ml. Heat the solution in steam at 100°C for 30 minutes.

To 200 ml of the base solution, melted and cooled to about 60°C add aseptically 0.6 ml of the neutral red solution and 0.2 ml of solution with crystal violet. Mix well and distribute into sterile Petri dishes.

Incubate the plates at 37°C for 24 hours (Figs 6.28 to 6.30) and examine for contamination. Inoculate four plates from the following stock culture *Salmonella typhi, Escherichia coli,* a mixture of *Salmonella typhi* and *E. coli* and *Shigella flexneri.* This will prove the efficacy of the culture media prepared and now it can be poured into petri dishes and refrigerated to be used on need for culture plates. It is advisable to keep them for 24 to 48 hours and to keep making fresh batches very often.

Nutrient Agar

A general purpose medium for the cultivation of microorganisms and a base for enriched or special purpose media. It can be made very simply by the powder available from Himedia laboratories by dissolving 28 gm of powder in 1000 ml of distilled water and boiling for 15 minutes. This would also sterilize the medium and it is ready for use after cooling. The powder contains

Peptic digest of animal tissue	5 gms/lit
Sodium chloride	5
Beef extract	1.5
Yeast extract	1.5
Agar	15
At 25°C the pH is 7.4	

Alternately if the powder is not available the separate entities can be taken, mixed and steamed for 2 hours. The pH should be adjusted first to 6.8 then clear the fluid with egg albumin. Filter and bottle. Autoclave at 15 1bs pressure for 20 minutes or steaming for 30 minutes each day on three successive days.

Blood Agar

An enriched medium for general use in routine cultivation of the more delicate microorganisms like *Neisseria meningitidis, N. gonorrhoeae* and

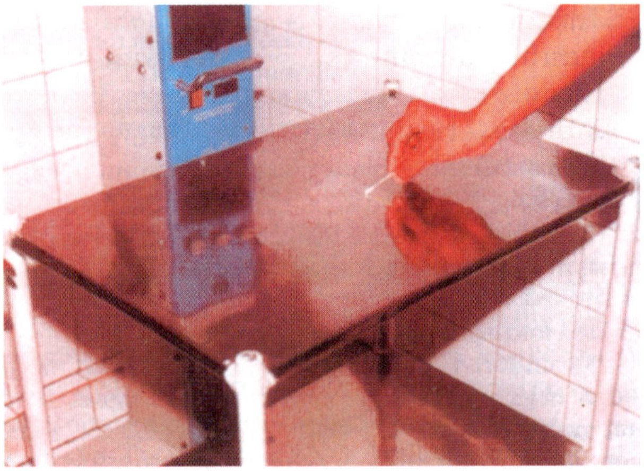

Fig. 6.28: Culture specimen taken using sterile swab stick from the instrument table

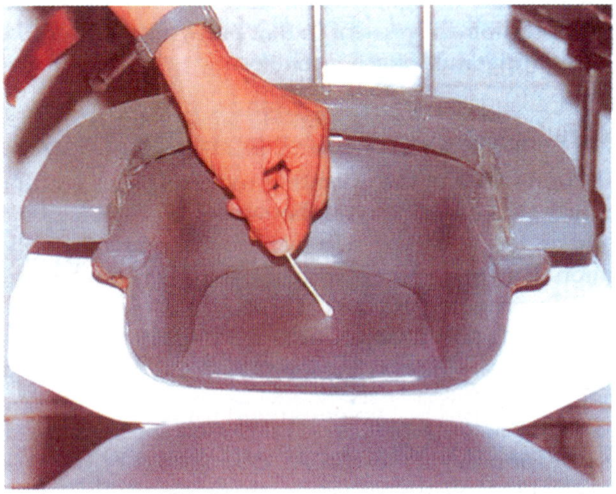

Fig. 6.29: Culture specimen taken using sterile swab stick from the operation table head rest

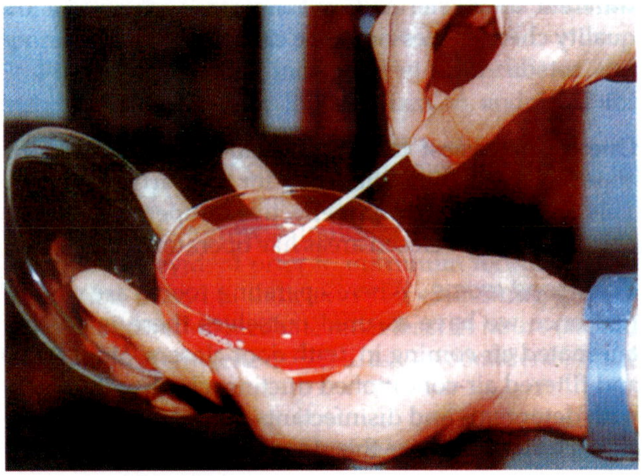

Fig. 6.30: Culture specimen taken using sterile swab stick being streaked on the MacConkey's blood agar culture plate

Diplococcus pneumoniae. The medium also serves as an indicator of hemolysin production by bacteria.

It is very simple to make. Add 6 to 10 percent defibrinated blood to melted nutrient agar and cool to 45 to 60°C. Pour plate or slant, incubate 24 hours to prove sterility.

STERILIZATION CONTROL

The infection control team which consists of a microbiologist must take regular samples from the different areas sterilized or disinfected. Some of the quality checks necessary to be carried out are:

Plate Test

One of the easiest to perform and tells us quite a bit about the cleaning tactics used for the particular room. This test would not be so effective in open areas but is quite reliable for closed areas like operating rooms.

For closed rooms Where operating rooms are concerned, once we have assured ourselves there is no contaminated air coming in, with door closers, air curtains and filtered air-conditioned ducting, cleaning the room with detergents and disinfectants should clear the air of all bacteria. However this does not remain so through out the day, and it is noticed that after a few surgeries due to human beings inside the operating rooms, bacteria do escape to contaminate the air. This can be effectively controlled by keeping a watch on the cleaning procedures and making sure a disinfectant mop is used after every procedure and on every item of the operating room.

However, testing for the efficacy of the cleaning procedures is devised by the PLATE TEST. Here a sterile bowl is used with sterile water and kept in the concerned room for 20 minutes. Should there be bacteria in the room they would settle down on the surface of the bowl of water. Thus skimming the surface a few drops are taken and placed on a Petri dish with culture media on it. This is incubated at 38°C for 48 hours and if this grows bacteria then we know our disinfectant procedures were not enough and we need to plough ourselves further. If it is negative then we can proceed with the same policy. This test should be ideally carried out everyday, before every procedure in every room of the operating area.

For open areas Lounges, where patients wait or the outside arenas are to be cleansed as well, if we would like to have a tight infection control in the operating area. After all these areas lead to the operating area—the most pious sanctum sanctorum of the hospital edifice.

The plate test is carried out everyday every few hours, and an optimum time interval given to the hospital authorities where it can be stated that every four hours the hospital lounges should be cleaned with disinfectant to maintain a clean bacteria-free atmosphere. This can now be controlled by taking plate test samples every four hours before cleaning procedures are done and making sure the tests remain negative for growth in all the tests taken. If not the program needs to be revised and the hours shortened.

This test should also be carried out in the consultation areas and optimum time intervals for cleaning prescribed by the microbiologist on the infection control team.

Culture Test from Walls, Floor, Fixtures, Furniture

Everyday the different areas should be taken for culture, it is advised to take eight different areas for culture from every room everyday. Methodology for taking culture is to take a moist swab, by dipping a cotton tip applicator in sterile water and rubbing it in a streak fashion on the culture plate.

The culture plates are made in Petri dishes about 3 inches in diameter. The back surface of the Petri dish can be stroked with a marker pen and each culture plate divided into eight parts.

One culture plate can be earmarked for each room, and 8 objects from the room can be cultured. It is preferrable to always include the floor of the room however different parts of the floor can be taken each day to ensure proper cleaning and disinfectant use. Other objects that can and should be cultured for are the fans, air-conditioners, lights, walls, tables, chairs, stools and all the equipment present in that particular room-like Boyles apparatus, phaco machines, etc.

All Fluids to be Cultured

All fluids used in the operating room must be sent for culture tests, sometimes this becomes less possible as the fluid is too little and necessary for parenteral application. However, every batch of fluids used can be sent for culture tests. This may not grow positive however its not growing positive itself is an indication of the efficacy of the program. This sets aside any debate that the fluid may have contained bacteria.

Of special importance is fluids used for intraocular use, or for intravenous use. As soon as each IV bottle is opened the first few drops from the IV set can be placed on a culture plate for incubation.

Many eye surgeons from our subcontinent have grown *E. coli* from the Ringer lactate used intraocularly. However, most often this has happened after a tragedy of multiple eyes have succumbed to postcataract surgery infection. Thus by performing this simple step we may be able to thwart further mishaps.

Should any one batch of fluids be found to be positive it is a good idea to report the matter so that others can be forewarned and to take every bottle from that batch.

All Fluids used Parenterally to be Checked for pH Value

Great importance should be given to the pH of fluids inside the body especially where the eye is concerned. We presume that all fluids marked for parenteral or intraocular use come at the pH close to 7.4, however, it is alarming to note the amount of times I have personally seen surgery go wary only due to the fact that the pH was either 5.6 or above 8. This can produce havock on the patient's cornea.

In 1992 over 300 cases were reported lost due to hazy opaque corneas following extracapsular cataract surgery in some states of India. This was followed by a widespread search for the culprit. What was found, was alarming to all concerned, a balanced salt solution (BSS) was sold in small bottles. It was learned that this solution carried an alkaline pH, because while cleaning the glass bottles the last rinse of soap solution (BSS) was not totally washed out and the remaining soap solution left behind an alkaline pH which recked havoc on the cornea producing total blindness.

It took the investigating authorities over six months to procure this data and cause by which time multiple surgeries had been carried out with much devastation.

A simple technology to avoid such future catastrophies is to check out the pH on table before the surgery. A few drops of the fluid can be dropped on a simple litmus strip and one minute later the color change noted with a rough estimate of the pH value noted.

This should be ideally carried out for all cases.

Specialized Equipment Cultures

Special tests are performed for special machines, like the one available for the ethylene oxide sterilizer.

Biological chemical indicator One or more biological chemical indicator can be placed in the steam or ethylene oxide test packs and the process passed through the sterilization cycles. If used to monitor a 270°F steam "flash" cycle, place a wire mesh bottom instrument tray and then proceed.

After sterilization processing has been completed, allow the biological chemical indicator to cool until safe to handle and open. Remove the indicators and allow to cool an additional 10 to 15 minutes. Observe chemical process exposure indicator on vial label to verify color change corresponding to sterilization cycle, i.e. ethylene oxide turns gas process indicator to gold and steam turns the steam process indicator to brown.

If chemical process indicator is unchanged, exposure to the sterilization process may not have occurred. Check the sterilization process.

If the chemical process exposure indicator on the vial label did change to the proper color and the indicator has cooled to touch, firmly seal the biological indicator by pushing the cap to close till the cap reaches second blue bar on the vial label.

Crush the inner ampoule from the outside wall of the plastic vial to ensure that the growth medium is released from the crushed ampoule and is in contact with the spore disk.

Place the activated indicators in an incubator and incubate it at 37°C for EO sterilization and 55°C for steam sterilization.

If there is a color change in the medium from deep blue to bright yellow and turbidity is evident, it means there is a positive growth. Indicators positive for growth will often be evident prior to maximum recommended incubation time, but indicators not evidencing growth must be allowed to incubate for at least 24 hours (steam) and 48 hours (ethylene oxide) to assure confidence in the negative reading.

When, where and why to use biologicals

When?

- Once a day in every sterilizer
- Once a week in steam sterilizer cycle used
- Every steam load with implants
- Every EO load.

Three consecutive times before using new sterilizer and after repairs.

Where?

All sterilization processes.

Why?

- To challenge your sterilizer's effectiveness
- To assure load sterilization parameters were up to standard.

Surgeons Hands Cultured

Right after scrubbing and ready for operation a surgeon's hands should be regularly swabbed and taken for culture so that a close check can be carried out to the efficacy of the cleaning and scrubbing solutions.

There are many surgeons who believe in different technologies of scrubbing. While some would swear with the pounding away of epithelial tissue by a brush, others would want to keep the epithelium intact at all times. While some would swear with a last dip into alcohol, others would keep alcohol well out of the way of surgeon's hands.

However it has been seen that three times to lather with soap and wash hands is a uniform tendency of most surgeons.

Linen and Textiles Cultured

Efficacy of sterilization on the different linens and textiles used in surgery should be tested by taking culture tests from these items just after surgery.

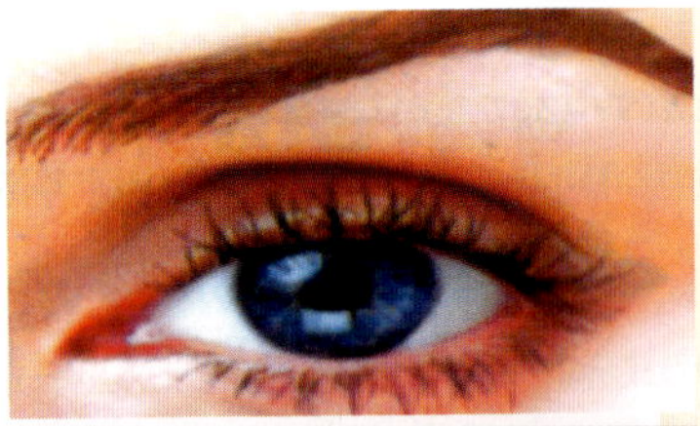

Seven

Anesthesia in Cataract Surgery

Ashok Garg (India)

INTRODUCTION

Anesthesia for Cataract Surgery has undergone tremendous changes and advancements in last century. In 1846 general anesthesia techniques were developed which were not found suitable and satisfactory for ophthalmic surgery. In 1884 Koller discovered surface anesthesia techniques using topical cocaine for cataract surgeries which found favor with the ophthalmologists. However, due to significant complications and side effects of cocaine Herman Knopp in 1884 described retrobulbar injection as local anesthetic technique for ocular surgery. He used 4 percent cocaine solution injected into the orbital tissue close to posterior part of the globe to achieve adequate anesthesia but in the subsequent injections patients experienced pain. In 1914 Van Lint introduced orbicularis akinesia by local injection to supplement subconjunctival and topical anesthesia. However, this technique found favor only after 1930 when procaine (Novocaine) a safer injectable agent made it feasible.

With the development of hyaluronidase as an additive to the local anesthetic solution Atkinson (1948) reported that large volumes could be injected with less orbital pressure and improved safety injections into the cone (retrobulbar) were recommended and gained rapid favor becoming anesthetic route of choice among ophthalmologists.

In mid 1970s, Kelman introduced an alternative technique of local anesthesia for ocular surgery known as peribulbar injection. However, till 1985 this new technique was not published in ophthalmic literature. In 1985 Davis and Mandel reported local anesthetic injection outside the cone into the posterior peribulbar space (periocular). Further modifications of both retrobulbar and periocular injection techniques were made by Bloomberg, Weiss and Deichaman, Hamilton and colleagues, Whitsett, Murdoch Shriver and coworkers. These modifications consisted of more anterior deposition of anesthetic solution with shorter needles and smaller dosages.

With the introduction of small incision cataract surgery, phaco emulsification and other microsurgical procedures in ophthalmology, use of shorter needles with smaller dosages became more common. Fukasawa and Furata *et al* reintroduced subconjunctival anesthetic techniques. Fichman in 1992 first reported the use of topical tetracaine anesthesia for phacoemulsification and intraocular lens implantation starting an era of topical anesthesia in ocular surgery.

With the advent of many ocular anesthetic techniques in past two decades indicates the need for the development of an ideal anesthetic and technique for ocular surgery. Every existing technique has its own advantages and disadvantages. General anesthesia for cataract surgery is virtually out of favor with ophthalmologists. Retrobulbar anesthesia, periocular (peribulbar, subconjunctival, orbital and epidural) and topical anesthesia or a combination of peribulbar and topical are being used in present day ocular sugery. Now with the advent of below 1 mm incision technique, foldable and rollable intraocular lenses, no anesthesia cataract surgery is becoming popular with increased frequency.

ANESTHESIA FOR CATARACT SURGERY

Cataract extraction may be performed under general anesthesia, local anesthesia or topical anesthesia, depending upon condition of patient cataract status and surgeon choice.

General Anesthesia

Usually for cataract surgery general anesthesia is not given. It is advisable only in highly anxious/nervous patient or when cataract surgery requires a long time for completion. Patients who are extremely apprehensive, deaf, mentally retarded, unstable or cannot communicate well with the surgeon are more suitable for general anesthesia. General

Table 7.1: Evolution of anesthetic techniques for cataract surgery

Technique	*Year*	*Author*
General anesthesia	1846	Morton
Topical cocaine	1884	Koller
Injectable cocaine	1884	Knapp
Orbicularis akinesia	1914	Van Lint, O'Briens, Atkinson
Hyaluronidase	1948	Atkinson
Retrobulbar (4% cocaine)	1884	Knapp
Posterior peribulbar	1985	Davis and Mandel
Limbal	1990	Furata and coworkers
Anterior peribulbar	1991	Bloomberg
Topical anesthesia	1992	Fichman
Pinpoint anesthesia	1994	Fukasaku
Topical plus intracameral	1995	Gills
No anesthesia	1998	Agarwal
Cryoanalgesia	1999	Gutiérrez Carmona
Xylocaine jelly	1999	Koch, Assia
Hypothesis, No anesthesia	2001	Pandey and Agarwal

Courtesy : Dr. F. Gutierrez Carmona (SPAIN)

anesthetic facilities with expert anesthetist are mandatory.

GENERAL ANESTHESIA PROCEDURE

Preoperative Preparation

A patient who is to be given a general anesthetic needs proper preoperative assessment and examination, preferably on the day before the anesthetic is to be administered, although preparation earlier on the day of surgery may be acceptable in many cases. Patients with cataracts are often elderly and not infrequently have other medical problems that must be considered before anesthesia is induced. These are—

Chronic (Obstructive) Respiratory Disease

These patients require more careful assessment. Their condition in severe cases can be adversely affected by anesthetic drugs and muscle relaxants. On the other hand, the inability to control obstructed respiration can lead to hazardous cataract surgery and a high incidence of failure. Preoperative preparation with antibiotics, bronchodilators, and physiotherapy often enable a sick patient to undergo a safe procedure with the benefit of a general anesthetic.

Cardiovascular Disease

Because many patients with cardiovascular disease will already be on diuretic treatment, preoperative assessment to detect and treat cardiac failure or hypokalemia is most important. The adequate control of hypertension is also an essential safety requirement, especially for the middle-aged.

Diabetes Mellitus

Diabetes mellitus is commonly found in those for whom cataract surgery is indicated. Preadmission stabilization is necessary, and when this is in doubt, a longer period of preoperative inpatient assessment and management is required to eliminate any ketonuria or gross hyperglycemia. Oral diabetic medication should be omitted on the day of surgery because the effects may persist for up to 24 hours. During surgery and throughout the early postoperative period, control is effected by using 5 percent glucose intravenously and insulin as required, as shown by the blood glucose levels. When the patient resumes normal oral intake postoperatively, the normal regimen is rapidly resumed.

Dystrophia Myotonica

These patients frequently require cataract surgery while they are quite young. They are particularly sensitive to anesthetic drugs and subject to prolonged respiratory depression. Suxamethonium is contraindicated; minimal doses of other drugs such as atracurium should be used.

Premedication

The aim of premedication is to allow a smooth induction of anesthesia. Most patients appreciate some sedation to alleviate the natural anxiety associated with any eye surgery. Opiates, however, are to be avoided because of their association with respiratory depression and postoperative vomiting. For the aged and anxious, oral premedication with diazepam, 5 to 10 mg, according to fitness and size or Lorazepam, 1 to 2 mg, works well. An antiemetic can then be administered during surgery.

For the younger and more robust, one can use a combination of pethidine, promethazine hydrochloride, and atropine. This is also a helpful combination for those with established respiratory disease.

Children over 1 year of age required sedation with trimeprazine tartrate syrup (3 to 4 mg per kg) 2 hours preoperatively. Younger babies should not require sedation. Atropine may be given either intramuscularly (0.2 to 0.6 mg 30 minutes preoperatively) or intravenously (0.015 to 0.02 mg with induction).

METHODS OF ANESTHESIA

Induction

A smooth induction avoids the problems of increased central nervous pressure with its consequent adverse effect on the intraocular pressure.

The drug most commonly used is thiopentone, which produces a rapid loss of consciousness. When it is used in doses of 3 to 4 mg per kg, the onset is relatively slow in the elderly, who frequently have a slower circulation time. For the very frail, methohexitone is useful, producing less change in blood pressure. More recently disoprofol (Diprivan) has been found to be useful; it also has a rapid onset of action and induces little nausea and vomiting.

Intubation of the trachea with a non-kinking endotracheal tube is achieved with suxamethonium. Its use is associated with a transient rise in the intraocular pressure due to choroidal expansion. Ventilation with nitrous oxide and oxygen with 0.5 to 1 percent halothane is continued until the effects of the suxamethonium have subsided.

More recently techniques have been described for rapid sequence induction with vecuronium. These methods do not seem to be associated with a significant rise in the intraocular pressure and they avoid the problems of suxamethonium.

Maintenance

A nondepolarizing muscle relaxant is used throughout the surgical procedure, dosages depending on the size, age, and health of the patient. Available drugs include tubocurarine, which is inclined to produce hypotension (occasionally severe), pancuronium, and more recently vecuronium and atracurium. Vecuronium has been demonstrated to lower intraocular pressure. Because both atracurium and vecuronium act and subside rapidly, their effectiveness must be monitored regularly by a peripheral nerve stimulator.

Intermittent positive pressure ventilation is maintained by nitrous oxide, oxygen, and an anesthetic drug. One-half percent halothane has long been considered effective and also lowers the intraocular pressure. Other anesthetic drugs include enflurane (associated with more postoperative vomiting and restlessness, though less hypotension) and isoflurane. The latter does not appear to adversely affect the stability of the cardiovascular system. Its effect on intraocular pressure has not been reported.

Throughout the procedure the pulse, blood pressure, electrocardiographic record, and arterial oxygen saturation must be regularly monitored, along with the nerve stimulation needed for the nondepolarizing muscle relaxant being used. All ventilators should be fitted with an alarm to warn of malfunction.

Completion of recovery from anesthesia after cataract surgery must be as smooth as the induction, care being taken to avoid gagging, coughing, and of course vomiting. Modern ophthalmic sutures are good but not foolproof! The neuromuscular blockade is reversed with atropine and prostigmine. Gentle extubation is associated with careful pharyngeal suction. Patients are encouraged to resume normal activity as soon as the effects of the anesthetic drugs have worn off.

ANESTHESIA FOR CHILDREN

Adequate premedication and careful handling should insure a calm and quiet child, and allow a smooth induction. Because the cataract is dealt with by using a closed system, the surgical risks of a rise in intraocular pressure are not so severe. Inhalational anesthesia using nitrous oxide and oxygen with halothane is usually sufficient.

COMPLICATIONS OF GENERAL ANESTHESIA

The complications associated with a general anesthetic range from death to the less serious but irritating nuisances of protracted nausea and vomiting or sore throats. This chapter covers only those complications producing serious morbidity or mortality and those peculiar to the patient with eye disease.

1. Hypoxemia (insufficient oxygen in the arterial blood to sustain life) is the most common cause of disaster, and failure to ventilate is the most common cause of hypoxemia. Unrecognized esophageal intubation, ventilator disconnection, and, most distressing of all, inability to ventilate after unconsciousness and paralysis have been obtained are all possible causes of failure to ventilate. Delivery of an inadequate oxygen concentration is a less common cause of hypoxemia. Most but not all of the foregoing are preventable with the monitoring and fail-safe devices available today, provided a competent anesthetist is monitoring the devices.

2. Aspiration of gastric contents remains a common complication despite such preventive measures as overnight fasting, the use of metoclopramide to enhance gastric emptying, and rapid sequence induction with cricoid pressure in emergency procedures. The two life-threatening results of aspiration are airway obstruction from large food particles and chemical pneumonitis from acidic gastric contents.
3. The two most serious cardiovascular complications, aside from cardiovascular collapse secondary to hypoxemia and acute anaphylaxis, are myocardial infarction and cerebrovascular accident. Surgery performed under general anesthesia within 3 months after a myocardial infarction carries a 40 percent incidence of repeat infarction. This figure decreases to about 10 percent at 6 months, after which the incidence is approximately the same as in the general population. All elective surgery is delayed until after 3 months, and a 6 month wait is encouraged unless poor visual acuity seriously limits activities.
4. Renal and hepatic toxic effects from anesthetic drugs are seldom seen in our practice. Careful preanesthetic screening identifies all patients with renal and hepatic disease. Halothane, which gained notoriety because of its hepatotoxicity, especially when administered repeatedly, is not used in adults and is usually used for induction only in children. The metabolic byproducts of methoxyflurane and enflurane are inorganic fluorides, which can produce nephrogenic diabetes insipidus. We no longer use these drugs because so many of our patients have diabetes and severe renal disease in our population.
5. Failure to resume respiration at the end of the surgery occurs often enough to merit mention. The most common causes are simple respiratory depression from the anesthetic drugs or narcotics, electrolyte disturbance (i.e., hypokalemia), hypothermia (particularly in infants), and the use of the combination of mycin antibiotics and nondepolarizing muscle relaxants. It also may occur after the administration of succinylcholine when there is a pseudocholinesterase deficiency. Respirations are main-tained until the cause is found and remedied.

Cardiovascular complications are the most commonly seen events in our practice. If diagnosed and treated properly, they need not result in a disaster. Hypertension is the most prevalent problem. The usual causes are apprehension, neosynephrine eyedrops, pain, distended bladder if mannitol was given, and autonomic nervous system imbalance secondary to the general anesthetic. Apprehension can be allayed with intravenous injections of 1 to 3 mg of Valium or 0.5 to 2 mg Zolpidem. Nitropaste applied to the skin and sublingual doses of nifedipine have proved invaluable, but an intravenous line should be in place before their use. Hypotension must be treated immediately and vigorously because it is tolerated less well than hypertension. Arrhythmias are the most frequent cause of cancellation on the day of surgery in the elderly patient with eye disease. The sudden onset of atrial fibrillation is the most common arrhythmia. An electrocardiographic monitor is mandatory for eye surgery.

Extrusion of ocular contents during administration of a general anesthetic is a serious complication in eye surgery. The entire anesthetic process is geared to minimize this possibility. Once the eye is opened, patients are kept deeply anesthetized or paralyzed with non-depolarizing relaxants to insure immobility.

Local Anesthesia

Local ocular anesthesia is the mainstay of cataract surgery. Local anesthesia minimises the risk of wound rupture a complication frequently associated with coughing during extubation and postoperative nausea and vomiting (in General Anesthesia) (Fig. 7.1). Generally, the use of 1:1 mixture of 2 percent Xylocaine and 0.50 percent Bupivacaine along with adrenaline and Hyaluronidase in facial, retrobulbar and peribulbar blocks achieve rapid anesthesia, akinesia and postoperative analgesia for several hours.

Care should be taken to avoid intravascular injections of anesthetic agents because refractory cardiopulmonary arrest may result from an inadvertent intravenous or intra-arterial injections.

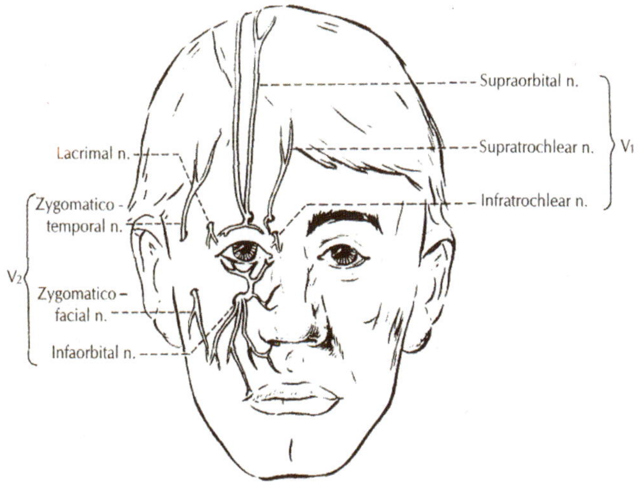

Fig. 7.1: Diagrammatic surface distribution of sensory nerves. Note branches derived from ophthalmic nerve (V_1) and maxillary nerve (V_2) a division of the trigeminal nerve

Many patients express pain of facial and retrobulbar injections so proper preoperative sedation and good rapport with the surgeon make them quite comfortable.

Following techniques are used for giving local anesthesia. These include:

Orbicularis Oculi Akinesia

Temporary paralysis of the orbicularis oculi muscle is essential before making section for the cataract surgery to prevent potential damage from squeezing of the lids. Following methods are used, for getting orbicularis oculi akinesia.

a. *O' Brien's technique* Usually 10 ml of mixture of 2 percent Lidocaine solution (5 ml) and 0.5 percent bupivacaine solution (5 ml) with 1:100,000 epinephrine and 150 units of hyaluronidase are infiltrated for local anesthesia.

O'Brien's method is the injection of above mentioned local anesthetic solution down to the periosteum covering the neck of the mandible where the temporofacial division of facial nerve passes forward and upwards (Fig. 7.2). A 10 ml syringe with preferably No. 17 or 18 needle and 2.5 cm in length is used. The patient is asked to open his mouth and the position of the condyle and temporomandibular

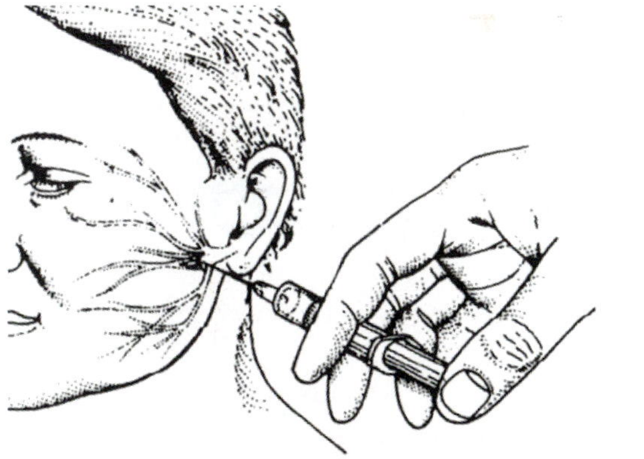

Fig. 7.2: Diagrammatic presentation of O'Brien technique of local anesthesia

joint is located by the forefinger of the operators' left hand. After closing the jaw, the injection is given on a horizontal line through the junction of the upper and middle third of the distance between the zygoma and angle of the mandible. The needle should pass straight down the periosteum. 2-3 ml of local anesthetic solution is injected and after withdrawing the needle firm pressure and massage are applied. Paralysis of orbicularis oculi should occur normally within 7 minutes. The injection is unlikely to injure the external carotid artery which lies posterior and at a deeper level. However, damage may be done to posterior facial vein and the transverse facial artery. Movement of jaws is sometime painful for few days after this injection.

b. *Van Lint's akinesia* Van Lint's method is a better alternative. The injection of local anesthetic solution is made across the course of branches of the seventh nerve as they pass over the zygomatic bone (Fig. 7.3).

In this technique a 5 cm in length and 25 gauge needle is passed through the wheal down to the periosteum of the zygomatic bone. The needle is then passed upward toward the temporal fossa without touching the periosteum (as it may be painful) and 4 ml of solution is injected and then forwards medially and downwards toward the infraorbital foramen to inject 2 ml and downwards and backwards along the lower margin of the zygoma for 2.5 cm where 3 ml of solution is injected. It is essential to massage the infiltrated area with a

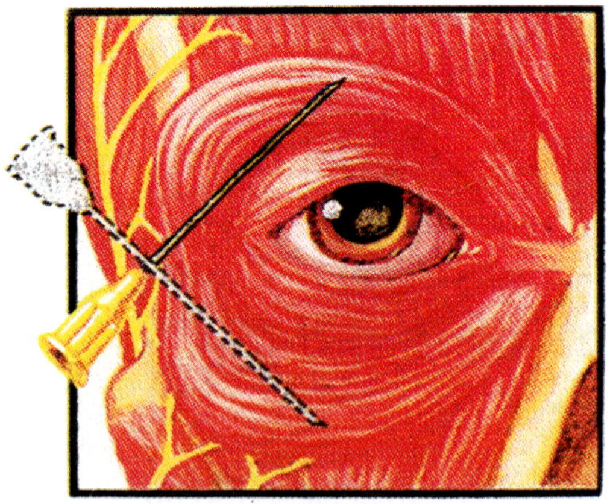

Fig. 7.3: Needle position for Van Lint akinesia (*Courtesy:* Ciba Geigy Clinical Symposia)

gauze swab. Motor nerves are less susceptible than sensory nerves to a block with local anesthetic agents.

The advantage of Van Lint's method is that it provides regional anesthesia as well as paralysis of the orbicularis muscle. After waiting for 5-7 minutes akinesia is tested by holding the eyelids open with a small swab on to a holder and asking the patient to close his eyelids. If slightest action is observed then injection may be repeated to obtain adequate akinesia.

c. *Atkinson block* The needle enters through a skin wheal at the inferior border of the zygoma just inferior to the lateral orbital rim. The path of the needle is along the inferior edge of the zygomatic bone and then superiorly across the zygomatic arch, ending at the top of the ear. 3 to 4 ml of the anesthetic is injected as the needle is advanced (Figs 7.4 and 7.5).

d. *Spaeth block* The Spaeth block avoids the inconsistencies of the O'Brien block as well as the postoperative discomfort caused by going through the parotid gland and entering the temporomandibular joint. An injection is made into the back of the mandibular condyle just below the ear, catching the facial nerve before it divides (Fig. 7.6). To locate the landmarks, the fingers are placed along the posterior border of the mandible as superiorly as possible. The needle is placed just anterior to the most superior finger. Bone should be reached shortly. If not, the needle is withdrawn and the position rechecked before a second attempt is made. After the bone is reached, the needle is pulled back slightly and suction is placed on the syringe to make sure that a vessel has not been punctured; 5 ml of anesthetic is then injected. Although rarely required, the needle can be redirected superiorly towards the outer canthus for 1.5 inches and an additional 5 ml is injected. After

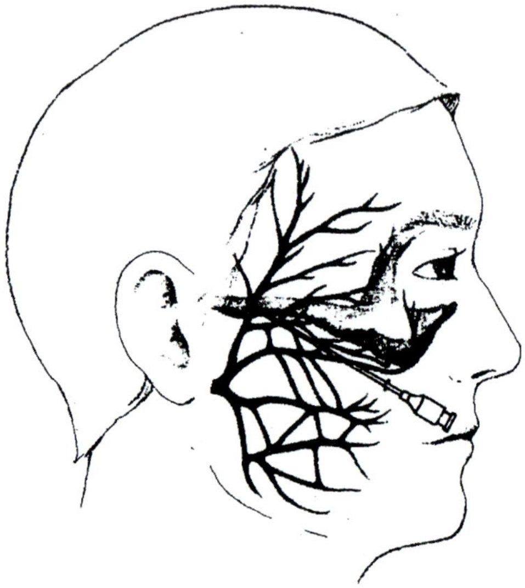

Fig. 7.4: Atkinson akinesia (Intercepting the facial nerve fibers as they cross the zygomatic arch)

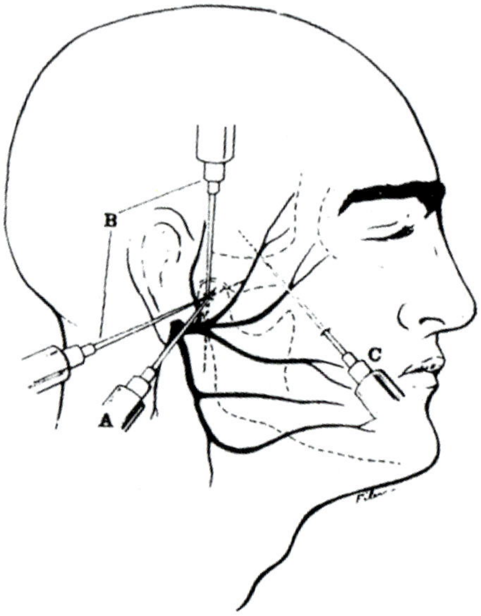

Fig. 7.5: Diagrammatic presentation of O'Brien and Atkinson techniques (A) Classic O'Brien technique (B) Modified O'Brien technique (C) Atkinson technique

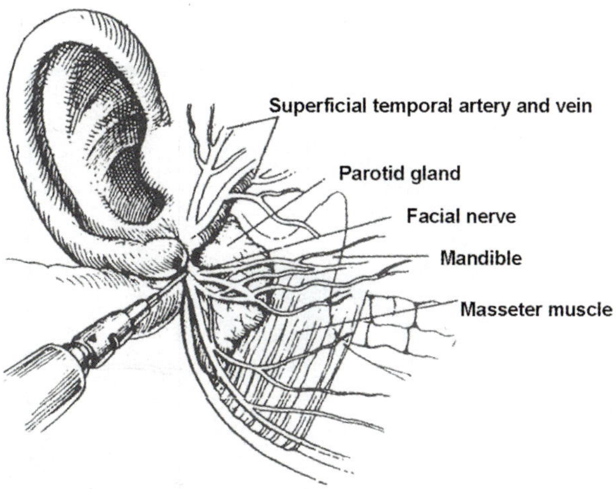

Fig. 7.6: Spaeth block (facial nerve is blocked where it crosses the posterior edge of the mandible)

30 seconds, nearly complete facial palsy should be evident.

e. *Nadbath block* An injection is made into the cavity between the mastoid process and the posterior border of the mandibular ramus. The skin is pierced, and a skin wheal is made 1 or 2 mm anterior to the mastoid process and inferior to the external auditory canal. A 12 mm, 26 gauge needle is used, with the injection of anesthetic extending from the skin wheal, passing through a taut membrane midway, to the full depth of the needle; 3 ml is injected (Fig. 7.7).

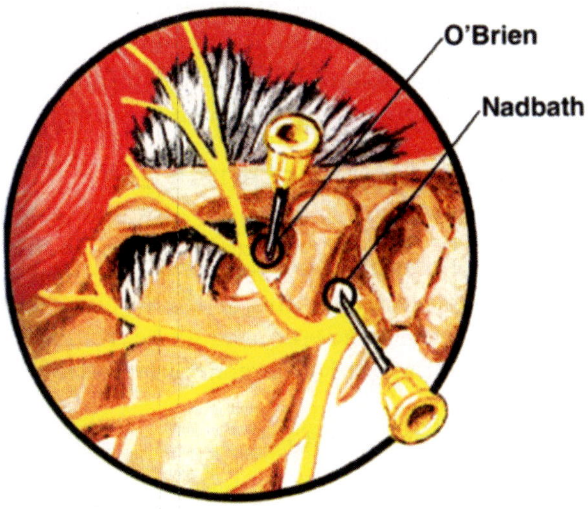

Fig. 7.7: Needle positions for O'Brien and Nadbath ocular akinesia. (*Courtesy:* Ciba Geigy Clinical symposia)

The Nadbath block insures ease of performance, and there are few complaints relating to the original injection or subsequent pain in the jaw area. The most common side effect is a bitter taste as the parotid gland secretes the anesthetic. Other problems reported are dysphonia, swallowing difficulty, and respiratory distress. Judging from the fact that these complications are seen predominantly in very thin patients and most certainly are secondary to the diffusion of anesthetic to the jugular foramen, 1 cm deeper than the stylomastoid foramen, the length of the needle, i.e. the depth of injection is critical.

Preexisting unilateral oropharyngeal or vocal cord dysfunction is a definite contraindication, as bilateral vocal cord paralysis could result. The Nadbath block should never be done bilaterally. If, after a unilateral Nadbath block, dysphonia or difficulty with swallowing or respiration occurs, lateral positioning will allow the paralyzed vocal cord to fall out of the way, clearing the airway.

Proper administration of local anesthesia requires knowledge of orbital anatomy, various anesthetic techniques, and the properties of the drugs used. Prompt recognition of side effects and complications following injection results in the best possible patient care.

f. *Retro-ocular (retrobulbar) injection* Anesthesia and akinesia of the eye are achieved by injecting a local anesthetic solution into the retrobulbar space within the muscle cone (Fig. 7.8).
   - In this method patient is asked to look upwards and to the opposite side. A 3.5 cm length 23 gauge sharp edge round tipped needle is inserted in the quadrant between the inferior and the lateral rectus muscles and directed posteriorly until the resistance of orbital septum is encountered. After it has penetrated the orbit the needle is directed towards the apex of the orbit and advanced until it meets the resistance of the inter-muscular septum. When this structure is penetrated, the needle tip is in the retrobulbar space. About 3-4 ml of local anesthetic mixture solution is injected taking care, to mini-

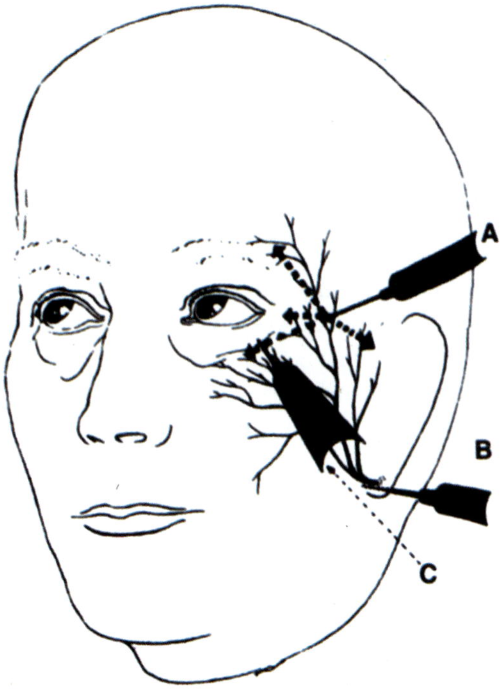

Fig. 7.8: Local anesthesia techniques (A) Van Lint akinesia (dotted arrows) (B) Nadbath facial nerve block (C) Retrobulbar needle position

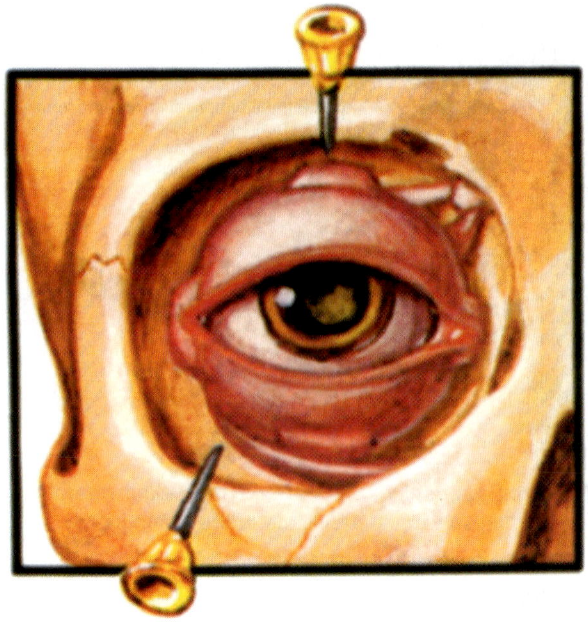

Fig. 7.9: Needle positions for retrobulbar and peribulbar anesthesia (frontal view) (*Courtesy:* Ciba Geigy clinical symposia)

mize the needle movement to prevent possible vessels lacerations. Following the injection the globe should be intermittently compressed for several minutes for distributing the anesthetic solution and to ensure hemostasis. A properly placed retrobulbar injection is effective within seconds. It blocks all extraocular muscles except superior oblique muscle, affects the ciliary ganglion and anesthetize the entire globe (Fig. 7.9).

Gills-Loyd Modified Retrobulbar Block

Before the anesthetic is administered, the patient's vision is checked and the A scan is done. Then, prior to the first injection, 2 drops of proparacaine 0.5 percent are given topically. The eyes are either fixed in primary gaze or directed slightly superiorly, avoiding the superonasal position. With sharp 27 gauge needle, enter is effected at LE 4:00, RE 8:00, 5 mm medial to the lateral canthus. The needle is inserted parallel to the optic nerve. A preretrobulbar injection of 1.5ml of pH adjusted Xylocaine is administered subconjunctivally. After 30 seconds, a 5 ml retrobulbar injection of pH adjusted Bupivacaine and Hyaluronidase is injected with a 25 gauge, 1¼ inch needle. After 8 to 9 minutes, the eye is checked for akinesia. A 1 to 3 ml supplemental injection of full strength anesthetic is given as needed to complete the block. 1.0 ml bolus is administered subdermally into the inferolateral lid to anesthetize the distal branches of the seventh cranial nerve; this technique does not require a total seventh nerve block. Next 0.5 ml of cefazole is injected subconjunctivally, and gentle eye compression is administered for 30 to 60 minutes with a Super Pinky Decompressor prior to surgery.

COMPLICATIONS OF RETROBULBAR INJECTION

A number of complications can occur as a result of retrobulbar injection, among them retrobulbar hemorrhage, perforation of the globe, retinal vascular obstruction, and subarachnoid injection.

Retrobulbar Hemorrhage

Retrobulbar hemorrhage probably occurs in 1 to 5 percent of the cases. It seems to occur less frequently if a blunt tipped needle is used, but this has not been demonstrated in any controlled study.

Retrobulbar bleeding may occur at a number of sites. The four vortex veins leave the globe approximately 4 mm posterior to the equator and could well be subjected to the shearing forces of an inserted needle, as could the central retinal or ophthalmic vein. An arterial source of bleeding must be postulated to explain severe hemorrhages that produce the rapid onset of proptosis, hemorrhage, chemosis, and immobility of the globe. The posterior ciliary arteries supplying the choroid, the central retinal artery, and other ophthalmic artery branches are all subject to damage. Even the ophthalmic artery can be reached in the area of the optic foramen with a $1^1/_2$ inch needle.

Most instances of retrobulbar hemorrhage resolve without complication, but should a complication arise, particularly during elective surgery, it is prudent to postpone the operation for at least 3 to 4 weeks and then consider general anesthesia if the patient can tolerate it.

Even when general anesthesia is employed, severe positive pressure can develop in an open eye if the operation is performed within several days after the hemorrhage.

Vision may be permanently decreased following a retrobulbar hemorrhage. This probably occurs as a result of closure of the central retinal artery or damage to the smaller vessels that supply the retrobulbar optic nerve.

If examination reveals that the central retinal artery has closed because of increased intraorbital and intraocular pressures, a lateral canthotomy should be performed. Other possible therapeutic modalities include anterior chamber paracentesis and orbital decompression. Prior of decompression of the orbit, computed tomographic scanning of the region should be undertaken to help localize the blood and rule out the possibility of bleeding within the optic nerve sheath, which also might have to be decompressed.

PERFORATION OFTHE GLOBE

This is another sight threatening complications of ophthalmic surgery with retrobulbar anesthesia. Highly myopic eyes are particularly suscepticle to this complication because of their long axial lengths. General anesthesia should be considered as an alternative in such eyes.

The scleral perforation should be repaired as soon as possible. Cryopexy or laser treatment of the break(s) may suffice, although vitreous traction that develops along the needle tract through the vitreous gel is better negated by a scleral buckling procedure. If the fundus view is obscured by vitreous hemorrhage, a pars plana vitrectomy is warranted to visualize the break(s). Although double scleral perforations probably have a worse prognosis than the single variant, the latter also can be devastating. I have seen one case in which the retina in the posterior pole was partially aspirated through the needle following a scleral perforation anterior to the equator.

Inadvertent injection of lidocaine into the vitreous cavity appears to be tolerated by the globe. However, it can cause an extreme elevation of the intraocular pressure and rapid opacification of the cornea.

RETINALVASCULAR OBSTRUCTION

Retinal vascular obstruction has been reported after retrobulbar anesthesia. The most common types are central retinal artery obstruction and combined central retinal artery-central retinal vein obstructions. Central retinal artery obstruction seems to occur more commonly in conjunction with diseases that affect the retinal vasculature, such as diabetes mellitus and sickling hemoglobinopathies. Nevertheless, it also can be seen in people with good health. Fortunately, the condition more often than not reverses spontaneously and the central retinal artery reperfuses within several hours. The causes are uncertain, but spasm of the artery, direct trauma to the vessel from the needle, and external compression by blood or an injected solution are possible mechanisms that could cause obstruction. Ophthalmic artery obstruction also can be induced, possibly by injection and subsequent compression within the optic foramen.

Therapy is directed towards relieving the obstruction and keeping the retina viable. Anterior chamber paracentesis may help, the aim being to lower the intraocular pressure and decrease the resistance to blood through the central retinal artery. Although paracentesis widens vessels narrowed by artery obstruction, fluorescein angiography shows that the filling occurs in a retrograde fashion, via the retinal veins. Hence, its value is questionable.

Combined obstruction of the central retinal artery and central retinal vein is a much more serious complication. Ophthalmoscopically a cherry-red spot is seen, as well as numerous intraretinal hemorrhages and dilated retinal veins. The Mechanisms of obstruction include direct trauma to the central retinal vessels from the needle or compression from blood or fluid injected into the nerve sheath. Blood within a dilated optic nerve sheath has been demonstrated in these cases.

The visual prognosis of these eyes is generally grim. Computed tomography of the retrobulbar optic nerve may be used to determine whether a nerve sheath hemorrhage is present. If an optic nerve sheath hematoma is discovered, decompression of the nerve sheath may be of limited benefit.

Neovascularization of the iris may develop after combined central retinal artery-central retinal vein obstruction. If the anterior chamber angle is not yet closed by a fibrovascular membrane, aggressive, full scatter panretinal photocoagulation treatment should be administered in an attempt to prevent neovascular glaucoma.

Injecting with the eye in the primary position may help prevent this complication. In contrast, injecting with the eye looking up and in, places the optic nerve and central retinal vessels more in the pathway of the needle and thus probably should be avoided.

Multiple emboli with the retinal arterial system have caused vascular obstruction following retrobulbar corticosteroid injection. No therapy is available for this visually devastating complication which likely results from injection into the central retinal or ophthalmic artery. In theory, the use of a needle shorter than $1^1/_2$ inches may help to prevent the complication, as can having the patient gaze in the primary position during the injection.

SUBARACHNOID INJECTION

Among the most recently recognized complications of retrobulbar, anesthesia, inadvertent injection into the subarachnoid space may be the most serious. The subarachnoid space extends around the retrobulbar optic nerve up to the globe and can be violated with a retrobulbar needle at any point along its course.

Optic atrophy and blindness have also been reported following retrobulbar blocks but they are fortunately rare. Due to these potential complications retro-ocular injection is out of favor with eye surgeon worldwide.

PERIBULBAR (PERIOCULAR)TECHNIQUE

Since, the exit of retrobulbar akinesia, peribulbar akinesia is considered a safe and effective technique of local anesthesia for cataract surgery. It is method of choice with eye surgeons for giving local anesthesia in cataract surgery. As the name indicates, peribulbar anesthesia is a technique in which a local anesthetic is injected into peribulbar space and is not aimed at blocking a perticular nerve.

Technique

Periocular anesthesia is administered at two site in lower temporal quadrant and nasal to caruncle (Fig. 7.10).

The required local anesthetics are Lidocaine 1 percent and Bupivacaine 0.75 percent with Hyaluronidase. Bupivacaine is preferred as it is a longer acting anesthetic agent which can provide prolonged anesthesia and analgesia.

In the first stage, injection of 0.5 cc of 1 percent lidocaine with a 26 gauge needle is done under the skin at about 1 cm away from the lateral canthus in the lower lid, along the orbital rim. The same needle is passed deeper to inject 0.5 cc of lidocaine into the orbicularis muscle and 1.0 cc into the muscle sheath. A second injection is done in the similar fashion in the upper eyelid just below the supraorbital notch. Pressure is applied at both for a minute using gauze pieces.

In the second stage, combination of 6.0 ml of 0.75 percent bupivacaine, 3 ml of 1 percent lidocaine and 0.25 cc of hyaluronidase is filled into a 10 ml disposable syringe fitted with a, 1-1/4 inch 23 gauge, hypodermic needle. The needle is first introduced deep into the orbit through the anesthetized site in the lower eyelid. One ml is injected just beneath the orbicularis muscle and then the needle is advanced upto the equator of the globe to inject

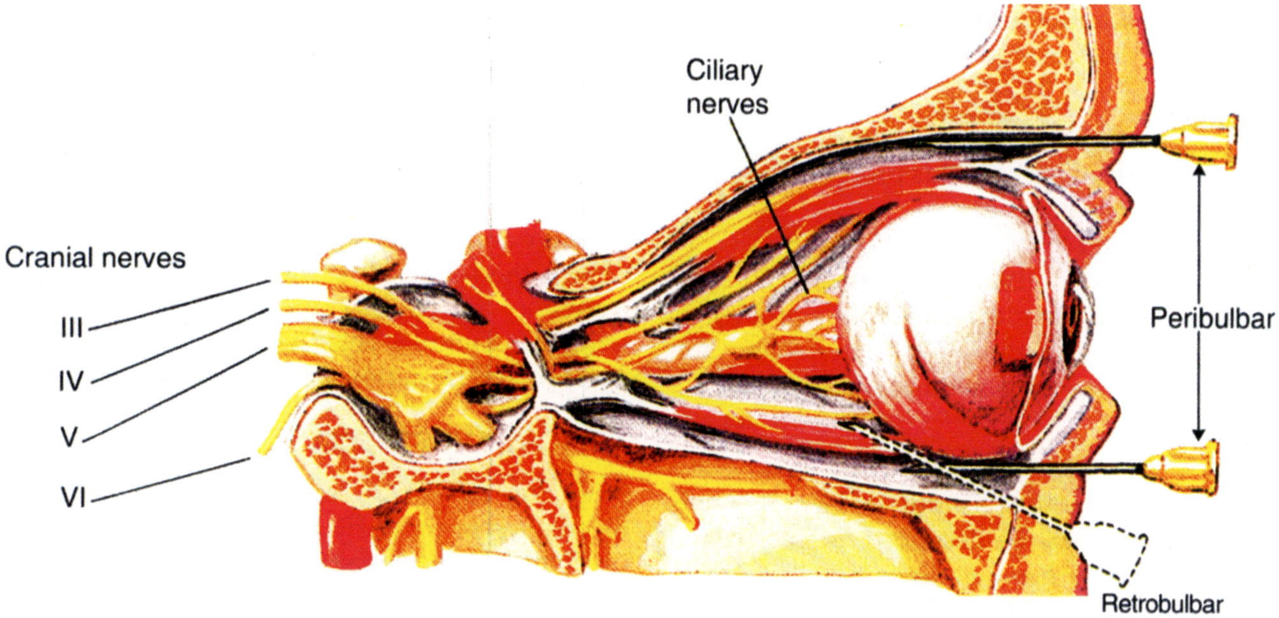

Fig. 7.10: Needle positions for peribulbar and retrobulbar akinesia (*Courtesy:* Ciba Geigy clinical symposia)

2 to 3 ml of the solution. The same procedure is followed in the upper nasal quadrant through the preanesthetised site to inject 1ml and another 1 ml may be injected around superior orbital fissure, by deeper penetration.

At the end of the procedure, fullness of the lids is noted due to the volume of the injected solution. Firm pressure with the flat of the hand is applied over the globe and is maintained for a minute. Then, before surgery, any pressure device as per the surgeon's choice like Honan's balloon, super pinky ball, balance weight or simple pad-bandage is applied for 20 to 30 minutes, to achieve the desire response of hypotony.

The efficacy of the anesthesia is evaluated after about 10 minutes of injection and if inadequate, 2 to 4 ml more can be injected. In case of persistent inferior or lateral movement injection lower temporal quadrant and in case of persistent movements upwards of nasally, the upper quadrant could be infiltrated in the same fashion.

Hyaluronidase is essential as it helps in the spread of the drug. Otherwise, there are chances of the eye being proptosed due to high orbital pressure induced by the large quantity of the fluid injected.

Single injection of 5 to 6 ml of anesthetic mixture injected from any site posterior to equator of the globe also achieves same results. For convenience, however, it may be done through lower lid the junction of lateral and middle one third, along the floor of the orbit.

Adequacy of akinesia is determined by the absence of ocular movements in all directions.

This technique is certainly better than retro-ocular technique and has least complications.

Advantages

The advantages reported are:

1. The injection is done outside the muscle cone and so, the inherent complications of passing the needle into the muscle cone is completely eliminated.
2. It does not enter the retrobulbar space and thereby avoids retrobulbar hemorrhage, injury to optic nerve and entry of anesthetic agents into subarachnoid space and other complications like respiratory arrest.
3. Since the needle is constantly kept parallel to the bony orbit, it avoids injury to globe and entry of anesthetic agents into the eyeball.
4. It causes less pain on injection.
5. The procedure is easier and can be performed without causing damage to vital structures.

6. It does not reduce vision on table.
7. No facial block is required.

Drawback

The possible drawbacks of this procedure are:
1. Chemosis of conjunctiva.
2. Delayed onset of anesthetic effect and
3. Potential risk of orbital hemorrhage. Though it occurs rarely, the magnitude of the problem is comparable to retrobulbar hemorrhage and necessitates postponement of surgery.

Mechanism

The exact mechanism is not known but this procedure may best be described as 'Infiltration anesthesia' where nerve endings in all tissues in the area of injection get anesthetised.

Peribulbar anesthesia is a safe and reliable technique for achieving akinesia and anesthesia of the globe. In case of inadequate anesthesia, repeat injections in the similar manner can be safely used to achieve the purpose.

Superior Rectus Injection

The induction of temporary paralysis of the superior rectus muscle is essential for any intraocular operation where the surgical field is upper half of the eye. This injection also affects the action of levator palpabrae superioris.

In this injection patient is asked to look down. The upper lid is retracted and 2.5 cm long needle is passed into Tenon's capsule at the temporal edge of the superior rectus muscle. The needle is directed posteromedially and about 1 ml of anesthetic mixture of 2 percent Xylocaine is injected around the muscle belly behind the equator. This injection can also be made through the skin of the upper orbital sulcus.

Tenon's Capsule Injection

The injection of anesthetic mixture can be given into Tenon's capsule around the upper half of the eyeball and into the belly of superior rectus muscle. It is considered safer than the retro-ocular injection across the postganglionic fibers of the ciliary body and may be effective in inducing extraocular muscle akinesia.

Parabulbar (Flush) Akinesia

Parabulbar (flush) administration is a new route for local anesthesia which is highly useful, safe, effective and technically easier (Figs 7.11 and 7.12). This method consists of a limbal sub-tenon administration of retrobulbar anesthesia using a blunt irrigating cannula. This technique can be used for anterior and posterior segment surgery.

TOPICAL ANESTHESIA

Since the advent of retrobulbar and peribulbar techniques in the early part of this century, both procedures are mainstay of local anesthesia for intraocular surgery till today. They do carry the risk of perforation of globe, optic nerve and the inadvertent injection of anesthetic at wrong places.

These accidents are mainly due to:
- Carelessness on the part of ophthalmologist who considers the procedures lightly and occurs more often with senior eye surgeons.
- Using long needles for these techniques endangers the perforation of globe, piercing the

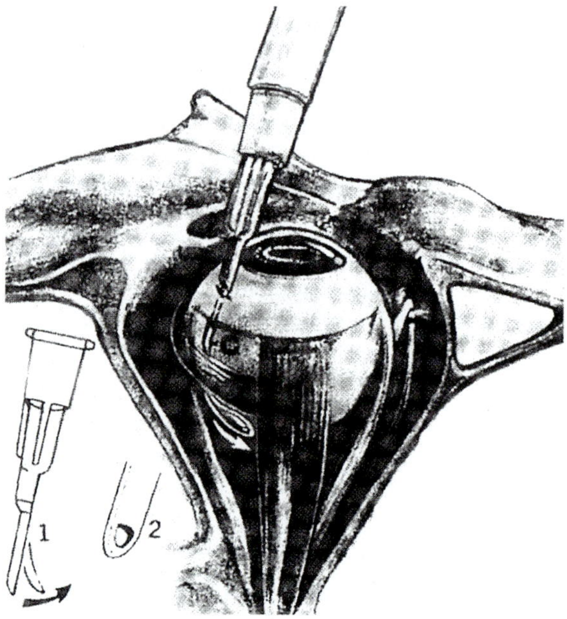

Fig. 7.11: Parabulbar (flush) local anesthesia (cross section view)

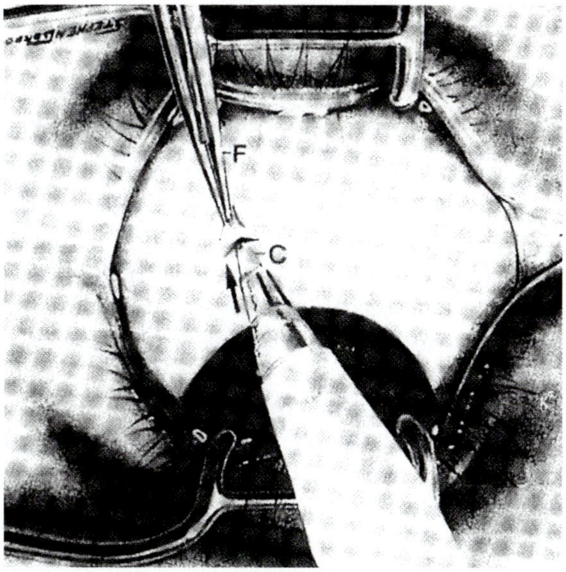

Fig. 7.12: Parabulbar (flush) local anesthesia (surgeon view)

optic nerve and entering crowded retrobulbar space and even touching the intracranial space on forceful injection of copious amounts.

- Anesthetics given through local injection with little knowledge of anatomy of this area.
- Retrobulbar hemorrhage with its adverse effects on nerve and globe is very common complication of this technique.
- Injury caused by perforation of globe can lead to hole formation, retinal detachment, vitreous hemorrhage and central and branch vein occlusions.

To overcome all these practical difficulties use of topical anesthesia in intraocular surgery has been widely suggested and used at an International ophthalmic level. Topical anesthesia meaning topical application of 4 percent Xylocaine or 0.5-0.75 percent proparacaine one drop 3-4 times at regular intervals in the eye has become increasingly popular and accepted. In present day high tech intraocular surgery specially phaco surgery topical anesthesia is the anesthesia of choice with the eye surgeons worldwide.

Indications to Use Topical Anesthesia

- Its indications in intraocular surgery are mainly when performing phacoemulsification and IOL implantation through a clear corneal tunnel and corneoscleral incisions.
- Topical anesthesia is ideally suited for small incision and stitchless cataract surgery. However, it is not a advocated to perform standard / manual extracapsular cataract extraction and IOL implantation.
- Proper selection of patient is of great importance in this technique. It is important to have a patient who will comply with the instructions given during surgery.
- Patients who are non-cooperative, hard of hearing, with language problem and anxious patients are poor candidates for surgery under topical anesthesia. Capsulorrhexis requires the maximum cooperation of the patient.
- Intraocular surgery likely to be problematic in patients with rigid small pupils responding poorly to dilating drops and eyes with lenticular subluxation and high grade nuclear sclerosis are relative contraindications for topical anesthesia.
- Eye surgeon operating with topical anesthesia should be proficient and experienced at phacoemulsification.
- This procedure requires the use of foldable IOL either as a silicone lens or an acrylic lens. This is essential because corneal tunnel suture lens incision cannot be larger then 3.5mm. Otherwise corneal complications may arise and the incision would not be self-sealing.

HOW TO ACHIEVE SURFACE ANESTHESIA FOR INTRAOCULAR SURGERY

Generally 3 applications of 4 percent Xylocaine or 0.4 percent Benoxinate HCL or 0.5-0.75 percent proparacaine 10 minutes apart starting 30 minutes before surgery are recommended. A drop is thereafter instilled prior to the incision. 1 CC of 4 percent Xylocaine or 0.4 percent Benoxinate HCI or 0.5-0.75 proparacaine (from fresh vail) is drawn into sterile disposable syringe and OT staff person is asked to instil a few drops of the same prior to cauterisation of bleeders and if required during surgery conjunctival anesthesia is used (pinpoint and mini pinpoint surface anesthesia)

Apart from giving topical anesthesia one has to give systemic analgesia. Besides it, surgeon should have a commanding hypnotic voice (vocal local anesthesia).

- Most surgeons doing corneal tunnel incision under topical anesthesia prefer to do it from temporal side.

CAN ONE CONVERT HALFWAY THROUGH SURGERY UNDERTOPICAL ANESTHESIA?

Intraoperative conversion from topical to peribulbar anesthesia can definitely be achieved if surgical situation warrants it. Since corneal tunnel incision is sutureless and self-healing a peribulbar injection can safely be given during the surgery.

Advantages of Topical Anesthesia

1. Phacoemulsification experts feel that use of topical anesthesia with a clear corneal tunnel self-healing incision is a significant advancement in intraocular surgery. With topical anesthesia visual recovery is immediate.
2. It prevents the well-known complications of retrobulbar and peribulbar injections as mentioned in the early part of this chapter.
3. It lessens the time of operating room use thereby lowering costs.
4. There is no immediate postoperative ptosis as seen in retrobulbar or peribulbar and Van Lint, O' Brien infiltrations lasts for 6-8 hours due to temporary akinesia of the lids.
5. With topical anesthesia photon laser intraocular surgery can be OPD procedure.
6. In practice we have seen the anxiety of patients to peribulbar and retrobulbar injections prior to surgery. With topical anesthesia this problem is over and patient compliance will be better during intraoperative period.
7. The need of qualified anesthesiologist is over in operation theater during the operation as a number of ophthalmologists have been seen to prefer anesthesiologist by their side for local anesthesia (retrobulbar and peribulbar anesthesia).
8. No risk of postponement of intraocular surgery as seen in cases of retrobulbar hemorrhage.

Again its main advantage is that it provides for immediate postoperative visual recovery.

Disadvantages of Topical Anesthesia

1. Only a highly experienced surgeon can operate with topical anesthesia. The eye can move which makes the operation more difficult. If the eye movement occurs when capsulorrhexis is being done, an undesirable capsular tear may take place leading to failure of this important step of the operation.
2. The chances of intraoperative complications with topical anesthesia can be high if the surgeon is not highly skilled. If such complications arise surgeon should be ready to convert to other methods of local anesthesia during the intraoperative stage, because topical anesthesia along may not be adequate to handle intraoperative complications. Surgeon should be of cool temperament who can handle such a situation without anxiety.
3. Topical anesthesia is not indicated in all patients specially in anxious stressed patients, people with hearing difficulties, children and very young patients.
4. As in our country a large number of patients come from rural areas who are illiterate and poor. Their compliance remains very poor and they do not respond adequately to the command during surgery with topical anesthesia.
5. The presence of very opaque cataract is a contraindication to the use of topical anesthesia. This is because surgeon depends on the patient ability to visually concentrate on the operating microscope light in order to avoid eye movement during the operation. Patients, who are not able to fix the eyes, may lead to complications.
6. Some patients may feel pain during surgery with topical anesthesia. One patient observed a lot more pain and felt as if a sword was being used to cut him up. The pain continued postoperatively for quite sometime.
7. In principle, adequate selection of patients is fundamental when considering the use of topical anesthesia.

In spite of these hurdles topical anesthesia will be a safe and common technique for local anesthesia during intraocular surgery in the near future.

NO ANESTHESIA CATARACT SURGERY

This is the latest technique of cataract surgery in which no anesthesia is required (whether local or topical). Neither the topical or intracameral anesthetics agents are used. This techniques is devised by Dr Amar Agarwal (India) and has been acclaimed and accepted worldwide and is being used routinely in phacoemulsification surgery.

REFERENCES

1. Arora R et al. Peribulbar anesthesia, J Cataract Ref Surg 1991; 17:506-08.
2. Bloomberg L. Administration of periocular anesthesia. J Cataract Ref Surg 1986; 12: 677-79.
3. Bloomberg L. Anterior peribulbar anesthesia. J Cataract Ref Surg 1991; 17: 508-11.
4. Davis DB. Posterior peribulbar anesthesia. J Cataract Ref Surg 1986; 12: 182-84.
5. Fichman RA: Topical anesthesia, Sanders DR, Slack 1993; 1661-72.
6. Furuta M et al. Limbal anesthesia for cataract surgery. Ophthalmic Surg 1990; 21: 22-25.
7. Garg A. Topical anesthesia: Current trends in ophthalmology. New Delhi: Jaypee Brothers Medical Publishers (P) Ltd., 1997;1-5.
8. Hay A et al. Needle perforation of the globe during retrobulbar and peribulbar injection. Ophthalmology 1991; 98: 1017-24.
9. Kimble JA et al. Globe perforation from peribulbar injection. Arch Ophthalmol 1987; 105: 749.
10. Shriver PA et al. Effectiveness of retrobulbar and peribulbar anesthesia. J Cataract Ref Surg 1992; 18: 162-65.
11. Zahl K et al. Ophthalmol Clin North Am. Philadelphia: WB Saunders, 1990.

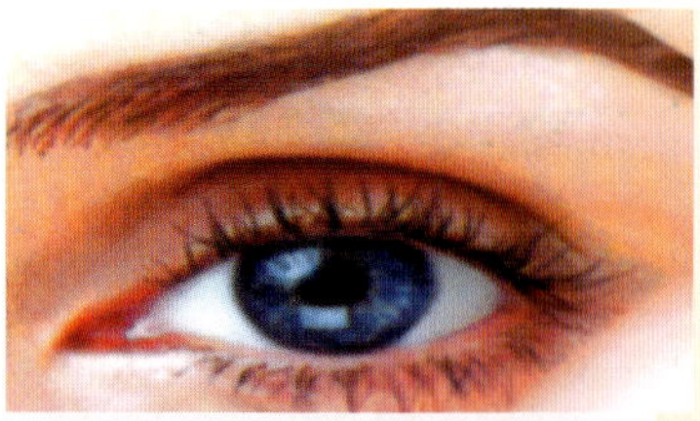

Eight

Viscoanesthetic Solutions for Small Incision Cataract Surgery: Experimental Studies and Clinical Applications

Suresh K Pandey
Liliana Werner
David J Apple
Rupal H Trivedi
Tamer A Macky
Andrea M Izak (USA)

OVERVIEW

Ophthalmic surgeons have witnessed a significant evolution in surgical techniques for cataract extraction in the 20th century (Fig. 8.1). The most remarkable advance is, of course, the considerable decrease in the size of the wound incision.[1] Anesthetic techniques for cataract surgery have also advanced significantly (Fig. 8.2).[2] General anesthesia was preferred in past years, followed by various techniques of injectable anesthesia including retrobulbar, peribulbar, sub-tenon, and subconjunctival anesthesia. Due to marked improvements in surgical techniques, it is no longer essential to ensure complete akinesia of the eye and as a consequence, the technique of topical anesthesia has been popularized as "phaco anesthesia" in the USA, according to recent survey of Leaming.[3] Topical anesthesia includes eye drops application, sponge anesthesia, eye drops plus intracameral injection, and most recently a combination of viscoelastic and anesthetic agent termed as- "viscoanesthesia".

Ciba Vision Corp. (Duluth, GA, USA) has recently developed a solution combining ophthalmic surgical devices (OVDs) with lidocaine that is marketed as **VisThesia™.** VisThesia is primarily a

Technique	Year	Author/Surgeon
Couching	800	Susutra
ECCE* (inferior incision)	1745	Daviel
ECCE (superior incision)	1860	von Graefe
ICCE** (tumbling)	1880	Smith
ECCE with PC-IOL***	1949	Ridley
ECCE with AC-IOL****	1951	Strampelli
Phacoemulsification	1967	Kelman
Foldable IOLs	1984	Mazzocco
Capsular Surgery	1992	Apple/Assia
Accommodating IOLs	1997	Cummings/Kamman
Phakonit/Microphaco/MICS	1998	Agarwal/Olson/Alio
Dye-enhanced Cataract Surgery	2000	Pandey/Werner/Apple

* ECCE: extracapsular cataract extraction
** ICCE: intracapsular cataract extraction
*** PC-IOL: Posterior chamber intraocular lens
**** AC-IOL: anterior chamber intraocular lens

Fig. 8.1: Evolution of techniques for cataract Surgery

Technique	Year	Author
General anesthesia	1846	—
Topical Cocaine	1884	Koller
Injectable Cocaine	1884	Knapp
Orbicularis Akinesia	1914	–Van Lint, O' Briens –Atkinson
Hyaluronidase	1948	Atkinson
Retrobulbar (4% cocaine)	1884	Knapp
Posterior peribulbar	1985	Davis and Mandel
Limbal	1990	Furata and coworkers
Anterior peribulbar	1991	Bloomberg
Pinpoint anesthesia	1992	Fukasawa
Topical	1992	Fichman
Topical plus intracameral	1995	Gills
No anesthesia	1998	Agarwal
Cryoanalgesia	1999	Guitierrez-Carmona
Xylocaine jelly	1999	Koch, Assia
Hypothesis, No anesthesia	2001	Pandey and Agarwal
Viscoanesthesia, La. Studies	2001	Werner, Pandey, Apple and Assia

Fig. 8.2: Evolution of Anesthetic Techniques for Cataract Surgery

viscoelastic substance, the thick, elastic gel used during eye surgery to protect the eye. The product also contains an anesthetic compound, which provides an ancillary, supportive anesthetic effect. The unique combination of viscoelastic and anesthesia, with topical and intracameral components, help shorten the procedure time and increase patient comfort. In addition, an intracameral injection has been shown to increase patient comfort over the use of a topical anesthetic alone. VisThesia™ is packaged with both topical and intracameral components with separate percentages of sodium hyaluronate and lidocaine hydrochloride. Topical: 2 percent Lidocaine, 0.3 percent HAc. Surgeons have the advantage of no longer needing to choose between a topical or intracameral anesthetic. In addition, they can save time by eliminating separate injections of viscoelastic and anesthetic. VisThesia is not yet approved by US FDA, however, it is available in the European Union and is CE Mark approved.

Combination of viscoelastic agent with visco-anesthetic would not only eliminate the necessity of extra surgical steps for intracameral injection of lidocaine, but also would help keeping the anesthetic effect longer. The indispensable role of OVDs in ophthalmic surgery, not only in maintaining the depth of the anterior chamber and keeping the capsular bag expanded but also in protecting intraocular structures, especially the corneal endothelium remain unchangeable. Nevertheless, by incorporating lidocaine to the OVD, the risk of toxicity to the corneal endothelial cells may increase, because of a direct and prolonged contact of lidocaine with these cells.

We have extensively evaluated the safety of viscoanesthetic solutions to intraocular structures. This work was divided into 3 parts:

1. We used the principles of vital staining of the corneal endothelium in an *in vitro* animal model to determine the toxicity of viscoanesthetic solutions to the corneal endothelium;
2. Toxicity of viscoanesthetic solutions to uveal tissues and retina were evaluated after phacoemulsification;
3. Surgical aspects such as injection and aspiration of the viscoanesthetic solutions were evaluated and compared to currently available OVDs.

VISCOANESTHESIA PART I

EVALUATION OFTOXICITY OF VISCOANESTHESIA SOLUTIONTO CORNEAL ENDOTHELIAL CELLS

Background

Intraocular lidocaine has recently gained attention as an effective adjunct to topical anesthesia during cataract surgery. Topical anesthesia was used in combination with intracameral lidocaine by 31 pecent of the respondents of the 1998 survey conducted by the American Society of Cataract and Refractive Surgery (ASCRS), by 37 percent of the 1999 ASCRS survey and by 40 percent of the 2000 ASCRS survey.[1-3] Its injection into the anterior chamber (AC) intraoperatively is claimed to be beneficial in reducing patient discomfort experienced during phacoemulsification and iris manipulation.[4] Literature has tested safety and efficacy of intracameral lidocaine.[5-19]

However, ophthalmologists who perform cataract surgery with the patient receiving topical and/or intracameral anesthesia must work quickly to finish the surgery before the anesthesia wears off and the patient starts reporting discomfort.[20] If a patient reports discomfort during the procedure, the surgeon may adopt one of the following strategies:

1. The surgeon can forge ahead and finish the procedure as quickly as possible, not providing additional anesthesia;
2. He may ask the anesthesiologist to administer an intravenous narcotic analgesic;
3. He can interrupt the procedure and administer a parabulbar or posterior orbital block, aware that this might generate unwanted external pressure on an open globe. Most surgeons consider supplementing the topical block with additional drops if this happens, or they might consider intracameral supplementation. If they choose either of the latter two options, they need to be aware about the likelihood of endothelial toxicity from any anesthetic agent that enters or is injected into the eye.

In viscoanesthetic solution ophthalmic surgical devices (OVDs) is combined with lidocaine. This would not only eliminate the necessity of extra surgical steps for intracameral injection of lidocaine, but also would help keeping the anesthetic effect longer. The indispensable role of OVDs in ophthalmic surgery, not only in maintaining the depth of the AC and keeping the capsular bag expanded but also in protecting intraocular structures, especially the corneal endothelium remain unchangeable.[21] Nevertheless, by incorporating lidocaine to the OVD, the risk of toxicity to the corneal endothelial cells may increase, because of a direct and prolonged contact of lidocaine with these cells.

Table 8.1: Solutions used in this study and number of corneas used in each group

Solution	*Number of corneas exposed*
1.5% Na hyaluronate / 0.5% lidocaine	5
1.5% Na hyaluronate / 1.0% lidocaine	5
1.5% Na hyaluronate / 1.65% lidocaine	5
1.5% Na hyaluronate (Ophthalin Plus®, Ciba Vision Corp., Duluth, GA)	5
No solution	2
BSS®	2
Mitomycin C (0.02%)	2
15% Dextran	2
Distilled water	2

In current study (Viscoanesthesia Part I), we used the principles of vital staining of the corneal endothelium in an *in vitro* animal model to determine the toxicity of the viscoanesthetic solution to the corneal endothelium.[5,22] The toxicity of viscoanesthetic solutions to uveal tissues and retina after phacoemulsification and surgical aspects such as injection and aspiration of the viscoanesthetic solutions will be discussed subsequently.[23,24]

In Vitro Animal Study for Evaluation of Endothelial Toxicity

A total of 15 Dutch Belted, pigmented rabbits weighing 2.0 to 2.5 kg were anesthetized with an intramuscular injection of xylazine (5-8 mg/kg) and ketamine hydrochloride (35-44 mg/kg). The care and treatment of animals conformed to the Association for Research in Vision and Ophthalmology (ARVO) statement for the use of animals in ophthalmic and vision research. They were sacrificed by injection of pentobarbitol sodium into an ear vein. The eyeballs were enucleated. This study used the model of Werner *et al*[5] to determine the toxicity of xylocaine to the corneal endothelium. Immediately after enucleation, their corneas and a 2.00 mm rim of sclera were removed with a blade, and a partial-thickness scleral section was created with scissors. Care was taken to avoid touching the center of the corneal endothelium during manipulation. The iris diaphragm was peeled from the cornea, which was then placed in a corneal cup, endothelial side up. The excavation of the cup corresponded to the corneal curvature.

Table 8.1 shows the different groups of solutions used in our study. We used viscoanesthetic solutions having 3 different concentrations of lidocaine. Table 8.2 presents some of the characteristic of these solutions, according to the manufacturer. Some corneas were also exposed to the same viscoelastic solution, without lidocaine (Ophthalin Plus®, Ciba Vision Corp., Duluth, GA, USA). Two negative controls (without toxicity) were used: the "no solution", where the corneas were stained immediately after excision, and BSS® (Alcon Laboratories, Fort Worth, TX). The positive controls used were 0.02 percent mitomycin C (toxic control), 15% Dextran (hyper-osmotic solution) and distilled water (hypo-osmotic solution). Each cornea was exposed to one of the solutions for 20 minutes at room temperature except in the no solution group, where the cornea was stained immediately after excision. The 20-minute exposure was selected because it is about the time the corneal endothelium is exposed to intracameral lidocaine during phacoemulsification and intraocular lens implantation.

Following rinsing of the cornea in 0.9 percent saline, the endothelium was immediately stained using a modification of the method of Spence and Peyman,[22] as follows: immersion in 0.25 percent trypan blue in saline for 90 seconds, 2 rinses in 0.9 percent saline, immersion in 1 percent alizarin red for 60 seconds and a final rinse in 0.9 percent saline.

Table 8.2: Characteristics of the viscoelastic and viscoanesthetic solutions used in this study

Formula	*OPHTHALIN Plus®*	*HA/ 0.5% Lidocaine*	*HA/ 1.0% Lidocaine*	*HA/ 1.65% Lidocaine*
[Na hyaluronate] mg/ml	14.9	15.4	15.7	16.1
[Lidocaine] %	0	0.49	0.97	1.65
[Chloride] as NaCl mg/ml	9.27	8.19	7.17	9.7
Osmolality mOsm/kg	335	309	288	380
pH	7.42	7.40	7.35	7.14

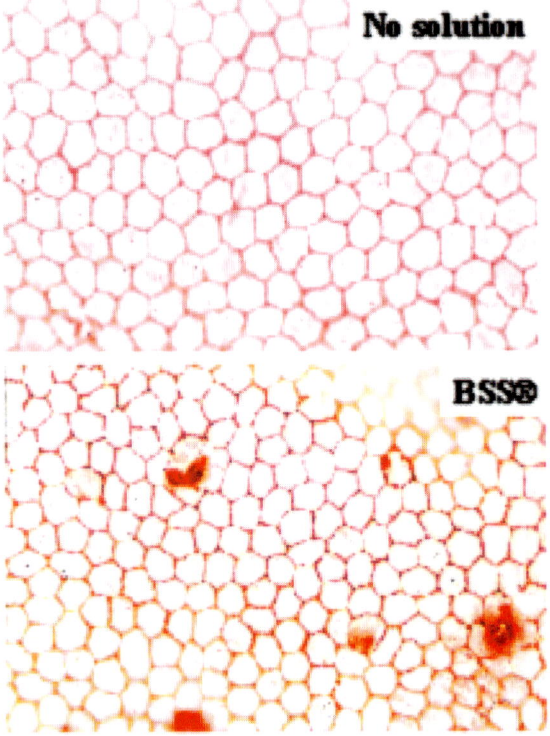

Fig. 8.3: Negative, non toxic control (No solution and BSS®). In the no solution group the corneas were stained immediately after excision

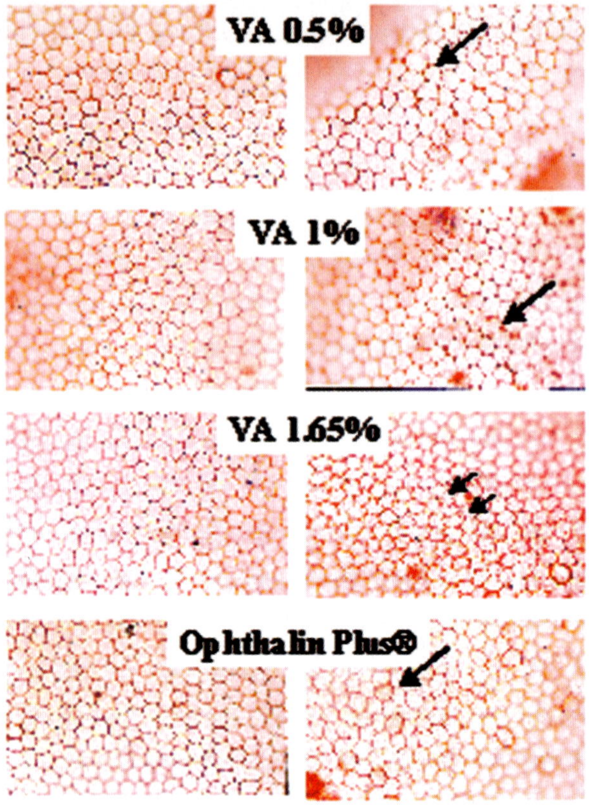

Fig. 8.4: Experimental solutions. In the majority of the corneas analyzed, the aspect of the corneal endothelial cells was similar to that in the negative controls. The large arrows indicate cells presenting slight edema. The small arrows indicate cells presenting irregular intercellular borders

Six to 8 peripheral radial incisions were made in each cornea, which was placed between a glass slide and a plastic cover slip for examination under a standard light microscope.

The amount of endothelial damage was assessed on photographs taken at a standard magnification of x 400. Five photomicrographs from the center of each cornea were required for analysis. The areas of damaged cells (trypan blue staining) and cell loss (alizarin red staining) were evaluated in each photomicrograph.

Results of *In Vitro* Animal Study

Figures 8.3 and 8.5 illustrate the status of endothelial cells in each group of corneas. With the visco-anesthetic solutions and Ophthalin-Plus® large areas of the corneal endothelium in all 5 corneas of each group were comparable to the negative controls (Figs 8.3 and 8.4). In some areas, the 6 corners of the endothelium cells presented a slight edema, appearing as dots (Fig. 8.4, big arrows). This was observed in the Ophthalin Plus® group and in all 3 viscoanesthetic groups. In some areas of the 1 percent and 1.65 percent viscoanesthetic groups, the corneal endothelial cells presented irregular intercellular borders (Fig. 8.4, small arrows). Nevertheless, staining of the cells with trypan blue, which indicates cellular damage, was just observed in some linear areas corresponding to corneal folds in all groups, including the no solution group (Fig. 8.5).

Figure 8.5 also demonstrates the effect on rabbit corneal endothelium after exposure to 0.02 percent mitomycin C, 15 percent Dextran and distilled water. Mitomycin caused an almost complete destruction of the endothelial cells. The intercellular

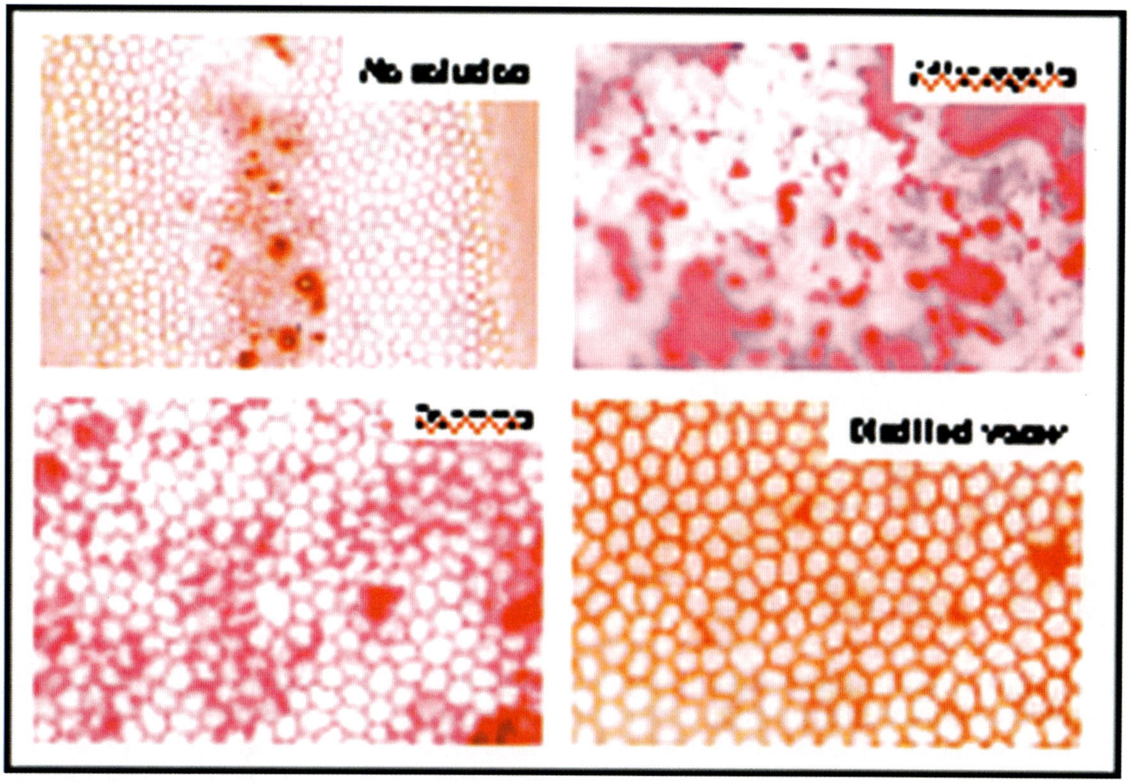

Fig. 8.5: Linear areas of staining with trypan blue were observed in all groups (arrows). Destruction of the endothelial cells was observed in the mitomycin C group. Osmotic effects were observed in the Dextran and distilled water groups

borders were irregular after exposure to Dextran, and thickened (edema) after exposition to distilled water.

PRESENT EXPERIMENTAL STUDY, REVIEW OF THE LITERATURE AND CLINICAL APPLICATIONS

Intraocular lidocaine theoretically diffuses into the iris and ciliary body to provide additional local anesthesia, which could be useful in cases in which manipulation of intraocular tissue (e.g., iris and lens) is required. However, intracameral lidocaine has the tendency to easily wash away during phacoemulsification. If the surgery is delayed for longer than a normal duration, its effect may wear off. As previously mentioned, the surgeon can repeat the injection of intracameral anesthetic solution. However, this may not be efficacious. The literature has reported a limited role of intracameral solutions once OVDs are injected into the AC, as they might not reach the target organs in sufficient concentration. Fenzl and Gills have reported that if patients were given an OVD before the introduction of the lidocaine, it significantly impedes this substance from accessing the iris root and the ciliary body.

If surgeons have anesthetic solutions pre-mixed in OVDs, in theory, the chances that they will reach the target organs would be maximized. This hypothesis is supported by the observation that the anterior capsule of white cataracts often does not stain well with trypan blue in the presence of an OVD in the anterior chamber. However, trypan blue pre-mixed with 1 percent sodium hyaluronate in a 2 ml syringe or in the viscoelastic disposable injector in a 1:1 ratio provides better visibility. Some authors have used this technique without significant surgical and postoperative adverse experiences. However, they noted that there might be potential risks of corneal decompensation after intraocular use of self-mixed solutions.[27]

The intracameral use of any new solution certainly raises the concern over its effect on the corneal endothelium. In this study we evaluated the safety of viscoanesthetic solutions to rabbit corneal endothelium. A rabbit model was chosen because of gross morphologic similarities between rabbit and human corneas, general familiarity of the medical community with this model and also, the effects of intracameral anesthesia have been previously tested in rabbit eyes.[5]

In this study, toxicity of viscoanesthetic solutions to the rabbit corneal endothelium was assayed using vital staining with trypan blue and alizarin red. In normal eyes, the endothelial cell is impervious to trypan blue and does not stain. However, in the presence of damage to the cell membrane, trypan blue will penetrate into the cells, producing blue-staining cytoplasms and nuclei. Exclusion of trypan blue suggests preserved cellular integrity. Alizarin red stains intercellular borders and bare Descemet's membrane. Therefore, combined staining with trypan blue and alizarin red allows the analysis of endothelium cell morphology and integrity, with determination of areas presenting cell damage or loss.[5,22]

No evidence of endothelial cell damage (staining with trypan blue) or endothelial cell loss (staining with alizarin red) was found with the viscoanesthetic solutions used in this study. Staining of the cells with trypan blue was only observed in some linear areas (Fig. 8.5, arrows), corresponding to corneal folds in all groups (controls and viscoanesthetic). These were probably caused during manipulation for corneal excision and staining.

The morphological aspect seen in Fig. 8.4 (irregular intercellular borders) is similar to the aspect of endothelium cells after exposition to lidocaine solutions as described by Werner *et al* in the literature.[5] We do not believe this effect is due to direct toxicity, but rather comes from differences in ionic composition, pH and osmolality of the solutions used. BSS® has a pH of 6.96 and an osmolality of 310 mOsmol/Kg. Also, its composition is close to that of the aqueous humor, with all the essential ions (potassium, calcium…). Thus, after 20 minutes of direct exposure with solutions having a composition different from that of the aqueous humor, some morphologic alterations could be expected to occur.[28,29]

Studies of irrigating solutions for intraocular surgery demonstrated their efficacy is critically dependent on their composition. Waring and coauthors[30] listed the factors that decrease barrier and pump functions of corneal endothelium. Among them, are the use of calcium-free solutions, substances such as diamide that cause oxidation of intracellular glutathione, solutions beyond the pH range of 6.8 to 8.2, preservatives such as sodium bisulfite, thimerosal, and benzalkonium chloride, substances such as Ouabain that cause inhibition of ATPase or bromacetazolamide that inhibits the carbonic anhydrase within the endothelial cells, bicarbonate-free solutions, and solutions with an osmolarity between 200 and 400 mOsm without the essential ions.

Our experimental model demonstrates that the morphological alterations in the experimental groups were not associated with cell nonviability (lack of trypan blue staining), but it did not assess how these alterations are associated with impaired endothelial functions. However, Yagoubi and coauthors[29] evaluated the effects of sodium chloride 0.9 percent, Hartmann's solution, BSS® and BSS® Plus on the corneal endothelium of rabbits. Irrigation with 1 of the solutions for 90 minutes was followed by a 6 hour perfusion with tissue culture medium, during which endothelial function was assessed by measuring the swelling and thinning rates of corneas, respectively, in the absence and presence of bicarbonate ions. All solutions caused some change in endothelial cell morphology, but none had an apparent effect on the barrier properties or pump function of the endothelium.

Our study showed that lidocaine pre-mixed with an OVD appears to be safe to the rabbit corneal endothelium. Effects of the prolonged contact of lidocaine contained in viscoanesthetic solutions with intraocular structures such as uvea and retina were evaluated in part II of this work. Further *in vivo* clinical studies are needed to determine the efficacy and long-term effects of viscoanesthesia on intraocular tissues.

VISCOANESTHESIA PART II

EVALUATION OF TOXICITY TO INTRAOCULAR STRUCTURES AFTER PHACOEMULSIFICATION

Background

The concept of using intracameral lidocaine as an adjunct to topical anesthesia during cataract surgery was introduced by Gills in 1995.[4] Since then, several studies have looked at the efficacy and safety profile of intracameral lidocaine and other anesthetic agents with respect to their effect on the corneal endothelium, aqueous flare and cells, and retinal photoreceptor cells.[4,3140] Most clinical studies suggest that the use of up to 0.5 ml of non-preserved 1% lidocaine intracamerally is safe.[31-33]

Anderson *et al*[8] found that the irrigation during phacoemulsification provides a washout effect and thereby limits the exposure of ocular tissues to lidocaine. Particularly, intracameral lidocaine injections occur in most surgeries after the use if viscoelastic to maintain the anterior chamber, thus allowing the corneal endothelium to be coated with viscoelastics, which will prevent direct contact with the lidocaine.

The aim of present study (Part II) was to assess the effects on intraocular structures of a solution combining 1.5 percent of sodium (Na) hyaluronate with 3 different concentrations of lidocaine, namely 0.5 percent, 1 percent and 1.65 perceny. Histological analyses of different ocular structures of rabbit eyes, in particular iris, lens capsular bag, ciliary body, and retina were performed at different time points after intraocular injection of the solutions.

In Vitro Animal Study

Twenty-nine Dutch Belted, pigmented rabbits weighing 2.0 to 2.5 kg were used in this study.[23] The care and treatment of animals conformed to the Association for Research in Vision and Ophthalmology (ARVO) statement for the use of animals in ophthalmic and vision research. Phacoemulsification was performed in both eyes of the 29 rabbits. For 21 rabbits, 1 of the viscoanesthetic solutions was used during the procedure (7 rabbits or 14 eyes/solution): (i) 1.5 percent Na hyaluronate/0.5 percent lidocaine, (ii) 1.5 percent Na hyaluronate/1.0 percent lidocaine and (iii) 1.5 percent Na hyaluronate/1.65 percent lidocaine. For 4 rabbits (8 eyes), BSS® was used as a control. For other 4 rabbits, 1.5 percent Na hyaluronate alone without lidocaine was used as a control. The 1.5 percent Na hyaluronate solution used in all groups was Ophthalin Plus® (Ciba Vision Corp., Duluth, GA, USA).

Surgical procedure

Table 8.3 shows the distribution of rabbit eyes according to the different solutions and surgical technique. The basic surgical technique used was as follows. The rabbits were anesthetized with an intramuscular injection of xylazine (5-8 mg/kg) and ketamine hydrochloride (35-44 mg/Kg). After pupil dilation with tropicamide and phenylephrine 10 percent eye drops, a 3.2 mm limbal incision was performed at 12 o'clock with a pre-calibrated keratome. The anterior chamber was entered and 1-2 ml of heparin (10,000 units/ml) was injected into the anterior chamber. This is required to control intraocular fibrin formation usually seen in this animal.

The viscoelastic/viscoanesthetic solution was injected into the anterior chamber and also behind the iris (according to the indications of the manufacturer). A 5 mm capsulorhexis was performed with an Utrata forceps, followed by hydrodissection and phacoemulsification/aspiration. For the control rabbits (n=8), capsulorhexis was performed under Ophthalin Plus®. After complete evacuation of the capsular bag, 0.2 ml of the viscoanesthetic solution (or BSS®, for 8 control eyes and Ophthalin Plus® for the other 8 control eyes) was injected into the capsular bag. The limbal incision was closed with a single 10-0 nylon suture. A subconjunctival injection of dexamethasone and gentamycin was performed at the end of the procedure.

Part (a) (Table 8.3); 24 rabbits or 48 eyes: The right eye of each rabbit was operated on as described above. The left eye underwent the same procedure, with one exception. The posterior capsule was intentionally perforated prior to injection of the viscoanesthetic solution (or BSS® or Ophthalin Plus) within the capsular bag.

Table 8.3: Distribution of rabbits in the study and control groups

a.	Lidocain			Concentration			Control		Control	
Enucleation (days)	*0.50%*	*0.50%*	*1%*	*1%*	*1.65%*	*1.65%*	*BSS®*	*BSS®*	*Ophthalin Plus*	
	PC perforation*		*PC perforation*		*PC perforation*		*PC perforation*		*PC perforation*	
	No	Yes	No	Yes	No	Yes	No	Yes	No	Yes
15	2**	2	2	2	2	2	1	1	1	1
30	2	2	2	2	2	2	1	1	1	1
60	2	2	2	2	2	2	1	1	1	1

b.	Lidocaine	Concentration		Control	Control
Enucleation (days)	*0.50% Intravitreous injection*	*1% Intravitreous injection*	*1.65% Intravitreous injection*	*BSS ® Intravitreous injection*	*Ophthalin Plus® Intravitreous injection*
15	0	0	0	0	0
30	0	0	0	0	0
60	2	2	2	2	2

*PC = posterior capsule.
** = number of rabbit eyes.

Part (b) (Table 8.3); 5 rabbits or 10 eyes: A separate group of 5 rabbits underwent the same procedure. After rupture of the posterior capsule in all of the 10 eyes, the same amount of viscoanesthetic solution (or BSS® or Ophthalin Plus®) was injected into the vitreous cavity.

Injection of solutions in the capsular bag after perforation of the posterior capsule (a) and direct intravitreal injection (b) were specifically done to analyze possible retinal toxicity secondary to retained viscoanesthetic solutions. Postoperative topical therapy included eye ointment containing dexamethasone, polymixin B and neomycin once a day for 2 weeks, and cyclopentolate eye drops once a day for 1 week. Slit-lamp examinations were performed weekly to evaluate the presence of corneal edema and inflammatory reaction of the anterior chamber.

Histopathological examination

Part (a) (Table 8.3); 24 rabbits or 48 eyes: After intramuscular anesthesia, as described above, 2 rabbits from each group of viscoanesthetic solutions were sacrificed with an intravenous injection of pentobarbital at 15, 30 and 60 days after the surgery. Two rabbits from the control group (1 of the BSS® group and 1 of the Ophthalin Plus® group) were sacrificed at each time point.

Part (b) (Table 8.3); 5 rabbits or 10 eyes: One rabbit from each group of viscoanesthetic solutions and two rabbits from the control group (1 of the BSS® group and 1 of the Ophthalin Plus® group) were sacrificed with an intravenous injection of pentobarbital at 60 days after the surgery.

After enucleation, all eyes were prepared for histological evaluation. Histological sections were stained with hematoxylin / eosin, PAS and Masson's trichome stains. Analyses focused on the presence of possible inflammatory reaction in structures such as iris, lens capsular bag, ciliary body, and retina, as well as signs of cell necrosis or degeneration.

Results of the Study

All of the surgeries were uneventful. In the first postoperative week, 9 rabbit eyes had moderate to severe inflammatory reactions, with cells and flare in the anterior chamber and corneal edema. These were: 1 eye in the group receiving 0.5 percent viscoanesthesia, 4 eyes in the group receiving 1 percent viscoanesthesia, 2 eyes in the group receiving 1.65 percent viscoanesthesia and 2 eyes in the group receiving Ophthalin Plus®. No eyes in the group receiving BSS® showed signs of moderate to severe inflammation. Most of these eyes had the inflammatory reaction and corneal edema resolved in the second postoperative week. Only 3 eyes developed permanent corneal opacities.

The other rabbit eyes (n=49) presented a mild inflammatory reaction in the first 2 days that resolved by the end of the first week leaving minimal posterior synechia in some cases. These eyes remained clinically quiet thereafter until the end of the 60-day follow up of the study.

Histopathologically all eyes in the study and control groups showed no signs of toxicity. Light microscopy examination of multiple sections from each eye showed normal iris tissue, ciliary body epithelium, lens epithelium, and neurosensory retina in all study and control groups. No differences were found among the various groups at 15, 30 and 60 days postoperatively (Figs 8.6 to 8.8). Also, there was no difference in the appearance of the neurosensory retina between eyes receiving intravitreal injections of the viscoanesthetic solutions in comparison to those that only received in the bag injections (with posterior capsule perforation or not).

Current Study, Review of Literature and the Clinical Applications

Although topical eye drop anesthesia alone has been shown to be safe and effective, various investigators have documented an increase in the patients' subjective experience of pain during parts of the surgery that involve iris manipulation, globe expansion, and intraocular lens (IOL) implantation.[11-13] Topically applied agents block the trigeminal nerve endings in the cornea and, to a lesser extent, the conjunctiva. The analgesic effect on the iris and ciliary body depends on penetration of the anesthetic agent into the anterior chamber. Bellucci *et al*[37] showed that topical lidocaine 4 percent eye drop administration results in intracameral penetration that increases with the number of applications. Behndig and Linden[12] measured aqueous humor concentrations of lidocaine after intracameral administration and found it to be 100 times higher than after topical administration. Hence, in an attempt to further decrease patient discomfort, it has been proposed that the anterior chamber should be irrigated with 1 percent unpreserved lidocaine at the beginning of surgery.

Lidocaine gel formulation has the potential advantage of increased contact time with the ocular surface, thus providing sustained release and a prolonged anesthetic effect. The safety of lidocaine 2 percent gel for ocular use during cataract surgery

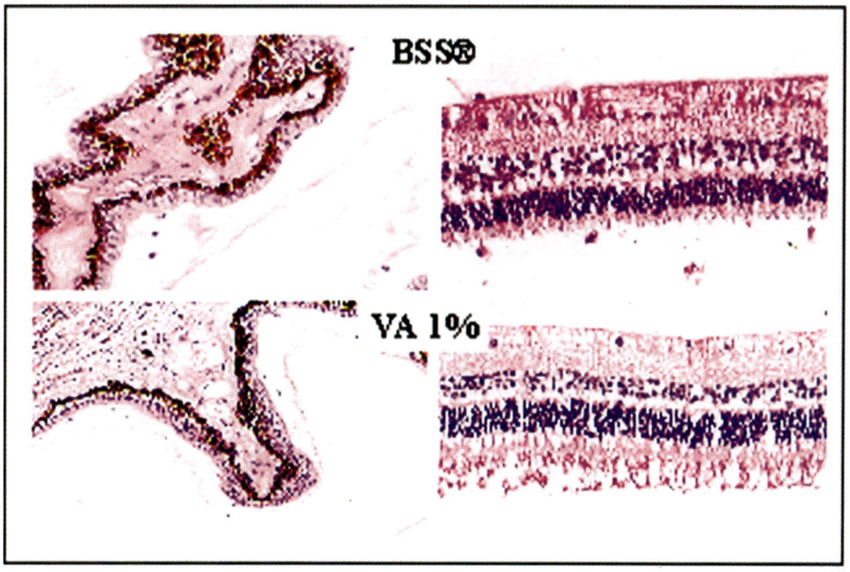

Fig. 8.6: Photomicrographs from the ciliary body (left) and retina (right) of rabbit eyes in the BSS® and 1% viscoanesthesia groups. Both rabbits had the posterior capsule purposely ruptured during the procedure and were sacrificed at 15 days postoperatively. PAS stain; original magnification x 100 and x 200

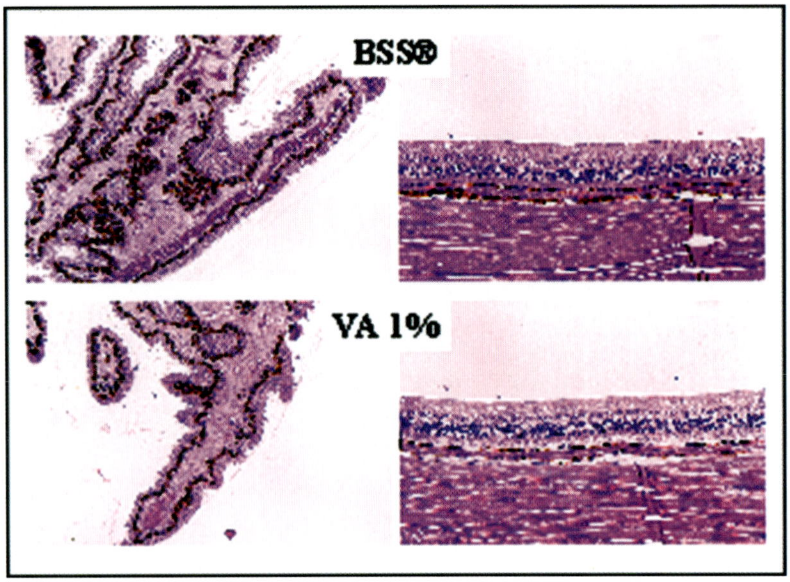

Fig. 8.7: Photomicrographs from the ciliary body (left) and retina (right) of rabbit eyes in the BSS® and 1% viscoanesthesia groups. Both rabbits were sacrificed at 30 days postoperatively. PAS stain; original magnification x100 and x 200

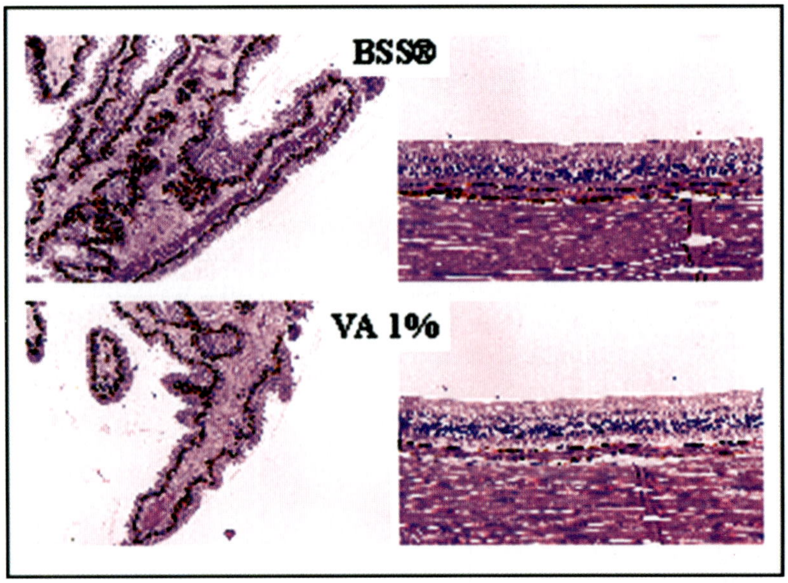

Fig. 8.8: Photomicrographs from the ciliary body (left) and retina (right) of rabbit eyes in the BSS® and 1% viscoanesthesia groups. Both rabbits had intravitreal injection of the solutions during the procedure and were sacrificed at 60 days postoperatively. PAS stain; original magnification x 100 and x 200

was investigated by Barequet *et al*[41] They demonstrated that an application of a 6.5 mm (0.25) strip of lidocaine 2 percent gel to the conjunctival fornix of rabbit eyes for up to 30 minutes did not cause any clinical or histopathologic changes to the corneal endothelium. Furthermore, intentional replacement of the aqueous humor with gel for 15 minutes, after which the rabbits were sacrificed, did not cause histopathologic corneal endothelial changes.

Barequet *et al*[41] also found in the clinical part of their study that a single application of 2 percent lidocaine gel was as effective as topical tetracaine 0.5 percent drops with respect to patients' subjective experience of pain. Koch[42] reported that a double application of 2 percent lidocaine gel was even more effective, making the pain scores comparable to topical proparacaine 1 percent plus 0.5 ml intracameral lidocaine 1 percent. Assia *et al*[43] used three to five applications of lidocaine 2 percent gel to demonstrate that this type of anesthesia can be used not only for phacoemulsification but also for manual extracapsular cataract extraction.

In our study we investigated the toxicity of a novel viscoanesthetic solution composed of 1.5

percent Na hyaluronate with different concentrations of lidocaine (0.5%, 1% and 1.65%) to ocular tissues, especially iris, lens capsular bag, ciliary body, and retina. The main objective of using such solutions is to maintain the anesthetic level of intraocular tissue by prolonging and maintaining the duration of ocular tissue exposure to lidocaine. This is expected to decrease patient discomfort and pain during intraocular manipulations, especially of the iris tissue either with surgical instruments or by the rapid change in anterior chamber depth during surgery. As a result of the prolonged exposure, a study investigating the toxicity of the new solution was essential. We purposely left 0.2 ml of the solutions in each rabbit eye at the end of the surgical procedure. This was done to evaluate the potential effects of having viscoanesthetic solutions in those eyes, after uncomplicated or complicated (posterior capsule rupture) cataract surgery.

Clinical and histopathological examinations showed no apparent toxicity to intraocular structures. There were no differences between the study and control groups at 15, 30 and 60 days postoperatively, or between the groups receiving in-the-bag injection and intravitreal injection. The viscoanesthetic solutions appeared to be well tolerated by intraocular tissues for 60 days. The moderate to severe inflammatory reactions and corneal edema observed in some of the eyes were probably due to the relatively large amount of residual viscoelastics material purposely left in the eye that caused a rise in intraocular pressure. This cannot be attributed to the lidocaine per se as it was observed in eyes receiving Ophthalin Plus® alone (without lidocaine) and not in eyes receiving BSS®. Unfortunately we were unable to check the intraocular pressure of the rabbit eyes during the first postoperative week to confirm this hypothesis.

Although not directly being one of the objectives of this study, it was observed that the viscoanesthetic solutions were of assistance in maintaining pupillary dilatation during surgery. Eyes operated on with viscoanesthetic solutions (0.5%, 1% or 1.65%) maintained better pupillary dilation during the phacoemulsification and up to the end of the surgery compared to eyes operated on with Ophthalin Plus®. We believe that pupillary dilation was significantly different between the study and control groups, but further scientific investigation of this phenomenon is essential before drawing definitive conclusions.

To summarize, the results of the present study indicate that intracameral or intravitreal administration of the newly proposed viscoanesthetic solutions induced no toxic effects to intraocular tissues. No histological evidence of toxicity to uveal tissue or neurosensory retina was observed in rabbit eyes at 15, 30 and 60 days postoperatively. Inflammatory reactions and corneal edema observed in some eyes were related to the presence of residual viscoelastic material. We cannot definitively rule out the possibility of sub-threshold toxic effects to the rabbit retina without electroretinogram and/or electron microscopic studies. Also, clinical trials are necessary to address the issue of efficacy of viscoanesthesia in providing long duration anesthetic effects in comparison to intracameral injection of aqueous lidocaine.

VISCOANESTHESIA PART III

EVALUATION OF THE REMOVAL TIME OF VISCOELASTIC/VISCOANESTHETIC SOLUTIONS FROM THE CAPSULAR BAG

Background

Viscoelastic agents or so-called ophthalmic viscosurgical devices (OVDs) have been widely used to increase the ease and safety of different ophthalmic surgeries.[44] Sodium hyaluronate was first used in 1972, when it was introduced as a replacement for vitreous and aqueous humor.[45] In recent years, the field of viscosurgery has broadened rapidly and viscoelastic agents have been used intraocularly, as well as extraocularly, for procedures including cataract, cornea, glaucoma, vitreoretinal, stra bismus, and oculoplastic surgeries. OVDs are used during the cataract surgery along with intraocular lens (IOL) implantation to maintain the anterior chamber depth and capsular bag distention, thus creating and preserving working space for the ophthalmic surgeon.[45-53] These substances were primarily designed to protect the delicate corneal endothelial cells during the surgery.

Researchers and vision scientists have been using OVDs as a vehicle to deliver capsular dyes for use during the cataract surgery (Akahoshi T, Soft shell stain technique for the white cataract, presented at the ASCRS symposium on Cataract, IOL, and Refractive Surgery, Boston, MA, May 2000).[27] Mixing these substances with the viscoelastic agent was attempted to prolong their effect and to limit adverse reactions on ocular tissues. Visthesia™ (Ciba Vision, Duluth, GA), was developed to prolong the anesthetic effect of intracameral lidocaine, as a complement to topical anesthesia. Also, the steps of intracameral injection of OVDs and of intracameral injection of lidocaine would be combined in only one step.

Since residual viscoelastic material is not metabolized in the eye, and its fate is unknown, a complete removal of these agents from the capsular bag and anterior chamber is recommended to avoid any adverse effects and complications, such as postoperative intraocular pressure (IOP) elevation.[2,3,7] Assia *et al*[54] have investigated the ease and the time necessary for complete removal of different OVDs from the capsular bag of human cadaver eyes, by using the Miyake-Apple posterior video technique.

We have recently performed an experimental work to investigate whether or not the addition of lidocaine to the OVD significantly changes its viscosity, and changes its intraoperative performance. We used the same model of Assia *et al*[54] focusing on the ease of injection and removal of 3 viscoanesthetic solutions containing different concentrations of lidocaine, in comparison to a currently available OVD.

In Vitro Experimental Study

Randomly accessioned post-mortem human eyes (n=6) obtained within 48 hours of death from Eye Banks nationwide were used to investigate and evaluate the removal time of various viscoelastic/viscoanesthetic solutions. The eyes were prepared according to the Miyake-Apple posterior video technique.[55,56] They were sectioned at the equator and the anterior segment was mounted on a glass slide to provide a posterior perspective of this portion of the eye. After the cornea and iris were removed, a capsulorhexis 5.0 to 5.5 mm in diameter was initiated using a 26-gauge needle and completed using a Utrata's forceps. A complete cortical-cleavage hydrodissection was performed by injecting balanced salt solution (BSS®, Alcon Ophthalmic, Fort Worth, TX, USA) between the lens capsule and the cortex with a 27-gauge cannula. This was followed by careful hydroexpression of the nucleus, avoiding damage to the posterior capsule. Cortical cleanup was performed using an irrigation/aspiration system.

Four solutions were investigated for time and ease of removal from the capsular bag. These included Ophthalin Plus® (Ciba Vision Corp., Duluth, GA, USA) (sodium hyaluronate 15 mg/ml), viscoanesthesia 0.5% (sodium hyaluronate 15 mg/ml mixed with 0.5% lidocaine), viscoanesthesia 1 percent (sodium hyaluronate 15 mg/ml mixed with 1.0 percent lidocaine), viscoanesthesia 1.65% (sodium hyaluronate 15 mg/ml mixed with 1.65% lidocaine). The injection and removal of each solution was performed in all of the 6 eyes. All the viscoelastic/viscoanesthetic solutions were dyed with fluorescein to facilitate complete removal from the capsular bag. For that, a fluorescein sodium ophthalmic strip (Fluor-I-Strip®-A.T., Bausch and Lomb, Rochester, NY, USA) was inserted into the syringe containing the solution, for 5 minutes. After filling the capsular bag with one of the viscoelastic solutions, a posterior chamber IOL was implanted (one piece, poly[methyl methacrylate], 5.0-mm optic, 12.0-mm loop diameter, Pharmacia 809P, Peapack, NJ, USA). The viscoelastic was then aspirated using an automated I/A device set at 250 mm Hg of aspiration. The same posterior chamber IOL and the same device setting were used in all cases by the same surgeon (SKP). The viscoelastic/viscoanesthetic solutions were aspirated continuously until complete removal was achieved. The "rock and roll" technique was used for viscoelastic removal (Arshinoff SA. Rock and roll removal of Healon® GV [video], presented at the American Society of Cataract and Refractive Surgery, Film Festival, Seattle, WA, USA, June 1-5,1996). The time required to remove most of the viscoelastic/viscoanesthesia solution and to remove all of the material was recorded. The terms "most" and "all" refer to the tip of the irrigation/aspiration probe being placed in front of the IOL (most) and behind the IOL (all), in order to completely remove all the viscoelastic from the capsular bag. Since the viscoelastic/viscoanesthetic solutions were dyed with fluorescein, even a residual amount could be detected. The entire surgical procedure was video tapped from posterior perspective (Figs 8.9A to 9F).

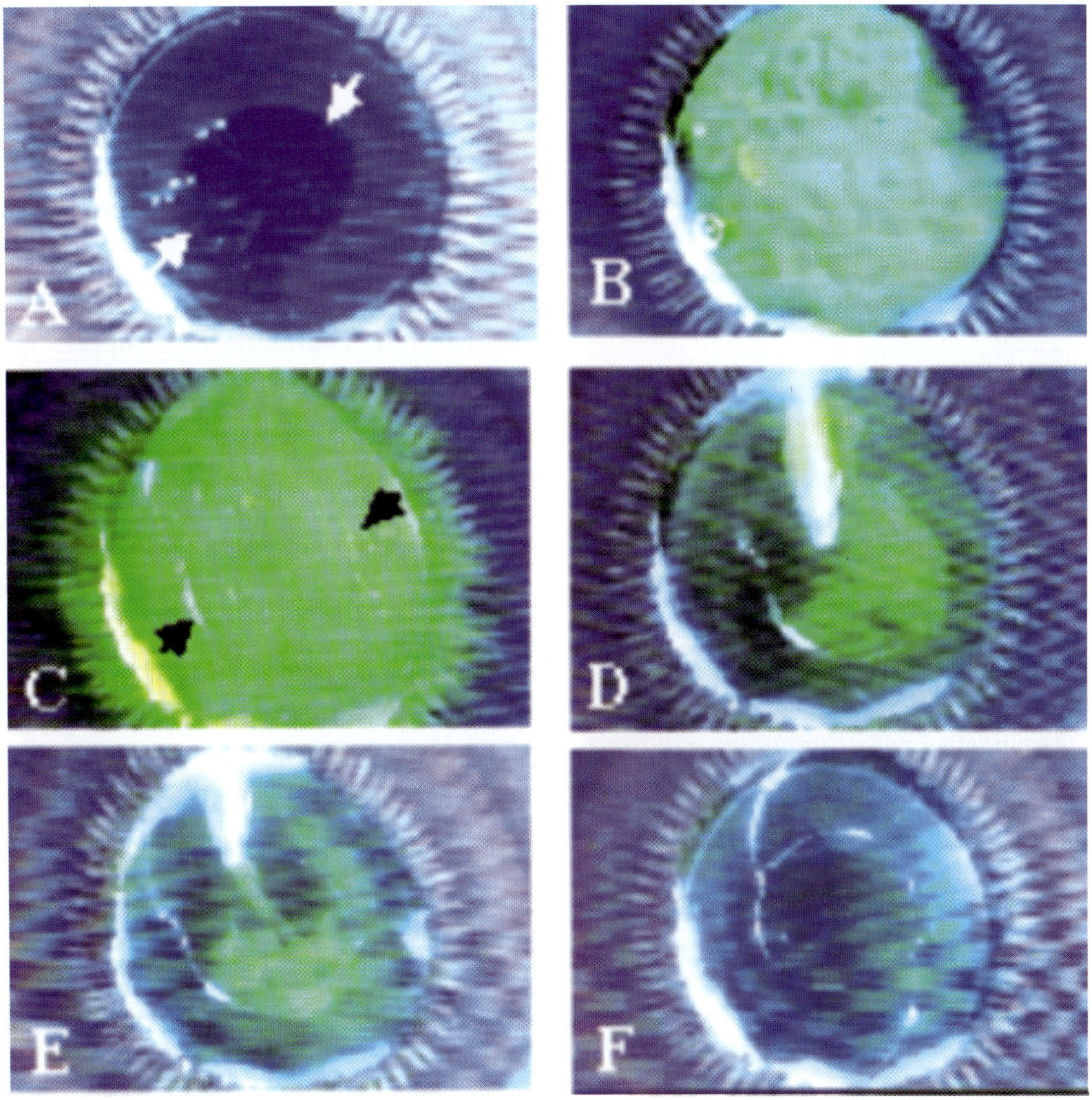

Fig. 8.9: Gross photographs from a human eye obtained postmortem (Miyake-Apple posterior view) showing the sequence of the experimental surgical technique. The removal of fluorescein-colored viscoelastic/viscoanesthetic solutions (green color as viewed with oblique illumination) from the capsular bag was documented by video taping. (A) This figure shows the eye after capsulorhexis and removal of lens substance (cortex and nucleus) by phacoemulsification. Note the edge of the anterior capsulectomy (arrows). (B) Capsular bag completely filled with viscoelastic/viscoanesthetic solution. C) Same eye after insertion of a one-piece, modified C-loop posterior chamber IOL in the capsular bag (arrows). (D) Viscoelastic/viscoanesthetic solution removal with automated aspiration, set at 250 mm Hg (Alcon Legacy 20,000). (E) Final removal of viscoelastic/viscoanesthetic substance. The surgeon reached behind the IOL optical edge to remove all the viscoelastic/viscoanesthetic material. (F) Aspect after complete removal of the viscoelastic/viscoanesthetic solution

Results of *In Vitro* Study

The results of the study are shown in Table 8.4. Mean time required for removal of most of the Ophthalin Plus®, viscoanesthesia 0.5 percent, viscoanesthesia 1 percent, and viscoanesthesia 1.65 percent solutions was 8.7±2.1, 7.7±1.1, 9.7±0.6 and 6.3±1.5 seconds, respectively (P = 0.1). It was possible to remove all of the solution of Ophthalin Plus®, viscoanesthesia 0.5 percent, viscoanesthesia 1 percent, and viscoanesthesia 1.65 percent after a mean time of 21.3±3.2, 19.7±2.5, 18.3±3.2 and 15.7±2.1 seconds, respectively (P = 0.166). No subjective difference was noted by the surgeon in relation to the viscosity and consistency of all solutions used, as well as in relation to the ease of injection and removal of the solutions.

Current *in vitro* Study, Review of Literature and Future Clinical Application

Residual viscoelastic material left in the eye after intraocular surgery is not metabolized, its fate being in fact unknown.[21] Undesired sequalae and complications of retained viscoelastic agents include increase in intraocular pressure, crystallization on the IOL surfaces, capsular block syndrome or capsular bag distension syndrome, and anterior uveitis.[57-62,] Also, an intraocular hemorrhage can be trapped between the vitreous space and the viscoelastic substances in the anterior chamber and mimic the appearance of vitreous hemorrhage.[63] Thus, complete removal of the OVDs is recommended and, in the case of viscoanesthesia, this appears to be even more reasonable as another agent is added (lidocaine).

Assia and associates[54] investigated the rate and ease of removal of various viscoelastic agents using the Miyake-Apple posterior video technique. Five viscoelastics were investigated: sodium hyaluronate (Healon®, Pharmacia Inc., Peapack, NJ, USA), Healon GV® (Pharmacia Inc., Peapack, NJ, USA), chondroitin sulfate / sodium hyaluronate (Viscoat®, Alcon laboratories, Fort Worth, TX, USA), hydroxypropylmethylcellulose (Occucoat®, Bausch and Lomb Surgical, Rochester, NY, USA), and polyacrylamide (Orcolon®, Optical Radiation Corporation, USA). The viscoelastics were also dyed with fluorescein and, after filling the capsular bag with one of the viscoelastic materials, a posterior chamber IOL was implanted. The viscoelastic was then aspirated using an automated irrigation/aspiration device. Healon® and Healon GV® were completely removed within 20 to 25 seconds. Viscoat® adhered to the lens capsule and to the posterior surface of the IOL and complete removal required approximately 3.5 minutes. Most Occucoat® and Orcolon® were aspirated within one minute; however, removal was completed only after three minutes. Removal of Healon® and Healon GV® was faster and more complete than removal of the other viscoelastics. Removal time for Viscoat®, Occucoat® and Orcolon® ranged from 3 minutes to 3.5 minutes. A possible explanation could be that viscoelastic solutions consisting of more than 1 type of molecules, such as Viscoat®/DuoVisc® (sodium hyaluronate and chondroitin sulfate) are less likely to entangle into massive molecules and thus less likely to come out as single mass. They tend to come out in pieces, and part of the gel often remains in the eye, thus requiring more time for complete removal from the capsular bag.

Table 8.4: Removal time (seconds) of viscoelatic/ viscoanesthetic solutions from the capsualr bag of human eyes obtained postmortem

Solution (eye#)	*Most**	*All***
Ophthalin Plus ®(1)	11	25
Ophthalin Plus ®(2)	8	19
Ophthalin Plus ®(3)	7	20
	(8.7 +/- 2.1)	(21.3 +/- 3.2)
Viscoanesthesia 0.5% (4)	7	20
Viscoanesthesia 0.5% (5)	9	17
Viscoanesthesia 0.5% (6)	7	22
	(7.7 +/-1.1)	(19.7 +/- 2.5)
Viscoanesthesia 1.0% (1)	10	22
Viscoanesthesia 1.0% (2)	10	17
Viscoanesthesia 1.0% (3)	9	16
	(9.7 +/- 0.6)	(18.3 +/- 3.2)
Viscoanesthesia 1.650% (4)	8	18
Viscoanesthesia 1.650% (5)	5	15
Viscoanesthesia 1.650% (6)	6	14
	(6.3 +/- 1.5)	(15.7 +/- 2.1)

* P = 0.100
** P + 0.166

Several techniques had been proposed for removal of viscoelastic agents, depending on their cohesiveness and physical properties.[21,44] These include the "rock and roll" technique, and the 2-compartment technique (Arshinoff SA. Rock and roll removal of Healon® GV [video], presented at the American Society of Cataract and Refractive Surgery, Film Festival, Seattle, WA, USA, June 1-5,1996). In our study the rock and roll technique was used for removal of viscoelastic solution in all eyes. However, the surgeon also attempted to go behind the IOL edge to clean the residual visoelastic agent trapped behind the implant (Fig. 8.9E). To minimize intraobserver variation the same surgeon performed the surgical maneuvers using the same I/A tip, machine parameters, and IOL.

According to the manufacturer, the addition of lidocaine to Ophthalin Plus® slightly changed some of its characteristics. The pH and osmolarity of the viscoanesthetic solutions had already been provided in Part I.[23] The intrinsic viscosity of Ophthalin Plus®, viscoanesthesia 0.5 percent and viscoanesthesia 1 percent were measured by the manufacturer as 29.9, 30.7, and 31.7 dl/g, respectively. However, no subjective difference in viscosity, ease of injection or removal was noted by the surgeon among the viscoelastic solutions, with or without lidocaine. Our results suggest that addition of lidocaine to the viscoelastic solution neither significantly altered the viscosity or consistency of the solution nor changed its removal time from the capsular bag. There was no statistically significant

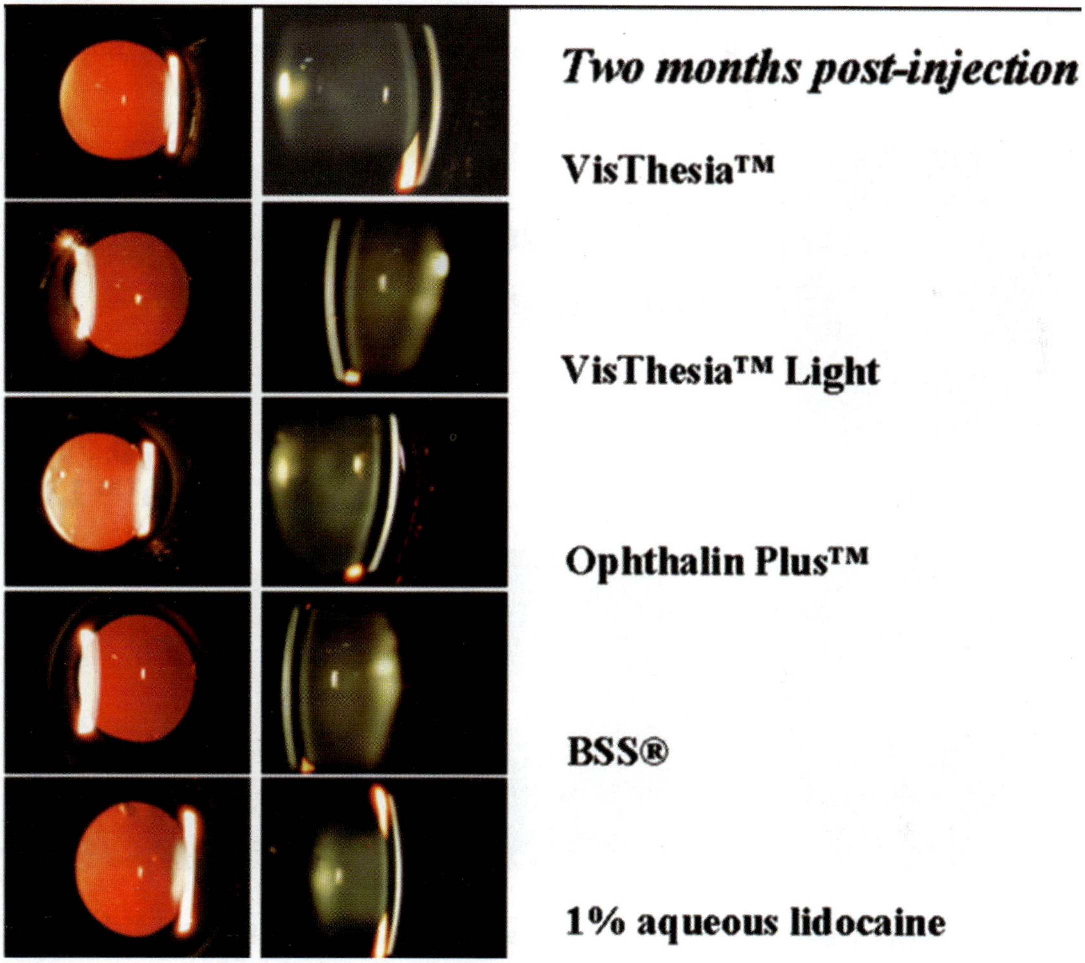

Fig. 8.10: Slit lamp photographs of rabbit eyes 2 months after injection of- VisThesia™, VisThesia™ Light, Ophthalin Plus™, BSS®, and unpreserved 1% lidocaine. Note the transparent crystalline lens in all groups

difference noted in the mean time required for removal of most or all of the Ophthalin Plus®, viscoanesthesia 0.5 percent, viscoanesthesia 1 percent, and viscoanesthesia 1.65 percent solutions (P = 0.1, P = 0.16, respectively, Table 8.4). Mean time for complete removal of standard viscoelastic solution (sodium hyaluronate 15 mg/ml) was 21.3±3.2 seconds. This was comparable to the result of the previous study done by Assia and associates[54] regarding a similar currently available OVD (Healon GV®).

Evaluation of the Toxicity of Viscoanesthetic Solutions in Phakic Rabbit Eyes

During this writing we are evaluating the toxicity of viscoanesthetic solutions in phakic rabbit eyes that will be relevant for use of viscoanesthesia for phakic IOL implantation. The purpose of this study is to evaluate any adverse effect of viscoanesthesia on the crystalline lens (eg. pacification). For this study, intracameral injection (0.1 ml) of the following agent was done in 40 phakic pigmented rabbit eyes:

a. VisThesia™ (N = 9 eyes),
b. VisThesia™ Light (N = 9 eyes),
c. Ophthalin Plus™ (N = 9 eyes),
d. BSS® (N = 9 eyes); and
e. Unpreserved 1% lidocaine (N = 4 eyes).

Clinical follow up was done till 3 months, with slit-lamp examinations. At the end of 3 months: sacrifice/enucleation was performed. All the globes were analyses from posterior or Miyake-Apple view as well as histopathological analyses. This analysis focused on crystalline lens opacification, which was not observed in any of the eye after a 3 months follow up. Figure 8.10 illustrates transparent crystalline lens in all the groups after slit lamp examination. Transparency of crystalline lens was also

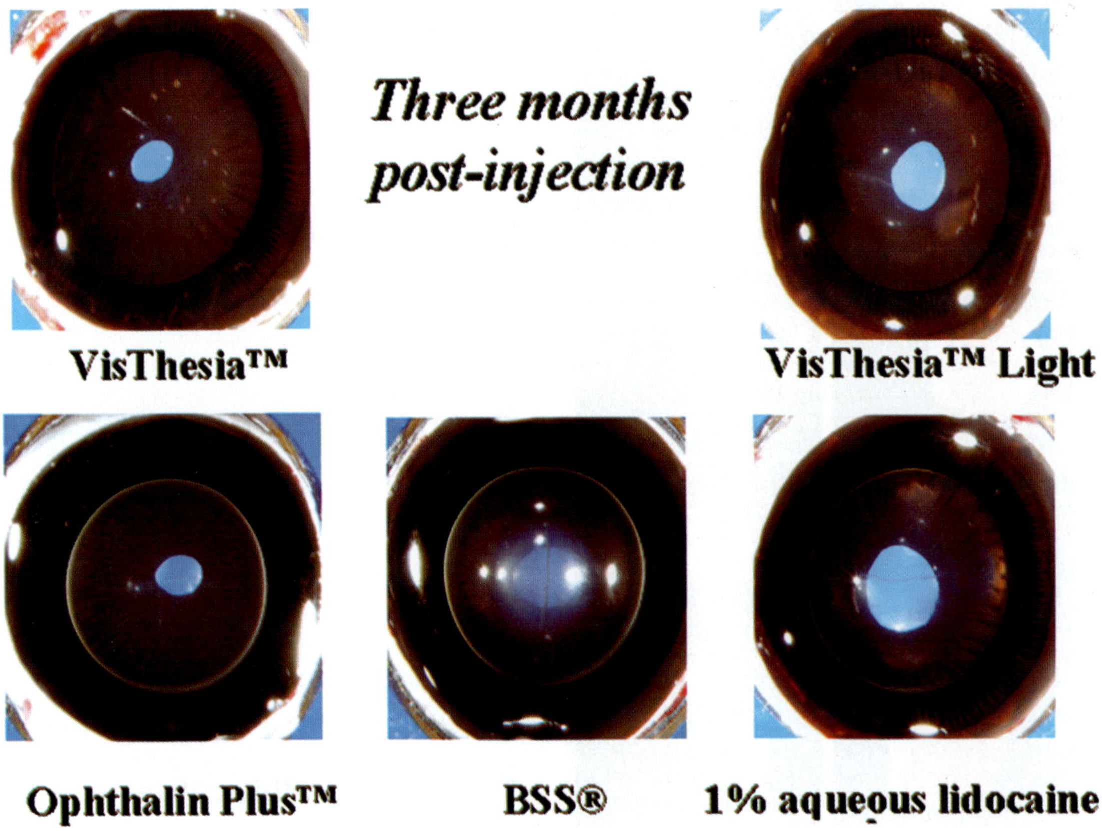

Fig. 8.11: Mipake-Apple view of enucleated rabbit eyes 3 months after injection of- VisThesia™, VisThesia™ Light, Ophthalin Plus™, BSS®, and unpreserved 1% lidocaine. Note the transparent crystalline lens in all groups from posterior views.

confirmed by posterior or Miyake-Apple view (Fig. 8.11) as well as histopathological analyses.

In summary, our experimental study demonstrated that addition of varying concentrations of lidocaine to Ophthalin Plus® neither significantly altered its viscosity or consistency nor changed its removal time from the capsular bag. Our previous studies on viscoanesthesia in rabbit eyes (viscoanesthesia Parts I and II)[23,24] had suggested that viscoanesthetic solutions with lidocaine concentrations up to 1.65 percent are not toxic for the corneal endothelium, uveal or retinal tissues. Our most recent study in phakic rabbit eyes suggested that the crystalline lens transparency was maintained after viscoanesthetic solutions with lidocaine concentrations up to 1.65 percent. The issue of efficacy of viscoanesthetic solutions in providing prolonged anesthesia needs to be addressed in clinical trails.

REFERENCES

1. Linebarger EJ, Hardten DR, Shah GK, Lindstrom RL. Phacoemulsification and modern cataract surgery. Surv Ophthalmol 1999;44:123-47.
2. Ram J, Pandey SK. Anesthesia for cataract surgery. In: Dutta LC, ed., Modern Ophthalmology, New Delhi, Jaypee Brothers, 2000;325-30.
3. Leaming DV. Practice styles and preferences of ASCRS members—2000 survey. American Society of Cataract and Refractive Surgery. J Cataract Refract Surg 2001;27:948-55.
4. Gills JP, Cherchio M, Raanan MG. Unpreserved lidocaine to control discomfort during cataract surgery using topical anesthesia. J Cataract Refract Surg 1997;23:545-50.
5. Werner L, Legeais JM, Obsler C, Durand J, Renard G. Toxicity of Xylocaine to rabbit corneal endothelium. J Cataract Refract Surg 1998;24:1371-76.
6. Masket S, Gokmen F. Efficacy and safety of intracameral lidocaine as a supplement to topical anesthesia. J Cataract Refract Surg 1998;24:956-60.
7. Pandey SK, Werner L, Apple DJ, et al. No-anesthesia clear corneal phacoemulsification versus topical and topical plus intracameral anesthesia. Randomized clinical trial. J Cataract Refract Surg 2001;27:1643-50.
8. Anderson NJ, Woods WD, Kim T, Rudnick DE, Edelhauser HF. Intracameral anesthesia: in vitro iris and corneal uptake and washout of 1% lidocaine hydrochloride. Arch Ophthalmol 1999;117:225-32.
9. Martin RG, Miller JD, Cox CC 3rd, Ferrel SC, Raanan MG. Safety and efficacy of intracameral injections of unpreserved lidocaine to reduce intraocular sensation. J Cataract Refract Surg 1998;24:961-63.
10. Kadonosono K, Ito N, Yazama F, et al. Effect of intracameral anesthesia on the corneal endothelium. J Cataract Refract Surg 1998;24:1377-81.
11. Tseng SH, Chen FK.A randomized clinical trial of combined topical-intracameral anesthesia in cataract surgery. Ophthalmology 1998;105:2007-11.
12. Carino NS, Slomovic AR, Chung F, Marcovich AL. Topical tetracaine versus topical tetracaine plus intracameral lidocaine for cataract surgery. J Cataract Refract Surg 1998;24:1602-08.
13. Crandall AS, Zabriskie NA, Patel BC, et al. A comparison of patient comfort during cataract surgery with topical anesthesia versus topical anesthesia and intracameral lidocaine. Ophthalmology 1999;106:60-66.
14. Anderson NJ, Nath R, Anderson CJ, Edelhauser HF. Comparison of preservative-free bupivacaine vs. lidocaine for intracameral anesthesia: a randomized clinical trial and in vitro analysis. Am J Ophthalmol 1999;127:393-402.
15. Elvira JC, Hueso JR, Martinez-Toldos J, Mengual E, Artola A. Induced endothelial cell loss in phacoemulsification using topical anesthesia plus intracameral lidocaine. J Cataract Refract Surg 1999;25:640-42.
16. Boulton JE, Lopatatzidis A, Luck J, Baer RM. A randomized controlled trial of intracameral lidocaine during phacoemulsification under topical anesthesia. Ophthalmology 2000; 107:68-71.
17. Schuster BL. Intracameral lidocaine for phacoemulsification. Ophthalmology 2001;108:833-34.
18. Karp CL, Cox TA, Wagoner MD, Ariyasu RG, Jacobs DS. Intracameral anesthesia: A report by the American Academy of Ophthalmology. Ophthalmology 2001;108:1704-10.
19. Pang MP, Fujimoto DK, Wilkens LR. Pain, photophobia, and retinal and optic nerve function after phacoemulsification with intracameral lidocaine. Ophthalmology 2001;108:2018-25.
20. Judge AJ, Najafi K, Lee DA, Miller KM. Corneal endothelial toxicity of topical anesthesia. Ophthalmology 1997;104:1373-79.
21. Liesegang TJ. Viscoelastic substances in ophthalmology. Surv Ophthalmol. 1990;34:268-93.
22. Spence DJ, Peyman GA. A new technique for the vital staining of the corneal endothelium. Invest Ophthalmol. 1976;15:1000-02.
23. Trivedi RH, Werner L, Apple DJ, et al. Viscoanesthesia Part I: Evaluation of the toxicity to corneal endothelial cells in a rabbit model. J Cataract Refract Surg 2003;29:550-55.
24. Macky TA, Werner L, Apple DJ, et al. Viscoanesthesia part II: Evaluation of toxicity to intraocular structures after phacoemulsification in a rabbit model. J Cataract Refract Surg 2003;29:556-62.

25. Pandey SK, Werner L, Apple DJ, et al. Viscoanesthesia part III: Evaluation of the removal time of viscoelastic/ viscoanesthetic solutions from the capsular bag of human eyes obtained postmortem. J Cataract Refract Surg 2003;29:563-67.
26. Eleftheriadis H, Liu C. Influence of ophthalmic visco-surgical device on the effects of intracameral anesthesia and stains. J Cataract Refract Surg 2001;27:11-12.
27. Kayikicioglu O, Erakgun T, Guler C. Trypan blue mixed with sodium hyaluronate for capsulorhexis J Cataract Refract Surg 2001; 27:970.
28. Werner L, Legeais JM, Durand J, et al. Endothelial damage caused by uncoated and fluorocarbon-coated poly (methylmethacrylate) intraocular lenses. J Cataract Refract Surg 1997;23:1013-19.
29. Yagoubi MI, Armitage WJ, Diamond J, Easty DL. Effects of irrigation solutions on corneal endothelial function. Br J Ophthalmol 1994; 78:302-06.
30. Waring GO 3rd, Bourne WM, Edelhauser HF, Kenyon KR. The corneal endothelium. Normal and pathologic structure and function. Ophthalmology 1982;89:531-90.
31. Garcia A, Loureiro F, Limao A, et al. Preservative-free lidocaine 1% anterior chamber irrigation as an adjunct to topical anesthesia. J Cataract Refract Surg 1998;24:403–06.
32. Martin RG, Miller JD, Cox CC III, et al. Safety and efficacy of intracameral injections of unpreserved lidocaine to reduce intraocular sensation. J Cataract Refract Surg 1998; 24:961–63.
33. Anderson NJ, Woods WD, Kim T, et al. Intracameral anesthesia, in vitro iris and corneal uptake and washout of 1% lidocaine hydrochloride. Arch Ophthalmol 1999; 117:225–32.
34. Liang C, Peyman GA, Sun G. Toxicity of intraocular lidocaine and bupivacaine. Am J Ophthalmol 1998; 125:191–96.
35. Behndig A, Linden C. Aqueous humor lidocaine concentrations in topical and intracameral anesthesia. J Cataract Refract Surg 1998;24:1598–1601.
36. Duguid IG, Claoue CM, Thamby-Rajah Y, et al. Topical anaesthesia for phacoemulsification surgery. Eye 1995; 9:456-59.
37. Bellucci R, Morselli S, Pucci V, et al. Intraocular penetration of topical lidocaine 4%. J Cataract Refract Surg 1999; 25:643–47.
38. Pandey SK, Werner L, Agarwal A. Anesthesia for cataract surgery. *In:* Phacoemulsification, Laser Cataract Surgery and Foldable IOLs- Second edition. Jaypee India, 2000, 217-25.
39. Naor J, Slomovic AR. Anesthesia modalities for cataract surgery. Curr Opin Ophthalmol 2000;11:7-11.
40. Greenhalgh D. Anesthesia for cataract surgery. In: Yanoff M, Ducker JS, eds, Ophthalmology. St Louis, Mosby-Yearbook, 1998;21.5-21.6.
41. Barequet IS, Soriano ES, Green WR, O'Brien TP. Provision of anesthesia with single application of lidocaine 2% gel. J Cataract Refract Surg 1999;25:626–31.
42. Koch PS. Efficacy of lidocaine 2% jelly as a topical agent in cataract surgery. J Cataract Refract Surg 1999; 25:632–34.
43. Assia EI, Pras E, Yehezkel M, et al. Topical anesthesia using lidocaine gel for cataract surgery. J Cataract Refract Surg 1999;25:635–39.
44. Arshinoff SA. New terminology: ophthalmic viscosurgical devices. J Cataract Refract Surg 2000;26:627-28.
45. Pandey SK, Thakur J, Werner L, Sharma V, Izak AM, Apple DJ. Update on ophthalmic viscosurgical devices. In: Garg A, Pandey SK, Sharma V, Apple DJ. *Advances in Ophthalmology*. Jaypee Brothers, New Delhi, India 2003, 198-213.
46. Pandey SK, Thakur J, Werner L, et al. Update on ophthalmic viscosugical devices. *In:* Phacoemulsification, Laser Cataract Surgery and Foldable IOLs- Third edition. Jaypee India., 2003 (in press).
47. Arshinoff SA, Hofmann I. A prospective randomized study comparing micro visc plus to Healon GV, and super prospective, randomized trial of Microvisc and Healon in routine phacoemulsification. J Cataract Refract Surg 1997;23:761-65.
48. Strobel J.Comparison of space maintaining capabilities of Healon and Healon GV during Phacoemulsification. J Cataract Refractive Surgery 1997; 23:1081-84.
49. Arshinoff SA. Dispersive–cohesive viscoelastic soft shell technique. J Cataract Refract Surg 1999;25:167-73.
50. Holzer MP, Tetz MR, Auffarth GU, Welt R, Volker H. Effects of Healon® 5 and 4 other viscoelastic substances on intraocular pressure and endothelium after cataract surgery. J Cataract Refractive Surg 2001;27:213-18.
51. Tetz MR, Holzer MP. Healon® 5 clinical performance and special removal technique (TCT). In: Viscoelastics in Ophthalmic Surgery, Eds, Buratto L, Giardini P, Belluci R,. Thorofare, NJ, USA Slack 2000;401-04.
52. Stegmann R, Pienaar A, Miller D. Viscocanalostomy for open angle glaucoma in black African patients. J Cataract Refract Surg 1999; 25:316-22.
53. Arshinoff SA. Dispersive and cohesive viscoelastics materials in phacoemulsification, revisited 1998. Ophthalmic Practice 1998; 16:24-32.
54. Assia EI, Apple DJ, Lim ES, et al. Removal of viscoelastic materials after experimental cataract surgery in vitro. J Cataract Refract Surg 1992; 18:3-6
55. Miyake K, Miyake C. Intraoperative posterior chamber lens haptic fixation in the human cadaver eye. Ophthalmic Surg 1985; 16:230-36.
56. Apple D, Lim E, Morgan R, et al. Preparation and study of human eyes obtained postmortem with the Miyake posterior photographic technique. Ophthalmology 1990;97:810-16.
57. Jensen MK, Crandall AS, Mamalis N, Olson RJ. Crystallization on intraocular lens surfaces associated with the use of Healon GV. Arch Ophthalmol 1994; 112:1037-42.

58. Olson RJ, Caldwell AS, Jensen MK, Huang SC. Intraoperative crystallization on the intraocular lens surface. Am J Ophthalmol 1998; 126:177-84.
59. Werner L, Shugar JK, Apple DJ, Pandey SK, et al. Opacification of piggyback IOLs associated to an amorphous material attached to interlenticular surfaces. J Cataract Refract Surg 2000;26:1612-19.
60. Miyake K, Ota I, Ichihashi S, et al. New classification of capsular block syndrome. *J Cataract Refract Surg* 1998; 24:1230-34.
61. Sugiura T, Miyauchi S, Eguchi S, et al. Analysis of liquid accumulated in the distended capsular bag in early postoperative capsular block syndrome. J Cataract Refract Surg 2000; 26:420-25.
62. Pandey SK, Thakur J, Werner L, et al. Ophthalmic viscosurgical devices: an update. In: Textbook of Ocular Therapeutics, Ed, Grag A. New Delhi, India, Jaypee 2002.
63. Nirankari VS, Karesh J, Lakhanpal V. Pseudo vitreous hemorrhage: A new introperative complication of sodium hyaluronate. Ophthalmic Sug 1981; 12:503-04.

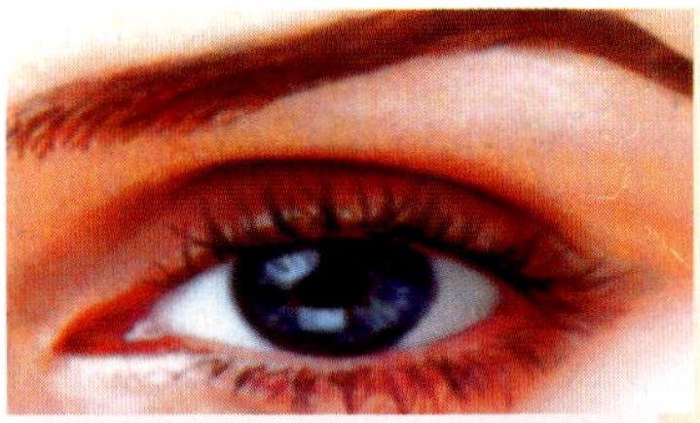

Nine

Dynamics of Ocular Surgical Adjuncts in Cataract Surgery

Ashok Garg (India)

INTRODUCTION

The ocular surgical adjuncts play an important role during Cataract Surgery regarding control of surgery, its quality and outcome. Fluid Dynamics are responsible for the flowing intraocular conditions specially related to AC depth fluctuations, AC turbulence, IOP status during surgery & fluid velocity. Thus fluidics is directly related to clinical and surgical outcome in any type of cataract surgery.

Viscoelastic agents, irrigating solutions and enzymes are adjuncts as fluidics to a variety of ophthalmological procedures and surgeries. These are vital components of any type of intraocular surgery.

First let me discuss various viscoelastic substances used in the cataract surgery.

VISCOELASTIC SUBSTANCES

The development of modern ophthalmic microsurgery has dramatically changed the facet of ocular surgery in many ways. But the increasing number of surgical steps also involves a greater risk of involuntary tissue damage. The field of microsurgery strategy is therefore not only the desired action on the tissue but also the prevention of undesired side effects on the surrounding tissue (Precision tissue specific action, PTSA). For this purpose space tactics are used.

Space tactics is a more active protection against touch by providing sufficient space for manipulation within the eye. It is accomplished by space maintaining or enlarging devices such as hydrodynamic flow systems or viscoelastic substances.

The term *viscosurgery* was coined by Prof. Endre Balasz of USA to describe the use of solutions with viscous elastic, pseudoplastic properties during and after ocular surgery. Viscosity makes a material protective and lubricating while elasticity provides protection from vibrating instruments and other mechanical impacts. Pseudoplasticity allows the material to deform and may be used to safely manipulate tissue. While we perform intraocular viscosurgery. We actually use a viscoelastic agent as a fluid or soft surgical instrument because the molecules of a true viscoelastic can deform and reform.

CRITERIA FOR SELECTION OF VISCOELASTIC MATERIAL

Optical Properties

Materials suitable for intraocular use should not impair the visibility of the operation field. Transparency is primary prerequisite. A color slightly different from aqueous is useful for distinction.

Surface Tension

The specific weight of the injected material determines whether the bubble will raise or descend in the aqueous and whether it can be used to elevate or to depress the surrounding tissue.

Viscosity

Viscous fluids are ideal surface tools since layers deposited onto tissue implant surface will remain there. As space tactical tools viscous fluids are suitable in walled off cavities with small orifices (anterior chamber).

Elasticity

Elastic materials are resistant against deformation and therefore stable as to their shape. They are ideal space tactical tools since their action is independent of flow conditions.

Viscoelasticity

The viscoelastic solutions, the viscous and elastic responses to a mechanical force depends on the velocity of the impact. The optimal solution for surgical purposes is a substance with a transition from viscous to elastic behavior at relatively low velocities.

Miscellaneous

Viscoelastic agent should be easy to inject, (inert, non-inflammatory, nontoxic). No particles or clumps, causes less rise of IOP with low molecular weight viscoelastics. It must be hydrophilic enough and able to be diluted and should not prevent the movement of metabolites and waste products.

ROLES OFVISCOELASTIC SUBSTANCES

Roles of viscoelastic substances in intraocular surgery are

- To maintain an anatomical situation created by surgeon and maintenance of anterior chamber
- To lubricate
- To protect and isolate newly created or restored tissue surfaces
- To prevent the formation of undesirable fibrin coagulum
- Protection of corneal endothelium from mechanical trauma
- To enable easy manipulation of tissues in the eye
- To provide coating ability to implants, instruments and corneal epithelial surface.

INDICATIONS FORVISCOELASTIC SUBSTANCES

- Phacoemulsification
- IOL implantation
- Congenital cataract surgery
- Extracapsular cataract surgery
- For breaking synechiae as a soft instrument
- Posterior segment surgery
- Penetrating trauma surgery
- Strabismus surgery
- Corneal surgery
- Plastic surgery for congenital ptosis surgery.

COMMERCIALLY AVAILABLE VISCOELASTIC SUBSTANCES

Hyaluronic Acid

It is a natural compound of connective tissue. In the ocular cavities it is a major component of the vitreous and occurs as covering layer on the tissue surface of the anterior segment. Hyaluronic acid is not metabolized or degraded within the eye. It passes unaltered through the trabecular meshwork as a large molecule and is transported then with the blood flow to the liver. Hyaluronic acid is a linear polysaccharide composed of sodium glucuronate and N-acetyl glucosamine. The chain is unbranched and contains no intermolecular bridges.

Sodium Hyaluronate

NaH, a large polysaccharide molecule is a viscoelastic substance. It is a natural biological product present nearly in all the connective tissues in living organisms from bacteria to human tissue. It stabilizes cells and tissues and hence protects cell from permanent deformation.

Various biological sources including the umbilical cord, bovine vitreous and rooster coomb contain a large amount of sodium hyaluronate. Low molecular weight sodium hyaluronate may also be produced from streptococci by microbial fermentation. It is component of capsular material around streptococcal organisms. In the eye concentration of sodium hyaluronate is highest in cortical gel and trabecular angle and low in the aqueous humor and covering the endothelium.

Sodium hyaluronate has two fractions H3 inflammatory (if-Na-Ha) and non-inflammatory (Nif-Na-Ha). For intraocular purpose non-inflammatory fraction is used.

The molecular weight of sodium hyaluronate varies dramatically depending on the sources. The viscosity of sodium hyaluronate solution is influenced by the molecular weight, concentration and shear rate. At higher shear rate, the resistance of flow decreases and it remains constant at low shear rate. This typical pseudoplasticity is exhibited by sodium hyaluronate only. In 1980, Mitter and Stegmann introduced sodium hyaluronate for anterior segment surgery.

One percent sodium hyaluronate is true viscoelastic agent. It is highly viscous, elastic and pseudoplastic of very high molecular weight ($1.1 - 1.8 \times 10)^{6.}$ Its viscosity is 100,000 – 300,000 centi poise and molecular weight is about 4 million Daltons. It is non-allergic and clear. It is 1 percent solution of highly purified sodium hyaluronate from dermis of roster coombs. It consists of very large hyaluronic acid chains with high molecular weight. One of its greater advantage is that the transition from viscous to elastic behavior occurs even at low concentration and low velocities. Owing to its elasticity it can be injected through a 30 G cannula and still retains its original shape in aqueous. Besides space tactics tools, sodium hyaluronate also inhibits migration of lymphocytes, granulocytes and macrophages. It also inhibits phagocytic activity, synthesis and release of prostaglandins by macrophages during phagocytosis.

Sodium hyaluronate preparation is a specific fraction development for use in anterior segment and vitreous procedures as a viscoelastic agent. It is non-antigenic, does not cause inflammatory or foreign body reactions and has a high viscosity.

The 1 percent solution is transparent and remains in the anterior chamber for less than 6 days. It protects chamber for less than 6 days. It protects corneal endothelial cells and other ocular strucutres. It does not interfere with epithelization and normal wound healing.

Indications

It is used as ophthalmosurgical aid in various anterior segment procedures like

- Phacoemulsification
- IOL implantation
- Facilitates capsulorrhexis
- Corneal transplant surgery
- Glaucoma surgery
- Reconstructive surgery following eye injury
- Various procedures of ocular microsurgery.
- Vitreous replacement after retinal detachment surgery.

It is also used as surgical aid in posterior segment surgery to gently separate, maneuver and hold tissues.

It also creates a clear field of vision therapy facilitating photcoagulation and intra- and postoperative inspection of the retina.

It has also been used in the treatment of refractory dry eye syndrome.

Administration and Dosage

It is available as preloaded syringe with 27 G or 30 G cannula containing sodium hyaluronate 10 mg/ml or 14 mg/ml strength (in 0.25, 0.50, 0.80, 2 ml and 4 ml syringes). Store at 2-8°C and remains unaltered after 3-5 years at this temperature. Do not freeze. Use the drug at room temperature (Acclimitization at room temperature is necessary).

Dosage

For phacoemulsification/IOL implantation/ECCE During cataract surgery as soon as the anterior chamber is entered, the role of viscoelastic begins. It fills, maintains and cushions the anterior chamber. During anterior capsulotomy it prevents scrolling up of margins.

Hydraulic separation of nucleus and cortex, synechiae (anterior or posterior) release can be easily done with sodium hyaluronate. When placed over the pupil, it gets dilated mechanically. It tamponades the bleeding vessels on iris or in wound. After capsulotomy it helps in viscoexpression of nucleus (after continuous curvilinear capsulorrhexis). It helps in plugging posterior capsule break and after dry aspiration. It makes phacoemulsification successful by coating corneal endothelial cells.

It protects anterior chamber angle during anterior chamber IOL insertion. It also acts as surgical instrument during anterior, posterior or iris clip lenses.

A sufficient amount is slowly introduced (using 27 G cannula or needle) into the anterior chamber.

Inject either before or after delivery of the lens. Injection before lens delivery protects the corneal endothelium from possible damage arising from removal of the cataractous lens. It may be used to coat surgical instruments and the IOL prior to the insertion.

Additional amount can be injected during surgery to replace any of the drug lost.

Sodium hyaluronate can be easily distinguished from vitreous. Vitreous sticks to cellulose sponge and cannot be washed out of anterior chamber.

Advantages of Hyaluronic Acid in Ophthalmic Viscomicrosurgery

- It ensures to maintain anterior chamber depth and visibility.

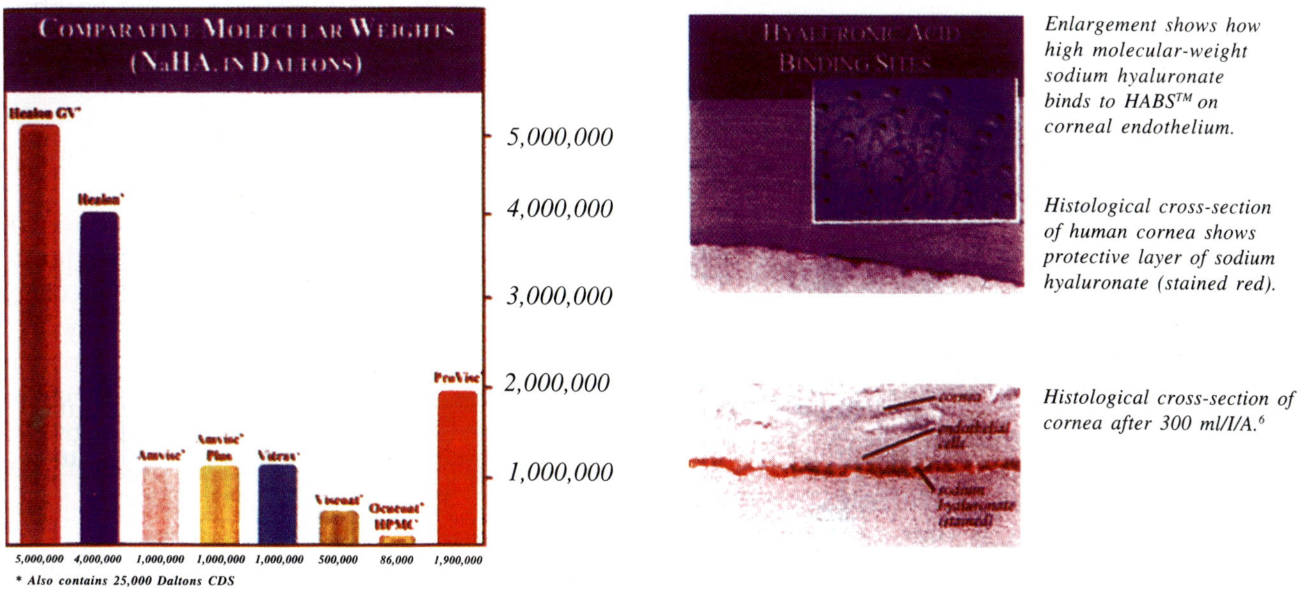

Fig. 9.1: Sodium hyaluronate and corneal endothelial protective mechanisms

- It minimises interaction between tissues and acts as temponade and vitreous substitute during retinal reattachment surgery.
- It also preserves tissue integrity and good visibility when use to fill the anterior and posterior segments of the eye following open sky procedures.
- It is a natural component of the tissues and is extremely well tolerated.
- It tends to counter-balance the vitreous thrust.
- It efficiently protects the intraocular structures.
- It is eliminated in relatively short time with no significant increase in postsurgical intraocular pressure.
- It does not have inflammatory reactions in the eye.
- It does not interfere with the physiological circulatory dynamics of the aqueous humor.
- It enhances the visibility of surgical field.
- It facilitates the insertion and the implantation of intraocular lenses and foldable lenses following phacoemulsification.
- Due to its lubricating and viscoelastic properties, transparency and ability to protect corneal endothelial cells is maintained.

At present there is no contraindications except for hypersensitivity reactions to the use of sodium hyaluronate solution when recommended for use in intraocular surgery.

Adverse Reactions

Although well-tolerated, a transient postoperative increase in IOP has been reported. Sometimes postoperative inflammatory reactions (iritis, hypopyon) corneal edema and corneal decompensation are also seen.

Precautions

Postoperative intraocular pressure may be elevated as a result of pre-existing glaucoma and by operative procedures and sequelae including enzymatic zonulysis, absence of an iridectomy, trauma to filtration structure and by blood and lenticular remanants in the anterior chamber.

- Do not overfill the anterior chamber, remove some of the preparation by irrigation or aspiration at the close of surgery (except in glaucoma surgery).
- Carefully monitor IOP specially during immediate postoperative period. Treat significant rise in IOP appropriately.
- In posterior segment surgery monitor rise in IOP after injection of large amounts of the drug (specially in aphakic diabetes).
- Hypersensitivity reactions as this preparation is extracted from avian tissues and contains minute amounts of protein, so potential risk of hypersensitivity may exist.

Other preparations of sodium hyaluronate available commercially are as follows:

Hyalectin (IAL)

It is highly viscous 1 percent solution of sodium hyaluronate of lower molecular weight—1 million Daltons. It is less viscous and less elastic than Healon. It has special features like:

- It is eliminated in relatively short time with no increase in postsurgical intraocular pressure. Therefore there is no need to remove IAL after the operation.
- It does not give inflammatory reactions.
- It is a specialty whose active ingradient is a specific fraction of the hyaluronic acid sodium salt which is obtained by unique methodology based on sequential molecular ultrafiltration stages. This procedure allows the exclusion of low molecular weight fractions and gives a product characterized by a mean molecular weight in the range of 500000-730000 and with a very high degree of purity.
- The isotonic 1 percent aqueous solution of hyalectin (20 mg/2 ml) exhibits particular viscous characteristics which make it specially suitable for intraocular viscomicrosurgery.
- It provides an effective protection to ocular tissues vulnerable to surgical manipulations and it allows to preserve anatomical form and relationship among the various structures of the eye.
- IAL favourably differentiates from hyaluronic acid with very high molecular weight whenever such substances are left in the anterior chamber.

IAL does not cause rise in postoperative IOP in comparison to hyaluronic acid with high molecular weight (which cause significant rise in postoperative IOP).

- It physically shields corneal endothelium, the lens and the angle structures during surgical procedures.
- IAL sets apart from each other traumatized tissues enhancing surgical repair and preventing formation of anterior and posterior synechiae.
- It helps in restoration and preservation of the ocular volume in reconstructive surgery following eye injury.

It is available as 1 percent solution in preloaded disposable syringes (2 ml).

Sodium Hyaluronate and Chondroitin Sulfate Solution

Viscoat

It is highly viscous but less elastic and pseudoplastic than 1 percent sodium hyaluronate. It is available as solution of (3:1 mixture of) 3 percent sodium hyaluronate and 4 percent chondroitin sulfate with 0.45 mg sodium dihydrogen phosphate hydrate, 2.65 mg disodium hydrogen phosphate and 4.3 mg NaCl (in 0.5 ml pack).

It is used as surgical aid in the anterior segment procedures including cataract extraction and IOL implantation. The molecular weight of sodium hyaluronate is 500000 and the chondroitin sulfate 50000. It is produced by genetic engineering. Because of its stickiness, it is claimed to be quite effective in protecting endothelium but does not maintain anterior chamber as healon.

The disadvantage is that it is difficult to aspirate, tends to trap small air bubbles, less cohesive and requires refrigeration.

Chondroitin Sulfate

It is a biological polymer and is a proteoglycan.

Chondroitin sulfate from shark cartilage was introduced in 1980 as a coating for intraocular lenses. It is a natural compound of hard connective tissue such as cartilage in humans and one of the major glycosaminoglycans of the corneal stroma.

The physical and chemical properties and molecular structure of chondroitin sulfate is quite similar to hyaluronic acid with the difference of presence of sulphur and double negative charges per molecular subunit.

The molecular size is 5 × 100 × 103 centistokes, thus being much smaller than hyaluronic acid. The sugar moieties occur as repeating disaccharide subunits consisting of glucuronic acid in B-1, 3 linkage with N-acetyl galactosamine for chondroitin sulfate.

Double negative charge of chondroitin sulfate coats the positively charged tissue or implant surface and thus decreases the electrostatic interaction between the implant and the endothelium.

Chondroitin sulfate alone has a low viscosity because of which it cannot maintain space. If concentration of chondroitin sulfate is increased to 50 percent, it improves the viscosity but causes endothelial cell damage due to dehydration, sticks of lens surface and does not wash away easily.

Due to these problem chondroitin sulfate is generally combined with another biological polymer-sodium hyaluronate. This formulation makes it a good viscous substance which increases its coating ability and cell protection.

When used alone it is available as 20 percent solution which can be injected through 30 G cannula. Chondroitin sulfate is more a surface than a space tactical tool. Chondroitin sulfate is available in combination with HPMC which has a good coating property and does not require refrigeration.

Methylcellulose

It was introduced in 1976 for coating of intraocular lenses. It is an artificial compound in the eye. Its viscosity is 3000-4000 centipoise approximately and an average molecular weight of 86000, an osmolarity of 285 mosm and a pH of 7.2.

It is somewhat viscous, low cost but not truly viscoelastic. It is water soluble, inert substance and nontoxic to the endothelium, transparent and nonpyrogenic. It is basically used as lubricant and maintain anterior chamber but not so well.

It is 2 percent solution of hydroxy propyl methyl cellulose suitable for intraocular use. It is highly purified brand of hydroxy propyl methyl cellulose. Hydroxy propyl and methyl groups increases the hydrophilicity of the compound. It is designed as such to serve as an acid in ophthalmic procedures of the anterior segment.

Injection of methyl cellulose serves to support a deep anterior chamber during intraocular surgery and allows through manipulation with less trauma to corneal endothelium and other surrounding tissues. It impedes vitreous leakage into the anterior chamber thereby decreasing the possibility of postoperative flat chamber.

Indications for Use of Methyl Cellulose

- Cataract surgery
- IOL implantation
- Keratoplasty
- Filtering surgery for glaucoma
- Vitrectomy
- Retinal detachment surgery
- Strabismus surgery
- Plastic surgery.

Precautions

- Do not overfill the anterior chamber with methyl cellulose
- Remove as much possible of methyl cellulose by irrigation/aspiration at the close of surgery for preventing corneal endothelial cell loss as a result of performed procedure
- Carefully monitor IOP specially during the immediate postoperative period
- Instillation of methyl cellulose should be done so as to avoid trapping of air bubble behind methyl cellulose
- Carefully examine the solution for rubber particles that may have been aspirated with repeated washing of sterile water for injection
- Concurrent presence of medication in the chamber or associated ocular structures should be avoided as it may interact with methyl cellulose to cause clouding.

Presentation

It is available as 2 percent HPMC solution in 2 ml vials or prefilled sterilised disposable. Syringes with sterile 27 G cannula. Administration route and technique is same as discussed in sodium hyaluronate section.

Adverse Reactions

Methyl cellulose is tolerated extremely well after injection into human eyes. However, transient rise in intraocular pressure postoperatively has been reported.

Isolated incidence of postoperative inflammatory reactions (Iritis, hypopyon) as well as corneal edema and corneal decompensation have been reported.

The main advantage of methyl cellulose is its availability at a very low cost in comparison to sodium hyaluronate specially in, developing countries. HPMC main advantages are its availability, ease of preparation, storage at room temperature, ability to with stand autoclaving and potential for low cost.

The disadvantage of this viscoelastic substance is its low viscosity because of which it is not able to maintain anterior chamber and requires large bore cannula.

Polyacrylamide

It is a linear, long chain and high molecular weight synthetic polpymer. It has repeated acrylamide units without protein or other molecular contamination. Acrylamide monomer units are highly reactive and toxic substances but in polymer form it is highly stable and nontoxic. Polyacrylamide has a low contact angle because of which it possesses good surface wetting and coating properties.

Orcolon (Low concentration poly acrylamide 4.5 mg/ml) is commercially available.

It has molecular weight of one million dalton and high and stable viscosity of approximately 40000 cps with good elastic and pseudoplastic properties. The osmolality is 340 mosm and the pH is 7.2. It is injected through 27 G cannula and can be stored at room temperature.

Delayed sustained increase in intraocular pressure secondary to the use of polyacrylamide in the anterior chamber has been reported. The cause may be related to presence of small particles of viscoelastic which could lead to compromised trabecular meshwork.

Collagen

Collagen constitutes an important bulk of connective tissues. There are different types of collagen, i.e. I, II, III and IV, etc. Collagel (1.4% collagen type IV) was viscoelastic introduced in 1990. It is obtained from human placental tissue.

It has a molecular weight of approximately one million daltons and a viscosity of 500,00 centipoise (Zero shear rate), an osmolality of 300 mosm and a pH of 6.2.

It has been clinically compared with healon and no significant difference in IOP, corneal thickness, endothelial cells and postoperative visual acuity have been observed. It is commercially available for use.

FUTURE VISCOELASTICS

A new polymer, poly-TEGMA 40 percent (triethylenglycol monomethacrylate) and poly-GLYMA (glycerol monomethacrylate) have been evaluated in rabbits and pre-clinical studies as potential viscoelastic substances for intraoperative use in anterior segment surgery. These are highly swelling and hydrophilic polymers. Poly- GLYMA and poly-TEGMA 40 percent are characterised by high biological tolerance after its implantation into the anterior chamber. Poly-TEGMA 40 percent is potential viscoelastic substance and shall be commercially available in short future.

Provisc has been recommended as a safe and effective visoelastic substance in modern surgery of cataract.

IRRIGATING SOLUTIONS

Irrigating solutions are aqueous solutions used to cleanse and to maintain moisture of ocular tissues. Ideally these solutions are isotonic. The optimum pH is 7.4. A pH less than 7 or greater than 8 has caused callular stress and death when the tissues have been exposed to prolonged period of time.

Two types of irrigating solutions are available for use in ophthalmolgoy.

Intraocular Irrigating Solutions

The commercially available intraocular irrigating solutions (e.g. BSS and BSS plus) are used during ocular surgery to protect the lens and cornea in patients. Unlike physiological saline and Ringer lactate solution, these balanced salt solutions provide magnesium and calcium ions as cellular nutrients.

These nutrients are required for intercellular and intracellular function during prolonged ocular, surgery. In addition to magnesium and calcium, bicarbonate, glucose and glutathione are present in these perfusion solutions (BSS plus). These components help to maintain a deturgesced or thin cornea by avoiding corneal clouding. Various commercially available intraocular irrigating solutions are:

BSS solution containing 0.64 percent NaCl, 0.075 percent KCl, 0.03 percent magnesium chloride, 0.043 percent calcium chloride, 0.39 percent sodium acetate, 0.17 percent sodium citrate and sodium hydroxide or hydrochloric acid in (15,30,300 and 500 ml sterile packs).

BSS plus (Mix aspastically just prior to use)

Part I—480 ml containing 7.44 mg NaCl, 0.395 mg KCl, 0.433 mg sodium phosphate, 2.19 mg sodium bicarbonate, hydrochloric acid or sodium hydroxide/ml.

Part II—20 ml containing 3.85 mg calcium chloridedihydrate, 5 mg magnesium chloride hexahydrate, 23 mg dextrose and 4.6 mg glutathione disulfide/ml.

It is preservative free (500 ml pack) and 30 ml pack. Its pH is at or near the optimal 7.4 level (pH of human aqueous humor).

Salient Features of BSS Plus Solution

- It is iso-osmotic with intraocular tissues
- BSS plus solution provides uncompromised endothelial nourishment even during phacoemulsification
- In addition to supplying fine essentials ions (Sodium, potassium, magnesium, calcium and chloride) this solution provides the endothelium with three additional constutuents
- Sodium bicarbonate for normal endothelial pump function to help reduce corneal swelling. It is vital for maintaining endothelial barrier integrity and is activating agent for endothelial cell metabolic pumps for maintaining corneal clarity
- Dextrose is an energy source for endeothelial cell metabolism and is essential for acrobic

metabolism of endethelial cells and helps to maintain transparency of cornea and lens
- Oxidized glutathione to protect cell against oxidative stress and maintain integrity of the blood aqueous barrier to minimise inflammation. It maintains functional complexes of endothelial cells
- BSS plus solution does not contain alien ingradients such as acetate or citrate which can chelate free calcium ions. Calcium ions help to maintain the corneal endothelium's vital barrier function.

Compound sodium lactate solution (in 500 ml pack) Compound sodium chloride solution (in 5 ml and 500 ml packs).

Extraocular Irrigating Solutions

Extraocular irrigating solutions are sterile isotonic solutions for general ophthalmic use.

Ocular uses include irrigating procedures following tonometry, gonioscopy, foreign body removal or use of Fluorescein. They are also used to soothe and clense the eye and in conjunction with hard contact lenses. As these solutions have short contact time with the eye, they do not need to provide nutrient to the cells. Unlike intraocular irrigants, irrigants for extraocular use contain preservatives which prevent bacteriostatic contamination. However, the preservatives are exceedingly toxic to the corneal endothelium and intraocular use of extraocular irrigating fluids is contraindicated.

Various commercial preparations of extraocular fluids available are:

Extraocular irrigating solution containing (EIS) 0.49 NaCl, 0.075 KCl, 0.048 percent calcium chloride, 0.03 percent magnesium chloride, 0.39 percent sodium acetate and 0.17 percent sodium citrate with 0.013 percent benzalkonium chloride (in 30 ml and 120 ml sterile packs).

EIS containing Boric acid and sodium borate with 0.004 percent phenylmercuric nitrate or 0.002 percent thimerosal (in 15,30, 120 and 180 ml packs).

EIS containing 0.49 percent NaCl, 0.075 percent KCl, 0.03 percent magnesium chloride, 0.048 percent calcium chloride, 0.39 percent sodium acetate, 0.17 percent sodium citrate, 0.013 percent benzalkonium chloride and sodium hydroxide or hydrochloric acid in (30 ml and 120 ml packs).

EIS containing 1.2 percent boric acid, 0.38 percent KCl, 0.014 percent sodium carbonate anhydrous, 0.05 percent EDTA and 0.01 percent benzalkonium chloride (in 30 ml and 120 ml packs).

EIS containing 0.05 percent tetrahydrozoline HCl with NaCl, sodium borate, boric acid, 0.01 percent benzalkonium chloride and 0.1 percent EDTA (in 15 ml pack).

EIS solution containing NaCl, sodium proprionate, sodium borate, boric acid, glycerin, rose and camphor water, extract of witch hazel, berbrine bisulfate and benzalkonium chloride (in 120 ml pack).

EIS solution containing 0.49 NaCl, 0.4 percent sodium biphosphate and 0.45 percent sodium phosphate with 0.005 percent banzalkonium chloride (in 180 ml pack).

SURGICAL ENZYMES

Various chemical enzymes used in ophthalmology are:

Alpha Chymotrypsin

It is a proteolytic enzyme. The principal proteolytic effect is exerted by the splitting of peptide bonds of amino acids in the zonular fibres and ocular tissues.

Indication It is mainly used for enzymatic zonulysis for intracapsular lens extraction particularly in young patients.

Destruction of the equatorial pericapsular membrane of the lens occurs in 5 minutes. Zonular fibers are lysed with in 10-15 minutes of application and complete lysis of the entire zonular membrane occurs in 30 minutes.

However, it does not have any effect on the vitreo-lenticular adhesions found in such patients in whom ECCE is the treatment of choice.

Contraindications Significant anterior displacement of lens-iris diaphragm with impending vitreous loss.

High vitreous pressure, gaping incisional wound, congenital cataracts, hypersensitivity to chymotrypsin or any componant of the preparation.

Administration and dosage Fresh solution of alpha chymotrypsin is prepared just before use.

Commercially it is available as powder for ophthalmic solution containing 150 units or 300 units with 2 ml sodium chloride diluent per dual chamber univial.

It is also available as 750 units per vial with 9 ml BSS diluent. Reconstitute solution before use. The 750 units vial may be reconstituted with 5 ml (150 units/ml) or 10 ml (75 units/ml) of the diluent provided. A solution of 150 units/ml is equivalent to a 1:5000 dilution. The 300 units vials reconstituted with 2 ml of diluent yield a 1:5000 solution.

When used for intracapsular cataract extraction, a fresh solution of alpha-chymotrypsin is injected into the anterior chamber immediately prior to the removal of lens (intracameral injection) and within 3-5 minutes will have sufficiently weakened the lens zonules. Usually 0.2-0.5 ml of freshly prepared 1:5000 solution injected slowly behind the lens into the posterior chamber. This enzyme is rapidly in activated in the presence of serum and blood however drugs used routinely in cataract surgery like adrenaline (1:100000) does not inhibit the enzyme activity.

Adverse reactions The adverse effects include transient rise in IOP, moderate uveitis corneal edema, striation. Delayed healing of incisions has also been reported. Other adverse effects are wound disruption, vitreous loss.

Urokinase

It is useful for dissolving blood clot of coagulated hyphaema. Usual dosage is: 5000 units of urokinase are dissolved in 2 ml of normal saline (pH 7.2–7.6) and injected into the anterior chamber through a small keratome incision. It causes liquefaction of the clot which can then be washed out with Ringer lactate solution.

Hyaluronidase

This enzyme is prepared from mammalian testes and acts by depolymerising hyaluronic acid an essential component of the intercellular ground substance which determines the permeability of tissue.

The enzyme hyaluronidase is commonly used in conjunction with local anesthetics lignocaine (2%) with adrenaline for infiltration and regional local anesthesia. Hyaluronidase is also indicated for subconjunctival hemorrhage for hasten reabsorption and for cortisone therapy when given subconjunctivally for early pterygium resolution. The advantages it brings to local injection are:

1. Quicker diffusion and a more effective action of lignocaine and adrenaline in promoting akinesia of orbicularis oculi and extraocular muscles.
2. The swelling at the site of injection is appreciably lessened by its presence. The duration of anesthesia is about the same as without the use of hyaluronidase provided that adrenaline is used.

   The effect of the injection is hastened by the massage of the infiltrated area.
3. Hyaluronidase increases the area of anesthesia by 40 percent.
4. It is nontoxic to the ocular tissues.

Dosage It is available as an odorless, fluffy powder containing 300 units of activity per mg.

It is freshly prepared just before use. For local anesthesia it is directly reconstituted in 2 percent lidocaine solution 1 ampoule of hyaluronidase containing 1500 IU (each ml) is directly mixed into 30 ml vial of 2 percent lidocaine and adrenaline. Hyaluronidase can also be obtained by dissolving the contents of one ampoule in 10 ml sterile distilled water and withdrawing 1 ml of it.

Adverse reactions Generally there are no signs of local or systemic tissue therapy.

Hyaluronidase is antigenic and may sometime produce allergic reactions. Because of danger of spreading the infection, the enzyme should not be injected into or around an infected area.

Ocular malignancy is also considered a contraindication for hyaluronidase for similar action.

Solutions of hyaluronidase rapidly lose their viscosity reducing activity at room temperature. Fresh solution should be used certainly within 12 hours.

REFERENCES

1. Agarwal Amar, Textbook of Ophthalmology, ed.1, New Delhi: Jaypee Brothers Medical Publishers, 2002.
2. Bartlett JD, Clinical Ocular Pharmacology, ed.4, Boston: Butterworth-Heinemann,2001
3. Bartlett. JD, Ophthalmic Drug facts, Lippincott–William and Wilkins, 2001.
4. Buratto Viscoelastics in Ophthalmic Surgery, Slack. Inc., 2000.
5. Crick RP, Trimble RB, Textbook of Clinical Ophthalmology, Hodder and Stoughton, 1986.
6. Dich Viscoelastics in Ophthalmic Surgery, Springer-Verlag, 2000.
7. Duane. TD, Clinical Ophthalmology, ed. 4: Butterworth – Heinemann, 1999.
8. Duvall, Ophthalmic Medications and Pharmacology, Slack Inc, 1998.
9. Ellis. PP, Ocular Therapeutics and Pharmacology, ed. 7: CV Mosby, 1985.
10. Fechner, Ocular Therapeutics, Slack Inc., 1998.
11. Fraunfelder, Current Ocular Therapy, ed. 5: WB Saunders, 2000.
12. Garg Ashok, Current Trends in Ophthalmology, ed. 1, New Delhi: Jaypee Brothers Medical Publishers, 1997.
13. Garg Ashok, Manual of Ocular Therapeutics, ed. 1, New Delhi: Jaypee Brothers Medical Publishers, 1996.
14. Garg Ashok, Ready Reckoner of Ocular Therapeutics, ed.1, New Delhi: 2002.
15. Goodman LS, Gilman A, Pharmacological Basis of Therapeutics, ed.7, New York: Macmillan, 1985.
16. Havener's, Ocular Pharmacology, ed. 6: C.V. Mosby, 1994.
17. Kanski, Clinical Ophthalmology, ed. 4: Butterworth – Heineman, 1999.
18. Kershner, Ophthalmic Medications and Pharmacology, Slack Inc, 1994.
19. Olin BR et al, Drugs Facts and Comparisons: Facts and Comparisons, St Louis, 1997.
20. Onofrey, The Ocular Therapeutics, Lippincott-William and Wilkins, 1997.
21. Rhee, The Wills Eye drug Guide, Lippincott–William and Wilkins, 1998.
22. Steven Podos, Textbook of Ophthalmology, New Delhi: Jaypee Brothers Medical Publishers, 2001.
23. Zimmerman, Textbook of Ocular Pharmacology, Lippincott and William and Wilkins, 1997.

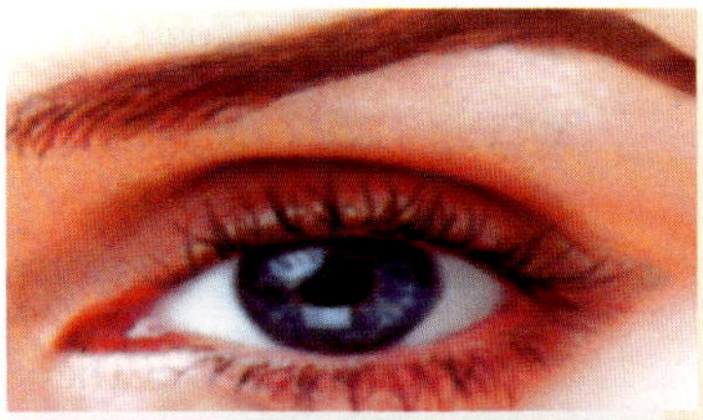

Ten

Suresh K Pandey
Liliana Werner
David J Apple
Andrea M Izak (USA)
Vidhushi Sharma
Ashok Garg (India)

Update on Ophthalmic Viscosurgical Devices

BACKGROUND

Viscoelastic substances are solutions with dual properties; they act as viscous liquids as well as elastic solids or gels. The ideal viscoelastic substance in ophthalmology should be viscous enough to prevent collapse of the anterior chamber at rest, yet liquid enough to be injected precisely through a small cannula. It should be elastic or shock absorbing and should enhance coating yet has minimal surface activity. It should be cohesive enough to be removed to be easily removed from the anterior chamber but not so cohesive that it is aspirated during irrigation and aspiration, which would provide no protection to endothelial cells during surgical manipulations. It should be eliminated from the eye in the postoperative period without an effect on intraocular pressure.[6-8,20,22,23]

Viscosurgery was a term coined by Balazs[10,11] to describe the use of these solutions that had viscous, elastic and pseudoplastic properties during and after surgical procedures. During viscosurgery, viscoelastic substances are used as a fluid or a soft surgical instrument. The viscoelastic sodium hyaluronate was first used in ophthalmic surgery in 1972, when it was introduced as a replacement for vitreous and aqueous humor.[10,11] Since then ophthalmic surgical procedures had undergone considerable advancement. The use of viscoelastic materials has become commonplace in anterior and posterior segment surgeries. These agents facilitate delicate and often difficult intraocular manipulations during various ophthalmic surgical procedures. They are used during cataract surgery and intraocular lens (IOL) implantation to maintain the anterior chamber depth and capsular bag distention, thus creating and preserving working space for the ophthalmic surgeon. These agents are designed to protect the delicate corneal endothelial cells during the surgery.[20]

The viscoelastic substances has been termed as "ophthalmic viscosurgical devices" (OVDs).[9] A detailed discussion regarding biocompatibilty, physical, and rheological properties of the OVDs are beyond the scope of this chapter. Interested readers may consult the excellent review article(s) published by Liesegang on this topic.[21,22] The viscoelastic substances must be non-toxic, non-pyrogenic, non-inflammatory, non-immunogenic, and sterile for use in the human eyes. The substance should not interfere with the normal metabolism of the cells in contact with it. Substances that are immunogenic, may cause granulation or capsule formation, stimulate cell invasion, or interfere with epithelization or blood coagulation cannot be used in the eyes. [17,22,23] Each viscoelastic substance has unique physicochemical properties which determines its clinical applications.[22,23,38,39,44] Figures 10.1A to C is a gross photograph showing physical characteristics (viscosity) of 3 different concentration of the sodium hyaluronate solution (Healon®, Healon-GV® and Healon-5®).

In this chapter, we will provide an update of currently used OVDs and will focus on the newly available viscoadaptive viscoelastics (e.g. Healon-5®), their clinical applications and complications. Some of the details related to OVDs had been discussed in the previous chapter of this textbook.[14] The current chapter is based on the review of the published literature on this topic and also derived from the information and illustrations available from the manufacturer. This chapter is divided in 4 sections:

Section 1: Classification of currently available OVDs;

Section 2: Clinical application of the OVDs;

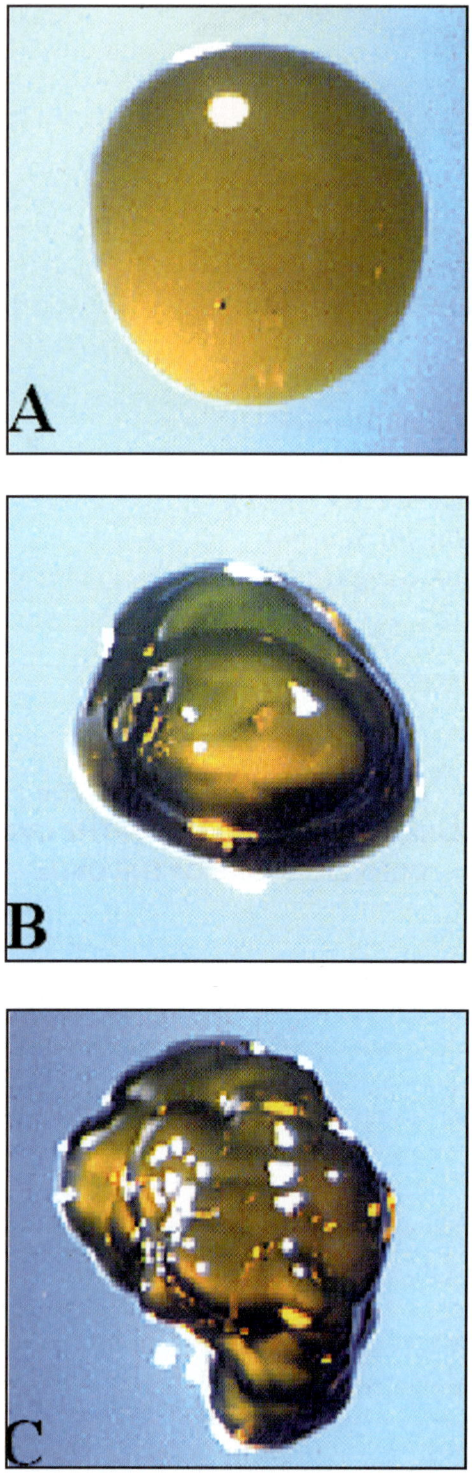

Figs 10.1A to C: Gross photograph showing physical characteristics (viscosity) of 3 different concentration of the sodium hyaluronate solution: (A) Healon®, (B) Healon-GV®, (C) Healon-5®

Section 3: Complications associated with OVDs;
Section 4: Summary and conclusions.

CLASSIFICATION OF THE OVDs

Table 10.1 presents summary of the currently available OVDs. OVDs can be classified according to their zero shear viscosity and cohesion. The zero shear viscosity is directly proportional to the molecular weight. This classification describes the surgical behavior of the viscoelastics and is as follows.[7]

1. *High viscosity –cohesive OVDs*
   a. Super viscous-cohesive OVDs (>1,000,000 mPs)
   b. Viscous–cohesive OVDs (Between 100,000 and 1,000,000 mPs)
2. Lower viscosity –dispersive OVDs
3. *Viscoadaptive OVDs (e.g. Healon-5®)*

High Viscous–cohesive OVDs

The super viscous-cohesive group includes Healon-GV® and I-visc plus® while the viscous–cohesive group includes products like I-visc®, Provisc®, Healon®, Amvisc®, Amvisc plus® and others. All these products contain sodium hyaluronate.

High viscous–cohesive OVDs are indicated in many routine procedures and are used to create space and also stabilize the surgical micro-environment. Examples of situations where they are used include deepening the anterior chamber, to enlarge small pupils, to dissect adhesions, and during IOL implantation to push back the iris and vitreous.

Super Viscous–cohesive OVDs

Healon-GV® (greater viscosity) is a sterile, non-pyrogenic agent produced from rooster coombs. It has a concentration of 1.4 percent sodium hyaluronate and a molecular weight of 5 million Daltons.

It is used as a surgical aid in various anterior segment procedures such as cataract extraction, IOL implantation, corneal transplant surgery and glaucoma surgery. In presence of high positive pressure, Healon-GV® has 3 times more resistance to pressure than Healon®. I-Visc® was introduced as a Healon-GV® clone. It has superior viscous and cohesive properties at low shear viscosity when compared to Healon-GV® (Table 10.1).

Super viscous-cohesive agents are better in current day techniques where topical and intracameral anesthesia are used and the surgeries are "entirely in-the-bag" phacoemulsification. High cohesiveness of superviscous and viscous materials result in easy removal as a single mass at the end of the surgical procedure, thus preventing the increased intraocular pressure postoperatively.

Lower Viscosity—Dispersive OVDs

Dispersive agents have low molecular weight and shorter molecular chains. *Medium viscosity, dispersive OVDs* possess zero shear viscosities between 10,000 and 100,000 mPs. *Very low viscosity, dispersive agents* include all of the unmodified hydroxypropyl-methycellulose (HPMC) agents.

These dispersive materials when injected into the eye have the property of fracturing and breaking into smaller bits and thus disperse in the anterior chamber. They include Viscoat®, Cellugel®, Vitrax®, Ocucoat® and others (Table 10.1).

Most of the dispersive OVDs are HPMC-hydroxypropyl methylcellulose, derived from wood pulp. Cellugel® is a chemically modified HPMC. Viscoat® is a combination of sodium hyaluronate and chondroitin sulphate. Vitrax® is a compound of low molecular weight molecular hyaluronate.

The clinical use of these agents is to hold back vitreous out of the surgical field especially in cases of zonular disinsertion. They are helpful in a compromised corneal endothelium conditions, as they are capable of dividing the anterior chamber into OVD-occupied space and surgical zone in which irrigation / aspiration can be continued without the mixing of the two areas—known as surgical compartilization.

The disadvantage of lower viscosity dispersive OVDs is that they do not maintain or stabilize spaces as compared to higher viscosity cohesive agents. They tend to be aspirated in smaller fragments during irrigation / aspiration thus leading to irregular viscoelastic aqueous interface, thus partially obscurring the surgical view of the posterior capsule. They also form microbubbles and can be trapped at the irregular interface thus

Table 10.1: Classification of ophthalmic viscosurgical devices (OVDs)

Viscosurgical agents	*Manufacturer*	*Molecular Wt (D)*	*Source*	*Chemical compound*	*Osmlality (mOsm/liter)*	*Viscosity*	*Vo(mPs)*
Higher viscosity: Cohesive OVDs							
Viscoadaptive (fracturable)							
Healon-5®	Pharmacia Inc.	5.0 M	Rooster Coombs	Hyaluronic Acid	322	2.3 Na Ha (23mg/ml)	7.0M
Super Viscous							
Healon-GV®	Pharmacia Inc.	5.0 M	Rooster Coombs	Hyaluronic Acid	310	1.4 Na Ha (14 mg/ml)	2.0M
I-Visc Plus®	I-Med Pharma	7.9M	Rooster Coombs	Hyaluronic Acid	—	1.4 Na Ha (14 mg/ml)	4.8 M
Viscous							
I-Visc®	I-Med Pharma	6.1 M	Roster Coombs	Hyaluronic Acid	336	1.0 Na Ha (10 mg/ml)	1.0 M
Healon®	Pharmacia Inc.	4.0M	Rooster Coombs	Hyaluronic Acid	302	1.0Na Ha (10 mg/ml)	230K
Provisc®	Alcon	2.0M	Microbial fermentation	Hyaluronic Acid	307	1.0Na Ha (10 mg/ml)	280K
Amvisc Plus®	IO lab (B and L surgical)	1.0M	Rooster Coombs	Hyaluronic Acid	340	1.6Na Ha (16 mg/ml)	100K
Amvisc®	IO Lab (B and L surgical)	1.0M	Rooster Coombs	Hyaluronic Acid	318	1.2 Na Ha (12 mg/ml)	100K
Biolon®	Biotech general corp	3.0M	Bacterial Fermentation	Hyaluronic Acid	279	1.0 Na Ha (12 mg/ml)	215K
Low viscosity: Dispersive OVDs							
Medium Viscosity							
Viscoat®	Alcon	500K	Bacterial Fermentation Shark Fin	Hyaluronic acid Chondriotin Sulphate	325	3.0 NaHa 4.0 CDS (40 mg/ml)	41K
Vitrax®	Allergan	500K	Rooster coombs	Hyaluronic Acid	310	3.0Na Ha (30 mg/ml)	25K
Cellugel®	Vision biology (Alcon)	100K	Synthetic	Hydrooxy-propyl methyl-cellulose	305	2.0 Chemically modified HPMC	38K
Ocucoat®	Storz (B and L surgical)	86 K	Wood pulp	Hydroxypropyl-methylcellulose	285	2.0 HPMC (20 mg/ml)	4K
Visilon®	Shah and Shah	86 K	—	—	—	2.0 HPMC (20 mg/ml)	4 K
Viscon	Dr. Agarwal's Pharma	86 K	—	Hydroxypropyl-methylcellulose		2.0 HPMC (20 mg/ml)	4 K
Visicrome®	Croma Pharma	—	—	—	—	2.0 HPMC (20 mg/ml)	—

Vo (mPs)= Zero shear Viscosity(milli Pascal Seconds); (D) = Daltons; M = Millions; K = Thousand; NaHa = Sodium hyaluronate; HPMC = Hydroxypropylmethylcellulose; CDS = Chondroitin sulphate

further obscurring visibility. Moreover they are difficult to remove at the end of the surgery because of low cohesion.

Soft Shell Technique

This technique was developed by Arshinoff, in order to take advantage of the best properties of both lower viscosity-dispersive agents and high viscosity-cohesive agents and to minimize the drawbacks of each by using them together. In this technique first the lower viscosity dispersive is injected into the anterior chamber, followed by high viscosity-cohesive agent, which is injected into the center of the lower viscosity-dispersive viscoelastic thus pushing it outwards and compressing it into a smooth, even layer against the corneal endothelium. This protects the endothelium during lens removal.

Prior to the implantation of the IOL, the reverse is done. High viscosity cohesive is injected first to partially fill the anterior chamber and the capsular bag, followed by injection of lower viscosity dispersive into the center of high viscosity cohesive agent. This allows the free movement of the IOL through the dispersive agent, with better stabilization of the surrounding iris and the capsular bag by the high viscosity agent.[48]

Removal of the OVDs is easily accomplished at the end of the surgery, since low viscosity dispersive OVA can be aspirated from the central anterior segment first, followed by higher cohesive agent. DuoVisc®-a combination of high viscocity–cohesive Provisc® and the lower viscosity dispersive Viscoat®.

Viscoadaptive OVD—Healon-5®

The existing viscoelastic products all have drawbacks. A cohesive viscous product used to create and maintain space may not stay in the eye during phacoemulsification. On the other hand, a less viscous dispersive product stays during phacoemulsification but often traps fragments or air bubbles and does not maintain adequate space during the surgical procedure.

Recently the new viscoadapative viscoelastic Healon-5® has been developed to change its behavior at different flow rates.[3] It acts as a viscous cohesive viscoelastic agent at lower flow rates and as a pseudodispersive viscoelastic agent at higher flow rates. It is all in one device that adapts its behavior to the surgeons' needs during the entire course of surgery.

This is a steam sterilized, non-pyrogenic solution. It is highly purified non-inflammatory, high molecular weight sodium hyaluronate at a concentration of 23 mg/ml (2.3%) dissolved in a physiological buffer. It has an osmolality and a pH similar to those of the aqueous humor. It has a viscosity at rest about 7 million times higher than aqueous humor. It is extracted from rooster coombs.

Hyaluronate is a polysaccharide made up of disaccharide units linked by glycosides bonds. It occurs naturally on the corneal endothelium bound to specific receptors. The natural hyaluronate is reduced during irrigation but can be restored by an exogenous one. Healon-5® has a high affinity to the receptors. It acts as a scavenger by neutralizing the free radicals formed during cataract surgery using ultrasound.

Characteristics and Advantages of the Viscoadaptive OVDs

1. Viscoadaptive OVD (Healon-5®) is specifically developed so that, at different flow rates it has different functions. At lower flow rates it behaves as a very cohesive viscoelastic like a Healon-GV®. At higher flow rates, e.g. in chopping techniques, it begins to fracture and behaves similarly to a dispersive viscoelastic, such as Viscoat®. Hence Healon-5® has features that can change according to the needs of the surgeon during various stages of cataract surgery.
2. It is crystal clear as pure water and has somewhat higher refractive index than the aqueous humor. Hence it increases the clarity within the surgical field.
3. It also has the ability to protect the delicate corneal endothelial cells from debris and turbulence during phacoemulsification, particularly with very low endothelial cell count. In a recent study by Holzer *et al.*,[16] the average loss of corneal endothelial cells was lowest for their surgeries using Healon-5® compared to other OVDs.
4. Viscoadaptive OVD (Healon-5®) is also helpful in patients with suboptimal pupil size because the viscomydriasis allows for a larger capsulorhexis and keeps the pupil larger during phacoemulsification thus increasing the visibility.

5. It also neutralizes the positive vitreous pressure and prevents capsulorhexis from extending by temporarily stopping all action, thus allowing the surgeon to determine what is going on inside the eye, analyze his or her options and effect the appropriate management.
6. The high viscosity of Healon-5® creates space and stabilizes the anterior segment. The elasticity absorbs shock and protects ocular tissues during IOL unfolding, which is slowed down and is more controlled.
7. Healon-5® is also easy to remove. The "Rock and Roll" technique[10] with suitable settings for each type of phacoemulsifications, was found to be a safe method for complete removal of it. In this technique there is sufficient turbulence created and this fractures Healon-5® into small pieces. The other method for Healon-5® removal is the two compartment technique (TCT).[50] Full advantage of the agent's viscoadaptive properties is taken in this technique. The superior space maintaining capacity of Healon-5® in the anterior chamber is utilized while removing the substance from the capsular bag. In the second step the anterior chamber is cleaned.

There is a learning curve for surgeons using Healon-5®, but as surgeons begin making a number of small procedural adaptations, the advantages of the viscoadaptive OVD will increasingly become apparent.

CLINICAL APPLICATIONS OF THE OVDs

In recent years the field of viscosurgery has broadened rapidly. It has been used both intraocularly as well as extraocularly, which includes cataract, cornea, glaucoma, viteroretinal, strabismus and oculoplastic surgeries.[7,22,23,30]

Use of OVDs in Cataract Surgery

OVDs are helpful in each step of modern cataract surgery using phacoemulsification with IOL implantation.[5,13,41,43] Some of these details are shown in the schematic photograph (Figs 10.2A to C and 10.3).

Capsulorhexis

In order to perform an intact and successful capsulorhexis, the contents of the anterior chamber have an important role. Till date balanced salt solution (BSS®), air and OVDs have been used. Out of these three the best is viscoelastic as it is considered the easiest, safest, and the most reproducible method in both routine and difficult cases (Figs 10.2A and B). To perform a good capsulorhexis, the viscoelastic to be used should have the four basic features:

1. High molecular weight and high viscosity at zero shear rate, which maintains the anterior chamber.
2. Excellent visibility provided by high transparency.
3. Make surgical maneuvers easy, due to high elasticity and pseudoplasticity.
4. It should gives a good capsular flap control, providing the soft and permanent spatula effect.

Cleavage of Lens Structure

It is best performed with the use of OVDs. The ideal viscoelastic material keeps the anterior chamber shape unchanged during BSS® injection and also avoids increase in pressure, which can be produced with excessive amount of BSS® known as capsular blockade.

Nuclear Emulsification

During phacoemulsification, the viscoelastic is likely to remain in the anterior chamber instead of leaking out of the eye (Fig. 10.2C). OVDs help in preserving the space and also because of their low cohesiveness, they remain in the anterior chamber despite high irrigation flow. Moreover OVDs adhere to the corneal endothelium, thus protecting the corneal endothelial cells. Healon® and Healon-GV® does not trap the air bubble and provide excellent endothelial protection (Fig. 10.2D). This is because of:

1. Scavenger effect—This effect captures the free radicals released during phaco with consequent inactivation.
2. Binding sites—There are chemical receptors for viscoelastic materials on the corneal endothe-

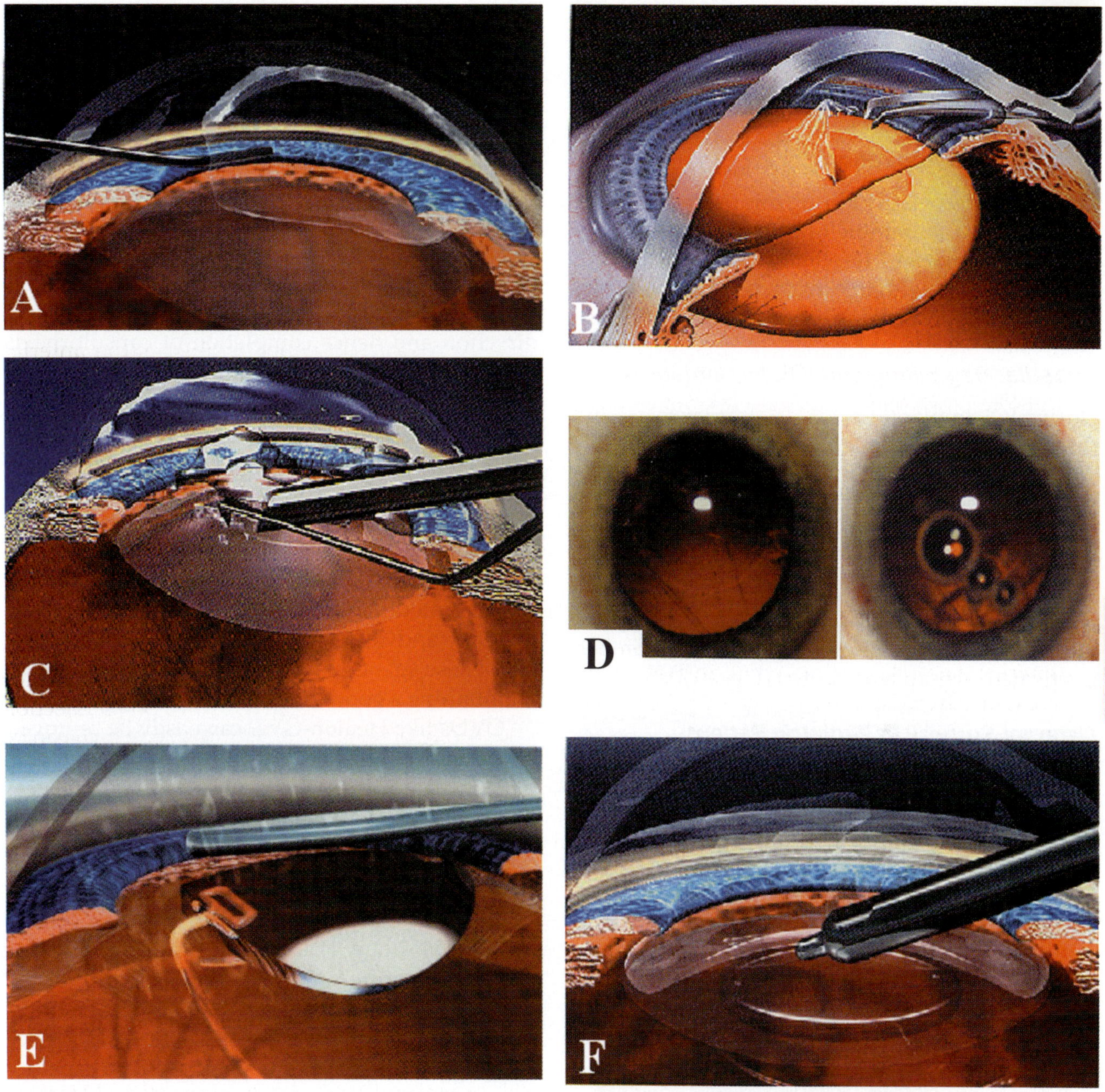

Figs 10.2A to F: Schematic photograph showing use of the OVD (viscoadaptive OVD-Healon-5® in this figure) during the various steps of the cataract surgery: (A) Injection of the viscoadaptive OVD in the anterior chamber through a 25 G cannula, (B) Capsulorhexis is in progress, (C) Phacoemulsification in progress, (D) Viscoadaptive OVD is transparent and easy to see during removal (left). Note the presence of the air bubbles within the anterior chamber after use of dispersive viscoelastic solution (right), (E) Implantation of a posterior chamber intraocular lens in the capsular bag, (F) Removal of the viscoadaptive OVD using irrigation-aspiration tip. (*Courtesy:* Pharmacia Inc. Peapack, NJ, USA)

lium. A molecular bond seems to occur between the viscoelastic solution and the corneal endothelium.

3. High elasticity—This also smoothes the possible impacts of the lens material against the endothelium.

The phaco tip being in a closed system, its vibrations are transmitted to the internal structures of the eye but viscoelastic provides a smothering shield against them.

Irrigation and Aspiration

The role of viscoelastic during this procedure is the protection of the endothelium. This is possible due to high adhesiveness. It remains where it is placed, without mixing with the cortex because of its low cohesiveness thus helping in easy removal of cortex.

Capsular Bag Filling and IOL Implantation

During IOL implantation, it is necessary to expand the capsular bag with a viscoelastic. It allows the surgeon to keep the bag well opened and formed thus allowing the easy IOL implantation. OVD is also helpful in correct positioning, centering and allowing for possible IOL rotation maneuvers (Figs 10.2E and F). Beside posterior chamber IOL implantation, OVD has also been used for implantation of other IOL designs (e.g. anterior chamber, iris fixated, artisan lenses, etc.) (Fig. 10.3).[52]

Cataract Surgery in Pediatric Patient

Pediatric cataract surgery like the adult surgery has undergone major changes in recent years with

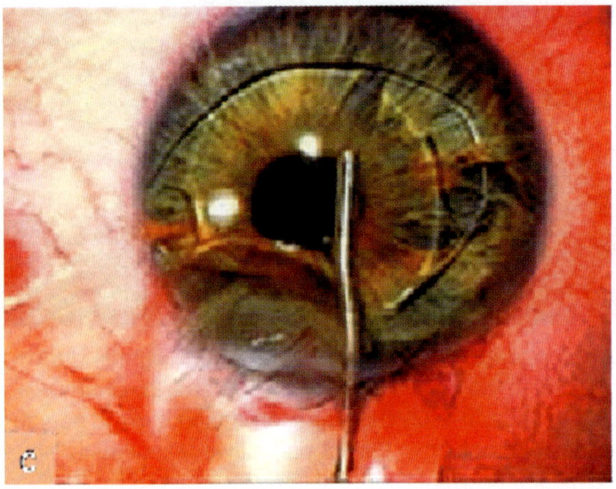

Fig. 10.3: Besides posterior chamber IOL fixation in the capsular bag, OVDs can also be used for implantation of the various phakic and aphakic IOL designs in the anterior chamber, ciliary sulcus, etc. Use of the OVD facilitated the implantation of the Artisan® IOL as shown in this photograph (*Courtesy:* Camil Budo, MD)

the evolution of techniques including small incision and the development of modern IOLs. The main principle lies in the control of the very elastic nature of ocular tissues.[42]

It is difficult to perform a good capsulorhexis in the presence of high capsular elasticity. Moreover there is low scleral rigidity, greater intravitreal pressure that makes the capsulorhexis even more difficult, as the pressure tends to curve the capsulorhexis. But with the use of viscoelastic, e.g. Healon-GV® the effective push is in the opposite direction and hence completion of capsulorhexis can be done.

In pediatric cases, the capsulorhexis must be started in the central portion and not towards the equator, in order to prevent radial extension. The high density viscoelastic agents stabilizes the posterior chamber and pushed back the vitreous face during the posterior capsulorhexis. During IOL implantation, the capsular bag is kept open and the anterior chamber is well formed thus ensuring easy and safe implantation of the IOL in the bag. These agents also help to dilate the pupil thus maintaining a good intraoperative mydriasis.[55-57]

OVDs like Healon-GV® can easily be removed at the end of the surgery including the position which is behind the IOL due to its high cohesiveness thus preventing capsular blockade.

Use of the OVDs in Glaucoma Surgery

Viscocanalostomy

Viscocanalostomy is a new surgical procedure for glaucoma therapy.[45] Viscoelastics play an important role in this procedure. Figures 10.4A to F illustrates the surgical steps of viscocanalosotomy. Viscocanalostomy literally means "opening of the canal by means of viscoelastic substance". This procedure is a non-penetrating and independent from external filtration. The advantages are decreased risk of infection, and decreased incidence of cataract, hypotony and flat anterior chamber as the anterior chamber is not opened, and moreover, with the absence of external filtration the bleb formation is prevented and also the related discomfort with it. It minimizes the risk of late infections and is independent from conjuntival and episcleral scarring.

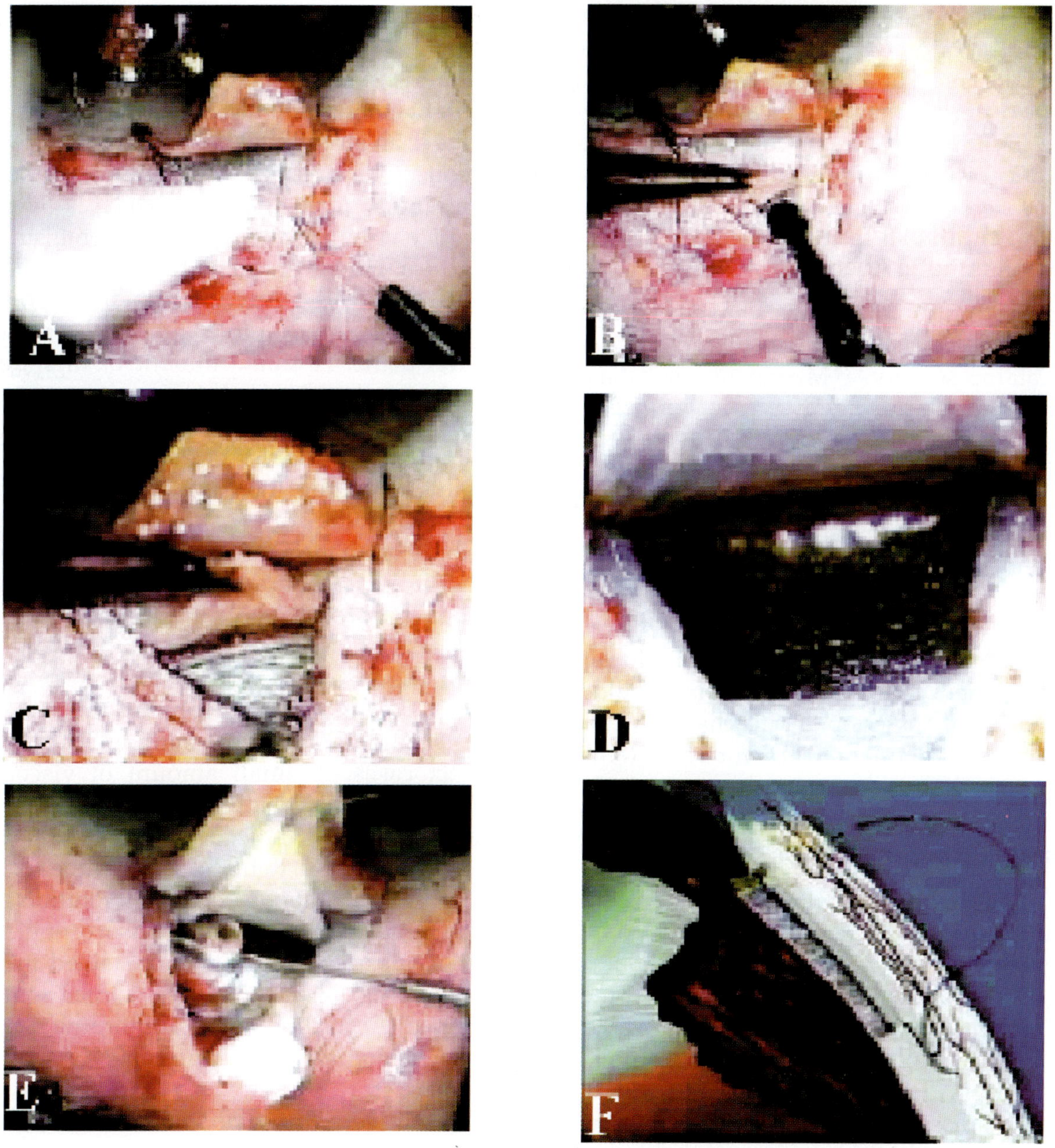

Figs 10.4A to F: Surgical steps of viscocanalosotomy. (A) Deep block construction incision, (B) Cutting the deep block in a single plane with a spoon blade, (C) Proximal to Schlemm's canal there is a subtle change in the scleral fibers, from a crossing pattern to a tangential pattern, with an increased opacity, (D) Descemet's window, (E) Cannulating Schlemm's canal with three puffs of viscoelastic directed at the osteum, (F) Tight closure suture of the flap. (*Courtesy:* Dr. med. Tobias Neuhann, M.D., Munich, Germany)

Viscocanalostomy allows the aqueous to leave the eye, through Schlemn's canal and episcleral veins thus restoring the natural outflow pathway. This procedure creates a bypass by which aqueous humor reaches Schlemn's canal, skipping the trabecular meshwork. A chamber is produced inside the sclera, which is in direct communication with the Schlemn's canal. There is also a communication through the Descemet's membrane with the anterior chamber.

The OVDs should have high pseudoplasticity to allow injection into Schlemn's canal through a small needle and should have high viscosity at shear rate of zero to maintain the spaces as long as possible. Healon-GV® and Healon-5® are viscoelastics of choice for this procedure.

OVDs for Intraocular Delivery of Dyes or Anesthetic Agents

Researchers and vision scientists have been using OVDs as a vehicle to deliver capsular dyes for use during cataract surgery.[1,25] Mixing these substances with the viscoelastic agent was attempted to prolong their effect and to limit the adverse effect on ocular tissues. Ciba Vision Corp (Duluth, GA, USA), has recently proposed mixing an OVD with lidocaine. This was termed "viscoanesthesia" and was intended to prolong the anesthetic effect of intracameral lidocaine, as a complement to topical anesthesia. Also, the steps of intracameral injection of OVDs and of intracameral injection of lidocaine, as a complement to topical anesthesia, would be combined in only one step. In this chapter we will briefly address the use of OVDs for viscostaining and viscoanesthesia.

Viscostaining of the Anterior Lens Capsule

Various non-toxic ophthalmic dyes have been extensively used as diagnostic agents for the detection and management of different ocular disorders. Dyes such as fluorescein sodium, indocyanine green (ICG), and trypan blue have been increasingly used for enhancing visualization by staining intraocular tissues during the adult and pediatric cataract surgery and vitreoretinal surgery. Staining of ocular tissues by using ophthalmic dyes makes visual differentiation and manipulation of tissues easier. Enhanced viewing of ocular tissues can assist a surgeon's ability to evaluate clinical structural relationships and may help attain surgical objectives with fewer complications.

Uses of various capsular dyes for staining the anterior lens capsule in white, mature cataracts have been reported.[31-37,46,53] The techniques originally reported for staining the anterior capsule using fluorescein sodium are: staining from above under an air bubble, as proposed by Nahra and Castilla[27] and intracameral subcapsular injection of fluorescein sodium (staining from below) with blue-light enhancement. The first technique (staining under an air bubble) is currently used by most surgeons. One benefit is the staining of the peripheral anterior capsular rim, which is otherwise difficult to visualize during the phacoemulsification procedure. However, air in the anterior chamber makes it unsteady. Any instrument entering the eye will cause some air to escape, with a rise of the lens-iris plane. A small amount of high-density viscoelastic placed near the incision can prevent the air bubble from escaping the anterior chamber, thus minimizing the risk of sudden collapse. Also, with this technique, there is a progressive dilution of the dye by the aqueous humor. This may be a possible explanation for the fainter staining observed with this technique in recent clinical reports, without compromising its usefulness. Most of the drawbacks of this technique can be avoided by careful use of a viscoelastic solution to seal the incision site. Akahoshi[1] proposed the "soft shell stain technique" for performing a CCC in white cataract cases. A small amount of viscoelastic (Viscoat®) was injected into the anterior chamber followed by high molecular weight viscoelastic material (Provisc®) to fill up the chamber completely. The author then injected ICG solution on the lens surface with a bent G27 viso cannula. The anterior capsule was uniformly stained in green and easily visualized while the cornea remained unstained. According to the author, the soft shell stain technique is extremely useful for CCC in white cataracts.

Alternatively, the dye solution can be mixed with viscoelastic agents a technique known as "viscostaining of the anterior lens capsule". Kayikicioglu and coworkers[19] proposed a technique for limiting the contact of trypan blue to corneal endothelium by mixing the dye with a viscoelastic solution. These researchers mixed 0.4 percent trypan blue with 1 percent sodium hyaluronate in a 2 mL syringe. The dye, mixed in a viscoelastic solution, is injected onto the anterior lens capsule, which covers the anterior capsule without coming in contact with the corneal endothelium. Trypan blue mixed with sodium hyaluronate greatly increases the visibility of the anterior lens capsule without significantly touching the adjacent tissues. There is always a potential risk of corneal decompensation after intraocular use of self-mixed solutions; however, these authors used this technique without significant surgical and postoperative adverse effects.

Use of OVDs in Topical Ophthalmic Anesthesia (Viscoanesthesia)

Anesthetic techniques for cataract surgery have also advanced significantly. General anesthesia was preferred in past years, followed by various techniques of injectable anesthesia including retrobulbar, peribulbar, sub-Tenon, and subconjunctival anesthesia. Due to marked improvements in surgical techniques, it is no longer essential to ensure complete akinesia of the eye and as a consequence, the technique of topical anesthesia has been popularized as "phaco anesthesia". This includes eyedrops application, sponge anesthesia, eyedrops plus intracameral injection, and most recently gel application.[15,40] Topical anesthesia is the preferred technique for the members of the American Society of Cataract and Refractive Surgery (ASCRS) in the United States (49%; range 37%-63%) according to a survey conducted by David Leaming in 2000.[21] It revealed that as high as 82 percent of the respondents using topical anesthesia preferred eye drops in association with intracameral injection of lidocaine.

We have recently completed some studies to evaluate the use of viscoelastic agents mixed with topical anesthetic solution (lidocaine). The aim of these studies was to evaluate the safety of this new solution (termed as viscoanesthesia) to intraocular structures.[24,32,51] Our animal and experimental studies were divided into 3 parts. In Part I,[24] we determined the toxicity of the viscoanesthetic solution to the corneal endothelium using a rabbit model. In Part II,[51] we evaluated the toxicity of viscoanesthetic solutions to uveal tissues and retina in a rabbit model after performing phacoemulsification. Finally, in Part III,[32] using postmortem human eyes, we evaluated and compared to currently available OVDs in regard to the surgical aspects such as injection and aspiration of the viscoanesthetic solutions. In brief, our experimental study demonstrated that addition of varying concentrations of lidocaine to sodium hyaluronate (Ophthalin Plus®) neither significantly altered its viscosity or consistency nor changed its removal time from the capsular bag. Our animal studies on viscoanesthesia (Part I, II) in rabbit eyes had suggested that viscoanethetic solution with lidocaine concentrations up to 1.65 percent are not toxic for the corneal endothelium, uveal or retinal tissues. Future clinical trails are necessary to address the issue of efficacy of viscoanesthetic solutions to provide prolonged topical anesthesia.

Removal of the OVDs

Several techniques has been reported in the literature for removal of the OVDs. These include: Rock and roll technique, two-compartment technique and bimanual irrigation/aspiration technique.[4] Figures 10.5A to H are photographs from a human eye obtained postmortem (Miyake-Apple posterior view) showing the sequence of the experimental surgical technique of the removal of fluorescein-colored viscoelastic solutions (green color as viewed with oblique illumination) from the capsular bag using the rock and roll technique.

An effective technique to remove Healon-5® is to create maximum turbulence to make it fracture into large pieces. This can be accomplished using rock and roll technique with standard I/A tip, 0.3 mm, with high settings; a flow rate of 25-30 ml/min., and vacuum 350-500 mm Hg, depending on the type of pump. If a peristaltic pump is used the vacuum should be set towards the lower limit. A bottle height of 60-70 cm above the eye level. Figures 10.6A to C summarizes the removal technique of viscoadaptive agent, Healon-5®.

An alternative technique has been developed allowing the use of less turbulence, using a standard I/A tip, 0.3 mm, with effectual flow at 20-25 ml and vacuum 250-3000 mm Hg. The bottle height should be 60-70 cm above eye level. Figures 10.7A and B present the steps of removal technique of the viscoadaptive agent, Healon-5®, using another technique.

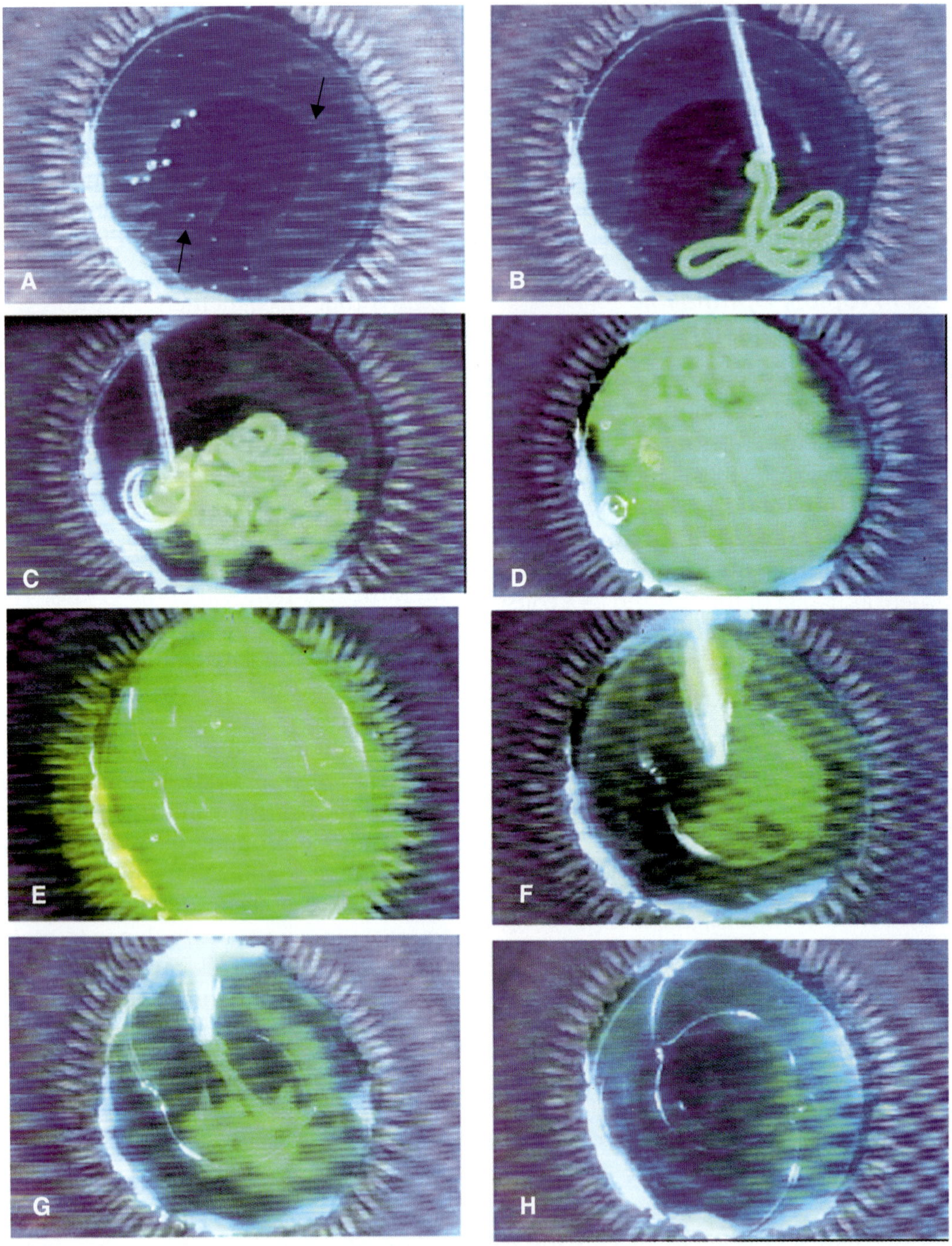

Figs 10.5A to H: Gross photographs from a human eye obtained postmortem (Miyake-Apple posterior view) showing the sequence of the experimental surgical technique of the removal of fluorescein-colored viscoelastic solutions (green color as viewed with oblique illumination) from the capsular bag was documented by video taping: (A) This figure shows the eye after capsulorhexis and removal of lens substance (cortex and nucleus) by phacoemulsification. Note the edge of the anterior capsulectomy (arrows), (B and C) Injection of fluorescein-colored viscoelastic solution (in this example, Ophthalin Plus®), with a 27-gauge Rycroft cannula through the orifice of the anterior capsulectomy, (D) Capsular bag completely filled with viscoelastic solution, (E) Same eye after insertion of a one-piece, modified C-loop posterior chamber IOL in the capsular bag (arrows), (F) Viscoelastic solution removal with automated aspiration, set at 250 mm Hg (Alcon Legacy 20,000), (G) Final removal of viscoelastic substance. The surgeon reached behind the IOL optical edge to remove all the viscoelastic material, (H) Aspect after complete removal of the viscoelastic solution

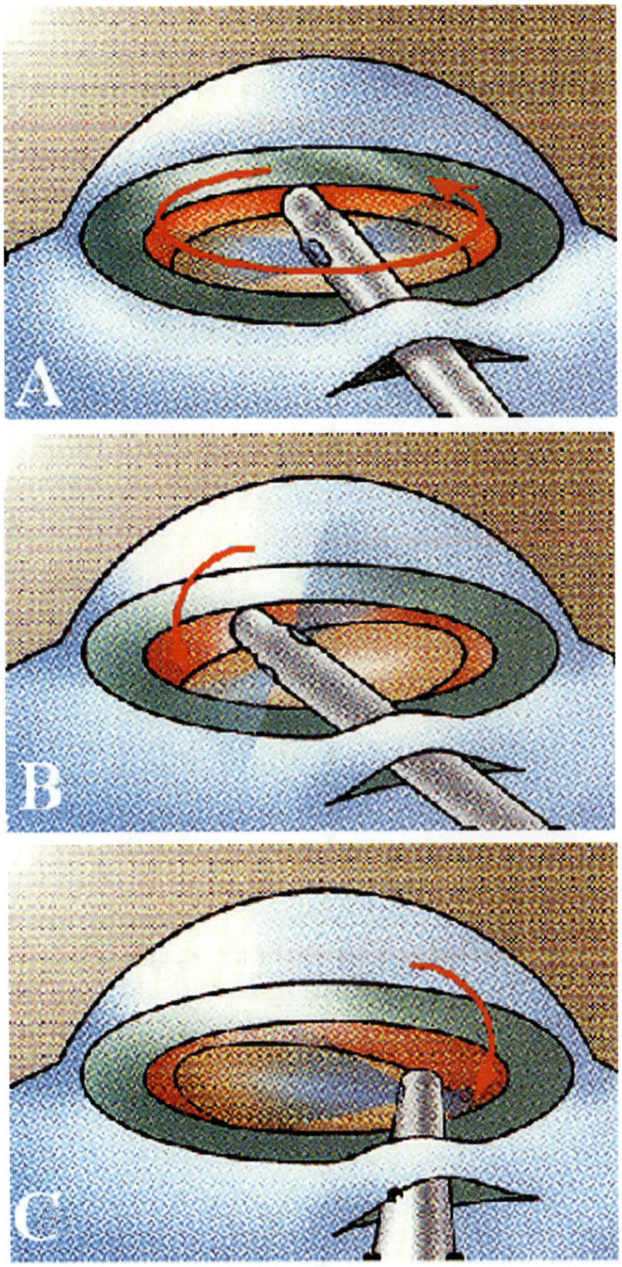

Figs 10.6A to C: Schematic photograph showing the one of the removal technique of viscoadaptive agent (Healon-5®), as recommended by the manufacturer: (A) The surgeon circle the I/A hand piece in the anterior segment at iris plane, (B and C) The surgeon gently rest the I/A hand piece on the anterior surface of the optic. Press gently on the IOL optic on one side and rotate the I/A hand piece directing the flow into the bag. Direct the hand piece port towards the equator of the capsular bag and stay in this position for a few seconds, and then repeat on the other side of the IOL optic until Healon-5® is completely removed. Finally sweep the anterior chamber including the angles and repeat the step, if necessary. (*Courtesy:* Pharmacia Inc. Peapack, NJ, USA)

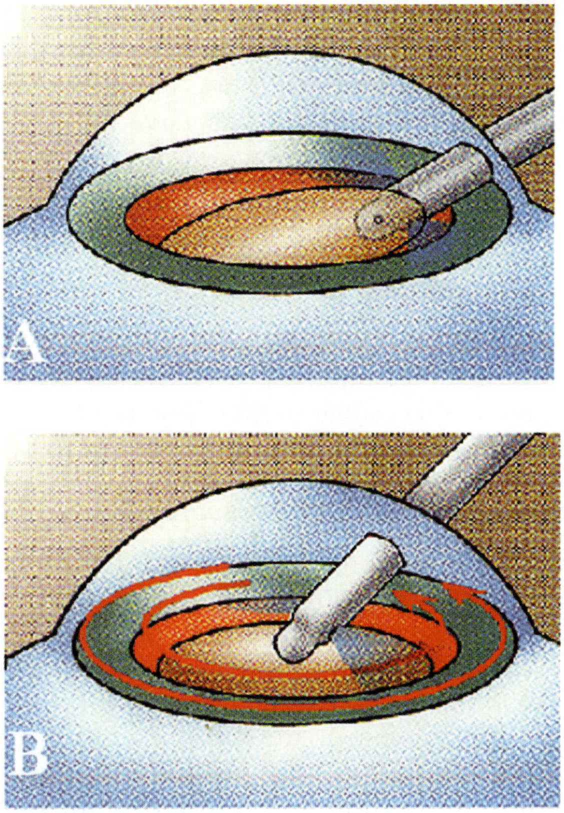

Figs 10.7A and B: Schematic photograph showing an alternative removal technique of viscoadaptive agent (Healon-5®), as recommended by the manufacturer: (A) Start the removal directly after IOL implantation, while the anterior chamber is still filled with Healon-5® and before the IOL has been centered. Go behind the IOL optic without engaging the flow of the I/A tip (port up) and then start flow. Remove Healon-5® from the capsular bag first and ensure that lens has adequately centered. During removal of Healon-5® from the capsular bag, the continuous flow of irrigation fluid keeps the bag inflated and reduces the risk of aspirating the capsular bag. While maintaining continuous flow remove the tip from behind the optic and place it on top of optic, (B) Continue the removal by circling the I/A tip at the iris plane, or on the optic surface, then make an additional sweep in the anterior chamber paying particular attention to angles. (*Courtesy:* Pharmacia Inc. Peapack, NJ, USA)

We would like to emphasize that a careful and thorough removal of the OVDs from the capsular bag and the anterior chamber of the eye is must after the end of the surgery. This is important to avoid complications such as rise in intraocular pressure, crystallization of the IOL surface (see later).[47] Studies have shown that complete removal of viscoelastic material from the capsular bag can be more difficult when some hydrophobic acrylic lenses are used because of the IOL's tacky surfaces (Apple DJ, Auffarth GU, Pandey SK. Miyake posterior view video analysis of dispersive and cohesive viscoelastics, video presented at the Symposium on Cataract, IOL, and Refractive Surgery, Seattle, WA, April 1999).

COMPLICATIONS OF THE OVDs

OVDs have many positive attributes but their drawbacks and complications must be given careful considerations. Some of the important complications are as follows.

Increase in Intraocular Pressure

Increase in intraocular pressure is the most important postoperative complication of OVDs. It was first noted with Healon®. The increase in pressure can be severe and prolonged, if the material is not thoroughly removed at the end of the surgery. The rise in pressure occurs in the first 6 to 24 hours and resolves spontaneously within 72 hours postoperatively.[2,12] The rise in pressure is due to the mechanical resistance of the trabecular meshwork to the large molecules of the viscoelastic material, which decreases the outflow facility. Hence to decrease the incidence of this complication, many have advocated removing and aspirating the viscoelastic material from the eyes at the end of the surgery.[16]

Crystallization on the IOL Surfaces

Olson *et al*[29] reported a physician survey, laboratory studies, and clinical observations of intraoperative crystallization on IOL surfaces. These authors sent a survey to all ophthalmologists in the states of Wyoming, Idaho, Montana, Utah, and Colorado (USA) asking whether crystallization on the IOL surface had occurred in any of their patients and what viscoelastics, IOLs, and other solutions were used. All returned surveys were tabulated and analyzed by standard statistical means. A sample of crystallization from an IOL submitted by a physician on a glass slide was analyzed to ascertain the relative elemental composition. During *in vitro* laboratory studies, BSS Plus® (Alcon Surgical, Fort Worth, Texas, USA) and BSS® (Alcon Surgical) were analyzed for precipitation. Healon-GV® (Pharmacia/Upjohn, Kalamazoo, Michigan, USA) and calcium chloride were combined in various solutions and examined for precipitate formation. Silicone IOLs were placed in different BSS® and BSS Plus® solutions with different viscoelastics and varying calcium concentrations. In seven patients, prominent crystallization on IOL surfaces was examined, photographed, and followed for up to 3 years. Results of this interesting survey showed that 206 surveyed ophthalmologists returned 181 surveys (88%) and reported 29,609 cataract surgeries with IOL implantation. In 22 eyes (0.07%) (22 patients) intraoperative crystallization was observed on the IOL surface during 1993. The survey indicated there was a correlation with BSS Plus® (chi-square = 4.9, P = .0268) and silicone IOLs (chi-square = 6.8, P = .0093). The analyzed sample submitted by one of the surgeons showed the cation to be calcium. The authors concluded that crystallization on the IOL surface during cataract surgery is a rare occurrence that may be associated with calcium as the cation. An osmotic gradient around the IOL is observed with increased calcium concentration. If encountered surgically, the lens should be exchanged in the operating theater after irrigating the anterior chamber with BSS® and completely filling the capsular bag with a low molecular weight viscoelastic.[18,29]

Since 1993 we received in our Center more than 9,000 IOLs explanted because of different complications. During gross and microscopic analyses of these lenses, it was not uncommon to find crystals on their surfaces, which exhibited some degree of birefringence (Figs 10.8A and B). Sometimes they had the typical fern-like appearance found after precipitation of viscoelastic or salt solutions. We believe those crystals correspond to precipitation of viscoelastic solutions used by the surgeons during the explantation procedure. These may crystallize on the surfaces of the IOLs sent to our Center in a dry state.

Many lenses sent to our Center were explanted because of the presence of crystalline deposits on their optical surfaces. They caused significant decrease in visual function requiring lens esplantation/exchange (Figs 10.8A and B). Our analyses demonstrated that these deposits were also composed of multiple confluent small crystals, which sometimes did not assume a fern-like appearance, but rather an amorphous arrangement.[54] Therefore, it could not be confirmed whether they were related to deposition/crystallization of viscoelastic material. Further studies are necessary to evaluate whether they may correspond to the crystallization of residual viscoelastics in an aqueous environment, late postoperatively. Most specifically, scanning electron microscopy coupled with a surface analysis technique such as energy-dispersive X-ray analysis could determine the elemental composition of the deposits observed on the surfaces of our explanted lenses. These observations highlight the fact that any viscoelastic agent should be thoroughly removed from the capsular bag and anterior chamber of the eye during cataract surgery.

Capsular Block Syndrome or Capsular Bag Distension Syndrome

Miyake and associates[26] proposed a new classification of capsular block syndrome (CBS), a newly described complication of cataract-IOL surgery, to improve understanding of the etiology and provide effective treatment. Three groups of eyes with CBS were reviewed by these authors: eyes originally reported and diagnosed as having CBS; eyes experiencing CBS after hydrodissection and luxation of the lens nucleus; and eyes with CBS accompanying liquefied after-cataract or capsulorhexis related lacteocrumenasia. These researchers noted that in all 3 groups, the CBS occurred in eyes with a capsulorhexis. It was characterized by accumulation of a liquefied substance within a closed chamber inside the capsular bag, formed because the lens nucleus or the posterior chamber IOL optic occluded the anterior capsular opening created by the capsulorhexis. Depending on the time of onset, CBS was classified as intraoperative (CBS seen at the time of lens luxation following hydrodissection), early postoperative (originally described CBS), and late postoperative (CBS with liquefied after-cataract or lacteocrumenasia). The etiology of the accumulated substance and the method of treatment are different in each type according to their study. These authors concluded that CBS is a complication of cataract/IOL surgery that can occur during and after surgery. Correctly identifying the type of CBS is crucial to understand the nature and effective treatment of this disorder.

Recently use of high-density viscoelastic agents, such as Healon-GV®, has been found to be associated with complication of late CBS. Sugiura and associates[49] analyzed the transparent liquid between the posterior lens capsule and the posterior chamber (PC) IOL in early postoperative capsular block syndrome and discussed the mechanism of posterior capsule distention. These authors evaluated 3 cases of capsular block syndrome presenting with transparent liquid in the distended capsular bag 1 day after cataract surgery. The transparent liquid material between the posterior capsule and PC IOL was aspirated and analyzed using high-performance liquid chromatography (HPLC). Also, sodium hyaluronate was diluted using a dialyzer to determine whether the aqueous humor was drawn into the capsular bag by an osmotic gradient across the capsule. Results of their study suggested that the elution time of the samples was almost the same as that of sodium hyaluronate 1.0 percent. The concentration of the samples ranged from 3.29 to 9.01 mg/mL by HPLC analysis. The sodium hyaluronate absorbed the physiological salt solutions through the dialyzer and expanded to 1.9 times its original volume. These results indicate that the main ingredient of the transparent liquid in capsular bags is sodium hyaluronate and that the distention is caused by aqueous humor being drawn into the capsular bag by an osmotic gradient across the capsule when the capsulorhexis diameter is smaller than that of the PC IOL and by viscoelastic material retained and trapped in the bag intraoperatively.

Pseudo-anterior Uveitis

The pseudo-anterior uveitis occurs because of the OVD's viscous nature and also the electrostatic charge of the materials.[28] The red blood corpuscles

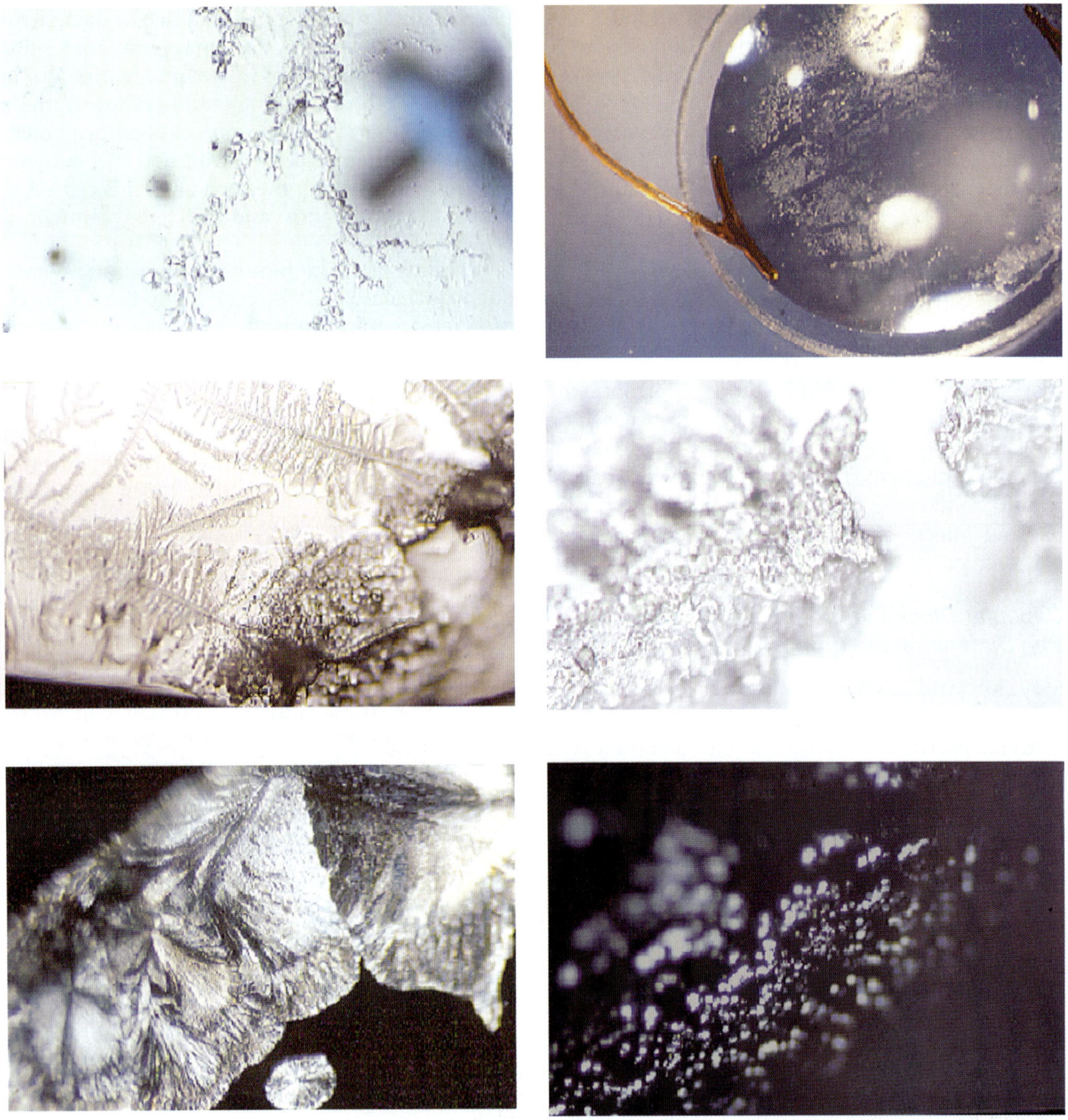

Figs 10.8A and B: Crystallization on the IOL surfaces secondary to precipitation of the OVDs on the surfaces: (A) Light photomicrographs taken from the anterior surface of intraocular lenses, which were explanted because of different complications (including error in power calculation) and sent to our center for analyses. A typical fern-like appearance of the crystals found on the surface of the lenses can be observed. Birefringence under polarized light is observed in the bottom picture, (B) Gross and light microscopic photographs taken from the posterior surface of a 3-piece silicone lens explanted because of opacification of the lens optic caused by a whitish deposit. The crystals found on the surface of the lens do not have a typical fern-like appearance, but exhibit birefringence under polarized light (bottom picture)

(RBCs) and inflammatory cells remain in the anterior chamber, thus giving it the appearance of uveitis. It spontaneously resolves within three days, requiring no treatment. Sometimes an intraocular hemorrhage gets trapped between the vitreous space and the OVD in the anterior chamber and mimics the appearance of vitreous hemorrhage.[28]

SUMMARY AND CONCLUSIONS

The choice of a viscoelastic substance depends largely on the intended surgical use. At the present time, no single viscoelastic agent is ideal under all circumstances. For any particular surgical task, the surgeon should consider the multiple physico-chemical characteristics of each viscoelastic material available as well as their desirable and undesirable clinical effects, then choose the most appropriate substance. As new materials are developed and as our knowledge of the physical properties, clinical effects, and surgical indications are better defined, the selection process for choosing the best product should improve.[20]

Widespread success in clinical situations has been achieved with pure hyaluronate and combination sodium hyaluronate chondroitin sulfate material. Although expensive, viscoadaptive agent-Healon-5®, has some distinct advantages. Methylcellulose posses special advantages of lower cost, no requirement of refrigeration, a larger quantity of the material per unit.

REFERENCES

1. Akahoshi T. Soft shell stain technique for the white cataract, presented at the ASCRS Symposium on Cataract, IOL, and Refractive Surgery, Boston, MA, 2000.
2. Anmarkrud N, Begaust B, Bulie T. A comparison of Healon and Amvisc on the early postoperative pressure after extracapsular cataract extraction with implantation of posterior chamber lens. Acta Ophthalmol Scand. 1996; 74:626-28.
3. Anna Densjo. Healon 5, The world's first Viscoadaptive. Ophthalmic express 1998; 6:4.
4. Arshinoff SA. Rock and roll removal of Healon® GV (video). Presented at the American Society of Cataract and Refractive Surgery Film Festival; Seattle, WA; 1996;1-5.
5. Arshinoff SA, Hofmann I. Prospective, randomized trial comparing Micro Visc Plus and Healon GV in routine phacoemulsification. J Cataract Refract Surg 1998;24:814-20.
6. Arshinoff SA, Opalinski YAV, Ma J. The pharmacology of lens surgery: Ophthalmic viscoelastic agents. In Yanoff M, Ducker JS, Eds, Ophthalmology. St Louis, Mosby-Yearbook, 1998;4:20.1-21.6.
7. Arshinoff SA. Dispersive and cohesive viscoelastics materials in phacoemulsification, Revisited 1998. Ophthalmic Practice 1998;16:24-32.
8. Arshinoff SA. Dispersive–cohesive viscoelastic soft shell technique. J cataract Refract Surg 1999;25:167-73.
9. Arshinoff SA. New terminology: Ophthalmic viscosurgical devices. J Cataract Refract Surg 2000;26:627-28.
10. Balazs EA, Freeman MI, Kloti R, et al. Hyaluronic acid and replacement of vitreous and aqueous humour. Mod Prob Ophthalmol 1972;10:3-21.
11. Balazs EA. The development of sodium hyaluronate (healon) as a viscosurgical material in ophthalmic surgery. In Eisner G, Ed. Ophthalmic Viscosurgery. Bern, Switzerland: Medicopia, 1986:1-19.
12. Barron BA, Busin M, Page C, et al. Comparison of the effects of Viscoat and Healon on postoperative intraocular pressure. Am J Ophthalmol 1985;100:377-84.
13. Cobo M, Beaty N. VITRAX? (sodium hyaluronate) in anterior segment surgery: a review and clinical study summary. Adv Ther 1990; 7:51-60.
14. Garg A. Viscoelastic substances and other surgical adjuncts. In Garg A, Ed., Textbook of Ophthalmology. New Delhi, Jaypee Brothers 2001;126-38.
15. Pandey SK, Werner L, Apple DJ, Agarwal A, Agarwal A, Agarwal S. No anesthesia clear corneal phacoemulsification versus topical and topical plus intracameral anesthesia: Randomized clinical trial. J Cataract Refract Surg 2001;27:1643-50.
16. Holzer MP, Tetz MR, Auffarth GU, Welt R, Volker H. Effects of Healon 5 and 4 other viscoelastic substances on intraocular pressure and endothelium after cataract surgery. J Cataract Refractive Surg 2001;27:213-18.
17. Hyndiuk RA, Schultz RO. Overview of the corneal toxicity of surgical solutions and drugs and clinical concepts in corneal edema. Lens Eye Toxic Res 1992; 9:331-50.
18. Jensen MK, Crandall AS, Mamalis N, Olson RJ. Crystallization on intraocular lens surfaces associated with the use of Healon-GV. Arch Ophthalmol 1994;112:1037-42.
19. Kayikicioglu O, Erakgun T, Guler C. Trypan blue mixed with sodium hyaluronate for capsulorhexis. J Cataract Refract Surg 2001; 27:970.
20. Larson RS, Lindstrom RL, Skelnik DL. Viscoelastic agents. CLAO J 1989;15:151-60.
21. Leaming DV. Practice styles and preferences of ASCRS members–2000 survey. J Cataract Refract Surg 2001; 27:948-55.
22. Liesegang TJ. Viscoelastics. Surv Ophthalmol 1990; 34:268-93.
23. Liesegang TJ. Viscoelastics. Int Ophthalmol Clin 1993; 33:127-47.

24. Macky TA, Werner L, Apple DJ, Izak AM, Pandey SK, Trivedi RH. Viscoanesthesia Part II: Evaluation of the toxicity to ocular structures after phacoemulsification in a rabbit model. J Cataract Refract Surg 2002.
25. McDermott ML, Edelhauser HF. Drug binding of ophthalmic viscoelastic agents. Arch Ophthalmol 1989; 107:261-63.
26. Miyake K, Ota I, Ichihashi S, et al. New classification of capsular block syndrome. J Cataract Refract Surg 1998;24:1230-34.
27. Nahra D, Castilla M, Capsulorhexis in no view cataract: Staining of the anterior capsule with 2 percent fluorescein, presented at the annual meeting of the American Academy of Ophthalmology, Chicago, Illinois,USA, 1996.
28. Nirankari VS, Karesh J, Lakhanpal V. Pseudovitreous hemorrhage: A new introperative complication of sodium hyaluronate. Ophthalmic Surg 1981;12:503-04.
29. Olson RJ, Caldwell AS, Jensen MK, Huang SC. Intraoperative crystallization on the intraocular lens surface. Am J Ophthalmol 1998; 126:177-84.
30. Pandey SK, Ram J, Werner L, Gupta A, Apple DJ. Persistent pupillary membrane. Br J Ophthalmol 2000; 84:554.
31. Pandey SK, Werner L, Apple DJ, et al. Dye-enhanced pediatric cataract surgery. J Pediatr Ophthalmol Strabismus 2002 (in press).
32. Pandey SK, Werner L, Apple DJ, Izak AM, Trivedi RH, Macky TA. Viscoanesthesia Part III: Evaluation of the removal time of viscoelastic/viscoanesthetic solutions from capsular bag of human eyes obtained postmortem. J Cataract Refract Surg 2002 (in press).
33. Pandey SK, Werner L, Apple DJ, et al. Update on dye-enhanced cataract surgery. In Chang DF, ed., Hyperguide Online Textbook of Ophthalmology, Thorofare, NJ, Slack, 2001, (http://www.ophthalmic.hyperguide.com).
34. Pandey SK, Werner L, Apple DJ. Capsular dye-enhanced cataract surgery. In Nema HV, Nema N, eds., Recent Advances in Ophthalmology, Volume 6, Jaypee Brothers, New Delhi, India, 11-29, 2002.
35. Pandey SK, Werner L, Apple DJ. Staining the anterior capsule. J Cataract Refract Surg 2001;27:647-48.
36. Pandey SK, Werner L, Escobar-Gomez M, Roig-Melo EA, Apple DJ. Dye-enhanced cataract surgery. Part I. Anterior capsule staining for capsulorhexis in advanced/white cataracts. J Cataract Refract Surg 2000; 26:1052-59.
37. Pandey SK, Werner L, Escobar-Gomez M, Werner LP, Apple DJ. Dye-enhanced cataract surgery. Part III. Staining of the posterior capsule to learn and perform posterior continuous curvilinear capsulorhexis. J Cataract Refract Surg 2000; 26:1066-71.
38. Poyer JF, Chan KY, Arschin SA. New method to measure the retention of viscoelastic agents on a rabbit corneal endothelial cell line after irrigation and aspiration. J Cataract Refract Surg 1998; 24:84-90.
39. Poyer JF, Chan KY, Arschin SA. Quantitative method to determine the cohesion of viscoelastic agents by dynamic aspiration. J Cataract Refract Surg 1998; 24:1130-35.
40. Ram J, Pandey SK. Anesthesia for cataract surgery. In Dutta LC, ed, Modern Ophthalmology. New Delhi, Jaypee Brothers, 2000;325-30.
41. Ram J, Pandey SK. Indications and contraindications of phacoemulsification. In Dutta LC, Ed., Modern Ophthalmology. New Delhi, Jaypee Brothers, 2000;437-40.
42. Ram J, Pandey SK. Infantile cataract surgery: Current techniques, complications and their management. In Dutta LC, ed., Modern Ophthalmology. New Delhi, Jaypee Brothers, 2000;378-84.
43. Saini JS, Pandey SK. Advances in techniques of penetrating keratoplasty. In Nema HV, Nema N, eds., Recent Advances in Ophthalmology, Volume IV, New Delhi, Jaypee Brothers, 1998;37-51.
44. Silver FH, Librizzi JJ, Benedetto D. Physical properties of model viscoelastic materials. J Appl Biomater. 1994; 5:227-34.
45. Stegmann R,Pienaar A, Miller D.Viscocanalostomy for open angle glaucoma in black African patients. J Cataract Refract Surg 1999;25:316-22.
46. Steinert RF. ICG dye aids in visualization of the anterior capsule. Ophthalmology Times, 1999.
47. Storr-Paulsen A. Analysis of the short-term effect of two viscoelastic agents on the intraocular pressure after extracapsular cataract extraction. Sodium hyaluronate 1% vs hydroxypropyl methylcellulose 2%. Acta Ophthalmol (Copenh) 1993; 71:173-76.
48. Strobel J. Comparison of space maintaining capabilities of Healon and Healon GV during Phacoemulsification. J Cataract Refract Surg 1997;23:1081-84.
49. Sugiura T, Miyauchi S, Eguchi S, et al. Analysis of liquid accumulated in the distended capsular bag in early postoperative capsular block syndrome. J Cataract Refract Surg 2000;26:420-25.
50. Tetz MR, Holzer MP. Healon® 5 clinical performance and special removal technique (Two Compartment Technique). In Viscoelastics in ophthalmic surgery, Eds, Buratto L, Giardini P, Belluci R, Thorofare, NJ, USA, Slack 2000;401-04.
51. Trivedi RH, Werner L, Apple DJ, Izak AM, Pandey SK, Macky TA. Viscoanesthesia Part I: Evaluation of the toxicity to corneal endothelial cells in a rabbit model. J Cataract Refract Surg 2002 (in press).
52. Werner L, Izak AM, Isaacs RT, Pandey SK, Apple DJ. Evolution and pathology of intraocular lens implantation. In Yanoff M, Ducker JS, eds, Ophthalmology. St Louis, Mosby-Yearbook, 2002 (in press).
53. Werner L, Pandey SK, Escobar-Gomez M, Hoddinott DSM, Apple DJ. Dye-enhanced cataract surgery. Part II.

An experimental study to learn and perform critical steps of phacoemulsification in human eyes obtained post-mortem. J Cataract Refract Surg 2000; 26:1060-65.

54. Werner L, Shugar JK, Apple DJ, Pandey SK, Escobar-Gomez M, Visessook N, Evans BB. Opacification of piggyback IOLs associated to an amorphous material attached to interlenticular surfaces. J Cataract Refract Surg 2000;26:1612-19.

55. Wilson ME, Trivedi RH, Apple DJ, Batholomew L, Werner L, Pandey SK. Ophthalmic viscosurgical agents (OVAs): A guide for the pediatric cataract surgeons. J Cataract Refract Surg 2002.

56. Wilson ME, Pandey SK, ThakurJ. Pediatric cataract surgery in the developing world. Br J Ophthalmol 2002.

57. Wilson ME, Pandey SK, Werner L, Ram J, Apple DJ. Pediatric Cataract Surgery: Current Techniques, Complications and Management. In Agarwal S, Agarwal A, Sachdev MS, Mehta KR, Fine H, Agarwal A, eds., Phacoemulsification, Laser Cataract Surgery and Foldable IOLs. New Delhi, Jaypee Brothers Medical Publishers, 2000;369-88.

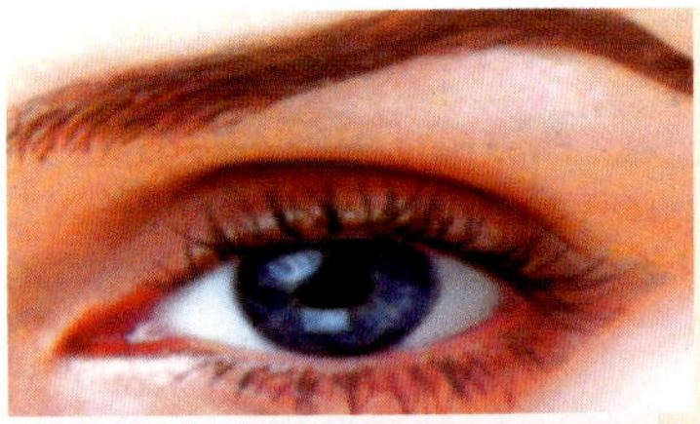

Eleven

Athiya Agarwal
Sunita Agarwal
Amar Agarwal
Ashok Garg
Nilesh Kanjani (India)

Corneal Topography in Cataract Surgery

INTRODUCTION

Topography is defined as the science of describing or representing the features of a particular place in detail. In corneal topography, the place is the cornea, i.e. we describe the features of the cornea in detail.

The word Topography is derived[1,2] from two Greek words:

TOPOS- meaning place
and
GRAPHIEN- meaning to write.

CORNEA

There are basically three refractive elements of the eye, namely: axial length, lens and cornea. The cornea is the most important plane or tissue for refraction. This is because it has the highest refractive power (which is about + 45 D) and it is easily accessible to the surgeon without going inside the eye.

To understand the cornea, one should realize that the cornea is a parabolic curve – its radius of curvature differs from center to periphery. It is steepest in the center and flatter in the periphery. For all practical purposes the central cornea, that is the optical zone is taken into consideration, when you are doing a refractive surgery. A flatter cornea has less refraction power and a steeper cornea has a higher refraction power. If we want to change the refraction we must make the steeper diameter flatter and the flatter diameter steeper.

KERATOMETRY

The keratometer was invented by Hermann Von Helmholtz and modified by Javal, Schiotz, etc. If we place an object in front of a convex mirror we get a virtual, erect and minified image (Fig. 11.1). A keratometer in relation to the cornea is just like an object in front of a convex reflecting mirror. Like in a convex reflecting surface, the image is located posterior to the cornea. The cornea behaves as a convex reflecting mirror and the mires of the keratometer are the objects. The radius of curvature of the cornea's anterior surface determines the size of the image.

The keratometer projects a single mire on the cornea and the separation of the two points on the mire is used to determine corneal curvature. The zone measured depends upon corneal curvature — the steeper the cornea, the smaller the zone. For example, for a 36-D cornea, the keratometer measures a 4 mm zone and for a 50-D cornea, the size of the cone is 2.88 mm.

Keratometers are accurate only when the corneal surface is a sphere or a spherocylinder. Actually, the shape of the anterior surface of the cornea is more than a sphere or a spherocylinder. But keratometers measure the central 3 mm of the cornea,

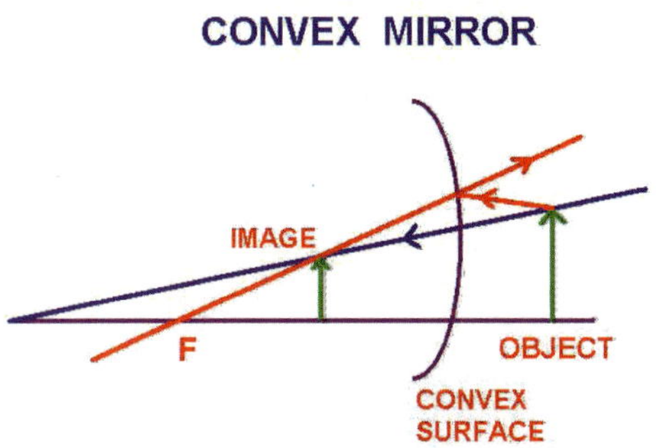

Fig. 11.1: Physics of a convex mirror. Note the image is virtual, erect and minified. The cornea acts like the convex mirror and the mire of the keratometer is the object

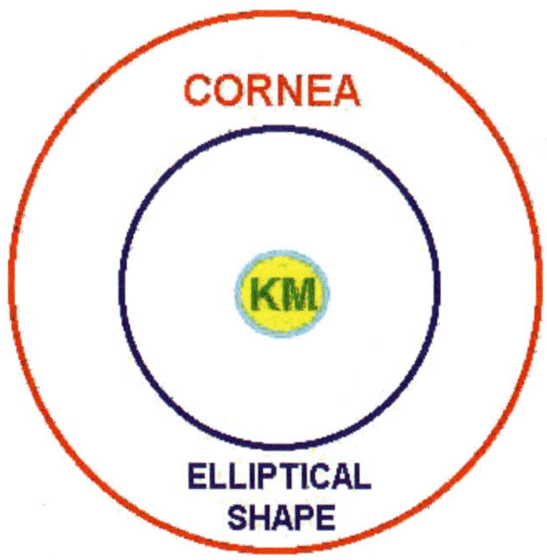

Fig. 11.2: Keratometers measure the central 3 mm of the cornea, which generally behaves like a sphere or a spherocylinder. This is the reason why keratometers are generally accurate. But in complex situations like in keratoconus or refractive surgery they become inaccurate

which behaves like a sphere or a spherocylinder. This is the reason why Helmholtz could manage with the keratometer (Fig. 11.2). This is also the reason why most ophthalmologists can manage management of cataract surgery with the keratometer. But today, with refractive surgery, the ball game has changed. This is because when the cornea has complex central curves like in keratoconus or after refractive surgery, the keratometer cannot give good results and becomes inaccurate. Thus, the advantages of the keratometer like speed, ease of use, low cost and minimum maintenance is obscured.

The objects used in the keratometer are referred to as mires. Separation of two points on the mire are used to determine corneal curvature. The object in the keratometer can be rotated with respect to the axis. The disadvantages of the keratometer are that they measure only a small region of the cornea. The peripheral regions are ignored. They also lose accuracy when measuring very steep or flat corneas. As the keratometer assumes the cornea to be symmetrical it becomes at a disadvantage if the cornea is asymmetrical as after refractive surgery.

KERATOSCOPY

To solve the problem of keratometers, scientists worked on a system called Keratoscopy. In this, they projected a beam of concentric rings and observed them over a wide expanse of the corneal surface. But this was not enough and the next step was to move into computerized videokeratography.

COMPUTERIZEDVIDEOKERATOGRAPHY

In this some form of light like a placido disk is projected onto the cornea. The cornea modifies this light and this modification is captured by a video camera. This information is analyzed by computer software and the data is then displayed in a variety of formats. To simplify the results to an ophthalmologist, Klyce in 1988 started the corneal color maps. The corneal color maps display the estimate of corneal shape in a fashion that is understandable to the ophthalmologist. Each color on the map is assigned a defined range of measurement. The placido type topographic machines (Fig. 11.3) do not assess the posterior surface of the cornea. The details of the corneal assessment can be done only with the Orbscan (Bausch and Lomb) as both anterior and posterior surface of the cornea are assessed.

ORBSCAN

The orbscan (Bausch and Lomb) corneal topography system (Fig. 11.4) uses a scanning optical slit scan that is fundamentally different than the corneal topography that analyses the reflected images from the anterior corneal surface. The high-resolution video camera captures 40 light slits at 45 degrees angle projected through the cornea similarly as seen during slit lamp examination. The slits are projected on to the anterior segment of the eye: the anterior cornea, the posterior cornea, the anterior iris and anterior lens. The data collected from these four surfaces are used to create a topographic map.

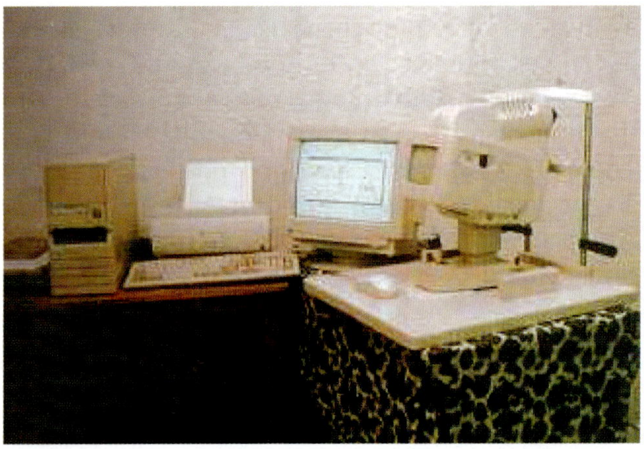

Fig. 11.3: Placido type corneal topography machine

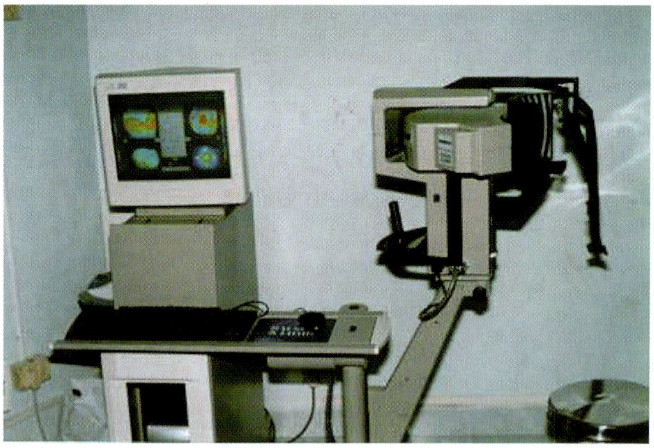

Fig. 11.4: Orbscan

NORMAL CORNEA

In a normal cornea (Fig. 11.5), the nasal cornea is flatter than the temporal cornea. This is similar to the curvature of the long end of an ellipse. If we see Figure 11.5 then we will notice the values written on the right end of the pictures. These indicate the astigmatic values. In that is written Max K is 45 @ 84 degrees and Min K is 44 @ 174 degrees. This means the astigmatism is + 1.0 D at 84 degrees. This is with the rule astigmatism as the astigmatism is plus at 90 degrees axis. If the astigmatism was

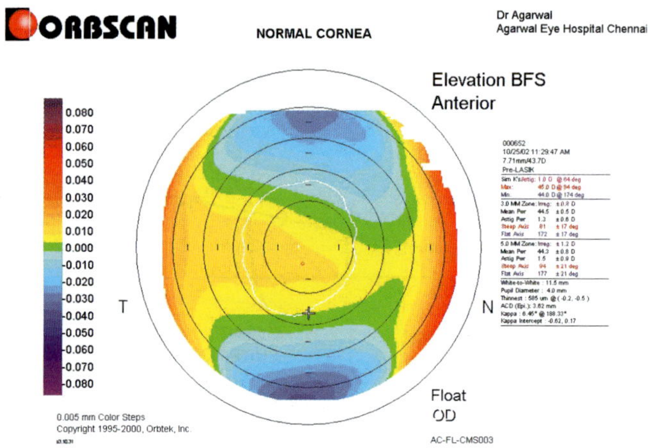

Fig. 11.5: Topography of a normal cornea

plus at 180 degrees then it is against the rule astigmatism. The normal corneal topography can be round, oval, irregular, symmetric bow tie or asymmetric bow tie in appearance. If we see Figure 11.6 we will see a case of astigmatism in which the astigmatism is + 4.9 D at 146 degrees. *These figures show the curvature of the anterior surface of the cornea. It is important to remember that these are not the keratometric maps. So the blue/green color denote steepening and the red colors denote flattening.* If we want the red to denote steepening then we can invert the colors.

CATARACT SURGERY

Corneal topography is extremely important in cataract surgery. *The smaller the size of the incision lesser the astigmatism and earlier stability of the astigmatism will occur.* One can reduce the astigmatism or increase the astigmatism of a patient after cataract surgery. The simple rule to follow is that- *wherever you make an incision that area will flatten and wherever you apply sutures that area will steepen.*

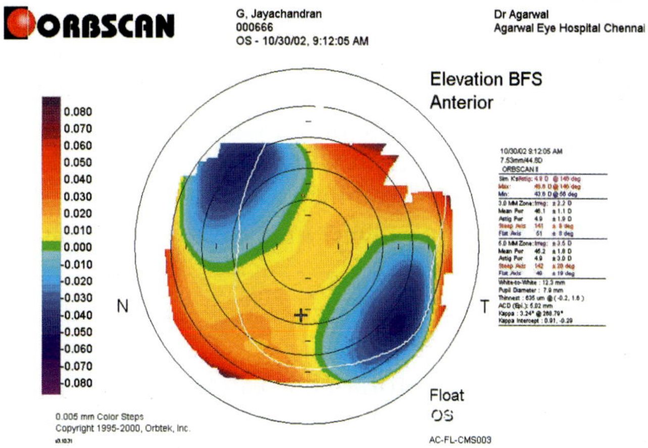

Fig. 11.6: Topography showing an astigmatic cornea

EXTRACAPSULAR CATARACT EXTRACTION

One of the problems in extracapsular cataract extraction is the astigmatism which is created as the incision size is about 10-12 mm. In Figure 11.7, you can see the topographic picture of a patient after extracapsular cataract extraction (ECCE). You can see the picture on the left is the preoperative photo and the picture on the right is a postoperative

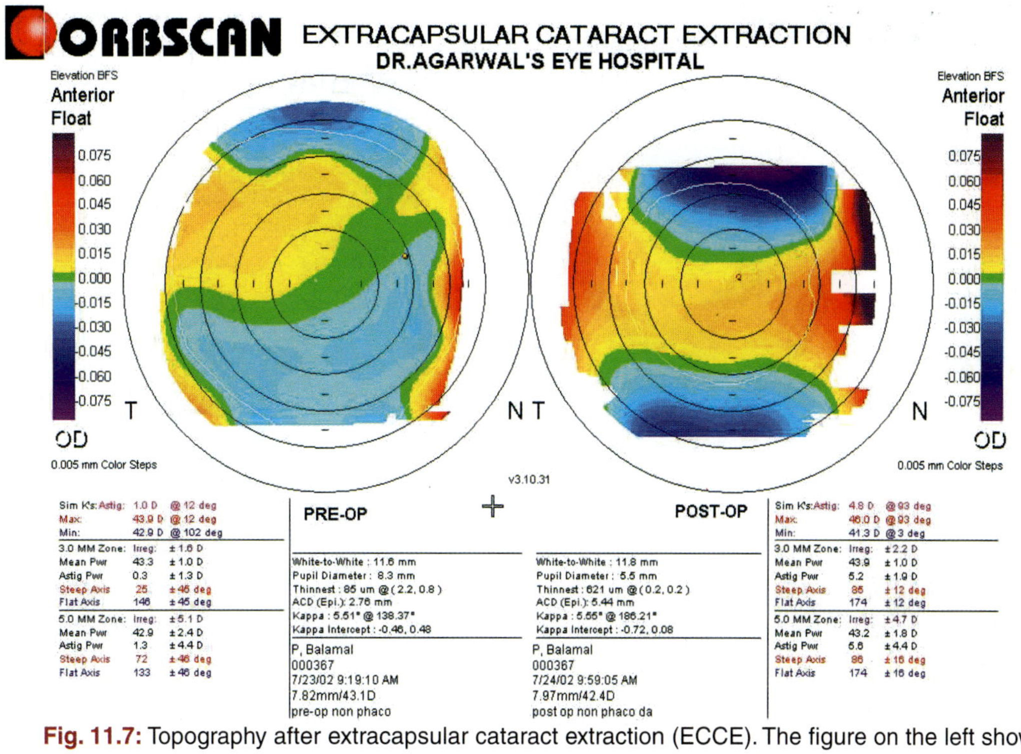

Fig. 11.7: Topography after extracapsular cataract extraction (ECCE). The figure on the left shows astigmatism of + 1.1 D at 12 degrees preoperatively. The astigmatism has increased to + 4.8 D as seen in the figure on the right

day 1 photo. Preoperatively one will notice the astigmatism is + 1.0 D at 12 degrees and postoperatively it is + 4.8 D at 93 degrees. This is the problem in ECCE. In the immediate postoperative period the astigmatism is high which would reduce with time. But the predictability of astigmatism is not there which is why smaller incision cataract surgery is more successful.

NON-FOLDABLE IOL

Some surgeons perform phaco and implant a non-foldable IOL in which the incision is increased to 5.5 to 6 mm. In such cases the astigmatism is better than in an ECCE. In Figure 11.8, the pictures are of a patient who has had a non-foldable IOL. Notice in this the preoperative astigmatism is + 0.8 D @ 166 degrees. This is the left eye of the patient. If we had done a phaco with a foldable IOL the astigmatism would have been nearly the same or reduced as our incision would have come in the area of the astigmatism. But in this case after a phaco a non-foldable IOL was implanted. The postoperative astigmatism one week postoperative is + 1.8 D @ 115 degrees. You can notice from the two pictures the astigmatism has increased.

FOLDABLE IOL

In phaco with a foldable IOL the amount of astigmatism created is much less than in a non-foldable IOL. Let us look now at Figure 11.9. The patient as you can see has negligible astigmatism in the left eye. The picture on the left shows a preoperative astigmatism of + 0.8 D at 166 degrees axis. Now, we operate generally with a temporal clear corneal approach, so in the left eye, the incision will be generally at the area of the steepend axis. This will reduce the astigmatism. If we see the postoperative photo of day one we will see the astigmatism is only + 0.6 D @ 126 degrees. This means that after a day, the astigmatism has not changed much and this shows a good result. This patient had a foldable IOL implanted under the no anesthesia cataract surgical technique after a phaco cataract surgery with the size of the incision being 2.8 mm.

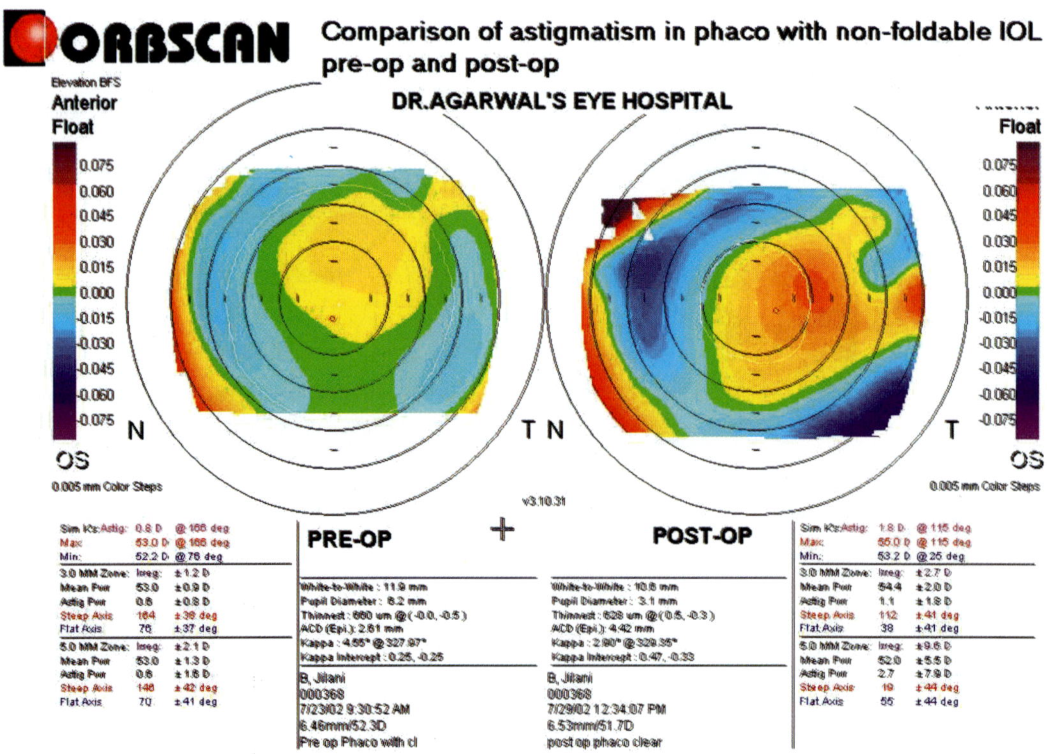

Fig. 11.8: Topography of a non-foldable IOL implantation

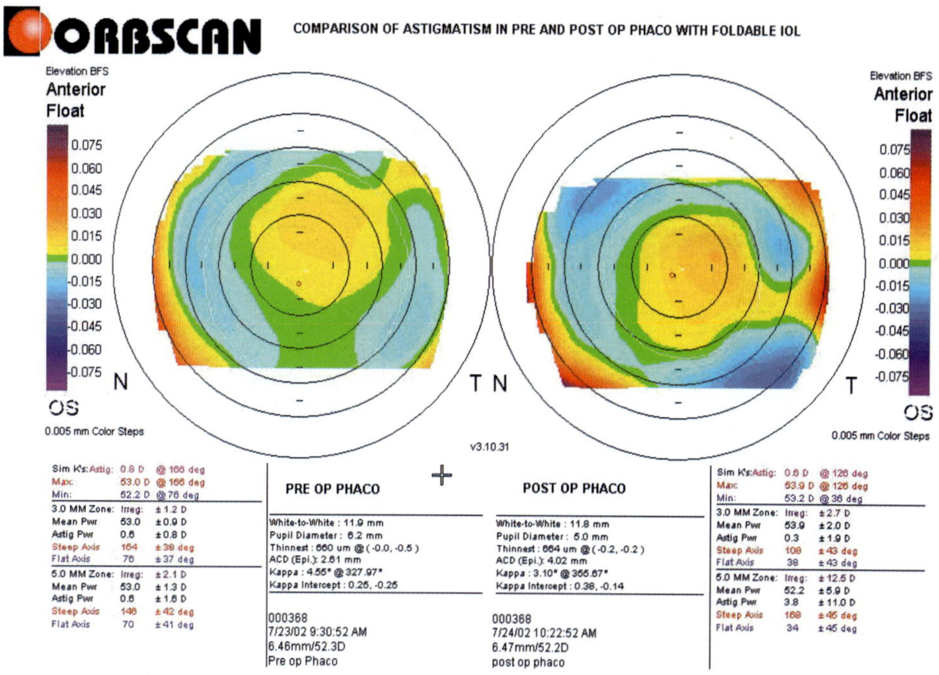

Fig. 11.9: Topography of phaco cataract surgery with a foldable IOL implantation

ASTIGMATISM INCREASED

If we are not careful in selecting the incision depending upon the corneal topography we can burn our hands. Figure 11.10, illustrates a case in which astigmatism has increased due to the incision being made in the wrong meridian. The patient had a 2.8 mm incision with a foldable IOL implanted after a phaco cataract surgery under the no anesthesia cataract surgical technique. Both the pictures are of the right eye. In Figure 11.10, look at the picture on the left. In the picture on the left, you can see the patient has an astigmatism of + 1.1 D at axis 107 degrees. As this is the right eye with this astigmatism we should have made a superior incision to reduce the pre-operative astigmatism. But by mistake we made a temporal clear corneal incision. This has increased the astigmatism. Now if we wanted to flatten this case, we should have made the incision where the steeper meridian was. That was at the 105 degrees axis. But because we were doing routinely temporal clear corneal incisions, we made the incision in the opposite axis. Now look at the picture on the right. The astigmatism has increased from + 1.1 D to + 1.7 D. This shows a bad result. If we had made the incision superiorly at the 107 degrees axis, we would have flattened that axis and the astigmatism would have been reduced.

BASIC RULE

The basic rule to follow is to look at the number written in red. The red numbers indicate the plus axis. If the difference in astigmatism is say 3 D at 180 degrees, it means the patient has + 3 D astigmatism at axis 180 degrees. This is against the rule astigmatism. In such cases, make your clear corneal incision at 180 degrees so that you can flatten this steepness. This will reduce the astigmatism.

UNIQUE CASE

In Figure 11.11, the patient had a temporal clear corneal incision for phaco cataract surgery under no anesthesia with a non-foldable IOL. Both the pictures are of the left eye. The figure on the left shows the postoperative topographic picture. The postoperative astigmatism was + 1.8 D at axis 115 degrees. This patient had three sutures in the site of the incision. These sutures were put as a

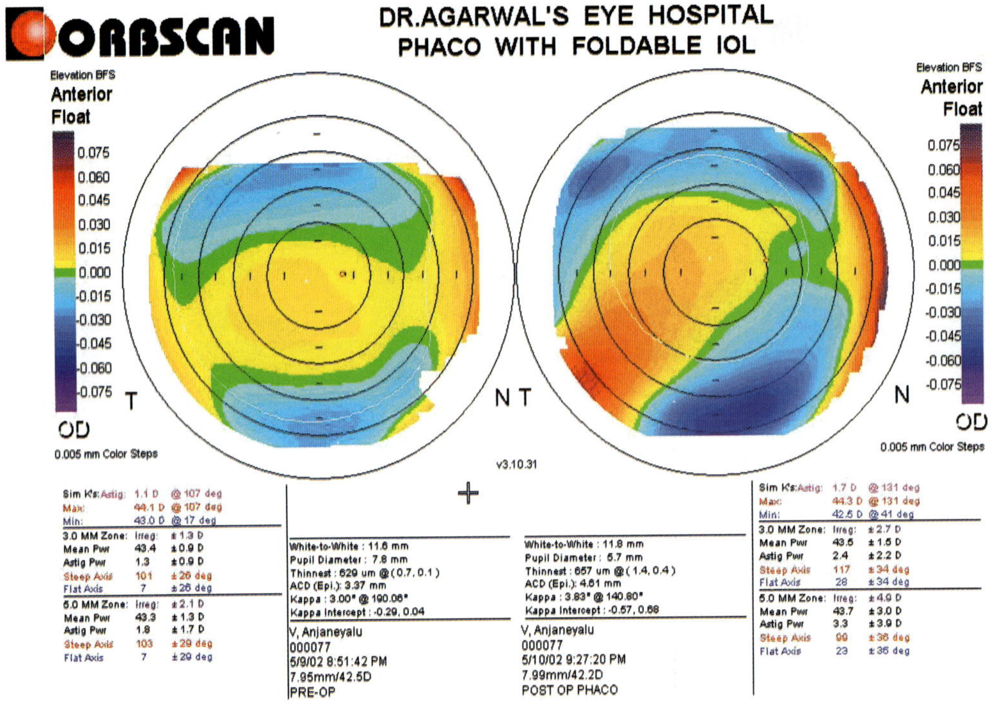

Fig. 11.10: Increase in astigmatism after cataract surgery due to incision being made in the wrong meridian. Topography of a phaco with foldable IOL implantation

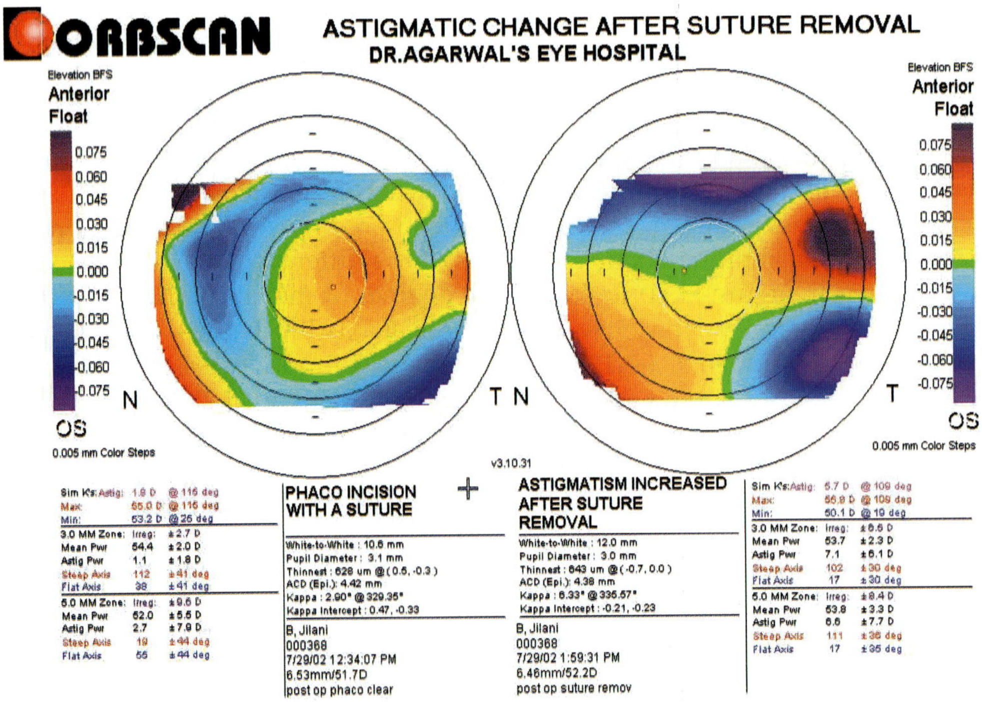

Fig. 11.11: Unique case- Topographic changes after suture removal

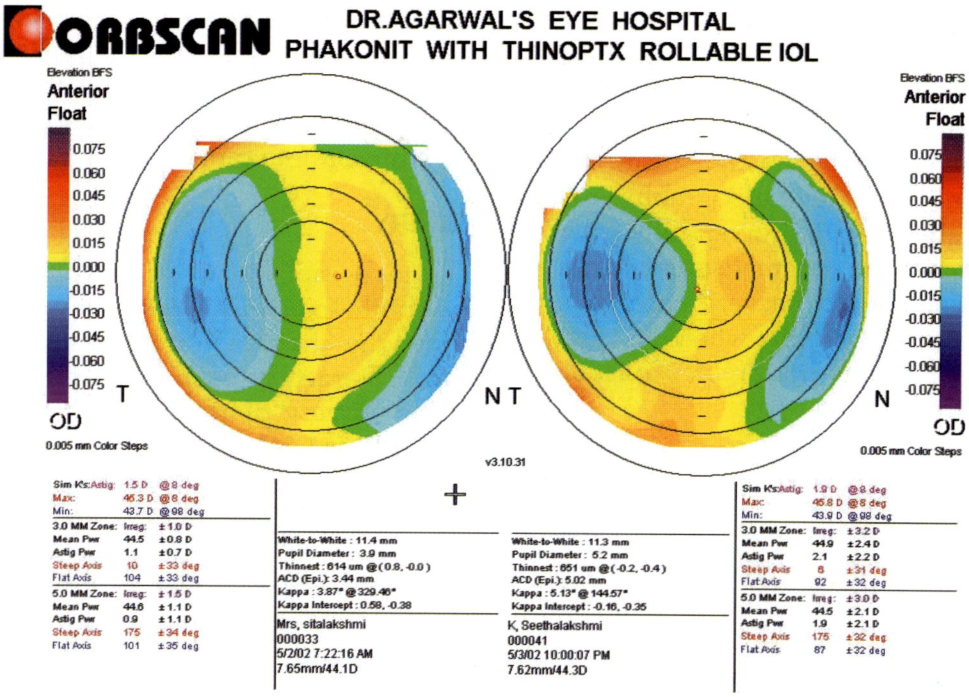

Fig. 11.12: Topography of a Phakonit with a rollable IOL

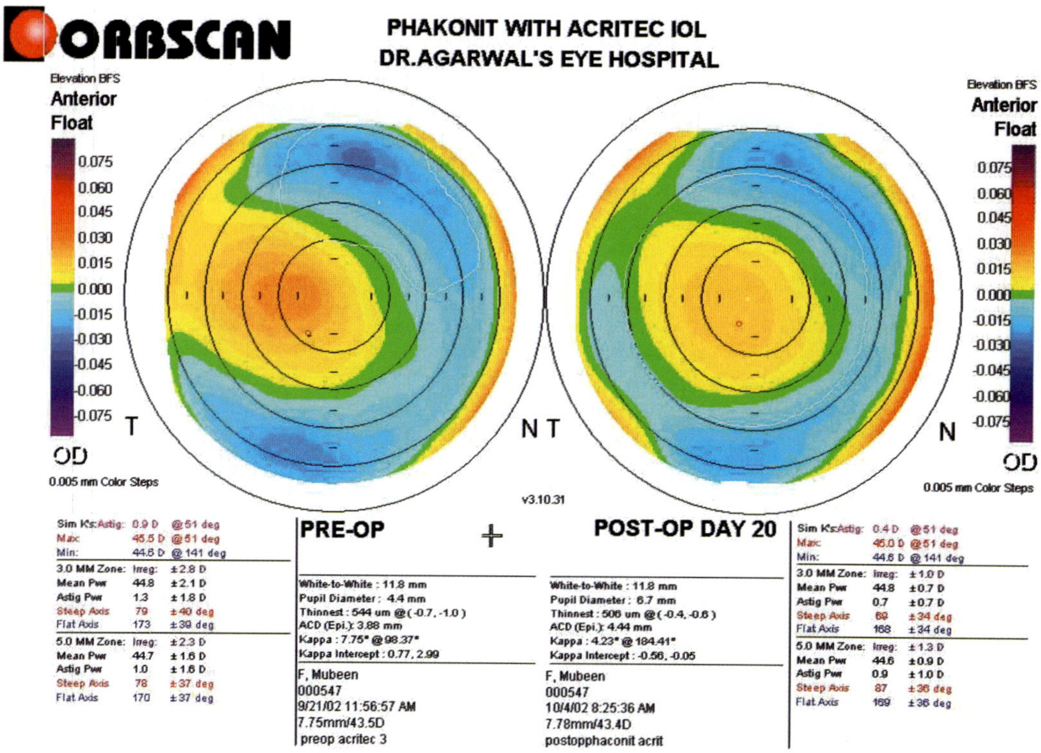

Fig. 11.13: Topography of a Phakonit with an Acritec IOL

nonfoldable IOL had been implanted in the eye with a clear corneal incision. When this patient came for a follow up we removed the sutures. The next day the patient came to us with loss of vision. On examination, we found the astigmatism had increased. We then took another topography. The picture on the right is of the topography after removing the sutures. The astigmatism increased to + 5.7 D. So, one should be very careful in analyzing the corneal topography when one does suture removal also. To solve this problem one can do an astigmatic keratotomy.

PHAKONIT

Phakonit is a technique devised by Dr Amar Agarwal in which the cataract is removed through a 0.9 mm incision. The advantage of this is obvious. The astigmatism created by a 0.9 mm incision is very little compared to a 2.6 mm phaco incision. Today with the rollable IOL and the Acritec IOL's which are ultra-small incision IOL's one can pass IOL's through sub 1.4 mm incisions. This is seen clearly in Figures 11.12 and 11.13. Figure 11.12 shows the comparison after Phakonit with a rollable IOL and Figure 11.13 with an Acritec IOL. If you will see the preoperative and the postoperative photographs in comparison you will see there is not much difference between the two. In this case a rollable IOL was implanted. The point which we will notice in this picture is that the difference between the preoperative photo and the one day postoperative photo is not much.

SUMMARY

Corneal topography is an extremely important tool for the ophthalmologist. It is not only the refractive surgeon who should utilize this instrument but also the cataract surgeon. The most important refractive surgery done in the world is cataract surgery and not Lasik (Laser-in-situ keratomileusis) or PRK (Photorefractive keratectomy). With more advancements in corneal topography, Topographic-Assisted Lasik will become available to everyone with an Excimer Laser. One might also have the corneal topographic machine fixed onto the operating microscope so that one can easily reduce the astigmatism of the patient.

REFERENCES

1. Gills JP et al: Corneal topography: The State–of-the Art. New Delhi: Jaypee Brothers, 1996.
2. Sunita Agarwal, Athiya Agarwal, Mahipal S Sachdev, Keiki R Mehta, I Howard Fine, Amar Agarwal: Phacoemulsification, Laser Cataract Surgery and Foldable IOL's (2nd Edn). New Delhi: Jaypee Brothers, 2000.

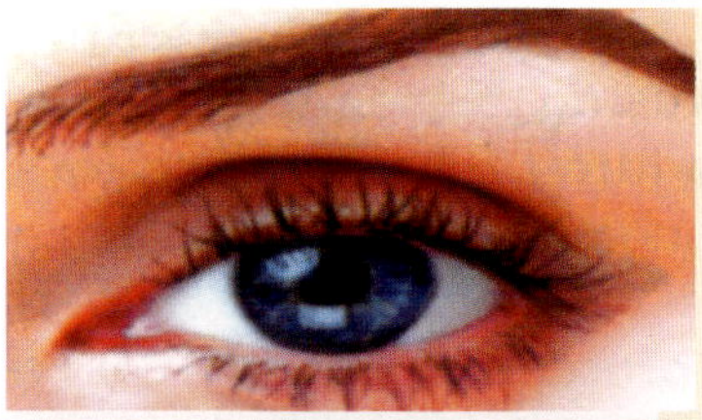

Twelve

Capsular Dye Enhanced Cataract Surgery

Suresh K Pandey
Liliana Werner
David J Apple (USA)
Ashok Garg (India)

INTRODUCTION
OPHTHALMIC DYES FOR ANTERIOR CAPSULORHEXIS
OPHTHALMIC DYES FOR PHACOEMULSIFICATION
OPHTHALMIC DYES FOR POSTERIOR CAPSULORHEXIS
OPHTHALMIC DYES FOR PEDIATRIC CATARACT SURGERY

INTRODUCTION

Various non-toxic ophthalmic dyes have been extensively used as diagnostic agents for the detection and management of different ocular disorders. Table 12.1 summarizes the use of various dyes in ophthalmology. Dyes such as fluorescein sodium, indocyanine green (ICG), have a long history of safety in humans.[1] There have been an increasing number of reports of enhanced visualization by staining intraocular tissues during cataract surgery and vitreoretinal surgery.[2-19] Staining of the ocular tissue by using the ophthalmic dyes makes visual differentiation and manipulation of tissues easier. Enhanced viewing of the ocular tissues can promote a surgeon's ability to evaluate clinical structural relationships and may help attain surgical objectives with fewer complications.[2-19]

Small incision cataract surgery using phacoemulsification has currently evolved into one of the most successful surgical techniques in ophthalmology and the visual sciences. Many modifications such as continuous curvilinear capsulorhexis (CCC),[20,21] hydrodissection,[22-25] hydrodelineation,[26] and various maneuvers for nuclear emulsification and cortical clean-up have been added to it, increasing its safety and efficacy. Posterior capsulorhexis,

Table 12.1: Use of dyes in ophthalmology

Segment	*Structure stained*	*Use*	*Dye*
Anterior segment			
	Cornea	Epithelial defects	FS*
		Contact lens fitting	FS
		Seidel's test	FS
		Dry eye	FS, RB**
		Diagnosis of keratitis	FS, RB
		Endothelial cell count	TB***
	Iris	Neovascularization	FS, ICG****
	Lens	Capsulorhexis (poor or no red reflex)	FS, ICG, TB
		Dye-enhanced cataract surgery	ICG, TB
Posterior segment			
	Retina	Angiography	FS, ICG
	Vitreous	Vitrectomy	FS, ICG
	Vitreoretinal surgery	IRM***** peeling	ICG

*:FS = Fluorescein sodium;**:RB = Rose Bengal;***:TB = Trypan blue; ****:ICG = Indocyanine green; *****:IRM = Internal limiting membrane

a technically challenging procedure, has also been recommended for delaying opacification of posterior capsule in pediatric cataracts and for managing the posterior capsule tears by several surgeons.[27-31]

We have extensively studied the use of non-toxic ophthalmic dyes (fluorescein sodium, ICG and trypan blue) to enhance visualization of various intraocular tissues while performing various critical steps of modern phacoemulsification procedure[7-9,12-14] (Pandey SK, Werner L, Escobar-Gomez M, Apple DJ. Anterior capsule staining in advanced cataracts: A laboratory study using postmortem human eyes; presented at the joint meeting of American Academy of Ophthalmology, Orlando, Florida, October 1999; Pandey SK, Werner L, Apple DJ, *et al.* Dye-enhanced cataract surgery in human eyes obtained postmortem: A laboratory study to learn critical steps of phacoemulsification: XVIIth Congress of the European Society of Cataract and Refractive Surgery, second prize: "Scientific Category," Vienna, Austria, September 1999). In this chapter we will address the use of non-toxic ophthalmic dyes to successfully stain the intraocular tissues during various steps of modern phacoemulsification procedure. For the convenience of readers, we have divided this chapter in 4 sections, adressing their use in adult and pediatric cataract surgery. To provide a brief detail to our readers, in Section 1, we will discuss the use of ophthalmic dyes to stain the anterior capsule while performing CCC in advanced/white cataracts. In Section 2, we will focus on the use of ophthalmic dyes to help enhance visualization to learn the critical steps of phacoemulsification surgery, which include: CCC, hydrodissection/hydrodelineation, nuclear emulsification, and cortical clean-up. In Section 3, we will address the use of ophthalmic dyes for posterior capsule staining to learn and perform technically challenging procedure of posterior capsulorhexis. Finally, in Section 4, we will focus on the use of ophthalmic dyes for pediatric cataract surgery.

OPHTHALMIC DYES FOR ANTERIOR CAPSULORHEXIS

Introduction

Cataract surgeons agree that an anterior CCC should be the goal of every opening of the anterior capsule. CCC has gained widespread popularity because it offers unquestionable advantages over other capsulotomy techniques.[20,21] Because of complications such as intraocular lens (IOL) asymmetrical fixation, decentration, or pea podding of the IOL haptics associated with the envelope or the can-opener capsulotomy techniques, CCC is preferred in PE or planned extracapsular cataract extraction.[20,21,32]

Capsulorhexis in Absence of Red Reflex

In today's clinical practice, white, mature and hypermature cataracts are still commonly seen, especially in the developing world (Figs 12.1A to C).[33] It is difficult to perform a CCC in the presence of mature cataracts because the red reflex, which is necessary to observe the actual tearing process, is

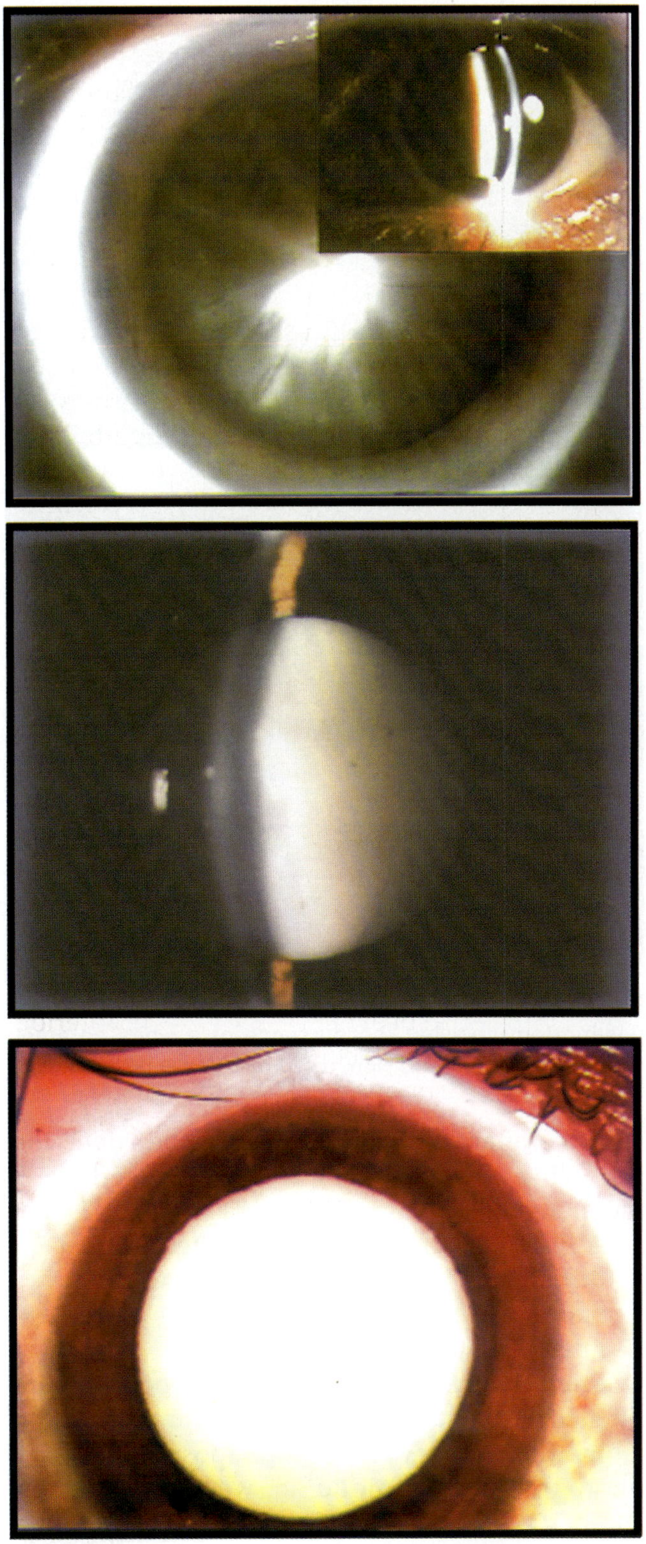

Figs 12.1A to C: Slit-lamp photographs showing 3 examples of advanced/white cataracts. (*Courtesy:* Abhay R Vasavada, MD, FRCS, Ahmedabad, India)

absent. With poor visibility, errant capsular tearing is very common and difficult to control, thus jeopardizing in-the-bag IOL implantation. The accepted recommendations to aid CCC in such cases are: dimming the operating room lights, increasing the operating microscope magnification and coaxial illumination, and using high-density viscoelastics. The use of air,[34] diathermy,[35] endoilluminator,[2] vitrectome, scissors,[36] and the two-stage CCC approach[33,37] have also been suggested.

Use of Ophthalmic Dyes in CCC

Ophthalmic dyes such as 2 percent fluorescein sodium, 0.5 percent ICG,[5,7,10] and 0.1 percent trypan blue[6,7,11,15] have been successfully used for staining the anterior capsule, for performing CCC. Two main surgical techniques have been used for fluorescein sodium: (a) staining from above, under an air bubble, and (b) intracameral subcapsular injection.[3,4] Use of 0.001 percent to 0.01 percent and gentian violet solutions and also 0.05 percent to 0.25 percent crystal violet solution have also been recently reported for staining the anterior capsule in animal models (albinos rats and rabbits respectively).[16,17] Gentian violet and crystal violet dyes are not preferred in human eyes due to adverse corneal effects and possible endothelial cell toxicity.

Study Comparing 3 Ophthalmic Dyes and 2 Surgical Techniques

We have evaluated in an experimental closed-system surgery, anterior capsule staining for performing CCC in postmortem human eyes with advanced / white cataracts, using 3 dyes.[7] These are fluorescein sodium, ICG, and trypan blue; and all have been clinically advocated for use with this procedure. We also compared the two commonly used methods of staining under an air bubble, and intracameral subcapsular injection (Pandey SK, Werner L, Apple DJ. ICG staining reduces your risk, compare three dyes. In *Clinical Update: Cataract. EyeNet* 2000; 4:25-26).[7]

Preparation of the Ophthalmic Dyes

A 2 percent fluorescein sodium solution was prepared by mixing 1 mL of 10 percent fluorescein for intravenous use (Alcon Ophthalmic, Fort Worth, TX, USA) with 4 mL of balanced salt solution (BSS®). ICG solution (Akorn, Inc., Buffalo Grove, IL, USA) was prepared by dissolving 25 mg of ICG in 0.5 mL of an aqueous solvent (provided with the ICG), which was mixed in 4.5 mL of an irrigating solution (BSS plus®, Alcon Ophthalmic, Fort Worth, TX, USA).[5] To obtain 0.1 percent trypan blue, we mixed 1 mL of a 0.4 percent solution (Life Technologies, Grand Island, NY, USA) in 3 mL of BSS®.

Surgical Technique

Randomly accessioned postmortem human eyes (n = 12) received within 4 days of death in the Center for Research on Ocular Therapeutics and Biodevices from Eye Banks nationwide, were used in this study. We only used eyes presenting advanced/white cataracts (Figs 12.2A and B). They were immersed in dextran solution for 30 minutes and prepared according to the technique of Auffarth *et al.*[38] After the eye was fixed in the training head, a self-sealing corneoscleral tunnel incision approximately 3.2 mm wide was made. The iris was pulled out from its attachment to allow better visualization of the anterior capsule. Two different techniques were used for the capsular staining. Initially in 6 globes, air was carefully injected using a 27 gauge cannula and a 2.0 cc syringe. Then, the dye was injected over the anterior capsule (0.10 ml) within the air bubble (2 globes/dye). After a few seconds, the air bubble was replaced with sodium hyaluronate (Healon®, Pharmacia Inc., Peapack, NJ, USA), and CCC was then performed (Figs 12.3A to E).

Alternatively, in the other 6 globes, we used the technique of intracameral subcapsular injection (Figs 12.4A to D and 12.5A and B). After the aqueous was replaced with Healon®, we carefully injected 0.05-0.10 mL of the dye beneath the anterior capsule (2 globes/dye) using a 30 gauge needle. A small leakage of dye from the subcapsular space was observed during this step. After the stained viscoelastic was replaced by clear Healon®, the point of injection was used for beginning the CCC with Utrata's forceps. Blue light enhancement was used during CCC for fluorescein sodium.

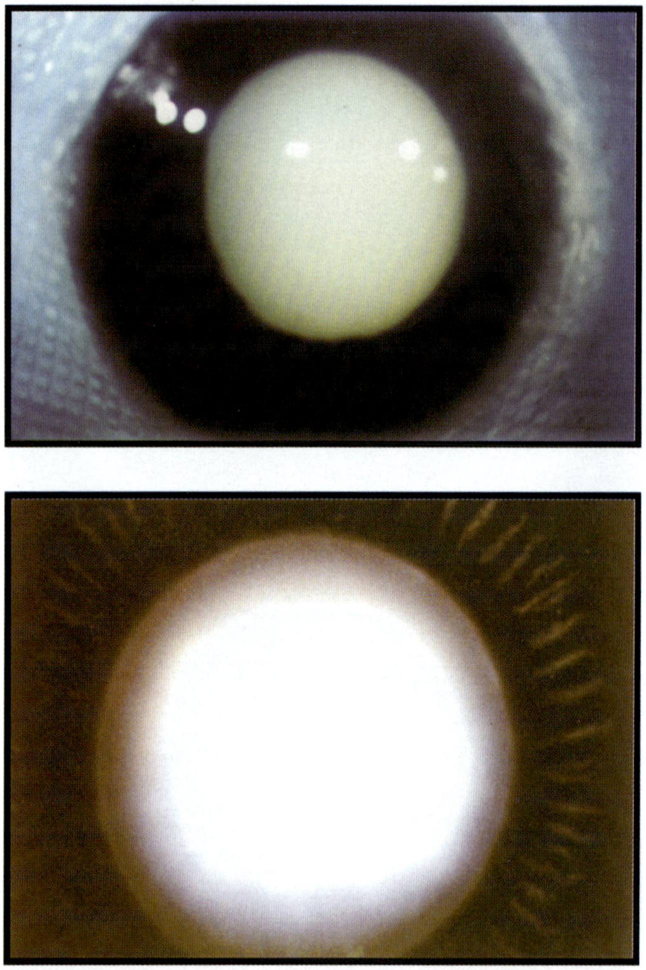

Figs 12.2A and B: Gross photographs of human eyes obtained postmortem showing the presence of a white cataract: (A) Anterior (surgeon's) view, (B) Miyake-Apple posterior view

To compare the 2 techniques and the 3 dyes, the following 2 parameters were evaluated by 2 independent surgeons (SKP, LW):

a. Ability to perform the staining technique (+ = difficult; ++ = intermediate; +++ = easy),
b. Staining of the anterior capsule (+ = faint; ++ = intermediate; +++ = good).

Photographs were taken using a Topcon camera fitted to the operating microscope, with and without a blue filter. The Miyake-Apple posterior video/photographic technique[39,40] was also used in another 3 globes to document any dye leakage into the vitreous cavity (1 globe/dye). We performed the staining of the anterior capsule under an air

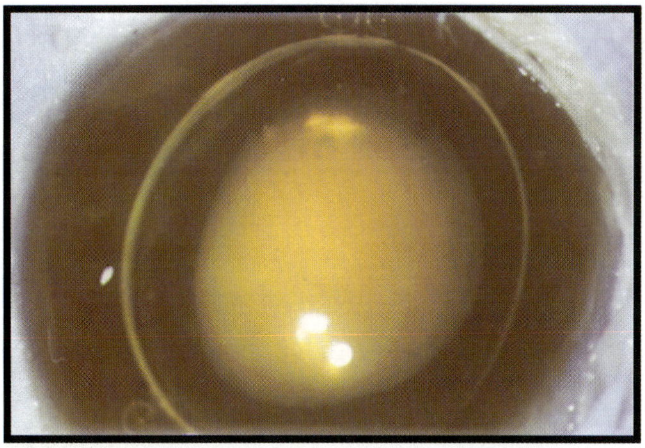

A. Fluorescein sodium

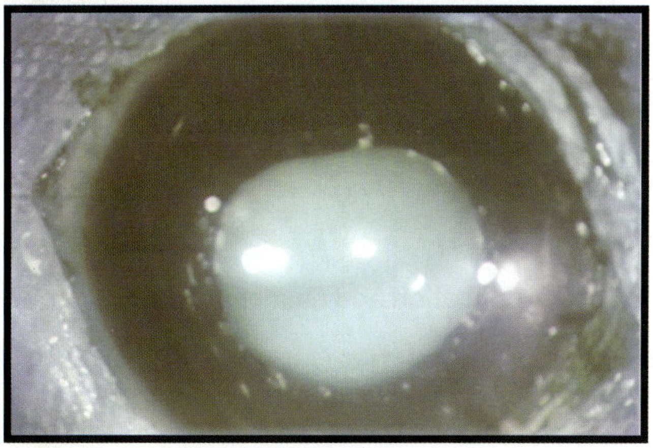

B. ICG

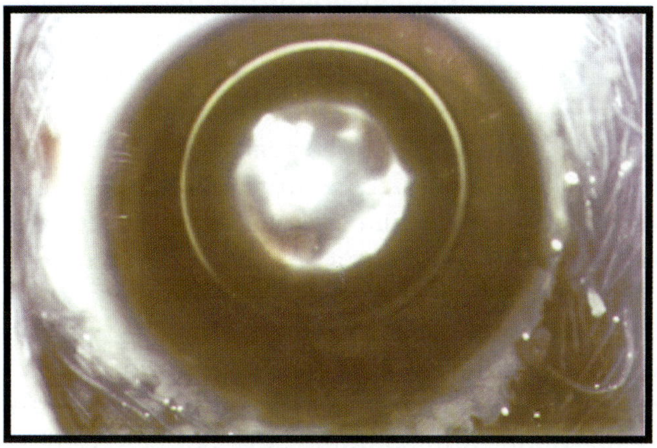

C. Trypan blue

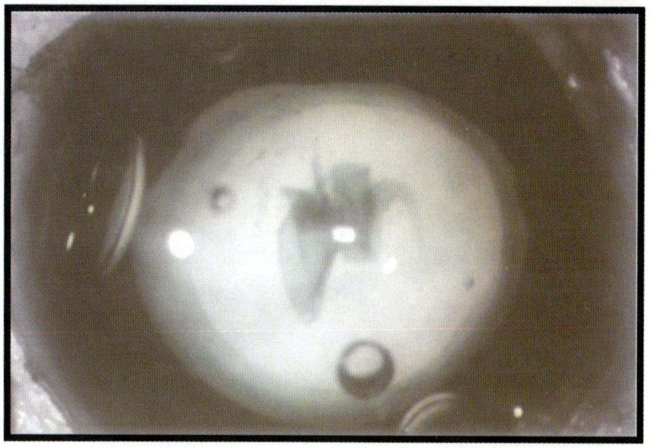

D. Visualization of the anterior capsule is enhanced after staining with ICG

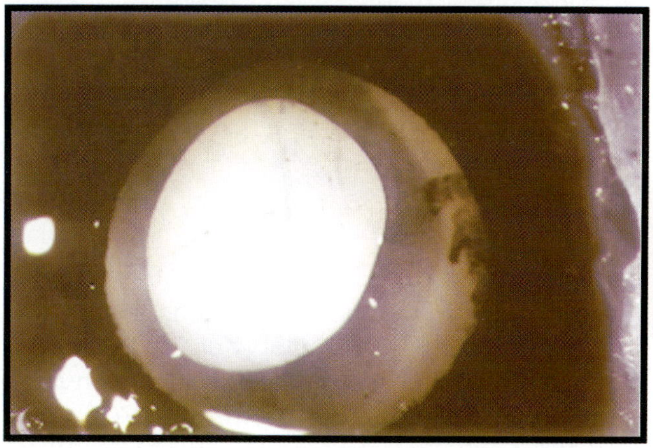

E. Visualization of the anterior capsule is enhanced after staining with trypan blue

Figs 12.3A to E: Anterior (surgeon's) view of a human eye obtained postmortem with advanced/white cataracts showing the staining of the anterior capsule under an air bubble

bubble using fluorescein sodium, ICG and trypan blue in 6 globes (2 globes each). Alternatively, the same dyes were used for intracameral subcapsular injection in the other 6 globes (2 globes each).

Results

Table 12.2 shows the results of our evaluation of the 2 staining techniques (under an air bubble, and intracameral subcapsular injection) and the 3 dyes (fluorescein sodium, ICG and trypan blue). In all globes, CCC was completed uneventfully. Of these 2 techniques, the intracameral subcapsular injection provided a slightly better staining of the anterior capsule. The dye remained trapped in the subcapsular space after the injection, in contact with the posterior surface of the anterior capsule, allowing enough time to perform any maneuver. Among the three dyes used in this study, the

Table 12.2: Evaluation of the dyes and techniques used for staining the anterior capsule

First surgeon					*Second surgeon*				
Eye	*Technique*	*Dye*	*Ability to perform the technique**	*Staining of anterior capsule***	*Eye*	*Technique*	*Dye*	*Ability to perform the technique**	*Staining anterior capsule***
1.	Under an air bubble	FS***	+++	+	7.	Under an air bubble	FS	+++	+
2.	Under an air bubble	ICG****	+++	++	8.	Under an air bubble	ICG	+++	++
3.	Under an air bubble	TB*****	+++	++	9.	Under an air bubble	TB	+++	+
4.	Subcapsular injection	FS	+++	++	10.	Subcapsular injection	FS	+++	++
5.	Subcapsular injection	ICG	+++	+++	11.	Subcapsular injection	ICG	+++	+++
6.	Subcapsular injection	TB	+++	++	12.	Subcapsular injection	TB	+++	++

*: + = difficult; ++ = intermediate; +++ = easy.
**: + = faint; ++ = intermediate; +++ = good.
***: FS = fluorescein sodium.
****: ICG = indocyanine green.
*****: TB = trypan blue.

staining provided by ICG, at the concentration used, was found to be slightly superior (Figs 12.4A to D and 12.5A and B). It was notably easier to localize the ICG stained posterior surface of the inverse anterior capsular flap while performing CCC, after the subcapsular injection of the dye (Figs 12.4C and D). The Miyake-Apple posterior video/ photographic technique demonstrated a leakage of fluorescein sodium into the vitreous after using both dye administration methods (under an air bubble and intracameral subcapsular injection). The intensity of this leakage increased progressively with time. Figures 12.6A to C illustrates the progressive leakage of the fluorescein sodium into the vitreous cavity after intracameral subcapsular injection. No vitreous leakage was observed with ICG or trypan blue after using any of the two aforementioned techniques of anterior capsule staining.

Tables 12.3 and 12.4 summarize the advantages and disadvantages associated with the use of dyes (fluorescein sodium, ICG and trypan blue) and the techniques of staining (under an air bubble, and intracameral subcapsular injection).

Clinical Application and Guidelines for Surgeons

Staining of the anterior capsule with ophthalmic dyes is a useful alternative for performing CCC in cases of advanced/white cataract. Fluorescein sodium was the first dye advocated for this use.[2-4] ICG and trypan blue were further recommended for this purpose.[5-7,10,11,15,18] ICG and trypan blue selectively stain dead corneal endothelial cells. Because the endothelial cells are alive in human cataract surgery, ICG and trypan blue neither stain these cells nor obstruct the surgeon's view. Because of its smaller molecular weight (376 d), fluorescein sodium can stain the cornea and also migrate to the vitreous cavity. We were able to demonstrate the leakage of fluorescein sodium into the vitreous cavity using the Miyake-Apple posterior video/ photographic technique. In the study of Horiguchi *et al.*,[5] fluorescein sodium could not be removed from the vitreous cavity by an irrigation-aspiration system. The reconstituted ICG dye is only good for 10 hours. Because the bottle of ICG is expensive (approximately US $ 90.00 for 25 mg ICG), it is

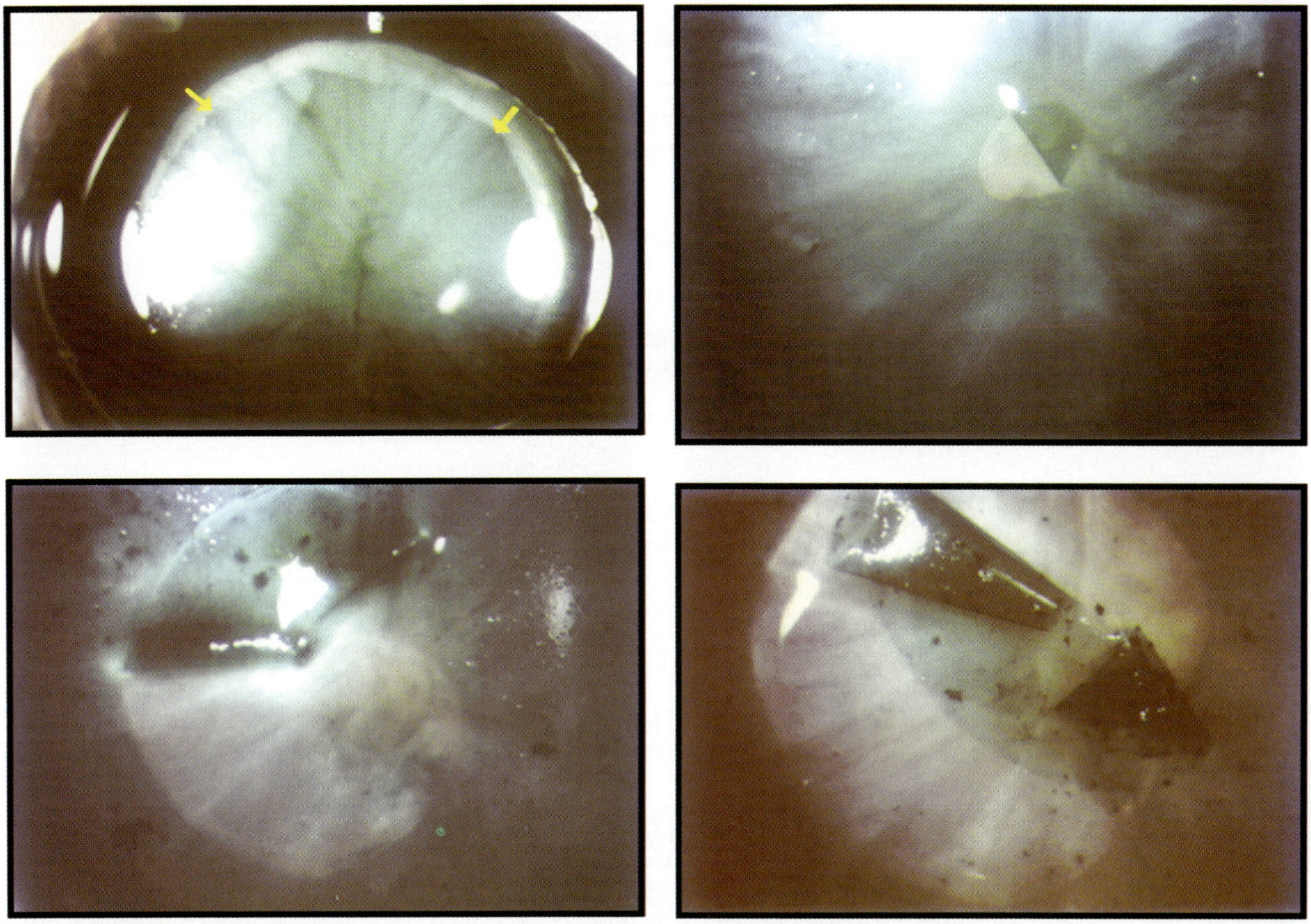

Figs 12.4A to D: Anterior (surgeon's) view of a human eye obtained postmortem with white cataract showing the staining of the anterior capsule using intracameral subcapsular injection of ICG. Cornea and iris were excised to allow better visualization of the anterior capsule: (A) Note the entrapment of the dye into the subcapsular space (arrows), (B) The capsulorhexis can be initiated by grasping the injection hole. (C and D) The visualization of the anterior capsule is enhanced by the staining of its posterior surface with the dye

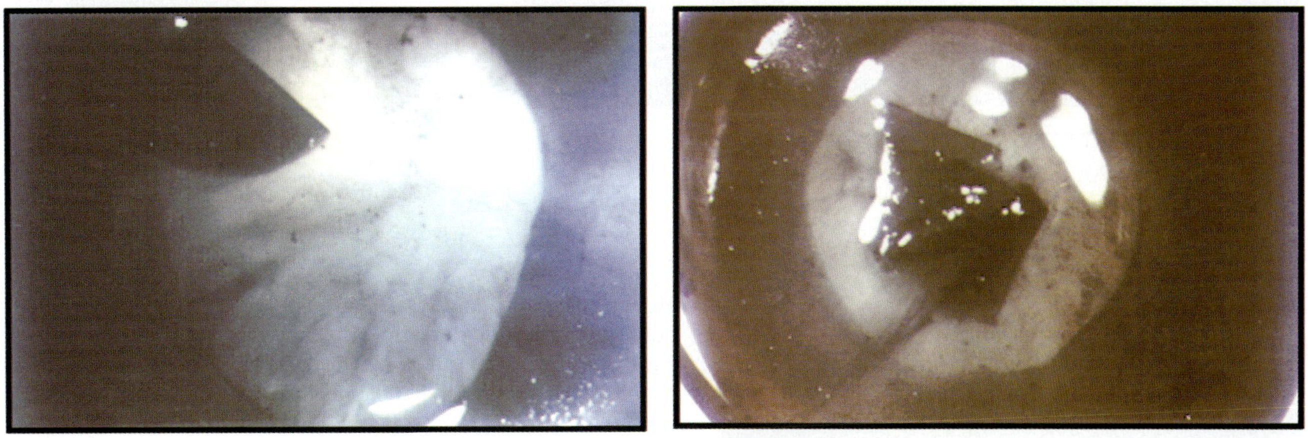

Figs 12.5A and B: Anterior (surgeon's) view of a human eye obtained postmortem showing the better contrast against the white cataract provided by the staining of the posterior surface of the anterior capsule with trypan blue

Table 12.3: Characteristics of the three dyes used for anterior capsule staining

Dye	*Concentration*	*Advantages*	*Disadvantages*
Fluorescein sodium	2%	Blue light enhancement can be used	Low molecular weight Vitreous leakage Staining of the cornea
Indocyanine green	0.50%	High molecular weight No vitreous leakage	Cost may be prohibitive
Trypan blue	0.10%	High molecular weight No vitreous leakage	Not indicated in pregnant/fertile females and children

Table 12.4: Characteristics of the two techniques used for anterior capsule staining

Staining under an air bubble		*Intracameral subcapsular injection*	
Advantages	*Disadvantages*	*Advantages*	*Disadvantages*
Technically less invasive	Air-filled anterior chamber is unsteady	Dye remains trapped in the subcapsular space	Technically more invasive
Staining of the peripheral anterior capsular rim, provides good visibility while performing phacoemulsification	Progressive dilution of the dye by aqueous	Good staining of the posterior surface of the capsular flap	Tear of the anterior capsule, if excessive injection of dye
Safer in intumescent hypermature cataracts		Injection hole can be used for initiating CCC	Anterior capsule tear in intumescent cataracts

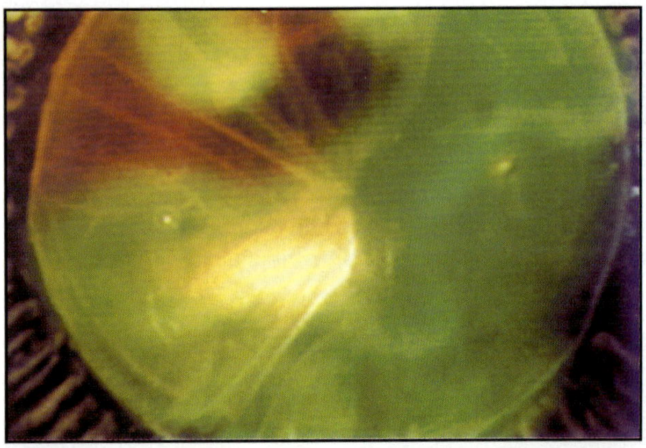

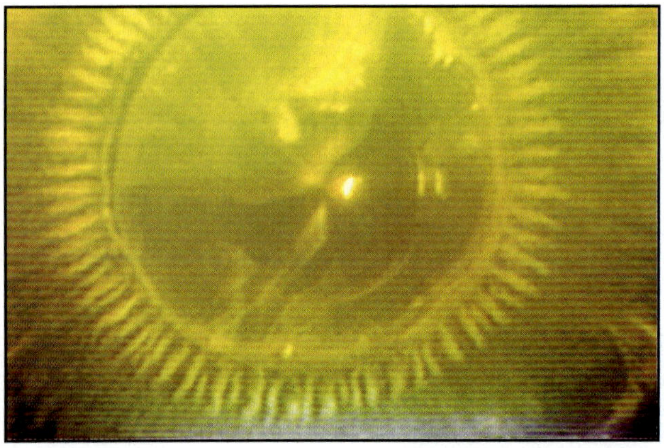

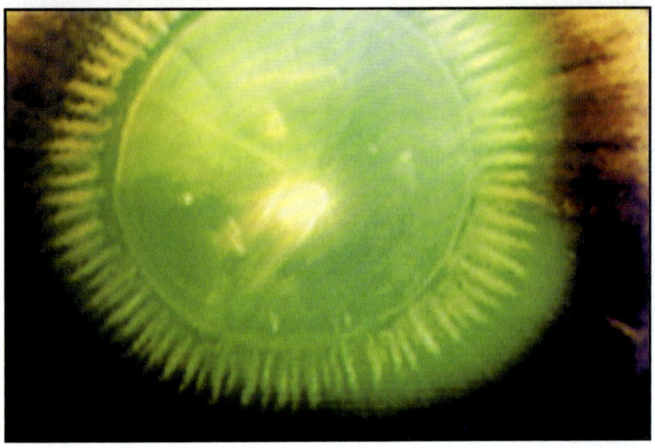

Figs 12.6A to C: Miyake-Apple posterior view of a human eye obtained postmortem showing the progressive leakage of fluorescein sodium into the vitreous cavity after intracameral subcapsular injection. Note that the intensity of the leakage increases as time progresses: (A) Five minutes after intracameral subcapsular injection, (B) Same globe, 15 minutes after intracameral subcapsular injection, (C) Same globe, 2 hours after intracameral subcapsular injection

better to schedule several patients with absent or poor red reflex on the same surgery day. Intraocular solutions of trypan blue have not yet been FDA approved and therefore are not currently available in the United States; thus, the solution has to be prepared before surgery. Trypan blue 0.1 percent solution (ready to be used) for capsular staining is commercialized by DORC International b.v. (Vn Zuidland, Holland) under the trade name of VisionBlue®, as it was proposed by Melles.[6] Recently, a 0.1 percent solution of trypan blue dye became commercially available from Dr Agarwal's Pharma Ltd. (Chennai, India) under the trade name of Blurhex®. Trypan blue is less expensive than ICG, and to the best of our knowledge, the cost of a 1 mL ampoule of trypan blue (Blurhex®) is approximately US $ 3, compared to the US $ 90.00 cost of 1 ampoule of 25 mg ICG powder.[18]

The surgeon should avoid using the trypan blue dye in fertile women, pregnant women, or children, because, in some animal studies, when this dye was given intravenously or intraperitoneally (more frequent applications, and at much higher concentrations), it induced neoplasms (Melles GRJ. Trypan blue dye helps to visualize capsulorhexis, Cataract and Refractive Surgery Eurotimes, May-June, 1999).

The surgeon should also be careful when using any ophthalmic dyes in cataract surgery combined with implantation of hydrophilic acrylic lenses having a high water content (73.5%), as this can lead to permanent staining (discoloration) of the IOL by ophthalmic dyes. This discoloration may also be associated with a decrease or alteration in the best-corrected visual acuity, eventually requiring IOL explantation / exchange. We have recently analyzed 2 Acqua® hydrophilic acrylic lenses explanted secondary to bluish discoloration after use of trypan blue dye.[41]

The techniques originally reported for staining the anterior capsule using fluorescent sodium are: staining from above under an air bubble, as proposed by Nahra and Castilla (Nahra D, Castilla M, Capsulorhexis in no view cataract: Staining of the anterior capsule with 2 percent fluorescein, presented at the annual meeting of the American Academy of Ophthalmology, October 1996, Chicago, Illinois, USA), and intracameral subcapsular injection of fluorescein sodium (staining from below) with blue-light enhancement.[3,4] The first technique (staining under an air bubble) is currently used by most surgeons. One benefit is the staining of the peripheral anterior rim, which is otherwise difficult to visualize during the phacoemulsification procedure.[6] However, air in the anterior chamber makes it unsteady. Any instrument entering the eye will cause some air to escape, with a rise of the lens-iris plane. A small amount of high-density viscoelastic placed near the incision can prevent the air bubble from escaping the anterior chamber, thus minimizing the risk of sudden collapse. Also, with this technique, there is a progressive dilution of the dye by the aqueous humor. This may be a possible explanation for the fainter staining observed with this technique in recent clinical reports, without compromising its usefulness (Steinert RF, ICG dye aids in visualization of the anterior capsule, Ophthalmology Times, May 15, 1999). Most of the drawback of this technique can be avoided by careful use of a viscoelastic solution to seal the incision site. Akahoshi proposed the "soft shell stain technique" for performing a CCC in white cataract cases (Akahoshi T, Soft shell stain technique fort white cataract, presented at the ASCRS symposium on Cataract, IOL, and Refractive Surgery, Boston, MA, May 2000). A small amount of viscoelastic (Viscoat®) was injected into the anterior chamber followed by high molecular weight viscoelastic material (Provisc®) to fill up the chamber completely. The author then injected ICG solution on the lens surface with a bent G27 viso cannula. The anterior capsule was uniformly stained green and easily visualize while the cornea remained unstained. According to author, the soft shell stain technique is extremely useful for CCC of white cataracts.

Alternatively, the dye solution can be mixed with viscoelastic agents. Kayikicioglu and coworkers[15] proposed a technique for limiting the contact of trypan blue by mixing the dye with a viscoelastic solution. These researchers mixed 0.4 percent trypan blue with 1 percent sodium hyaluronate in a 2 mL syringe. The dye, mixed in a viscoelastic solution, is injected onto the anterior lens capsule, which covers the anterior capsule without coming in contact with the corneal endothelium. Trypan blue mixed with sodium hyaluronate greatly increase the visibility of the anterior lens capsule without significantly touching the adjacent tissues. There is a potential risk of corneal decompensation after intraocular use of self-mixed solution; however, these authors used this technique without significant surgical and postoperative adverse effects.

Intracameral subcapsular injection is another, but less commonly used, technique of anterior capsule staining. It has the advantage of trapping the dye in the subcapsular space, mostly in the center and in the midperipheral part. It gives sufficient time for the surgeon to perform any maneuver until the CCC releases it. Meanwhile, the dye remains in contact with the posterior surface of the anterior capsule. This may be a possible explanation for the better staining observed in our laboratory study on postmortem human eyes.[7] The capsule and cortex are both stained by the dye used, but they can be clearly distinguished from the feathery appearance of the cortex and the smooth staining of the capsule. The CCC is fairly easy to perform by grasping the injection hole. This technique was originally proposed for fluorescein with blue-light enhancement, but we also used it with ICG and trypan blue. When the capsular flap is inverted, the stained posterior surface of the anterior capsule enhances visualization and thus facilitates tearing during CCC. In our study, this was more obvious with the intracameral subcapsular injection of ICG.[7] Further, this can be performed without the need for any special type of illumination, such as a cobalt blue-filter. We would like to emphasize that there is the risk of anterior capsule tear formation after subcapsular injection of dye. However, we did not observe this complication (anterior capsule tear) in any postmortem human eyes used in our laboratory study.[7] We would certainly not recommend the intracameral subcapsular injection technique for performing CCC in intumescent and hypermature cataracts owing to the high intralenticular pressure and fragile anterior lens capsule that may easily result in radial tear formation.

Horiguchi *et al*,[5] reported the technique of staining the anterior capsule using a 2 percent solution of ICG in patients with mature cataracts. They compared the results of phacoemulsification and IOL implantation in 2 groups of 10 eyes. In the first group, the anterior capsule was stained with ICG before CCC, and in the second, no dye was used. There was no statistically significant difference reported in their study between both groups concerning specular-microscopy endothelial cell counting, and laser flare-cell photometry, thus the staining procedure was considered to be safe.

Clinical experience with ICG and trypan blue for anterior capsule staining in mature white or brunescent cataracts was first reported by David Chang[42] in two consecutive, non-randomized series of mature or brunescents cataracts. The technique of dye injection under an air bubble, ICG dye was used in the first series, and trypan blue in the subsequent series. According to author, both dyes provided consistently excellent visualization and clinical results without any adverse effects. However, trypan blue created a more intense and persistent staining, and provided superior visualization when compared with ICG, according to this first clinical study (Chang DF, MD. Compare two dyes. *EyeNet* 2000; 4:22).[42]

We would like to provide some recommendations and guidelines for ophthalmic surgeons regarding suitable ophthalmic dyes and the anterior capsule staining technique. These are based on our experience in postmortem human eyes, as well as published clinical reports from several other surgeons. Both ICG and trypan blue are currently preferred over fluorescein sodium dye, due to better staining of the anterior capsule and the absence of vitreous leakage (due to high molecular weight). Both these dyes provide excellent visualization of the anterior capsule flap during CCC, without causing any toxic effects on the corneal endothelium. Trypan blue has the advantage of being less costly when compared to the cost of ICG. However, trypan blue should be avoided in fertile/pregnant females and in children due to the possible teratogenic and/or mutagenic effects observed in animal studies when using this dye. Further studies may be helpful to determine the least available concentration of the trypan blue dye that can be used to stain the anterior lens capsule in order to perform the CCC. ICG remains a valuable alternative for these special patients (children and pregnant females). Staining under the air bubble technique is safer and therefore recommended for intumescent and hypermature cataract patients presenting with high intralenticular pressure and a fragile anterior lens capsule. Viscoelastic solutions can be used to visco-seal the incision site in order to avoid escape of the air bubble, and to minimize any anterior chamber fluctuations. Alternatively, mixing the dye with a viscoelastic solution may also be used for better anterior capsule staining, and for limiting the contact with adjacent ocular tissues.

OPHTHALMIC DYES FOR PHACOEMULSIFICATION

Introduction

It is important to practice the phacoemulsification (PE) procedure in a wet laboratory setting in order to reduce the learning curve and enhance the safety margin before operating on the real patient.[42-46] Human eye bank or animal eyes are commonly used for this purpose. The surgeon must be familiar with the critical steps of the PE procedure. Each step is therefore to be learned independently and carefully in order to achieve a successful outcome and reduce complications. This is even more important when dealing with advanced/white cataracts in a clinical setting. The absence of a red reflex in such cases renders CCC as well as nucleus sculpting maneuvers difficult, if not impossible.[47]

In the first Section, we have discussed a detailed evaluation of the staining of the anterior capsule for CCC in advanced cataracts, comparing 3 dyes (fluorescein sodium, ICG, and trypan blue dyes), and two injection techniques, in postmortem human eyes. All dyes provided satisfactory staining of the anterior capsule for CCC. However, fluorescein sodium progressively leaked into the vitreous.[7] In this Section we report our experience with the application of 0.5 percent ICG and 0.1 percent trypan blue to obtain complete hydrodissection/delineation, to stain the nuclear substance during nuclear emulsification, and to stain capsular bag during the cortical clean-up. Application of the ophthalmic dye for performing phacoemulsification is termed *Dye-enhanced Phacoemulsification* and this section will focus on the use of dye to enhance visualization for learning, and performing critical steps of the phacoemulsification procedure.

Study of Dye-enhanced Phacoemulsification

Surgical Technique

Randomly accessioned postmortem human eyes (n = 16) obtained within 4 days of death from eye banks nationwide were used in our study.[8]

They were prepared according to the Miyake-Apple posterior video technique.[39,40] Two independent surgeons (LW, SKP) evaluated the use of 0.5 percent ICG and 0.1 percent trypan blue to perform the critical steps of PE in 8 eyes (2 eyes/dye/surgeon). Dye solutions were prepared as previously described in this chapter (Section 1). In 8 other eyes used as controls, the PE procedures were performed without the use of dye. After the cornea and iris were removed, a CCC (4.5 to 5.5 mm in diameter) was initiated using a 26 gauge needle cystitome and completed using Utrata's forceps. A complete cortical cleaning hydrodissection was performed by injecting 2-3 cc of the dye solution (0.5% ICG or 0.1% trypan blue) between the lens capsule and the cortex with a 27 gauge cannula. This was followed by hydrodelineation: placement of a 27 gauge cannula deep into the nucleus and injection of the dye solution created the colored fluid-wave marking the separation of the nucleus and the epinucleus. Balanced salt solution (BSS®) was used to perform hydrodissection/delineation in the control group. Nuclear emulsification (Alcon Legacy 20,000, Alcon Surgical, Fort Worth, TX) was performed using the divide-and-conquer nucleofractis technique.[47] One to two microdrops of the dye solution were instilled into the capsular bag, and cortical clean-up was performed using the irrigation and aspiration system.

The enhancement of visualization while performing each step of the surgery using the dyes was evaluated by the two independent surgeons. They particularly noted:

a. If the use of a colored solution helped in visualizing the fluid waves and the plane of cleavage during hydrodissection/delineation,

b. If the staining of the nucleus substance helped in appreciating the depth of the phaco tip and its position in relation to the posterior capsule during the nuclear emulsification, and
c. If the staining of the inner surface of the capsular bag helped in identifying residual cortical material during the cortical clean-up procedure using the irrigation-aspiration system.

Results

Our experimental study suggested that both dyes (0.5% ICG, and 0.1% trypan blue) successfully enhanced visualization while performing critical steps of the PE procedure, when compared to the control group.[8] During hydrodissection/hydrodelineation, the use of dye helped to visualize the formation of a complete cleavage between the capsule and cortex, as well as between the nucleus-epinucleus complex (Figs 12.7A and B). Incomplete cleavage could be easily identified by using a colored solution, and promptly completed by reinjection in the appropriate quadrant.

During the nuclear emulsification procedure, the use of dye helped in appreciating the position of the phaco tip and its relation with the posterior capsule, thus increasing the safety of the procedure (Figs 12.8A and B).

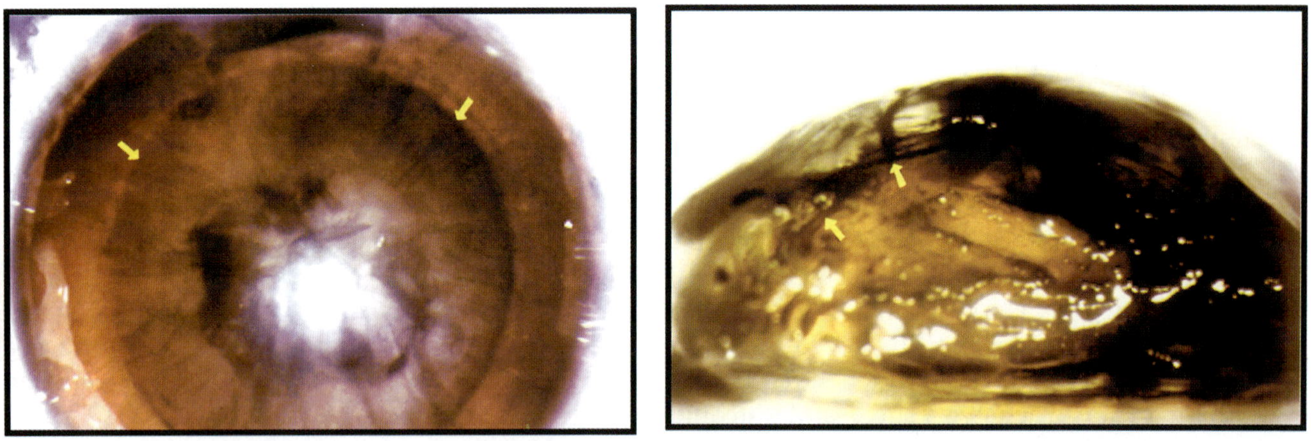

Figs 12.7A and B: Gross photographs of a human eye obtained postmortem. Cornea and iris were excised to allow better visualization: (A) Anterior (surgeon's) view showing hydrodissection/hydrodelineation enhanced by trypan blue. Notice the complete (360 degrees) blue-colored fluid wave indicating separation of the nucleus/epinucleus complex, (B) Sagittal section of the same crystalline lens, showing the demarcation zone between the nucleus/epinucleus complex (arrows)

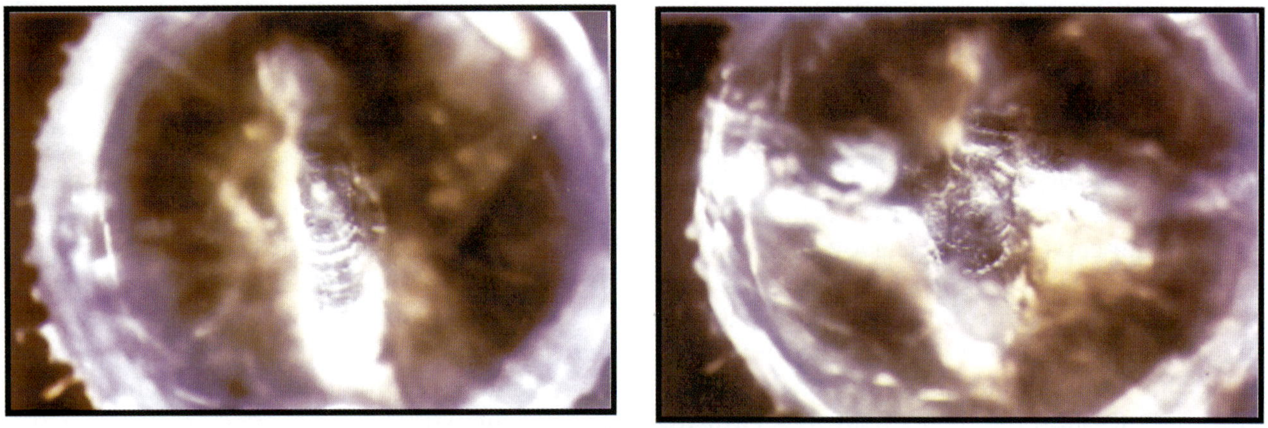

Figs 12.8A and B: Gross photographs of a human eye obtained postmortem taken from an anterior (surgeon's) view while performing nucleus sculpting. Cornea and iris were excised to allow better visualization: (A and B) Gimbel's divide-and-conquer nucleofractis technique. Notice that trypan blue dye enhances visualization of the groove. This is helpful to judge the position of the phaco tip and its relation with the posterior capsule

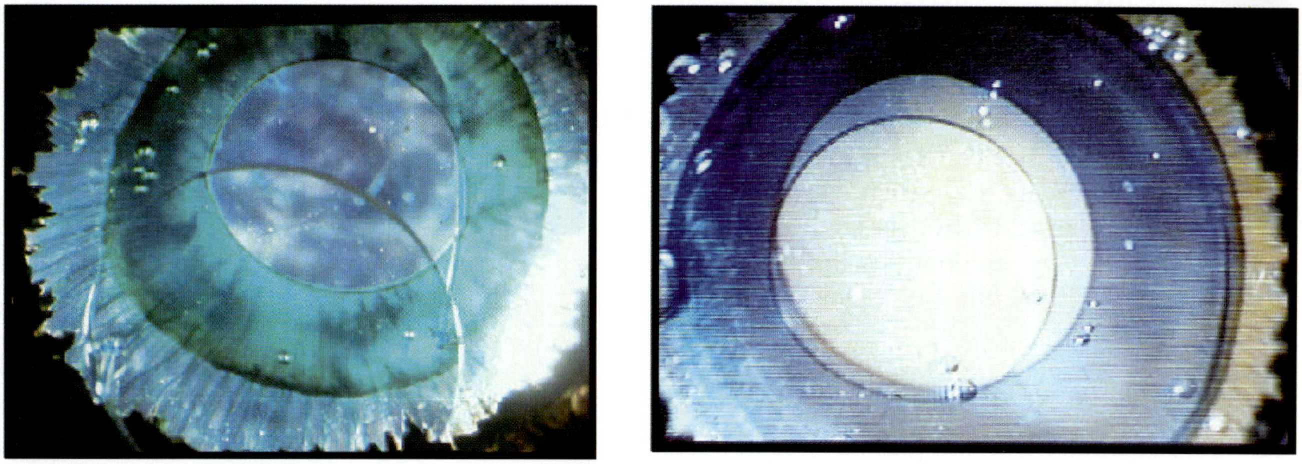

Figs 12.9A and B: Gross photographs of human eyes obtained postmortem taken from an anterior (surgeon's) view after the completion of irrigation/aspiration. Cornea and iris were excised to allow better visualization. Note the cleaned capsular bags, stained green and blue after the use of ICG and trypan blue dyes, respectively. The arrows demonstrate in both cases the staining of the minimal residual cortical material. (A) ICG (B) Trypan blue

For the complete cleaning of the capsular bag, the use of dye provided better visualization of the residual cortical material during the irrigation-aspiration procedure (Figs 12.9A and B). It was easy to differentiate the feathery, irregular staining of the cortex from the smooth staining of the capsule.

Learning Critical Steps of Phacoemulsification

It is important to learn the critical steps of the PE procedure, which include CCC, hydrodissection, hydrodelineation, nuclear emulsification maneuvers, and cortical clean-up. In a series of 7,169 patients undergoing phacoemulsification, Gimbel reported 36 peroperative posterior capsule tears.[48] Of these, 19 (53%) occurred during the irrigation/aspiration step and 13 (36%) occurred during the phacoemulsification itself. Five and six percent of the posterior capsule tears occurred during the IOL implantation and the hydrodissection, respectively. Visualization while performing each step can be enhanced by the use of different dyes, thus increasing their safety margin.

CCC

We have addressed the techniques of anterior capsule staining for anterior capsulorhexis using fluorescein sodium, ICG, and trypan blue dyes. In addition to the staining of the anterior capsule when performing CCC, ICG and trypan blue can also be successfully used to learn other critical steps of the PE procedure in a laboratory setting. We believe that the use of dye would not only be useful during the anterior capsule management in white cataracts, but also for learning and practicing the other critical steps of phacoemulsification procedure as discussed here.

Hydrodissection/Hydrodelineation

Hydrodissection is an important step of small incision cataract surgery using phacoemulsification. The use of this procedure was first reported by Faust.[22] Fine[24] added the concept of cortical cleavage hydrodissection to separate the superficial cortex from the lens capsule. The use of dye (instead of BSS®) helps in the localization of the complete (360 degree) cortical cleavage plane, separating the equatorial and posterior capsule from the cortex. It is much easier to visualize a dye-colored fluid wave of hydrodissection. Therefore, it helps in achieving complete separation between capsule and cortex. Hydrodelineation,[26] associated with the formation of a golden ring, is sometimes difficult to notice. With the injection of a capsular dye solution, however, the surgeon can successfully visualize the demarcation between the nucleus and the epinucleus (Fig. 12.7A). In this situation, an incomplete hydrodissection/delineation can be easily identified and completed by injecting more stained fluid in that particular quadrant, if needed. After achieving complete hydrodissection and hydrodelineation, it is easier to perform nuclear emulsification with less ultrasound power and time, decreasing the need for cortical clean-up and the risk of posterior capsule tears. Recent studies from our laboratory suggest that hydrodissection-enhanced cortical clean-up is an unidentified but important factor for delaying the onset of posterior capsule opacification.[49]

Nuclear Emulsification

A number of different techniques have been used by surgeons for nuclear emulsification of hard and soft cataracts. While performing nuclear emulsification maneuvers, visualization of the depth at which the phaco tip is sculpting is crucial. Its significance cannot be overemphasized for preventing complications like unnoticed posterior capsular tears, vitreous loss and dislocation of the nucleus into the vitreous cavity. When a good red reflex is present, the surgeon can rely on an increasingly brighter-red reflex to gauge proximity to the posterior capsule while sculpting the nucleus. However, the absence of a red reflex (e.g. in advanced, white, mature or hypermature cataracts) complicates nucleus emulsification because it is difficult to judge the depth of the phaco tip during sculpting (Chang D. Solutions offered for mature white cataracts. *Ocular Surg News* 1999; 6:8). The staining of the nucleus (lens substance) helps in visualizing the position of the phaco tip and its relation with the posterior capsule, thus enhancing the safety margin of the procedure.

Cortical Clean-up

Studies have shown that at least half of the cases of capsular tears and vitreous loss occur at the time of cortical clean-up.[48] Staining of the capsular bag enhances its visualization and the surgeon can distinguish feathery, irregular staining of residual cortex from smooth staining of the anterior, equatorial and posterior capsule. Thus, the staining facilitates the cleaning of residual cortical matter from the capsular bag. Posterior capsule staining can also be very useful to learn and perform the PCCC procedure, details of which will be provided in Section 3 of this chapter .

Possible Clinical Application and Future Trials

Our laboratory study provides evidence that both dyes (ICG and trypan blue) can be used in the clinical setting of living human eye operations to achieve a complete hydrodissection / delineation.[8] They can also be used to visualize the depth of the phaco tip during sculpting and its relation to the posterior capsule, especially in patients with a poor or absent red reflex (advanced / white cataracts). It is easier to differentiate the cortical matter from the anterior or posterior capsules after the staining of the capsular bag. This would be helpful in achieving a complete cortical clean-up during the irrigation / aspiration steps, with lower incidence of posterior capsule tear.

In summary, the use of dyes (ICG and trypan blue) during small-incision adult cataract surgery using PE facilitated complete hydrodissection and hydrodelineation, nuclear emulsification maneuvers and a complete cortical clean-up. We believe that, in addition to practicing an anterior capsulorhexis, these dyes can also be used to enhance visualization for learning other important steps of the phacoemulsification procedure in a wet laboratory setting.[8] This study also suggests the need for future clinical trials using these dyes in a clinical setting of living human eye operations.

OPHTHALMIC DYES FOR POSTERIOR CAPSULORHEXIS

Introduction

Posterior continuous curvilinear capsulorhexis (PCCC) is a posterior continuous central capsulotomy technique described by Gimbel and Blumenthal and coworkers in 1990.[27,28] PCCC is recommended for converting an irregular tear of the posterior capsule into a circumscribed cut not extending to the equator.[27,29] It can also be used for the removal of posterior capsular plaques in posterior subcapsular or polar cataracts.[50]

Recently, the use of PCCC combined with optic capture of an IOL[30,31] and / or anterior vitrectomy[51-54] successfully evolved for delaying the development of posterior capsule opacification (PCO) or secondary membrane formation in pediatric cases. Primary posterior capsulotomy, in the form of PCCC, is especially important in younger children for maintaining a long-term clear visual axis in order to prevent the development of amblyopia.[55] Besides children, some surgeons also recommend to perform PCCC during extracapsular cataract extraction or during the PE procedure in adults, because this is a more effective and safer procedure than the Nd: YAG laser capsulotomy for the management of PCO.[56,57]

However, to learn and perform PCCC is technically challenging due to the thin and transparent nature of the posterior capsule. Further, it should not be attempted if visibility is mediocre and/or vitreous pressure is assessed to be high.

Study on Dye-enhanced Posterior Capsulorhexis

Considering the wide clinical implications of PCCC and keeping the difficulty to learn and perform this important procedure in mind, we carried out a study in human eyes obtained postmortem.[9] We evaluated if the staining of the posterior capsule with different dyes could be useful to facilitate PCCC, similar to the anterior capsule staining for performing anterior capsulorhexis in cataracts with poor or no red glow.

Surgical Technique

Randomly accessioned postmortem human eyes (n = 12) obtained within 4 days of death from eye banks nationwide were used in this study. The eyes were prepared according to the Miyake-Apple posterior video technique.[39,40] They were sectioned at the equator and the anterior segment was mounted on a glass slide to provide a posterior perspective of this portion of the eye. After the cornea and iris were removed, a capsulorhexis 5.0 to 5.5 mm in diameter was initiated using a 26 gauge needle and completed using a Utrata's forceps. A complete cortical-cleavage hydrodissection was performed by injecting balanced salt solution (BSS®, Alcon Ophthalmic, Fort Worth, TX, USA) between the lens capsule and the cortex with a 27 gauge cannula. This was followed by careful hydroexpression of the nucleus, avoiding damage to the posterior capsule. Cortical clean-up was performed using an irrigation/aspiration system.

Two independent surgeons (SKP, LW) evaluated the use of dye to enhance visualization of the posterior capsule during PCCC (4 eyes/surgeon). Both surgeons were inexperienced with the PCCC procedure and performed it for the first time in their professional career. PCCC was also performed in 4 other eyes (2 eyes/surgeon) without the use of dye. The posterior capsule was stained by instilling 1 microdrop of the dye solution into the capsular bag. We used 0.5 percent ICG and 0.1 percent trypan blue solutions (4 eyes/dye). The dye solutions were prepared as described by us earlier in this chapter. After waiting 1-2 minutes, the excessive dye was washed out. The capsular bag was filled with a viscoelastic agent (Healon®, Pharmacia Inc., Peapack, NJ, USA) and PCCC was initiated by using a 26 gauge needle cystotome and completed using a Utrata's forceps. Optic capture of a posterior chamber intraocular lens (PC-IOL), as well as an anterior vitrectomy, were also practiced.

Results

Our laboratory study in 8 postmortem human eyes confirmed that the posterior capsule can be successfully stained using ICG and trypan blue (Figs 12.10A to D and 12.11A to D). For both surgeons, it was much easier to initiate and complete PCCC successfully after staining of the posterior capsule, when compared to the control (non-stained) eyes. PCCC was completed fairly easily in all globes, due to better visualization of the stained posterior capsule flap (PCF) against the transparent (non-stained) anterior hyaloid phase (AHP) of the vitreous (Figs 12.10A to C and 12.11A to C). It was simpler to perform optic capture of PC-IOLs after staining the posterior capsule (Figs 12.10D and 12.11D). Both dyes used in this study provided satisfactory visualization when performing PCCC.

Clinical Application and Future Trials

PCCC is currently getting more and more attention due to its clinical implication in the prevention of

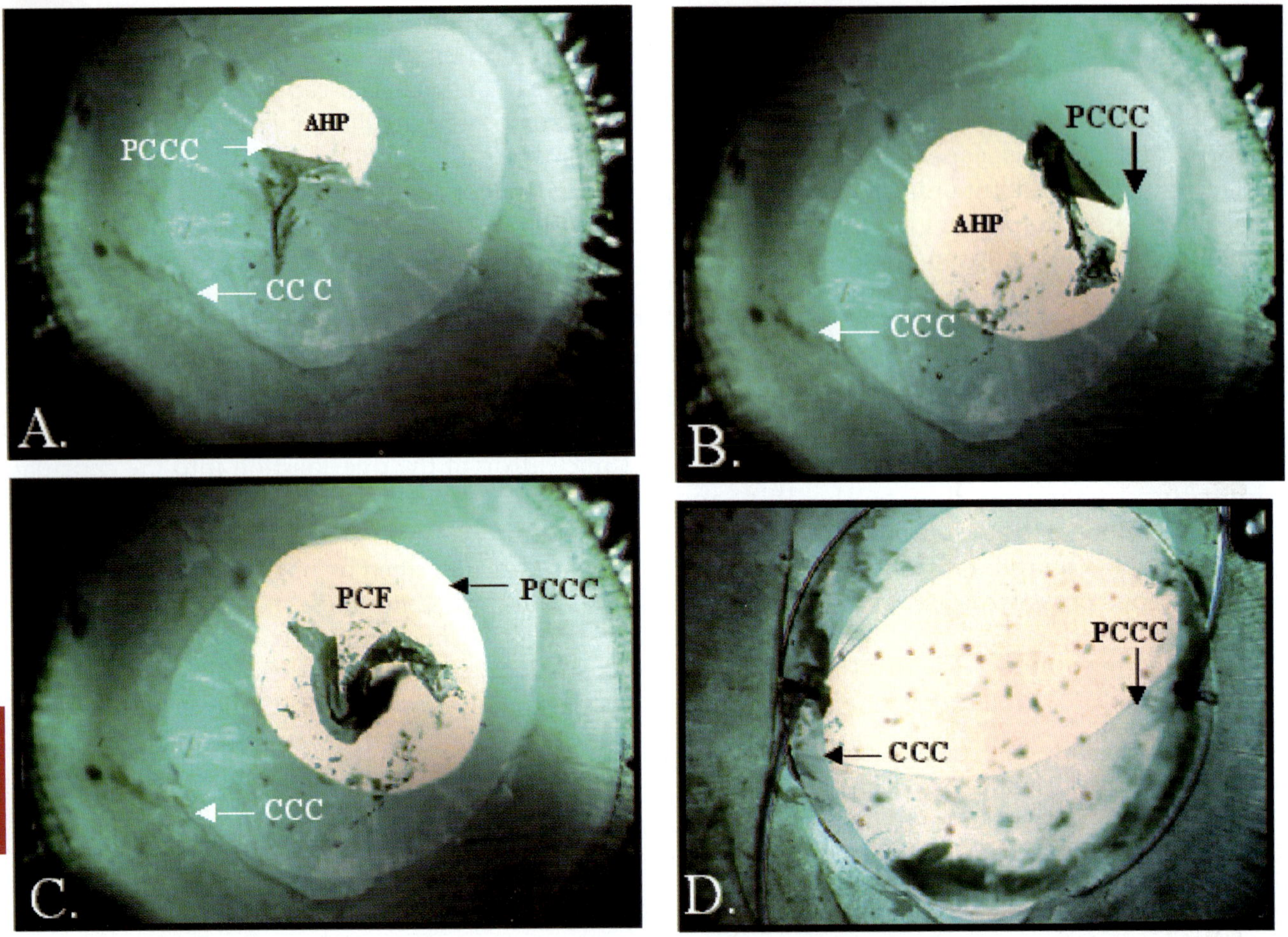

Figs 12.10A to D: Gross photographs of a human eye obtained postmortem showing posterior continuous curvilinear capsulorhexis (PCCC) after the staining of the capsular bag with indocyanine green (ICG). Cornea and iris were excised to allow better visualization: (A) Anterior (surgeon's) view of the cleaned and stained capsular bag showing initiation of the PCCC. Note that it is easier to visualize the stained posterior capsule flap (PCF) against transparent (non-stained) anterior hyaloid phase (AHP) of the vitreous, (B) The PCCC is in progress, (C) The PCCC is completed. Note the stained PCCC margin; PCF: posterior capsule flap, and (D) Higher magnification of the optic-haptic junctions after intraocular lens (IOL) optic capture. Both haptics are present in the capsular bag and the IOL optic is captured behind the posterior capsule

the PCO development primarily in children, and to some extent in adults. Additionally, this procedure is also important in the management of posterior capsule tears of congenital, traumatic or surgical origin, and the pealing of plaques associated with posterior polar and posterior subcapsular cataracts.[50] As mentioned before, learning PCCC is technically challenging due to the thin, transparent, and elastic nature of the posterior capsule. Attempting PCCC in the presence of poor visibility associated with positive vitreous pressure is difficult, and may cause an inadvertent radial tear extending toward the equator. Cauwenberge, Rakic and Galand[58] recently reported the etiology, management and outcome of complicated posterior capsulorhexis. In a 1-year retrospective analysis of 650 patients, they identified 32 (5%) cases of complicated PCCC. According to them, the most frequent problem was the performance of a central capsulorhexis within the optimum size (< 5 mm in diameter). This was not possible in 14 (44%) cases in their series. In 12 (37%) cases, a PCCC was carried out with great difficulty because of either insufficient visibility during the procedure or an anatomically

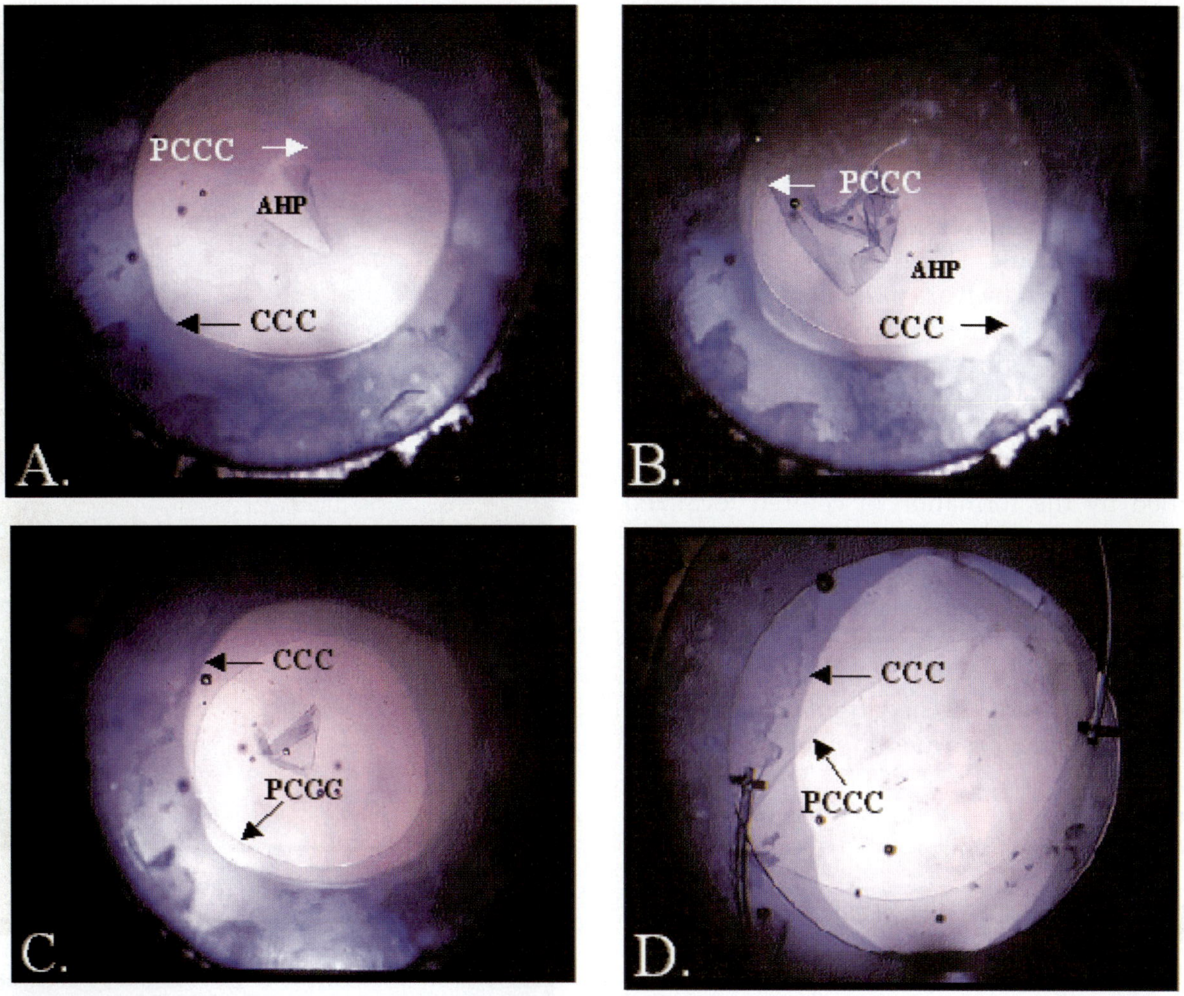

Figs 12.11A to D: Gross photographs of a human eye obtained postmortem showing posterior continuous curvilinear capsulorhexis (PCCC) after the staining of the capsular bag with trypan blue. Cornea and iris were excised to allow better visualization: (A) Anterior (surgeon's) view of the cleaned and stained capsular bag showing initiation of the PCCC. Note that it is easier to visualize the stained posterior capsule flap (PCF) against transparent (non-stained) anterior hyaloid phase (AHP) of the vitreous, (B) The PCCC is in progress, (C) The PCCC is completed. Note the stained PCCC margin; PCF: posterior capsule flap, (D) Higher magnification of the optic-haptic junctions after intraocular lens (IOL) optic capture. Both haptics are present in the capsular bag and the IOL optic is captured behind the posterior capsule

changed capsule (floppy or fibrotic in its center). Vitreous loss occurred in 6 (19%) cases during the PCCC procedure. All the aforementioned complications were reported by these authors despite their 4-year experience with the PCCC procedure, performed on more than 1,300 patients.

Posterior capsulorhexis, which is considered technically difficult and challenging, became easier to learn and perform after staining the posterior capsule with ICG or trypan blue. Staining enhances visualization of the posterior capsule flap, which can be easily recognized against the transparent anterior hyaloid phase of the vitreous.

OPHTHALMIC DYES FOR PEDIATRIC CATARACT SURGERY

Beside in adults, ophthalmic dyes can also be used to facilitate anterior and posterior capsulorhexis during pediatric cataract surgery. We have evaluated the use of 2 ophthalmic dyes, 0.5 percent ICG, and 0.1 percent trypan blue for staining the posterior capsule, while performing PCCC in pediatric eyes obtained postmortem (Figs 12.12A to C).[14] As we have mentioned before, learning the posterior capsulorhexis procedure, and achieving a consistent size of the posterior capsule opening for performing the optic capture, can be difficult for the beginning surgeon due to the thin and transparent nature of the posterior capsule. This is especially important in pediatric eyes, which are particularly associated with a thin sclera and a positive vitreous pressure, thus making PCCC difficult, if not impossible.[52,53,55] Gimbel's technique of PCCC with IOL optic capture can be successfully practiced after staining the posterior capsule.[30,31] Vitreous loss can be easily identified by the formation of colored localized clumps, depending on the type of dye used.

In brief, results of our laboratory study in postmortem human eyes revealed that posterior capsule staining using ICG or trypan blue is very helpful when performing the PCCC procedure both in adults and children. The need remains for future clinical trials using these dyes to stain the posterior capsule when performing PCCC. This technique can be helpful for the beginning surgeon, or in the presence of poor visibility.

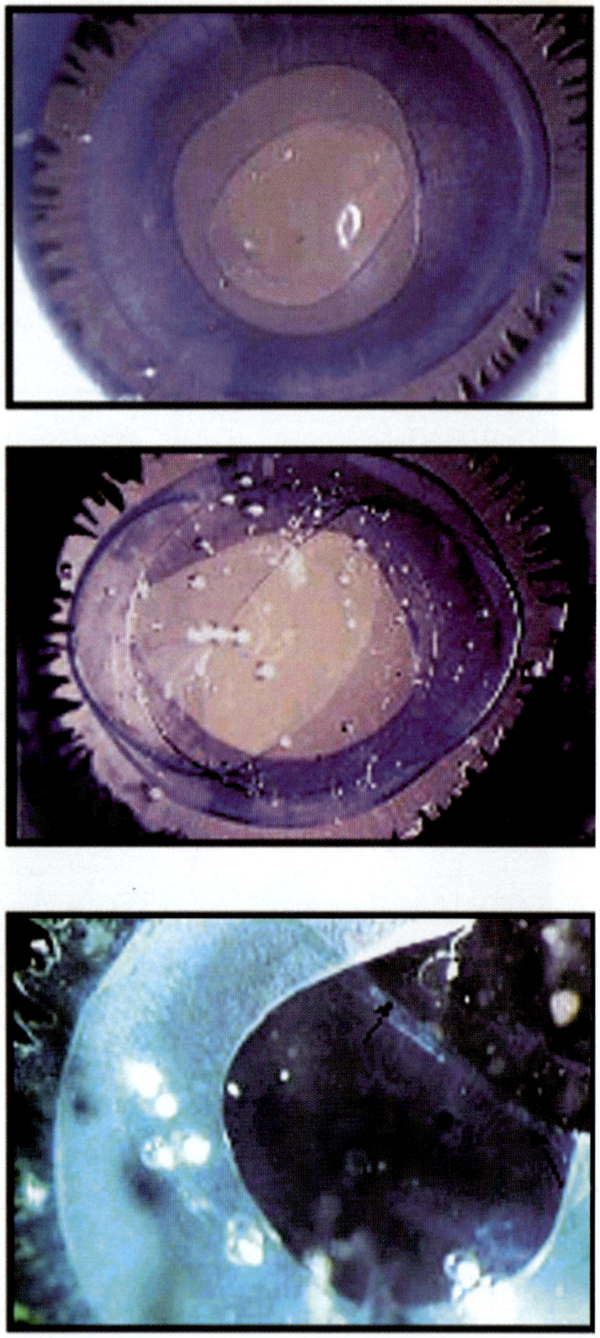

Figs 12.12A to C: Photographs of a pediatric eye obtained postmortem, taken from anterior (surgeon's view) illustrating the use of the capsular dye to enhance visualization during various steps of the pediatric cataract surgery: (A) Posterior capsulorhexis after the staining of the capsular bag with trypan blue, (B) Posterior capsulorhexis and optic capture of a foldable IOL after the staining of the capsular bag with trypan blue, (C) Visualization of a posterior capsule tear after staining of the capsular bag with ICG (arrows)

SUMMARY AND CONCLUSIONS

The use of non-toxic ophthalmic dyes to enhance visualization during the various steps of cataract surgery has been summarized in Table 12.5. Based on our experience of ophthalmic dyes for cataract surgery, we confirm that capsule staining using various dyes in cataractous eyes with poor or no red reflex, helps create an intact anterior capsulorhexis.[7] Several laboratory and clinical studies suggested that both ICG and trypan blue are safe and provide excellent visualization of the anterior capsule flap during CCC.[5-7,10,12,13,59] The trypan blue dye has the advantage of being less expensive than ICG. However, trypan blue dye should not be used in fertile / pregnant females nor in children due to the possibilty of a teratogenic and / or mutagenic effect. ICG remains a valuable alternative for these special patients. Anterior capsule staining under the air bubble technique provides good visualization without the possibility of an anterior capsule tear formation, thus suitable

Table 12.5: Summary of ophthalmic dyes in adult and pediatric cataract surgery

Step	*Dye*	*Study*	*Structure stained*	*Indication*
*CCC	2% FS**		Anterior lens capsule	Patients with poor or no red reflex
	a. Under an air bubble	Mansour[2]	(anterior surface)	
	b. Intracameral subcapsular inj.	Hoffer/McFarland[3]	(posterior surface)	
	0.5% ICG*** Under an air bubble	Horiguchi et al[5]	(anterior surface)	
	0.1%TB**** Under an air bubble	Melles et al[6]	(anterior surface)	
	2% FS, 0.5% ICG, and 0.1% TB	Pandey/Werner et al[7,13]		
	a. Under an air bubble		(anterior surface)	
	b. Intracameral subcapsular inj.		(posterior surface)	
Hydro-dissection/delineation	0.5% ICG, 0.1%TB	Pandey/Werner et al[8, 13]	Interfaces capsule-cortex epinucleus-nucleus	Visualization of the cortical cleavage planes and nucleus dimensions
Nucleus sculpting	0.5% ICG, 0.1% TB	Pandey/Werner et al[8, 13]	Nuclear substance	To judge phaco tip depth and relations with post capsule
Capsular bag cleaning	0.5% ICG, 0.1% TB	Pandey/Werner et al[8, 13]	Inner surface of capsular bag	Complete cleaning of capsular bag
*****PCCC	0.5% ICG, 0.1%TB	Pandey/Werner et al[9,13]	Anterior surface of posterior capsule	Posterior capsule staining for PCCC

*: CCC = Continuous curvilinear capsulorhexis; **: FS = Fluorescein sodium; ***: ICG = Indocyanine green; ****: TB = Trypan blue; *****: PCCC = Posterior continuous circular capsulorhexis

in intumescent and hypermature cataract patients. In addition, our laboratory studies demonstrate that the ophthalmic dyes can be successfully used to enhance visualization while learning the other critical steps of phacoemulsification.[8] Also the technically more challenging procedure of posterior capsulorhexis can be performed with more facility.[9]

REFERENCES

1. Hogan RN, Zimmerman CF. Sodium fluorescein and other tissue dyes. In Zimmerman TJ, et al (Eds): Textbook of Ocular Pharmacology. Philadelphia, PN, Lippincott-Raven, 1997; 849-63.
2. Mansour AM. Anterior capsulorhexis in hypermature cataracts (letter). J Cataract Refract Surg 1993; 19:116-17.
3. Hoffer KJ, McFarland JE. Intracameral subcapsular fluorescein staining for improved visualization during capsulorhexis in mature cataracts (letter). J Cataract Refract Surg 1993; 19:566.
4. Fritz WL. Fluorescein blue light assisted capsulorhexis for mature or hypermature cataract. J Cataract Refract Surg 1998; 24:19-20.
5. Horiguchi M, Miyake K, Ohta I, Ito Y. Staining of the lens capsule for circular continuous capsulorhexis in eyes with white cataract. Arch Ophthalmol 1998; 116:535-37.
6. Melles GRJ, Waard PWT, Pameyer JH, Beekhuis WH. Trypan blue capsule staining in cataract surgery. J Cataract Refract Surg 1999; 24:7-9.
7. Pandey SK, Werner L, Escobar-Gomez M, Roig-Melo EA, Apple DJ. Dye-enhanced cataract surgery. Part 1: Anterior capsule staining for capsulorhexis in advanced/white cataract. J Cataract Refract Surg 2000; 26:1052-59.
8. Werner L, Pandey SK, Escobar-Gomez M, Hoddinott DSM, Apple DJ. Dye-enhanced cataract surgery. Part 2: Learning critical steps of phacoemulsification. J Cataract Refract Surg 2000; 26:1060-65.
9. Pandey SK, Werner L, Escobar-Gomez M, Werner LP, Apple DJ. Dye-enhanced cataract surgery. Part 3: Posterior capsule staining to learn posterior continuous curvilinear capsulorhexis. J Cataract Refract Surg 2000; 26:1066-71.

10. Newsom TH, Oetting TN. Indocyanine green staining in traumatic cataract. J Cataract Refract Surg 2000; 26:1691-93.
11. Nodarian M, Feys J, Sultan G, Salvanet-Bouccara A. Capsulorhexis staining by trypan blue in mature cataract surgery. J Fr Ophtalmol 2001; 24:274-76.
12. Pandey SK, Werner L, Apple DJ. Staining the anterior capsule (Letter to the Editor). J Cataract Refract Surg 2001; 27:647-48.
13. Pandey SK, Werner L, Apple DJ, et al. Update on dye-enhanced cataract surgery. In Chang DF, ed, Hyerguide Online Textbook of Ophthalmology, Thorofare, NJ, Slack, 2001.
14. Pandey SK, Werner L, Apple DJ, et al. Dye-enhanced pediatric cataract surgery. J Pediatr Ophthalmol Strabismus 2001 (submitted).
15. Kayikicioglu O, Erakgun T, Guler C. Trypan blue mixed with sodium hyaluronate for capsulorhexis. J Cataract Refract Surg 2001; 27:970.
16. Unlu K, Askunger A, Soker S, et al. Gentian violet solution for staining the anterior capsule. J Cataract Refract Surg 2000; 26:1228-32.
17. Gamal Eldin SA, el Mehelmy EM, el Shazli, Mostafa YM. Experimental staining of the anterior lens capsule in albino rabbits. J Cataract Refract Surg 1999; 25:1289-94.
18. Agarwal A, Agarwal A, Agarwal S. Trypan blue in the management of mature cataracts. In Agarwal S, Agarwal A, Sachdev MS, Mehta KR, Fine IH, Agarwal A, (Eds): Phacoemulsification, Laser Cataract Surgery and Foldable IOLs. New Delhi, Jaypee Brothers 2000; 618-23.
19. Burke SE, DaMata AP, Snyder ME, et al. Indocyanine green-assisted peeling of the internal limiting membrane. Ophthalmology 2000; 107:2010-14.
20. Gimbel HV, Neuhann T. Development, advantage, and methods of the continuous circular capsulorhexis technique. J Cataract Refract Surg 1990; 16:31-37.
21. Assia EI, Apple DJ, Barden A, et al. An experimental study comparing various anterior capsulotomy techniques. Arch Ophthalmol 1991; 109:642-47.
22. Faust KJ. Hydrodissection of soft nuclei. Am Intraocular Implant Soc J 1984; 10:75-77.
23. Anis AY. Origin of hydrodissection (reply – letter to the editor). J Cataract Refract Surg 1995; 21:6.
24. Fine IH. Cortical cleaving hydrodissection. J Cataract Refract Surg 1992; 18:508-12.
25. Koch DD, Liu JF. Multilamellar hydrodissection in phacoemulsification and planned extracapsular surgery. J Cataract Refract Surg 1990; 16:559-62.
26. Gimbel HV. Hydrodissection and hydrodelineation. Int Ophthalmol Clin 1994; 34:73-90.
27. Gimbel HV. Posterior capsule tears using phacoemulsification causes, prevention and management. Eur J Implant Refract Surg 1990; 2:63-69.
28. Blumenthal M, Assia E, Neumann D. The round capsulorhexis capsulotomy and the rationale for 11.0 mm diameter IOL. Eur J Implant Refract Surg 1990; 2:15-19.
29. Castaneda VE, Legler UF, Tsai JC, et al. Posterior continuous capsulorhexis. An experimental study with clinical applications. Ophthalmology 1992; 2:63-69.
30. Gimbel HV, DeBroff BM. Posterior capsulorhexis with optic capture: Maintaining a clear visual axis after pediatric cataract surgery. J Cataract Refract Surg 1994; 20:658-64.
31. Gimbel HV. Posterior capsulorhexis with optic capture in pediatric cataract and intraocular lens surgery. Ophthalmology 1996; 103:1871-75.
32. Pande M. Continuous curvilinear (circular) capsulorhexis and planned extracapsular cataract extraction: are they compatible? Br J Ophthalmol 1993; 77:152-57.
33. Vasavada AR, Singh R, Desai J. Phacoemulsification of white cataracts. J Cataract Refract Surg 1998; 24:270-77.
34. Brusini P. Capsulorhexis in mature cataracts: Why not? Doc Ophthalmol 1992; 81:281-84.
35. Hausmann N, Richard G. Investigations on diathermy for anterior capsulotomy. Invest Ophthalmol Vis Sci 1991; 32:2155-59.
36. Vajpeyee RB, Angra SK, Honavar SG, et al. Capsulotomy for phacoemulsification in hypermature cataracts. J Cataracts Refract Surg 1995; 21:612-15.
37. Gimbel HV. Two stage capsulorhexis for endocapsular phacoemulsification. J Cataract Refract Surg 1990; 16:246-49.
38. Auffarth GU, Wesendahl TA, Solomon K, et al. A modified preparation technique for closed system ocular surgery of human eyes obtained postmortem: An improved research and teaching tool. Ophthalmology 1996; 103:977-88.
39. Miyake K, Miyake C. Intraoperative posterior chamber lens haptic fixation in the human cadaver eye. Ophtalmic Surg 1985; 16:230-36.
40. Apple DJ, Lim ES, Morgan RC, et al. Preparation and study of human eyes obtained postmortem with the Miyake posterior photographic technique. Ophthalmology 1990; 97:810-16.
41. Werner L, Apple DJ, Crema A, Izak A, Pandey SK, Trivedi RH, Ma L. Permanent bluish discoloration of a hydrophilic intraocular lenses caused by intraoperative use of trypan blue. J Cataract Refract Surg 2001 (in press).
42. Chang DF. Capsule staining and mature cataracts: A comparison of indocyanine green and trypan blue dyes. Br J Ophthalmol (video report) July 2000.
43. Pandey SK, Werner L, Escobar-Gomez M, Apple DJ, et al. Creating cataracts of varying hardness to practice extracapsular cataract extraction and phacoemulsification. J Cataract Refract Surg 2000; 26:322-29.
44. Pandey SK, Werner L, Vasavada AR, Apple DJ. Induction of cataracts of varying degrees of hardness in human eyes obtained postmortem for cataract surgeon training. Am J Ophthalmol 2000; 129:557-58.

45. Synder RW, Donnenfeld ED. Teaching phacoemulsification to residents and physicians in transition. Int Ophthalmol Clin 1994; 34:191-99.
46. Synder RW, Allinson RW, Fante RG, et al. Learning phacoemulsification surgery. Ophthalmology 1992; 99:448-53.
47. Gimbel HV. Divide and conquer nucleofractis phacoemulsification and variations. J Cataract Refract Surg 1991; 17:281-91.
48. Gimbel HV. Posterior capsule tears using phacoemulsification causes, prevention and management. European J Implant Refract Surg 1990; 2:63-69.
49. Peng Q, Apple DJ, Visessook N, Werner L, Pandey SK, et al. Surgical prevention of posterior capsule opacification. Part II. Enhancement of cortical clean up by focusing on hydrodissection. J Cataract Refract Surg 2000; 26:188-97.
50. Vasavada A, Singh R. Phacoemulsification in eyes with posterior polar cataract. J Cataract Refract Surg 1999; 25:238-45.
51. Basti S, Ravishankar U, Gupta S. Results of a prospective evaluation of management of pediatric cataracts. Ophthalmology 1996;103:713-20.
52. Pandey SK, Wilson ME, Trivedi RH, Izak AM, Macky TA, Werner L, Apple DJ. Pediatric cataract surgery and intraocular lens implantation: Current techniques, complications and management. Int Ophthalmol Clin 2001;41:175-96.
53. Wilson ME, Pandey SK, Werner L, Ram J, Apple DJ. Pediatric Cataract Surgery: Current Techniques, Complications and Management. In Agarwal S, Agarwal A, Sachdev MS, Mehta KR, Fine H, Agarwal A, (Eds): Phacoemulsification, Laser Cataract Surgery and Foldable IOLs. New Delhi, Jaypee Brothers Medical Publishers (P) Ltd, 2000; 39:369-88.
54. Ram J, Pandey SK, Infantile cataract surgery: Current techniques, complications and their management. In Dutta LC, (Ed): Modern Ophthalmology. New Delhi, Jaypee Brothers Medical Publishers (P) Ltd, 2000; 378-84.
55. Vasavada A, Desai J. Primary posterior capsulorhexis with and without anterior vitrectomy in congenital cataracts. J Cataract Refract Surg 1997; 23.
56. Galand A, Cauwenberge VF, Moosavi J. Posterior capsulorhexis in adult eyes with intact and clear capsules. J Cataract Refract Surg 1996;22:458-61.
57. Galand A. Primary posterior capsulorhexis in adults. In Nema HV, Nema N (Eds) Recent Advances in Ophthalmology 4. New Delhi, Jaypee Brothers Medical Publishers (P) Ltd, 1998, 157-61.
58. Cauwenberge VF, Rakic JM, Galand A. Complicated posterior capsulorhexis: Aetiology, management, and outcome. Br J Ophthalmol 1997; 81:195-98.
59. Sharma N, Pangtey MS, Dada VK. Experience with indocyanine green dye (letter). J Cataract Refract Surg 2001; 27:1342.

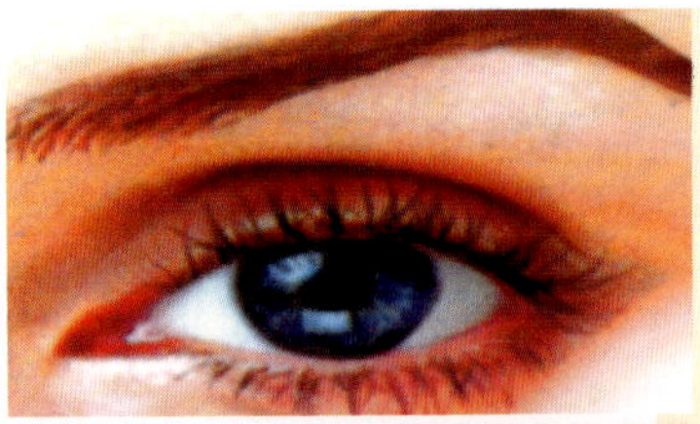

Thirteen

Relevance and Clinical Significance of SICS (Manual Phaco) in Modern Cataract Surgery

RD Ravindran
Haripriya Aravind
Minu Mathen (India)

OBJECTIVE IN MODERN CATARACT
–SURGERY
–SIZE OF INCISION
MANUAL SICS AS AN EFFECTIVE ALTERNATIVE TO PHACOEMULSIFICATION

Cataract is the main cause of avoidable blindness worldwide, with the developing world accounting for three quarters of blindness.[1] Despite the 10 to 12 million cataract operations performed globally, cataract blindness is still thought to be increasing by 1-2 million/year.[2] In order to effectively address this increasing backlog, significant efforts are being undertaken to increase the output of cataract surgical services in many developing countries[3] and to make cataract surgery affordable to all people irrespective of their economic status. The transition from intracapsular cataract surgery to extracapsular surgery with IOL implantation has effected a dramatic change in the postoperative visual outcome, quality of life and increased acceptance of surgical intervention by the community.

The main objective in modern cataract surgery is to achieve a better-unaided visual acuity with rapid post surgical recovery and minimal surgery related complications. Early visual rehabilitation and better-unaided vision can be achieved only by reducing the incision size. The size of the incision in turn depends on mode of nucleus delivery and type of intraocular lens (rigid or foldable). In standard extra capsular cataract extraction, the incision needs to be 10-12mm for safe delivery of nucleus. In manual small incision cataract surgery (SICS). it is between 5.5 to 7mm and in instrumental phaco, it varies from 3 to 6 mm depending on the technique and implant. The use of smaller incision with advantages of faster rehabilitation, less astigmatism and better postoperative vision without spectacles led to phacoemulsification becoming the preferred technique where resources are available.

Despite excellent facilities and skilled surgeons, the poor in the developing world are even deprived of the visual benefits of the IOL because of their inability to afford them.[4] With this background phacoemulsification with all its benefits may not be an affordable technique due to the cost involved in the developing countries. Alternatively manual SICS with its relatively smaller incision has similar advantages to phacoemulsification and is affordable.

Manual SICS has evolved as an effective alternative to phacoemulsification in the present times. Recent studies have proved that Manual SICS is cost-effective and has more benefits than conventional ECCE.[5] To list a few of them

- Better and early wound stability
- Less postoperative inflammation
- Can avoid suture and suture related complications (e.g. iris prolapse, suture infiltrate, bleeding)
- Less postoperative visits
- Early reduction and stability of surgically induced astigmatism.

Moreover, manual SICS can be performed in almost all type of cataracts in contrast to phacoemulsification where case selection is extremely important for an average surgeon. The duration of surgery and phaco power varies with the nucleus density, as also the incidence of intraocular complications, where as in manual SICS, the time spent on nucleus delivery does not vary from case to case. In cataracts with dense nuclei, with the incision enlarged to 7 mm, the nucleus can be delivered with an irrigating vectis. An alternative technique for extraction through a smaller wound is by phacosandwich technique. This is a bimanual technique where under the cover of viscoelastics the nucleus is delivered bimanually with a vectis and Sinskey hook. Phacofracture is another technique used in manual SICS to bring out nuclei of varying grades through a smaller tunnel up to 4 or 5 mm.

Hypermature cataracts with liquefied cortex and hard nuclei can get excellent results with manual SICS. To handle hypermature cataracts in phaco becomes difficult because of the fibrosed capsule, weak zonules, hard mobile nucleus etc., Again traumatic cataracts following penetrating trauma, colobomas, cataract following RD surgery, etc. are better tackled by this procedure.

Capsulorhexis is mandatory for phaco but manual SICS can also be done with the canopener technique. In a study where the learning curve in residents learning phaco was analyzed four patients had to convert to extra capsular cataract extraction and in three patients the reason for 'bailing out' was the absence of an intact rhexis.[6] In MSICS the conversion to ECCE due to an absence of capsulorhexis is not necessary as the nucleus is delivered comfortably even with a canopener capsulotomy.

Incidence of intraoperative complications like posterior capsule rupture is less common in MSICS when compared to phaco. Yet another recent study compared the safety of ECCE, MSICS and phaco, and reported a lower intraoperative and immediate postoperative complication in the MSICS group, when compared with the rest.[7] Certain phaco related complications such as corneal burns due to the phaco probe and iris chaffing are not encountered in manual SICS. The endothelial cell counts on this subgroup of patients are no different from those who have had phacoemulsification.[8] Endothelial cell loss in phaco depends on the density of the nucleus[9] in contrast to manual SICS, where, the skill of the surgeon plays an important role.

Published evidence points out that surgically induced astigmatism following ECCE is 3.91 times higher than MSICS.[6] Their results show that the difference in surgically induced astigmatism between MSICS and phaco with rigid IOL was not statistically significant. Implantation of foldable IOL though a standard procedure in the developed countries, is used only among the affluent society in developing countries. This is because the foldable IOL costs as much as 10 times as that of a rigid IOL. The final visual acuity between these two groups is also comparable. Our own unpublished data shows that the final postoperative visual acuity in both MSICS and phaco are similar.

Surgical time in phacoemulsification is dependent on the type of cataract. In a study performed in a rural eye camp in India manual SICS was performed within 3.8 to 4.2 minutes.[7] Being a faster procedure, manual SICS can be performed in a high volume set up. In an Indian study where cost comparison between the two procedures was done, the average cost for the provider was US$15.82 for ECCE and US$15.68 for SICS.[10] Both these surgeries are thus economical. Yet another study points out the cost to be US$17 for ECCE, US$18 for MSICS and US$ 26 for phacoemulsification.[6] Though the provider costs are similar for MSICS and ECCE, Patient's costs might be lower for SICS patients considering the fewer postoperative medications, follow up visits and spectacles and the total cost may thus work out to be more economical. Another major advantage of manual SICS is that, it is not a machine dominated procedure. The surgical skills and experience of the surgeon play a significant role in the results. Also considerable expense in acquiring and maintaining a machine is not required.

Transition to phacoemulsification is easier if one has mastered Manual SICS, as he is familiar with steps such as scleral pocket incisions, capsulorhexis, hydroprocedures, etc. Familiarity with these steps helps reduce the incidence of complications while learning phaco.[11] There are instances where we have to convert form phacoemulsification to extra capsular cataract surgery. One study reports the conversion rate from phaco to extra capsular by an experienced surgeon to be 3.7 percent.[12] Converting to an extra capsular result in a larger, unstable wound than manual SICS. If one is familiar with the manual nucleus delivery technique with the self-sealing wound one can reduce suture induced astigmatism and other complications.

Phacoemulsification being an expensive technique cannot be employed as the standard procedure in developing countries with a cataract backlog and is a strain on the economy. High quality, high volume cataract surgery has been popularized in eye care centers in India to effectively manage the large backlog of cataract blindness.[13]

In an era where advances are linked to expensive innovative technology, it is exciting to witness the evolution of simplified, low cost alternatives. Manual small incision cataract surgery offers the smaller incision size of phacoemulsification and the added advantage of not requiring expensive equipment. Manual SICS offers all the merits of phacoemulsification with the added advantages of having wider applicability, better safety, with a shorter learning curve and lower cost.

REFERENCES

1. Thylefors B, Negrel AD, Pararajasegaram R, et al. Global data on blindness: An update. Bull World Health Organ 1995;73:115-21.
2. World Health Organisation. Global initiative for the elimination of avoidable blindness. Geneva: WHO, WHO/PBL/97.61
3. Limburg H, Vasavada A, Muzumdar G et al. Rapid assessment of cataract blindness in urban district of Gujarat. Indian J ophthalmol 1999;47:135-41.
4. Malik AR, Qazi ZA, Gilbert C, Visual outcome after high volume cataract surgery in Pakistan. Br J ophthalmol 2003;87:937-940.
5. Gogate PM, Deshpande M, Wormald RP. Is manual small incision cataract surgery affordable in the developing countries? A cost comparison with extracapsular cataract extraction.Br J Ophthalmol. 2003; 87(7):843-6.
6. Muralikrishnan R, Venkatesh R, Babu B Manohar, Prajna N Venkatesh. A comparison of the effectiveness and cost effectiveness of three different methods of cataract extraction in relation to the magnitude of postoperative astigmatism. Asia Pacific J Ophthalmology 2003;15:5-12.
7. Balent LC, Narendran K, Patel S, Kar S, Patterson DA High volume sutureless intraocular lens surgery in a rural eye camp in India. Ophthalmic Surg Lasers. 2001;32(6):446-55.
8. Mathew Ana et al. Manual nucleo fragmentation and endothelial cell loss. J Cataract Refract Surg1997;23:995-99.
9. Hayashi K, Hayashi H, Nakao F, Hayashi F Risk factors for corneal endothelial injury during phacoemulsification. J Cataract Refract Surg. 1996;22(8):1079-84.
10. Gogate PM, Deshpande M, Wormald RP. Is manual small incision cataract surgery affordable in the developing countries? A cost comparison with extracapsular cataract extraction. Br J Ophthalmol. 2003;87(7):843-6.
11. Thomas R, Naveen S, Jacob A, Braganza A Visual outcome and complications of residents learning phacoemulsification. Indian J Ophthalmol. 1997;45(4):215-19.
12. Dada T, Sharma N, Vajpayee RB, Dada VK., Conversion from phacoemulsification to extracapsular cataract extraction: Incidence, risk factors, and visual outcome. J Cataract Refract Surg. 1998;24(11):1521-24
13. Natchiar G, Robin AL, Thulasiraj R. Attacking the backlog of India's curable blind; the Aravind Eye Hospital model Arch Ophthalmol. 1994;112:987-93.

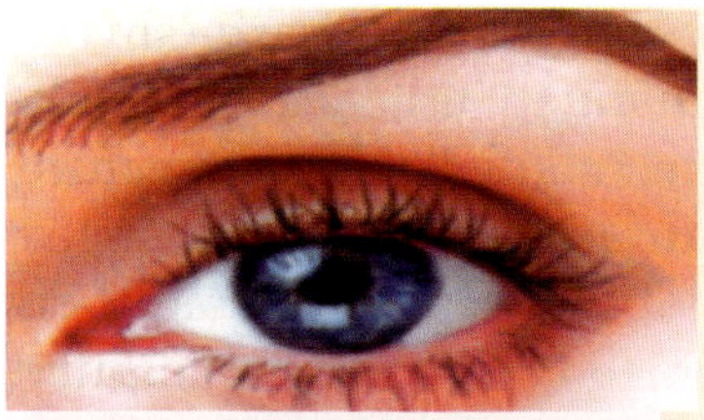

Fourteen

Learning Curve in Small Incision Cataract Surgery

Nikhilesh Trivedi
(India)

MSICS
LEARNING CURVE

The speed at which new techniques are evolving in Ophthalmology, those who like to keep abreast of the latest will soon find themselves emerging out of one learning curve only to plunge down another! However, not all of us are compelled to try out every new fad. Small Incision Cataract Surgery techniques are here to stay. Even in the developed nations in the world, there is an awakening, however late, regarding this modality. MSICS is more and more being looked upon, not as a 'Poor man's Phaco' but rather as a viable, and in some societies a preferable, alternative to Phacoemulsification. There are pros and cons to both the techniques. But the learning and practicing of one does not preclude or forbid dabbling in the other! As per my personal experience, a background in MSICS will ease the learning curve for Phaco, as many steps are common. And being adept at MSICS will also help to "salvage" a Phaco surgery case if one is forced to bail out, and still come out with a respectable sutureless outcome to the surgery!

A far more preferable alternative to having to convert to ECCE, as can happen even in the hands of experienced Phaco surgeons, what to say about learners!

The issue of learning curve in any technique needs to be viewed from at least two perspectives.

The first deals with the process of 'learning' as in the case of the Residents and PGs. The second involves the process of 'unlearning' as in the case of Senior Practitioners, who were trained in more dated and basic techniques like ECCE, or even ICCE, as in my own case!!

We envy the Residents and PGs today, who have a wide choice of training programs, fellowships, and such, to impart excellent training in many modalities. Most of the training institutions in this country now impart sound training to their students in Phacoemulsification as well as, happily, in MSICS. It is a rich and rewarding experience to be trained at the hands of versatile and caring teachers. The future Ophthalmic Surgeons of this country are definitely headed for a brighter and better time. The outcomes of such methodical and planned training are evident. Witness the resident house surgeon who, 3 months after joining Ophthalmology, deftly does an MSICS case in such places. An ongoing study at Sankara Nethralaya has compared the learning curve among the residents between Phaco and SICS. Early findings were presented at an International Workshop on SICS recently. They have found the two learning curves to be almost identical! Though the number of cases studied so far is small and the findings not conclusive, nevertheless a trend is perceptible. These findings speak volumes about the meticulous training programs being conducted by the training institutions. On this front, one does not foresee much difficulty.

The difficulties arise when one was trained, during one's residency and Post-graduation, in more basic techniques like ICCE and ECCE. A lot many of us belong to that era when a trainee's best opportunity was Eye camps, with hoards of ICCE cases to be done. Those among us, who have been fortunate enough to be affiliated to training/teaching institutions, have managed to adapt themselves to the latest advances, as they were supposed to teach the same to their juniors! But imagine the plight of a Private Practitioner. This Surgeon is in his prime, having established a modest or flourishing practice, having learnt, with trepidation and some difficulty, the ECCE+PCIOL, even mastering it in these years. Now he is faced with the daunting task of having to 'unlearn' old habits to adapt to the newer technique!! At this juncture, no aid or assistance is unwanted. Publications like these are our best hope. That, and the many workshops being organized all round the country. There is also some merit in going as an observer to places/surgeons doing volume work in one particular technique. But the most rewarding method for learning MSICS can be condensed in two words: PATIENCE AND PERSEVERENCE.

Indeed, much can be achieved individually, and without systematic training, by following these tenets, while remembering that our first duty is towards restoring sight to the patient. And, that no learning can take precedence over this responsibility. Modifying 1-2 steps at a time can be considered, as also experimenting on Goat's eyes, which are easily available. The biggest roadblock, I believe is the **mental block**. It is the very step involving making an incision on Sclera that holds us back initially!! But then, who said learning is easy? Believe me, the rewards of learning MSICS are worth more than all the effort you might have put in. And remember, learning MSICS will only make learning phaco later that much easier.

Another important point is: USE GOOD/ EXCELLENT INSTRUMENTS, BLADES etc.!!!

A poor instrument or blade will only make your task that much more unpleasant and difficult. It is always wiser to invest in instruments initially so that you get used to your personal set early on. (Also, the pressure of having spent money will help you in persevering with the learning!!)

As far as possible, follow one technique only, and go step by step, as taught by a learned master. Only after a reasonable trial, switch over to another technique of MSICS. There are many. Each has its own merits and demerits. No one technique is absolutely the best universally! One has to decide, by trial and error, as to which will suit one the best.

Many good textbooks, atlases, and videos or CDs are available for most techniques. And many experienced surgeons are willing to share their experiences and opinions with a patient listener. It is always advisable to consult regarding instruments, materials to be used, etc. with somebody who uses them on a daily basis. The primary objective should be to adapt oneself to a technique that will give 'better' results in ones own hands.

To begin with, those converting from ECCE to MSICS should focus on the making of a tunnel, which is a step that mostly differentiates between ECCE and MSICS. A cool head is an important ingredient for success. I'd even suggest choosing a Sunday, posting 2-3 cases, and inviting an experienced colleague to stand beside you for moral support. Contrary to the steps as described in the text, it is prudent for the beginner to *make the tunnel first and foremost,* so that one can easily convert to ECCE should one fail to fashion a satisfactory tunnel wound. Practicing tunneling on a Goat's eye, particularly with an AC Maintainer, would also be a good idea. There should be no ego involved, and no hesitation in converting to ECCE in case of any doubt or loss of confidence. For the same reason, there should be no advance 'publicity' of providing 'sutureless' surgery (or Phaco surgery, for that matter!) to one's patients, till one has mastered the technique. It will only add to the pressures on the hapless learner. Being relaxed in the OT is very important. Perhaps important enough to sacrifice a couple of Sundays for learning!

There is no substitute to visual learning. Attending workshops, watching videos/CDs, and reading textbooks can be of great help. Even after one does a few cases successfully, this relearning will help in ironing out wrinkles, and help in solving some practical difficulties one may have faced during actual surgery.

The learning curve for MSICS is, perhaps for most of us, less steep and less expensive than that for phaco. Nevertheless, there is a learning curve. One should not lose sight of this fact! But rest assured, this is much easier to learn and master, provided you approach it with an open mind.

REFERENCES

1. Thomas R, Kuriakose T, George R: Efficient Small Incision Cataract Surgery, Indian Journal of Ophthalmology 2000;48:145-51.
2. Dada T, Sharma N, Vajpayee RB, Dada VK: Conversion from phacoemulsification to extracapsular cataract extraction: Incidence, risk factors, and visual outcome. J Cataract Refract Surg 1998;24:1521-24.
3. Thomas R, Braganza A, Raju R, Lawrence, Spitzer KH: Phacoemulsification- A Senior surgeon's learning curve. Ophthalmic Surgery 1994; 24(8): 504-9.
4. Thomas R, Naveen S, Jacob A, Braganza A: Visual outcome and complications of residents learning phacoemulsification. Indian Journal of Ophthalmology 1997;45: 215-19.

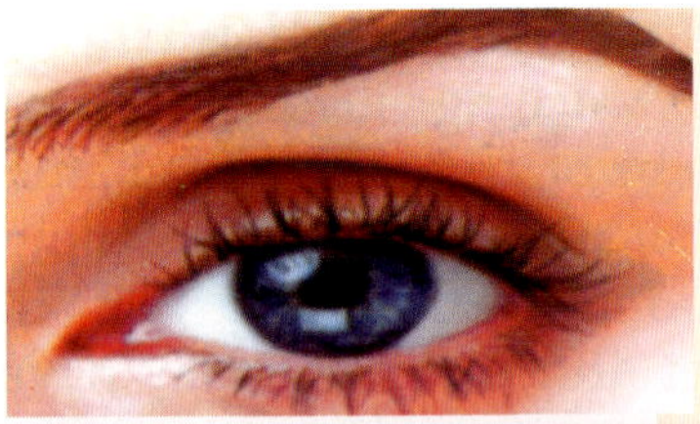

Fifteen

Preoperative Preparation of the Patient in Small Incision Cataract Surgery

Ashok Garg (India)

INTRODUCTION

In manual small incision cataract surgery (SICS) there is obvious need to adequately asses the patient ophthalmic suitability preoperatively through ophthalmic and general medical history as well as complete ocular examination and several special investigations. Complete ophthalmic check up and investigations results are analysed to ensure that surgical plan does not breach any surgical technical exclusions and to ensure best postoperative results.

In clinical practice it is seen that many patients are at a heightened risk of developing an intra-operative or postoperative complications, which can be, identified preoperatively due to the presence of one or more risk factors. A comprehensive history and detailed clinical examination needs to be a part of every preoperative assessment to ensure any such risk factors are identified.

Some risk factors like external ocular infections can be modified allowing the surgery to proceed. It is not necessary that all patients with a risk factor will develop a complication however good clinical management shows that with such an visually important elective procedure, it is better to exclude some patients who may have a successful outcome to protect those at a heightened risk of significant complications.

In clinical practice we have seen that it is always easier to explain to the patient why they can not have surgery than why they have developed a significant complication. To a greater extent criteria of a good SICS surgery practice is the rigor of its exclusion criteria.

Most eye surgeon hold the general principals of good cataract surgery. However, the exact numerical value at which patients are counselled not to have surgery often varies depending upon.

PREOPERATIVE ASSESSMENT AND CONSIDERATIONS

First of all detailed history of the patients should be taken.

History

A directed ocular and general history should be taken to identify any ophthalmic instability or the presence of any specific risk factors. It is necessary to exclude the presence of serious systemic diseases like hypertension, diabetes mellitus, cardiac problems, obstructive lung, disorders and any potential source of infection in the body like urinary tract infection (UTI), septic gums etc. The necessary testing depends upon the patient age and prior medical history.

A preoperative ophthalmological evaluation should include a complete ocular history specially related to recurrent redness, pain, discharge or previous ophthalmic treatment if any Refractive history should be taken to assess whether the patient is ammetropic or emmetropic at the age of +40 years. It is essential in relation to IOL power calculation and status of scleral rigidity as it is directly related to nucleus delivery during SICS.

Past ocular history is quite important specially in relation to previous corneal grafts, previous microbial Keratitis, previous herpes simplex Keratitis or previous retinal surgery, family history specially in first degree relatives should be taken for any ocular disorder which may hamper visual out come after SICS.

Clinical Examination

Complete and thorough ocular examination is necessary to rule out comorbid conditions such as long standing amblyopia, pseudo exfoliation, retinal tears or holes, macular lesions or optic nerve abnormalities that may affect the visual or surgical outcome. The following useful information is required before the patients is declared fit for SICS.

An accurate refraction of both eyes, measurement of corneal refractive power by Keratometer and measurement of axial length by A–Scan ultrasonography are necessary to calculate appropriate IOL power should be done.

Good assessment of corneal endothelium should be made by examining cornea by Eisner lens or by specular Microscopy (whenever available). It helps in excluding patients with low endothelial cell count specially in conditions like glaucoma, chronic iritis, Fuch's Dystrophy, trauma and old age. Keratic precipitates (KP) should also be examined.

Retinal Function Tests

The retinal functions should be thoroughly evaluated as if it is faulty even a good quality operation shall be useless from vision angle and patient must be warned about the prognosis to avoid unnecessary disappointment and medicolegal problem. A few important retinal functions are described here.

- Perception of light (PL) must be present for potential useful postoperative vision.
- Marcus-Gunn pupillary response test should be done routinely because in its presence visual prognosis is poor.
- Projection of light (PR) is an important test for functions of peripheral retina and should be done routinely. A poor PR inference shall indicate towards the poor visual prognosis.
- Two light discrimination test should be done to know about macular function. If the patient perceive two normal lights in this test it indicates normal macular function.
- Maddox rod test : An accurate perception of red line indicates normal function.
- Color perception indicates macular function is present and optic nerve is relatively normal.

- Entopic visualization is done to know about retinal functions.
- Laser interferometry (wherever possible) is a good test for measuring the macular potential for visual acuity in the presence of opaque media.
- Objective tests for evaluating retina are essential when some retinal pathology is suspected. These tests include:
  B.Scan ultrasonography of the posterior segment of the eye.
  — Electroretinogram (ERG).
  — Electro oculogram (EOG)
  — Visually evoked response (VER)
  — Indirect ophthalmoscopy
  — Color Doppler ultrasonography.

Potential local source of infection should be checked by ruling out conjunctival infections, meibomitis, Blepharitis, Lacrimal sac infection and chronic dacryocystitis. Thorough Lacrimal sac examination including syringing should be done. In case of presence of chronic dacryocystitis DCR (Dacryocystorhinostomy) or DCT (Dacryo cystectomy) should be performed prior to SICS.

Complete anterior segment examination by slit lamp biomicroscopy should be done in each case routinely to rule out any Keratic precipitate present at the back of cornea, subtle uveitis etc.

Iris pupil examination under slit lamp should be done under mesopic condition to see for any evidence of posterior synchiae, pigment on lens or pupil abnormalities. Pupil examination should also be done after dilatation to know details about iris and pupil status (whether dilating easily or not). Small contracted pupil makes capsulorrhexis very difficult and nucleus prolapse into anterior chamber become impossible.

- Complete lens examination should be done by pupil dilation to ascertain the cataract grading.
- Thorough Fundus Examination is necessary to rule out macular degeneration, diabetic maculopathy and optic atrophy.
- Hypotonic eye is not fit for SICS as it is very difficult to make scleral tunnel wound construction in hypotonic eye. It is also difficult in nucleus prolapse in AC expression of nucleus in hypotonic eye. It is generally advised not to put pinky ball or any other IOP lowering gadget prior to SICS. Instead gentle massage of the eye with finger can be done after peribulbar anesthesia.
- Age of patient is quite important because nucleus hardness increase with advancing age. Hence, very old patients with very hard and big nucleus should be avoided for SICS.
- Preoperative IOP measurement should be done in each case. The presence of raised IOP shall require a prior management before cataract surgery.

Patients who had undergone glaucoma filtering surgery are not ideal for manual SICS due to hypotony factor.

- Patients who had recurrent episodes of anterior or posterior uveitis with synechiae formation are not suitable for SICS for the following rationale.
- It is difficult to perform capsulorrhexis as the pupil does not dilate full because of synechiae adhesions between Iris and capsule.
- Nucleus prolapse into AC becomes difficult.
- Due to weak posterior capsule there are increased chances of vitreous prolapse and PC rent.
- Iatrogenic inflammation is more intense in uveitic patients.
- Increased chances of Zonular weakness, high IOP, miosis and Cystoid macular edema.

There are certain absolute contraindications in which SICS should not be performed. These include:

- Fuch's endothelial dystrophy.
- Microphthalmos
- Extensive congenital anomalies
- Rubella iridis
- Lens subluxation
- Preoperative counseling for surgery should include a full explanation of the potential risks and benefits of proposed SICS and anesthesia as well as the technique for instilling eye drops and ointments and other postoperative care.
- Both Out patients and indoor surgical facilities are used for SICS, with the latter reserved for patients at risk for medical complications well equipped outpatients surgical facilities offer the

patient the shortest possible surgical experience and reduce to a minimum the disruption of the patients normal life routine.

PREOPERATIVE MEDICATIONS AND PREPARATIONS

Topical antibiotics such as levofloxacin(0.5%) or tobramycin(0.3%) three to four times a day 72 hours before SICS should be started as prophylaxis against infections.

- Systemic antibiotics such as ciprofloxacin 500mg twice daily is advised by some ophthalmic surgeons at previous night and in the morning before surgery.
- Preparation of the eye to be operated includes trimming of eye lashes of upper eyelid at previous night and eye to be operated should be properly marked to avoid last minute confusion.
- Each patient should be advised to take scrub bath including face and hairwash with soap and water before surgery.
- Preoperative IOP lowering is done by giving oral acetazolamide tablety 500mg stat 2 hours before the surgery preoperative IOP reduction prevent operative complications such as vitreous loss, expulsive choroidal hemorrhage and shallowing of the anterior chamber.
- Mydriasis is essential for SICS. It is crucial that pupil is widely dilated throughout the procedure time. This is most achieved with a preoperative combination of an adrenergic agent (Phenylephrine 5-10%), an anticholinergic agent (tropicamide-1%) and a cyclo-oxygenase inhibitor (flurbiprofen). Intraoperative mydriasis may also be maintained with the use of dilute epinephrine in the irrigating solution.
- Some times highly anxious and nervous patients are also given oral diazepam in small dose (2.5-5.0mg) one hour before surgery to alleviate the anxiety.
- Mental preparation of patient for the surgery is essential. A written consent should be taken from the patient or from his near relative regarding full explanation of pros and cons of surgery to the patient by the operating doctor.
- Preoperative prepping–antibiosis is used to prevent postoperative endophthalmitis. Most surgeons prepare the lids and facial skin with 10 percent povidone iodine and placing a drops of 5 percent povidone iodine into the conjunctival cul-de-sac.

In summary, the key to successful small incision cataract surgery is proper selection of cases, efficient counseling of the patients and meticulous preoperative preparation of the patients. A well planned SICS (Step by step) can ensure satisfactory postoperative visual acuity to the patients without any complications.

REFERENCES

1. Garg Ashok. Cataract in text book of ophthalmology, New Delhi: Jaypee Brothers 3:1620-59.
2. Singh Kamaljeet : Small incision cataract surgery, New Delhi: Jaypee Brothers 2002.
3. Natchair G. In Manual small incision cataract surgery, Arvind Publication, India: 2000.
4. Shah Anil: In small incision cataract surgery, Bhalani Publishing House, India: 2000.
5. Rozakis GW, In cataract surgery, Alternative small incision technique, Ist Ed. Thordofare Inc 1995.

Section Two

Manual Small Incision Cataract Surgery (MSICS) Techniques

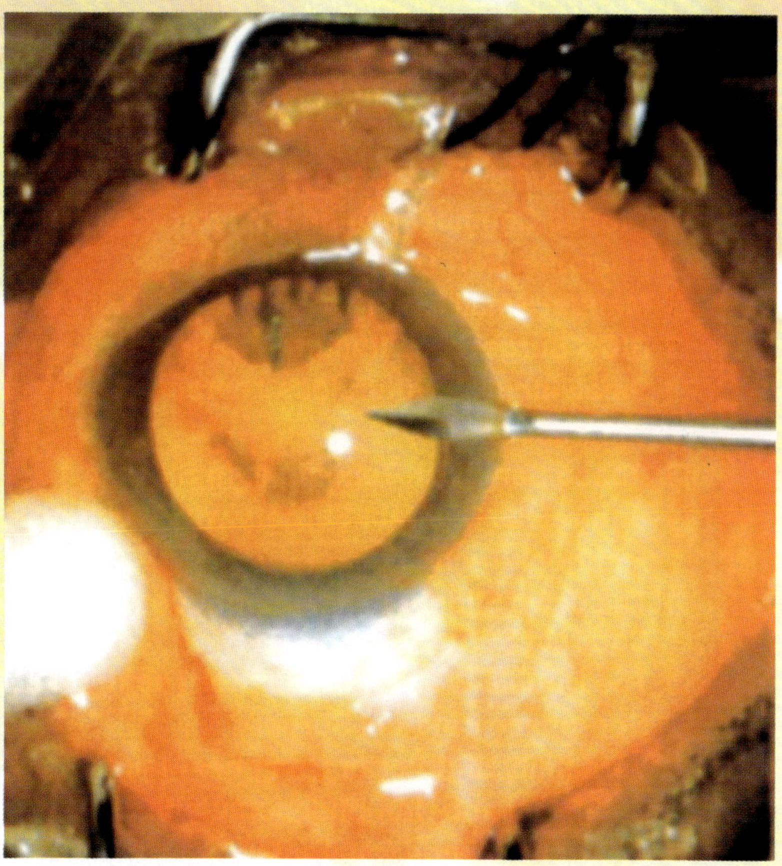

- The Dynamics of Sutureless Cataract Incisions
- Small Incision Planned Extra
- Dynamics of Incision and Wound Construction in SICS
- Capsulorhexis
- Dynamics of Hydroprocedures in Manual Small Incision Cataract Surgery
- Dynamics of Cortex and Epinucleus Aspiration in Manual Small Incision Cataract Surgery
- Dynamics of Nucleus Management in SICS
- IOL Implantation Techniques in Manual Small Incision Cataract Surgery
- Materials for Intraocular Lenses
- Blumenthal's Technique in MSICS: A 100% Approach
- Phacofracture Technique in SICS
- Manual Multiphacofragmentation (MPF) Allows for Small Incision Cataract Surgery
- Closed Chamber Manual Phacofragmentation
- Phacosection Technique in SICS
- Manual Small Incision Cataract Surgery Using Irrigating Vectis
- SICS Surgery in Difficult Situations
- Small Incision Sutureless Temporal Approach Extracapsular Cataract Surgery
- Phaco Sandwich Technique in SICS
- Sutureless Cataract Surgery with Nucleus Extraction—Fishhook Technique
- The Jaws Slider Pincer Technique for Small Incision Non-phaco Cataract Surgery
- The Double Wire Snare Splitter Technique for Small Incision, Non-phaco Cataract Surgery
- Versatility of Anterior Chamber Maintainer in SICS
- Small Incision Non-phacoemulsification Surgery and Glaucoma
- SICS in Pediatric Cataracts
- Mini Nuc Cataract Surgery Under Topical Anesthesia
- Ocular Pharmacokinetics in Manual Small Incision Cataract Surgery

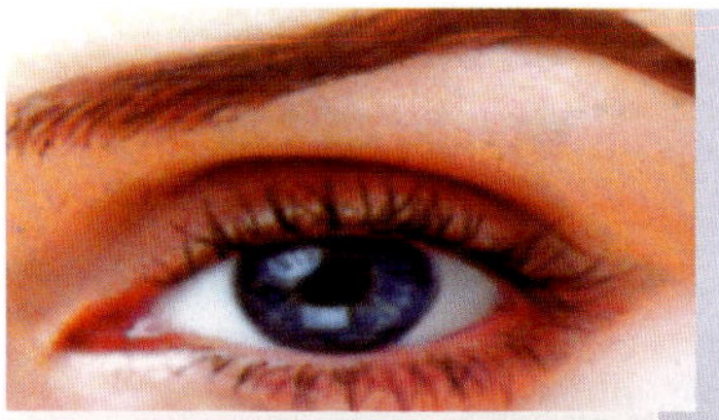

Sixteen

The Dynamics of Sutureless Cataract Incisions

Samuel L Pallin (USA)

HISTORY

Prior to the advent of silk sutures, sutureless cataract incisions were the norm of necessity in ophthalmology but they were not self-sealing for obvious reasons relating to technique and instrumentation. Many advances in technique and technology have taken us through several stages in the evolution of modern cataract operations. The earliest mentions of self-sealing cataract incisions were made by Richard P Kratz in 1980[1] and by Louis J Girard in 1984.[2,3] Dr Kratz viewed the scleral tunnel incision as an astigmatism-neutral method of entering the anterior segment and felt that the sutures which he routinely used provided a "belt and suspenders" secure closure. In 1980s, a mention was made by Jim Gills at a meeting in Atlanta, Georgia, USA, that a sutureless cataract closure should be possible. In March, 1990, Steven B Siepser described a radial transverse incision which admitted only foldable implants.[4] This was a workable but technically difficult incision, and was potentially dangerous in inexperienced hands. A brief published report in *Ocular Surgery News* in March, 1990 quoted Michael McFarland[5] who indicated he had developed a sutureless incision for foldable implants which was based on a series of relaxing incisions in

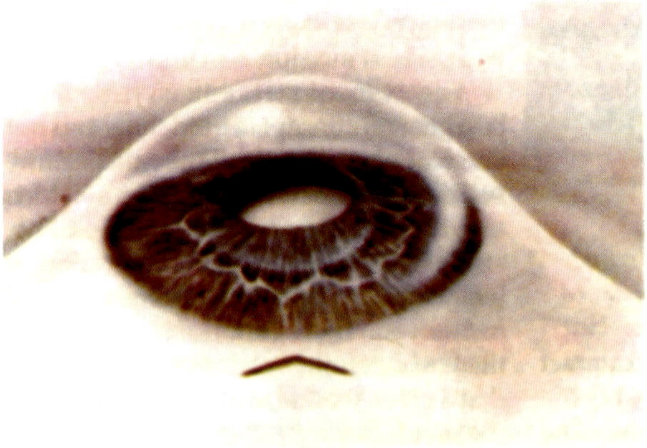

Fig. 16.1: Artist's depiction of the author's Chevron® incision

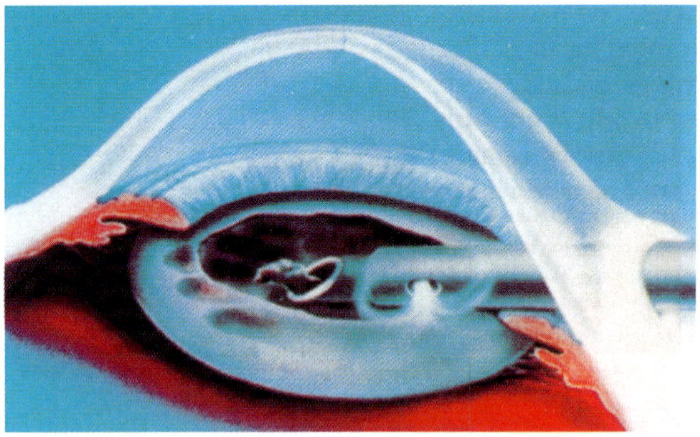

Fig. 16.2: Artist's depiction of a corneal incision

the bed of a scleral tunnel. In April, 1990 a Chevron-shaped sutureless scleral tunnel incision (Fig. 16.1) was described by the author in a letter to the Editor of the *Journal of Cataract and Refractive Surgery*.[6] The Chevron® incision was designed to admit not only foldable but rigid lenses as well, and was practical and easily adopted by cataract surgeons. Preliminary results with the Chevron® incision[7] were presented at the 1991 American Society of Cataract and Refractive Surgeons (ASCRS) meeting in Boston, Massachusetts. A similar incision called the Frown incision was widely popularized by Jack Singer. Dr. Singer initially closed with one suture and later adapted the Frown incision to sutureless cataract surgery.[8]

Sutured wounds were not all bad. Like all stages in the advancement of technology, they participated in a cascade of improvements to the field, not the least of which was the use of the operating microscope. It was the quest for finer sutures and better wounds that stimulated the transition to modern microsurgery in ophthalmology.

The incision preferred by the majority of ophthalmologists in the United States today is the clear-corneal incision (Fig. 16.2). Most current incisions are designed to be suture free and self-sealing.[9] It has become clear that the more corneal the placement of the incision, the certainty of self-sealing without sutures decreases. **A scleral tunnel incision or a limbal tunnel incision in most hands will seal if the geometry is correct. Corneal incisions still require sutures in some cases because of the nature of corneal tissue which resists stretching, and because of the tendency of the incision to tear during implant insertion.**[10,11] According to Nick Mamalis, [12] corneal incisions measured pre- and post- insertion of folded implants show a mean increase in internal width of 4.4 to 6.2 percent, depending upon whether forceps or injector insertion technique is used.

COMMON DENOMINATOR

Having come to this point in the history of the cataract incision, it is appropriate to see what might be the common denominator of self-sealing incisions. The earliest theory proposed was called the "corneal flap mechanism." In this therapy, a layer of deep cornea seals from the interior against the wound creating a trap-door effect when the eye is reinflated. This was a popular theory to explain self-sealing incisions until April, 1995. In that year at the annual meeting of the ASCRS in San Diego, California, this author presented gonioscopic photographs (Fig. 16.3) showing insertion of an implant through the angle with a slit-like internal incision and no corneal flap.[13] The incision was in fact self-sealing, as have been many others like it.

PROPERTIES

So, to what factors can we ascribe the self-sealing quality of a cataract incision? **One theoretical principle which seems to stand the test of time is the so-called "square incisional geometry." This means that the length of the tunnel must be equal to or exceed the width of the incision.** In other

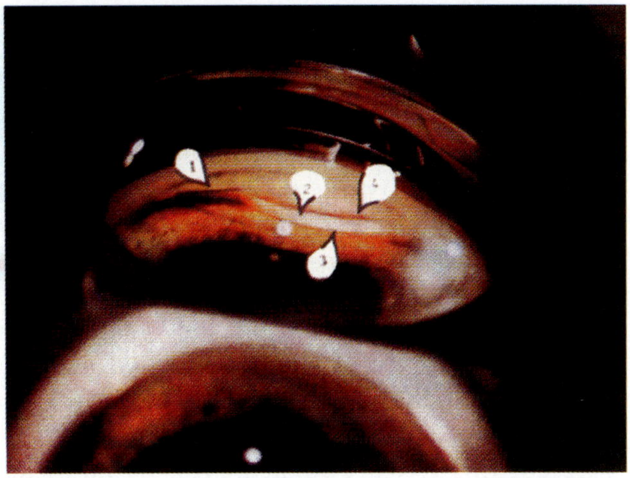

Fig. 16.3: Internal view through gonioscopic lens: 1—IOL haptic, 2—wound, 3—leading edge of optic, and 4—trabecular meshwork

words, a short tunnel with a long incision is less likely to be self-sealing than a long tunnel with a short incision.

Square incisional geometry should be understood to be a general concept, a guideline, and not a strict rule for surgical planning. While the theoretical ideal of a self-sealing tunnel would be a figure in which length is equal to width, in the real world self-sealing incisions only strive to approach that configuration. Rarely does the length of the tunnel actually equal the width of the entry incision and more commonly is marginally smaller. But there is a definite relationship in which the probability that a given wound will be self-sealing is proportional to the successful approximation of square geometry.

It is pertinent to discuss two incisions, one at either end of the tunnel: the first is the external entry wound to the tunnel, and the second is the internal communication between the tunnel and the anterior chamber. The reason for the importance of this distinction is that one can make an incision into becoming a self-sealing wound by making the external incision small and the internal incision larger. Lest the reader assume this configuration violates the square geometry rule, bear in mind that the tunnel is still nearly as long as the internal incision and longer than the external incision. In fact a smaller external incision is more reliably self-sealing than a larger external incision. Since a small incision presents an obstacle to the insertion of lens implants, the *external* incision can be made in a geometric shape which lends itself to stretching and thus will admit a lens implant without difficulty (e.g. Chevron or Frown). The *internal* incision located in corneal territory does not lend itself to stretching and tearing can be dangerous. Therefore, the internal incision must be of a size to admit the chosen lens implant. So, the properties of the reliable self-sealing incision are

- Square incisional geometry
- Relatively short external incision, with a tunnel that flares to a larger internal incision
- A geometric external incision *shape* which lends itself to stretching.

Incisions which do not meet these criteria are subject to tearing or are problematic when required to be self-sealing.

Given the above answers to the question, "What constitutes the essential elements of a self-sealing cataract incision?" One also might like to know what explanation we have for the fact that a pressurized sphere refrains from ejecting its contents through an incision to the atmosphere? In practical terms one can think about the globe as a double-walled structure, at least in the vicinity of the wound. For the purposes of a cataract incision, one wall is the roof of the tunnel and one is the floor of the tunnel. It is these two layers acting in a predictable manner when pressure is applied from within during reformation of the anterior chamber that results in closure of the wound. Visualize for example two latex balloons of the kind we see at children's parties. One balloon is inserted inside the other balloon. One can make an incision in the outer balloon and then inflate the inner balloon and no air escapes. This is intuitively obvious. If on the other hand, one were to make an incision in the inner balloon as well but place that incision in a remote location away from the incision in the external balloon, and then inflate the internal balloon, one can imagine that the two disparate incisions would fail to communicate and inflation would still be viable. This mechanism is similar to what occurs in the globe after reinflation of the anterior chamber following cataract removal and lens implantation. The internal incision in the anterior chamber, whether it be in clear cornea or at the limbus, is remote from the external incision on the sclera, the limbus, or the cornea. The two incisions do not communicate directly. Communication can be forced by accessing the tunnel between them. When the internal pressure of the eye is re-established and the tunnel reacts to increased pressure from the interior as compared with ambient atmospheric pressure on the exterior surface of the globe, the tunnel collapses and the two incisions, in disparate locations, no longer communicate.

The current popularity of clear-corneal incisions is understandable considering several advantages

- Topical and intracameral anesthesia have been shown to be most effective in clear-corneal procedures.[14, 15]
- Corneal incisions are usually located at the temporal aspect of the anterior segment which tends to counteract against-the-rule (ATR) astigmatism found in the elderly population most commonly.[16,17]
- The lack of the necessity to incise conjunctiva and cauterize blood vessels saves time and is esthetically pleasing to the surgeon.

However, there are some disadvantages also to corneal incisions:

- It is difficult to obtain square incisional geometry since a long tunnel through cornea presents a problem during manipulations in the anterior chamber.[18,19] This phenomenon has been called "oarlocking" (Fig. 16.4).

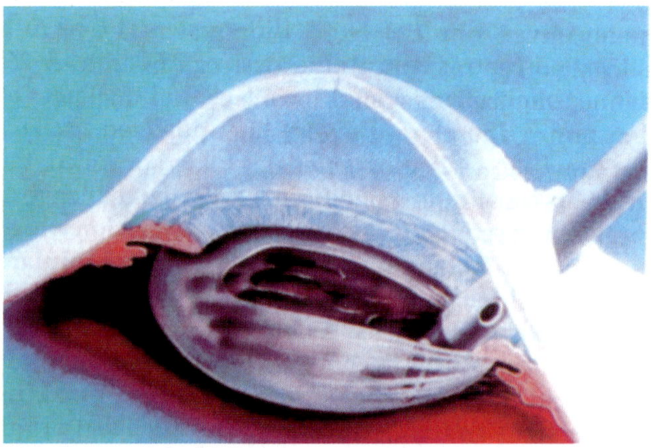

Fig. 16.4: Artist's depiction of an example of oarlocking

- Since the tunnel in a clear-corneal incision cannot be very long, square geometry dictates the external incision be limited in length. Short external corneal incisions tend to tear when a lens implant is forced through an incision of marginal size.[11,12,20,21]
- Corneal tissue does not heal quickly, is not usually subject to fibrosis, and forms relatively weak adhesive bonds making the incisions less secure.[11,22]
- Corneal incisions depend for their integrity upon swelling of the lips of the incision initially. However, swelling is a transient phenomenon and the incision which appears to be self-sealing at surgery may be easily induced to leak in the postoperative period.

According to Kurt Buzard, "It is by no means certain that the shift of the external opening of the incision toward the cornea [from the sclera] is beneficial, and in fact it is our contention that it is a negative development with disadvantages that are hidden by the smaller size routinely used for clear-corneal incisions.[23]

With respect to iatrogenic astigmatism—there is a controversy over whether a superior scleral tunnel incision or a temporal clear-corneal incision induces less astigmatism. If there is a difference, it appears to be a small one. But there is agreement over the fact that earlier stabilization occurs with scleral tunnel incisions. [24-26]

A few words about folding lens implants versus rigid implants—since small incisions in general and clear-corneal incisions in particular are favored based upon the premise that smaller and smaller incisions are preferable, it is necessary to regard the lens implant as the limiting factor in the tendency to decreasing size of incision. Bear in mind that the geometry of a lens implant is three-dimensional. One has to account for the diameter of the implant, but what is often forgotten is that one must also account for the thickness. For example, a planoconvex implant of 15 diopters might have a calculated central optical thickness of 0.64 mm. A 25-diopter similar lens would have a central thickness of 0.98 mm.[27] Therefore if a very high-powered implant (for example, a +25 diopter lens) is folded or rolled, the thickness constitutes a significant part of the challenge in the insertion sequence. **In other words, an incision which is sufficient in length to admit a 15-diopter implant**

which is folded, may *not* be sufficiently large to admit a 25-diopter folded lens. As a result there is a law of diminishing returns in choosing folding lens implants over rigid implants solely for the purpose of making the incision smaller. It is possible to imagine that a rigid implant of say, 15 diopters may actually require a smaller incision than a very thick folded implant of 25 diopters. **Add to this the fact that some soft lens materials have a lower index of refraction than the polymethylmethacrylate (PMMA) of hard implants. With a lower index of refraction, the foldable implant must be thicker than its hard counterpart of the same power.**

It is also true that the "smaller is better" dictum as applies to incisions has limitations. Transitioning from a large planned extracapsular incision to a small phacoemulsification incision does provide increased wound integrity and decreased iatrogenic astigmatism. But it is not clear that the same advantage applies, for instance, when the transition is from a scleral tunnel incision of 4.0 or 4.5 mm to a clear-corneal incision of approximately 3.2 mm (note—the author's Chevron incision stretches from approximately 4.0 mm to more than 5.5 mm).[7]

Nevertheless, clear-corneal incisions and folded lens implants have become the most popular combination of choice by United States surgeons today.[9] **With the burgeoning numbers of clear-corneal procedures it is not surprising that some of these are subject to tearing during implant insertion and may require a suture for security more often than a scleral tunnel or limbal tunnel incision does.**

CONCLUSION

In conclusion, it is proper to say that many variations of incisional design and incisional closure are viable and successful. Modern cataract incisions vary in geographic and anatomical location from superior to temporal and from scleral to clear corneal in position and location. There is agreement in two areas: (i) it is generally accepted that a smaller incision is better than a larger incision—this is true for reasons of wound integrity and the control of iatrogenic astigmatism, and (ii) there seems to be agreement among surgeons and patients that self-sealing incisions are preferred to sutured incisions. No doubt there will be continued progress in the area of wound construction and there is a plethora of solutions and more on the horizon with respect to management of astigmatism. Wound length, wound placement, tee-cuts, relaxing incisions, toric intraocular implants, and laser ablations in the photorefractive keratectomy (PRK) and in the LASIK configurations are available to modify astigmatism at the present time. Astigmatism historically has been the greatest stimulus to the exploration of cataract wound design. It is possible that with laser ablation and wavefront analysis the treatment of first order and higher order aberrations will be accomplished as a distinct and separate procedure making the astigmatism concern of very little significance in cataract wound design. The one challenge that will always attend cataract surgery is a secure suture-free closure. In this discussion a description of those principles which lead to reliable self-sealing closures is presented.

REFERENCES

1. Kratz RP, Colvard DM, Mazzocco TR et al: Clinical evaluation of the Terry surgical keratometer. Am Intraocular Implant Soc J 1980;6:249-51.
2. Girard LJ, Hofmann RF: Scleral tunnel to prevent induced astigmatism. In Emery JM, Jacobson AC (Eds): Current Concepts in Cataract Surgery: Proceedings of the Eighth biennial Cataract Surgical Congress Norwalk: Appleton-Century-Crofts 1984;101-02.
3. Girard LJ: Origin of the scleral tunnel incision (letter). J Cataract Refract Surg 1995;21:7.
4. Radial Incision Helps Reduce Astigmatic Forces. Ocular Surgery News 1990;1.
5. Surgeon Undertakes Phaco, Foldable IOL Series Sans Sutures. Ocular Surgery News 1990;1.
6. Pallin SL: Chevron incision for cataract surgery (letter). J Cataract Refract Surg 1990;16:779-81.
7. Pallin SL: Chevron sutureless closure—a preliminary report. Proceedings American Society of Cataract and Refractive Surgery Annual Symposium Boston, MA, 1991, and later published J Cataract Refract Surg 1991;17:706-09.
8. Singer JA: Frown incision for minimizing induced astigmatism after small incision cataract surgery with rigid optic intraocular lens implantation. J Cataract Refract Surg 1991;17:677-88.

9. Leaming DV: Practice styles and preferences of ASCRS members—1998 survey. J Cataract Refract Surg 1999;25:851-59.
10. Ernest PH: Cataract incisions—rationale for the limbus. EyeWorld 1997;2(9):56.
11. Radner W, Amon M, Mallinger R: Diamond-tip versus blunt-tip caliper enlargement of clear corneal incisions. J Cataract Refract Surg 1997;23:272-76.
12. Mamalis N: Incision width after phacoemulsification with foldable intraocular lens implantation. J Cataract Refract Surg 2000;26:237-41.
13. Pallin SL: Self-sealing versus corneal flap. Proceedings of the American Society of Cataract and Refractive Surgery Annual Symposium San Diego, CA. 1995
14. Gills J: The Use of Intraocular Xylocaine to Control Intra-operative Discomfort During IOL Surgery. Proceedings from the Fifth Annual Ocular Surgery News Symposium Cataract and Refractive Surgery (Suppl) 1997;22.
15. Koch P: Anterior chamber irrigation with 1% unpreserved lidocaine for anesthesia for cataract surgery—a prospective sutdy of 400 cases. Proceedings from the Fifth Annual Ocular Surgery News Symposium Cataract and Refractive Surgery (Suppl) 1997;32.
16. Fine IH: Corneal tunnel incision with a temporal approach. In Fine IH, Fichman RA, Grabow HB (Eds): Clear-Corneal Cataract Surgery and Topical Anesthesia Slack: Thorofare 1993;5-28.
17. Fine IH: Self-sealing corneal tunnel incision for small-incision cataract surgery. Ocular Surgery News 1992;38-39.
18. Ernest PH, Lavery KT, Kiessling LA: Relative strength of scleral corneal and clear corneal incisions constructed in cadaver eyes. J Cataract Refract Surg 1994;20:626-29.
19. Mackool RJ, Russell RS: Strength of clear corneal incisions in cadaver eyes. J Cataract Refract Surg 1996;22:721-25.
20. Kohnen T, Lambert RJ, Koch DD: Incision size for foldable intraocular lenses. Ophthalmology 1997;104:1277-86.
21. Steinert RF, Deacon J: Enlargement of incision with phacoemulsification and folded intraocular lens implant surgery. Ophthalmology 1996;103:220-25.
22. Ernest P, Tipperman R, Eagle R et al: Is there a difference in incision healing based on location? J Cataract Refract Surg 1998;24:482-86.
23. Buzard KA, Febbraro JL: Transconjunctival corneoscleral tunnel "blue line" cataract incision. J Cataract Refract Surg 2000;26:242-49.
24. Lyhne N, Krogsager J, Corydon L et al: One year follow-up of astigmatism after 4.0 mm temporal clear corneal and superior scleral incisions. J Cataract Refract Surg 2000;26:83-87
25. Olse T, Dam Johansen M, Bek T et al: Corneal versus scleral tunnel incision in cataract surgery: a randomized study. J Cataract Refract Surg 1997;23:337-41.
26. Huang FC, Tseng SH: Comparison of surgically induced astigmatism after sutureless temporal clear corneal and scleral frown incisions. J Cataract Refract Surg 1998;24:477-81.
27. Naeser K, Naeser EV: Calculation of the thickness of an intraocular lens. J Cataract Refract Surg 1993;19:40-42.

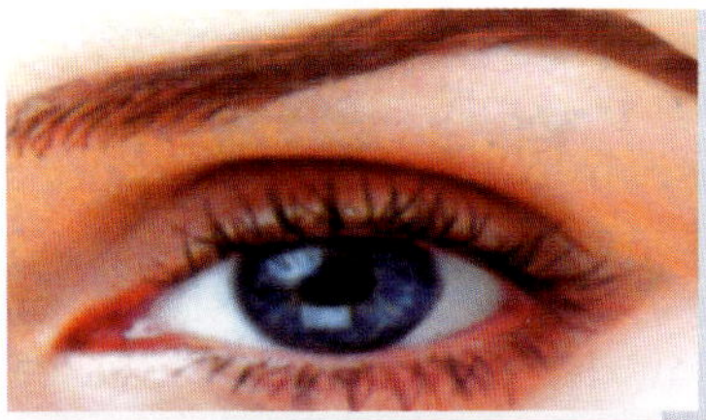

Seventeen

Small Incision Planned Extra

Luther L Fry (USA)

INTRODUCTION

In this chapter, I would like to describe a small incision manual technique which I have used since 1985. It involves "sandwiching" the nucleus out between a lens loop and spatula. This technique uses an incision of 7.0 mm. It can be used with capsulorhexis or with any other type of capsulotomy, such as can-opener. This 7.0 mm "frown" incision is self-sealing in the majority of cases, and does not require a suture. This larger incision does give more astigmatic shift than a 3.0 mm phaco incision, however this can be of benefit if one operates on the steep axis of K.

This technique works as well with rock-hard nuclei as with soft nuclei. It can be done with inexpensive reusable instruments, and may be more appropriate than phaco in situations where finances are limited. It might also be helpful for the phaco surgeon to use for the occasional very hard nucleus. My endothelial cell loss for the procedure is around 2 percent (Fry LL Yee, RW: Healon GV® in extracapsular cataract extraction with intraocular lens implantation. *J Cataract Refractive Surg* 19(3): 409-12, 1993). This is less than my loss with phaco, and certainly less than the loss when I emulsify a very hard nucleus.

This is my present technique (Please note that I am left handed).

Topical anesthesia with intracameral lidocaine is used. I presently prefer 2 percent lidocaine gel. The 1 percent nonpreserved intracameral lidocaine seems to sting less if it is made-up by diluting 2 percent nonpreserved lidocaine 50/50 with BSS (We did, on one occasion, inadvertently use preserved 1 percent lidocaine for 12 cases until the error was discovered. Although I would not recommend this, these corneas all looked fine the next day).

INCISION

A side-port is made with a 15° blade. A few tenths cc of 1 percent nonpreserved lidocaine are instilled (Figs 17.1 and 17.2). The eye is filled with viscoelastic through the side-port (Healon GV® is presently my preferred viscoelastic).

An 8.0 mm peritomy is made with scissors and bleeding is cleared up with wet-field cautery (under topical anesthesia, this may cause a slight sting. This, and the cauterization closure of conjunctiva at the end are normally the only times the patient feels anything. The discomfort is minor, and not a problem if the patient is forewarned). A superior rectus suture is not used. The incision site is on steep axis of "K" for cylinder 1.0 diopter or greater. For less than 1.0 diopter cylinder, temporal approach is preferred. Deep set eyes are also approached temporally. A limbal relaxing incision opposite the incision is added for cylinder greater than 2 diopters (Figs 17.3 to 17.5).

A "frown" incision is made with a guarded diamond knife set at 0.25 mm. The incision is dissected forward into clear cornea with a bevel-up crescent blade (Figs 17.6 and 17.7). Superior incisions are dissected about 1.0 mm into clear cornea and temporal about 1½ mm into clear cornea (the initial groove can also be free-handed with either the crescent blade or other blade, I feel the guarded diamond gives a better and more reproducible groove).

The anterior chamber is entered with a 3.2 mm keratome at the depth of this scleral flap, giving a

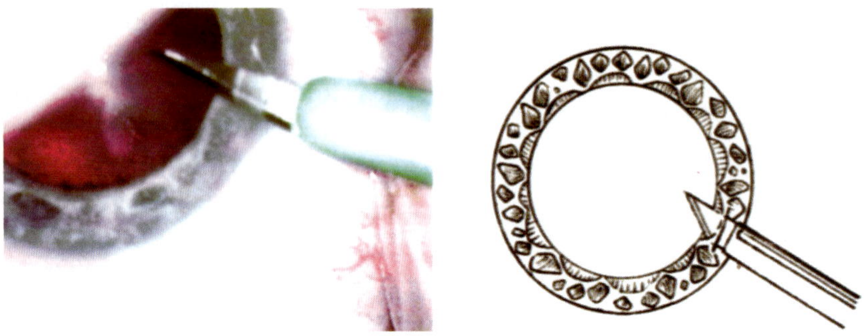

Fig. 17.1: Side port

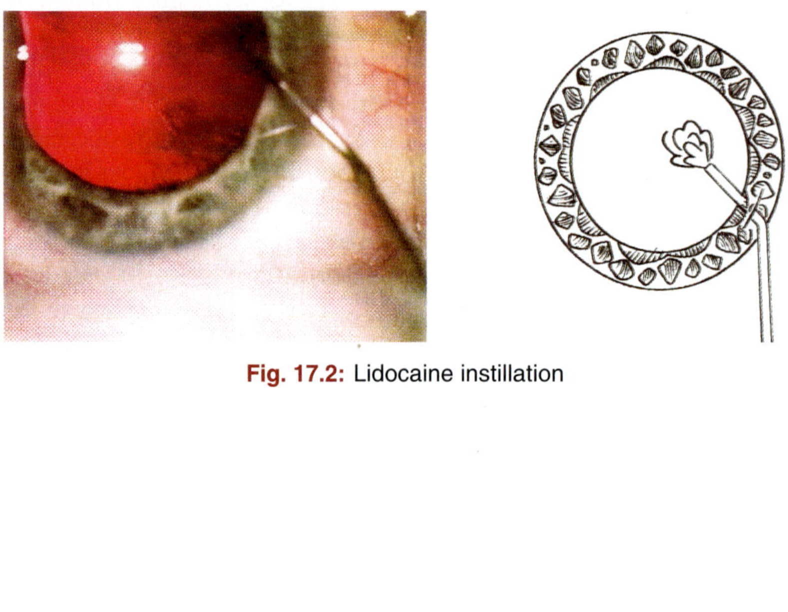

Fig. 17.2: Lidocaine instillation

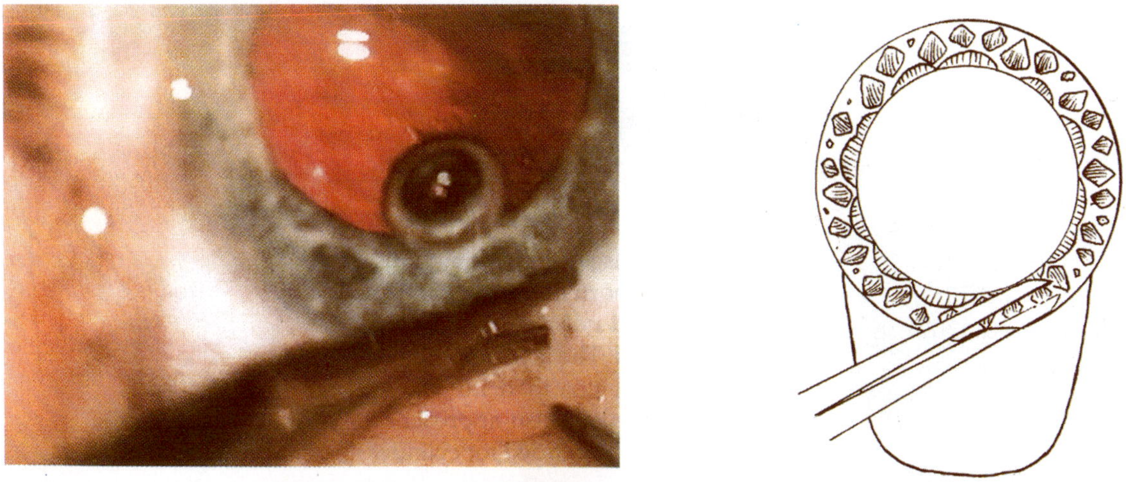

Fig. 17.3: Peritomy

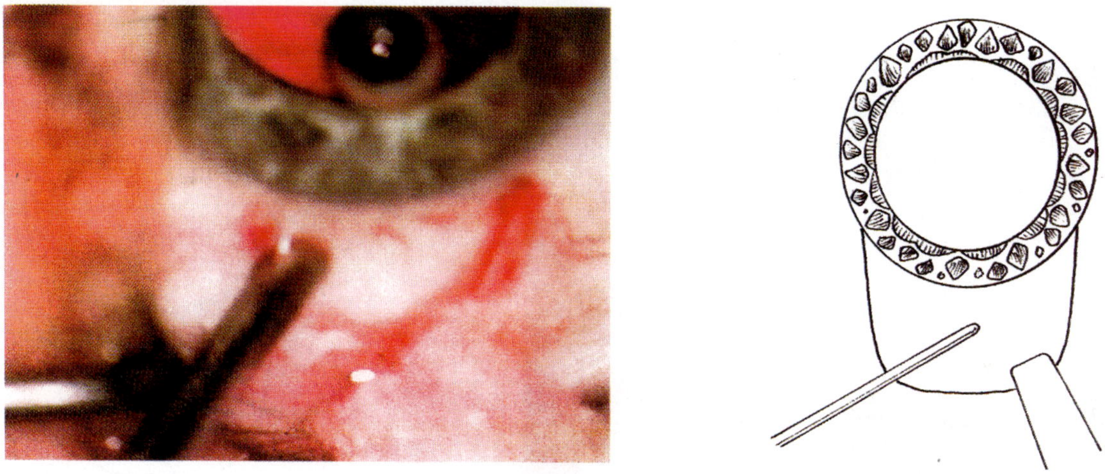

Fig. 17.4: Cautery

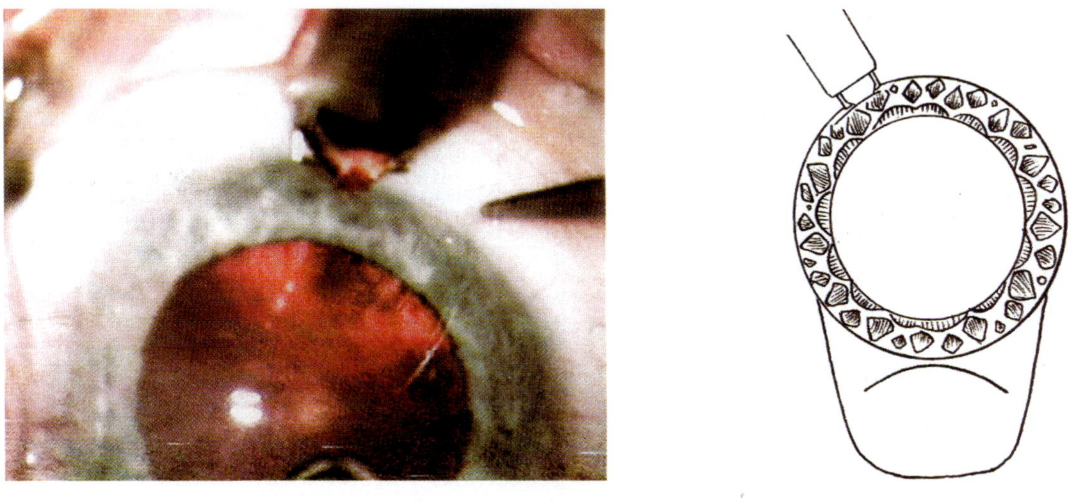

Fig. 17.5: Limbal relaxing incision

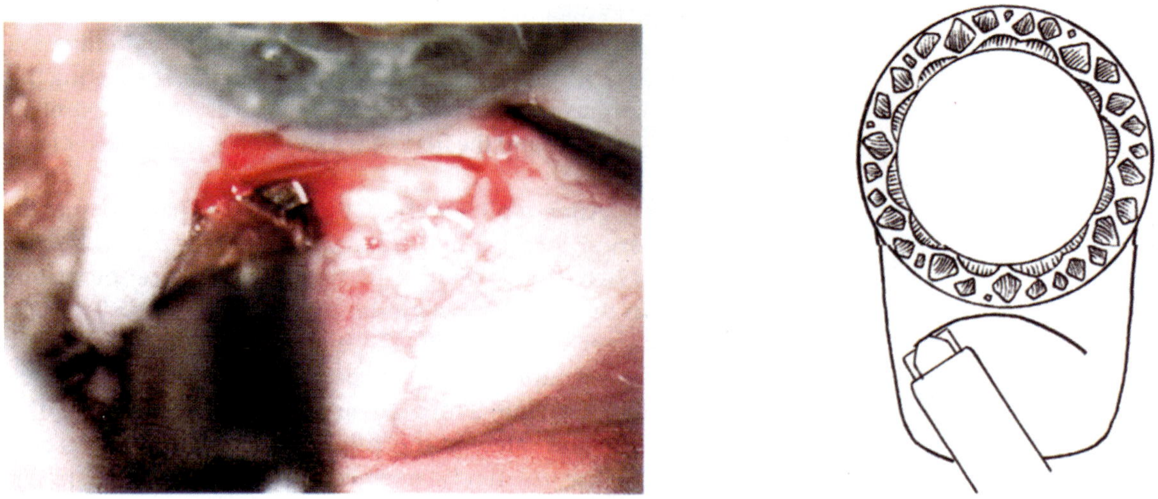

Fig. 17.6: "Frown" incision

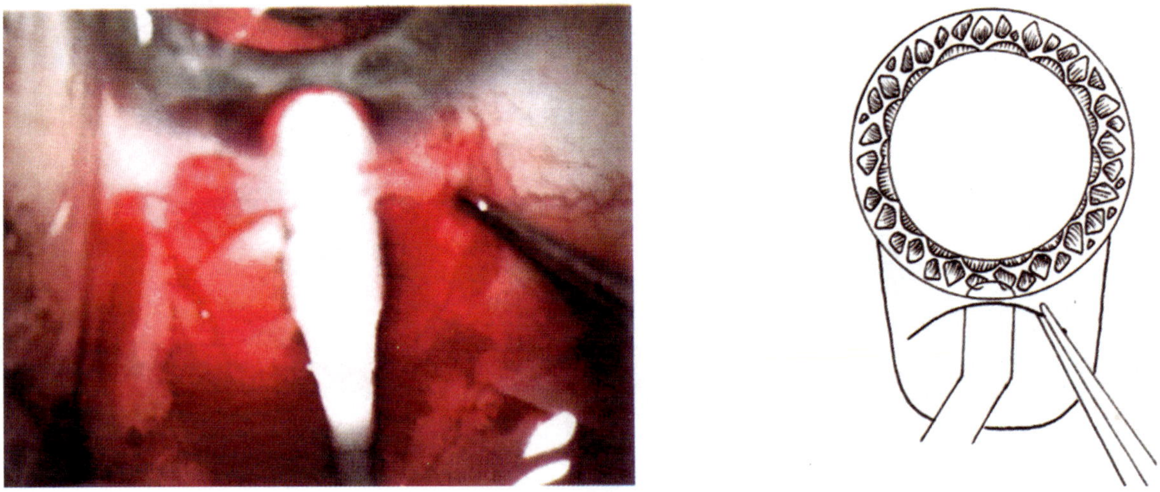

Fig. 17.7: Dissect into clear cornea

self-sealing internal flap. Additional viscoelastic is placed (Figs 17.8 and 17.9).

SMALL PUPILS

Small pupils are managed by stretching them out with two Kuglen hooks. One stretch, limbus-to-limbus, is all that is necessary. Additional stretches give little additional effect. Stretching slowly may help to avoid rupturing the sphincter. Hold for a second or two at maximal stretch. Then expand the iris out with viscoelastic (Figs 17.10 to 17.13).

After pupil stretching, the pupil may be permanently larger than before, with crenated edges, particularly if it was very small and nondilatable preoperation. In these cases, it might be advisable to use a 6.0 mm or larger optic (I prefer 7.0 mm optics in all cases). This larger pupil is actually a benefit in allowing easier fundus viewing. I think you will be impressed by the ease and safety of this pupil stretching maneuver, and by the relatively normal appearance of the pupil postoperation.

ANTERIOR CAPSULOTOMY

Any type of capsulotomy works well with this procedure. I prefer a capsulorhexis. The capsulorhexis, however, needs to be made as large as possible to allow nucleus tip-up. A can-opener

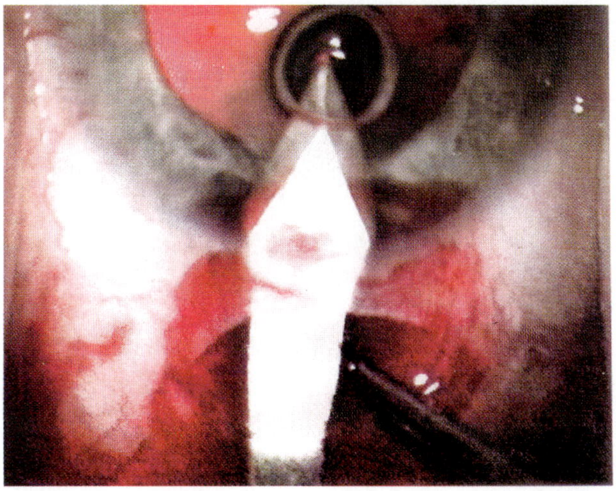

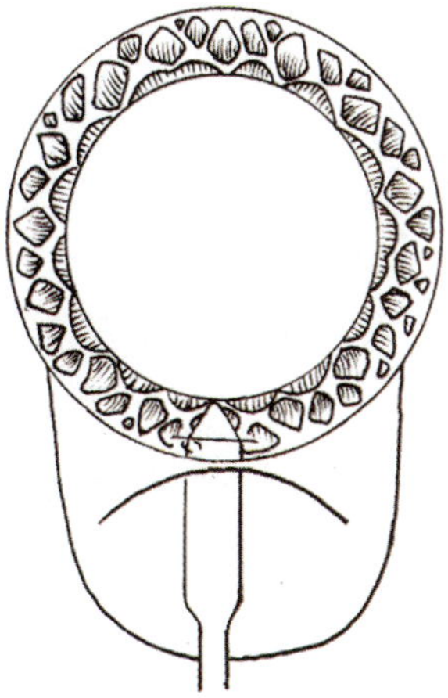

Fig. 17.8: Keratome entry

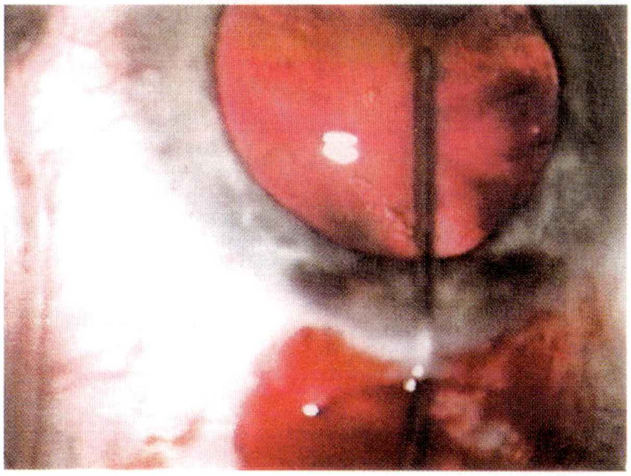

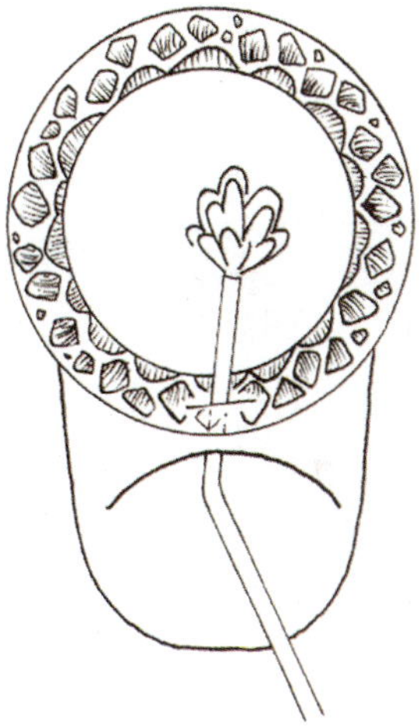

Fig. 17.9: Additional viscoelastic

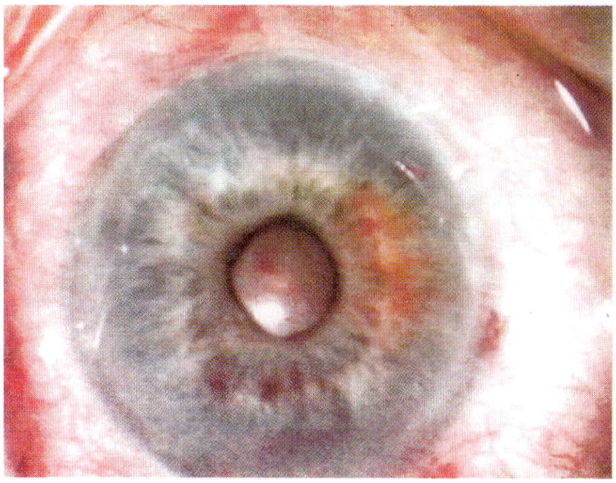

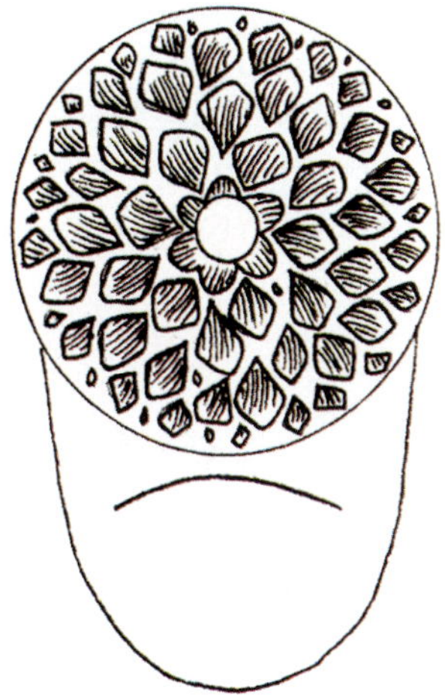

Fig. 17.10: Small pupil

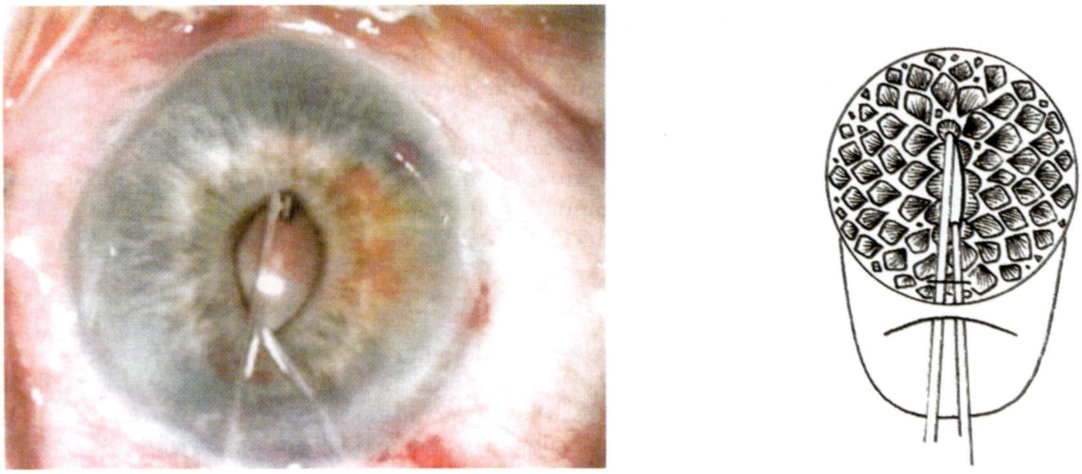

Fig. 17.11: Stretch beginning

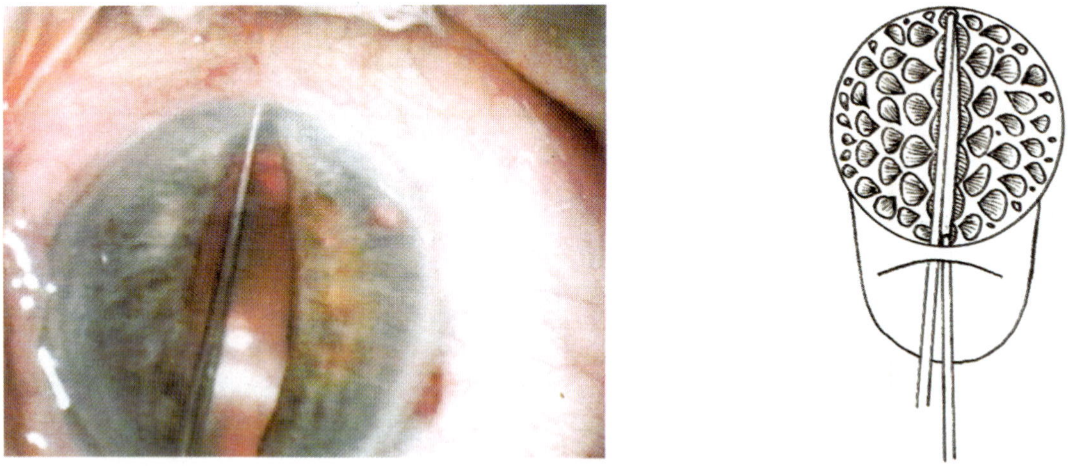

Fig. 17.12: Fully stretched

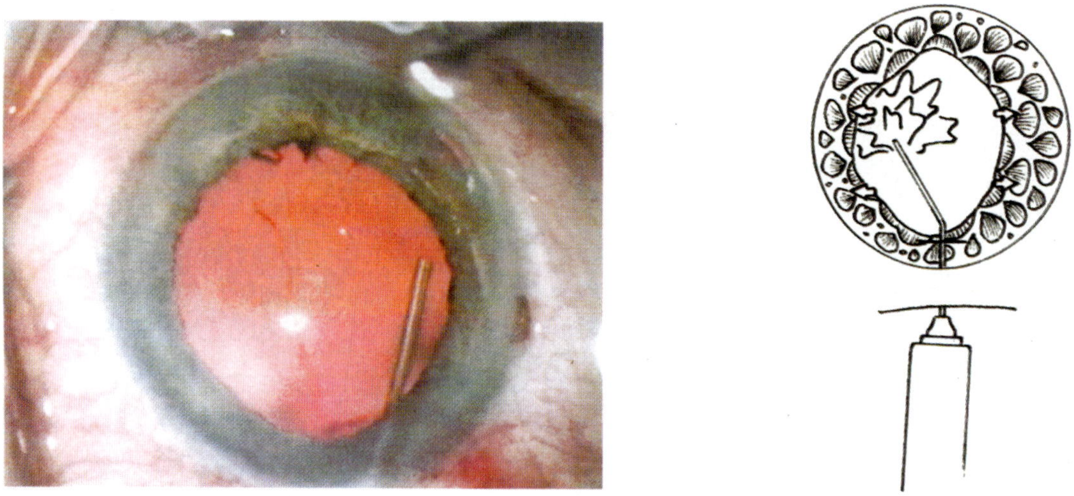

Fig. 17.13: Expand with viscoelastic

capsulotomy works well also and is used if there is difficulty with the capsulorhexis. For mature cataracts, capsular staining under an air-bubble with either ICG or Trypan Blue (Vision Blue®, from Dutch Ophthalmic) makes the capsulorhexis much easier (Figs 17.14A to D).

I prefer a Gimbel Utrata forceps for the capsulorhexis. This forceps has sharp tips so the capsule can be penetrated and the rhexis completed without changing instruments. I start in the middle and spiral out. Re-deepen with viscoelastic anytime the tear wants to "head south" (Figs 17.15 and 17.16).

HYDRODISSECTION

Complete hydrodissection is done, with the cannula just beneath the anterior capsule, to loosen the nucleus and get it rotating freely. Generally one fluid wave to the right and one to the left will be adequate. I like to use a spatula through the sideport and the hydrodissection cannula through the incision to bimanually rotate the nucleus after hydrodissection (Fig. 17.17).

NUCLEUS DELIVERY

After capsulotomy, the 3.2 mm incision is enlarged to 7.0 mm. I find that a 5.2 mm keratome works best for this. The crescent blade also works fairly well. Attempt to maintain the internal self-sealing incision all the way across (Fig. 17.18).

The chamber is refilled with viscoelastic. A Kuglen hook in the left hand nudges the nucleus gently away from the incision. The spatula catches

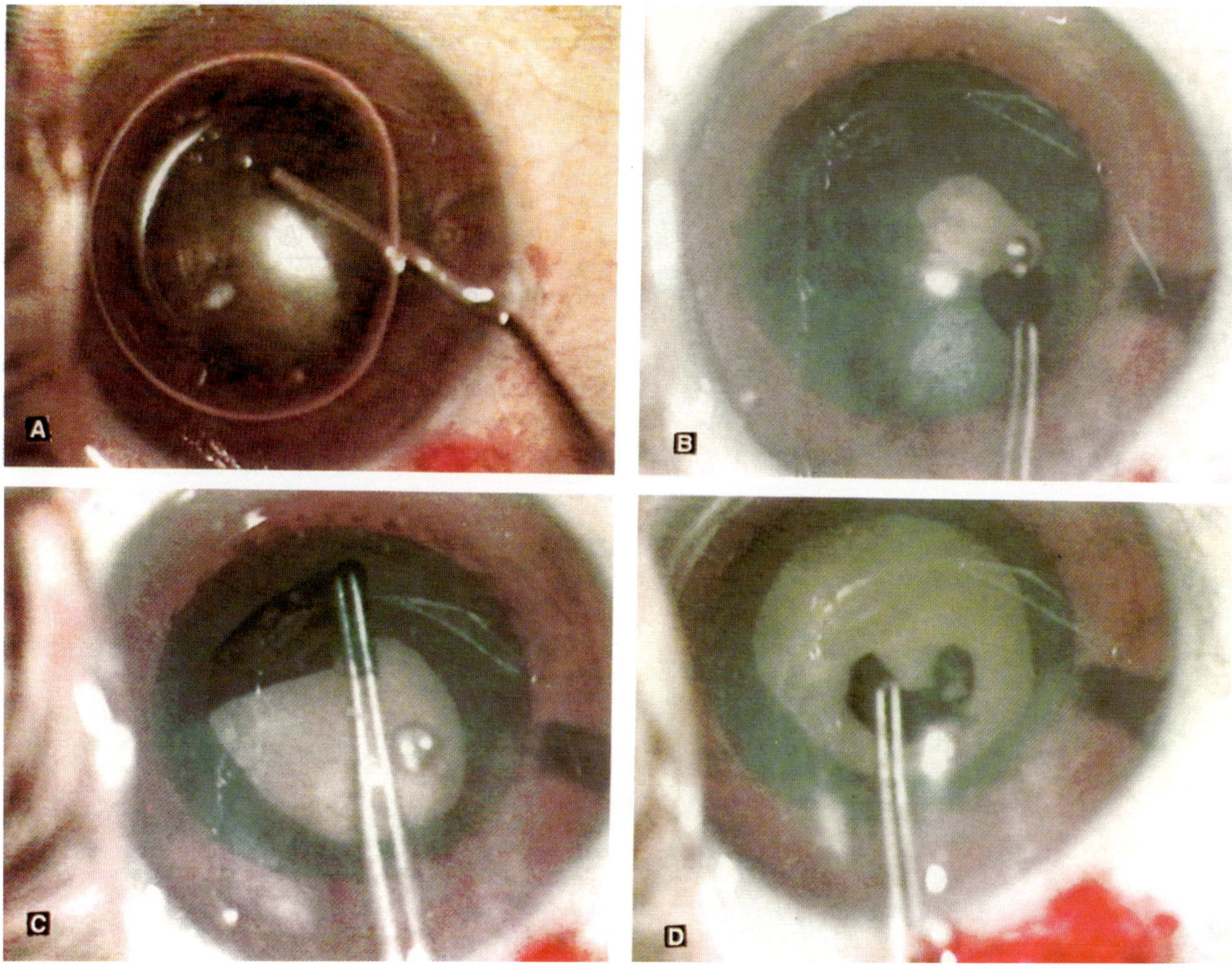

Figs 17.14A to D: Use of Trypan Blue (Vision Blue®)

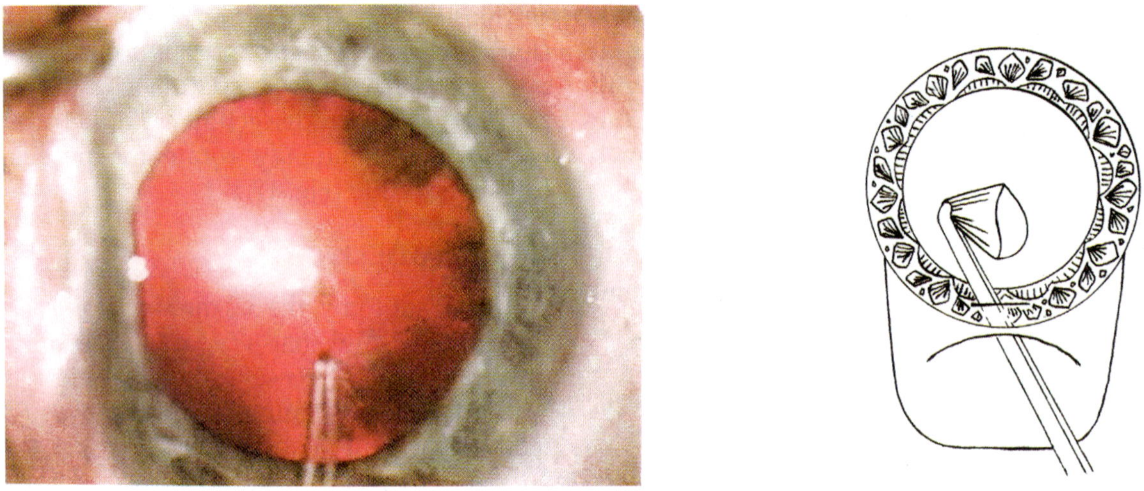

Fig. 17.15: Start of capsulorhexis

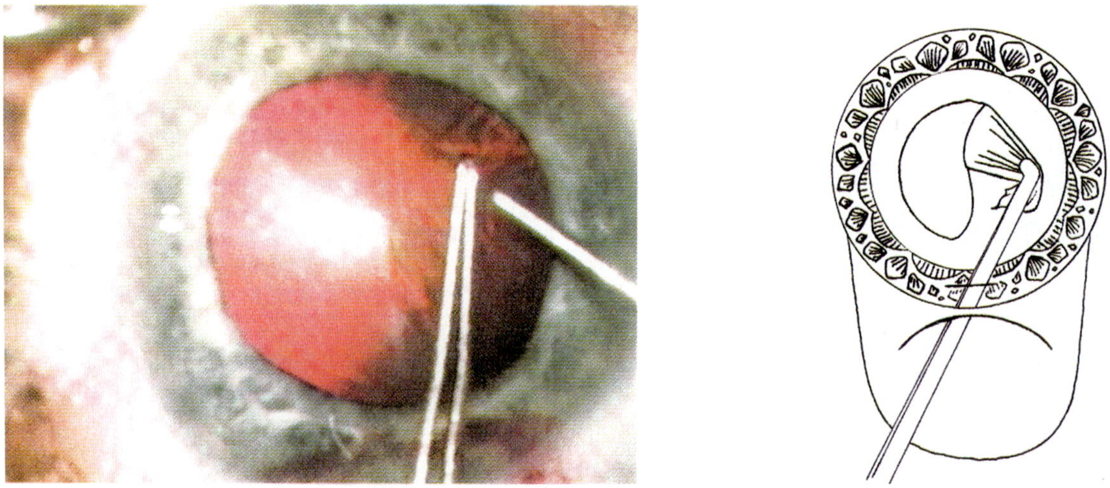

Fig. 17.16: Completion of capsulorhexis

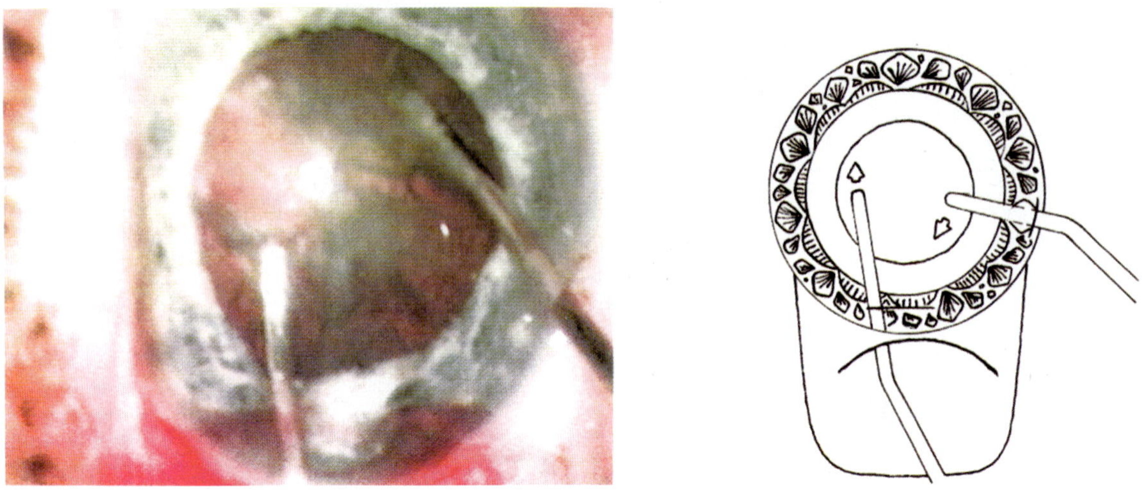

Fig. 17.17: Bimanual nucleus rotation

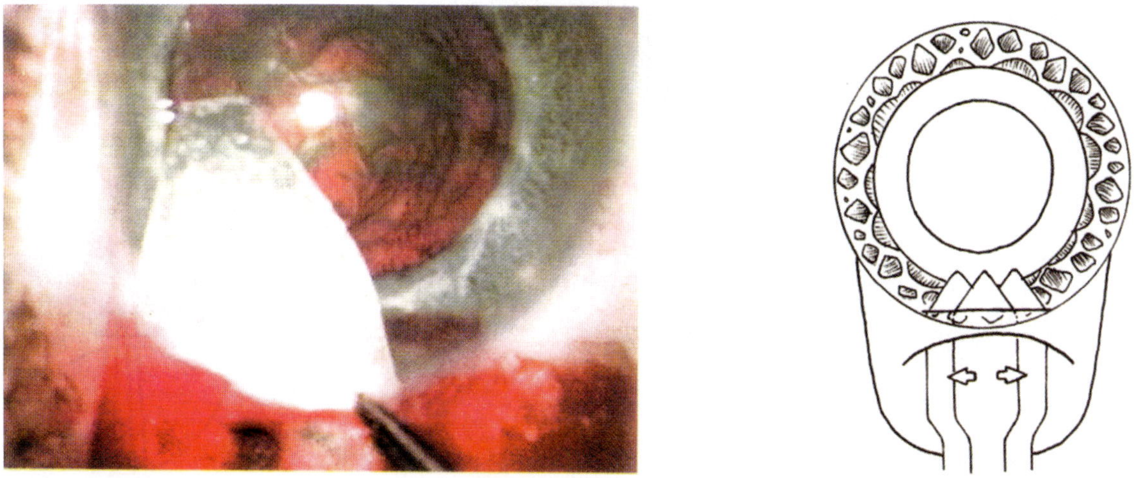

Fig. 17.18: Enlarge to 7.0 mm

the superior pole of the nucleus at the equator and tips it up. Using the two instruments, the nucleus is then cartwheeled through the capsulorhexis and pupil (Figs 17.19 to 17.22) into the anterior chamber (as an alternative, it may be "somersaulted" end-over-end into the anterior chamber).

If nucleus tip-up is difficult, aspirate the cortex off the top of the nucleus with the 0.3 IA tip, refill with viscoelastic, and attempt tip-up again.

Additional viscoelastic is placed beneath the nucleus. The lens loop is placed beneath the nucleus and the spatula on top. The nucleus is extracted, "sandwiched" between the two instruments. The outer portion of the nucleus will be sheared off with this technique, but it is soft and easily aspirated or irrigates out of the self-sealing incision with gentle pressure on the posterior wound lip (Figs 17.23 to 17.26).

If the nucleus breaks in two during removal, rotate the residual fragment so it is oriented with its long axis perpendicular to the incision. Add additional viscoelastic to blow the iris back and resandwich it (Figs 17.27 to 17.29).

Large brunescent nuclei may be extracted through a 7.0 mm incision by purposely breaking off a superior wedge, then rotating 90° and removing. This is done by placing the lens loop and spatula one-third of the way down the nucleus and pinching off a fragment, reducing its diameter. Then, rotate long axis perpendicular to the incision and sandwich (Figs 17.30 to 17.33).

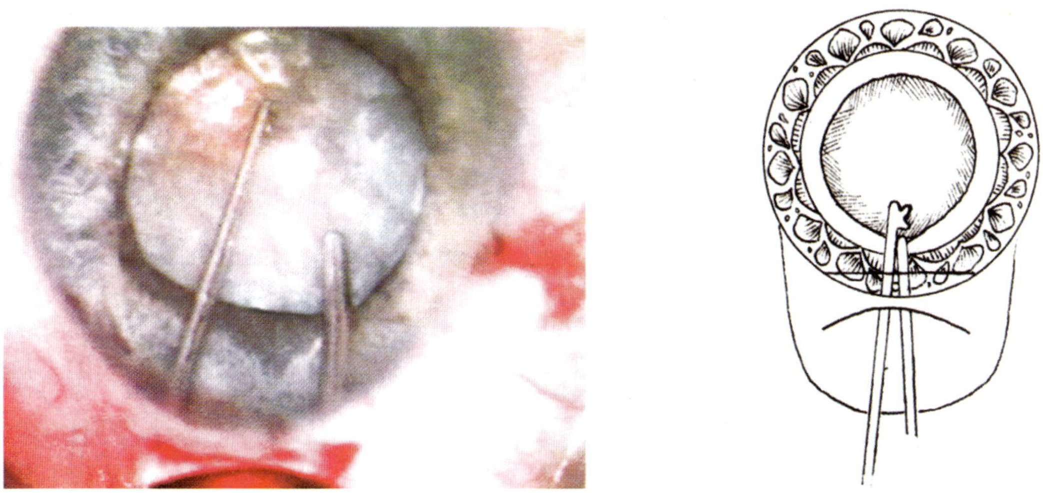

Fig. 17.19: Nudge nucleus away from incision with spatula, retract capsulorhexis edge slightly with Kuglin hook

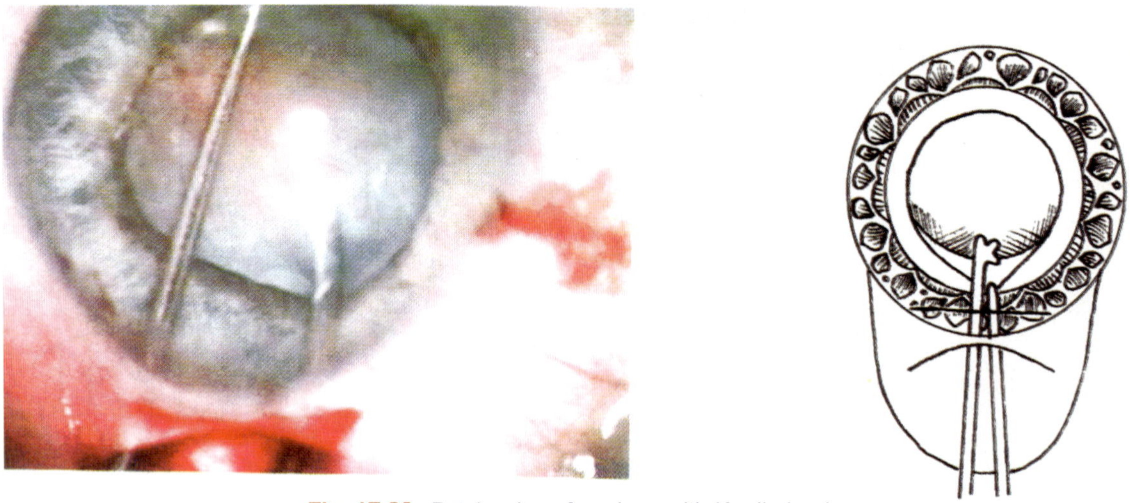

Fig. 17.20: Catch edge of nucleus with Kuglin hook

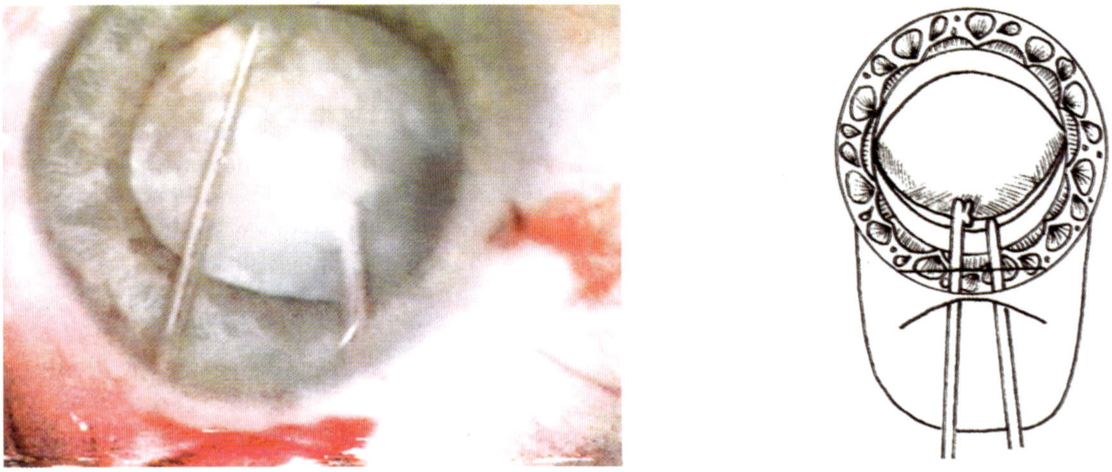

Fig. 17.21: Rotate nucleus through rhexis

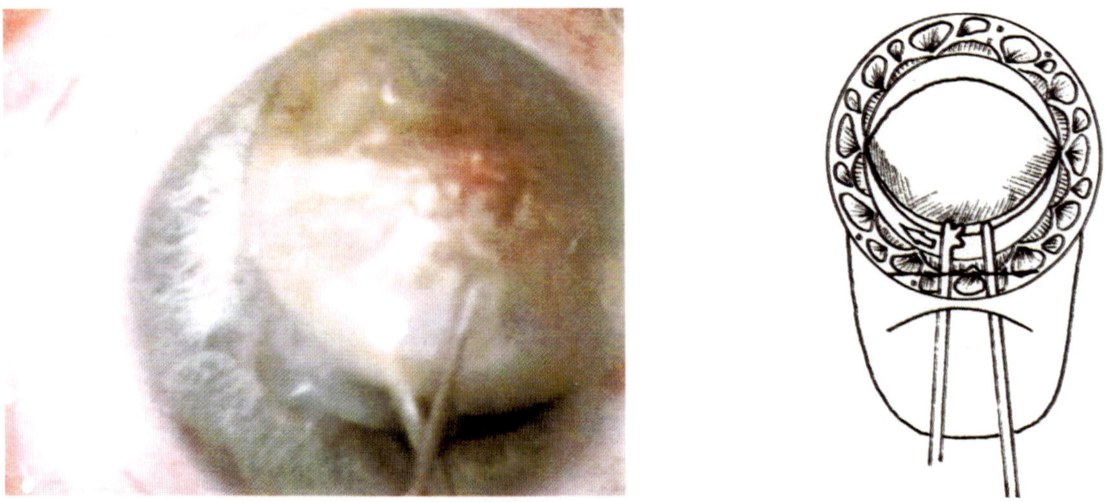

Fig. 17.22: Continue to rotate until nucleus is anterior to capsule and iris

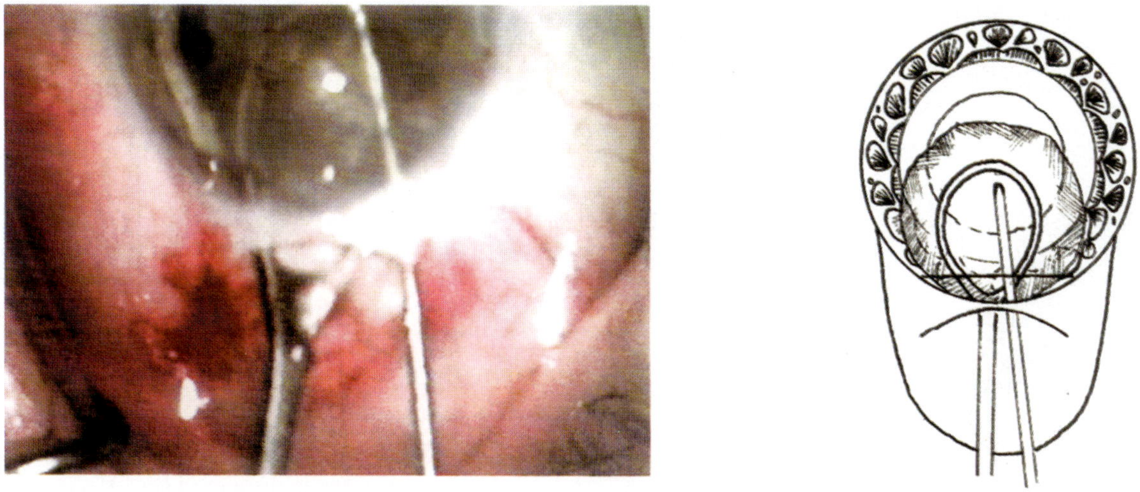

Fig. 17.23: Sandwich the nucleus between the lens loop and spatula

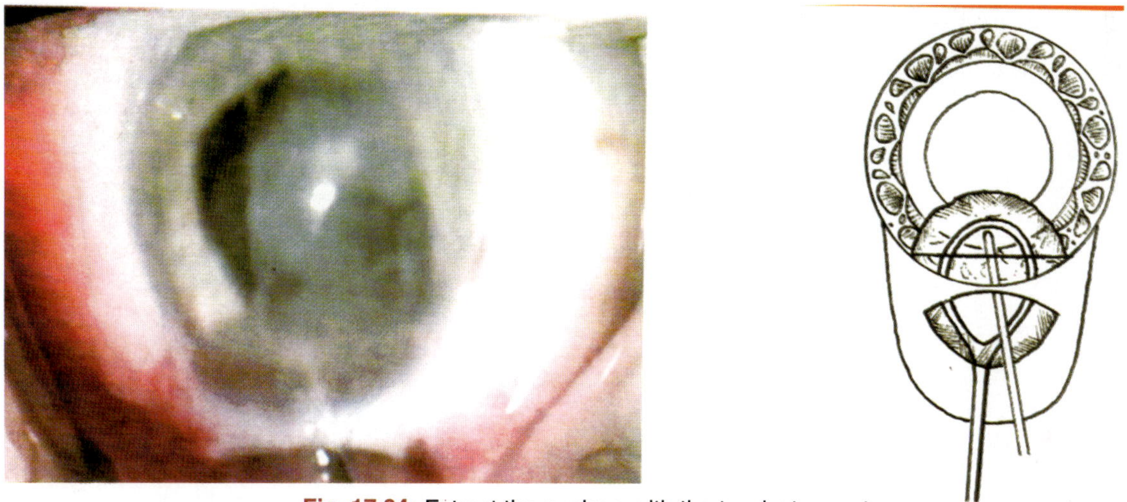

Fig. 17.24: Extract the nucleus with the two instruments

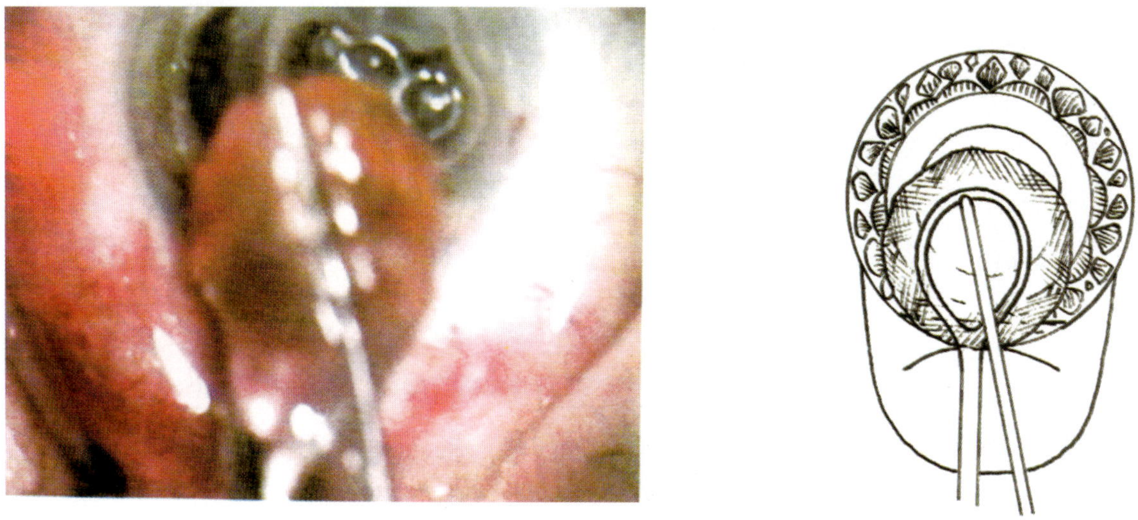

Fig. 17.25: Nucleus out, between the two instruments

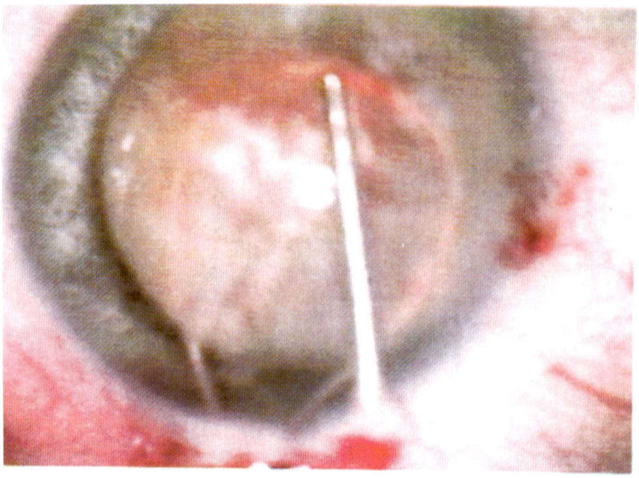
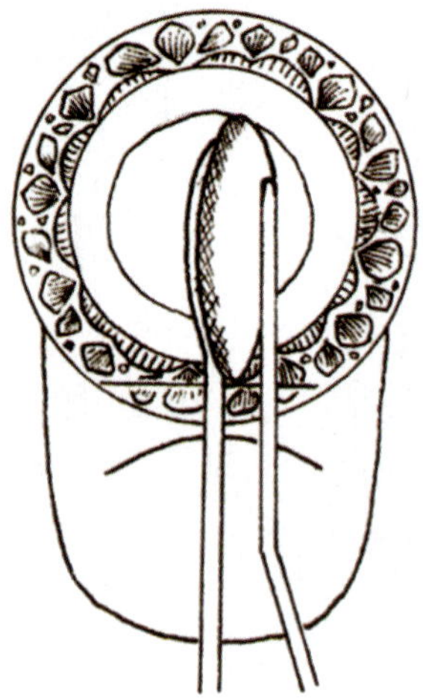

Fig. 17.26: Two instruments holding nucleus, side view

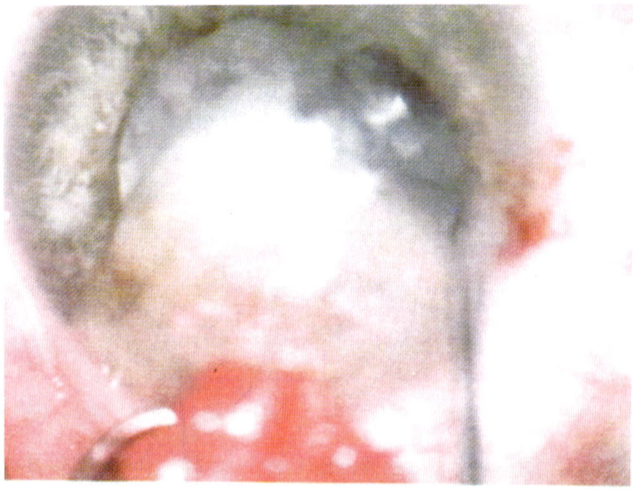
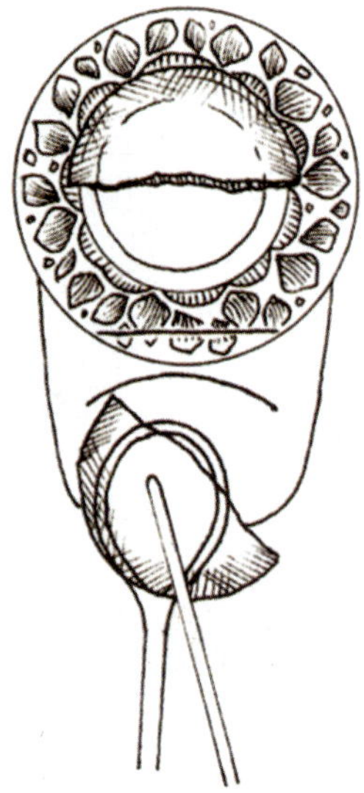

Fig. 17.27: Piece of nucleus breaks off

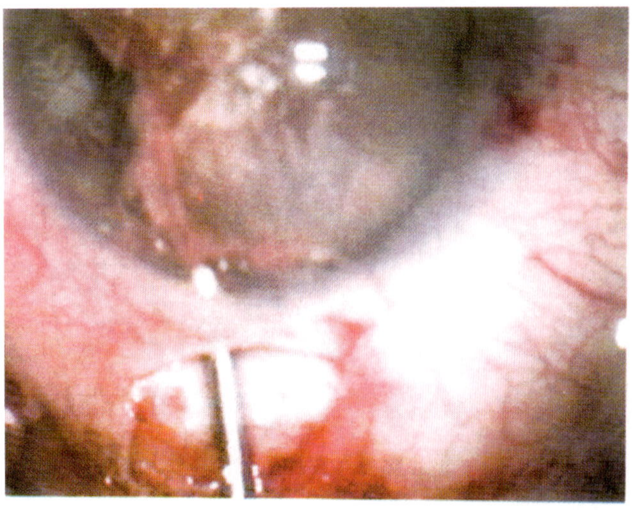
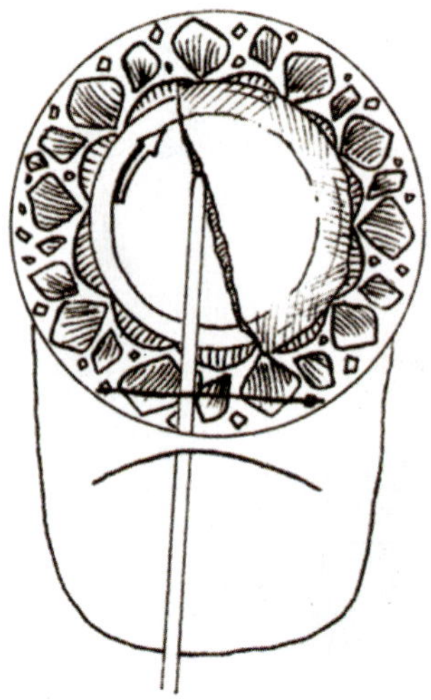

Fig. 17.28: Rotate residual nucleus

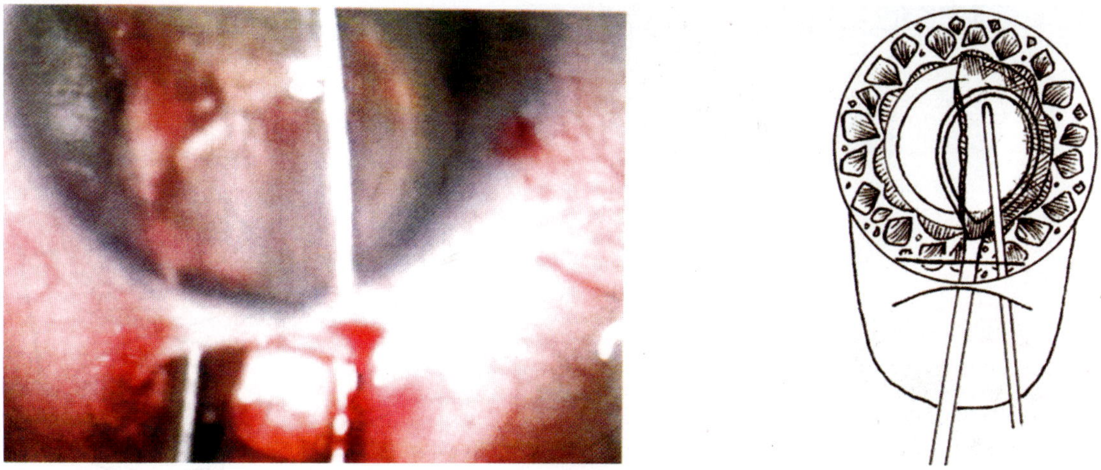

Fig. 17.29: Add viscoelastic and resandwich

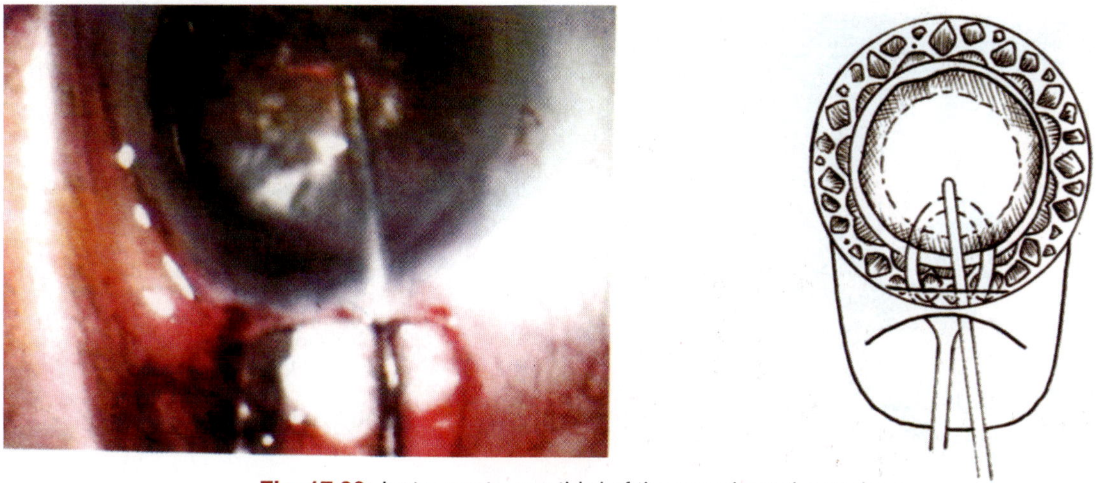

Fig. 17.30: Instruments one-third of the way down the nucleus

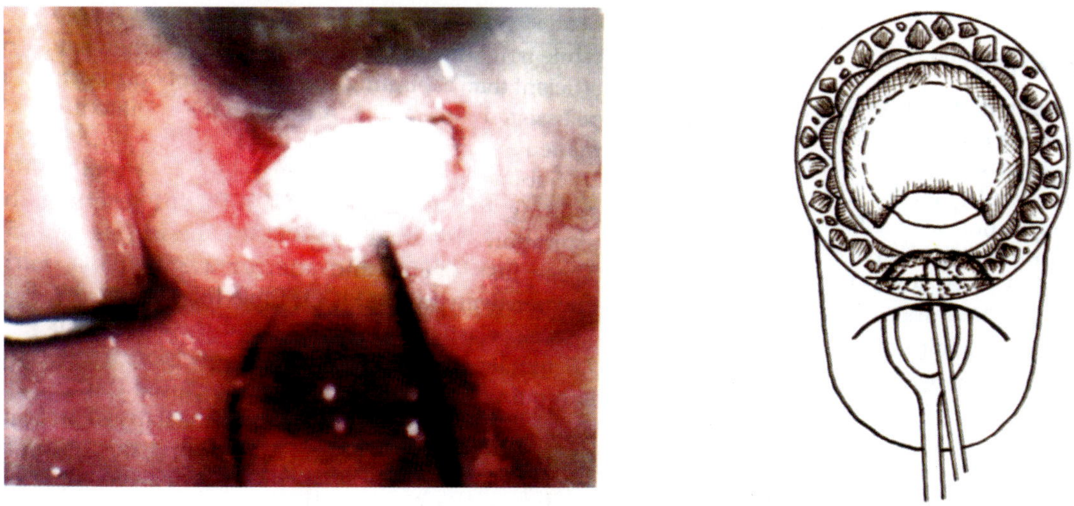

Fig. 17.31: Break-off a wedge

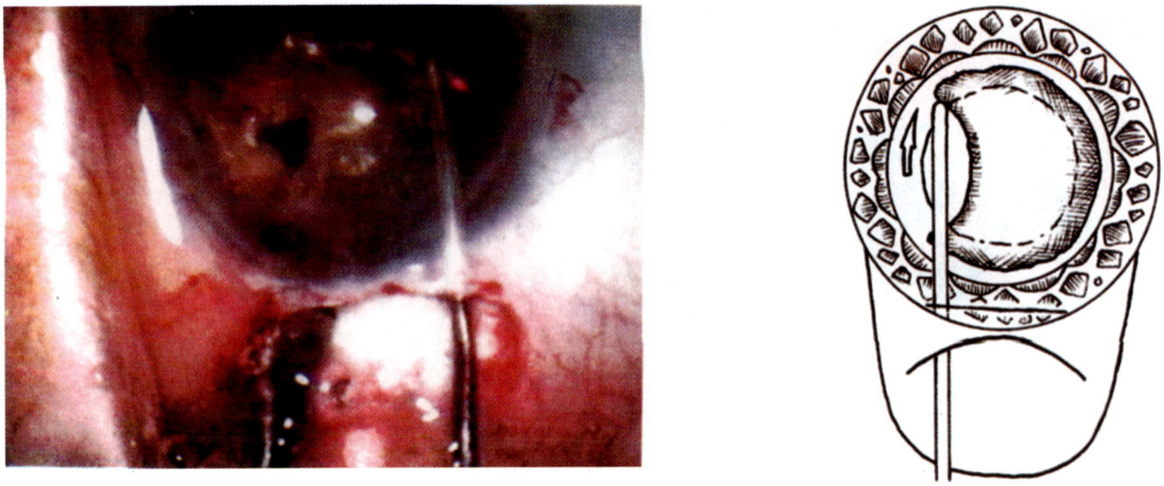

Fig. 17.32: Rotate the nucleus

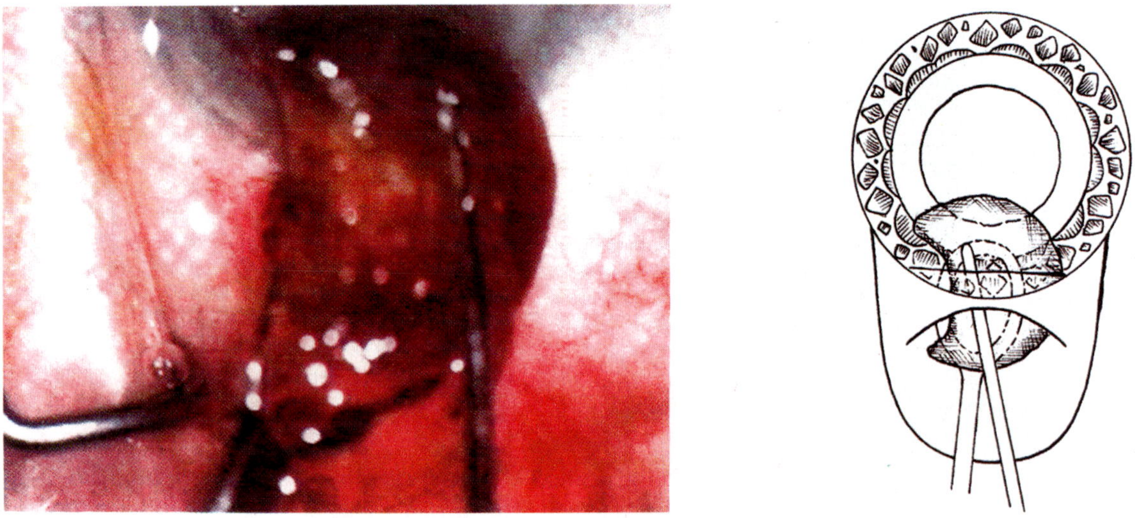

Fig. 17.33: Add viscoelastic and resandwich

CORTEX ASPIRATION

Cortex is aspirated with the technique of your choice. I prefer automated technique with 0.3 IA tip. Manual technique also works well. If there are damaged zonules or a break in the capsule, I go to a "dry" technique, with manual cortex aspiration with a 27 gauge cannula on a 3 cc syringe under viscoelastic. A noncohesive viscoelastic, such as Viscoat, works better in this situation than Healon. A Morcher capsular support ring is helpful in cases with damaged or absent zonules.

A safety suture is not necessary. If there is a tendency to iris prolapse, this usually means a self-sealing incision has not been obtained and an "X" suture will be required at the end of the case. Residual epinucleus can be washed out of the wound by slightly depressing the posterior lip while irrigating with the IA tip. This is somewhat more efficient than aspirating epinucleus. Stubborn cortex can be assisted into the 0.3 IA tip with the "potato masher" maneuver (Fig. 17.34).

Subincisional cortex can be more easily removed by splitting irrigation and aspiration and inserting the aspiration cannula through the side-port (Fig. 17.35). These instruments and adaptor are available fairly inexpensively from ASICO (Table 17.1).

Viscoelastic is used to expand the capsular bag. A 7.0 mm lens fits snugly through the incision. If

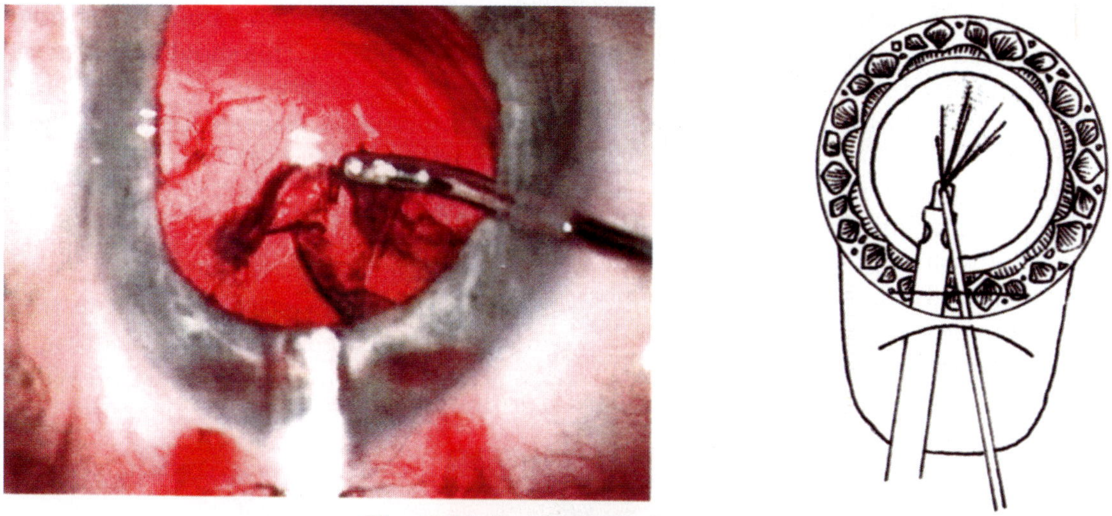

Fig. 17.34: "Potato masher" maneuver

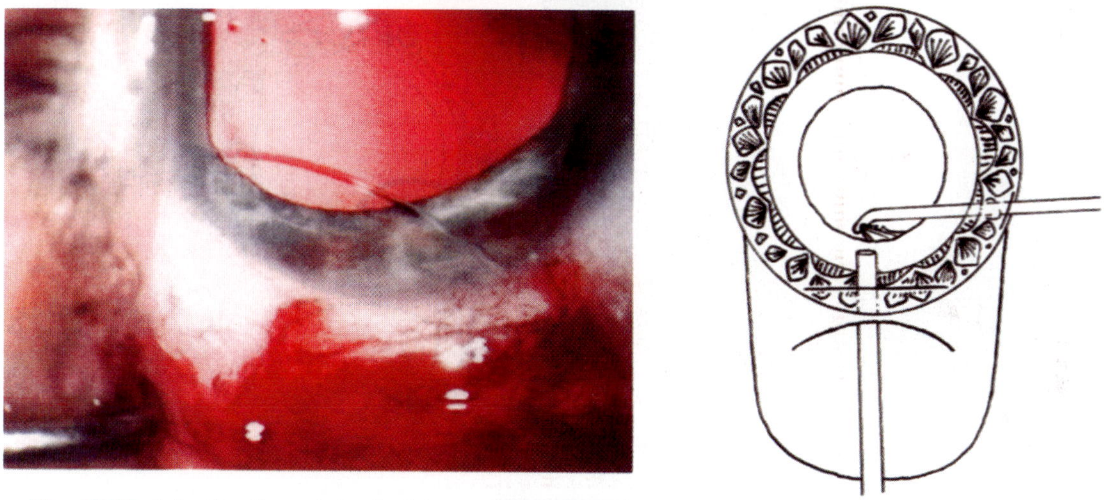

Fig. 17.35: Irrigation through the incision and aspiration through the side-port for subincisional cortex

Table 17.1: Instruments list

LENS LOOP	Morrison Lens Loop–ASICO #AE2545 ($97.00)		
SPATULA	Fry Spatula ½ mm–ASICO #AE2052 ($78.00)		
KUGLEN HOOK	Kuglen Iris Hook and Lens Manipulator Straight–ASICO #AE2230 ($113.00)		
	BIMANUAL I-A SET		
SIDE-PORT ADAPTOR	Fry Infusion Handle–ASICO #AE7389 ($24.00)		
ASPIRATING CANNULA	Anis Cortex Aspirating Cannula–ASICO #AE7403 ($45.00)		
IRRIGATING CANNULA	Fry Cannula–ASICO #AE7190 ($17.50)		
	DISPOSABLE INSTRUMENTS (can be reused until dull) (Available from many manufacturers–these are the ones I use)		
Crescent Knife	Alcon #8006594002 (bevel up)	$133.00 (6)	$22.17 ea
Slit Knife–3.2 mm	Alcon #8065992961	$127.00 (6)	$21.17 ea
15° blade–#75 beaver blade			
5.2 mm Keratome	Medical Sterile Products–Keratome Blade 5.2 mm, rounded tip #55B-5.20 RT	$14.00	

(I have no financial interest in any manufacturer mentioned in this chapter, and get no royalties from any instrument)

squeezing is required, hold the eye with the closed 0.12 forceps inserted into the side-port (holding the flap risks tearing it). Insert the leading loop of the lens first, then the optic to avoid loop crimping (Figs 17.36 to 17.38).

Aspirate viscoelastic. The internal flap is sealed by pressurizing the eye with BSS through the side-port. Blood in the wound gives a Seidel effect to demonstrate any leak. The chamber depth can also be observed to demonstrate no leak. If the chamber deepens with pressurization and does not shallow once the pressurization cannula is removed, self-sealing is indicated. This should occur in 95 percent + of cases (Fig. 17.39).

Conjunctiva is brushed over the wound and sealed with wet-field cautery (Fig. 17.40).

CAVEATS

This technique is viscoelastic dependent. Be sure to have plenty of viscoelastic both in front of the nucleus and behind it when sandwiching. Attempting to remove the nucleus under air will result in

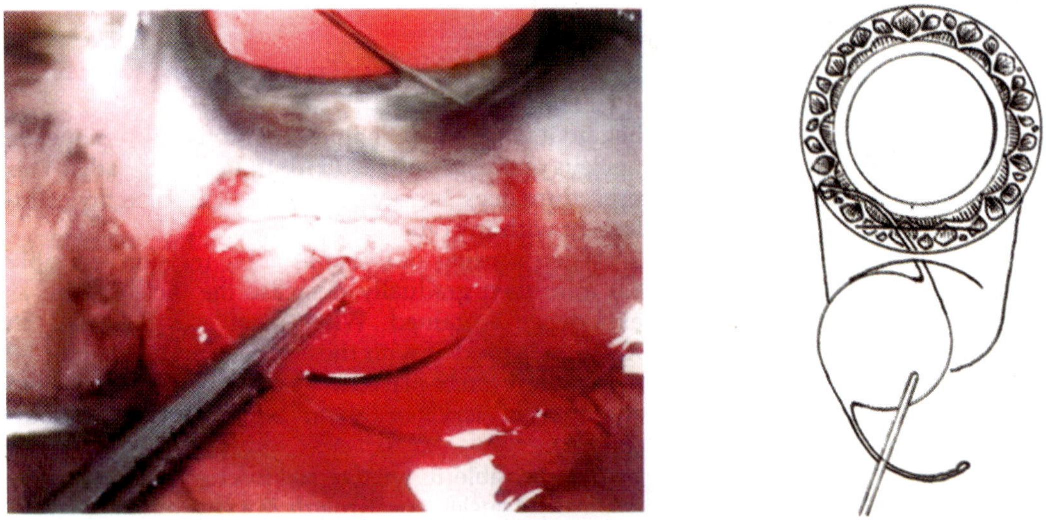

Fig. 17.36: Loop in first

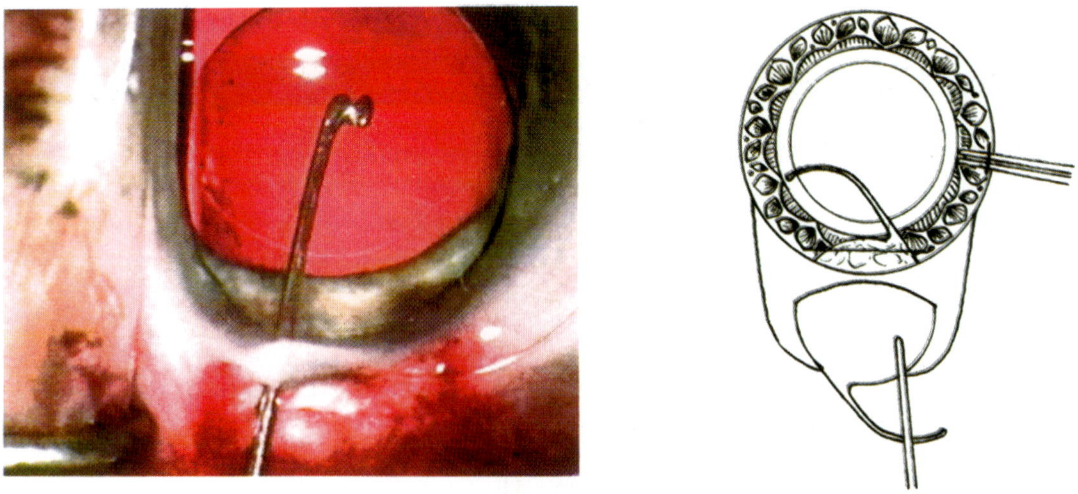

Fig. 17.37: Hold through side-port

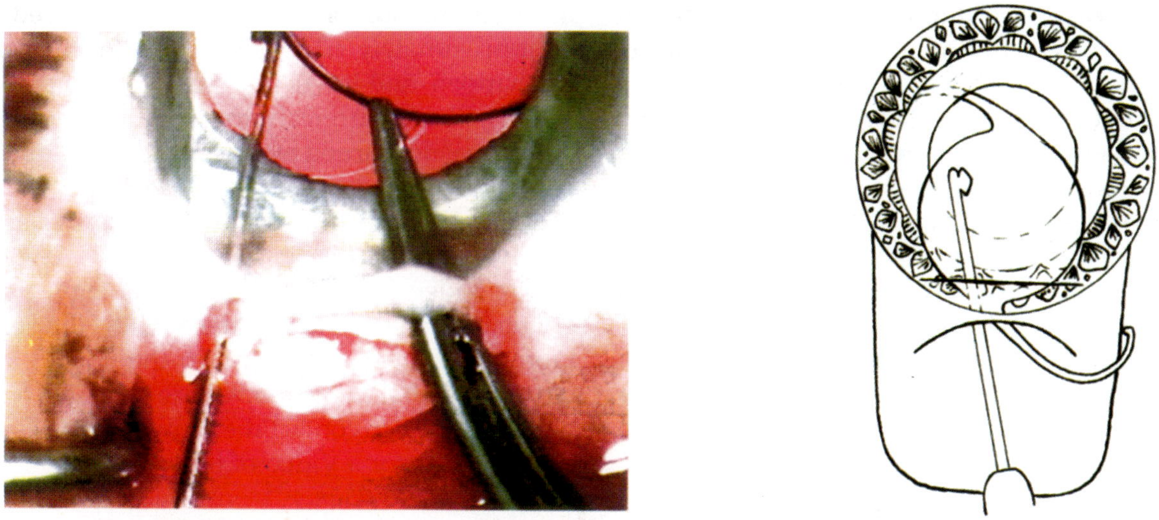

Fig. 17.38: Lens into bag

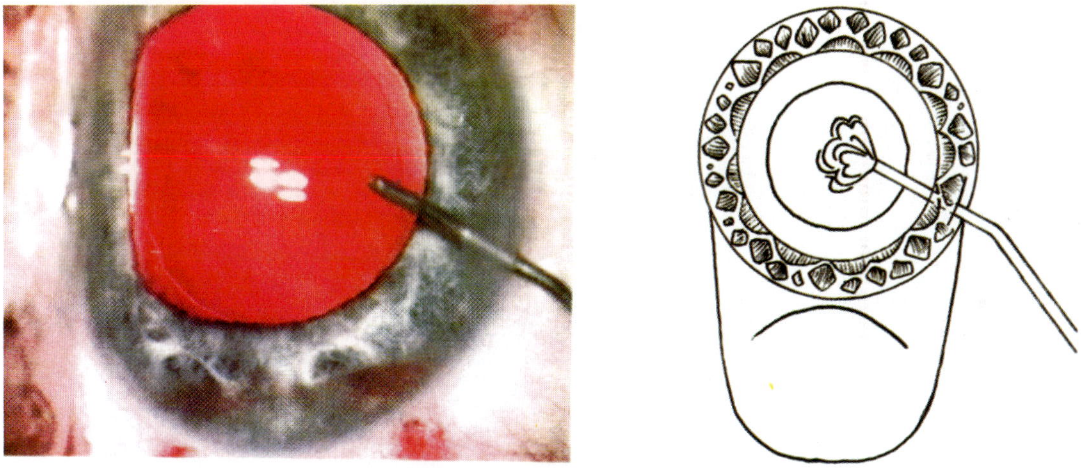

Fig. 17.39: Fill through side-port

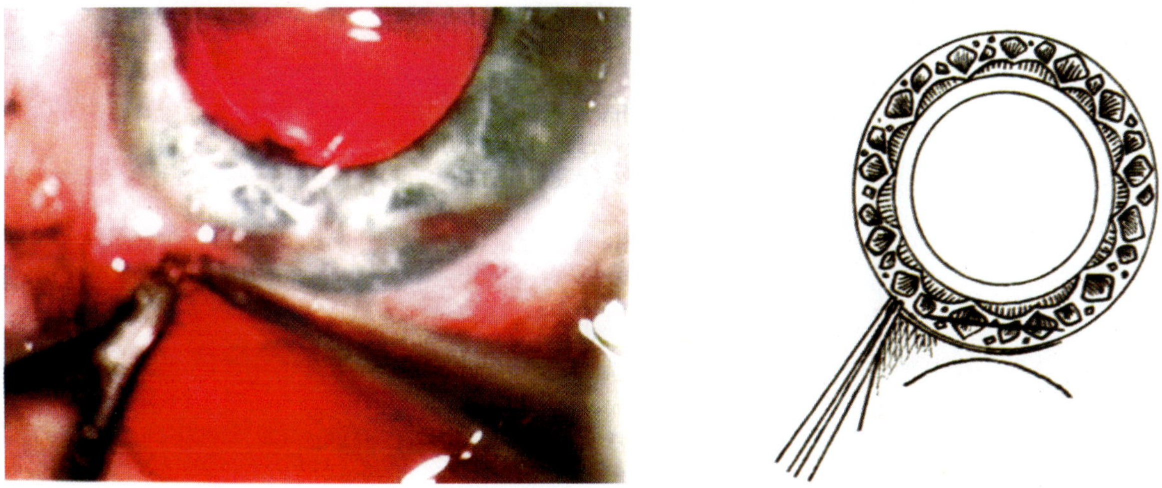

Fig. 17.40: Seal conjunctiva with wet field cautery

striate keratopathy. This procedure does, however, work well with methylcellulose, or with any other viscoelastic.

When starting out, use a larger incision, possibly 8.0 mm; then gradually decrease the incision size as experience is gained. Where cost is a factor, if an X-suture is needed with these larger incisions, the 10-0 nylon suture can be placed in a 4 × 4 and can be autoclaved and reused (Vicryl® or Dexon® will not withstand autoclaving).

It is possible to engage iris inferiorly between the spatula and nucleus, particularly in a very mature cataract where you cannot see the lens loop through the nucleus. This can result in an iridodialysis. This has occurred to me 3 times out of approximately 10,000 cases. Just be aware this can happen, and it will not happen to you.

As with any surgical procedure, this procedure is more easily learned by watching video tape than with a written description. This procedure was shown on Bobby Osher's Video Journal of Cataract and Refractive Surgery Vol IV, Issue 1, 1988, and on the Video Journal of Ophthalmology, Vol IV, Number 4, 1988. It is also in the ASCRS Film Festival Library 1987 and 1991, and in the ESCRS Video Library, 1999. If none of these are available to you, please feel free to contact me at my office in Garden City, Kansas, for a Video of the procedure.

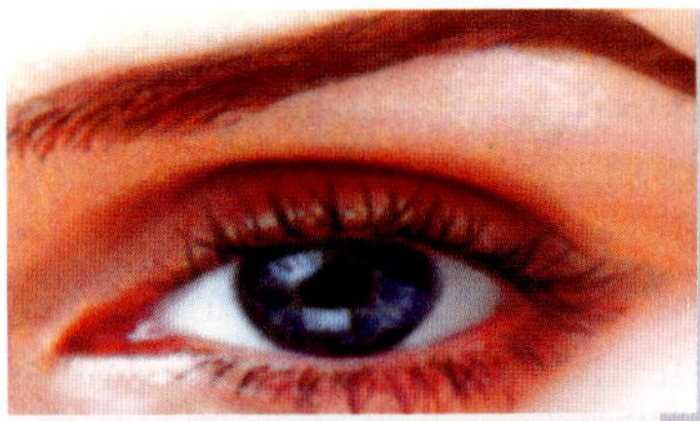

Eighteen

Dynamics of Incision and Wound Construction in SICS

Yogesh Shah
Gaurav Shah
Shushmita (India)

INCISIONS FOR CATARACT SURGERY
WOUND CONSTRUCTION FOR SMALL INCISION MANUAL SURGERY
PRE-EXISTING ASTIGMATISM
STABILITY OF THE WOUND
PROCEDURE OF WOUND CONSTRUCTION
COMPLICATIONS DURING WOUND CONSTRUCTION
CONVERSION TO STANDARD ECCE WOUND

INCISIONS FOR CATARACT SURGERY

From the time that "SHUSHRUT–Father of Surgery" performed cataract surgery for the first time, revolutionary changes have taken place in the management of cataract. And still, if one studies these changes little more in detail, there are many similarities in the surgery performed then and what we intend to achieve today. Shushrut performed couching without any anesthesia and today we are marching towards minimal anesthesia. He performed surgery as outdoor procedure and again today we talk of day care surgery. His incision was just a small puncture wound and today we are looking at small incision surgery and trying to make every effort to reduce the incision size and make it as much safe as possible.

As we progressed in our surgical approach to treat cataract we evolved Ab-interno incision with Von-Grafe's knife. Here we created the wound from inside out and this needed a great deal of surgical expertise. But, though difficult, it gave clean edges and was very quick in the hands of the expert.

This was further modified into Ab-externo incision. Here the wound is created from out side inwards. Though slow, in this incision the skill required is relatively less and the surgeon has much greater control on the incision. Most of the incisions designed today for various techniques of cataract surgery basically are Ab-externo incisions. The edge of the incision may be vertical, slopping or like a step. The shape of incision may be a straight line or curved upwards (frown) or downwards parallel to limbus. Curved incisions help us reduce the width of the incision in comparison to the length. This helps in controlling astigmatism.

The incision depending on its anatomical position may be divided into scleral, anterior-limbal, posterior-limbal or corneal. In small incision manual surgery, scleral incision is the standard choice.

WOUND CONSTRUCTION FOR SMALL INCISION MANUAL SURGERY

Wound forms the foundation for any type of cataract surgery. Accuracy in wound construction and its closure are inversely proportional to the rate of complications both in intra and post-operative stages. Though wound construction is important step in any technique of cataract surgery it is of vital importance in SICS. The ultimate outcome and the ease of delivering the nucleus are dependant on wound architecture.

In last decade cataract surgery has gained popularity as a mode of refractive surgery also.

The goal at the end of cataract surgery is Emmetropia. Two factors, which are of paramount importance for achieving Emmetropia, are

- Accurate IOL power calculation, which takes care of spherical element.
- Wound construction, which takes care of cylindrical component.

The factors which one needs to look at for choosing any type of wound are

- Site of wound
- Dimensions of wound
- Design and Architecture of wound
- Pre-existing astigmatism
- Stability of the wound

Site of wound

Surgeon's comfort and pre-existing astigmatism are two most important factors, which govern the location of wound. Though in most cases we prefer 12 o'clock position mainly because we are more familiar with this location, there are surgeons who are equally comfortable with temporal location. Recently some surgeons have resorted to topical or sub-conjunctival anesthesia for SICS and they prefer temporal approach. Though in clear corneal temporal approach for phacoemulsification, there are reports of slightly higher incidence of endophthalmitis, no such authentic study has been reported for SICS. In view of larger size of wound and conjunctival dissection, one must keep in mind the possibility of higher incidence of endophthalmitis, if the incision site is temporal. If patient has had previous glaucoma operation at superior limbus, one may be forced to take a limbal incision.

Dimensions of Wound

The size of wound varies from surgeon to surgeon. Though initially almost all surgeons started with 5 to 6 mm external incision, many individual variations have come into existence. It is possible to reduce width of the incision to 3.5 to 4 mm by changing the nucleus delivery technique. Many factors play role in deciding size of incision.

- Type of cataract that the patient has
- Technique of nucleus delivery
- Skill of the surgeon
- Design of wound

Design and Architecture of Wound

Size of the nucleus can be assessed fairly well pre-operatively on slit lamp examination. If one dislodges the nucleus (through side port) in anterior chamber before main wound construction then the size of the tunnel can be decided by seeing the actual size of the nucleus. Minification of the nucleus by hydrodelineation, Phaco sandwich technique, snare or pre-chopper will help surgeon reduce the width of incision. Use of additional instrument like Vectis to deliver full size nucleus will need larger width of incision. In the initial phase of learning curve, it is better to have slightly larger incision than what you think is necessary.

The dimensions of wound will alter depending upon the design and the architecture of wound. It will also depend on the length of the tunnel, that is, how far you go from the limbus and how deep in the cornea. It is usually 3 to 3.5 mm depth of the tunnel that gives optimum results. Most surgeons now prefer 5 mm wide incision with backward extension creating side pockets (as shown in the diagram). In most cases this section allows easy delivery of large brown nucleus also.

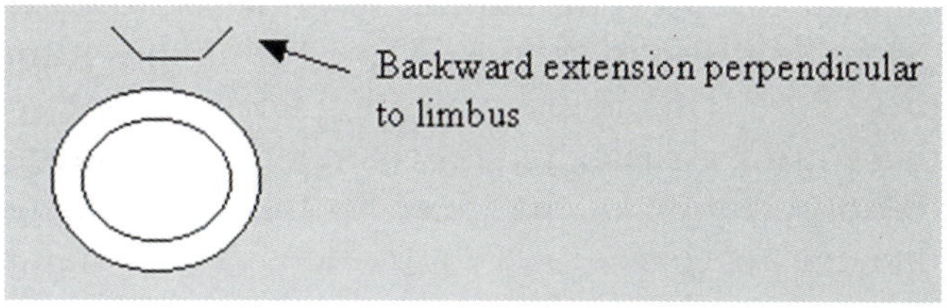

The internal incision is always larger than the outer one giving a shape of funnel to the wound. Inner lip of the wound normally has a width of 8 to 9 mm. Dr. Bluementhal prefers the inner lip to be parallel to the limbus and not a straight horizontal line. It is the integrity of inner lip that is most important rather than its width. The inner lip should extend almost upto the limbus but should not cut the limbus on either side. This reduces induced astigmatism as described by Dr. Bluementhal.

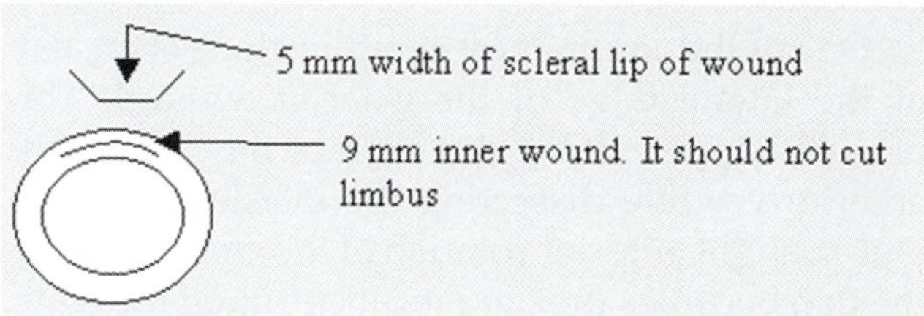

The design of the wound varies from surgeon to surgeon. Besides what is described above as standard Bluementhal technique of wound construction, the external wound can be

- Horizontal
- Curved – frown
- V-shaped
- M-shaped
- Horizontal with straight backward extension

PRE-EXISTING ASTIGMATISM

The wound, which induces minimum astigmatism, also has minimum capacity to correct pre-existing astigmatism. Thus standard Bluementhal type of

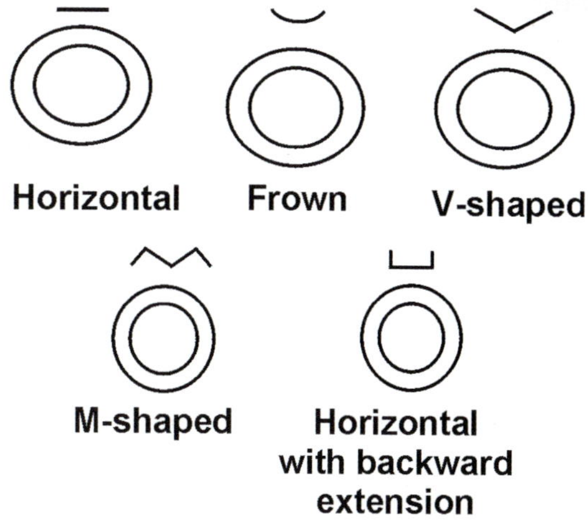

section has very small effect on pre-existing astigmatism and it cannot be used to correct more than 0.75 to 1.0 D of pre-existing astigmatism. If patient has pre-existing astigmatism with steep meridian in horizontal plain and if surgeon takes 12 o'clock incision the additive effect of two factors may give rise to substantial astigmatism, finally making patient unhappy. Every surgeon should evaluate his cases and establish the nomogram about the surgically induced astigmatism in his hand with his technique. By and large most scleral tunnel sections are astigmatically neutral as compared to clear corneal wounds.

STABILITY OF THE WOUND

Stability and integrity of wound is single most vital factor that controls intra and postoperative complications. The surgeon's comfort in intraoperative phase has been greatly increased by invention of close wound technique. The stability of wound directly depends on the good architectural design and skilful construction of the wound. Good knowledge of the technique, use of sharp instruments and adhering to the standard norms in every case will certainly help the surgeon to achieve reproducibility of good stable wound.

PROCEDURE OF WOUND CONSTRUCTION

We will discuss this under 3 headings

- Anesthesia used
- Instruments used
- Technique of wound construction

Anesthesia

Most surgeons prefer peri-bulbar anesthesia for small incision manual surgery. However, various modifications depending upon the surgeons choice are not uncommon. Topical anesthesia with 4% paracain drops, sub-conjunctival injection of 2% Xylocain with Sensorcain, sub-tenon perfusion with canula, application of wet cotton plaque dipped in Xylocain at the site of wound, intracameral preservative free Xylocain are some of the alternatives practised by different surgeons.

Instruments used

For making external scleral incision one can use Diamond knife, 15 or 11 no Bard Parker blade or angled keratome. The desired length of the incision is marked with calliper. The tunnel is constructed with metal or diamond crescent. It is very important to use good sharp instrument so that proper plane of dissection is maintained and architecture of wound is not destroyed. 3 mm sharp tip angled keratome is used for construction of inner lip of the wound.

Technique of Wound Construction

After dissecting fornix based conjunctival flap, superficial vessels are cauterized preferably with wet-field cautery. It is important not to apply deep cautery to prevent induced astigmatism. Deep cautery may also interfere with creation of uniform tunnel. Desired size of external wound is measured with calliper about 3 mm behind limbus and external wound created with diamond or steel blade. Dissection is then carried out with crescent knife going towards the limbus. As one goes laterally a scleral pocket is created by taking the cutting blade posteriorly such that the backward extension of the cut remains perpendicular to the limbus. The dissection, anteriorly, extends for about 1mm in the stroma of the cornea. Once the tunnel is created along with lateral scleral pockets on either side, a sharp tip 3 mm angled kerotome is taken to enter the anterior chamber and the inner lip of the wound is created. The inner lip extends on either side for about 9mm width. To create the inner lip one should extend the cut as keratome enters the chamber (during the forward stroke). However, while withdrawing the blade no attempt should be made to create the inner lip. As one cuts the inner lip on lateral side the direction of the blade turns more sideways to create funnel shaped wound. The inner lip should be extended almost up to the limbus on the either side but it should not cut the limbus. This prevents induced astigmatism to some extent. It is best to keep ACM on during the entire procedure. This helps in creating tense eyeball so that cutting is easier and the chamber remains deep during creation of the inner lip thus preventing damage to cornea, iris or the lens. The wound construction is an art and it can be acquired with some practice. There is a definite learning curve for this procedure.

COMPLICATIONS DURING WOUND CONSTRUCTION

While creating a conjunctival flap haematoma may occur. It is best left alone unless it comes in the way of future steps of the operation. At times one may create a buttonhole in the conjunctival flap. This also can be left alone or sutured at the end of the operation.

One of the commonest complications is the tear of the lateral edge of the external wound. This usually happens if the direction of the knife turns anteriorly while dissecting the incision laterally. Due to slight anterior rotation of the crescent knife, the flap becomes thin and it cuts through the edge. This can also happen if the crescent blade is blunt and the surgeon has to use undue force. This can be easily repaired with one or two 10-0 sutures at the end of the surgery. One has to remember that the integrity of the inner wound is more important than the outer one.

Too sharp a knife or too quick movements can result in to premature entry in to the anterior chamber. This can cause problem in future steps of the operation like iris prolapse, shallow chamber, injury to the angle of the chamber and intraocular bleeding. It is best to prevent this from happening. At times it may become necessary to close this wound and create a new incision at other site. If one is able to complete the procedure but the inner lip is not well constructed, it is best to take sutures at the end of the surgery to prevent post-operative complications. This complication is most likely to increase the quantum of induced astigmatism.

CONVERSION TO STANDARD ECCE WOUND

Surgeon may need to convert to standard extra-capsular surgery in the event of any complication occurring during the surgery or the wound construction it self is defective. If the integrity of the wound is lost during its construction and further steps become difficult it may be wise to convert to standard ECCE at least during the learning curve. If one edge of the wound is torn it is best to extend the wound in that direction while converting. This will maintain the integrity of the wound on the other side. If both sides of wound are intact and surgeon has to convert to ECCE, than he can do it in any one direction or both the directions. The guideline here could be pre-existing astigmatism (move towards the steeper axis) and the quadrant,

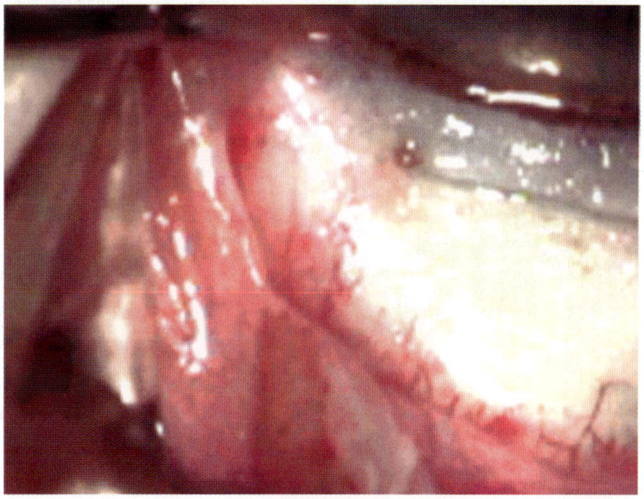

Fig. 18.1: Horizontal incision

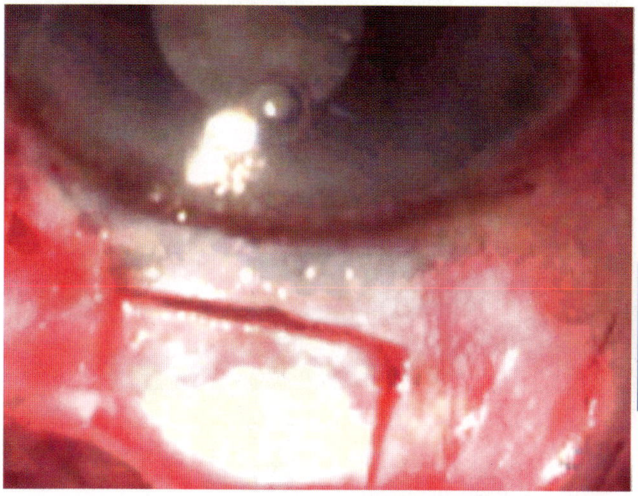

Fig. 18.2: Backward extension

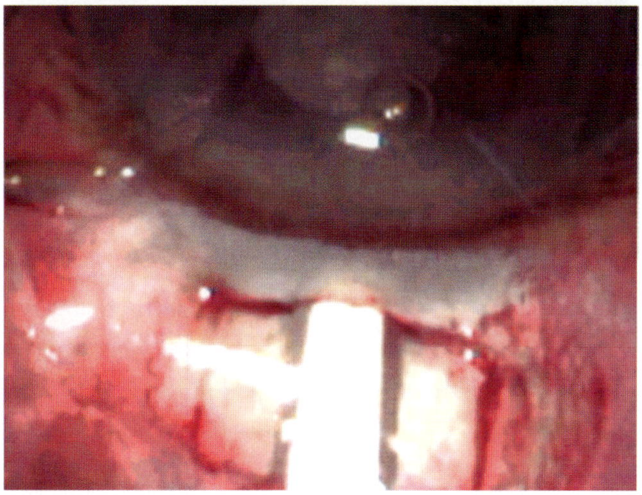

Fig. 18.3: Initial tunnel with crescent

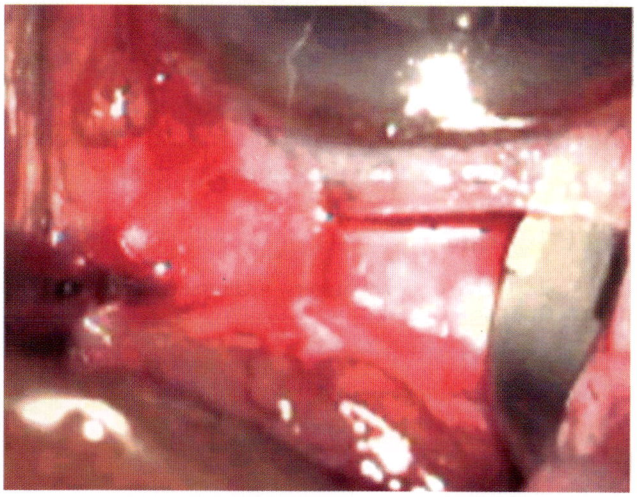

Fig. 18.4: Tunnel extended up to limbus

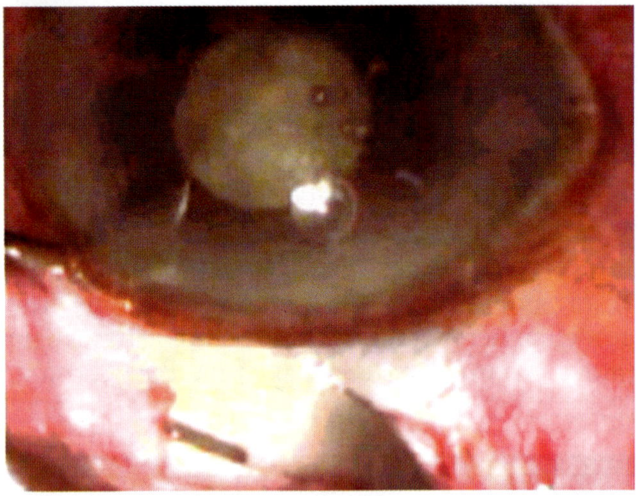

Fig. 18.5: Scleral pocket

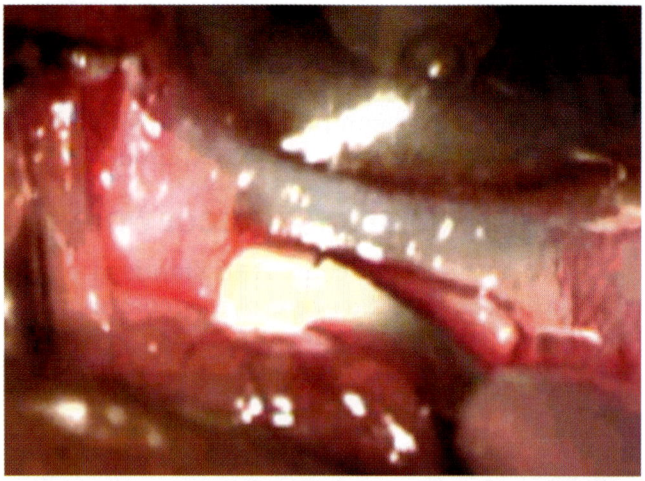

Fig. 18.6: Scleral pocket

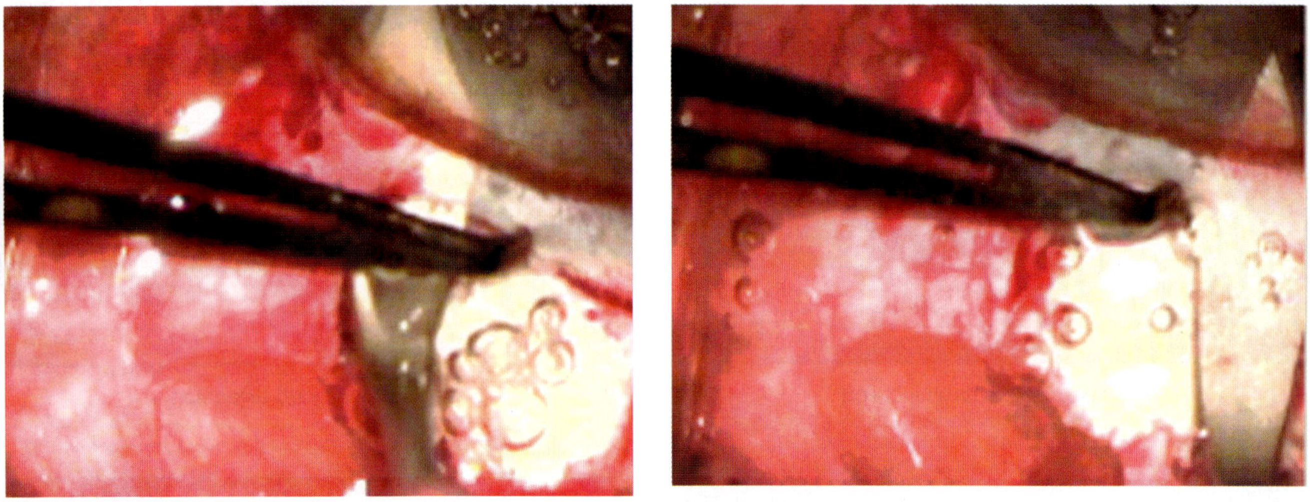

Figs 18.7A and B: Construction of the inner lip of the wound

which will be more comfortable for the surgeon to take care of remaining part of the surgery.

REFERENCES

1. Rozakis GW: Cataract surgery—Alternative small incision techniques.
2. Stainer GA, Binder PS, Parker WT, Perl T: The natural and modified course of post cataract astigmatism. OS 1982;10:822-27.
3. Troutman RC: Corneal astigmatism*-aetiology, prevention and management. Mosby Year Book, 1992.
4. Samuelson SW, Koch DD, Kuglen CC: Determination of maximal incision length for true small incision surgery.

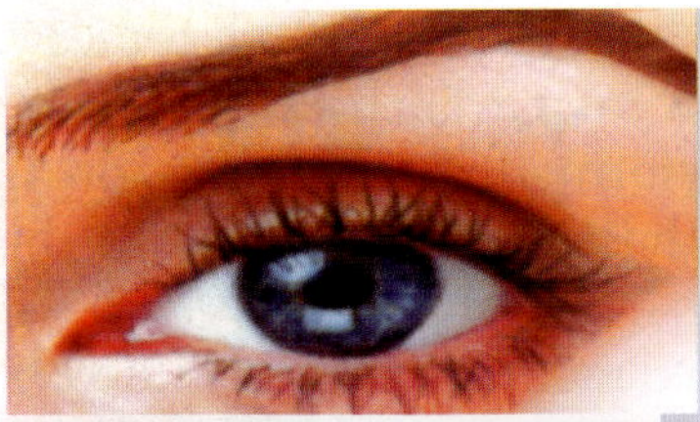

Nineteen

Tobias H Neuhann
(Germany)

Capsulorhexis

HISTORY

The problems originating in sulcus implantation of posterior chamber intraocular lenses in the late 1970s and early 1980s caused the members of today´s American Society of Cataract and Refractive Surgery (ASCRS), to discuss and favor the idea of intraocular lens (IOL) implantation into the capsular bag to achieve a better centration of the implants and accordingly a reduction of postoperative complications. The Simcoe loops (modified C-loop), a new design of that time, provided a considerable improvement in intracapsular centration compared to the generally used J-loops. However, decentration remained common.

The analysis of this decentration showed that in spite of targeted and correct endocapsular implantation, tears of the anterior capsule originated, so that at least one loop luxated into the sulcus, mostly forming the precondition for later decentration. Realizing that the Kelman Christmas-tree and also the Galand letter-box technique as well as the most frequently applied can-opener technique produced jagged edges which were a locus minoris resistentiae the idea of the continuous curvilinear capsulorhexis (CCC) was born.

Based on mutual experiences and observations my brother, Thomas F Neuhann, who was the first to describe a reproducible method for a capsulorhexis[1] and I in the course of time developed the needle and forceps technique, the capsulorhexis technique which is still applied today.

At the same time and completely independent of our development, Howard Gimbel worked on the same idea, produced the same result and called his new technique continuous tear capsulotomy. In the attempt to find the most suitable and precise term for the new technique and to take the original terminological approach of both inventors into account Neuhann and Gimbel finally decided to call their mutual development "continuous curvilinear capsulorhexis" (CCC),[2] which was soon to become a standard technique in cataract surgery. The fact that two independent developments had been made in the "old" as well as in the "new world" already at that time indicated that the CCC simply presented the most logical conclusion summing up the experiences of the past (Fig. 19.1).[3,4]

NEEDLE TECHNIQUE

Today the two-step needle technique has become history—with this approach the capsule is first opened peripherally with the needle below the incision, and the incision is enlarged curve-shaped to the right and left applying the sharp edges of the needle accordingly, which results in a larger flap. The same needle is now bent in such a way that the flap which was transformed into an incision is flipped around, and the tear is completed in the known way.

The currently applied method of the needle technique first requires an initial puncture of the anterior capsule within the central area to be removed, which is then extended in a curve-shaped manner to the targeted eccentric circle to be described. The circular tear is started by either pushing or pulling the central anterior capsule in either direction, while the flap to be created is gently lifted. The next step is to turn over the flap and apply the vectorial forces in tearing with the needle in such a way that a more or less concentric opening originates. Once the full circle is almost completed, the end will automatically join the beginning of the curve outside in (Figs 19.2 to 19.4). It is also possible to place the first puncture directly within the planned curvature and start the rhexis with a curved enlargement of this tiny hole. In this case, the tear is brought around on both sides, until finally the ends join together as already described.

Advantages of Needle Technique

Advantages of the needle technique are that it is economical, since it can be performed with appli-

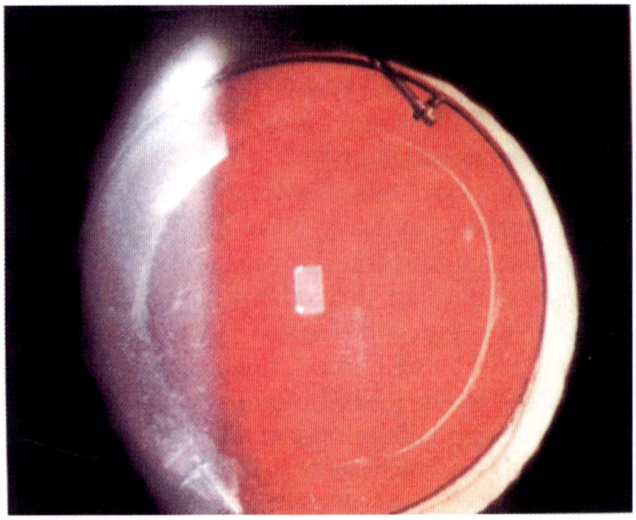

Fig. 19.1: The ideal continuous curvilinear capsulorhexis (CCC)

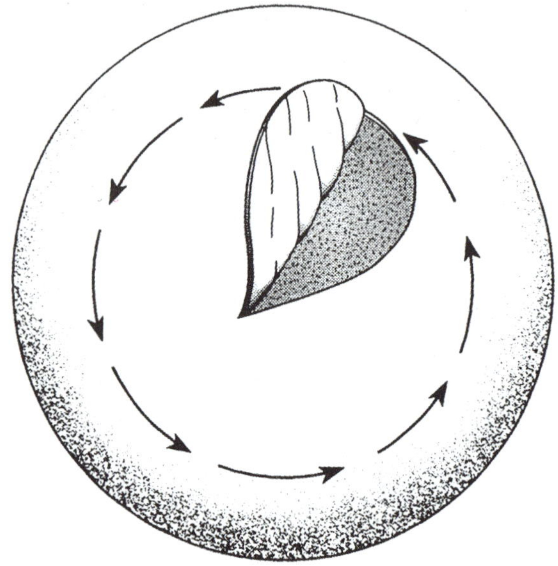

Fig. 19.2: Basic principle of the CCC

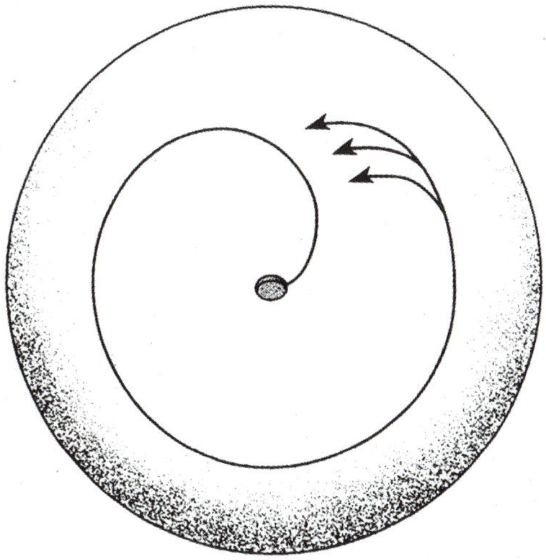

Fig. 19.3: The right and safe way to perform the CCC

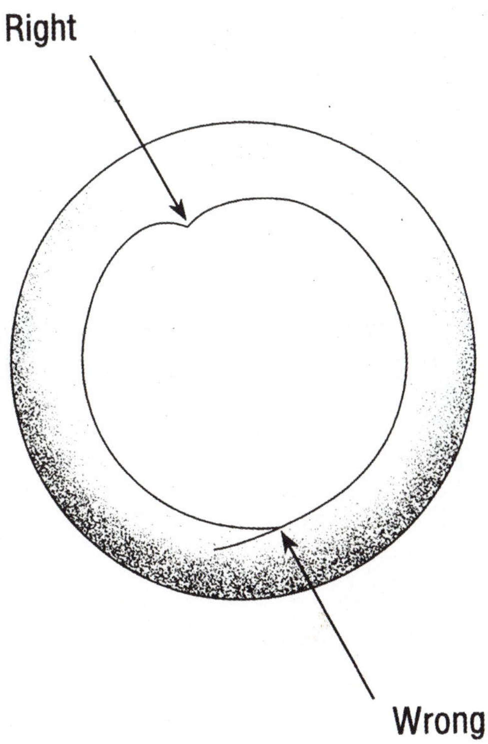

Fig. 19.4: Right and wrong approach to close the CCC

cation, of balanced salt solution (BSS) as well as viscoelastics and the cost of the needles is negligible. In addition, the following factors are essential for the success of the needle capsulorhexis.

Needle

- Even though many different needles are available, only the 23-gauge needle can be recommended. The lumen of this type of needle is just sufficient to produce a pressure exchange between anterior chamber and BSS irrigating bottle.
- The metal of such a cannula supplies just enough rigidity to provide the necessary resistance for difficult manipulations. Needles with higher gauge do not meet the described requirements, and although this is unfortunately not generally known, this alone can cause CCC failure.

A higher, i.e. positive pressure in the anterior chamber compared to the intracapsular pressure is mandatory. This becomes especially noticeable with intumescent lenses, where the lens protein is hydrated resulting in a volume increase inside the capsular bag, so that also the endocapsular pressure is considerably increased. Only if the anterior chamber pressure is greater than or equal to that inside the capsular bag can a successful capsulorhexis be performed. The pressure in the anterior chamber can be adjusted by varying the height of the infusion bottle.

The needle tip should be as sharp as possible, since a blunt needle creates stellate burst, which is more difficult to handle (Figs 19.5 and 19.6).

FORCEPSTECHNIQUE

The forceps technique is easier to learn. For this reason, it is also the most frequently applied capsulorhexis technique, which, however, can only be performed using viscoelastics. The principle of the forceps capsulorhexis exactly corresponds to the principle of the needle technique. In addition to the known Utrata forceps, there are mini forceps which are similar in construction to the forceps developed for the posterior segment of the eye. The advantage of these newly designed forceps is that they can be inserted into the anterior chamber via a paracentesis, so that the incision is not exposed to needless strain.

To point out the difference between the needle and the forceps technique, the following example might be appropriate—to turn over a page of a book you can take the sheet between two fingers

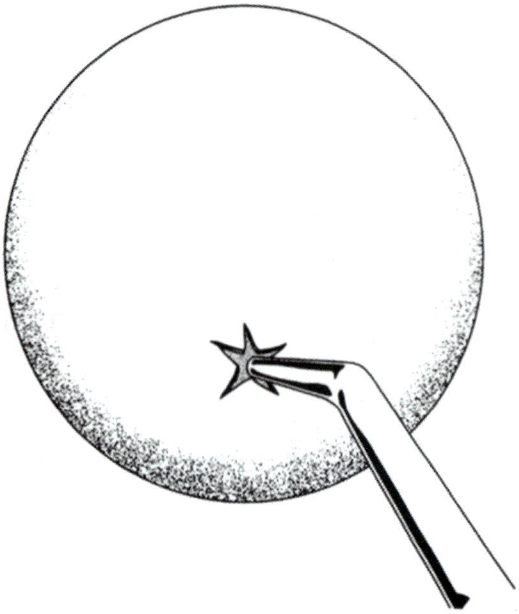

Fig. 19.5: Stellate burst created by a blunt needle

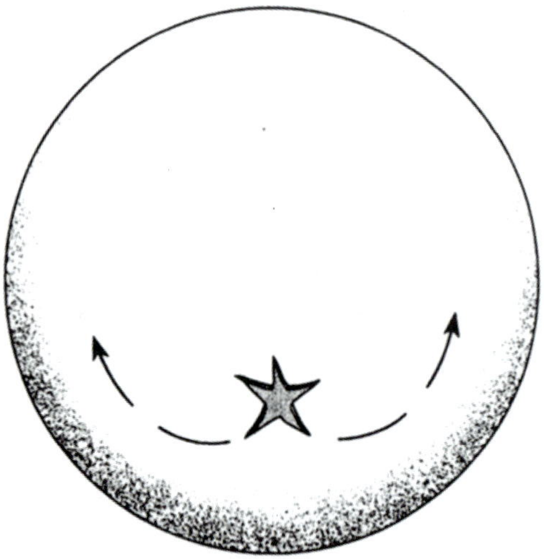

Fig. 19.6: Completion of the CCC in the presence of stellate burst

and turn it from one side to the other (this is what you do with the forceps), or you take a moistened finger, press the page a bit down and then turn it over (i.e. what you do with the needle, the counterhold is the cortex). With this in mind, the consequences appear quite clear-cut. I always use a needle technique, the initial puncture peripheral or central, for the great majority of my cases. The forceps I use in those situations where the needle, so to say, lacks the other branch. This is mainly the case when liquefied cortex is apparent or secondary enlargement of the capsulorhexis diameter is necessary.

Capsulostripsis

Capsulostripsis is a relatively new technique, which was invented by F Rentsch and described by JH Greite at the 1995 ASCRS meeting (Fig. 19.7). This technique is specifically designed for difficult cases, where the intracapsular pressure exceeds that of the anterior chamber. With this method, a vitrector with infusion sleeve is used to create an irregular opening in the anterior capsule. Experience shows that a cutter is preferrable to a rotating system. Extremely slow motion is essential to avoid tears of the capsule. The result is a jagged but stable edge, since the mouse bite-like cuts of the vitrector tip are rounded. The method is rather time-consuming compared to conventional CCC performed by an experienced surgeon, however, it is easy to perform and provides a promising alternative approach for hypermature or even milky cataracts without sufficient red reflex and other cases with difficult CCC, such as subluxated lenses or cataracts in children with elastic capsules.[5]

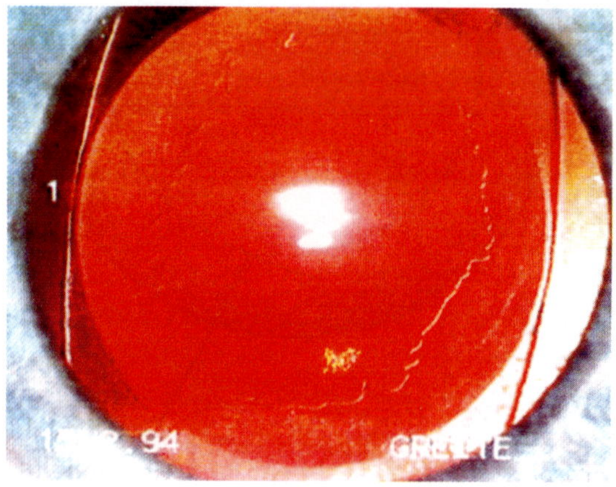

Fig. 19.7: Capsulostripsis opening and IOL *in situ* (*Courtesy:* JH Greite)

Diathermy Capsulotomy

Another alternative method to create a circular and stable aperture of the anterior capsule which lately has been quite frequently discussed is diathermy capsulotomy. This technique must be performed under viscoelastics. The method is especially recommended for intumescent cataracts, but a number of surgeons find it easier to perform than the CCC in general. However, even though the postoperative result may resemble that of a capsulorhexis, it should not be neglected that comparative studies demonstrated that the CCC is more stable and has a perfectly smooth edge compared to multiple irregularities, less stability and less elasticity of the diathermy opening, so that the application of diathermy in routine cataract surgery cannot be recommended.[6-8]

Capsulorhexis Size

The author prefers a capsulorhexis which is somewhat smaller than the optic diameter of the IOL to be implanted. In fact, no study has ever been able to show that a larger CCC diameter relative to the IOL optic is more advantageous. Supporting this preference, comparative studies found that in addition a slightly smaller capsulorhexis diameter seems to reduce posterior capsule opacification.[9,10] When it comes to rhexis-fixated IOL implantation, this type of IOL is completely excluded with an excessive rhexis diameter, for instance in case of damage of the posterior capsule, which is another reason for keeping the rhexis size smaller than the optical part of the lens.

DIFFICULT CASES

Small Pupil

Now, that several different methods are available to intraoperatively extend a narrow pupil, capsulorhexis has become easier in such cases. The generally applied measures in such cases are:

- removal of the pupillary membrane
- bimanual stretching
- removal of synechiae
- iris hooks
- pupil dilator.

To perform a capsulorhexis in the usual way, first the pupil is extended using one of these methods, then the CCC can be made with needle or forceps, according to the preference of the operating surgeon.

Pseudoexfoliation Syndrome, Uveitis and Pigmentosa

With these patients often a thickened anterior capsule can be clinically observed, which is hard to tear. Another common finding in such cases is also a subluxated lens, which is only diagnosed intraoperatively. An important aspect of surgery in such patients is to strictly refrain from a rather small capsulorhexis, as the result of this might be an undesired shrinkage of the anterior capsule.

Capsules of Infants, Children and Juveniles

Due to the high elasticity of the anterior capsule, a smaller rhexis must be performed in such patients than is the case with adults. Here it must be taken into account that the rhexis opening still enlarges by 0.5 to 1.0 mm after conclusion of the rhexis. Regarding pediatric posterior capsulorhexis, the necessity of an accompanying anterior vitrectomy is controversially discussed. Here, in a number of cases, a self-sealing closure provided by the IOL could be successfully achieved.[11]

Capsulorhexis in Calcified Capsules or Anterior Flaps

These cases mostly require a completely individual CCC, where Ong or Vannas scissors or the like must be applied in addition.

Posterior Capsulorhexis

A series of indications, such as large-scale capsular fibrosis, damage of the posterior capsule[12] or less frequent conditions like persisting arteria hyaloidea as shown by Greite at the 1990 European Society of Cataract and Refractive Surgery (ESCRS) meeting may require a primary or secondary posterior capsulotomy. In the same way as the anterior CCC, the posterior capsulorhexis also offers the preservation of a stable capsule. First the anterior capsulorhexis is performed using forceps or needle in the usual way, and phacoemulsification or IOL explantation are carried out as preferred. The anterior segment is filled with viscoelastics to stabilize the posterior capsule. Then, the posterior capsule is first only perforated, and viscoelastics are injected prior to further manipulations. This instillation of viscoelastics behind the capsule is vital to prevent a vitreous prolapse. The posterior CCC can then be carried out with needle or forceps in the same way as an anterior CCC. In some cases, a successive vitrectomy may be necessary to prevent the vitreous from invading the capsular bag via the posterior opening. The remaining tire-like capsular residue provides a stable and secure site for IOL fixation. Gimbel especially recommends a posterior capsulorhexis in pediatric cataract surgery to avoid secondary membrane formation after cataract extraction (Figs 19.8 and 19.9).[13]

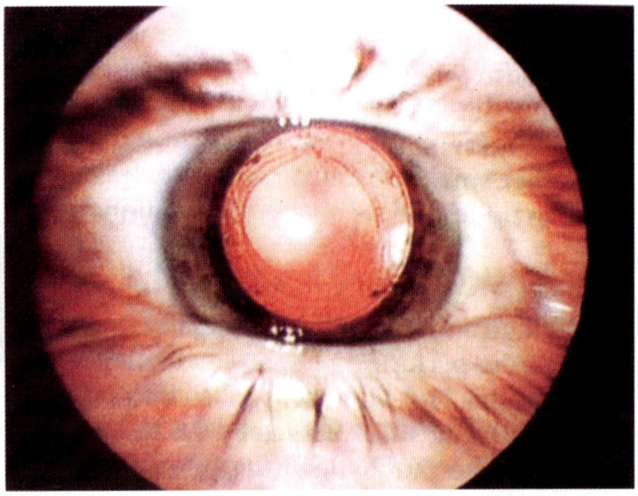

Fig. 19.8: Smaller posterior capsulorhexis size compared to the normal-sized anterior CCC

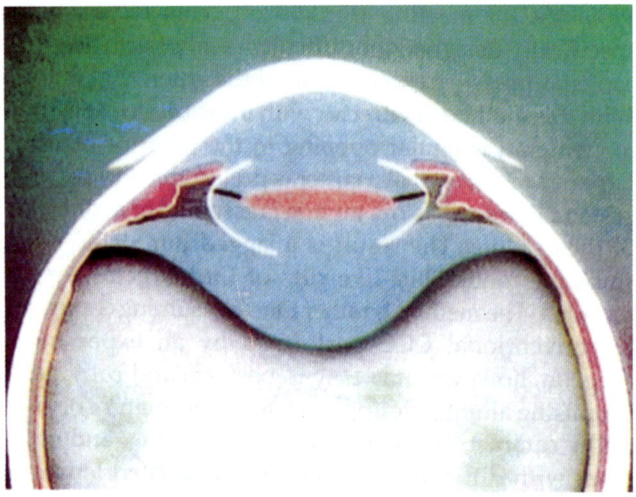

Fig. 19.9: Principle of the posterior CCC

Capsulorhexis in the Presence of a Broken Posterior Capsule

If ruptures of the posterior capsule occur intraoperatively and cannot be transformed into a posterior CCC, placement of the IOL in the ciliary sulcus with the known disadvantages of this fixation as listed below seems to be the only option. To avoid this, rhexis fixation of the IOL is the possible solution. The applicable technique was first presented by the author at the 1991 ASCRS Film Festival. The precondition for this method is an intact anterior capsulorhexis with a smaller diameter compared to the IOL optic. Here the lens optic is manipulated behind the anterior capsulorhexis rim with a spatula, while the loops remain in the sulcus ciliaris (Fig. 19.10). This approach leaves the IOL optic securely positioned inside the capsule in a button-like manner (Fig. 19.11). This method is also possible in pediatric surgery, where mostly a posterior capsulorhexis is performed as well to prevent secondary cataract formation.[14,15] The only restriction with this method is the implied exclusion of plate-haptic IOLs. This kind of fixation provides several advantages:

- no sunset or sunrise syndrome are possible
- rotation and decentration are excluded
- the calculated lens power is effective because of the reliable location of the optic
- iris chaffing cannot occur

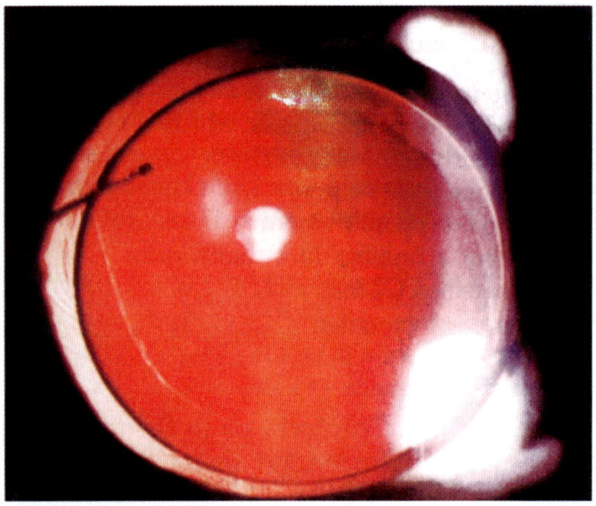

Fig. 19.10: Endocapsular fixation of the IOL optic in the presence of a broken posterior capsule—rhexis/fixation

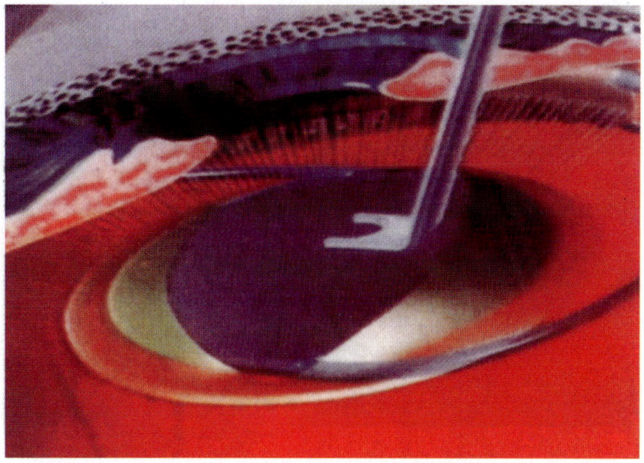

Fig. 19.11: Principle of button-like IOL fixation—rhexis/fixation

- vitreous prolapse is prevented by stable endocapsular placement of the implant
- secondary cataract formation is avoided due to removal of the posterior capsule.

A variation of this technique was recently described by Howard Gimbel. He uses the opened posterior capsule as support/fixation location in infantile or juvenile lens implantation, thus, trying to prevent a vitreous prolapse.[13]

COMPLICATIONS AND PITFALLS

There are three major potential intraoperative problems so an ophthalmic surgeon may find himself confronted with in performance of the CCC.

Discontinuity of the Capsulorhexis

To avoid this complication, the capsulorhexis should never be completed from inside out. But also stellate bursts originating from initial puncturing attempts with a blunt needle may destroy an intact capsular margin in the course of surgery to form a discontinuity which presents a most critical source for a radial tear down into the peripheral capsule. In the presence of such a discontinuity, the entity of mechanical forces inside the capsular bag concentrate on this weakest point, and the only effective remedy is to repair the discontinuity immediately (Fig. 19.12). If such a repair by transformation of the tear into a smooth edge is no longer possible, utmost care must be employed in the remaining intracapsular manipulations.

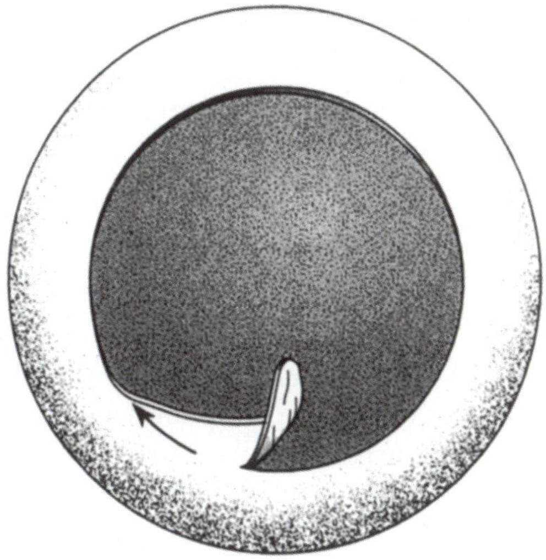

Fig. 19.12: Repair of a discontinuity by creation of a smooth edge

Tear into the Zonula

If a tear has already reached a zonular fiber, a conventional repair of the capsulorhexis is too hazardous, as it might result in further rupture right along the zonular fiber toward the equator. This critical situation can be coped with using two different approaches. One way is to follow the end of the respective zonule down to its origin, gently free it with the forceps and use this singled-out zonular fiber to tear a smooth-edged curve to unite with the otherwise intact capsulorhexis. The other and more risky approach is to firmly and briskly pull the flap toward the center.

Insufficient Capsulorhexis Size

Realizing during the process of circular tearing that the capsulorhexis will be smaller than originally planned is not really an intraoperative problem. In such cases all the surgeon has to do is to direct the vector forces in such a way that the circle is not closed but rather proceeds further into the periphery. With this kind of spiral-shaped enlargement, the CCC diameter can be increased to the desired size. Once the capsulorhexis is large enough, the circle is closed in the usual way.

CAPTUREDVISCOELASTICS

If the anterior capsular rim tightly covers the anterior IOL surface after implantation, viscoelastic residues may be trapped behind the lens. Usually this problem does not occur if the viscoelastics are carefully removed. If it does, mostly the lens blocks the passage for the viscoelastics into the anterior chamber and at the same time allows the aqueous to invade the area behind the implant, thus, pushing the IOL against the cornea. In such a situation, an additional puncture of the peripheral anterior or—in comparably narrow pupils—posterior capsule is required to provide for a release of the visco-elastics into the anterior chamber or the vitreous, respectively (Fig. 19.13).

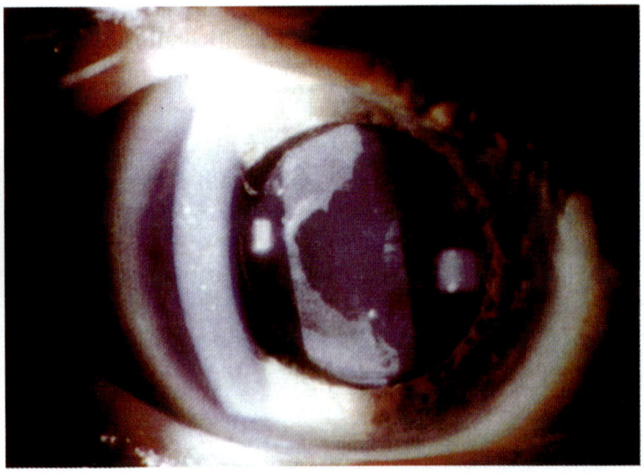

Fig. 19.13: Lens epithelial cell (LEC) growth on the surface of an IOL—only seen with capsulorhexis

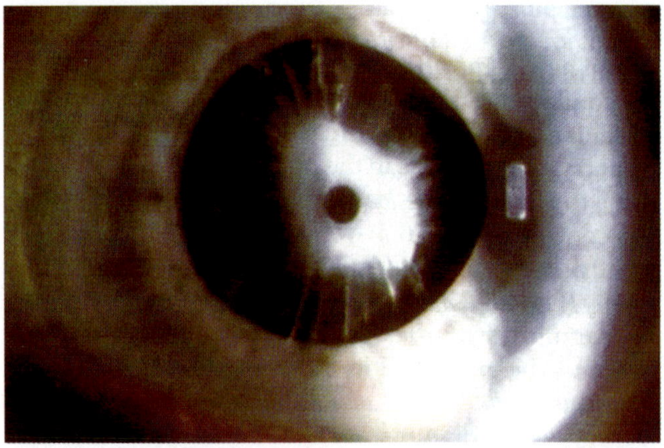

Fig. 19.14: Capsular phimosis before YAG-laser treatment

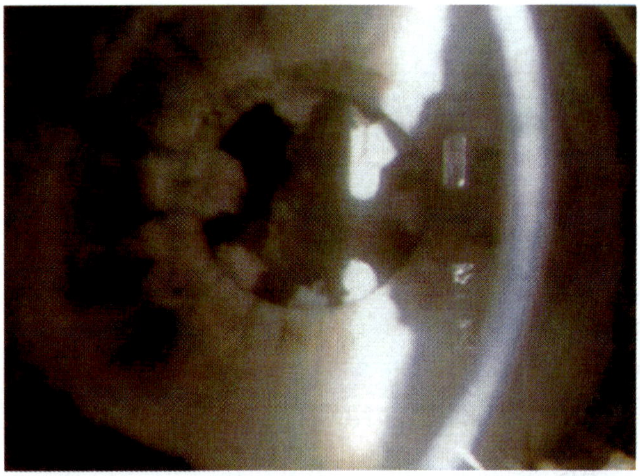

Fig. 19.15: Capsular phimosis after YAG-laser treatment

DISADVANTAGES OFTHE CCC

Since capsulorhexis was introduced, a new problem was described over time, which is the capsular shrinkage syndrome or capsular phimosis (Figs 19.14 and 19.15).[16] This was never seen before in other capsulotomy techniques. The genuine patho-mechanism could not be clarified until today. Clinically, this problem can be observed especially in patients suffering from pseudoexfoliation syndrome (PEX), uveitis, retinopathia pigmentosa or subluxatia lentis in combination with polymethylmethacrylate (PMMA) or silicone IOL implantation. All these diseases have a considerably reduced number of zonular fibers in common. The fact that up to now this complication has not been described in patients suffering from these diseases in context with an acrylic IOL implantation allows the conclusion that a certain mechanical interaction of acrylic lens surface and capsule successfully prevents this problem, so that the acrylic IOL is presently the lens of choice in such cases. This, however, is not valid for low-water acrylics (Fig. 19.16).

The aim of every surgeon is to provide the greatest degree of stability for the longest period of time possible. The other important goal is to restore the patient´s condition closest to that found in a healthy person. The development of the capsulo-rhexis definitely introduced a new age in small

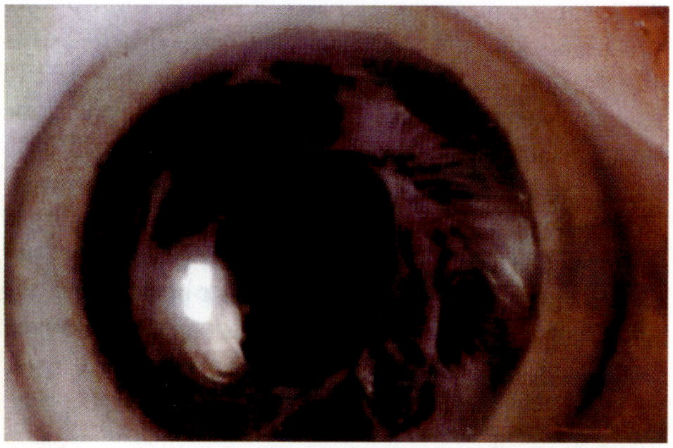

Fig. 19.16: Postoperative contracture of the CCC

incision cataract surgery. This applies both for the development of new phaco techniques and for the important role phacoemulsification plays in modern cataract surgery in general.

While capsulorhexis as a principle is well-established, its technical performance is being refined and advanced. In this context, I would like to stress once again that capsulorhexis in essence really is not a technical procedural detail but a fundamental surgical principle. Its theory needs to be well understood—then its technical details emanate as a logical consequence. In other words, you should be convinced that this anterior capsular opening is what you want to have.

Also secondary surgery including IOL exchange benefits from the specific properties of the capsulorhexis aperture. Today´s ophthalmic market is booming with a multitude of capsulorhexis tools to offer maximum comfort at the individual surgeon´s preference and for the broadbend of anatomical conditions and intraoperative situations.[17] Intraocular manipulations in the anterior as well as posterior segment of the eye which could not even be dreamed of some 20 years ago are feasible today, now that circular apertures at any required number and dimensions in both the anterior and the posterior capsule can be created securely and without taking the risk of tear originating from intraoperative manipulations. And what is more, the structural integrity of the capsule is not only maintained throughout the course of surgery but also postoperatively, thus, forming the precondition for stable, safe and permanent IOL placement. Stability of the manipulated capsular bag as well as perfect centration of an IOL as provided by the CCC are a must on the way to emmetropia.

REFERENCES

1. Neuhann T: Theorie und Operationstechnik der Kapsulorhexis. Klin Monatsbl Augenheilkd 1987;190:542-45.
2. Gimbel HV, Neuhann T: Continuous curvilinear capsulorhexis (letter). J Cataract Refract Surg 1991;17:110-11.
3. Assia EI, Apple DJ, Barden A et al: An experimental study comparing various anterior capsulectomy techniques. Arch Ophthalmol 1991;109(5):642-47.
4. Krag S, Thim K, Corydon L et al: Biomechanical aspects of the anterior capsulotomy. J Cataract Refract Surg 1994;20(4):410-16.
5. Wilson ME, Bluestein EC, Wang XH et al: Comparison of mechanized anterior capsulectomy and manual continuous capsulorhexis in pediatric eyes. J Cataract Refract Surg 1994;20(6):602-06.
6. Morgan JE, Ellingham RB, Young RD et al: The mechanical properties of the human lens capsule following capsulorhexis or radiofrequency diathermy capsulotomy. Arch Ophthalmol 1996;114:1110-15.
7. Krag S, Thim K, Corydon L: Mechanical properties of diathermy capsulotomy versus capsulorhexis—a biomechanical study. J Cataract Refract Surg 1997;23:86-90.
8. Sugimoto Y, Kuho E, Tsuzuki S et al: Histological observation of anterior capsular edges produced by continuous curvilinear and diathermy capsulorhexis. J Jpn Ophthalmol Soc 1996;100(11):858-62.
9. Ravalico G, Tognetto D, Palomba M et al: Capsulorhexis size and posterior capsule opacification. J Cataract Refract Surg 1996;22(1):98-103.
10. Hollick EJ, Spalton DJ: Capsulorhexis size? Smaller seems better. J Cataract Refract Surg 1997;2(5):12.
11. Gimbel HV, Chin PK, Ellant JP: Capsulorhexis, Ophthalmol Clin North Am 1995;8(3):441-45.
12. Galand A, Van Cauwenberge F, Moossavi J: Le capsulorhexis posterieur chez l´adulte. J Fr Ophtalmol 1996;19(10):571-75.
13. Gimbel HV, DeBroff BM: Posterior capsulorhexis with optic capture—maintaining a clear visual axis after pediatric cataract surgery. J Cataract Refract Surg 1994;20(6): 658-64.
14. Behrendt S, Wetzel W: Vollständige Okklusion der Kapsulorhexisöffnung durch Vorderkapselschrumpfung. Ophthalmologe 1994;91(4):526-28.
15. Neuhann T: When posterior capsule tears, use capsulorhexis for IOL fixation. Phaco and Foldables 1991;4(6): 1-3.
16. Sabbagh LB: Rhexis can hold IOL when posterior capsule breaks. Ocular Surgery News 1992;3(3):1-10.
17. Wilson ED: Capsulorhexis tools—from fancy forceps to mock pizza cutters, ASCRS Ophthalmic Services Corp 1997.

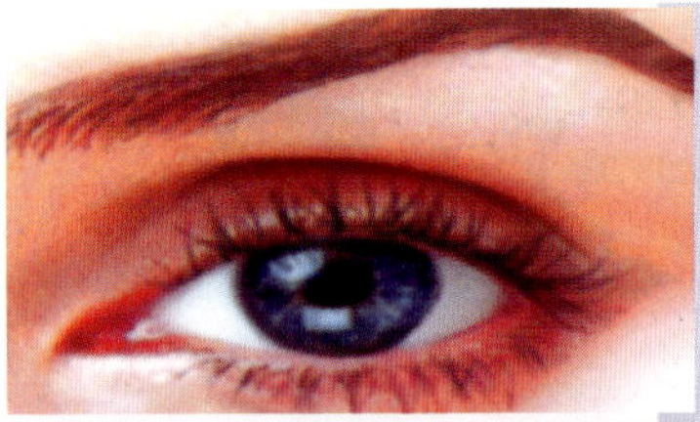

Twenty

Dynamics of Hydroprocedures in Manual Small Incision Cataract Surgery

Ranjit S Dhaliwal
(India)

HISTORY OF HYDROPROCEDURES
HYDRODISSECTION
HYDRODELINEATION
COMPLICATIONS OF HYDROPROCEDURES

Hydroprocedures in Manual Small Incision Cataract Surgery constitute hydrodissection and hydrodelineation. These procedures are performed by injecting irrigation fluid / balanced salt solution into the various anatomical layers of the cataractous lens with a cannula. These are performed to divide the various components of the lens, to separate the cortico-nuclear mass of the lens from the capsule, the nucleus from the epinucleus and cortex and to strip the nucleus bare of its different layers, to its hardest kernel.

The dynamics of hydrodissection and hydrodelineation in Manual Small Incision Cataract Surgery are essentially the same as in phaco or planned extracapsular surgery.

For a proper study and understanding of the hydroprocedures, even at the cost of duplication elsewhere, a brief sketch of the anatomy and surgical anatomy of the lens would not be out of place.

Anatomy of the Human Lens

The human crystalline lens is a bi-convex, encapsulated, transparent, avascular body of cells, which are ectodermal in origin. It is suspended between the iris and the vitreous within the eyeball, by the zonular fibres or the zonules. The zonules arise from the ciliary body and are attached to the lens all around its periphery.

The adult lens measures about 9-10 mm in diameter in the equatorial region and is 4.75-5 mm antero-posteriorly. The axial length of the lens may be up to 7 mm in an intumescent cataract and may shrink to 2.5-3 mm in a hypermature cataract. The axial diameter of the lens varies markedly with accommodation.

The lens remains optically transparent due to its avascularity, specific fiber pattern and complex metabolism. The avascularity provides the lens a relative immunity, from primary inflammatory reactions and pathological hyperplasia. However, the epithelial cells in the equatorial zone possess mitotic activity. The newly formed fibers form the outer most peripheral layers, while the older fibers form the deeper layers of the lens. This heterogeneous pattern of fibers is the reason for a variable refractive index of the lens in different zones. The lens has an approximate dioptric power of 20D.

Histologically, with reference to Manual Small Incision Cataract Surgery the human lens can be divided into:

- Capsular bag,
- Superficial cortex,
- Intermediate epinucleus, and
- Deep nucleus.

The *capsule,* which forms the capsular bag, is transparent, homogeneous and highly elastic, and is made up of type IV collagen fibers of variable thickness. The capsule is thicker in the anterior pre-equatorial region (14 –21 μm) and thinner posteriorly, especially so in the center of the posterior capsule (4 μm). The capsule gives support to the lens substance.

The lens *cortex* is made up of 10-15 layers of homogeneous structure with a specific fiber pattern.

The lens *nucleus* is made up of compact and compressed cortical fibers. This zone does not have a definite pattern of cell nuclei. There is no demarcation of cortex and nucleus since transition is gradual and intermediate fibers retain their histological pattern.

Surgical Anatomy of the Human Lens

From a surgical point of view, the human lens is anatomically classified into:

1. *Capsular bag:* The capsule envelops the whole lens substance. Immediately behind the anterior lens capsule is a layer made up of single layer of cubical cells, known as the lenticular epithelium.
2. *Superficial cortex:* Cortex is the white, soft lens matter, which surrounds the epinucleus and the nucleus. It is aspirated or irrigated out during surgery.
3. *Epinucleus:* Epinucleus is the semi-soft lens matter, which surrounds the nucleus, and which is either hydro- or visco- expressed out or is aspirated with a large cannula during cataract surgery.
4. *Nucleus:* Nucleus or the hard kernel has a well-defined configuration, and is fractured or fragmented and hydro- or visco-expressed during Manual Small Incision Cataract Surgery.

History of Hydroprocedures

Michael Blumenthal of Israel was the first to describe hydroprocedures. The aim of hydroprocedures in Manual Small Incision Cataract Surgery was originally to reduce the nuclear size to the smallest hard core endonucleus. Hydroprocedures facilitate the rotation of the nucleus in the bag, its subsequent prolapse into the anterior chamber and its hydro- or visco- expression or manual removal through the self sealing sclero corneal tunnel. Thorough hydroprocedures play a pivotal role in Manual Small Incision Cataract Surgery and may be performed with the anterior chamber maintainer in on or off state.

Faust coined the term hydrodissection

Instruments for Hydroprocedures

1. *Syringe:* One may use a glass or a plastic syringe of 1 – 2 cc capacity. A 2 cc syringe gives a good grip and adequate amount of fluid for injection. But a 1 cc tuberculin syringe gives a better control over the amount of fluid injected. A glass syringe is easier to handle as it is smoother. But if the piston is ill fitting there may be fluid leak. Always

use same type and size of syringe as a tactile feedback of the syringe and the plunger is important, particularly when the red glow is insufficient or the pupil is narrow.

2. *Cannula:* The cannula to be used, may be 26 – 30 G in size, may be straight or bent, but should have a smooth rounded tip.

Before starting the hydroprocedures the patency of the cannula and the smooth functioning of the syringe must be checked personally by the surgeon.

HYDRODISSECTION

Hydrodissection is essentially the complete dissection of the cortico-nuclear mass from the capsule with the mechanical help of a fluid wave produced by injecting BSS, exactly in-between the anterior capsule and the cortex. This frees the nucleus, epinucleus and cortex from the entire capsular bag, simplifying in the process the later manipulations on the nucleus.

Classification of Hydrodissection

1. *Conventional Hydrodissection:* Originally hydrodissection was essentially the separation of the superficial cortex from the epinucleus.
2. Cortical cleavage Hydrodissection: Howard Fine was the first to describe cortical cleavage hydrodissection. In cortical cleavage hydrodissection, the cannula is slightly lifted up, tenting the capsule a little in the process and small amount of the fluid is injected with a jerk (Fig. 20.1).
3. *Hydro-free dissection:* Hydro-free dissection was described by Gimbel and is more or less like cortical cleavage hydrodissection. Before injecting the fluid the cannula is first swept along the plane of cleavage.

Technique of Hydrodissection

Before beginning hydrodissection, remove a part of the viscoelastic, which had been introduced into the anterior chamber to facilitate capsulorhexis. This makes the procedure safe and helps to prevent repeated prolapse of the iris during the hydroprocedure and undue pressure on the posterior capsule. A 26-G blunt tipped hydrodissection cannula mounted on a 1cc syringe filled with irrigation

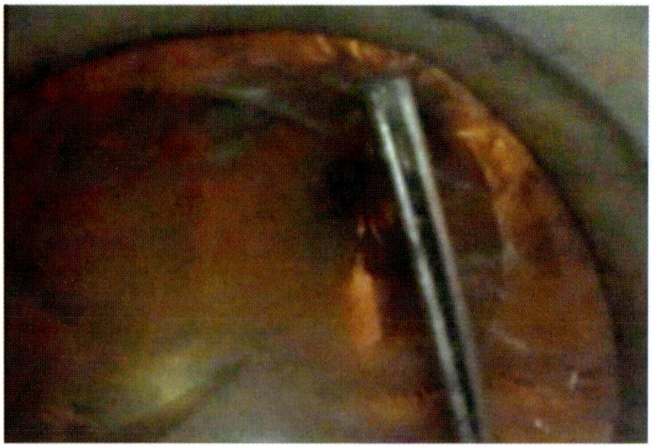

Fig. 20.1: Cortical cleavage hydrodissection (*Courtesy:* Dr Ravijit Singh, Amritsar)

fluid / BSS is guided a mm behind the rhexis margin in the subcapsular plane first at 12 o'clock and then in all the other quadrants (Figs 20.2 to 20.4). Lift up the cannula slightly, tenting the capsule a little in the process and inject a small amount of the fluid with a jerk to produce fluid wave (Figs 20.5 to 20.8). Fluid injected slowly and smoothly, and not with a jerk does not produce a wave and comes back into the anterior chamber. For hydrodissection at 12 o'clock, the cannula maybe inserted through one of the side ports. Otherwise, a J-shaped cannula may also be used to inject the fluid to the right and left of 12 o'clock meridian.

Hydrodissection separates the cortex from the capsule all around. Most of the times, a fluid wave can be seen traversing the field of vision as it

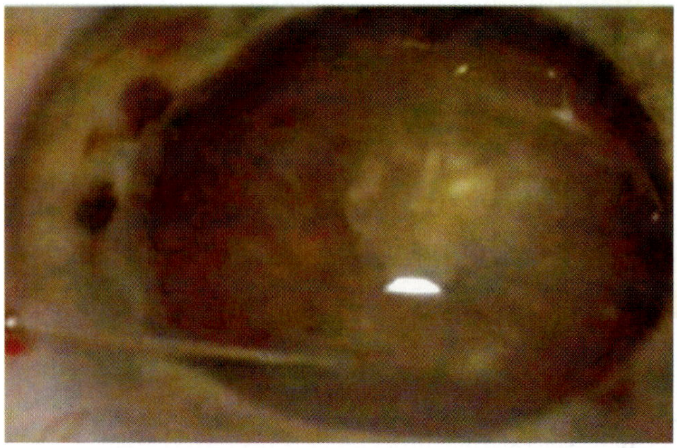

Fig. 20.2: Sub Incisional Hydrodissection (*Courtesy:* Dr Ravijit Singh, Amritsar)

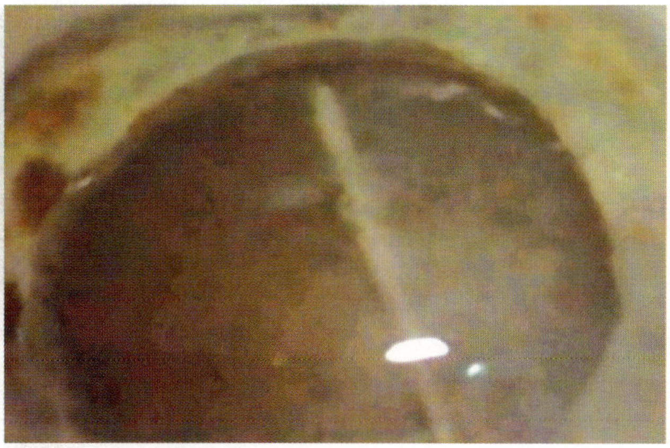

Fig. 20.3: Hydrodissection at 6 O' clock
(*Courtesy:* Dr Ravijit Singh, Amritsar)

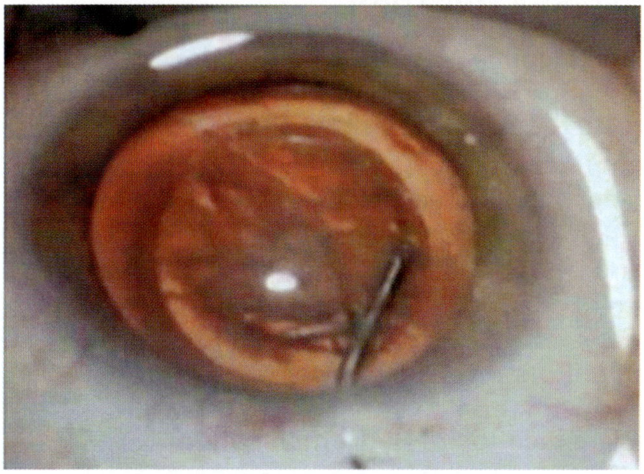

Fig. 20.4: Hydrodissection at 9 O' clock
(*Courtesy:* Dr Ravijit Singh, Amritsar)

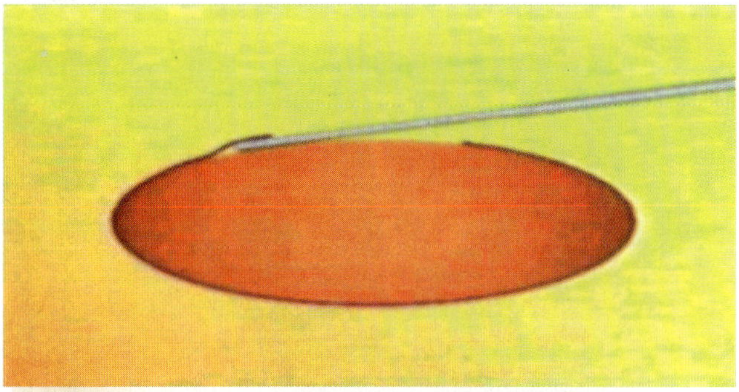

Fig. 20.5: Insert the cannula and tent the capsule

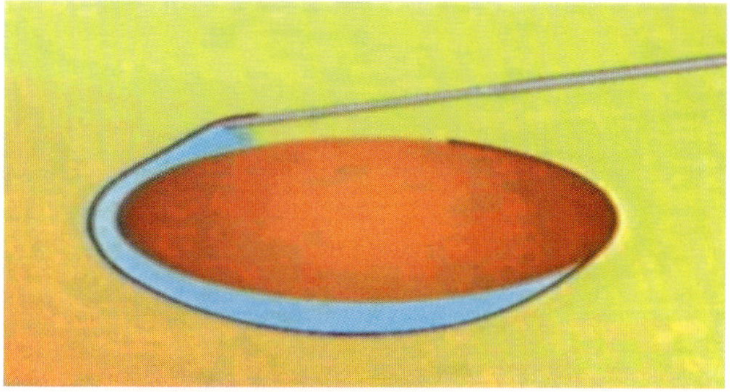

Fig. 20.6: Inject BSS under the capsule

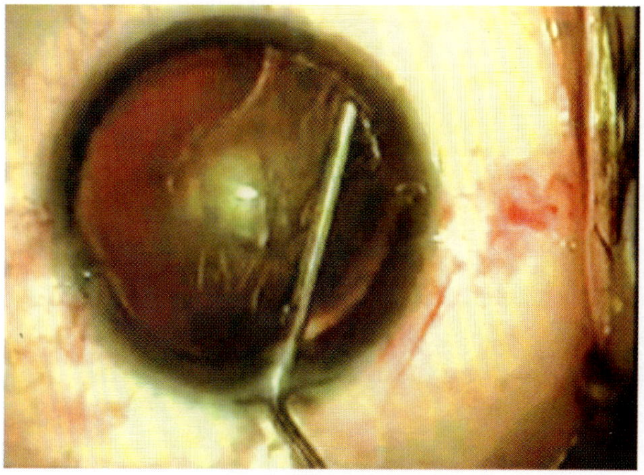

Fig. 20.7: Fluid wave in hydrodissection
(*Courtesy:* Dr Ravijit Singh, Amritsar)

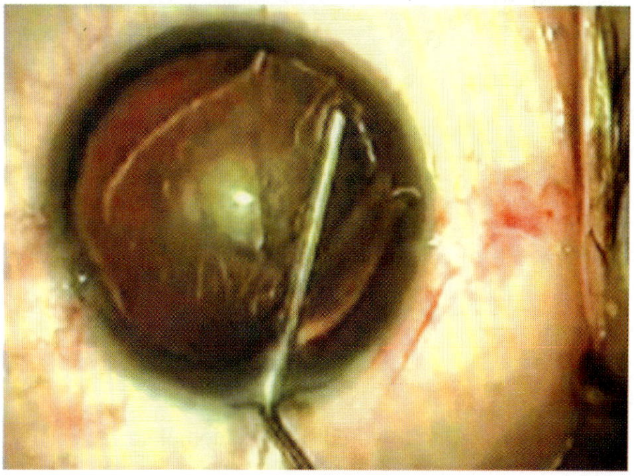

Fig. 20.8: Progress of the fluid wave
(*Courtesy:* Dr Ravijit Singh, Amritsar)

separates the posterior capsule from the cortex. A shallowing of the anterior chamber also indicates the dissection and is because of the entrapped fluid behind the nucleus in the subcapsular space. A gentle tap on the nucleus (Figs 20.9 and 10) in the shallow part of the anterior chamber completes the hydrodissection and deepens the chamber (Fig. 20.11). This is called compression hydrodissection.

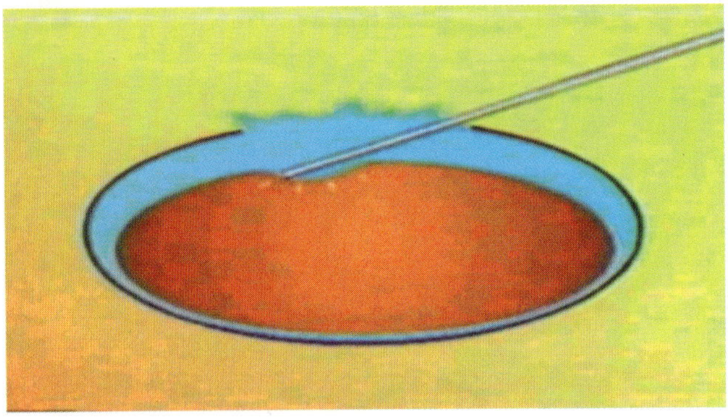

Fig. 20.9: Tap the nucleus

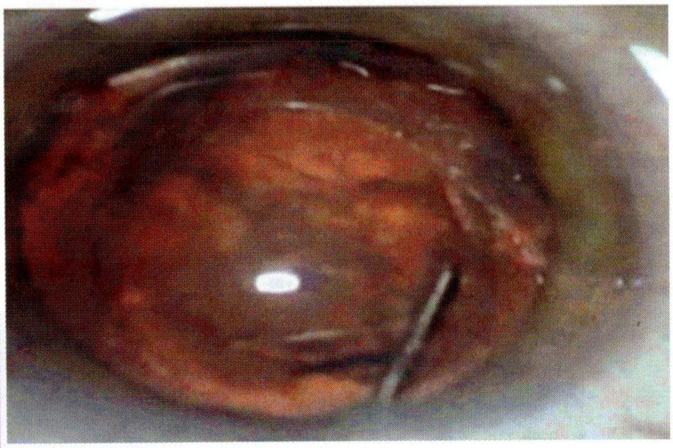

Fig. 20.10: Tapping the nucleus
(*Courtesy:* Dr Ravijit Singh, Amritsar)

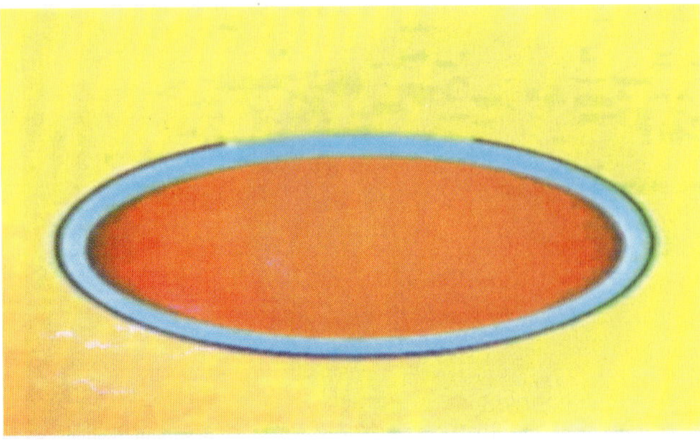

Fig. 20.11: Hydrodissection complete

Nucleus is then rotated, both clockwise and anticlockwise. Free rotation is suggestive of a successful hydrodissection.

Advantages of Hydrodissection

In Manual Small Incision Cataract Surgery hydrodissection makes the nuclear manipulations safer. It separates the nucleus from the capsular bag so that the nucleus will be free to rotate within the bag. Having hydrodissected the cortico-nuclear mass from the capsular bag, the rotation of the nucleus and its subsequent prolapse into the anterior chamber does not exert any tug on the zonular ligaments because of the reduced resistance to the expression of the nucleus from the capsular bag. Good hydrodissection is very essential before nucleus removal.

This reduces the risk of:

- zonular dialysis,
- posterior capsular rupture and
- posterior dislocation of the nucleus.

HYDRODELINEATION

Hydrodelineation has been called hydrodelamination or hydrodemarcation by many. Hydrodelineation, is essentially the separating of the epinucleus from the nucleus by injecting the irrigating fluid between these two (Figs 20.12 and 13). The fluid wave, which goes around the nucleus, appears like a golden ring (Figs 20.14 and 15) under the operating microscope. In Manual Small Incision Cataract Surgery hydrodelineation helps in the minification of the nucleus by debulking.

Classification of Hydrodelineation

1. Manual hydrodelineation.
2. Hydrosonic delineation, devised by Aziz Anis in USA, is left out of this text on Manual Small

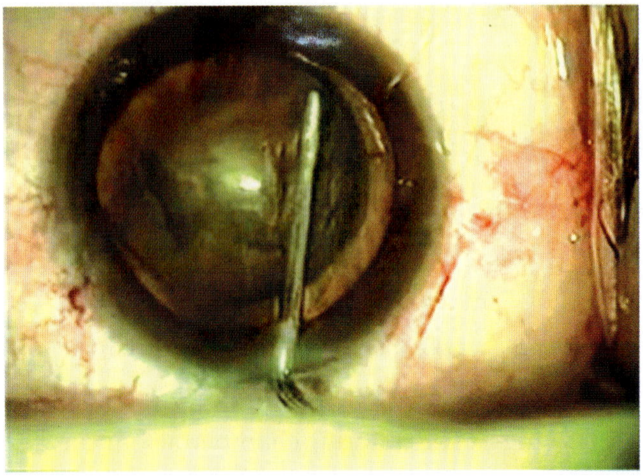

Fig. 20.12: Hydrodelineation
(*Courtesy:* Dr Ravijit Singh, Amritsar)

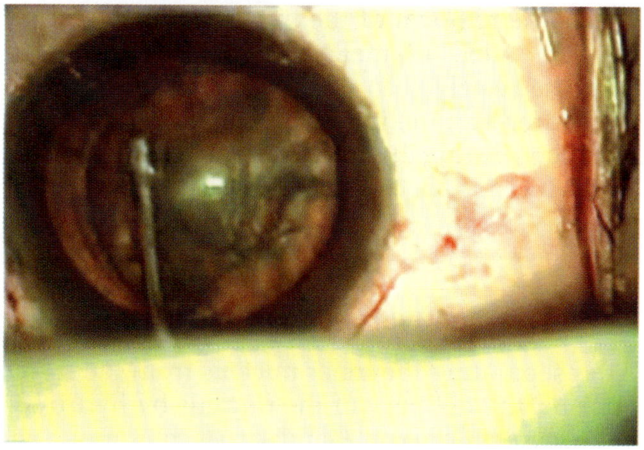

Fig. 20.13: Hydrodelineation
(*Courtesy:* Dr Ravijit Singh, Amritsar)

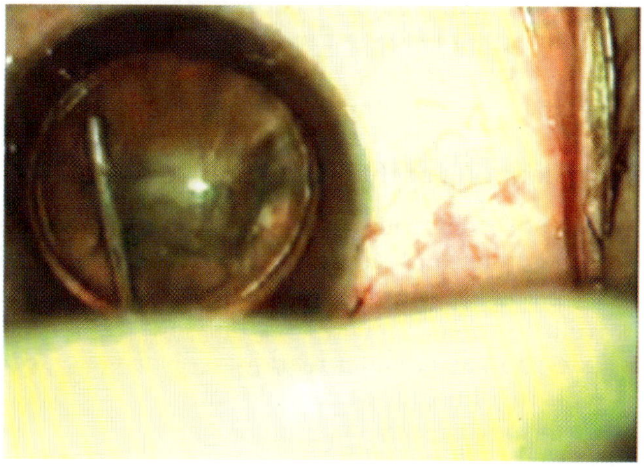

Fig. 20.14: Partial golden ring
(*Courtesy:* Dr Ravijit Singh, Amritsar)

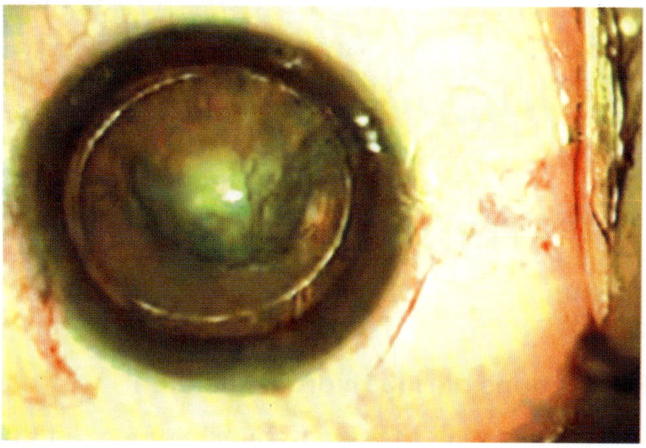

Fig. 20.15: Complete golden ring
(*Courtesy:* Dr Ravijit Singh, Amritsar)

Incision Cataract Surgery for description by texts on phacoemulsification.

Technique of Manual Hydrodelineation

As in hydrodissection, remove a part of the viscoelastic introduced into the anterior chamber. This prevents repeated prolapse of the iris during the hydroprocedure.

After the capsulotomy the focus of the microscope is shifted from the anterior capsule to the posterior capsule. Other than in cases of mature white cataracts and very dark brunescent cataracts, it is almost always possible to bring the concavity of the surface of the posterior capsule into focus. This is sometimes possible even in dense nuclear sclerosis. In the presence of wedges of cortical cataract, posterior capsule is focussed through clear spaces between the wedges. Visualization of the whole lens including the nucleus is easiest in posterior subcapsular cataract. Retro-illumination is used to visualize the posterior capsule in very dense cataracts and also in mature white cataracts, by switching off all the other lights in the operation theatre.

The major advantage of beginning hydrodelineation posteriorly and proceeding anteriorly is the ability to see the anterior layers and visually monitor the depth of penetration to avoid puncturing the posterior capsule.

A narrow gauge cannula, usually 26 to 30 G is attached to a 1 cc syringe filled with irrigating fluid / BSS. When the posterior capsule is focused, the hydrodelineation cannula is introduced through the capsulotomy into the cortex and nucleus until its tip is posterior to the central hard core of the nucleus, just in front of the posterior capsule. No fluid is injected until this point is reached. Small amount of irrigation fluid / BSS is now injected in jerky pulsed doses while simultaneously withdrawing the cannula along the track. This will give rise to concentric golden rings, which assure the completion of hydrodelineation.

Pulsed injection of the irrigation fluid should be undertaken not during movement of the cannula, but on reaching the required depth. While effecting the required hydrodelineation, care must be taken while injecting fluid into the nucleus, by pressing on the posterior lip of the incision. This is necessary to prevent entrapment of the fluid within the capsular bag.

In cases where the posterior capsular surface cannot be visualized the cannula is pushed into the nucleus until it meets with resistance. At this point of impediment, the cannula is withdrawn a fraction of a millimeter and the irrigating fluid is injected. The fluid advances into the body of the cataract and a plane of cleavage, usually identified by the appearance of a golden ring, appears around the inner nucleus. Sometimes, only a dark separation plane or a gray reflex appears.

If the ring appears only partially, it is necessary to reintroduce the cannula in a different zone and inject the irrigating fluid again. The goal is to totally separate the outer from the inner nucleus.

Beginners can start by aspirating the anterior cortex and epinucleus with a 5/10 cc syringe and 20/21G cannula. The anterior chamber maintainer may be kept on. The anterior surface of hard core nucleus is exposed and one can see the cleavage between epinucleus and hard core. Then one can go ahead with the hydrodelamination, with the whole procedure fully visible to the surgeon. Once experienced, this extra step is not necessary. One can just feel the resistance of the hard core and proceed.

Encountering of resistance marks the end of the soft outer nucleus and the beginning of the firm inner nucleus. In certain cataracts this is a distinct boundary of the inner hard nucleus, whereas in others it is not so evident. This demarcation is evident in the young and difficult to find in the elderly. Hydrodelineation is also useful in highlighting the line of demarcation between the fetal and the adult nucleus.

In extremely hard cataracts, the inner nucleus extends right up to the capsule. The cleavage plane cannot be identified. So hydrodelineation cannot be performed in such cases. In these cases what actually is effected is hydrodissection. But the hydroprocedure in such cases should be undertaken extremely carefully.

In very soft cataracts, when several cleavage planes are isolated, delamination of the cataract makes the removal of the nucleus very easy, and the outer nuclear lamellae can be visco- or hydro-expressed easily.

Hydrodelamination is performed for increasing the safety, during the removal of nucleus in Manual Small Incision Cataract Surgery. The inner hard nucleus, the firm structure is very small and can easily be removed.

Advantages of Hydrodelineation

After separating the inner nucleus from the softer nucleus, the delivery of the nucleus by hydro- or visco- expression or the sandwich technique is easy through a 5-6 mm wide tunnel.

The hydro procedures thus form an integral part of Manual Small Incision Cataract Surgery, and help in mobilizing the nucleus. Further, they debulk the hard core nucleus so as to facilitate evacuation through the narrowest tunnel.

Complications of Hydroprocedures

In Manual Small Incision Cataract Surgery, all the complications that occur during hydrodissection are possible complications during hydrodelineation as well.

1. Extension of capsular tear,
2. Rupture of posterior capsule, and
3. Posterior dislocation of the nucleus,

These complications may occur if a large quantity of irrigation fluid / BSS is injected with too much of force during the hydroprocedures. One should be careful not to inject a large volume of fluid in the bag, as it may jeopardize its integrity.

These are especially possible when the hydro-procedure is being carried out through the side port. With an anterior chamber filled with visco-elastic during the hydroprocedures through the side port, the fluid may not flow around the nucleus and there can be a rapid rise of the intracapsular pressure, leading to any or all of these complications.

Precautions during Hydrodelineation

In Manual Small Incision Cataract Surgery all the precautions that are necessary during hydro-dissection are adhered to during hydrodelineation as well.

1. *Successful Capsulorhexis:* Though a successful capsulorhexis is not much emphasized in Manual Small Incision Cataract Surgery, it is a prerequisite for hydroprocedures. The integrity of the capsulorhexis margin makes these procedures absolutely safe. The irrigating fluid is injected beneath the capsulorhexis margin, so that the fluid injected does not regurgitate into the anterior chamber without completing the hydrodelineation all around. Capsulorhexis in Manual Small Incision Cataract Surgery should not be very small.
2. *Viscoelastic in anterior chamber:* Before the hydroprocedures, the viscoelastic in the anterior chamber should be removed. This is very important especially when hydrodissection is being done through the side port. Unlike hydrodissection, where viscoelastic is completely evacuated before the procedure, in hydrodelineation the viscoelastic in the anterior chamber is only partially removed. Viscoelastic over the capsulorhexis helps in directing the fluid wave into the lens substance and delineation of the nucleus.
   Removal of the viscoelastic is effected by exchanging it through the sclero corneal tunnel with irrigating fluid, by injecting the fluid into the pole opposite the main entry, while simultaneously pressing the posterior lip of the tunnel.
3. *Use of the side port:* If hydroprocedure is carried out through the side port and the anterior chamber is formed with a viscoelastic, it is absolutely necessary to use very small amount of the irrigating fluid. A 1 cc glass syringe attached to a cannula is used. A larger syringe is to be avoided, as a sudden gush of irrigation fluid / BSS in the crystalline lens might burst the posterior capsule. The cannula should be introduced first under the anterior capsule at the 12 o'clock position. Not more than 0.1 cc to 0.3 cc of irrigation fluid is injected.
   Use of the side port for hydroprocedures is best avoided and is to be used only by the beginners to work in the sub-incisional area.
4. *Use of an anterior chamber maintainer:* In the presence of an anterior chamber maintainer and the fluid flowing, hydroprocedures are easily performed through the tunnel (Figure 20.16 and 20.17), but these may be performed even through one of the two paracenteses located at 10 and 2 o'clock. This is possible because the anterior chamber is filled with the irrigation fluid / BSS and any excess therein easily flows out of the side port from around the cannula. Another explanation is that an anterior chamber maintainer keeps replenishing any loss of the fluid from the chamber. But when an excess of the fluid comes through the hydrodissection or

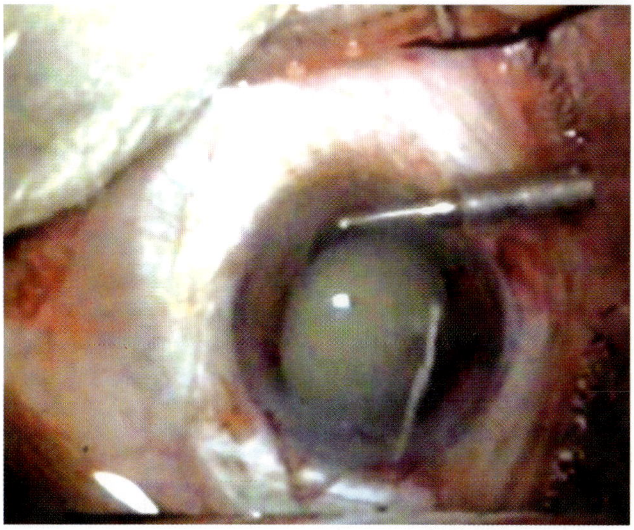

Fig. 20.16: Hydrodissection with ACM on (*Courtesy:* Dr Nikhilesh M Trivedi, Balaghat)

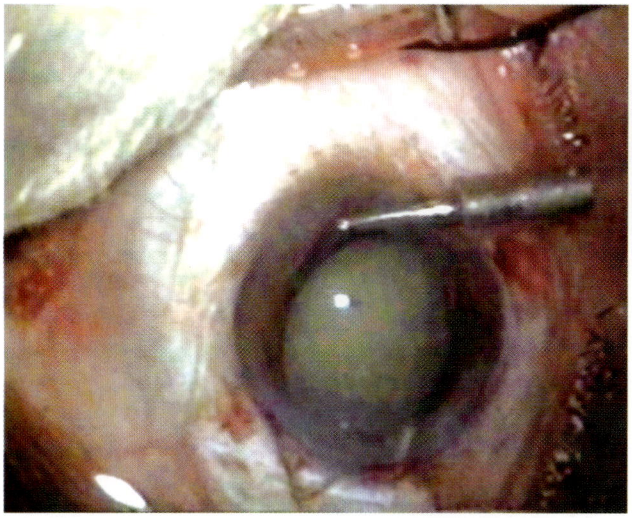

Fig. 20.17: Hydroprocedure with ACM on (*Courtesy:* Dr Nikhilesh M Trivedi, Balaghat)

Section 2

hydrodelineation cannula, the replenishment slows down (rather there is a relative back flow into the anterior chamber maintainer). This buffers the effect of the excess fluid through the cannula.

5. *Preoperative conditions:* Certain conditions which necessitate extraordinary care during hydro-procedures are
   - High myopes
   - Post vitrectomy
   - Traumatic cataract
   - Pseudoexfoliation syndrome
   - Posterior polar cataract
   - Posterior lenticonus
   - Complicated cataract and
   - Hypermature cataract.

Hydrodissection should be avoided in cases of posterior polar cataract and Hydrodelineation is not required in hard cataracts.

Hydroprocedures are not necessary in hypermature cataracts.

REFERENCES

1. Duke Elder S: System of Ophthalmology, Normal and Abnormal Development, Vol. III, Part I and II, Henry Kimpton, London, 1964.
2. Duke Elder, S: System of Ophthalmology, Diseases of Lens and Vitreous, Glaucoma and Hypotony, Vol. XI, St. Louis, CV Mosby, 1969.
3. Warwick, Roger: Eugene Wolff's Anatomy of the Eye and Orbit, 7th Edition, Lewis, London, 1976.
4. Ropper Hall, MJ: Stallard's Eye Surgery, IV Edition, Bombay, KM Verghese Company, 1980.
5. Koch D. Advanced Phacoemulsification Techniques, Slack Inc., New Jersey, 1991.
6. Sachdev MS, Venkatesh P. Hydro Procedures Related to Phacoemulsification, Phacoemulsification–A Practical Guide, New Delhi, New Age International Ltd., 1996.
7. Blumenthal M, et al: Small Incision Manual Extracapsular Cataract Extraction using selective Hydro dissection, Ophthalmic Surgery, 1992;23(10):699-701.
8. Boyd, Benjamin F. The Modern Manual Small Incision Extra-capsular with Mini-Nuc Technique, Highlights of Ophthalmology, No. 1, 2000.
9. Saha S. Non Phaco Small Incision Cataract Surgery, Nucleus Removal–Tips and Tricks, Delhi Journal of Ophthalmology, 2000;8:(2).
10. Bidaye, Vilas: Non Phaco Small Incision Cataract Surgery, Delhi Journal of Ophthalmology, 2000;8(2):
11. Malik KPS, Goel R. Manual Small Incision Cataract Surgery, CME Series, No. 8, All India Ophthalmological Society.
12. Shah Anil. Small Incision Cataract Surgery (Manual Phaco) Best out of Waste, Mumbai, Bhalani Publishing House, 2000.
13. Titiyal JS. Phacoemulsification: Complications, DOS Times, 2001;7(6).

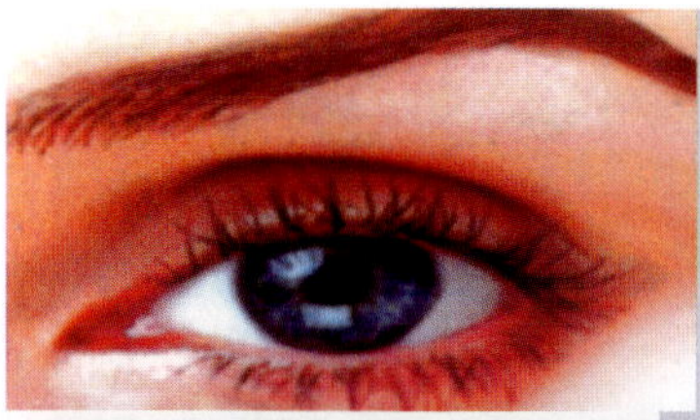

Twenty one

Dynamics of Cortex and Epinucleus Aspiration in Manual Small Incision Cataract Surgery

Ranjit S Dhaliwal
(India)

The epinucleus and cortex aspiration is performed immediately after the complete removal of the nucleus. Thorough and complete removal of the epinucleus and cortical material is a very important part of successful Manual Small Incision Cataract Surgery. Removal of the epinucleus and cortical aspiration is not the bag and anterior chamber clean up alone. To preserve the capsular bag without causing zonular dialysis and causing least damage to the corneal endothelial endothelium is of paramount importance.

Removal of the cortical matter in toto helps reduce early and late postoperative uveitis, contraction of the capsular bag, and incidence of posterior capsular opacification (PCO) and cystoid macular edema. Iris distortion and Intraocular Lens Implant (IOL) decentration because of remnant cortex is best avoided. Posterior segment visibility is improved immediately and visual acuity recovery is faster, where there is no cortex in the eye after surgery.

METHODS

1. Epinucleus Removal.
   A. Expression.
   i. Hydro-expression.
   ii. Visco-expression.

B. Aspiration.
   i. Automated Aspiration
   ii. Manual Aspiration.
2. Cortex Removal.
   A. Expression.
   i. Hydro-expression.
   ii. Visco-expression.
   B. Aspiration.
   i. Automated Aspiration.
   ii. Manual Aspiration.

EPINUCLEUS REMOVAL

Expression

Hydro-expression

Epinucleus is hydro-expressed out of the eye in Michael Blumenthal's Mini-Nuc Technique. In this the continuous flow of the irrigating fluid from the anterior chamber maintainer and the resultant positive intraocular pressure (IOP), inflate the capsular bag after the hydro-expression of the nucleus. The soft epinucleus left behind in the anterior chamber is usually hydro-expressed spontaneously, immediately after the hydro-expression of the nucleus. To facilitate this maneuver a spatula maybe introduced through the tunnel to create an outflow channel. If the epinucleus is left behind in the capsular bag, it is manipulated out. Right and left movements of the spatula in the bag will release the epinucleus from its connections with the cortex, and allow it to be flushed out.

Visco-expression

The epinucleus is visco-expressed from the anterior chamber using a 24-26G cannula on a syringe filled with a viscoelastic. As the viscoelastic is injected into the capsular bag and the anterior chamber the posterior lip of the sclerocorneal tunnel is slightly depressed to facilitate the visco-expression of the epinucleus. A slight tug on the superior rectus bridle suture is helpful. It provides the counter pressure. Viscoelastic is injected into all the quadrants of the capsular bag and anterior chamber (Figs 21.1 to 21.3).

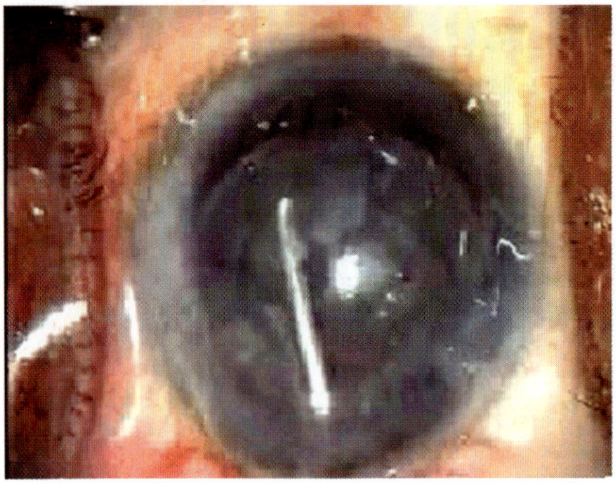

Fig. 21.1: Visco-expression of epinucleus (*Courtesy:* Dr G Natchiar, Aravind Eye Hospital)

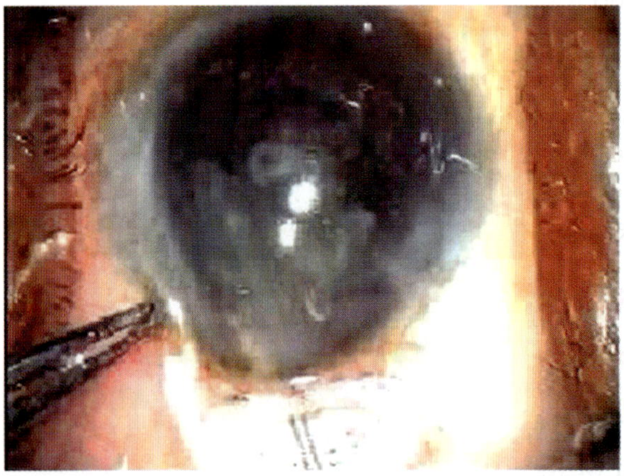

Fig. 21.2: Visco-expression of epinucleus (*Courtesy:* Dr G Natchiar, Aravind Eye Hospital)

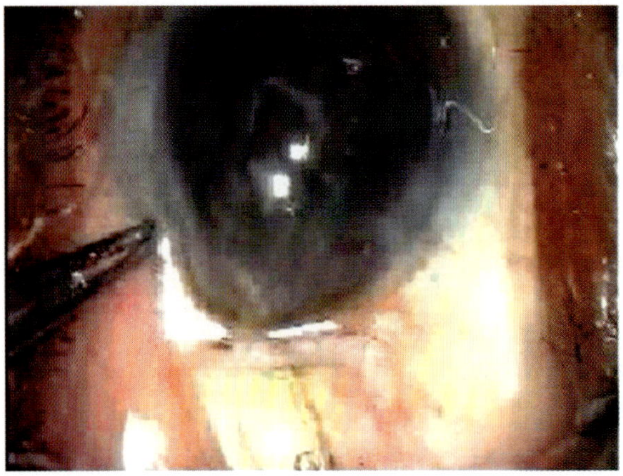

Fig. 21.3: Visco-expression of epinucleus (*Courtesy:* Dr G Natchiar, Aravind Eye Hospital)

Aspiration

Automated Aspiration

The main advantage of automated systems includes irrigation and aspiration of epinucleus in a tightly closed anterior chamber. Less irrigation is required and normal anatomic relations are maintained, i.e. deep anterior chamber, open and accessible fornices. There is no forward movement of vitreous and posterior capsule. There are very little chances of endothelial damage.

Manual Aspiration

This technique consists of capturing the epinucleus by aspiration exerted by a coaxial cannula connected to a syringe containing irrigating fluid / BSS and mobilizing the mass out of the bag. In this case, the cannula has an orifice at the top. The epinuclear mass is then aspirated with the coaxial I/A cannula inserted through the side port incision. The disadvantage with manual aspiration is that a large aspiration port is required.

CORTEX REMOVAL

Expression

Hydro-expression

Most of the free cortex in the anterior chamber or the capsular bag is hydro-expressed out of the eye in Michael Blumenthal's Mini Nuc Technique (Fig. 21.4). In this the continuous flow of the irrigating fluid from the anterior chamber maintainer and the resultant positive IOP, inflate the capsular bag after the hydro-expression of the nucleus and the epinucleus. The soft cortex left behind in the anterior chamber is usually hydro-expressed spontaneously. As in hydro-expression of the epinucleus, to facilitate this maneuver a spatula maybe introduced through the tunnel to create an outflow channel. Right and left movements of the spatula in the bag will bring out any free cortex, and allow it to be flushed out.

Visco-expression

The cortex is not usually visco-expressed from the anterior chamber. When undertaken this procedure

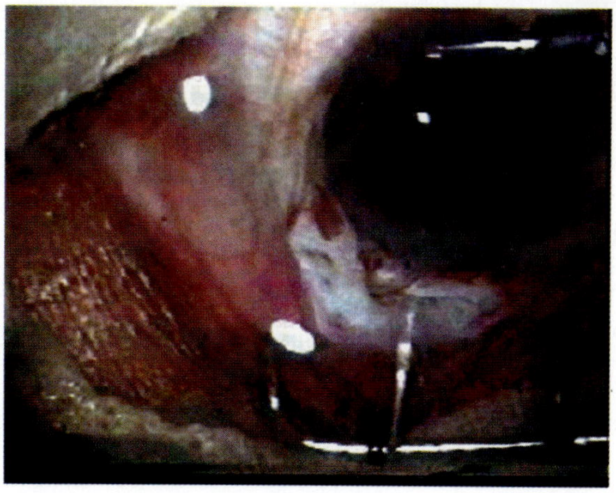

Fig. 21.4: Hydro-expression of free cortex with ACM (*Courtesy:* Dr G Natchiar, Aravind Eye Hospital)

is performed using a 24-26G cannula on a syringe filled with a viscoelastic. As the viscoelastic is injected into the capsular bag and the anterior chamber the posterior lip of the sclerocorneal tunnel is slightly depressed to facilitate the visco-expression of the epinucleus. A Viscoelastic is injected into all the quadrants of the capsular bag and anterior chamber to move any recalcitrant cortex.

Aspiration

Cortical aspiration may be undertaken, using either the automated system or manual irrigation aspiration (I/A) devices or both may be required in special situations. Every method has got its merits and demerits. No single technique can be labeled

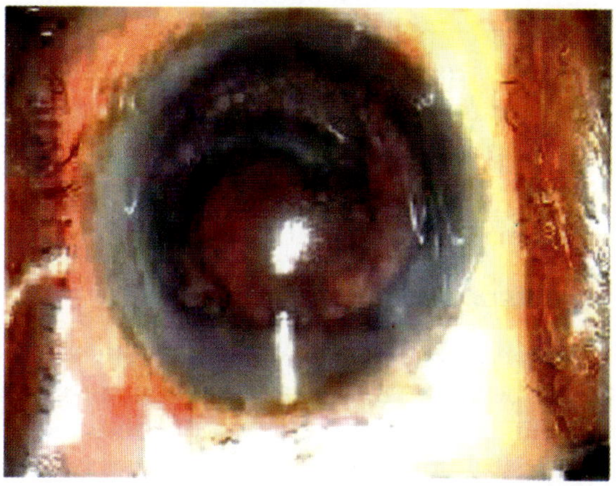

Fig. 21.5: Hydro-expression of free cortex with ACM (*Courtesy:* Dr G Natchiar, Aravind Eye Hospital)

to be suitable for all circumstances. Each surgeon may have his own likes and dislikes. He would know his circumstances, and would know what suits him the best and would select a technique accordingly.

Automated Aspiration

The main advantages of an automated system comprise

- Irrigation and aspiration of cortex is performed in a closed anterior chamber.
- Less of irrigation is required.
- Normal anatomical relations are maintained, i.e. deep anterior chamber, open and accessible fornices.
- There is no forward movement of vitreous and capsulo-zonular structure.
- Chances of choroidal effusion or hemorrhage are few.
- Endothelial damage is less with a deep anterior chamber.

But the automated system is, nonetheless, not free of disadvantages. These include

- It is difficult to perform during learning stage.
- A difficult procedure requiring preoperative settings.
- Changing of bottle height is essential to alter the flow, which is dependent on gravity. But it lacks instantaneously variable intraoperative control by the surgeon.
- The posterior capsule, zonules or both may rupture, if there is a sudden surge of machine controlled infusion pressure.
- Outflow around the cannula in a less tightly closed anterior chamber increases the volume of irrigation fluid required and may cause more corneal endothelial damage, in spite of the fact that it decreases the chances of capsular rupture.

Manual Aspiration

All surgeons must be conversant with such manual systems because if a sophisticated automated system fails or malfunctions, one does not feel helpless and may switch over to manual irrigation and aspiration devices. The advantages of manual cortical aspiration are that

- It can be easily mastered.
- It is not machine dependent and ensures independence.
- It is very safe, flexible and reliable.

CORTICAL ASPIRATION IN MANUAL SICS

An experienced implant surgeon will not find much difficulty in cortical aspiration in Manual Small Incision Cataract Surgery, for he is already accomplished in cortical aspiration during conventional extracapsular cataract surgery. As in phaco, very little cortex remains in the anterior chamber and the capsular bag, after expression or evacuation of the nucleus. Some of the cortex is washed out during hydrodissection, while most is removed with the hydro- or visco- expression of the epinucleus.

A deep anterior chamber during Manual Small Incision Cataract Surgery keeps the capsular bag ballooned. Cortical aspiration is easy in an inflated capsular bag. The residual cortex is already hydrated and so it can be aspirated with ease.

Manipulation of the iris in Manual Small Incision Cataract Surgery is minimal. This and the positive pressure in the anterior chamber reduce any chances of pupillary constriction. A fully dilated pupil assists cortical aspiration.

If Manual Small Incision Cataract Surgery is accompanied by continuous circular capsulorhexis, the absence of any loose capsular tags further eases the process of cortical aspiration. The capsular tags keep occluding the aspiration port and interfere in cortical aspiration.

Removal of cortex from the sub-incisional 12 O'clock region is arduous because of the difficult approach due to the small incision and capsulorhexis.

Before starting cortical aspiration every SICS surgeon must remember the following points:

1. In young patients below 25 years of age, the nucleus is soft and may be aspirated with the irrigation aspiration hand piece directly after the hydrodissection.
2. The 0.3 mm irrigation aspiration tip is most commonly used, though these are available in a choice of four sizes: 0.2, 0.3, 0.5 and 0.7 mm.
3. SICS surgeon should select the I/A cannula most suitable in his hand.

4. To avoid frustration one must check the functioning of I/A cannula and hand piece before starting the procedure.
5. Lifting the anterior lip of the incision and slightly depressing the posterior lip of the incision facilitates entry of the probe into anterior chamber.
6. The aspiration port of the tip should face anteriorly and the irrigation openings horizontally. If the aspiration port is oriented posteriorly, the aspiration port catches the posterior capsule.

METHOD OF CORTICAL ASPIRATION

Aspiration with I/A Cannula

The basic method of irrigation and aspiration process in Manual Small Incision Cataract Surgery is described here. Different surgeons might opt for some variations according to their experiences.

I prefer a reverse Simcoe irrigation and aspiration cannula attached to a BSS fluid line through an irrigating handle. But one may use any available cannula one is comfortable with.

The cannula is inserted into the anterior chamber with irrigation on. Aspiration is started later, after entering the anterior chamber. The cannula is gently guided into the capsular fornix, keeping it as close as possible to the posterior capsule, thereby avoiding the possibility of tugging the free capsulorhexis edge. The idea is to bring the aspiration port in contact with the cortex. The cortex plugs the aspiration port, preventing thereby, undesirable adherence of the anterior capsule to the tip of the cannula. Aspiration is started at this stage.

The cortex engages in the tip in a second or two. Draw the tip of the cannula into the pupillary space, stripping with it the cortex from the posterior capsule and the capsular fornix. Cortex should always be engaged in the periphery and aspirated in the central area.

This procedure is started at 6 O'clock position. It is then repeated both, clockwise and anti-clockwise at all clock hour positions, till only the cortex at 10 to 2 O'clock is left. The cortex in the 12 O'clock, subincisional region, immediately beneath the sclerocorneal tunnel is aspirated in the end.

However, some surgeons find it easiest to remove 12 O'clock cortex in the beginning as adjacent cortex helps in keeping the capsular bag open. Moreover, approaching 12 O'clock cortex first allows its aspiration as a single sheet.

A Simcoe cannula made of 21G needle with a 0.3mm orifice is routinely used. A smaller orifice provides a better vacuum grip on the cortex, but it prolongs the aspiration time. The reverse is true for a cannula with a larger orifice measuring 0.5 to 0.7mm.

Aspiration with Anterior Chamber Maintainer in Place

This technique of manual aspiration has been described, mastered, practiced and recommended by Michael Blumenthal. Cortex is aspirated with a single one way 21G/23G cannula. The tip of the cannula is rounded and sand blasted. It has a 0.3 or 0.4mm aspiration hole. It is attached to a 2 cc glass syringe for controlled aspiration through one of the side ports. If attempted through the tunnel it may allow the (Fig. 21.6) irrigation fluid/BSS to escape. The resulting instability of the posterior capsule would not be favourable for smooth aspiration of the cortex.

Using the paracentesis port for aspiration allows the amount of irrigation fluid/BSS aspirated or lost, to be instantaneously replaced, through the anterior chamber maintainer (Fig. 21.7). Subincisional cortex is aspirated first. The under surface of the anterior capsule is polished as a routine.

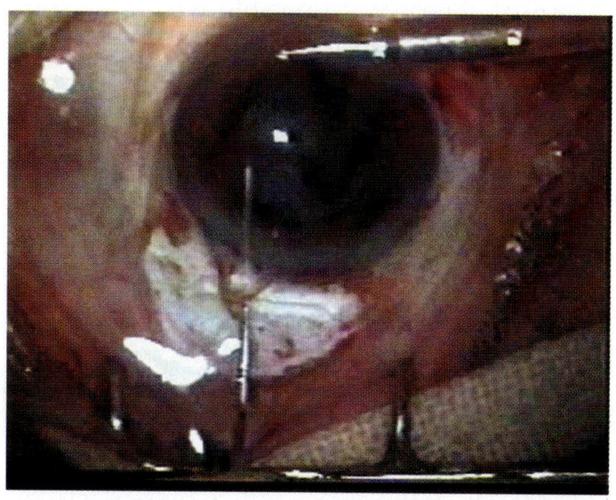

Fig. 21.6: Cortex Aspiration through tunnel with ACM (*Courtesy:* Dr G Natchiar, Aravind Eye Hospital)

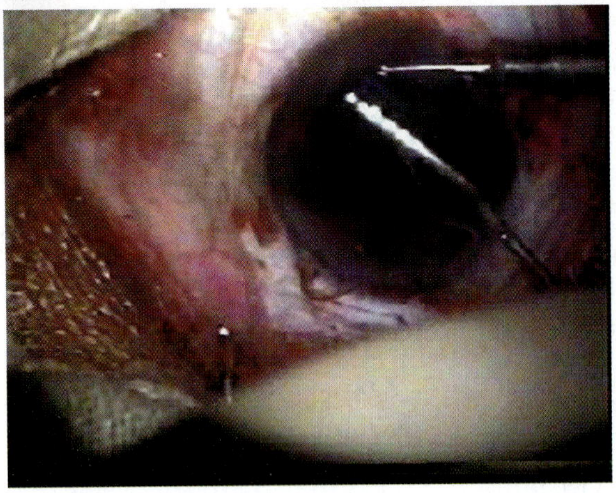

Fig. 21.7: Cortex Aspiration through side port (*Courtesy:* Dr G Natchiar, Aravind Eye Hospital)

With the anterior chamber maintainer on the posterior capsule is way behind and the fornices are fully open. One can aim for a 100% cortical clean-up with this technique.

Finally, a hydrodissection cannula is introduced through the side port. It is used to create water jet bursts of irrigation fluid/BSS directed on to the posterior capsule, to forcefully free any cortical material left over, from its attachments to the capsule, either on the posterior capsule or in the equator of the lens bag.

Advantages of 1cc Glass syringe with 26/27G Cannula are:

1. Glass syringe is more controllable; rotating motion is better than pushing of the piston.
2. Cortical clearing is possible with ease without tenting the posterior capsule.
3. 26/27G cannula is ideal because of the firmness and size.

Close chamber irrigation and aspiration has following advantages:

1. Endothelial damage is minimal, due to a deep and well-maintained anterior chamber.
2. Anterior chamber remains deep and pushes the vitreous back, ensuring its safety.
3. Aspiration of the cortex is easy because of open and accessible capsular fornices.
4. Protects against choroidal hemorrhage.
5. Hydration of the cortex which helps easy cortical aspiration.

Aspiration of Subincisional Cortex

Subincisional cortex situated below and around the incision, in the 12 O'clock region, is the most difficult to aspirate. This is particularly difficult if the rhexis is small or distally decentered. One approach to the 12 O'clock cortex is aspiration through a separate side port incision. There are various other methods used to remove the subincisional cortex and we will discuss these one by one for their advantages and drawbacks. Various methods to aspirate the cortex in this location are:

Verticalization of the Cannula Tip

To perform this procedure, the bottle of irrigating fluid/BSS is raised, to increase the depth of the anterior chamber and balloon the capsular bag. The cannula is held vertically so as to bring the aspirating aperture in contact with cortex at 1 O'clock or on either side of it. Once the cortex is engaged, the tip is moved peripherally to strip the cortex off the capsule and aspirate it as it is brought into the middle of the capsular bag. Likewise the cortex in other superior locations is aspirated.

In this technique of verticalization, abnormal pressure is exerted on both edges of the incisions, upward on the anterior edge resulting in the formation of corneal folds with consequent reduction in visibility, and downward on the posterior edge resulting in abnormal pressure on the iris tissue. There is an increased loss of the irrigating fluid in this maneuver due to the distortion of the incision. This causes a forward movement of the posterior capsule and an increased risk of posterior capsular capture and rupture.

If this procedure is attempted through the sclerocorneal tunnel and we have a narrow pupil with a small rhexis, successful aspiration of the subincisional cortex is almost impossible.

Manual Mobilization of the Cortex with a J or U Shaped Cannula

This technique consists of engaging the cortical material by aspiration exerted through a narrow J or U - shaped cannula having the aspiration hole at the tip. It is mounted on a 2 cc syringe containing irrigation fluid/BSS and inserted into the incision sideways, rotated and the tip is guided under the anterior capsule. The cortex engaged is pulled into the central part of the capsular bag. The cortical mass is then aspirated out with a reverse Simcoe cannula inserted through a side port.

Side Port Cannulation

In this technique either of the stab side ports, made away from the sclerocorneal tunnel is used. A Reverse Simcoe Cannula attached to an irrigating fluid line is used to aspirate the 12 O'clock cortex under viscoelastic cover (Figs 21.8 to 10).

Iris Prolapse or Retraction Technique

In this technique direct aspiration of the subincisional cortex is performed after prolapsing the iris through the wound or by retracting the 12 O'clock iris with an iris hook. In these techniques the chances of damage to zonules and the iris are greatly increased.

Ice Cream Scoop Maneuver

The aspiration orifice of the Simcoe cannula is turned to the side at 1 O'clock position, guided a little under the iris, to engage the cortex. As the aspiration is initiated, the tip of the cannula is simultaneously turned anteriorly and moved towards the middle of the capsular bag. This step is repeated to aspirate the subincisional cortex from all the adjacent areas.

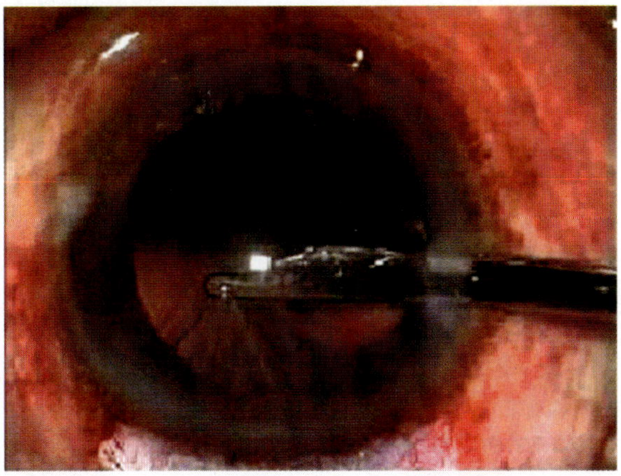

Fig. 21.8: Simcoe cannula for subincisional cortex (*Courtesy:* Dr G Natchiar, Aravind Eye Hospital)

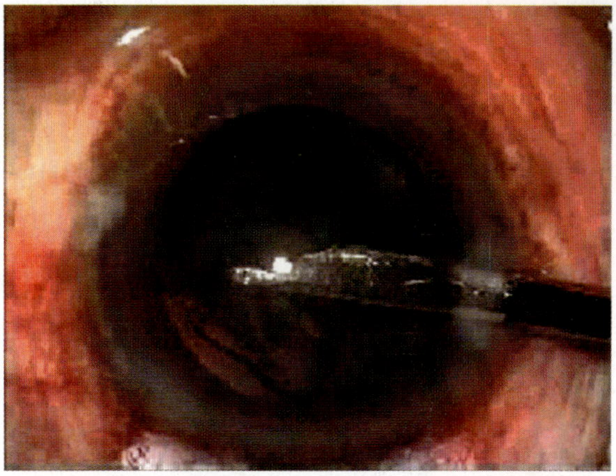

Fig. 21.9: Subincisional cortex stripped off (*Courtesy:* Dr G Natchiar, Aravind Eye Hospital)

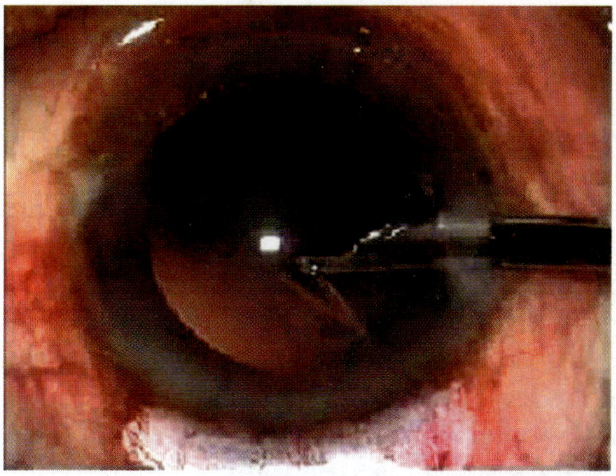

Fig. 21.10: Subincisional cortex aspiration completed (*Courtesy:* Dr G Natchiar, Aravind Eye Hospital)

Iris Massage Maneuver

The tip of the irrigation aspiration cannula is used to gently massage the iris at 12 O'clock with the irrigating fluid flowing. The cortex thus loosened is aspirated by the ice cream scoop maneuver. This technique invariably results in damage to the iris, zonules and endothelium.

Post IOL Implantation Aspiration

This technique involves the implantation of an intraocular implant in the capsular bag, even while the subincisional cortex is still in the bag. Do not remove the viscoelastic that was injected for the implant. The lens is rotated 360°. The mechanical action exerted first by one haptic and then by the other, mobilizes the cortical mass. It is then aspirated together with the viscoelastic using a reverse Simcoe irrigation aspiration cannula.

Drawbacks of this technique are:

- Rotating the IOL may be difficult because of the presence of the cortex,
- Mobilizing the cortex may be difficult,
- Extensive zonular stress because of repeated rotation of the implant, which is not a smooth procedure every time, and
- It does not remove the residual cortex completely.

Bi-manual Irrigation Aspiration (Manual)

This procedure is somewhat similar to the one described by Blumenthal, except for the fact that in Blumenthal's technique the anterior chamber maintainer is fixed at 6 O'clock. In this the anterior chamber maintainer is fixed in either of the side ports and is connected to the irrigation fluid line.

Aspiration cannula with the opening facing upward is connected to 1 cc syringe for cortical aspiration. Start the irrigation and aspirate through the other side port. Due to the closed chamber, the anterior chamber remains deep and the capsular fornices remain open. Insert the aspiration cannula into the anterior chamber and start aspirating by placing the tip of the aspiration cannula in contact with the cortex. Engage the cortex and move the tip of the cannula from periphery to the center. This strips off cortex from the capsular bag. Aspirate the cortex when in the center.

Interchange the anterior chamber maintainer cannula and aspiration cannula and aspirate other half of the cortex as above.

Manual I/A has more advantages than automated I/A. Advantages of manual I/A are

- better flexibility
- easy learning
- better safety margin and
- better surgeon control.

Precautions during Cortical Aspiration

Management of Anterior Capsular Tags

i. At times when a can opener capsulotomy has been performed or the capsular margins are torn or ragged, the anterior capsular tags tend to plug the aspiration port and create problems in aspirating the cortex. If a tag has a narrow base it can be held with a McPherson forceps and pulled with a jerk to free it, as if tearing away a piece of toilet tissue. Slow pull on the tag pulls the posterior capsule, resulting in zonular dehiscence. This maneuver is not performed if the tag has a broad base.

ii. Another maneuver to handle anterior capsular tags is that the base of tag is partially engaged into the port and the capsule is held between the I/A port and a sharp iris hook, and torn with a quick movement.

Posterior Capsular Adherence

To minimize the occurrence of the posterior capsular adherence to the aspiration tip, it should always be kept facing anteriorly. However, at times the posterior capsule may inadvertently adhere to the tip, giving rise to appearance of folds or stress lines in the posterior capsule, converging on to the aspiration port. The irrigation and aspiration must be stopped immediately. If the capsule is not released swiftly, it will be ruptured.

In Difficult Situations the following Steps May be of Great Help

i. Raising the height of infusion bottle to deepen the chamber.
ii. Stab incision at 3 to 9 O'clock allows a spatula to loosen 12 O'clock cortex. These incisions can also be used for side port cannulation.
iii. Speed of irrigation may be increased.
iv. Capsule polisher may 'fluff up' the cortex which may be washed using side port infusion.
v. Mini I/A tip with 0.2 mm port may be used for fine cortical matter.
vi. Small amount of cortex is better left alone, than to struggle and cause a posterior capsular rent or zonular dialysis.

Management of the Capsule

A. *Posterior Capsule Vacuuming:* Having removed the entire visible cortex, the 0.3 mm irrigation aspiration tip is placed on, and moved across the surface of the posterior capsule, away from the direction the aspiration port is facing. This forms a drumhead across the aspiration port. This in effect tents the posterior capsule up, almost up to, but not into the port, thereby helping free the debris. The tip is moved rapidly across the posterior capsule to aspirate the fine cortical material on the capsule. It is not allowed to stop or slow down for the fear that the port may get completely occluded with posterior capsule. This is accompanied by the appearance of stress lines. Aspiration is immediately stopped, to resume again, preventing in the process a capsular rupture.

B. *Posterior Capsular Polishing:* There are many instruments available to polish the posterior capsule. These include scratchers, squeezes, curettes, and olive tips. Kratz scratcher is a curved irrigating needle roughened by sand blasting or coated with particles of diamond dust, for polishing the posterior capsule. Kratz scratcher is attached to a 2 cc syringe filled with irrigation fluid to polish the posterior capsule. Charles Kelman uses a blunt air injection cannula or an olive tipped needle attached to a 5ml syringe, for polishing the posterior capsule. The posterior capsule is gently burnished with this cannula.

Technique of Posterior Capsular Polishing

Through a good coaxial microscope, evaluate the posterior capsule. A good view of the red glow is a must. The posterior capsule is focussed. On touching and slightly pressing with a posterior capsule polisher, in the center of the slightly convex posterior capsule, a halo is seen around the tip of the polisher. A halo, 4 mm in size, shows that the amount of pressure exerted is just right. A higher pressure with the polisher shows up in the form of radial stress lines. The posterior capsule is gently rubbed to remove adherent fine cortical material (Fig. 21.11).

In the Blumenthal technique, the posterior capsule is polished with a blunt cannula with an aspiration pore on the under surface of the tip. This cannula is fitted to a 2 cc glass syringe with the piston removed. This exhibits a negative pressure at the tip thus vacuuming the surface of the posterior capsule.

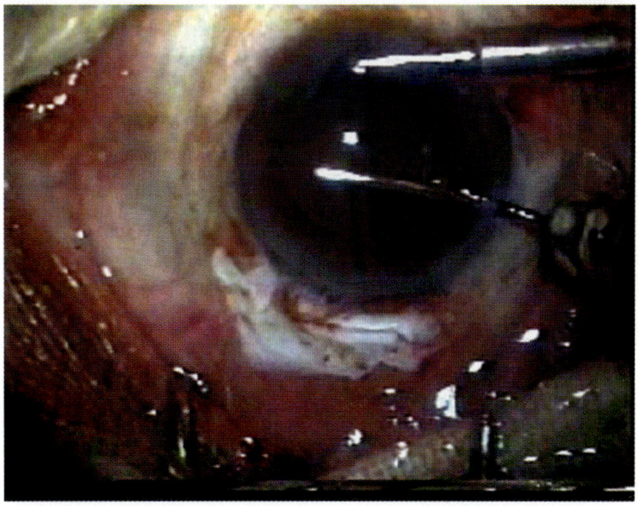

Fig. 21.11: Posterior capsular vacuuming and polishing (*Courtesy:* Dr G Natchiar, Aravind Eye Hospital)

Anterior capsule polishing: Howard Gimbel has stated that complete removal of epithelial cells lining the anterior capsule reduces the incidence of postoperative uveitis and posterior capsular opacification. Vacuuming of anterior capsule is performed with 0.3mm. I/A tip. Vacuuming removes 50-60 percent of subcapsular epithelial cells. Anterior capsule vacuuming and polishing is particularly useful in young patients.

Cortical Aspiration in Presence of Posterior Capsular Tear

In the case of a posterior capsule rupture, which is small and has an intact vitreous face, while cortical aspiration is still in progress, the area in the vicinity of posterior capsular tear is left untouched. And the cortex is manually aspirated from the other areas with very low irrigation and aspiration. The exposed vitreous is not traversed. Cortex is aspirated towards the tear, rather than away from it.

Dry aspiration under viscoelastic, described by Anis Aziz is most appropriate. The anterior chamber is filled with viscoelastic material to open up the capsular bag and to push back the vitreous. A Simcoe irrigation and aspiration cannula, with little or no irrigation, is used to gently aspirate the cortex from the capsular fornices. The entire cortex can be aspirated without disturbing the vitreous, with this technique.

Vitrectomy is not required, if the tear in posterior capsule is small and aspiration is complete or if the tear occurs while polishing the capsule.

Air can be injected to determine the amount of vitreous in the anterior chamber. If the air moves freely in all parts of the angle of the anterior chamber, nothing needs to be done. But if it is not freely mobile in certain areas, it means sufficient cortex remains and/or vitreous is in the angle of the anterior chamber or the wound. This warrants an anterior vitrectomy. Anterior vitrectomy is preferably performed with irrigation from a separate port to avoid direct pressure on the tear.

REFERENCES

1. Jaffe. Cataract Surgery and its complications, 4th Edition, Mosby Jaypee Bros, 1989.
2. Gupta VP. Adequate Cortical Clean Up, Phacoemulsification–A Practical Guide, New Delhi, New Age International Ltd, 1996.
3. Vasavada AR, Desai JP. Phacoemulsification, Iladevi Cataract and Intraocular Lens Research Center, Ahmedabad, 1996.
4. Boyd Benjamin F. The Modern Manual Small Incision Extra-capsular with Mini-Nuc Technique, Highlights of Ophthalmology, No. 1, 2000.
5. Saha S. Non Phaco Small Incision Cataract Surgery, Nucleus Removal–Tips and Tricks, Delhi Journal of Ophthalmology, 8(2): June 2000.
6. Malik KPS, Goel R. Manual Small Incision Cataract Surgery, CME Series, No. 8, All India Ophthalmological Society.
7. Shah Anil. Small Incision Cataract Surgery (Manual Phaco) Best out of Waste, Bhalani Publishing House, Mumbai, 2000.
8. Titiyal JS. Phacoemulsification: Complications, DOS Times, 7(6): 2001.

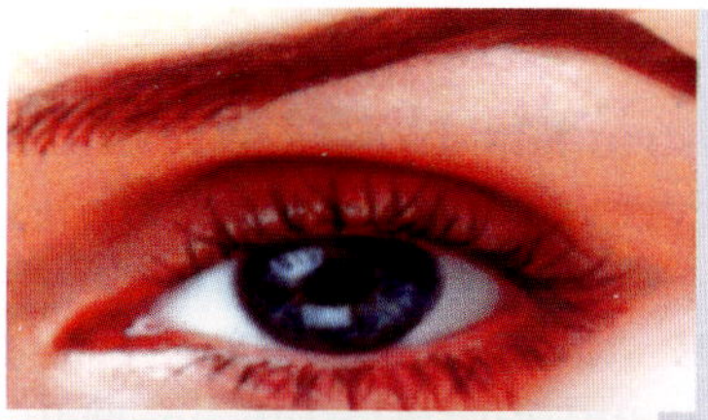

Twenty two

Yogesh Shah
Gaurav Shah
Shushmita (India)

Dynamics of Nucleus Management in SICS

It is interesting that CCC developed after Phacoemulsification was invented. And similarly SICS came into existence after Phacoemulsification. Two vital steps in SICS are wound construction and Nucleus management. Both these steps also differ a great deal from Phacoemulsification surgery. Just as Phacoemulsification surgery aims at management of various types of nuclei using minimum energy, SICS has many variations to tackle the nucleus with smallest possible size of wound and with minimum damage to the endothelium of cornea and the posterior capsule.

The steps of nucleus delivery after doing hydro procedure are

- Dislocating equator of the nucleus out of the bag
- Delivering the nucleus into the anterior chamber
- Minification of the nucleus may be attempted
- Delivery of the nucleus out of the eye.

DISLOCATING EQUATOR OF THE NUCLEUS OUT OF THE BAG

Nucleus delivery starts with dislodging any one part of the equator of the lens out of the bag. This is achieved by manoeuvring the canula from the CCC margin, going underneath the edge of the nucleus and pushing fluid underneath to dislodge the equator out of the bag. It is important to do all the steps through side port except the actual delivery of nucleus. Some surgeons use viscoelastic material for this step.

DELIVERING THE NUCLEUS INTO THE ANTERIOR CHAMBER

Once the equatorial edge of the lens is seen out of the CCC margin, it is best to rotate lens in clockwise and anti-clockwise direction to separate it from the capsule and bring it in front of CCC. If required one can use additional viscoelastic material. However, most surgeons prefer to do this step with the AC maintainer on. Once again this step should be done through the side port. Either a dialler or 26 number bent needle can be used for this purpose. Both above procedures need some learning curve but, once learnt, are not difficult.

MINIFICATION OF THE NUCLEUS

In an attempt to complete the surgery through smaller incision many surgeons have resorted to various techniques either to divide the nucleus or reduce its bulk. Commonly used procedures include:

- Use of snare
- Use of pre-chopper
- Phaco sandwich technique
- Mechanical debulking of prolapsed nucleus

Use of Snare

Snare is a steel wire loop which passes through a small steel lumen and opens up as it comes out. The method is simple. As the snare is introduced in the eye the loop passes all around the nucleus engaging it firmly within the loop. As the loop is withdrawn it cuts the nucleus into two. If required, the lens nucleus can be divided in to three parts by using the snare twice cutting one third of the nucleus every time. Each piece can then be removed with Mac-pherson forceps. This enables the surgeon to perform the surgery from 3.5 to 4 mm incision. During the entire procedure it is best to fill up the chamber with viscoelastic material.

Use of Pre-chopper

Pre-chopper is an instrument like Mac-pherson forceps, but has a reverse action, i.e. its blades open up when surgeon attempts to press two blades. After filling the chamber with viscoelastic material pre-chopper is introduced from the main wound and is pushed within the nuclear substance. If required the nucleus can be stabilised with the second instrument, like a dialler, introduced from the side port. When an attempt is made to open up the blades a cleft is created in the centre of the nucleus. This cleft then can be enlarged dividing the nucleus into two parts. Each part can be subsequently removed by holding it with the forceps.

Phaco Sandwich Technique

Here the instrument having a plate posteriorly and a wire vectis-like ring anteriorly grabs the nucleus between two prongs and crushes it in to smaller fragments. These can then be removed keeping the wound size small.

Mechanical Debulking of Prolapsed Nucleus

It is often difficult to remove large hard-brown nucleus through standard 5mm tunnel. To remove such nucleus one can cut the part of the nucleus that jets out of the wound with any sharp instrument. Then push the nucleus back in the chamber, dial it and attempt to remove diagonally opposite edge of the nucleus. As this edge jets out of the wound, cut it. Thus , when either side of the lens is cut of it will take up an oval shape, which can then be expressed out with ease.

FLUIDICS OF HYDRO-EXPRESSION

In a classical way of Bluementhal technique of nucleus delivery, a glide is introduced through the main wound till it goes and supports the nucleus posteriorly. The nucleus is then allowed to get engaged in the inner lip of the tunnel as one presses the glide and the posterior lip of wound to open the tunnel. Moment the nucleus is engaged in the inner lip, the escape of fluid through the wound is stopped and the pressure in the chamber rises depending on the height of bottle to which ACM is connected. Once the nucleus presents at the outer wound, it is slowly expressed out by rotating it from side to side while the positive pressure in the chamber pushes it out. Throughout the entire procedure, the ACM is kept on which maintains adequate positive pressure to push the nucleus out of the eye. The height of the bottle to which ACM is connected, is normally kept 50 cm. above patient's eye. It is possible to deliver the nucleus without the use of glide also. In an event of rupture of posterior capsule, glide is of a great help to prevent nucleus being dropped in vitreous cavity. The glide need not go right up to 6 o'clock position as that itself can lead to rupture of the posterior capsule.

FLUIDICS OFVISCO-EXPRESSION

Though in a classical Bluementhal technique hydro-expression of the nucleus is done with the help of ACM, similar results can be obtained with visco-expression. The ACM, if used, is kept off and viscoelastic is injected from the side port to express the nucleus out of the wound. Like in typical Bluementhal technique a glide can be used. The wound is kept open to engage the nucleus in the inner lip of wound and slowly extracted by side-to-side movement. If required the nucleus delivery can be assisted with vectis or 26 number bent needle cystitome. It is the positive pressure created in anterior chamber by viscoelastic which pushes the nucleus towards the wound, which is the path of least resistance.

In both above techniques, where minification of the nucleus is not performed and the delivery of the whole nucleus is done through 5 mm wound, the epi-nucleus is shelled off as the nucleus passes through the wound. This to some extent reduces the volume of nucleus.

ROLE OF ACM

The use of AC Maintainer has made the SICS surgery safe, stable and reproducible. ACM has grossly reduced the complication rate and has given ease to the surgeon during all the steps of SICS. The role of ACM is multifold

- It maintains the stability of anterior chamber throughout the procedure.
- It creates positive pressure in the chamber once the nucleus is engaged in the wound which helps in hydro expression.
- In case of rupture of posterior capsule it prevents sudden collapse of wound and hence does not allow the tear to expand.
- It pushes the vitreous phase posteriorly in an event of posterior capsular rupture thus preventing vitreous loss.
- It allows the surgeon to perform the entire surgery without the use of viscoelastic material.
- Lens can be implanted and dialled easily in presence of well formed chamber and dilated capsular bag due to the flow from ACM.
- It maintains the pupillary dilatation throughout the surgery due to its positive pressure effect in the chamber.

COMPLICATIONS DURING NUCLEAR MANAGEMENT

Prolapse of Iris During Nuclear Management

It is not uncommon to find iris getting prolapsed in the wound as one attempts the nucleus delivery. If the nucleus gets well engaged in the inner lip of the tunnel then Iris has no chance to get into the wound. Some of the reasons why Iris prolapses in the wound before the nucleus gets engaged in the wound are

- Premature entry of the tunnel in the anterior chamber
- Too big a tunnel (like 7 mm horizontal diameter)
- Loss of integrity of wound (cutting of lateral edge of the wound)
- Positive pressure behind the Iris pushing it forward
- Small Pupil
- Laxity of iris tissue

If the wound is too big or its architecture is damaged with loss of integrity of the wound it may be advisable to take one stitch. The positive pressure from behind the Iris must be removed. It is important not to inject too much of viscoelastic in anterior chamber as this it self may go behind Iris and push it forward. While injecting visco-elastic, care must be taken to inject small quantity

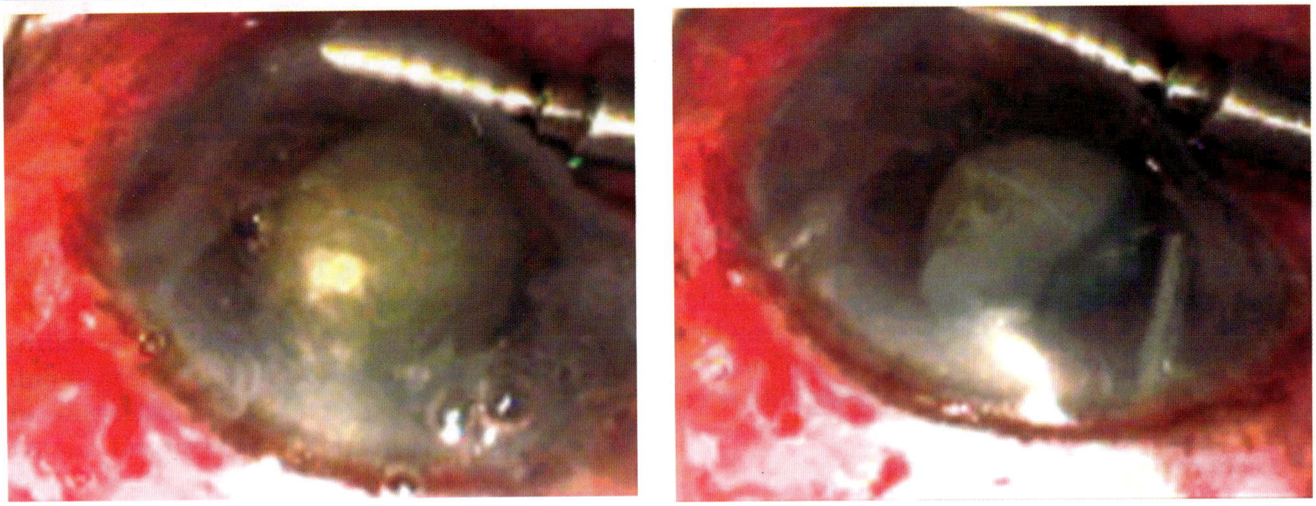

Fig. 22.1A and B: Forward tilt of the edge of the nucleus out of CCC

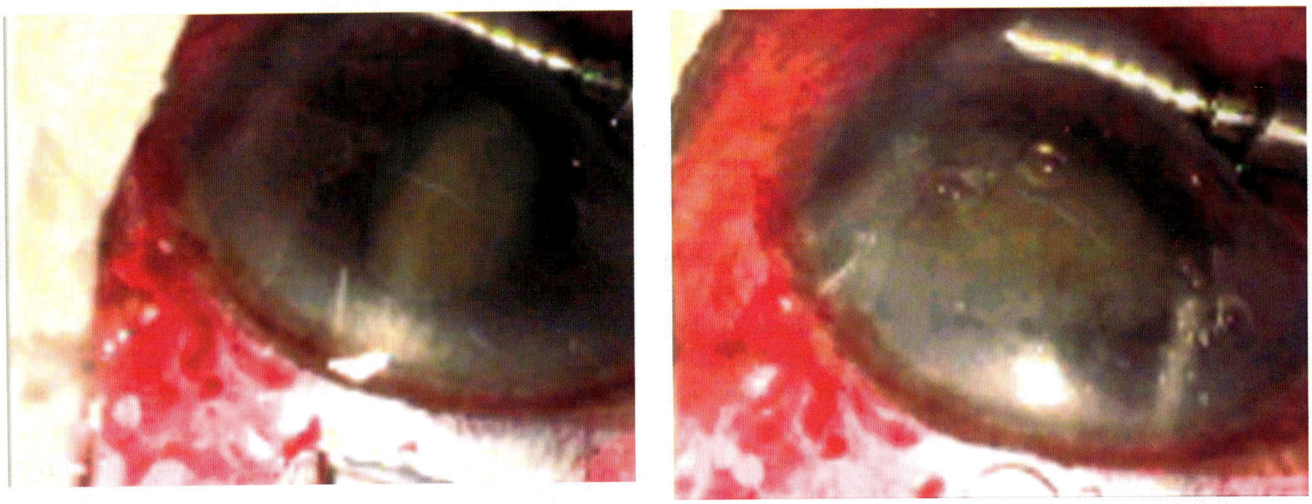

Fig. 22.2A and B: Nucleus delivered in AC

starting just underneath the wound well above the Pupil and Iris. Bottle height may be adjusted to adjust pressure in chamber. One can use a spatula to avoid the iris from jetting forward. Once the nucleus fills the inner lip of wound nothing can prolapse except the nucleus in spite of high pressure within the chamber.

POSTERIOR CAPSULAR RUPTURE

There are many causes which can lead to rupture of the posterior capsule during various stages of surgery, and it is being tackled elsewhere in this book. However, few important points to remember are:

- Do not get upset and try to compose yourself in event of the complication.
- One must first establish the extent of damage to posterior capsule.
- Find out whether the vitreous phase is intact or not.
- Do not stop ACM, but you can lower the height of the bottle.
- If one has to inject viscoelastic material, it should be injected while the flow from ACM is slowly cut off.
- At no stage sudden lowering of IOP should occur in presence of tear.

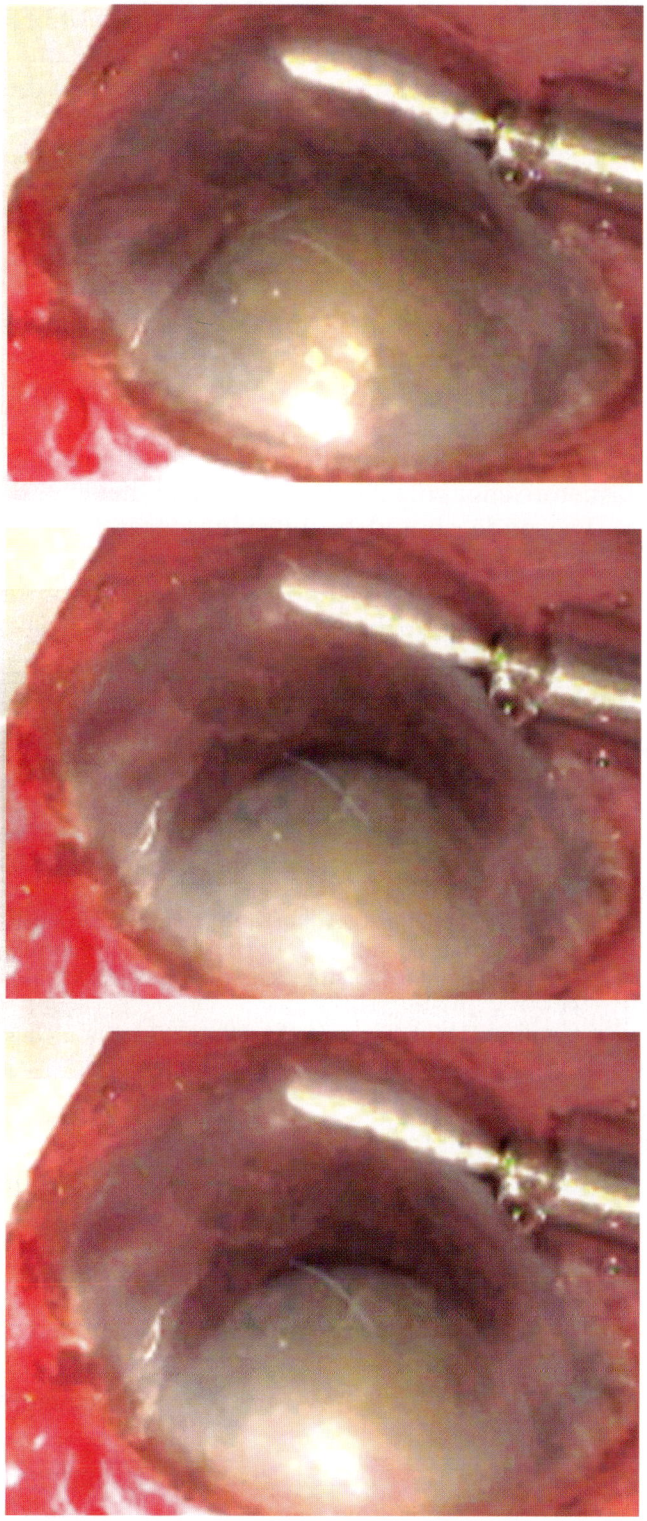

Figs 22.3A to C: Nucleus engaged in the inner lip of the wound and entering the tunnel

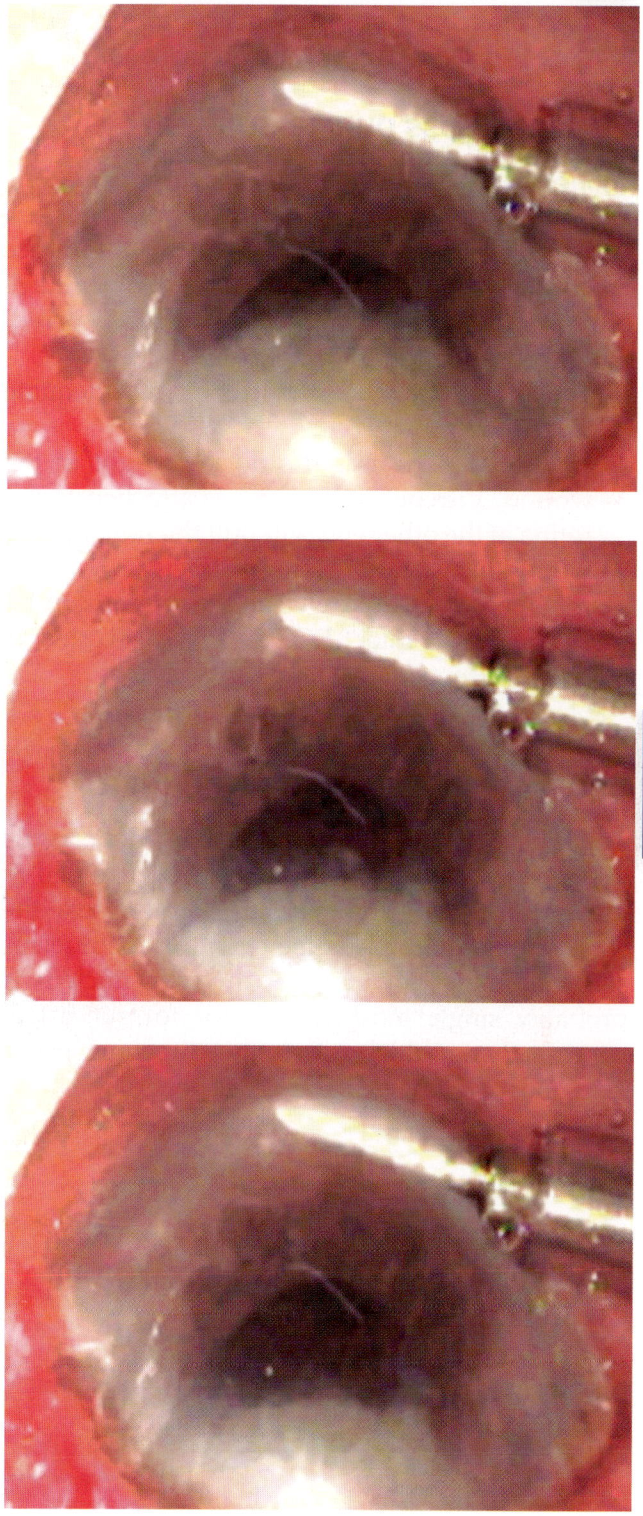

Figs 22.4A to C: Nucleus being delivered from the tunnel

The detailed management of posterior capsular rupture is discussed elsewhere in this book.

VITREOUS LOSS DURING SURGERY

Alongwith the rupture of posterior capsule one may find that the anterior vitreous phase is broken and vitreous prolapses out of the wound. Once again the treatment will depend on at what stage of the surgery the complication has occurred. However, minimum that one needs to do is

- Thorough clean up of vitreous by adequate vitrectomy
- No vitreous strands should be caught in the wound. Vitreous jelly which is attached to the retina at the other end will pull the retina as the wound heals and the scar contracts.
- If one has been able to clean the vitreous and if the Rhexis is intact PC IOL can be fixated in sulcus.
- Scleral supported IOL.

DROPPED NUCLEUS DURING SURGERY

Zonular rupture or rupture of the posterior capsule is pre-requisite for the nucleus to get dropped in vitreous cavity. However, in some cases, the surgeon may not realise the event till the nucleus starts sinking. Prevention of dropped nucleus is probably single most vital factor for successful surgery. Steps, which help in this direction, are –

- Good adequate size C.C.C. without a notch
- Proper hydrodissection and prevention of BSS getting trapped behind the nucleus. If the fluid gets trapped, one will suddenly notice that the eye becomes tense, the chamber becomes shallow and the pressure in chamber suddenly rises pushing the iris in the wound. This can be easily relieved by gently tapping the nucleus posteriorly which allows the trapped BSS to flow out.
- Keeping the capsular bag ballooned all throughout the procedure. This can be achieved by adjusting the height of bottle to which ACM is connected.
- Deliver the nucleus fully in anterior chamber before engaging it in the inner lip of the wound.
- The glide should be introduced carefully to avoid damage to the capsule.

However, if surgeon finds that there is a rupture of capsule then further steps have been described elsewhere.

Once learnt this technique is consistent, easy and rewarding.

REFERENCES

1. Thomas R, Kuriakose T, George R. Towards achieving small incision cataract surgery 99.8% of the time. Ind J Ophthalmol 2000;48(2):145-51.
2. Menapace R, Radax U, Amon N, Papapanos P. No stitch, small incision cataract surgery with flexible intraocular lens implantation. J Cataract Refract Surg 1994;20(5):534-42.
3. Blumenthal M, Ashkenazi I, Fogel R, Assia EL: The gliding nucleus. J Cataract Refract Surg 1993;19(3):435-37.
4. Jaffe N: Cataract Surgery and its Complications.

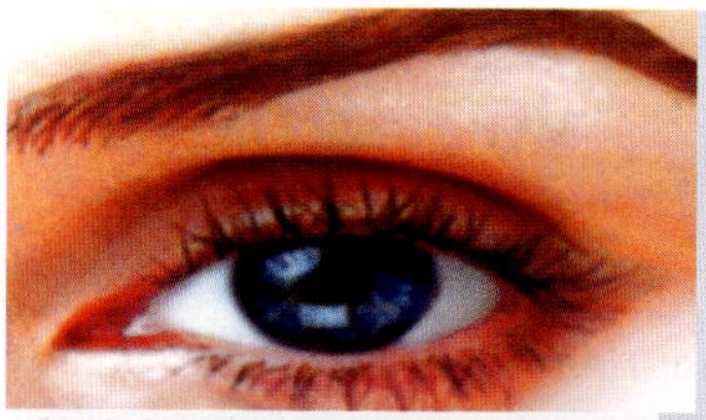

Twenty three

IOL Implantation Techniques in Manual Small Incision Cataract Surgery

Arun Kshetrapal
Ramesh Kshetrapal
(India)

INTRODUCTION

Once the nucleus has been removed, cortex has been meticulously cleaned up and capsule has been polished, we are ready to implant an IOL. Using a proper technique can lead to smooth insertion of an IOL through the tunnel into the bag but, at the same time certain principles are to be kept in mind while inserting an IOL for its uneventful delivery into the bag.

The most commonly used IOL after non phacoemulsification small incision cataract surgery is an all PMMA 6 mm optic sized IOL.

Intraocular lens insertion techniques differ in a case of small incision cataract surgery (SICS) from that of a conventional extra capsular cataract extraction (ECCE). In a case of SICS an IOL has to be manipulated through a 3 to 4 mm long sclerocorneal tunnel before reaching the anterior chamber. The width of the tunnel in most of the cases is almost equal to the diameter of the optics of an IOL. Since the IOL has to be passed through a snugly fitting tunnel it cannot be manipulated much, while it is traveling through the tunnel. So in a case of SICS the insertion of an IOL is slightly difficult as compared to conventional ECCE.

An intraocular lens can be inserted in the bag after inflating it with a viscoelastic or anterior chamber maintainer can be used to keep the anterior chamber formed and bag inflated during the procedure of IOL implantation. In this chapter we will discuss both the techniques of IOL implantation.

Before we proceed to discuss about the techniques of IOL insertion, we must prepare our tunnel to accept the IOL so as to face minimum complications during insertion of an IOL. The width of the sclero-corneal tunnel should be sufficient enough to let pass the IOL smoothly without the need to push it forcefully. The incisions that are too small to let an IOL pass through intensify the corneal trauma.[1] A 6 mm sized IOL should be preferred as the incidence of glare from the margins will be less as compared to 5.0 or 5.5 mm sized IOL when the pupil dilates. The glare problem will be more so with sharp edge intraocular lenses.[2] Increasing the width of incision from 5.5 mm to 6.0 mm to let the smooth passage of IOL through the tunnel will increase the ease of IOL insertion and the increased size of the incision to 6.0 mm will not lead to any significant difference in visual acuity or astigmatism as compared to 5.5 mm incision.[3]

The size of capsulorhexis has to be such that it covers the IOL from all side to prevent the lens from getting decentered in future, but again the size of capsulorhexis will depend on the size of the nucleus to be prolapsed out. Prolapsing out an over sized nucleus through a small capsulorhexis can result into zonulodialysis and sometimes accidental intracapsular extraction of cataract. So the size of the capsulorhexis has to be balanced according to the size of nucleus and the size of the IOL to be implanted.

INSTRUMENTS

Since the IOL has to traverse through a tunnel, it requires an IOL holding forceps which has strong arms such as a Shepard lens holding forceps which has duckbill shaped jaws with a gentle curve (Fig. 23.1) or a Kratz lens holding forceps which has narrow curved jaws. The curved forceps is required as the entry into the tunnel is about 2 mm posterior to the limbus and there is limited space available for manipulation.

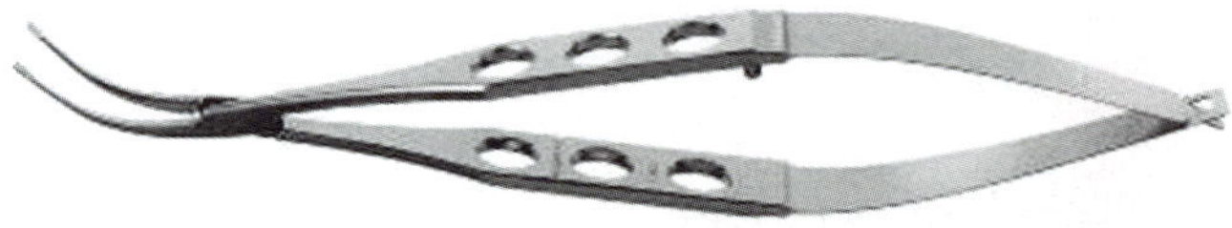

Fig. 23.1: Shepard lens holding forceps

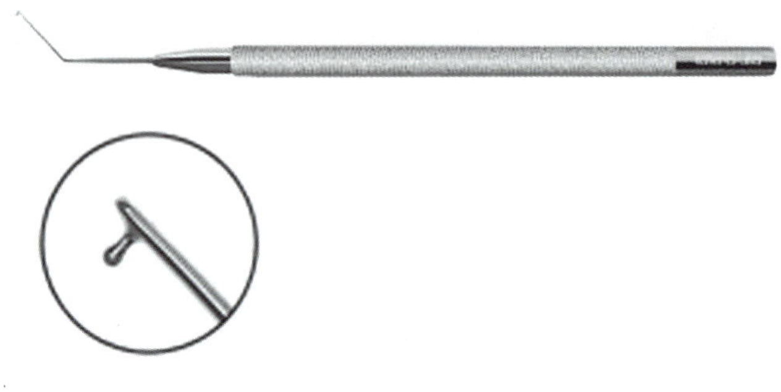

Fig. 23.2: Lester Lens Manipulator

Once the IOL is inside the anterior chamber a lens manipulator such as Lester lens manipulator or a forked manipulator is desired for easy manipulation into the bag.

Technique

Once the cortical clean up and capsule polishing has been done the anterior chamber maintainer if being used is removed and the capsular bag is inflated and anterior chamber formed with a viscoelastic. The viscoelastic is injected at the 6 o'clock position and the cannula is withdrawn as the anterior chamber fills up with viscoelastic from 6 to 12 o'clock. Some viscoelastic is left inside the tunnel for smooth passage of IOL. The area adjacent to the tunnel is cleaned of all the debris and blood lest, they should stick with the IOL and may be carried into the anterior chamber. The desired power IOL is held longitudinally in between the arms of the forceps and is manipulated through the tunnel into the anterior chamber (Fig. 23.3). The IOL is held slightly tilted upwards at the time the leading haptic is entering the sclero-corneal tunnel lest, it should touch the lid margin. As the haptic enters the tunnel, the IOL is made horizontal and brought into the plane of the tunnel and pushed gently through the tunnel. If you find any resistance during the insertion of IOL; do not force it through

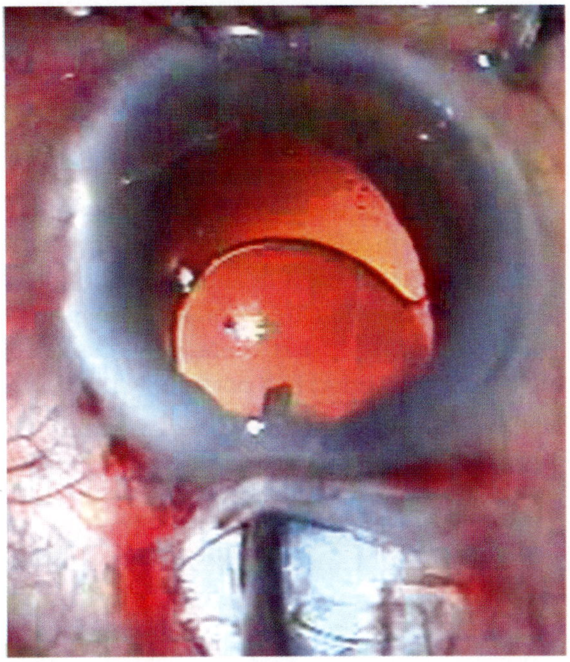

Fig. 23.3: IOL is pushed through the tunnel into the anterior chamber with a forceps

the tunnel as it may cause trauma to the tunnel and may damage the self sealing nature of the tunnel. It is advisable to enlarge the tunnel by 0.5 mm in such cases.

Once the leading haptic has reached the margin of capsulorhexis at 6 o'clock position the IOL is pushed back slightly so that the leading haptic goes beneath the capsulorhexis margin. Generally the lower loop of the IOL will go right into the capsular bag, but if it is riding forwards then gently lifting the trailing haptic will tilt the leading haptic posteriorly into the capsular bag. Once the IOL is inside the tunnel and the leading haptic is below the anterior capsule, the IOL is released gently and forceps withdrawn out (Fig. 23.4).

A lens manipulator is then used to manipulate the IOL into the bag. The lens manipulator is engaged in between the haptic optic junction and the lens is rotated in a clockwise direction and simultaneously pushed back until the trailing haptic snaps into the bag (Fig. 23.5).

Alternatively, instead of a lens manipulator a Kelman-McPherson forceps can be used to insert the trailing haptic. The trailing haptic is grasped with the help of Kelman- McPherson forceps and the IOL is pushed and rotated and simultaneously

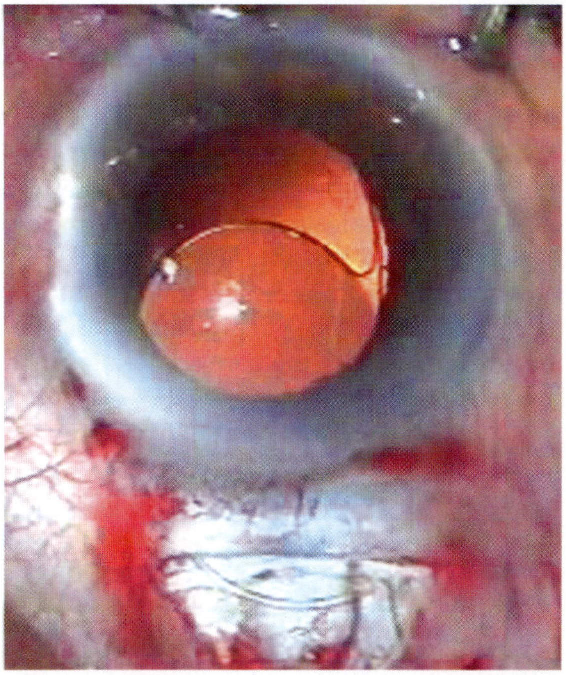

Fig. 23.4: IOL inside the anterior chamber but the trailing haptic still outside the tunnel

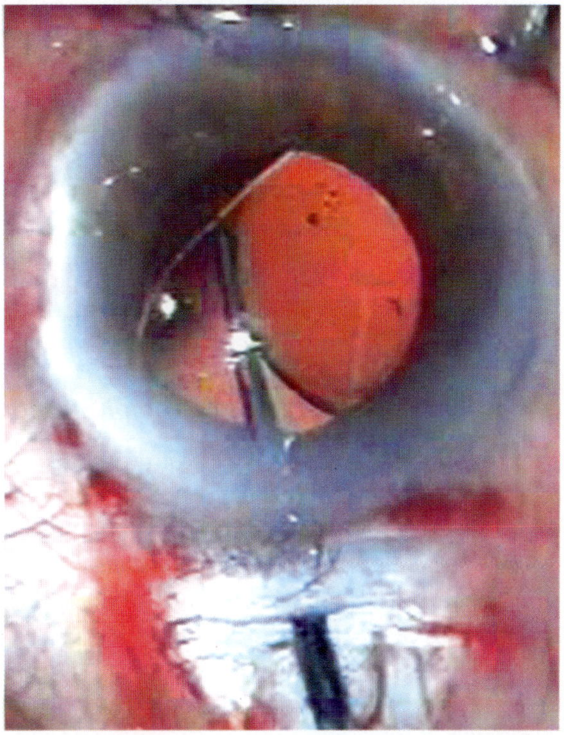

Fig. 23.5: IOL being dialed into the bag with Lester Manipulator engaged in optic haptic junction

the haptic is bent inferiorly so that the elbow of the haptic is below the anterior capsule and it is tucked underneath the capsule and released so that the haptic snaps into the capsular bag.

Many a times when the IOL is being pushed through the tunnel or when the forceps is withdrawn some of the viscoelastic gets leaked out resulting into shallowing of anterior chamber. If the viscoelastic has leaked out or at any time during the IOL insertion the anterior chamber becomes shallow, viscoelastic is replenished to reform the anterior chamber. The viscoelastic is injected in between the IOL and the cornea so as to push the IOL backwards.

Once the lens is in the bag, all the viscoelastic is removed from the bag. The viscoelastic is removed from under the IOL either by lifting it up slightly with the irrigation aspiration cannula or by tilting the lens on to the side.

An intraocular lens can also be inserted into the bag without the use of viscoelastic and making the use of anterior chamber maintainer to keep the bag inflated. The insertion technique basically remains the same when inserting an IOL using an anterior chamber maintainer. Alternatively when using an anterior chamber maintainer the IOL can be placed into the tunnel with the help of a forceps and then pulled into the anterior chamber with the help of a Sinskey hook inserted through a side port. This technique prevents the shallowing of anterior chamber while pushing the IOL through the tunnel.[4] The only advantage an anterior chamber maintainer over viscoelastic for implantation of an IOL is a lower IOP on the first postoperative day[5].

Intraocular Lens Insertion in Special Situations

Sometimes IOL has to be inserted in the absence of capsulorhexis or when there is a posterior capsular tear or when the posterior capsule is absent.

Intraocular lens insertion in absence of capsulorhexis It is not possible to achieve capsulorhexis in all the cases. When a capsulorhexis is not present it becomes slightly difficult to implant an IOL into the bag. The technique of IOL insertion does not differ much. Before insertion all the anterior capsule flaps are trimmed and the bag is well inflated with viscoelastic. During insertion at all the times the IOL is kept pressed downwards. It is slightly difficult to insert the IOL into the bag in the absence of capsulorhexis as the haptics keep springing back out of the bag where the anterior capsule is deficient in the periphery.

Intraocular lens insertion in the presence of posterior capsular rent In the case of posterior capsular rent the decision to implant a lens lies entirely on the operating surgeon. The site and the size of the rent are assessed and then a decision is made regarding implantation of a lens. If there is a small central rent it can be converted to a posterior capsulorhexis and an IOL can be implanted into the bag with the use of viscoelastic. If the rent is too large and if you have a good capsulorhexis margin to support the IOL then the IOL can be implanted into the sulcus above the anterior capsulorhexis. The technique of insertion of IOL in such a case will consist of injecting viscoelastic in between the anterior capsule and the iris to lift it up slightly. Now a Sheet's glide[6] is inserted in between the anterior capsule and the iris. The IOL is now glided over the Sheet's glide, so that, it is directed towards the ciliary sulcus. Once the leading haptic is under the iris and in the sulcus the glide is withdrawn out and the IOL is dialed into the sulcus with the help of a lens manipulator. Care is taken not to push the IOL backwards.

Intraocular lens implantation in the anterior chamber When the posterior capsular is absent or the rent in posterior capsule is too big for the safe implantation of an IOL in the posterior chamber or the anterior capsulorhexis is absent then IOL can be implanted into the anterior chamber. In such cases a scleral fixated IOL can also be implanted. A Kelman lens can be implanted very safely into the anterior chamber in a case of SICS. After constriction of pupil, the anterior chamber is deepen with viscoelastic and a Sheet's glide is inserted over the iris to cover the pupil. The Sheet's glide will prevent the accidental passage of IOL into the posterior chamber through the pupil. The Kelman lens is inserted over the glide and then dialed in anticlockwise direction into its place. Once the IOL is in its place the Sheet's glide is withdrawn and viscoelastic removed.

CONCLUSION

If the IOL is inserted through the tunnel keeping the basic principles in mind, the insertion will be very smooth and effort less. At all the time during insertion of IOL, the anterior chamber should be well formed with viscoelastic. It is important to balance rotational and backward push forces during manipulating an IOL into the bag with the help of a lens manipulator. If these forces are not balanced, then one will just keep on rotating the lens over the iris without pushing it into the bag.

REFERENCES

1. Radner W, Menapace R, Zehetmayer M, Mallinger R. Ultrastructure of clear corneal incisions. Part I: Effect of keratomes and incision width on corneal trauma after lens implantation. J Cataract Refract Surg. 1998;24(4):487-92.
2. Ellis MF. Sharp-edged intraocular lens design as a cause of permanent glare. J Cataract Refract Surg. 2001; 27(7):1061-64.
3. el-Maghraby A, Anwar M, el-Sayyad F, Matheen M, Marzouky A, Gazayerli E, et al: Effect of incision size on early postoperative visual rehabilitation after cataract surgery and intraocular lens implantation. J Cataract Refract Surg. 1993;19(4):494-98.
4. Ttivedi N. The technique of IOL implantation in SICS. In Singh K (Ed): Small incision cataract surgery (manual phaco), New Delhi, Jaypee Brothers, 2002;155-57.
5. Shingleton BJ, Mitrev PV. Anterior chamber maintainer versus viscoelastic material for intraocular lens implantation: Case-control study. J Cataract Refract Surg. 2001; 27(5):711-14.
6. Blumenthal M, Ashkenazi I, Fogel R, Assia EI. The gliding nucleus. J Cataract Refract Surg. 1993;19(3):435-37.

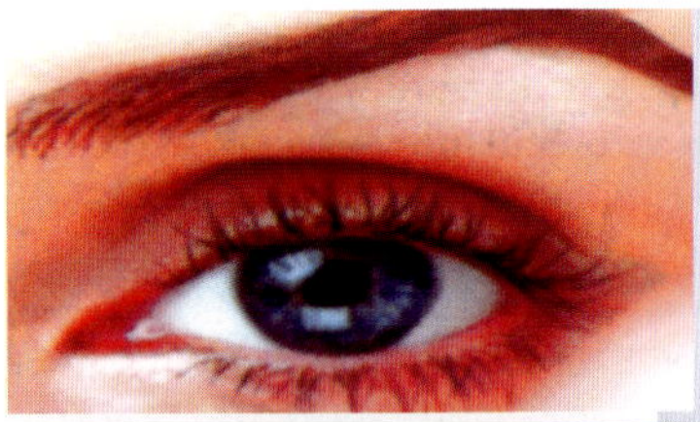

Twenty four

Materials for Intraocular Lenses

Jean-Marc Legeais
(France)

POLYMETHYLMETHACRYLATE AND INTRAOCULAR LENSES

Polylethylmethacrylate (PMMA) is a polyacrylic derivative marketed under the brand names Plexiglas, Perspex, Diakon, Lucite, etc. The optical and organoleptic properties of PMMA have established it as the standard material for the manufacture of intraocular lenses (IOLs). It is amorphous, transparent and colorless. It has a refractive index of 1.49 to 1.50 and transmits 92 percent of the incident light. Chromophores can be incorporated into it and it is easily tinted. PMMA is rigid at room temperature. It has a vitreous transition temperature (i.e. the temperature at which it becomes flexible) of 105°C. It has a specific density of 1.19 gm/cm^3. PMMA is fairly water-repellent, has an angle of contact of 70° and a water absorption index of 0.25 percent.

It is insoluble in water and aliphatic hydrocarbons and stands up well to exposure to oils, fats, alkaline solutions and dilute acids. The manufacturing process for the optical part of the PMMA IOLs involves turning or molding. Leaves of PMMA are used in the manufacturing method that requires turning. The lenses are cut by rotating the slab of PMMA or by rotating the cutting tool.

The thickness of the lens depends on the intended optical power and the edges are then polished until a satisfactory surface finish is obtained. Molding can be carried out by injection or by compression. In the injection method, the PMMA is heated to a temperature of 160 to 200°C until it melts and it is then injected into a mold with a compression pressure of about 140 kg/cm^2. The edges of the lens are polished after the mold has been opened. In the compression molding method, a steel mould is filled with PMMA and subjected to a pressure of 500 kg. It is then heated to a temperature of 20°C and the pressure raised to 2600 kg. The pressure is then brought back to normal and the mold is cooled by ventilation. Cast molding is a more recent method in which a mixture of methylmethacrylate monomer and a polymerization initiator are injected into the mold. This improves the reproducibility of the manufacturing process.

PMMA has to be sterilized at a low temperature, ethylene dioxide is therefore used to sterilize PMMA IOLs.

Biocompatibility and PMMA

When a foreign material is introduced into a biological medium, the first phenomenon observed is the adsorption of macromolecules and particularly of proteins. Protein adsorption occurs rapidly and the layer deposited is of the order of 100 nm thick. This adsorption seems to result from acid/base and dipole/dipole interactions. These are directly related to the surface energy of the material, its chemical structure and the distribution of binding sites on the surface of the material. This layer of proteins mediates the chemical reactions that occur at the material-tissue interface over the next few minutes or hours.

Removing the natural lens and implanting the artificial IOL ruptures the blood/eye barrier. Adsorption of protein onto the implanted lens occurs immediately. Complement is then activated by the alternative pathway. Polymorphonuclear cells and monocytes are attracted, giving rise to macrophages and giant cells, and the IOL becomes the focus of a reaction to a foreign body. Kochounian *et al* used the Western blot method to identify the proteins adsorbed onto the surface of PMMA IOLs that had been incubated for 3 hours in rabbit plasma (*in vitro*) or implanted for 48 hours in the capsule of rabbits (*in vivo*). The protein layer consisted of at least 6 different proteins: albumin, complement fraction C_3, IgG, fibrinogen/fibrin, fibronectin and transferrin. The main proteins adsorbed *in vitro* were albumin IgG, fibronectin and fibrinogen. The dominant types adsorbed *in vivo* were fibronectin and fibrinogen.

Studies have also demonstrated the effect of surface properties on cell adhesion. These studies covered several factors, such as the free energy of the interface (FEI), the surface energy (SE) and the angle of contact (AC). If the FEI is used as the assessment criterion, the most hydrophilic materials, with a low FEI (< 5 ergs/cm^2) and the most water-repellent materials, which have a high FEI (> 40 ergs/cm^2) resulted in much lower cell adhesion than does PMMA. The intermediate FEI values (5 to 40 ergs/cm^2) of a PMMA make it favorable to cell adhesion and cell proliferation. The same conclusions were reached from a study of the SE and AC. The more hydrophilic (higher SE and lower AC), or more water-repellent (lower SE and higher AC) a material, the greater will be the adhesion of cells to its surface. The study of Tamada and Ikada showed that the adhesion and proliferation of rat fibroblasts is greatest on substrates with an AC of about 70° (the angle of contact of PMMA). Reich *et al* have developed a system for measuring the adhesive force between a material and the corneal endothelium of the rabbit and showed that these forces of adhesion were greater for PMMA.

The surface properties affect the opacification of the posterior capsule (OPC). Pathogenic aspects of OPC include the formation of Elschnig pearls, from equatorial epithelial cells that proliferate along the posterior capsule, and capsular fibrosis, due to anterior cuboid epithelial cells that undergo fibrous metaplasia. The epithelial cells of the lens require a surface on which to proliferate and the surface properties of the implanted lens determine the degree of postoperative OPC. Epithelial cells from rabbits, cattle, pigs and humans adhere *in vitro* less well to IOLs that are more hydrophilic or more hydrophobic than PMMA. However, no direct relationship was found *in vivo* between the surface properties and the degree of postoperative OPC.

PMMA IOL AND SURFACE PROCESSING

The surface properties of a polymer can be altered by various methods, known collectively as surface treatment. These treatments make it possible to modify the surface energy of the polymer (hydrophilic-hydrophobic balance) by three methods

- Treatment of the surface proper
- Coating with a deposit
- Grafting by the attachment of new molecules.

Treating of the Surface Itself

Various methods can be used to modify the surface of the polymer. The main ones are:

- Chemical techniques (chemical oxidation—exposure to ozone)
- Flaming
- Electromagnetic radiation (bombardment with ionizing radiation, bombardment with light rays; low-pressure cold plasma: crown discharges).

They are intended to create new chemical functions on the surface of the backing, which are then used to graft molecules or to alter some characteristics or the surface, such as roughness, hardness or slipperiness, without grafting molecules. The thickness treated is of the order of a few nanometers. Examples of the use of this method in ophthalmology tend to be linked to placing functional groups on the backing.

Coating with a Deposit

Another polymer (deposit) with the desired properties is deposited on the backing to form a layer, which may reach a thickness of about 10 microns. The method usually is that known as the "soaking method", in which the backing is soaked in a solution of the deposit. The deposit is not made to adhere by chemical means and the two materials can have very different mechanical properties.

Teflon-coated Lenses

Polymethylmethacrylate intraocular lenses can be coated with a layer of a transparent fluorocarbon, Teflon AF. This is the first transparent, Amorphous Teflon, which can be dissolved in fluoridized solvents (liquid fluorocarbons). This property means that it can be applied in very thin layers to substrates, rendering them entirely hydrophobic. The main steps in this process are:

- Soaking the PMMA lenses is a solution of Teflon AF in C8F18 for 3 seconds
- Drying the lenses under vacuum at 37°C until the C8F18 has evaporated.

Teflon-coated lenses have been implanted in animals after phacoemulsification. No synechiae was observed between the iris and these implants over a follow-up period of 3 months. A significantly smaller number of cell deposits were found on the IOLs coated with Teflon than with those that were not. Another study, using a model of endothelial contact, demonstrated that the trauma induced by the implantation of Teflon-coated lenses was reduced, with less adhesion of the endothelial cells to their surface.

Grafting on New Molecules

This method is used to bind one or more molecules (ligands) to the surface of a polymer (backing) by a covalent bond. The ligand is selected on the basis of specific new properties that the backing is required to have to make it more suitable for its final purpose. The grafting process includes the placing of functional groups on of the backing and the binding of the ligand to them.

Heparin Surface-modified Lenses

The surface of PMMA lenses is heparin surface-modified by attaching heparin via covalent bonds in a series of chemical reactions.

- The lens surface is treated with sulfuric acid and potassium permanganate to create carbonyl and sulfate groups
- They are then incubated with polyethylene-amine, a polymer that contains high levels of amines. This polymer reacts strongly with the surface of the treated lenses
- The heparin is partially depolymerized with nitrous acid. The resulting molecular fragments have terminal aldehydes

- The molecules containing aldehyde groups react with the primary amines to form bases, which can be reduced to form secondary amines. In this way the fragments of aldehydes of the partially degraded heparin are coupled to the amine groups on the surface of the PMMA IOLs. Stable covalent bonds are then obtained by reduction with sodium cyanoborohydride. Larsson *et al* showed that the concentration of heparin on the surface of the lenses, obtained by this process was 0.6 mg/cm^2. It was found to have very satisfactory chemical stability.

Several studies have demonstrated the greater antiadhesive effect of heparin surface-modified lenses compared to untreated PMMA IOLs.

Pekna *et al* showed that the grafting of heparin reduces complement activation by PMMA IOLs. In a model of endothelial injury using the rabbit cornea, heparin surface-modified lenses caused significantly fewer lesions and there was less adhesion of the endothelial cells to these lenses. Versura and Caramazza cultured human fibroblasts, monocytes and platelets on 4 types of IOLs: PMMA; heparin surface-modified PMMA, hydrogen and plasma-treated PMMA lenses. Electron microscopy identified reduced cell adhesion to heparin surface-modified IOLs and hydrogel lenses. A similar finding was reported by Joo and Kim for various cell models. Activation of the granulocytes by heparin surface-modified IOLs (assessed by the production of superoxide anions by exposed cells) was also reduced. Power *et al* followed by Cortina *et al* have demonstrated *in vitro* reduced adhesion of human epithelial cells to heparin surface-modified IOLs compared to PMMA IOLs. Power also compared the behavior of hydrogel IOLs, which had degrees of cell adhesion similar to those of heparin surface-modified lenses. Milazzo *et al* used organotypic cultures of chick embryo corneas and demonstrated that the surface of heparin surface-modified lenses is less propitious for cell adhesion and migration than the surface of unmodified PMMA lenses.

The antiadhesive property of heparin surface-modified IOLs seems to extend to bacteria, such as *Streptococcus epidermidis*, *Staphylococcus aureus* and *Pseudomonas aeruginosa*.

Rabbits were implanted with a heparin surface-modified or control artificial IOL and the number of leukocytes in the anterior chamber one day later was significantly lower in rabbits given heparin surface-modified lenses. The same thing was found in a similar type of study in which uveitis had been induced. The fibrinous reaction on heparin surface-modified IOLs was significantly less marked than that on PMMA intraocular lenses that had been implanted in monkeys for 4, 8 and 18 weeks. Larsson *et al* have shown that the concentration of heparin grafted to the surface of the PMMA IOLs by covalent bonding remained stable for 2 years after implantation in the anterior chamber of the rabbit.

These experimental findings have been confirmed in human studies. In a prospective study carried out by Borgioli *et al* 260 patients were given a heparin surface-modified lens and 264 a control lens. The number of patients presenting with cell deposits and posterior synechiae was reported to be lower in the group that had received heparin surface-modified lenses after 3 months and one year. In a group of 54 patients who had undergone surgery for cataract with phacoemulsification Shah and Spalton found that there were fewer giant cells (counted by reflection microscopy) on the heparin surface-modified lens during the first year after surgery. Amon and Menapace, in a study involving 50 patients, found that 8 percent of the patients had giant cells on the lenses (mean follow-up time of 16 months versus one-third of cases after the implantation of conventional PMMA lenses). Zetterström carried out a study involving 40 patients with exfoliation syndrome. Two years later, the incidence of pigment and cell deposits was lower in the group of patients who were given a heparin surface-modified lens, opacification of the posterior capsule was also less marked in this group. Percival and Pai implanted heparin surface-modified lenses in 36 patients with a history of chronic uveitis. Cell deposits were found on only 16.6 percent of the lenses versus 22 percent in patients who also had a history of uveitis but had been given conventional lenses. Linn *et al* studied a group of patients with diabetes, glaucoma or chronic uveitis, found that the inflammatory reaction was less severe in the patients who were given heparin surface-modified lenses.

Damage to the heparin surface-modified surface has been caused by an Nd:YAG laser and by surgical instruments. The clinical consequences of this damage are not known.

Surface Passivated Intraocular Lenses

Gupta and Van Osdel developed surface passivated IOLs in 1987. According to their patent, the process by which these lenses are produced consists of three steps:

- PMMA intraocular lenses are subjected to surface treatment (or functionalization) consisting of exposure to ozone. This results in oxidation of the outer surfaces of the lenses.
- The intraocular lenses are then exposed to a moist atmosphere, such as air, leading to hydrolysis of the outer, oxidized surfaces and the formation of hydroxyl groups.
- The treated intraocular lenses are then soaked in a solution containing fluorocarbon (CF2) x, where x is between 6 and 12 and the binding agents. As a result, a layer of fluorocarbons is chemically bound to the outer layer of the lenses and reduces their energy. However, according to the marketing literature issued by Ioptex-Allergan, the purpose of the lens surface-passivation process is to lower the energy and reduce the irregularity of the surface. Many studies have given disappointing results. Koch *et al* did not find any significant difference between the surface energy of surface-passivated lenses and unprocessed PMMA lenses. In this same study, ESCA (Electron Spectroscopy for Chemical Analysis) and SIMS (Static Secondary Ion Mass Spectroscopy) identified the presence of fluoride ions on the surface of only 1 of the 5 IOLs tested. Kochounian *et al* have shown that the passivated lenses activate the complement cascade, generating the same levels of C3a and C5a fractions as the conventional PMMA lenses. In a human study, Umezawa and Shimizu did not find any significant difference between the postoperative flare (measured using a laser flare cell meter) in the patients who had received surface-passivated and unprocessed PMMA lenses. However, using a model of endothelial contact in the cat, Balyeat *et al* have shown that passivated IOLs are associated with less epithelial injury and less adhesion of endothelial cells to their surface than unprocessed PMMA intraocular lenses.

Intraocular Lenses treated with Cold Plasma CF4

Another PMMA IOL was developed in 1990. These lenses are fluoridated by cold plasma treatment. The term "plasma" is used in physics to describe an ionized and electrically neutral gas. It can be produced artificially by confining the gas to a closed, high-frequency electromagnetic field under low pressure (1 mbar). The gas is placed in an unpolymerizable or polymerizable reactor. The gas used may be CF4 CF3H or CF3Cl, which contain a single carbon atom. It produces a chemical change in the surface of the polymer by substituting atoms of fluorine or CF2 or CF3 groups for hydrogen atoms. The thickness affected is no more than 0.01 mm.

The findings of the study of PMMA IOLs treated with CF4 plasma carried out by Eloy *et al* were as follows: ESCA of their surfaces detected the grafting of the fluorine and the *de novo* appearance of carbon-containing functions, particularly CF, CF2 and CF3; measurement of the angle of contact with water showed that the surface energy of the treated lenses was lower than that of the processed lenses; the adhesion of human granulocytes to the surface of treated IOLs was reduced after incubation. The granulocytes in contact with the treated IOLs were less active, and this was reflected by the rate of superoxide production by these cells.

Despite the excellent optical and physicochemical properties of PMMA, it is not totally inert. Surface treatment of PMMAs improves their acceptability. According to the literature, heparin surface-modified IOLs are more effective, particularly in high-risk patients. However, the data for surface-passivated IOLs is disappointing, because no significant difference between treated and untreated PMMA IOLs has been demonstrated *in vivo*. The efficacy of cold plasma CF4-treated IOLs *in vivo* remains debatable.

SILICONE FOR IOL

The use of soft intraocular lenses (IOLs) for cataract surgery has been growing since the 1980s. These lenses can be folded and inserted through small incisions, and may cause less postoperative astigmatism and allow quicker visual rehabilitation. The advantage of using small incisions has been demonstrated on several occasions by Oshika *et al*. The extent of the inflammatory reaction in the anterior chamber depends on the length of the incision and the differences remain statistically significant for one month after surgery. Postoperative astigmatism was found to be directly related to the length of the incision in most studies, except in that carried out by Neumann *et al*.

The first silicone soft IOL was used in 1984. This new generation of IOLs was accompanied by the development of various types of silicone materials with increasing refractive indices and types of IOLs that have been influenced by advances in surgical techniques. Capsulorhexis, for instance, was developed long after IOL of this type were first implanted.

The first elastomer used in the manufacture of the optical part of the soft IOLs was polydimethylsiloxane (-Si(CH_2)3O-)n. The main drawback of this material is its low refractive index (1.412 at 25°C), which makes it necessary to produce relatively thick lenses to achieve a given refractive index. These thick lenses are more difficult to fold. A second generation of silicone elastomers was then developed using a copolymer of diphenyl- and dimethylsiloxane, which has a refractive index of 1.464 (-$CH_3Si(C_6H_5)O$-)n. Silicones with even higher refractive indices have been developed, but have proved to be mechanically unsuitable for use as soft IOLs. Intraocular lenses made of various types of polydimethylsiloxane and polydimethyldiphenylsiloxane materials have been exhaustively assessed and subjected to numerous tests. They have been shown to be very resistant to artificial aging in tests including exposure to ultraviolet light equivalent to 20 years of exposure under normal conditions of use. According to the study carried out by Kborz *et al*, polydimethylsiloxane and PMMA IOLs seem to have equivalent optical qualities.

Molding Flash and Silicone IOL

The most commonly used method for manufacturing silicone intraocular lenses is injection molding. This method often results in surface irregularities at the junction of the two sides of the lens, which take the form of a rough line visible all around the edges of the lens. This defect is known as molding flash, and it has been clearly identified by scanning electron microscopy. This defect can impair the biocompatibility of the lens. Newman *et al* have reported the case of a patient fitted with an early Staar silicone intraocular lens in the ciliary sulcus. The onset of glaucoma made it necessary to carry out explantation. Scanning electron microscopy identified severe molding flash all round the edge of the lens.

The quality of the lenses available has gradually improved, and routine assessment of this defect by various teams has shown that the quality of the finish of most IOLs is acceptable. In 1992, Tsai *et al* assessed the most commonly used IOLs, and although they found that the surface was smooth and regular and the finish acceptable, most of the lenses had molding flash. Similarly, in 1996, Omar *et al* compared these silicone IOLs with single-piece PMMA IOLs, which these authors, like many others, consider to set the standard for their quality of finish. Scanning electron microscopic examinations revealed that most of the silicone lenses had molding flash plus some irregularities at the optic loop junctions.

Investigation of the effects of folding these lenses sometimes detected surface changes, but these were usually temporary. So although Brady *et al* have reported finding creases on the anterior surface of polydimethylsiloxane immediately after folding, these were no longer detectable by scanning electron microscopic examination ten minutes later.

The effects of the Nd:YAG laser have also been investigated by Newland *et al* who examined 17 silicone IOLs under the scanning electron microscope after standardized Nd:YAG exposure. The mean depth of the surface damage caused to these lenses was 143 (13.4 μm). According to the authors, these regions looked darker when viewed under a slit lamp, and looked very much like pigment deposits.

Biocompatibility and Silicone IOL

Silicone intraocular lenses were first used in 1984 by Mazzocco. Several studies of cell adhesion have subsequently been carried out both *in vivo* and *in vitro* and have shown that their safety is similar to that of IOLs made of PMMA.

Mondino *et al* incubated PMMA and silicone IOLs in serum. Using radioimmunological techniques, they demonstrated that the PMMA lenses activated the alternative complement pathway, whereas the silicone ones did not.

In vitro studies using cell models to evaluate the adhesion and toxicity of these materials have demonstrated better outcomes than those for standard PMMA.

Joo and Kim compared the adhesion of cells (platelets, human granulocytes, macrophage-like RAW 264.7 and rat fibrosarcoma L 929) to PMMA, heparin surface-modified PMMA, silicone and hydrogel. Less cell adhesion was found with the heparin surface-modified and hydrogel IOLs. There was slightly less cell adhesion to the silicone lenses than to the untreated PMMA lenses. In the same study, the authors evaluated granulocyte activation and measured the production of superoxide anions. Heparin surface-modified lenses and silicone lenses produced degrees of granulocyte activation intermediate between those found for PMMA and hydrogel IOLs.

In vitro animal studies carried out by Menapace *et al*, Kulnig *et al* found no differences between the numbers or types of cells deposited on PMMA and silicone IOLs. According to these authors, the prevalence of cell deposits was not directly linked to the nature of the polymer, but depended on the severity of the postoperative inflammatory reactions. Several methods have been proposed to avoid between-animal differences, which could impair the validity of the data.

Okada *et al* developed a model for comparing the cell populations on PMMA and silicone IOLs. This system eliminates between-animal differences due to the surgical trauma or the postoperative inflammatory reaction. They coated half of the PMMA IOLs with polydimethylsiloxane and implanted them in albino rabbits. Examinations carried out 1, 2 and 3 weeks after surgery using a reflecting microscope found significantly fewer cells on the surfaces of the lenses coated with silicone. Similar conclusions were drawn from the study carried out by Cook *et al*, who implanted silicone-coated or PMMA-coated posterior chamber lenses (PCLs) in rabbits.

Carlson *et al* used fluorophotometric and histological methods to evaluate the inflammatory response in brown rabbits after phacoemulsification and the implantation of intraocular PMMA, silicone and hydrogel lenses. All 3 types of IOL showed good biocompatibility during a 16-week follow-up. The only difference identified was the occurrence of non-granulomatous, chronic inflammation of the conjunctiva in the limbus of those rabbits which had been given a soft lens, although the authors did not identify any clinically significant repercussions.

No signs of toxicity were detected after implanting silicone PCLs in monkeys or cats. Both studies found that the cell loads deposited on the silicone lenses were significantly lighter than those on the PMMA lenses.

Endothelial contact models confirmed this tendency towards lower cell adhesion to Herzog *et al* demonstrated that the silicone IOLs caused less trauma of the endothelial cells.

Bacterial adhesion to this type of material is also an important factor. This is particularly relevant because cultures of the aqueous humor were positive for 29 to 43 percent of the patients who had undergone surgery for cataract. Cusamo *et al* cultivated coagulase-negative staphylococci on PMMA, silicone and hydrogel intraocular lenses. Bacterial growth was greatest on the silicone lenses, least on the PMMA and intermediate on the hydrogel IOLs. An increase in the incidence of endophthalmia after the implantation of soft lenses has not been confirmed, except in a context of suspected bacteriological risk arising from the use of polypropylene loops. The first clinical trials demonstrated good biocompatibility of silicone IOLs. The complications associated with them consisted essentially of decentering, which sometimes called for surgical repair. These problems are linked to the geometry of the lens and the operating technique, rather than to the materials of which they are made. The earliest silicone IOLs were initially implanted in the ciliary sulcus. The first silicone IOL was designed by Mazzocco. The first implantations of these lenses into the capsular bag did not yet use the capsulorhexis technique, and the incidence of decentering was very high. Once capsulorhexis had been introduced by Neuhann and Gimbel, the shapes of the silicone IOLs were soon changed to make them more suitable for implantation in the capsular bag. At present, some authors believe that this decentering is primarily attributable to shortcomings in the capsulotomy technique, and that the shape and material is a secondary factor.

Silicone IOLs can be arbitrarily divided into three main groups: single-piece or "spindle" or "boat-shaped" lenses, three-piece lenses with polypropylene loops and lenses with PMMA loops.

The implantation of silicone IOLs of all three types calls for regular capsulorhexis and an intact posterior chamber. The nature of the single-piece and of the attached loops affect the risk of decentering and secondary lens deformity. Single-piece IOLs have no real anchor within the capsular bag. Secondary symphysis of the anterior chamber to the posterior chamber holds the loops in place. Fibrosis and contraction of the capsular bag can also lead to decentering and horizontal distortion of the lens. This seems to be particularly true of silicone single-piece IOLs and those with polypropylene loops, in which the forces brought to bear by the capsular bag on the loops are more readily transmitted to the ocular part of the lens. Polypropylene is very flexible and has a tendency to lose its "memory", becoming permanently distorted during implantation. A few cases of pupillary capture have been reported involving silicone IOLs with polypropylene loops. The flexibility of polypropylene seems to facilitate the forward shift of the lens during contraction of the capsular bag, particularly if the loops have no anterior angulation.

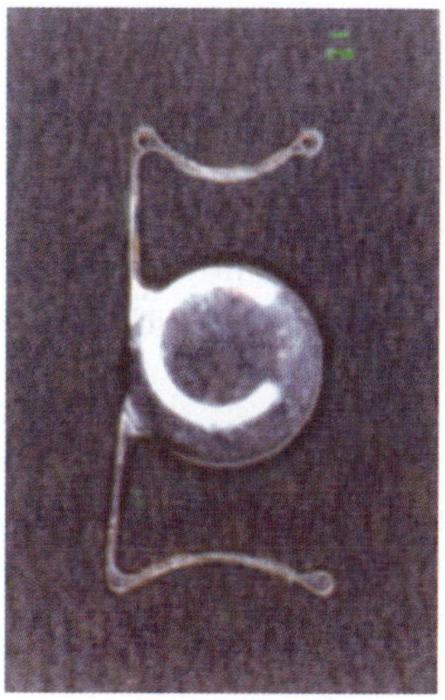

Fig. 24.1: Anterior chamber lens (PMMA). Kellman IOL

Studies have demonstrated that silicone lenses are not statistically significantly more often decentered than PMMA lenses: Blotnick *et al* examined 7 eyes obtained postmortem 6 weeks to 13 months after surgery for cataract during which a 3-piece silicone intraocular lens (AMO SI-18NB/silicone lens, polypropylene loops) had been implanted. This IOL was the first 3-piece lens to come onto the market, hence the importance of this study. Macroscopic examination showed that the lenses were all located in the capsular bags, with minimal decentering except in two cases, in which significant decentering was associated with radial tearing of the capsulorhexis and secondary contraction of the capsular bag. Histological examination did not reveal any inflammatory reaction of the iris, ciliary body capsular bag or anterior chamber. An FDA report on this IOL investigated the behavior of these lenses in 500 patients over a period of 3 years. The clinical safety and visual acuity were similar to those of the PMMA IOLs. The complication rate after 3 years did not seem to be directly related to the lens type.

Auffarth *et al* studied the anchoring and centering of single-piece silicone IOLs (boat-shaped) and 3-piece lenses in 30 cadaver eyes. The mean displacement from the center observed for single-piece lenses was 0.26 (0.13 mm), while that for 3-piece lenses was 0.37 (0.31 mm) this difference was not statistically significant. The difference between them and PMMA single-piece or 3-piece IOLs was also not significant.

In another group of 100 explanted silicone IOLs (63 three-piece lenses with polypropylene loops) and 37 (boat-shaped lenses) Auffarth *et al* once again found no difference between these lenses and the PMMA IOLs with regard to the reasons for explantation (42% decentering, 27.7% inflammation). The authors think that the long-term clinical prognosis depends mainly on the quality of the surgery and above all on the anchoring of the lens in the capsular bag.

Disk-shaped silicone IOLs were produced at the same time as these boat-shaped IOLs and the three-piece lenses with separate loops. Some people thought that this shape would have the theoretical advantage of ensuring better centering. In a study of 35 eyes, Duncker *et al* found that 25 percent were located at least 1 mm off center, and decided to stop using this type of lens (FK-1 and Adatomed 90-D).

Other authors recommend the use of 3-piece silicone lenses with PMMA loops, which are stiffer than polypropylene loops and less sensitive to the forces exerted by the capsular bag. Egan *et al*, monitored for 4 months, 100 patients fitted with an AMO SI-40NB IOL. They found that this IOL provided excellent centering during surgery and after 4 months.

Surface Modification

Like PMMA IOLs, silicone lenses can also be surface-modified to alter their characteristics. Hettlich *et al* exposed polydimethylsiloxane lenses to oxygen plasma, which made their surfaces less water-repellant (the contact angle fell from 121.86 to 96.5°). They intended to evaluate the impact of these surface modifications on the foreign-body reaction induced by the IOL. The only difference observed was the significantly lower incidence of posterior synechiae in the rabbits that had been given a surface-modified lens. Similarly, several attempts were made to carry out surface-modification using heparin.

Discoloration and Capsular Opacification of Silicone IOL

Miauskas was the first to report secondary discoloration of silicone lenses. In 1991, he reported 15 cases monitored for between 15 and 60 months after being implanted. The presence or absence of UV-blocks did not seem to affect the discoloration, as this occurred both in the IOLs manufactured by the Staar Surgical Co., which do not contain a UV block, and those manufactured by Iolab Co., which do. In the most severe instances (the surface of the lenses turned brown), there was an associated loss of contrast. Milauskas has subsequently identified another 9 cases involving these two types of lens. This discoloration was attributed to the presence of impurities, which could account for the granular, brownish appearance under the slit-lamp. The manufacturing process of these lenses has since been modified by adding an extra filtration of the silicone to remove all traces of impurity. In 1991, Watt also reported a case of brown discoloration of the center of a silicone lens (AMO Model S-18NGB) 6 weeks after surgery. In view of the location of the discoloration and the short interval since surgery, the author thought that this abnormality might already have been present when the IOL was implanted. In 1992, Koch and Heit reported two similar cases involving the same model of IOL. Allergan Medical Optics researchers have suggested that the brownish haze at the center of the lenses could have been due to diffusion of the light due to water vapor in the silicone immersed in an aqueous medium. This was attributed to defective polymerization or to the incomplete elimination of fractions of unpolymerized silicone. Kershner suggested that eyedrops may have affected the silicone. In 1992, Chapman *et al* investigated the possible interactions with compounds used before or after surgery. They found that none of the materials tested (PMMA, silicone and hydrogel) could have acted as a reservoir of these drugs (pilocarpine, gentamicin, dexamethasone, norepinephrine / noradrenaline) as the adsorption and desorption of these drugs was insufficient by any of the routes used (topical, subconjunctival and intravenous). It is unlikely that interactions of this type could contribute to the discoloration of silicone IOLs. No case has been recorded or reported in the literature since 1993.

The incidence of opacification of the anterior and posterior chamber after implantation of silicone IOLs has undergone considerable investigation. Fibrosis and opacification following surgery for cataract appears to be less frequent in the anterior chamber than in the posterior chamber. These effects are generally linked to a severe postoperative inflammatory reaction, promoted by capsular pseudoexfoliation or small-incision capsulorhexis. They can severely hinder the detailed examination of the fundus, taking retinographs and laser or surgical treatment of the retina. They may be combined with contraction of the capsular bag and lead to subsequent tilting or even folding of the lens. The material and shape of the lens may produce combined or independent effects. Auer and Gonvers studied two groups of 17 patients. Opacification of the anterior chamber occurred much more often when the lens was a single-piece silicone lens with flat loops (Staar® AA4203) (70%) rather than a PMMA lens (18%). It was suggested that this might have been due to the greater area in contact with the anterior chamber, which could have facilitated the proliferation of epithelial cells in the anterior chamber. Fibrosis and opacification of the posterior chamber appears to occur less frequently with single-piece silicone lenses with flat loops, because of the small area of contact between the IOL and the posterior chamber. Watts and Pearce demonstrated that a disk lens could act as a mechanical barrier, inhibiting the opacification of the posterior chamber. However, this was not observed in the study carried out by Duncker, in which 33 percent of the eyes displayed opacification of the posterior chamber after a mean follow-up time of 20.5 months.

The clinical results obtained with silicone IOLs are similar to those obtained with PMMA lenses. There is a considerable follow-up time, as the first implantations were carried out in 1984. Improvements in the manufacturing process have made it possible to solve the problems of lens discoloration which occurred in the early 1990s. But it is still possible to improve the surface finish of these lenses, as most of the models available have surplus material at the loop / lens junctions (molding flash). However, a recent circular from the DASS [French Social Security Authority] recommends avoiding the use of this type of material if there is silicone in the posterior segment, or if there is a risk of a slipped retina, because the adsorption of silicone to the surface of these lenses is irreversible.

SOFT ACRYLIC IOL

Silicone elastomers are some of the most frequently used materials in the manufacture of soft IOLs. Other materials are also used, including hydrogels and acrylics. The term "hydrogel IOLs" is generally taken to mean polyhydroxyethylmethacrylate (PHEMA) IOLs. In fact, the term encompasses a large group of polymers, of which PHEMA is just one. These materials all have a moisture content of at least 20 percent.

Soft "acrylic" IOLs are somewhat arbitrarily divided into groups. However, they all belong to the same group of chemicals, which includes stiff, hydrophobic polymethylmethacrylate (PMMA) and soft hydrophilic hydrogels, such as PHEMA. This large group of materials consists of monomers of esters of acrylic and methacrylic acids.

One important characteristic of the acrylics or acrylates is their vitreous transition temperature (VTT). This is the temperature at which the material undergoes a phase change and softens. The VTT of PMMA is 110°C. This means that it is stiff at room temperature, but becomes flexible from 110°C. Methacrylate monomers have much higher VTT values than acrylates. A polymer with an intermediate VTT can be obtained by selecting an appropriate combination of acrylates and methacrylates. For example, a copolymer containing 50 percent methacrylate (VTT = 10°C) and 50 percent methylmethacrylate (VTT = 105°C) would have a VTT of about 55°C. The materials used in the manufacture of soft IOLs, usually known as "acrylics", are copolymers synthesized from combinations of acrylics or acrylates. These ingredients are carefully selected to produce soft acrylic IOLs with high refractive indices and a VTT around room temperature while still having the optical properties of PMMA. These copolymers have a three-dimensional molecular structure, which enables them to retain a memory of shape. In view of the large number of possible combinations, the various copolymers synthesized have differing refractive indices, moisture contents, folding and unfolding properties and surface properties. These materials can be synthesized by copolymerization using 0.5 to 2.0 percent of a cross-linking agent, such as ethyleneglycol dimethacrylate (EGDMA). PHEMA is synthesized from the monomers 2-hydroxyethylmethacrylate (HEMA) and HEGDMA.

The hydrophilicity of these materials, like that of PHEMA, is linked to the inclusion of an (OH) group which enables them to absorb water into the polymer mesh. This mesh is rigid when dry, but becomes soft in an aqueous medium. The molecules of water have a plasticizing effect which renders the material flexible.

HYDROGEL INTRAOCULAR LENSES

PHEMA is the hydrogel most commonly used in the manufacture of IOLs. It contains 38 percent water. The earliest models were single-piece IOLs, with a biconvex lens and flanged flat loops. Their rear surface has a continuous convex arc of curvature, giving it a "taco-like" appearance.

These materials are highly hydrophilic, which theoretically gives them the advantage of having a lower cell adhesion capacity than PMMA. The endothelial trauma caused by PMMA IOLs and hydrogel IOLs as a result of *in vitro* contact with the endothelium is nearly 20 times greater (3.6% of an endothelial area of 0.25 mm^2 for the hydrogels versus 62% for untreated PMMA IOLs and 27 to 57% for PMMA IOLs coated with a 1% solution of sodium hyaluronate Healon®). Reich *et al* have shown that the cell adhesion force is about 7 times lower than that of PMMA [0.09 (0.02 g/cm^2 or hydrogel vs. 0.66) (0.11 g cm^2 for PMMA and 0.19) (0.05 gm/cm^2 for the Healon®-coated PMMA)]. Similarly, Power *et al*, who compared the *in vitro* adhesion of human lenticular epithelial cells to PMMA, heparin surface-treated PMMA and hydrogel, also demonstrated lower cell adhesion to the hydrogels. This has been confirmed for porcine, and bovine lenticular epithelial cells, as well as for human fibroblasts, monocytes and platelets. Bacterial adhesion to these IOLs remains controversial. Cusumano *et al* cultured coagulase-negative staphylococci on PMMA, silicone and hydrogel IOLs. Bacterial growth was greatest on the silicone lenses, least on the PMMA lenses and intermediate on the hydrogel lenses. In contrast, Ng *et al* demonstrated that the *in-vitro* adhesion of *S. epidermidis* to PMMA was 20 times greater than to hydrogel ($p < 0.001$). These results are confirmed by those of a study carried out by Hogt *et al*, who showed that the adhesion of *S. epidermidis* decreases as the HEMA content of the materials increases, and is therefore related to its hydrophilicity. This discrepancy between the findings of Cusumano *et al* and Ng *et al* is attributable to their use of differing methods, particularly involving different strains and concentrations of bacteria and the methods used to count the bacteria adhering to the materials. These materials cause little inflammatory reaction. Packard *et al* showed that implanting hydrogel IOLs in the rabbit for 2 months did not trigger any significant inflammatory reactions. Similarly, Amon and Menapace and Ravalico *et al* studied the cell deposits on PMMA and PHEMA IOLs and found that there was little cell reaction on the latter. Giant cells induced by foreign bodies were detected on only 9 percent of the PHEMA IOLs.

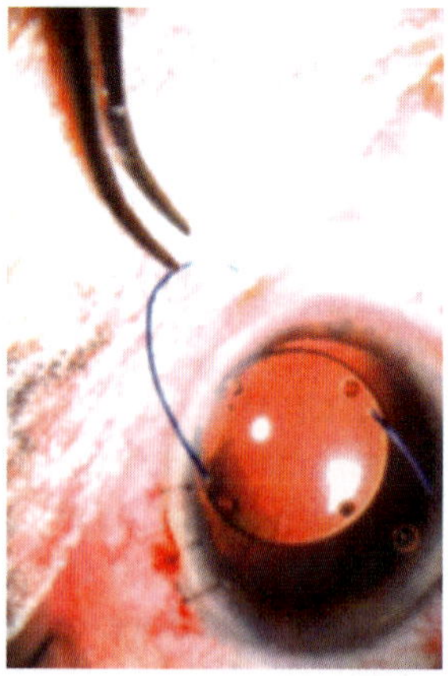

Fig. 24.2: Manual extracapsular surgery. Posterior chamber lens. Optic in PMMA, haptic with prolene

Hydrogel IOLs seem to be more resistant to the Nd:YAG laser than those made of PMMA or silicone. This has been demonstrated in several studies, including the *in vitro* study of Keates *et al* and a human study after discission of the posterior chamber. Skelnik *et al* compared hydrogel and PMMA IOLs immersed in a culture medium and exposed to an Nd:YAG laser and found that the PMMA lenses were always more severely damaged.

Despite their advantage in terms of biocompatibility, the earliest hydrogel IOLs had two drawbacks essentially linked to their design. The first posterior-chamber intraocular lens (PCL) made of poly-HEMA was developed and designed by Barrett, the IOGEL PC-12 model (Alcon). This was first implanted in 1983 in Perth, Australia. IOLs made of hydrogels with a higher water content than PHEMA, and hydrogel iris-supported IOLs had already been used in the 1970s. The PC-12 measured 6 mm wide and 12 mm long, and was intended for implantation in the sulcus or the capsular bag. This lens was often too long or too short, depending on whether it was implanted in the sulcus or the capsular bag, which is sometimes associated with a high degree of pigment dispersal. The design of the IOL was therefore modified to make it more suitable for implantation in the capsular bag. A second model, 1103, has a total length of 11.3 mm. The loops were shorter, and therefore less likely to be squashed once the IOL was positioned in the capsular bag. At the time, this single-piece lens was considered to be one of the best single-piece IOLs.

A more recent model, 1003, is supplied with a half-disk 6.5 mm wide and 10.3 mm long. It has a larger optical zone than the models mentioned above, which makes the center of the lens thicker. This IOL is smaller than the other models, and severe decentering has resulted from attempts to implant it in the capsular bag. Its wider and thicker optical zone resulted in more frequent contact between the iris and the anterior chamber, increasing the risk of fibrosis and iridocapsular synechia.

Many studies have shown that the visual acuity obtained with hydrogel IOLs is as good as that of PMMA IOLs. The only study in which the results for PMMA IOLs were significantly better than those for hydrogel IOLs (Alcon, Iogel PC-1103) was that of Lowe and Easty who investigated the sensitivity to contrast. This was not confirmed in the study of Weghaupt *et al*. They measured the contrast sensitivity of patients who had a PMMA implant in one eye and a hydrogel (Alcon, Iogel PC-1103) in the other. They did not find any significant difference.

Posterior chamber opacification (PCO) appears to be increased. Several studies have shown that the incidence of PCO is lower for PHEMA IOLs. Conflicting data have been obtained. Menapace evaluated the incidences of PCO and capsulotomy associated with PHEMA IOLs (PC-12, 1103, 1003) and found that 75 percent of these patients had impaired visual acuity and concomitant PCO over a period of 3 years. Theoretically, the posterior convexity of these lenses should prevent the migration of epithelial cells to lenses implanted in the capsular bag. However, the taco-style single-piece structure of these IOLs made it impossible to fuse the anterior and posterior chambers. A space developed behind the lens in 1/3 to 1/2 cases, within which there were numerous Elschnig pearls. According to the author, lens design was not the only factor responsible for this, and the properties of PHEMA were also implicated. The presence of Elschnig pearls in the capsular bag could have resulted in an osmotic pressure differential because fluid and nutrients pass through the IOL, which explains why Elschnig pearls filled the space behind the lens.

Levy *et al* have abandoned the use of hydrogel IOLs after the occurrence of two cases of this backward displacement of the IOLs into the vitreous humor during posterior capsulotomy using an Nd:YAG laser. The authors think that the lack of adhesion of the PHEMA to eye tissues and the design of these IOLs are responsible for these complications. This tendency has not been observed in any other study. The displacements reported by Levy *et al* led the FDA (Food and Drug Administration) to prohibit their use from September 1989.

Given the risk of backward displacement of the implant during YAG laser capsulotomy, Menapace and Yalon have recommended surgical aspiration of the Elschnig pearls if PCO occurs and substituting a PMMA IOL for the hydrogel IOL. The authors pointed out that it is easy to explant the soft and non-adhesive IOL and insert the PMMA lens because the anterior and posterior chambers are not attached.

The use of hydrogel IOLs has dwindled in the light of these incidents of decentering, backward displacement and pigment dispersal. The taco-style single-piece design is no longer considered suitable for hydrogel IOLs due to the symphysis of the anterior and posterior chambers. Barrett has recently produced a new design of PHEMA IOL intended to improve their attachment, eliminating the risk of backward displacement after YAG laser capsulotomy. The actual lens had a diameter of 6 mm and forms a continuous entity with the "C"-shaped loops. This design makes it possible to fuse the anterior and posterior chambers between the loops. The fixing and centering performance of these new IOLs obtained by Barrett in a group of 67 patients was excellent. Similar results were also obtained in Condon's study of 20 patients followed up for 6 months. However, Percival and Jafree reported one case of decentering caused by incomplete fusion of the bottom of the anterior and posterior capsules.

Another drawback often attributed to hydrogel IOLs is the fact that they do not incorporate UV filters. Despite this, the PC-12 model was monitored for 5 years after being implanted in 125 eyes and compared to a group of patients implanted with a PMMA PCL. The incidence of macular disease in these 2 groups were similar, despite the lack of incorporated UV-blocking chromophores in the hydrogel. Subsequently, Chirila was able to produce hydrogel IOLs containing melanin, which absorbs UV. These IOLs are currently undergoing experimental evaluation.

Bucher *et al* recently, reported a case of a PHEMA implant totally opacified by white deposits. Histological and physical examination showed that these deposits were due to calcification. These calcifications occurred even in patients without hypercalcemia. The authors suggested that the calcium was derived from residual lens fragments and the phosphorus from a solution of phosphated thymoxamine used preoperatively to induce miosis. This suggests that phosphated solutions should not be used with a PHEMA IOL.

SOFT ACRYLIC IOLS

The copolymers used in the manufacture of the soft acrylic IOLs discussed here are 3D chains synthesized from an ester of acrylic acid and an ester of methyacrylate acid (AcrySof® / Acrylens®) or from two esters of methacrylate acid (Memorylens®). A primer and a UV filter were included in their composition.

They have higher refractive indices than the PCLs. Despite being soft, they still have many of the advantages of PMMA, including its excellent optical characteristics. As a result of the three-dimensional arrangement of their chains, these lenses return to their initial shape and size after being inserted into the eye. They unfold more slowly than soft silicone IOLs. Only slight pressure is required to alter their shape. The forceps may often leave an imprint while they are being folded, but this disappears within a few minutes. However, their surface is fragile, and folding and insertion maneuvers can leave permanent marks. Soft acrylic IOLs are growing in popularity, and in Japan they are now preferred to silicone IOLs.

Hydrophilic Soft Acrylic IOLs

Memory Lens®

Two models are currently supplied: the U780A, with an optical diameter of 7 mm and a total diameter of 14 mm, and the U940 A, with an optical diameter of 6 mm and a total diameter of 13 mm. Both models have a three-piece design with C-shaped polypropylene loops.

In the initial clinical trials, the Memory Lens had to be folded before being inserted. To do this it had to be attached to a folding device and heated in a heat exchanger supplied by the manufacturer. The heated IOL was folded and then cooled in a second chamber of the heat exchanger. These are complicated operations, and damage was sometimes caused at this stage. Prefolded IOLs are now available. These have to be kept at 8°C before use. Once implanted, they slowly unfold (10 to 15 minutes) under the influence of body heat, and the folds have all disappeared by the day after the operation. The polypropylene loops on the prefolded IOL reach their normal position in the capsular bag as soon as they have been implanted. The hydrophilicity of the Memory Lens means that, unlike "hydrophobic" soft acrylic IOLs, its surfaces show no tendency to stick to each other or to the surgical instruments.

Pötzsch and Lötzsch implanted and compared 36 Memory Lens and 36 PMMA IOLs over a period of 4 years. The results for visual acuity, inflammatory reactions and opacification of the posterior chamber in the two groups were similar. There was less postoperative astigmatism in the Memory Lens group, and this IOL was also found to be more resistant to the YAG laser. This was confirmed by Johnson and Henderson, in a study in which MemoryLens and PMMA IOLs immersed in sterile physiological solution were exposed to the Nd:YAG laser. The Memory Lens IOLs suffered less damage.

Other hydrophilic soft acrylic IOLs are available in Europe, including the Hydroview® (Storz: 3 piece, PMMA loops, 18% water content, refractive index 1.47) and the EasAcryl® (Chiron Vision: single-piece, 26% water content, refractive index 1.46). Akreos Disc® and First®, from the Chauvin group. The Haptibag® from Holtech and the ACR 6D® from corneal are some of the best known of these. Clinical trials involving these IOLs are in progress.

Hydrophobic Soft Acrylic IOLs

The choice of material is controlled to some extent by patents (Allergan and Neslé/Alcon) which prevent the use of hydrophobic materials.

AcrySof was the first of the hydrophobic soft acrylic lenses to come onto the market. The MA60BM model has an optical diameter of 6 mm and a total diameter of 13 mm. The C-shaped loops are made of PMMA and have an anterior angle of 10°. The folding and unfolding of AcrySof depends on temperature. They are more flexible at higher temperatures which makes them easier to fold. Shugar has described a method for facilitating the implantation of AcrySof lenses without damaging them that is based on this characteristic. The IOLs are heated and coated with viscoelastic before being folded. It is advisable to handle AcrySofs using folding and insertion instruments and grasping them by the edges. The folding axis recommended by Shugar[48] corresponds to 6 O'clock to 12 O'clock, but Oh and Oh maintain that folding along the 4 O'clock to 10 O'clock axis makes it easier to handle the loops. Miller *et al* used the Staar 1-MTC-45 injection system to implant AcrySofs MA30BA through 2.8 mm incisions. This is not recommended, because this system has been specially designed for Staar silicone IOLs. However, the results of Miller *et al* show that a similar system for AcrySofs would make it easier to insert them through very small incisions, with less risk of damaging the optical part. A specific injector is now available. Several studies have reported creases or even cracks on the lens itself, all of which were produced during the folding and insertion maneuvers. Milazzo *et al* have shown that the marks produced on AcrySofs during folding are still visible under a slit lamp after a follow-up time of 17.75 (1.89 months, but have no impact on the visual recovery of the patients. Oshika and Shiokawa have shown that the procedures generally used for folding acrylic lenses do not affect their optical performance. In their study, damage to the material with deterioration of its optical properties was seen only after harsh treatment.

Shugar *et al* implanted 2 AcrySofs (1 in the capsular bag and 1 in the sulcus) in patients presenting with severe preoperative hypermetropia. The authors think that the AcrySof is appropriate for these multiple implantations because of its high refractive index, which makes it possible to produce thinner and flatter IOLs than with PMMA or silicone. AcrySof has a refractive index of 1.55 (37°C-550 nm), which is higher than that of any of the other materials used for IOLs. A 24D AcrySof lens is 0.3 mm thick. The fact that the AcrySof is flatter reduces the space between the two implanted lenses to a minimum. Where there is a space, lenticular epithelial cells can proliferate in it, leading to the formation of Elschnig pearls.

If the AcrySof IOL has to be explanted during or after surgery, it can be cut using Vannas scissors and the two halves removed as demonstrated by Koo *et al*. A special instrument has had to be devised to cut silicone IOLs. Neuhann has proposed an alternative method of intraocular folding for removing acrylic lenses without enlarging the incision. This preserves the advantages of small incisions.

Kohnen *et al* studied visual function in patients implanted with PMMA PCLs (n = 19), silicone (n = 20) and AcrySofs (n = 16). The outcome in terms of visual acuity was excellent in all three groups. However, significantly better results were obtained with regard to glare and contrast sensitivity with the PMMA lenses and AcrySofs. Oshika *et al* implanted AcrySofs in 64 patients who were monitored for 2 years. The intensity of postoperative "flare" was measured using a flare cell meter and was significantly higher in these patients than in those who had been given a PMMA or silicone lens. As a result of a burst capsule, one AcrySof was implanted in the ciliary sulcus with no adverse effect. Seven patients underwent YAG laser capsulotomy and the damage to the AcrySof lenses caused by this procedure was similar to but less severe than that incurred by the PMMA lenses. In the same study, the authors observed that AcrySof tended to stick to the forceps while it was being freed from the capsular bag. Sometimes the surfaces that came into contact with each other during folding stuck together. It was often necessary to introduce a second instrument through a lateral working incision to free the lens completely.

There have been some recent reports of glistening in the AcrySof lenses, which was first seen one week after surgery. In the study of Dhaliwal *et al* 17 of the 56 patients investigated displayed some glistening. Nine out of 10 patients with a silicone IOL in the other eye exhibited a loss of contrast sensitivity due to glistening in the eye fitted with the AcrySof. There was never any reduction of visual acuity and the glistening decreased with time in many of the patients. According to Alcon, this phenomenon is linked to hydration of the IOLs. Water vacuoles form in the lens and are visible as a result of the difference in the refractive indices of the polymer and of water. Placing AcrySof in BSS® at body temperature for 48 to 72 hours produced the same surface appearance. Other complications with the AcrySofs reported by Omar *et al* consisted of 9 cases of distension of the capsular bag. This distension was not specific to this type of IOL and had already been reported for hydrogel IOLs.

Sensar® IOL consists of a reticulated hydrophobic acrylic polymer that is now on the market in France. It has a lower refractive index than PMMA (1.47 versus 1.49) and a low melting point (13°C). This lower refractive index has the drawback of making it necessary to have a thicker lens for a given number of diopters, but it does cause less glare and reflection. An injection system is also provided.

The AcryLens (model ACR360) is a three-piece IOL with an optical diameter of 6 mm and a total diameter of 13.65 mm. C-shaped polypropylene loops have a forward angulation of 5°. Sanchez and Artaria implanted an AcryLens in each of 50 patients and monitored them for 12 months. The clinical outcomes were very similar to those obtained with other foldable IOLs. Two of these patients had preoperative complications (a radial tear of the capsulorhexis in one case and a burst posterior chamber in the other). Despite this, the AcryLens® was successfully implanted in the ciliary sulcus (as the AcrySof had been). This is an advantage over the spindle-shaped lenses, for instance, which cannot be implanted in the sulcus as they require a regular capsulorhexis and an intact capsular bag. Sanchez and Artaria also found the same tendency to stick to the surgical instruments as had been seen with AcrySof. The marks visible immediately after inserting these lenses were still visible by slit-lamp throughout the follow-up period. According to the authors, an injection system would simplify the insertion of these IOLs into the eye by preventing them from sticking to surgical instruments and protecting their fragile optical surfaces.

Surface Quality

Kohnen *et al* used scanning electron microscopy to analyze the quality of the surface of several acrylic, hydrogel and soft acrylic IOLs before and after folding. All the IOLs had smooth, uniform optical surfaces of excellent quality, in particular in the case of those containing HEMA (PHEMA, MemoryLens and Hydroview lenses). In the case of the Hydroview, the scan showed perfect fusion between the acrylic polymer (the optical part) and the PMMA (loops). There was no sign of the molding flash which is often associated with silicone IOLs, and the finish of the edges of all the lenses was thought to be generally of good quality. The AcryLens ACR360 had some fine irregularities on the polypropylene loops. Small gaps were found at the lens / loop junctions in the AcrySof MA60BM (PMMA loops) and the MemoryLens U940A (propylene loops). Minute linear defects were found in both hydrophobic acrylic IOLs (AcryLens ACR360 and AcrySof MA60BM) that had been folded for 1 minute. They were visible under very high magnification in the areas that had been

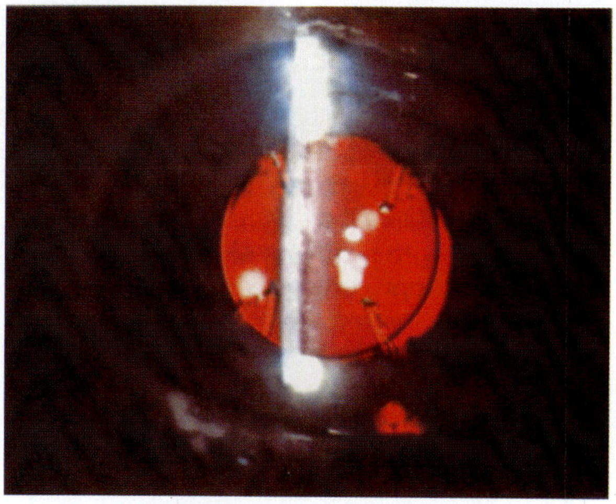

Fig. 24.3: Binkhorst (B4)

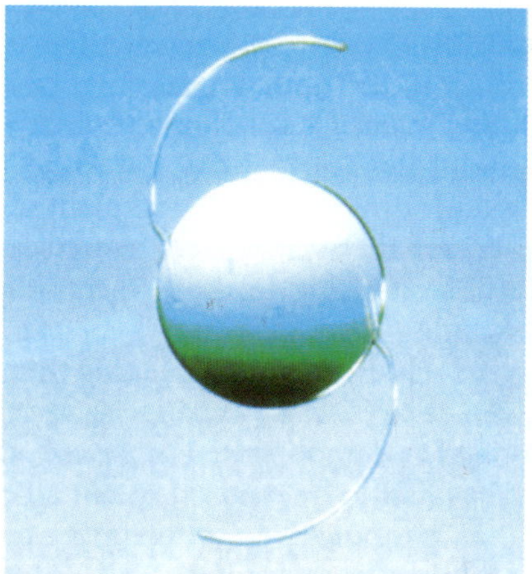

Fig. 24.4: PMMA intraocular lens

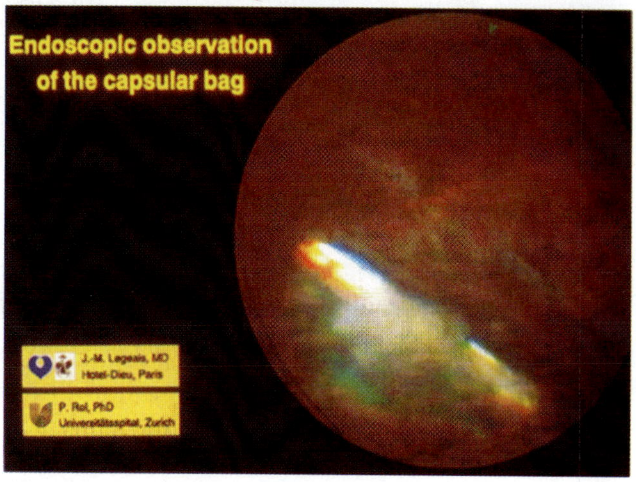

Fig. 24.5: Endoscopic observation of the capsular bag with PMMA haptic

gripped by the forceps. This confirmed the findings of other authors concerning the greater fragility of these lenses.

The main chemical constituents of the materials currently available for the manufacture of IOLs fall into just two groups: acrylate/methacrylate polymers and silicone elastomers. PMMA, hydrogel, PHEMA and the various copolymers used for the manufacture of soft acrylic IOLs all actually belong to the same group. It is the different chemical groups attached to the main chain of the standard polymer which produce the differing properties observed. Soft acrylic IOLs are becoming increasingly popular, and in some countries they are the most frequently used soft IOLs. Acrylic copolymers, in addition to those mentioned here, are also currently under investigation.

FURTHER READING

1. Absolom DR, Thomson C, Hawthorn LA et al. Kinetics of cell adhesion to polymer surfaces. J Biomed Mater Res 1988;22:215-29.
2. Allmer K, Hilborn J, Larsson PH et al. Surface modification of polymers. V. Biomaterial applications. J Appl Polym Sci Pol Chem 1990;28:173-83.
3. Allmer K, Hult A, Ranby B. Surface modification of polymers. III. Grafting of stabilizers onto polymer films. J Appl Polym Sci Pol Chem 1989;27:3405-17.
4. Amon M, Menapace R. Cellular invasion on hydrogel and poly(methyl methacrylate) implants; *in vivo* study. J Cataract Refract Surg 1991;17:774-79.
5. Amon M, Menapace R. Evaluation of a one-piece poly (methyl methacrylate) intraocular lens with a 7 mm biconvex optic and a total diameter of 10 mm. J Cataract Refract Surg 1993;19:16-21.
6. Amon M, Menapace R. Long-term results and biocompatibility of heparin-surface-modified intraocular lenses. J Cataract Refract Surg 1993;19:258-62.
7. Anderson C, Koch DD, Gree G et al. Alcon AcrySof™ acrylic intraocular lens. In Martin RG, Gills JP, Sanders DR (Eds): Foldable Intraocular Lenses. Thorofare: NJ Slack 1993;161-77.
8. Apple DJ, Mamalis N, Loftfield K et al. Complications of intraocular lenses. A historical and histopathological review. Surv Ophthalmol 1984;29:1-54.
9. Apple DJ, Mamalis N, Olson RJ et al. Intraocular lenses: evolution designs, complications, and pathology. Williams and Williams: Baltimore, 1989;429.
10. Arciola CR, Caramazza R, Pizzoferrato A. In vitro adhesion of Staphylococcus epidermidis on heparin-surface-modified intraocular lenses. J Cataract Refract Surg 1994;20:158-61.

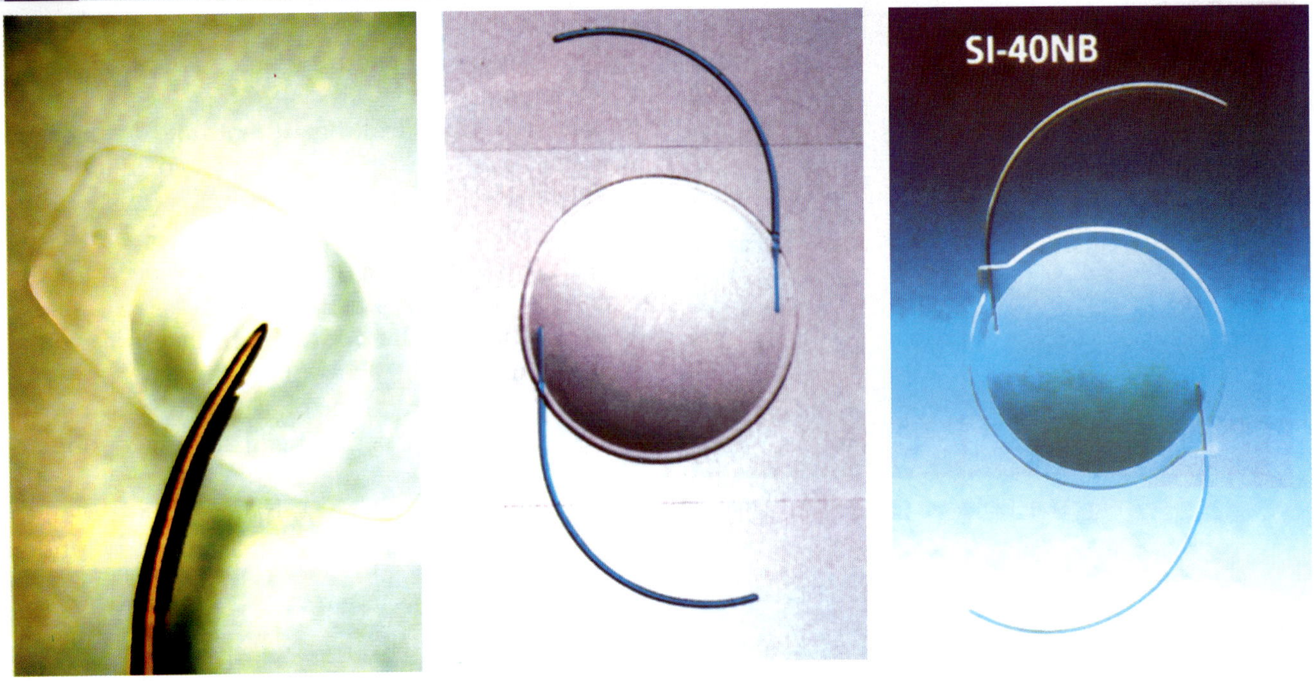

Figs 24.6A to C: Silicone IOL

Fig. 24.7: Silicone optic IOL observation by SEM (scanning electron microscopy)

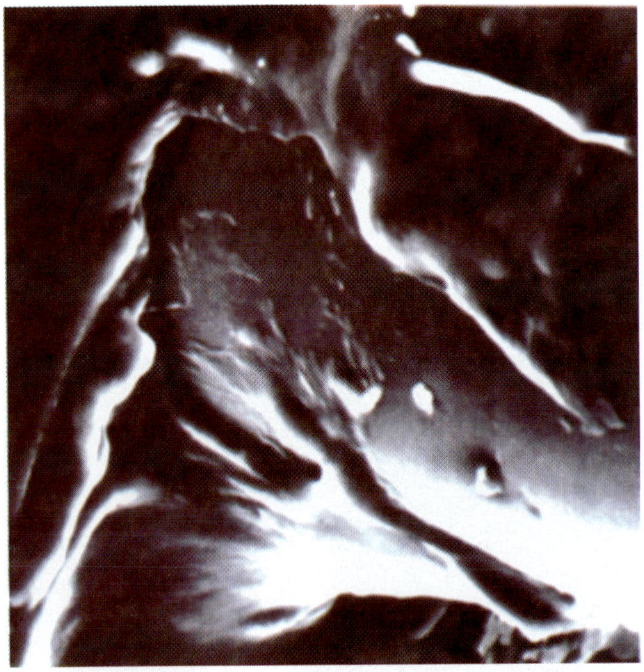

Fig. 24.8: Silicone IOL molding flash at the junction optic/haptic

11. Auer C, Gonvers M. Implant intraoculaire monobloc en silicone et fibrose de la capsule antérieure. Klin Monatsbl Augenheilkd 1995;206:293-95.

12. Auffarth GU, McCabe C, Wilcox M et al. Centration and fixation of silicone intraocular lenses: Clinicopathological findings in human autopsy eyes. J Cataract Refract Surg 1996;22:1281-85.

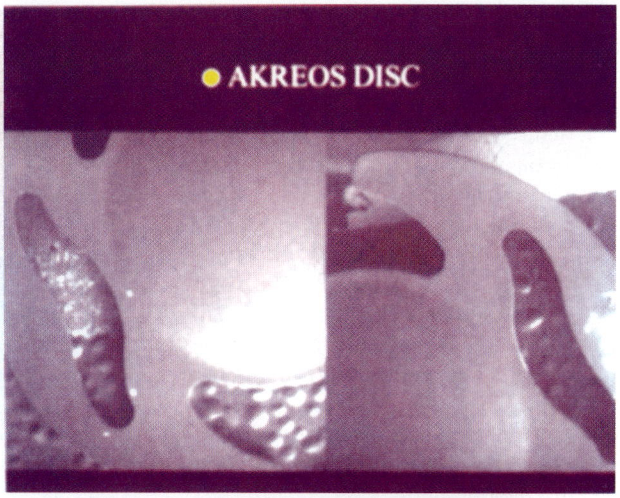

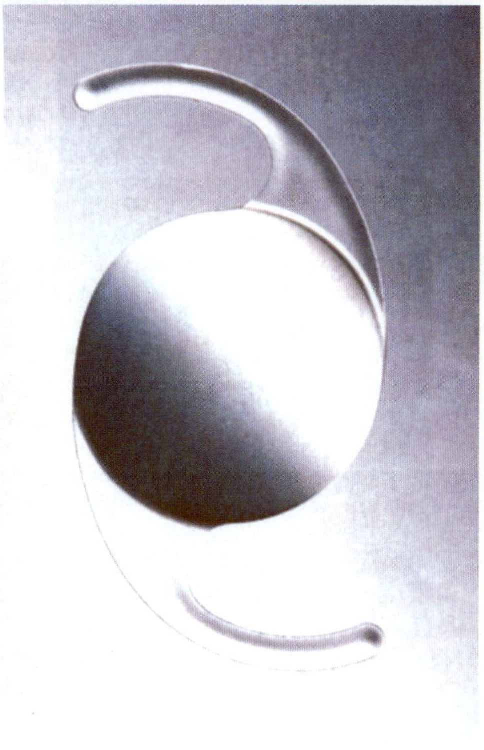

Figs 24.9A and B: Hydrophilic acrylic IOL

13. Auffarth GU, Wilcox M, Sims JCR et al. Analysis of 100 explanted one-piece and three-piece silicone intraocular lenses. Ophthalmol 1995;102:1144-50.
14. Babizhayev MA, Chumayevskii NA: Tinting effect of ultraviolet radiation on intraocular lenses of polymethyl methacrylate. Biomed Mater Eng 1994;4:1-16.
15. Baldeschi L, Rizzo S, Nardi M. Damage of foldable intraocular lenses by incorrect folder forceps. Am J Ophthalmol 1997;124:245-47.
16. Balyeat HD, Nordquist RE, Lerner MP et al. Comparison of endothelial damage produced by control and surface modified poly(methyl methacrylate) intraocular lenses. J Cataract Refract Surg 1989;15:491-94.
17. Barrett G, Constable IJ. Corneal endothelial loss with new intraocular lenses. Am J Ophthalmol 1984;98:157-65.
18. Barrett GD, Beasley H, Lorenzetti OJ et al. Multicenter trial of an intraocular hydrogel lens implant. J Cataract Refract Surg 1987;13:621-26.
19. Barrett GD, Constable IJ, Stewart AD: Clinical results of hydrogel lens implantation. J Cataract Refract Surg 1986;12: 623-31.
20. Barrett GD: A new hydrogel intraocular lens design. J Cataract Refract Surg 1994;20:18-25.
21. Barrett GD: The evolution of hydrogel implants. Dev Ophthalmol 1991;22:70-71.
22. Bechetoille A, Legeay G, Legeais V et al. Dispositif à usage ophtalmologique formé d'un substrat polymérique comportant des groupements fluorés en surface, et procédé d'obtention. Brevet d'invention No. FR 51035 A, déposé le 21/11/90, Paris.
23. Blotnick CA, Powers TP, Newland T et al. Pathology of silicone intraocular lenses in human eyes obtained postmortem. J Cataract Refract Surg 1995;21:447-52.
24. Borgioli M, Coster DJ, Fan RFT et al. Effect of heparin surface modification of polymethylmethacrylate intraocular lenses on signs of postoperative inflammation after extracapsular cataract extraction. Ophthalmol 1992;99:1248-54.
25. Bourne WM, Kaufman HE: Endothelial damage associated with intraocular lenses. Am J Ophthalmol 1976;81:482-85.
26. Boyd W, Peiffer RL, Siegal G et al. Fibronectin as a component of pseudophakic acellular membranes. J Cataract Refract Surg 1992;18:180-83.
27. Brady DG, Giamporcaro JE, Steinert RF. Effect of folding instruments on silicone intraocular lenses. J Cataract Refract Surg 1994;20:310-15.
28. Brinen JS, Greenhouse S, Pinatti L. ESCA and SIMS studies of plasma treatments of intraocular lenses. Surf Interface Anal 1991;17:63-70.
29. Brint SF, Ostrick DM, Bryan JE. Keratometric cylinder and visual performance following phacoemulsification and implantation with silicone small-incision poly(methyl methacrylate) intraocular lenses. J Cataract Refract Surg 1991;17:32-36.
30. Bronner A, Baikoff G, Charleux J et al. La correction de l'aphakie, Masson et Cie éditeurs, Paris, 1983;287-89.
31. Bucci FA, Lindstrom Rl. Total pupillary capture with a foldable silicone intraocular lens. Ophthalmic Surg 1991;l22:414-15.
32. Buchen SY, Richards SC, Solomon KD et al. Evaluation of the biocompatibility and fixation of a new silicone intraocular lens in the feline model. J Cataract Refract Surg 15: 545-53, 1989.

33. Bucher PJM, Buchi ER, Daicker BC. Dystrophic calcification of an implanted hydroxyethylmethacrylate intraocular lens. Arch Ophthalmol 1995;113:1431-35.
34. Carlson KH, Cameron JD, Lindstrom RL: Assessment of the blood-aqueous barrier by fluorophotometry following poly(methyl methacrylate), silicone, and hydrogel lens implantation in rabbit eyes. J Cataract Refract Surg 1993;19: 9-15.
35. Carlson KH, Johnson DW: Cracking of acrylic intraocular lenses during capsular bag insertion. Ophthalmic Surg Lasers 1995;26:572-73.
36. Champetier G, Monnerie L: Introduction à la chimie macromoléculaire, Masson et Cie éditeurs, Paris, 1969;505-06.
37. Chapman JM, Cheeks L, Green K: Drug interaction with intraocular lenses of different materials. J Cataract Refract Surg 1992;18:456-59.
38. Chasset R, Legeay G, Touraine JC et al. Fluoration du polyéthylène par plasma froid: mouillabilité, indice d'oxygène, coefficient de frottement. Eur Polym 1988;24:1049-55.
39. Chen TT: Clinical experience with soft intraocular lens implantation. J Cataract Refract Surg ;13:50-53.
40. Chirila TV, Vijayasekaran S, Constable IJ et al. Melanin-containing hydrogel intraocular lenses: a histopathological study in animal eyes. J Biomater App 1995;9:262-74.
41. Chirila TV: Melanized poly (HEMA) hydrogels: basic research and potential use. J Biomater App 1993;8:106-45.
42. Christ FR, Buchen SY, Deacon J et al. Biomaterials used for intraocular lenses. In Wise DL, Trantolo DJ, Altobelli DE et al (Eds): Encyclopedic Handbook of Biomaterials and Bioengineering. Part B: applications Marcel Dekker, Inc: New York, 1995;2:1261-1313.
43. Christ FR, Buchen SY, Fencil A et al. A comparative evaluation of the biostability of a poly (ether urethane) in the intraocular, intramuscular, and subcutaneous environments. J Biomed Mater Res 1992;26:607-29.
44. Christ FR, Fencil DA, Van Gent S et al. Evaluation of the chemical, optical, and mechanical properties of elastomeric intraocular lens materials and their clinical significance. J Cataract Refract Surg 1989;15:176-84.
45. Cobo LM, Ohsawa E, Chandler D et al. Pathogenesis of capsular opacification after extracapsular cataract extraction; an animal model. Ophthalmol 1984;91:857-63.
46. Condon PI: Initial results with the IOGEL 1000 IOL. Eur J Implant Refract Surg 1994;6:176.
47. Cook CS, Peiffer RL, Jr, Mazzocco TR: Clinical and pathologic evaluation of a flexible silicone posterior chamber lens design in a rabbit model. J Cataract Refract Surg 1986;12:130-34.
48. Cortina P, Gomez-Lechon MJ, Navea A et al. In vitro test of intraocular lens biocompatibility. Cataract Refract Surg 1995;21:112-13.
49. Crawford JB, Faulkner GD. Pathology report on the foldable silicone posterior chamber lens. J Cataract Refract Surg 1986;12:297-300.
50. Cumming JS, Ophth FC. Surgical complications and visual acuity results in 536 cases of plate haptic silicone lens implantation. J Cataract Refract Surg 1993;19:275-77.
51. Cumming JS: Postoperative complications and uncorrected acuities after implantation of plate haptic silicone and three-piece silicone intraocular lenses. J Cataract Refract Surg 1993;19:263-74.
52. Cunanan CM, Tarbaux NM, Knight PM: Surface properties of intraocular lens materials and their influence on in vitro cell adhesion. J Cataract Refract Surg 1991;17:767-73.
53. Cusumano A, Busin M, Spitznas M: Bacterial growth is significantly enhanced on foldable intraocular lenses. Arch Ophthalmol 1994;112:1015-16.
54. Davison JA: Capsular bag distension after endophacoemulsification and posterior chamber intraocular lens implantation. J Cataract Refract Surg , ;16:99-108.
55. Davison JA: Capsule contraction syndrome. J Cataract Refract Surg 1993;19:582-89.
56. Davison JA: Modified insertion technique for the SI-18NB intraocular lens. J Cataract Refract Surg 1991;17:849-53.
57. deGottrau P, Chevalley G, Dosso A et al. Les implants pliables dans la chirurgie de la cataracte à la Clinique Ophtalmologique de Genève. Klin Monastsbl Augenheilkd 1995;206:296-99.
58. Dhaliwal DK, Mamalis N, Olson RJ et al. Visual significance of glistenings seen inthe AcrySof intraocular lens. J Cataract Refract Surg 1996;22:452-57.
59. Dick B, Jacobi KW, Kohnen T: Alterations of heparin coating on intraocular lenses caused by implantation instruments. Klin Monatsbl Augenheilkd 1995;206:460-66.
60. Dickey JB, Thompson KD, Jay WM: Anterior chamber aspirate cultures after uncomplicated cataract surgery. Am J Ophthalmol 1991;112:278-82.
61. Duncker GIW, Westphalen S, Behrendt S: Complications of silicone discs intraocular lenses. J Cataract Refract Surg 1995;21:562-66.
62. Egan CA, Kottos PJ, Francis IC et al. Prospective study of the SI-40NB foldable silicone intraocular lens. J Cataract Refract Surg 1996;22:1272-76.
63. Elias HG: Macromolecules: Synthesis, Materials and Technology Plenum Press: New York 1984;2:926-27.
64. Eloy R, Parrat D, Due TM et al. In vitro evaluation of inflammatory cell response after CF_4 plasma surface modification of poly(methyl methacrylate) intraocular lenses. J Cataract Refract Surg , ;19:364-70.
65. Fagerholm P, Koul S, Trocmé S: Corneal endothelial protection by heparin and sodium hyaluronate surface coating of PMMA intraocular lenses. Acta Ophthalmol 1987;65:110-14.

66. Faulkner GD. Early experience with STAAR™ silicone elastic lens implants. J Cataract Refract Surg 1986;12:36-39.
67. Faulkner GD. Folding and inserting silicone intraocular lens implants. J Cataract Refract Surg 1987;13:678-81.
68. Fishkind WJ. ORC MemoryLens™: A thermoplastic IOL. In Martin RG, Gills JP, Sanders DR (Eds): Foldable Intraocular Lenses Slack: Thorofare, 1993;161-77.
69. Fogle JA, Blaydes JE, Fritz KJ et al. Clinicopathologic observations of a silicone posterior chamber lens in a primate model. J Cataract Refract Surg 1986;12:281-84.
70. Francese JE, Pham L, Christ FR. Accelerated hydrolytic and ultraviolet aging studies on SI-18NB and Si20NB silicone lenses. J Cataract Refract Surg 1992;18:402-05.
71. Gimbel HV, Neuhann T. Development, advantages, and methods of the continuous circular capsulorhexis technique. J Cataract Refract Surg 1990;16:31-37.
72. Gupta A, van Osdel RL. Surface passivated intraocular lens. U.S. Patent No. 4,655,770. Ioptex, Inc: California 91702, 1987.
73. Hansen SO, Tetz MR, Solomon KD et al. Decentration of flexible loop posterior chamber intraocular lenses in a series of 222 postmortem eyes. Ophthalmol 1988;95:344-49.
74. Herzog WR, Peiffer RL, Hill C. Comparison of the effect polymethylmethacrylate and silicone intraocular lenses on rabbit corneal endothelium in vitro. J Cataract Refract Surg 1987;13:397-400.
75. Hettlich HJ, Kaufmann R, Harmeyer H et al. In vitro and in vivo evaluation of a hydrophilized silicone intraocular lens. J Cataract Refract Surg 1992;18:140-46.
76. Hettlich HJ, Kaufmann R, Otterbach F et al. Plasma-induced surface modifications on silicone intraocular lenses; chemical analysis and in vitro characterization. Biomaterials 1991;12:521-24.
77. Hoffman AS: Ionizing radiation and gas plasma (or glow) discharge treatments for preparation of novel polymeric biomaterials. In Dusek K (Ed). Advances in Polymer Science Springer-Verlag: Berlin,1984;57:142-57.
78. Hogt AH, Dankert J, Feijen J. Adhesion of coagulase-negative staphylococci to methacrylate polymers and copolymers. J Biomed Mater Res 1986;20:533-45.
79. Holladay JT, Ting AC, Koester CJ et al. Silicone intraocular lens resolution in air and in water. J Cataract Refract Surg 1988;14:657-59.
80. Holladay JT, Van Gent S, Ting AC et al. Silicone intraocular lens power vs temperature. Am J Ophthalmol 1989;107:428-29.
81. Humphry RC, Ball SP, Brammall JE et al. Lens epithelial cells adhere less to HEMA than to PMMA intraocular lenses. Eye 1991;5:66-69.
82. Ichijima H, Kobayashi H, Ikada Y. In vitro evaluation of biocompatibility of surface-modified poly(methyl methacrylate) plate rabbit lens epithelial cells. J Cataract Refract Surg 1992;18:395-401.
83. Inoue H, Kohama S. Surface photografting of hydrophilic vinyl monomers onto diethyldithiocarbamated polydimethylsiloxane. J Appl Polym Sci 1984;29:877-89.
84. Janssen S: Biocompatibility and IOL. Bull Soc belge Ophtalmol 1992;245:103-07.
85. Johnson SH, Henderson C. Neodymium: YAG laser damage to VU-absorbing poly (mythyl methacrylate) and UV-absorbinb MMA-HEMA-EGDMA polymer intraocular lens materials. J Cataract Refract Surg 1991;17:604-07.
86. Joo CK, Kim JH. Compatibility of intraocular lenses with blood and connective tissue cells measured by cellular deposition and inflammatory response in vitro. J Cataract Refract Surg 1992;18:240-46.
87. Kaufman HE, Katz J, Valenti J et al. Corneal endothelium damage with intraocular lenses: contact adhesion between surgical materials and tissue. Science 1977;198:525-27.
88. Keates RH, Erdey RA, Ringel DM et al. Seventy-six consecutive cases of IOGEL intraocular lens implants. J Cataract Refract Surg 1990;16:47-50.
89. Keates RH, Sall KN, Kreter JK. Effect of the Nd:YAG laser on polymethylmethacrylate, HEMA copolymer, and silicone intraocular materials. J Cataract Refract Surg 1987;13:401-09.
90. Kershner RM. In reply to: Milauskas AT. Silicone intraocular lens implant discoloration in human. Arch Ophthalmol 1991;109:913-14.
91. Knight PM. In reply to: What RH. Discoloration of a silicone intraocular lens 6 weeks after surgery. Arch Ophthalmol 1991;109:1494-95.
92. Knorz MC, Lang A, Hsia TC et al. Comparison of the optical and visual quality of poly(methyl methacrylate) and silicone intraocular lenses. J Cataract Refract Surg 1993;19:766-71.
93. Koch DD, Heit LE. Discoloration of silicone intraocular lenses. Arch Ophthalmol 1992;110:319-20.
94. Koch DD, Samuelson SW, Dimonie V. Surface analysis of surface-passivated intraocular lenses. J Cataract Refract Surg 1991;17:131-38.
95. Koch HR. Lens bisector for silicone intraocular lens removal. J Cataract Refract Surg 1996;22:1379-80.
96. Kochounian HH, Kovacs SA, Sy J et al. Identification of intraocular lens-adsorbed proteins in mammalian in vitro and in vivo systems. Arch Ophthalmol 1994;112: 395-401.
97. Kochounian HH, Maxwell WA, Gupta A: Complement activation by surface modified poly(methyl methacrylate) intraocular lenses. J Cataract Refract Surg 1991;17:139-41.
98. Kohnen S, Ferrer A, Brauweiler P. Visual function in pseudophakic eyes with poly (methyl methacrylate), silicone, and acrylic intraocular lenses. J Cataract Refract Surg 1996;22:1303-07.
99. Kohnen T, Jacobi KW, Dick B. Effects of Nd:YAG microexplosions on heparin-coated PMMA intraocular lenses. Ophthalmol 1995;92:293-96.
100. Kohnen T, Magdowski G, Koch DD. Scanning electron microscopic analysis of foldable acrylic and hydrogel

intraocular lenses. J Cataract Refract Surg 1996;22:1342-50.
101. Kohnen T. The variety of foldable intraocular lens materials. J Cataract Refract Surg 1996;22:1255-58.
102. Koo EY, Lindsey PS, Soukiasian SH: Bisecting a foldable acrylic intraocular lens for explantaion. J Cataract Refract Surg 1996;22:1381-82.
103. Korinek P. Nouvelle génération de polymères fluorés. Matériaux et Techniques 1991;2:1-3.
104. Kulnig W, Menapace R, Skorpik C et al. Tissue reaction after silicone and poly(methyl methacrylate) intraocular lens implantation: a light and electron microscopy study in a rabbit model. J Cataract Refract Surg 1989;15:510-18.
105. Kulnig W, Skorpik C. Optical resolution of foldable intraocular lenses. J Cataract Refract Surg 1990;16:211-16.
106. Larm O, Larsson R, Olsson P. A new non-thrombogenic surface prepared by selective covalent binding of heparin via a modified reducing terminal residue. Biomat Med Dev Art Org 1983;11:161-73.
107. Larsson R, Selén G, Björklund H et al. Intraocular PMMA lenses modified with surface-immobilized heparin: evaluation of biocompatibility in vitro and in vivo. Biomaterials 1989;10:511-16.
108. Larsson R, Selén G, Formgren B et al. Long-term stability of heparin-surface-modified intraocular lenses in vivo. J Cataract Refract Surg 1992;18:247-51.
109. Legeais JM, Hallegot P, Chabala J et al. Trifluorothymidine localization in the rabbit cornea by secondary ion mass spectrometry imaging microanalysis. Cur Eye Res 1989;8:971-73.
110. Legeais JM, Legeay G, Werner LP et al. Teflon AF pour implant intraoculaire. Brevet d'invention INSERM No. FR 9604267, déposé le 04/04/96, Paris.
111. Legeais JM, Renard G. La microanalyse en Ophthalmologie. J Fr Ophtalmol 1991;14:415-21.
112. Legeais JM, Werner LP, Legeay G et al. In vivo studies—A fluorocarbon polymer for intraocular lenses. J Cataract Refract Surg 1998;24:371-79.
113. Lerman S. Assessing the biostability of intraocular lenses. Lens Eye Toxicity Res 1992;9:395-410.
114. Levy JH, Pisacano AM, Anello RD. Displacement of bag-placed hydrogel lenses into vitreous following neodymium: YAG laser capsulotomy. J Cataract Refract Surg 1990;16:563-66.
115. Levy JH, Pisacano AM. Initial clinical studies with silicone intraocular implants. J Cataract Refract Surg 1988;14:294-98.
116. Liesegang TJ, Bourne WM, Ilstrup DM. Short and long term endothelial cell loss associated with cataract extraction and intraocular lens implantation. Am J Ophthalmol 1984;97:32-39.
117. Lin CL, Shieh G, Chou JC et al. Heparin-surface-modified intraocular lens implantation in patients with glaucoma, diabetes, or uveitis. J Cataract Refract Surg 1994;20:550-53.
118. Lindstrom RL. Foldable intraocular lenses. In Steinert RF (Ed): Cataract Surgery: Technique, Complications and Management WB Saunders: Philadelphia, 1995;279-94.
119. Lowe KJ, Easty DL. A comparison of 141 polymacon (IOGEL) and 140 poly(methyl methacrylate) intraocular lens implants. Br J Ophthalmol 1992;76:88-90.
120. Lundgren B, Holst A, Tärnholm A et al. Cellular reaction following cataract surgery with implantation of the heparin-surface-modified intraocular lens in rabbits with experimental uveitis. J Cataract Refract Surg 1992;18:602-06.
121. Lundgren B, Ocklind A, Holst A et al. Inflammatory response in the rabbit eye after intraocular implantation with poly(methyl methacrylate) and heparin surface modified intraocular lenses. J Cataract Refract Surg 122;18:65-70.
122. Lundgren B, Selén G, Spangberg M et al. Fibrinous reaction on implanted intraocular lenses. A comparison of conventional PMMA and heparin surface modified lenses. J Cataract Refract Surg 1992;18:236-39.
123. Mackool RJ: Ioptex Acrylens^{TM} acrylic IOL. In Martin RG, Gills JP, Sanders DR (Eds): Foldable Intraocular Lenses. Thorofare: NJ Slack 1993;191-97.
124. Marcus DM, Azar D, Boerner C et al. Pupillary capture of a flexible silicone posterior chamber intraocular lens (letter). Arch Ophthalmol 1992;110:609.
125. Martin RG, Sanders DR, van Der Karr MA et al. Effect of small incision intraocular lens surgery on postoperative inflammation and astigmatism; a study of the AMO SI-18NB small incision lens. J Cataract Refract Surg 1992;18:51-57.
126. Martin RG, Sanders DR. Visual, astigmatic, and inflammatory results with the Staar AA-4203 single-piece foldable IOL: a randomized, propective study. Ophthalmic Surg 1992;23:770-75.
127. Mazzocco TR. Early clinical experience with elastic lens implants. Trans Ophthalmol Soc UK 1985;104:578-79.
128. Menapace R, Amon M, Radax U: Evaluation of 200 consecutive IOGEl 1103 capsular-bag lenses implanted through a small incision. J Cataract Refract Surg 1992;18:252-64.
129. Menapace R, Juchem M, Skorpik C et al. Clinicopathologic findings after in-the-bag implantation of open-loop polymethylmethacrylate and silicone lenses in the rabbit eye. J Cataract Refract Surg 1987;13:630-34.
130. Menapace R, Papapanos P, Radax U et al. Evaluation of 100 consecutive IOGEL 1003 foldable bag-style lenses implanted through a self-sealing tunnel incision. J Cataract Refract Surg 1994;20:432-39.
131. Menapace R, Skorpik C, Wedrich A. Evaluation of 150 consecutive cases of polyHEMA posterior chamber lenses implanted in the bag using a small-incision technique. J Cataract Refract Surg 1990;16:567-77.
132. Menapace R, Skorpik Ch, Juchem M et al. Evaluation of the first 60 cases of polyHEMA posterior chamber lenses

implanted in the sulcus. J Cataract Refract Surg 1989;15:264-71.
133. Menapace R, Yalon M. Exchange of IOGEL hydrogel one-piece foldable intraocular lens for bag-fixated J-loop poly (methyl methacrylate) intraocular lens. J Cataract Refract Surg 1993;19:425-30.
134. Menapace R. Posterior capsule opacification and capsulotomy rates with taco-style hydrogel intraocular lenses. J Cataract Refract Surg 1996;22:1318-30.
135. Milauskas AT. Capsular bag fixation of one-piece silicone lenses. J Cataract Refract Surg 1990;16:583-86.
136. Milauskas AT. In reply to: Watt RH. Discoloration of a silicone intraocular lens 6 weeks after surgery. Arch Ophthalmol 1991;109:1495.
137. Milauskas AT. Posterior capsule opacification after silicone lens implantation and its management. J Cataract Refract Surg 1987;13:644-48.
138. Milauskas AT. Silicone intraocular lens implant discoloration in humans. Arch Ophthalmol 1991;109:913-15.
139. Milazzo S, Sigot-Luizard MF, Borhan M et al. In vitro organotypic culture method to evaluate the biocompatibility of heparin-surface-modified intraocular lenses. J Cataract Refract Surg 1994;20:638-42.
140. Milazzo S, Turut P, Blin H. Alterations to the AcrySof intraocular lens during folding. J Cataract Refract Surg 1996;22: 1351-54.
141. Miller KM, Grusha YO, Ching ECP. Injecting the Alcon MA30BA lens through a STAAR 1-MTC-45 cartridge. J Cataract Refract Surg 1996;22:1132-33.
142. Mondino BJ, Nagata S, Glovsky MM. Activation of the alternative complement pathway by intraocular lenses. Invest Ophthalmol Vis Sci 1985;26:905-08.
143. Mondino BJ, Rajacich GM, Summer H. Comparison of complement activation by silicone intraocular lenses and polymethylmethacrylate intraocular lenses with polypropylene loops. Arch Ophthalmol 1987;105:989-90.
144. Neuhann T: Theorie and Operationstechnic der Kapsulorhexis. Klin Monatsbl Augenheilkd 1987;190: 542-45.
145. Neuhann TH. Intraocular folding of an carylic lens for explantation through a small incision cataract wound. J Cataract Refract Surg 1996;22:1383-86.
146. Neumann AC, Cobb B: Advantages and limitations of current soft intraocular lenses. J Cataract Refract Surg 1989;15: 257-63.
147. Neumann AC, McCarty GR, Osher RH. Complications associated with STAAR silicone implants. J Cataract Refract Surg 1987;13:653-56.
148. Neumann AC, McCarty GR, Sanders DR et al. Small incisions to control astigmatism during cataract surgery. J Cataract Refract Surg 1989;15:78-84.
149. Newland TJ, Auffarth GU, Wesendahl TA et al. Neodymium: YAG laser damage on silicone intraocular lenses. A comparison of lesions on explanted lenses and experimentally produced lesions. J Cataract Refract Surg 1994;20:527-33.
150. Newman DA, McIntyre DJ, Apple DJ et al. Pathologic findings of an explanted silicone intraocular lens. J Cataract Refract Surg 1986;12:292-97.
151. Ng EWM, Barrett GD, Bowman R. In vitro bacterial adherence to hydrogel and poly(methyl methacrylate) intraocular lenses. J Cataract Refrct Surg 1996;22:1331-35.
152. Nishi O, Nishi K: Intraocular lens encapsulation by shrinkage of the capsulorhexis opening. J Cataract Refract Surg 1993;19: 544-45.
153. Noble BA, Hayward JM, Huber C. Secondary evaluation of hydrogel lens implants. Eye 1990;4:450-55.
154. Obstbaum SA: Development of foldable IOL materials (editorial). J Cataract Refract Surg 1995;21:233.
155. Obstbaum SA. The Binkhorst Medal Lecture—Biologic relationship between poly (methyl methacrylate) intraocular lenses and uveal tissue. J Cataract Refract Surg 1992;18: 219-31.
156. Oh KT, Oh KT. Simplified insertion technique for the SI-26NB intraocular lens. J Cataract Refract Surg 1992;18:619-22.
157. Oh KT. Optimal folding axis for acrylic intraocular lenses. J Cataract Refract Surg 1996;22:667-70.
158. Okada K, Funahashi M, Iseki K et al. Comparing the cell population on different intraocular lens materials in one eye. J Cataract Refract Surg 1993;19:431-34.
159. Omar O, Eng CT, Chang A et al. Capsular bag distension with an acrylic intraocular lens. J Cataract Refract Surg 1996;22:1365-67.
160. Omar O, Mamalis N, Veiga J et al. Scanning electron microscopic characteristics of small-incision intraocular lenses. Ophthalmol 1996;103:1124-29.
161. Oshika T, Shiokawa Y. Effect of folding on the optical quality of soft acrylic intraocular lenses. J Cataract Refract Surg 1996l;22:1351-54.
162. Oshika T, Suzuki Y, Kizaki H et al. Two-year clinical study of a soft acrylic intraocular lens. J Cataract Refract Surg 1996;22:104-09.
163. Oshika T, Yoshimura K, Miyata N. Postsurgical inflammation after phacoemulsification and extracapsular extraction with soft or conventional intraocular lens implantation. J Cataract Refract Surg 1992;18:356-61.
164. Oshika T. Intraoperative complications of foldable IOL. 2. Soft acrylic IOL. Jpn J Clin Ophthalmol 1995;49:1614-15.
165. Packard R. European clinical results with the AcrySof IOL. Eur J Implant Refract Surg 1994;6:178-79.
166. Packard RBS, Garner A, Arnott EJ: Poly-HEMA as a material for intraocular lens implantation: a preliminary report. Br J Ophthalmol 1981;65:585-87.
167. Pekna M, Larsson R, Formgren B et al. Complement activation by polymethylmethacrylate minimized by end-point heparin attachment. Biomaterials 1993;14:189-92.
168. Percival P. Capsular bag implantation of the hydrogel lens. J Cataract Refract Surg 1987;13:627-29.
169. Percival P. Prospective study comparing hydrogel with PMMA lens implants. Ophthalmic Surg 1989;20:255-61.

170. Percival SPB, Jafree AJ. Preliminary results with a new hydrogel intraocular lens. Eye 1994;8:672-75.
171. Percival SPB, Pai V. Heparin-modified lenses for eyes at risk for breakdown of the blood-aqueous barrier during cataract surgery. J Cataract Refract Surg 1993;19:760-65.
172. Percival SPB. Five-year follow-up of a prospective study comparing hydrogel with PMMA single piece lenses. Eur J Implant Refract Surg 1994;6:10-13.
173. Pfister DR. Stress fractures after folding an acrylic intraocular lens. Am J Ophthalmol 1996;121:572-74.
174. Philipson B, Fagerholm P, Calel B et al. Heparin surface modified intraocular lenses. Three-month follow-up of a randomized, double-masked clinical trial. J Cataract Refract Surg 1992;18:71-78.
175. Portolés M, Refojo MF, Leong FL. Reduced bacterial adhesion to heparin-surface-modified intraocular lenses. J Cataract Refract Surg 1993;19:755-59.
176. Potzsch DK, Losch-Potzsch CM. Four-year follow-up of the MemoryLens. J Cataract Refract Surg 1996;22:1336-41.
177. Power WJ, Neylan D, Collum LMT. Adherence of human lens epithelial cells to conventional poly(methyl methacrylate), heparin-surface modified, and polyHema lenses. J Cataract Refract Surg 1994;20:440-45.
178. Ravalico G, Baccara F, Lovisato A et al. Postoperative cellular reaction on various intraocular lens materials. Ophthalmol 1997;104:1084-91.
179. Redbrake C, Salla S, Becker J et al. Immunological reactions against PMMA lens material? Graefe's Arch Clin Exp Ophthalmol 1993;231:238-41.
180. Reich S, Levy M, Meshorer A et al. Intraocular-lens-endothelial interface: adhesive force measurements. J Biomed Mater Res 1984;18:737-44.
181. Ridley H: Intraocular acrylic lenses. Trans Ophthalmol Soc UK 1951;71:617-21.
182. Saika S, Kobata S, Yamanaka O et al. Cellular fibronectin on intraocular lenses explanted from patients. Graefe's Arch Clin Exp Ophthalmol 1993;231:718-21.
183. Saika S, Tonoe O, Kanagawa R et al. Immunohisto-chemical study of deposits on intraocular lenses explanted from human eyes. Jpn J Ophthalmol 1991;35:96-101.
184. Saika S, Uenoyama S, Kanagawa R et al. Phagocytosis and fibronectin of cells observed on intraocular lenses. Jpn J Ophthalmol 1992;36:184-91.
185. Sanchez E, Artaria L: Evaluation of athe first 50 ACR360 acrylic intraocular lens implantations. J Cataract Refract Surg 1996;22:1373-78.
186. Schrage NF, Reim M, Burchard WC et al. Scanning electron microscopic and energy-dispersive X-ray analysis findings on two brand new intraocular lenses. Ophthalmic Res 1992;24:51-54.
187. Shan SM, Spalton DJ. Comparison of the postoperative inflammatory response in the normal eye with heparin-surface-modified and poly(methyl methacrylate) intraocular lenses. J Cataract Refract Surg 1995;21:579-85.
188. Shan SM, Spalton DJ. Natural history of cellular deposits on the anterior intraocular lens surface. J Cataract Refract Surg 1995;21:466-71.
189. Shephard JR. Induced astigmatism in small incision cataract surgery. J Cataract Refract Surg 1989;15:85-88.
190. Shepherd JR. Capsular opacification associated with silicone implants. J Cataract Refract Surg 1989;15:448-50.
191. Shepherd JR. Continous-tear capsulotomy and insertion of a silicone bag lens. J Cataract Refract Surg 1989;15: 335-39.
192. Shugar JK, Lewis C, Lee A. Implantation of multiple foldable acrylic posterior chamber lenses in the capsular bag for high hyperopia. J Cataract Refract Surg 1996;22:1368-72.
193. Shugar JK. Implantation of AcrySof acrylic intraocular lenses. J Cataract Refract Surg 1996;22:1355-59.
194. Skelnik DL, Lindstrom RL, Allarakhia L et al. Neodymium:YAG laser interaction with Alcon IOGEL intraocular lenses: an in vitro toxicity assay. J Cataract Refract Surg 1987;13:662-68.
195. Skorpik C, Menapace R, Gnad HD et al. Evaluation of 50 silicone posterior chamber lens implantations. J Cataract Refract Surg 1987;13:640-43.
196. Smetana K, Sulc J, Krcoca Z et al. Intraocular biocompati-bility of hydroxyethyl methacrylate and methacrylic acid copolymer partially hydrolyzed poly (2-hydroxyethyl methacrylate). J Biomed Mater Res 1987;21:1247-53.
197. Spangberg M, Kihlström I, Björklund H et al. Improved biocompatibility of intraocular lenses by heparin surface modification: a 12-month implantation study in monkeys. J Cataract Refract Surg 1990;16:170-77.
198. Steinert RF, Bayliss B, Brint SF et al. Long-term clinical results of AMO PhacoFlex model SI-18 intraocular lens implantation. J Cataract Refract Surg 1995;21:331-38.
199. Steinert RF, Brint SF, White SM et al. Astigmatism after small incision cataract surgery; a prospective, rando-mized, multicenter comparison of 4- and 6.5 mm incisions. Ophthalmol 1991;98:417-23.
200. Stoy V: Intraocular Lenses. US Patent No. 4,731,079. Kingston Technologies: Dayton 935224, 1988.
201. Tamada Y, Ikada Y. Fibroblast growth on polymer surfaces and biosynthesis of collagen. J Biomed Mater Res 1994;28:783-89.
202. Tamada Y, Ikada Y. Fibroblast growth on polymer surfaces and biosynthesis of collagen. J Biomed Mater Res 1994;28:783-89.
203. Tsai JC, Castaneda VE, Apple DJ et al. Scanning electron microscopic study of modern silicone intraocular lenses. J Cataract Refract Surg 1992;18:232-35.
204. Umezawa S, Shimizu K. Biocompatibility of surface-modified intraocular lenses. J Cataract Refract Surg 1993;19:371-74.
205. Uyama Y, Ikada Y. Electrostatic properties of UV-irradiated and surface-grafted polymers. J Appll Polym Sci 1990;41:619-29.

206. Versura P, Caramazza R. Ultrastructure of cells cultured onto various intraocular lens materials. J Cataract Refract Surg 1992;18:58-64.
207. Vrabec MP, Syverud JC, Burgess CJ. Forceps-induced scratching of a foldable acrylic intraocular lens (letter). Arch Ophthalmol 1996;114:777.
208. Wasserman D, Apple DJ, Castaneda VE et al. Anterior capsular tears and loop fixation of posterior chamber intraocular lenses. Ophthalmol 1991;98:425-31.
209. Watt RH. Discoloration of a silicone intraocular lens 6 weeks after surgery. Arch Ophthalmol 1991;109:1494.
210. Watts MT, Pearce JL: Implantation of a disc lens in the capsular bag. Ophthalmic Surg 1988;19:546-48.
211. Weghaupt H, Menapace R, Wedrich A. Functional vision with hydrogel versus PMMA lens implants. Graefe's Arch Clin Exp Ophthalmo 1993;231:449-52.
212. Werner LP, Legeais JM, Durand J et al. Endothelial damage produced by uncoated and fluorocarbon-coated polymethylmethacrylate intraocular lenses. J Cataract Refract Surg 1997;23:1013-19.
213. Werner LP, Legeais JM. Les matériaux pour implants intraoculaires. Partie I. Les implants intraoculaires en polyméthylmétacrylate et modifications de surface. J Fr Ophthalmol 1998;21:515-24.
214. Werner LP, Legeais JM. Les matériaux pour implants intraoculaires. Partie II. Les implants en silicone. J Fr Ophthalmol 1999;22:492-512.
215. Wolter JR. Cytopathology of intraocular lens implantation. Ophthalmol 1985;92:135-42.
216. Zeigler JM, Fearon FWG. Silicon-based polymer science. A comprehensive resource. American Chemical Society, Washington DC. 1990.
217. Zetterström C. Incidence of posterior capsule opacification in eyes with exfoliation syndrome and heparin-surface-modified intraocular lenses. J Cataract Refract Surg 1993;19:344-47.
218. Ziemba SL. In reply to: Milauskas AT. Silicone intraocular lens implant discoloration in humans. Arch Ophthalmol 1991;109:914-15.

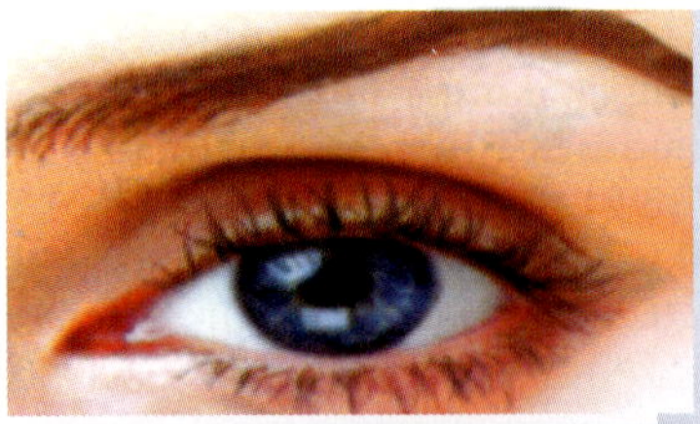

Twenty five

Blumenthal's Technique in MSICS: A 100% Approach

Nikhilesh Trivedi
(India)

INTRODUCTION

It was probably in 1990 that we were shown the videos of Blumenthal's technique. Many surgeons took an instant liking to the concept of 'Hydrodynamic' delivery of the nucleus. There has been no looking back since then. The band of followers of this particular technique has been steadily growing. As Manual Small Incision Cataract Surgery (MSICS) gains more popularity, several techniques have emerged, only to be tried and discarded later. Blumenthal's technique is among the few to have withstood the test of time. Perhaps because of it's tremendous 'replicability'. I mean that if the steps are followed correctly, there is no reason why every surgeon's results would not be comparable! There also is a wonderful flexibility to the whole technique. Each surgeon can adapt or modify steps to suit his "comfort zone". And adaptability with the times is a feature too. Initially doing it under peribulbar, Dr.Blumenthal himself is now performing this surgery under topical anesthesia plus a little superior subconjunctival lidocaine!

My personal experience has been very rewarding. The quality of surgery that I was able to obtain in ECCE after 10 years, I could achieve the same in 1 year with Blumenthal's technique!

PRINCIPLE

The principle underlying this technique is that BSS is the nearest physiologically to the natural aqueous humor, and it should be used under pressure to carry out all the surgical maneuvers in a close chamber Surgery. The judicious use of the Anterior Chamber Maintaining system, using the Anterior Chamber Maintainer (ACM) connected to a bottle of BSS elevated to the required height provides a comfortably formed AC for doing the procedure of Cataract Extraction and IOL Implantation. The nucleus delivery is BSS assisted, thereby removing the need to introduce any other instrument inside the eye. At no stage does the IOP rise beyond 40 mm of Hg., that too for brief periods of time. Use of Sheet's glide makes delivery of the nucleus smooth and effortless. Because of a deeply formed chamber at all times, viscoelastic materials are not needed.

ANTERIOR CHAMBER MAINTAINER (ACM)

This is a very versatile instrument comprising of a canula 2.5mm long, with 1mm external diameter and 0.6mm internal opening, with a beveled tip. It is slightly flattened, giving the lumen an oval shape. The tip is rounded, and not sharp, to prevent damage to the Descemet's membrane or the endothelium. It is attached to a bottle of BSS via silicon tubing and IV Set. The height of the bottle should be adjustable for different steps in the surgical protocol. In my personal opinion, this instrument is to MSICS what Simcoe's Canula is to ECCE. Except, perhaps that while Simcoe's Canula can be used only for cortical aspiration, the ACM plays a pivotal role in ALL steps of surgery. The advantages of the use of ACM in different maneuvers will be highlighted at each stage in the following account, and again at the end.

We will now proceed step by step through the surgery, mentioning alternatives wherever required.

SIDE PORTS AND ACM PORT

Always use an MVR blade for this. The 20G MVR will give you a side port able to comfortably take most of the instruments needed to be introduced inside, as well as an ACM port adequate for the 20 G ACM. Ensure that the blade is sharp, to avoid Descemet's detachment. The side ports can be one or two, at 9.30 o'clock, and at 2.30 o'clock. Their length should be roughly 1mm intra-stromal, to ensure self-sealing nature (Fig. 25.1). The ACM port should be at 6 o'clock, **directed horizontally** (from Temporal to Nasal). The intra-stromal length in this case should be 1.5-2mm, to accommodate the ACM and keep it stable during surgery (Fig. 25.2). The ACM is introduced **without flow with bevel up.** After it has entered the AC, the bevel is rotated down, and BSS flow is resumed (Fig. 25.3).

CAPSULOTOMY

In the interest of In-the-bag placement of IOL, a CCC should be the aim in every case. But the technique is NOT rhexis dependant. In all MSICS techniques, one should aim for a 6-6.5mm rhexis. Here, the BSS bottle should be raised to 70-75 mm to get as deep a chamber as possible, and as flat and relaxed an anterior capsule as possible. A standard 26G needle cystitome should be used, mounted on a BSS filled syringe. Optionally, this step may be undertaken with the ACM closed and AC filled with a viscoelastic material if that is more comfortable for the surgeon. I've found it much better to use the ACM. The advantages are as follows:

a. The Capsular flap moves a little with the turbulence in the AC thereby making it easier to identify.
b. Cortex, if disturbed by the cyst tome, stays in its place instead of floating free in the chamber.
c. In hypermature and mortgaging cataracts, the milky fluid is either expelled from the side port, or can be aspirated with the same syringe, the fluid in the AC being instantly replaced from the ACM, without causing turbidity. In case the rhexes runs out, one can easily convert to can-opener capsulotomy. The only problem, as I see it, may arise for those used to using forceps for CCC. Well, they will just have to learn to use a cystitome!! Once the capsulotomy is completed, removing the capsular fragments is very easy. Most often, the fragment presents itself at the side port as the cystitome is being withdrawn.

If not, a canula may be introduced to suck it out. Sometimes, a canula can also be used to "catch" the capsular flap and perform the rhexis after the initiation with a cystitome!

Scleral Incision

A fornix based Conjunctival flap is made, and underlying blood vessels cauterized with Bipolar Cautery.

The scleral incision is placed 1-2 mm behind the limbus. A horizontal 5.5 mm partial thickness groove is fashioned in a straight line. From the 2 ends of this, 2 cuts of 1-1.5 mm are made **radially,** i.e., directed towards the center of the cornea, but going away from the main incision into the sclera (Fig. 25.4). A carefully handled Razor blade fragment can be as good as an expensive pre-set knife. The groove should be about half thickness of the

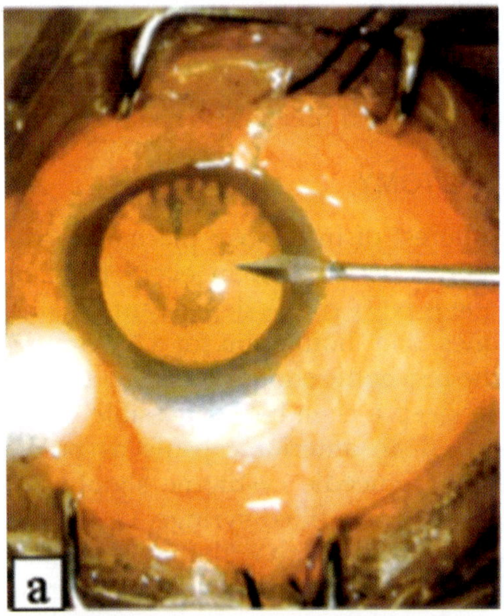

Fig. 25.1: side port making with MVR

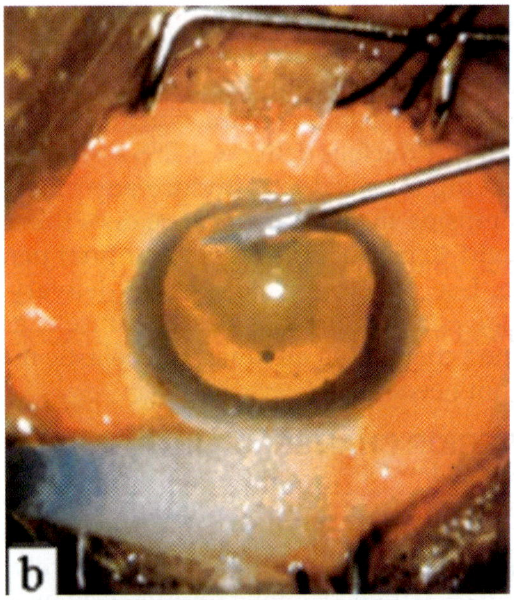

Fig. 25.2: ACM port making with MVR

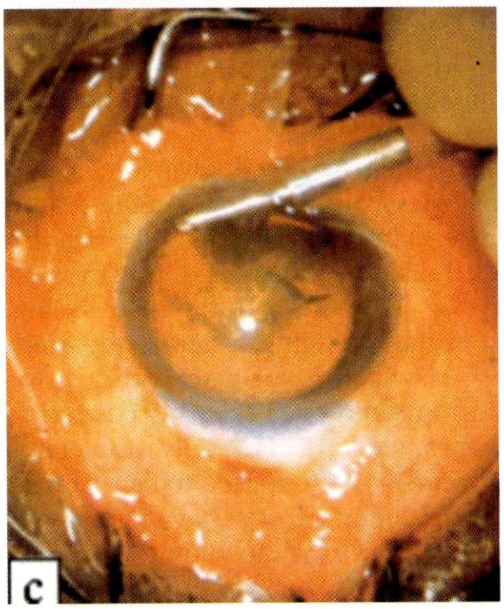

Fig. 25.3: ACM fitting

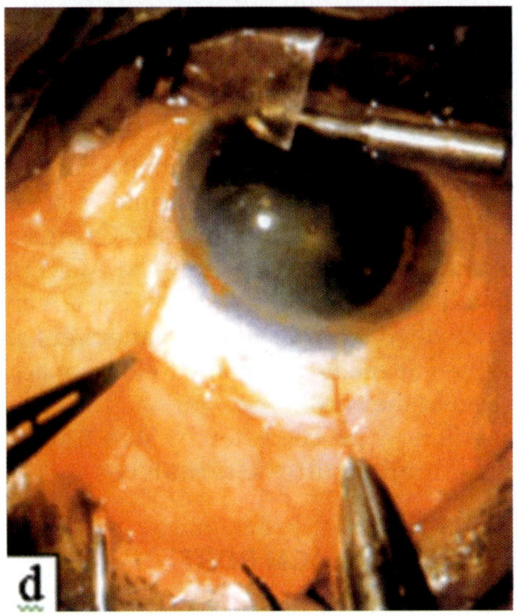

Fig. 25.4: Scleral incision

Sclera. In the unfortunate situation of accidentally going too deep, Uveal tissue will become visible, or may even bulge through. In that case, lower the bottle height or close the ACM, suture the wound, and try the same at a different location!

TUNNEL AND INTERNAL OPENING

Using a sharp Crescent blade, start the tunnel at any point along the horizontal incision (preferably at the center) and take it into clear cornea straight to about 2-2.5 mm, with a wriggling movement of the blade. Extend the tunnel on either side to include the side-cuts, by slightly angling the blade (Fig. 25.5). Ensure that the corneal end of the pocket is larger than the outer, scleral end, and the inner edge is almost parallel to the limbus, i.e., it is Crescent-shaped. This gives us a 'pocket' which is about 6mm by 4.5mm, with an internal end of about 7-8mm (Fig. 25.6). Make sure that the tunnel is uniplaner and adequate by once more sweeping the crescent blade through it. AVOID holding the Scleral lip of the tunnel with forceps at any stage!! You may hold the neighboring limbal conjunctiva or subconjunctival tissue with an atraumatic forceps to stabilize the eyeball during this maneuver. Use of a SHARP crescent every time will reduce the drag on the tissues, and give you a smooth tunnel and a lesser astigmatism!

The Anterior Chamber is now entered from the center of the internal edge of the tunnel using a sharp keratome angled downwards, pointing towards the center of the pupil. As soon as the tip of the keratome becomes visible in the AC, the blade is made parallel to the Iris plane, and the entry completed. This is now enlarged in either direction, using the same instrument, or switching to a blunt tip enlarging keratome. Remember to 'cut' only while entering, and not while withdrawing the instrument from the AC. If the keratome is angled to cut forward and sideways, you can fashion an internal opening which will be parallel to the limbus, instead of a straight line incision. Do not cut UPTO the limbus, but stop just short of it (Fig. 25.7). This ensures a 'true' self-sealing incision, as well as helps in reducing Post-op. Astigmatism. The presence of ACM gives you a turgid, 'normal' feeling eyeball, making it easy to do these steps. You may 'experience' the difference, by trying the Tunnel and Entry step in one case, with ACM off, and the eye filled with Visco-elastic material!!

It will be prudent to always bear in mind that this step, the designing of the Scleral Tunnel and the internal opening, will play a major role in giving

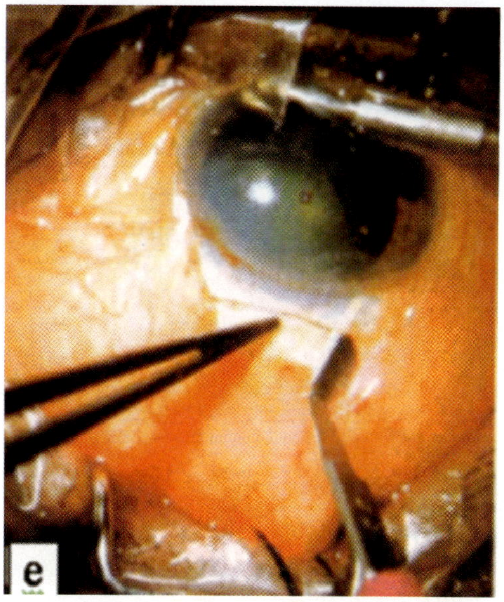

Fig. 25.5: Scleral tunnel

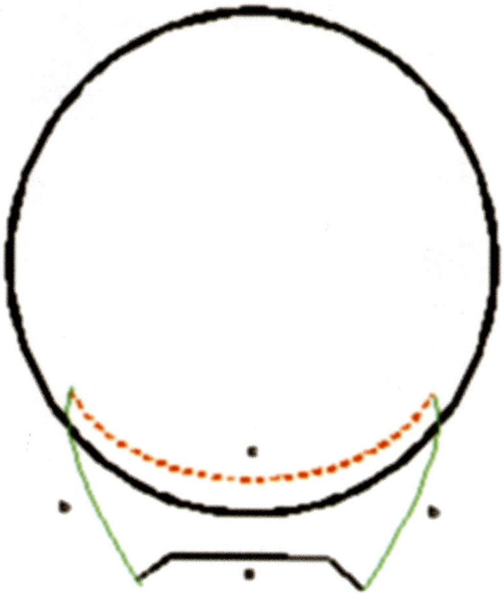

Fig. 25.6: Diagrammatic skethc of incision and tunnel. (a) scleral incision (b) side pockets; (c) internal corneal opening

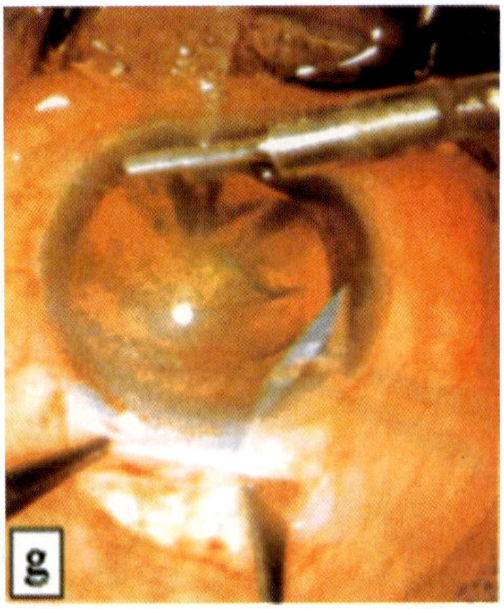

Fig. 25.7: Enlarging internal opening

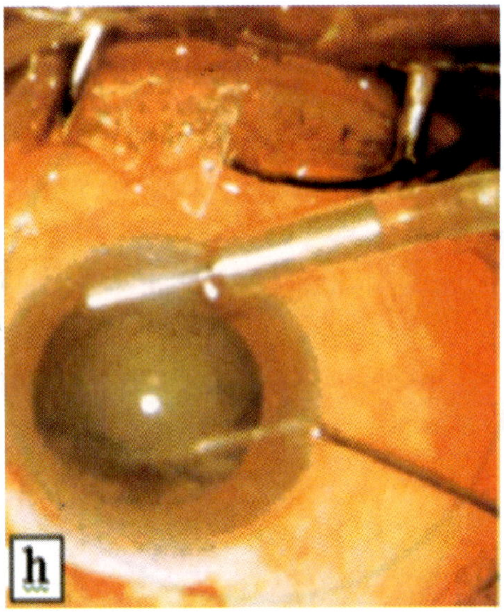

Fig. 25.8: Hydroprocedures and nucleus prolapse

you minimum Post-op. Astigmatism and a true self-sealing wound. Therefore, stick to using the best and sharpest blades, thereby ensuring sound sleep for you!!

HYDROPROCEDURES AND NUCLEUS PROLAPSE

This step is best undertaken at this stage. I used to do hydroprocedures soon after CCC. The benefit was that it gives us a fair idea of the size of the nucleus before we start making our incision, thereby allowing us to tailor our incision size according to the nucleus. But very enthusiastic hydro-dissection before opening the chamber has the risk of putting undue stress on the zonules, as well as on the posterior capsule. Also, in some cases, the nucleus immediately prolapses into the AC, increasing the risk of endothelial touch during Tunneling or wound enlargement. Hence, it is better to do this step at this stage. Also, it may be more prudent for the beginner to use a little Visco-elastic material (with the ACM closed) to coat the endothelium at this point, before starting hydroprocedures. The ACM may then be opened. A small quantity of BSS from a syringe with an appropriate canula is now injected between the rim of the anterior capsule and the cataract till a 'fluid wave' becomes visible. The canula is now relocated by withdrawing, and reinserting obliquely into the soft cortex, till resistance is felt in the form of hard core of the nucleus. Again injecting about 0.5ml of BSS will, hopefully, produce the 'Golden Ring', completing the separation between the hard-core nucleus and the epinucleus. Most often, with this, one edge of the nucleus 'pops-up' out of the capsular bag. This part of the equator of the lens is engaged gently with the tip of the canula, and 'cart wheeled', to loosen the remaining attachments of the nucleus, and to induce it to prolaps out of the capsular bag. More gentle irrigation beneath this edge may be of further help. The aim is not necessarily to completely bring the entire nucleus into the AC, but only to ensure that the nucleus is indeed 'free'. Also, to rotate the prolapsed pole of the nucleus to the 12 o'clock position (Fig. 25.8).

NUCLEUS EXPRESSION

The Sheet's Glide is a transparent plastic strip, about 3-4mm wide, 0.3mm thick, and about 3 cm long, with rounded and smoothened tip (Fig. 25.9). This is gently introduced in the eye through the tunnel, passing its tip under the up tilting pole of the nucleus, up to about 1/3rd of the way. The function of the glide is twofold. One is to guide the nucleus into the tunnel. The other is to provide a smooth surface for the 'gliding' nucleus!

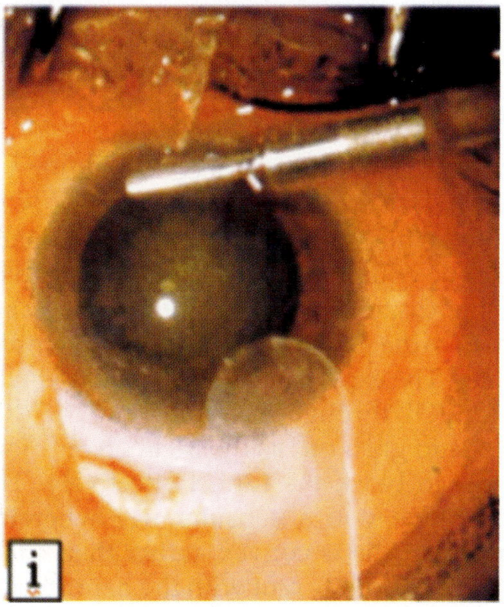

Fig. 25.9: Sheet's glide

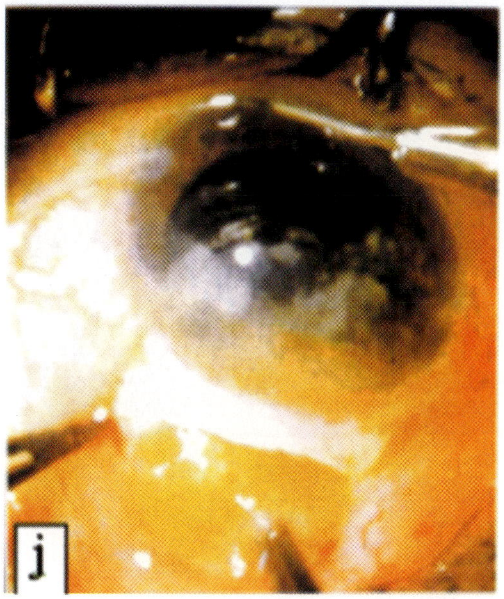

Fig. 25.10: Sheet's glide

Once the glide is in position, place the Mcpherson forceps tip just inside the tunnel, resting on the glide, and exert gentle pressure downwards. The nucleus will engage in the corneal end of the tunnel, thereby effectively blocking it, and reducing the outflow of BSS to almost nil. Further, continued pressure, will cause the nucleus to 'shave-off' epi-nucleus and mould itself into the tunnel till it is finally expelled in a gush of BSS (Fig. 25.10). If necessary, after the nucleus engages, one can raise the BSS bottle height again to 70cms., as had been done for CCC (presuming that it had been lowered after CCC), to raise the expulsion pressure being exerted on the nucleus. Most nuclei, irrespective of color, size, and hardness, can be removed this way!

(The experience is akin to the normal 'delivery' of a baby!!)

It is really very difficult to produce a PC rent with the glide unless one is very rough, or pushes the glide too far inside. One must aim at insinuating it just beneath the nucleus and advancing it a little. The direction of push should be towards the 6 O'clock position, and not downward.

In a few cases, the nucleus may engage in the tunnel, its pole may present itself at the Scleral end of the incision, but the body of the nucleus may get stuck at the corneal end of the tunnel. In such cases, the nucleus can be engaged with the Cystitome, or the Sinsky hook, and gently dialed out. Either the whole nucleus will get dialed out, or a Pie-shaped piece will break from it. In that case, one can rerotate the nucleus so that the now reduced diameter engages and the nucleus is expelled. A little 'tapping' at the scleral incision at this stage will expel the remaining free epinucleus, part of which may have got stuck in the tunnel itself.

CORTICAL CLEANUP

This part is the most enjoyable in this technique! Because of the ACM, the irrigation aspect is automatically taken care of, and a deep, closed chamber ensures easy accessibility of cortical remnants. I prefer using a J-shaped, round tipped, top opening 23G canula attached to a disposable 5cc syringe for this job. It is introduced through one side port and cortex is sucked, drawn free, and aspirated by gentle movements and changes in aspiration pressure. Because of the ACM, the chamber remains constantly deepened, and even the equatorial cortex becomes easy to hold (Fig. 25.11). If the freed cortex chunks appear difficult to aspirate, just release them in the AC. One tap at the outer lip of the incision will expel them in a second!

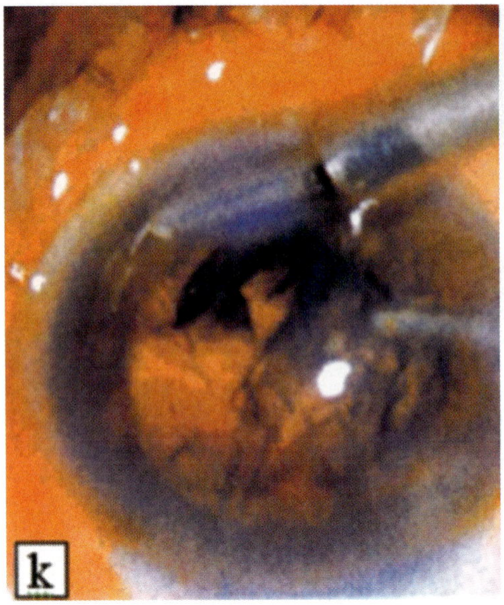

Fig. 25.11: Sheet's glide

This is the magic of ACM. One should not try to bring them out through the side port, as they're sure to get stuck there, and you'll be busy removing these from the second side port!

The two side ports together provide a complete 360-degree reach for Cortex Extraction. One can use a sand blasted tip to polish the under-edge of the anterior capsule. Alternatively, just aspirating with the regular canula can also help denuding the remaining epithelial cells from the anterior capsule.

There are wonderful alternatives for polishing the posterior capsule in this technique. Attaching a J-shaped, round tipped, bottom opening canula to a Glass Syringe without the plunger, one gently moves it over the posterior capsule. The positive pressure in the AC created by the ACM combines with the negative pressure in the Glass Syringe (because of the absence of the plunger) to produce a 0-degree suction at the tip of the canula. This bottom opening of the tip, when it is gently moved over the posterior capsule, sucks up whatever debris may be remaining there! Alternatively, one can employ the technique of 'Water-jetting', wherein gentle puffs of water from a 26G canula are directed at different parts of the posterior capsule to effectively dissect out the adhering remnants, sometimes even plaques! Small leakages of BSS from the side port engaging the 26G canula prevent the pressure from rising to dangerous levels.

IOL INSERTION

The step now being described is specific to the Blumenthal's Technique where the lens is being implanted without the use of visco-elastic material, but may be equally beneficial in other modalities too. I like to describe this as "Pull and Dial", in contrast to the "Push and Dial" step employed generally. The explanation being that as you try to 'push' an IOL through the tunnel into the AC, the BSS tends to gush out as the McPherson's forceps is unable to block the tunnel effectively. This is likely to give you a capsular bag wherein the Posterior capsule is convex, rather than concave. The likelihood of PC rent with the haptic becomes very high!

To prevent this, I insert the inferior haptic followed by the body of the optic into the tunnel, holding it with the forceps. At this point, the haptic and the lower dialing hole on the optic are visible in the chamber. I now release the optic, only using a plane forceps in the left hand to hold the superior haptic, preventing it from altering the angle of the IOL. With the right hand, I enter from the side port with a Sinsky hook and engage the lower dialing hole on the optic which is lying within the AC (Fig. 25.12). This is now dragged down and towards 6 o'clock position till the lower haptic and lower part of the optic is safely in the capsular bag. As the optic gently slides in, the tunnel keeps closing over it, thereby preventing any shallowing of the AC. The upper dialing hole is now engaged with the same hook, and the upper haptic is dialed into the bag (Fig. 25.13).

CLOSING UP

There isn't much left to do in this! The wound is checked for leaks, i.e., the chamber of the IV set is viewed while gently pressing on the eye, near the 9 o'clock or 3 o'clock limbus. If there is excessive outflow of BSS, it suggests a leaking wound. The tunnel is checked for residual debris which may be the cause. Removing the ACM now will produce a slight shallowing of the anterior chamber and

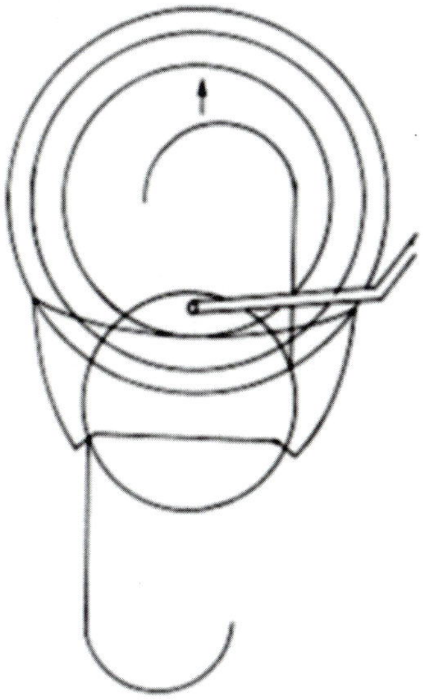

Fig. 25.12: Implantation technique engaging lower dialing hole

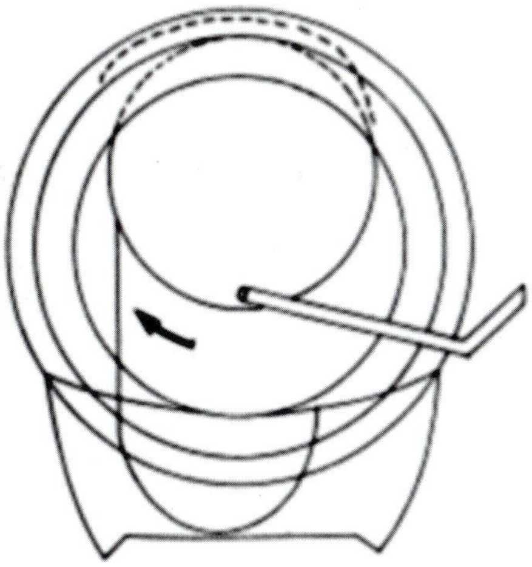

Fig. 25.13: Implantation technique drawing the lens downwards from upper hole

narrowing of the pupil (Fig. 25.14). If felt necessary, the chamber may be deepened by injecting some BSS from a side port. The side ports and the ACM port may be sealed tighter with Stromal hydration if needed (more so for the surgeon's sound sleep!). The slight corneal haze that appears as a result is of no risk, and would vanish by the next morning.

The conjunctiva may be apposed with Bipolar Cautery, or simply drawn down over the wound and left there.

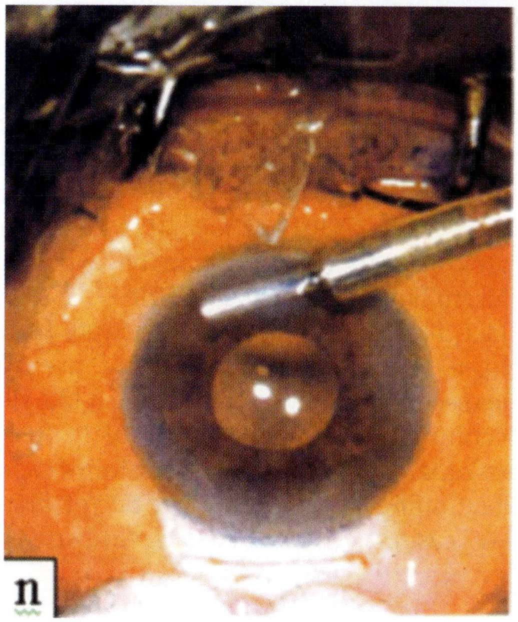

Fig. 25.14: Checking for leaks

ADVANTAGES OF THE TECHNIQUE

The advantages of the Blumenthal's technique are the same as those of using an Anterior Chamber Maintainer. I'd like to list them out systematically here:

1. The use of BSS exclusively maintains the normalcy of the AC to a larger extent throughout the surgery, thereby decreasing the release of Prostaglandins and such, which is evident in the lower inflammatory reaction in the Anterior Chamber the next day. The reduction in the Chamber depth fluctuation and turbulence are also contributory factors.
2. During all steps, as mentioned earlier with each step, the presence of the ACM eases the maneuvers, particularly for one converting from ECCE to MSICS.
3. In cases of PC rent, the ACM pressure prevents a break in the vitreous face, allowing you to convert the rent into a posterior capsulorrhexis. If Vitreous face does break, it is still prevented from prolapsing much into the AC. If anterior vitrectomy is needed, the ACM provides the irrigation, leaving one hand of the surgeon free to hold another instrument, like the light-pipe.
4. Playing with the height of the BSS bottle, you

can control the pressure in the eye, making this technique a truly 'Controlled' surgery. For example, you can raise the height to 70 cms for CCC and nucleus expulsion, lowering it to about 45-50 cms for the other steps. It can be lowered even further, to 20 cms or so, in case of a break in the Anterior Vitreous face. It is known as to approximately what IOP can be expected at different heights of the BSS bottle.

In fact, for most of us who've adapted to this technique whole-heartedly, fitting the ACM becomes second nature, reflexly doing it like fitting the speculum before starting surgery!!

From repairs, to repolishing of posterior capsule, to repositioning of an errant haptic (of another surgeon's case), we find the ACM an indispensable tool. It acts as a third hand for the surgeon, justifying the extra few seconds spent in fitting it, as well as creating an extra opening in the eye.

(Illustrations/photographs Courtesy Indian Journal of Ophthalmology and Jaypee)

REFERENCES

1. Thomas R, Kuriakose T, George R. Efficient Small Incision Cataract Surgery, Indian Journal of Ophthalmology. 2000;48:145-51.
2. Blumenthal M, Askenazi I, Fogel R, et al. The Gliding Nucleus, J Cataract Refract Surg 1993;19:435-37.
3. Blumenthal M: Surgical principles and techniques for Small Incision ECCE, Mini Highlights of Ophthalmology 1993.;21:5(1-8).
4. Trivedi N: The techniques of IOL Implantation in SICS, Small Incision Cataract Surgery 155-157,(K.Singh; Jaypee)

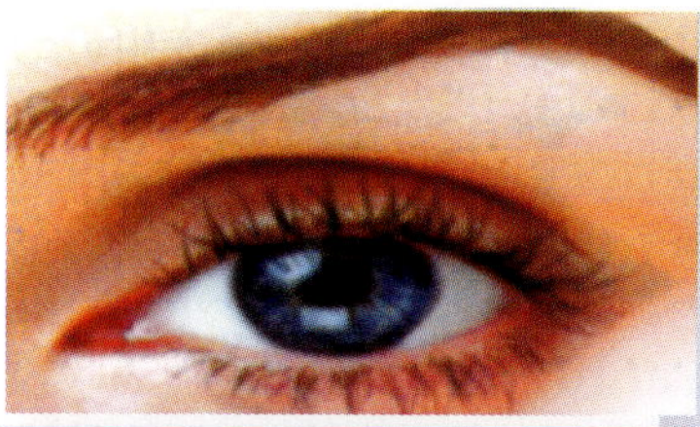

Twenty six

Phacofracture Technique in SICS

Kamaljeet Singh
(India)

ANESTHESIA
INCISION
CAPSULORHEXIS
HYDROPROCEDURE
NUCLEAR LUXATION
NUCLEUS DELIVERY
COMPLICATION

In the last two decades the cataract surgery has seen tremendous advancements. With the advent of phacoemulsification, Kelman predicted that incisions 3 mm wide be astigmatism-neutral because of their reduced size. However, within a very short time after the introduction of phacoemulsification, intraocular lens (IOL) implants became more common. This necessitated enlargement of the phacoemulsification incision to 6.5 to 7 mm for lens implantation.

Kratz is generally credited as the first surgeon to move from the limbus posteriorly to the sclera, increasing appositional surfaces to enhance wound healing and attempt to exert less traction on the cornea, thereby controlling surgically induced astigmatism. Girard and Hoffman were the first to call the posterior incision a 'scleral tunnel incision' and were perhaps the first to make a point of actually entering the anterior chamber from a slightly corneal location.

The 7.5 mm incision continued for long till foldable lenses became available. Before that the 3 mm incision was increase to 5.5 mm in order to implant a nonfoldable IOL of 5.5 mm optics.

There are various techniques of manual phaco like phacosandwich, Blumenthal's technique, microvectis technique and fishhook technique, in which the nucleus is removed as a whole. Although surgeons claim that they can remove the nucleus through a 5.5 mm incision, but Indian cataracts are hard and their nucleus is large, which necessitates the enlargement of incision to 6.5 mm to 7.0 mm to prevent the damage to corneal endothelium during delivery of nucleus. Decrease in the size of wound can be achieved by reduction of the nuclear volume within the anterior chamber by fracturing nucleus in smaller pieces or fragments. Kansas introduced the technique of phacofracture using his vectis and trisector. The technique involves breaking the nucleus into smaller pieces in anterior chamber by two instruments and then viscoexpressing them.

My method combines elements of phacosandwich as made popular by Luther fry and the phacosection as practiced by Peter Kansas.

ANESTHESIA

Peribulbar anesthesia is used.

INCISION

The aim is achieving a 6mm-selfsealing-corneoscleral wound. I use a crescent, 3.2 mm keratome and 5.5 mm extending keratome. A half thickness depth incision is fashioned with a razor fragment 6 mm in length and 1.5 mm behind the limbus. Crescent is then moved in this half depth thickness in the sclera towards the cornea. Once we reach the cornea the direction of the movement is changed slightly anteriorly taking care of the contour of the cornea. It goes about 1.5 mm in the cornea. Then a sweeping movement is made in the cornea laterally. The crescent is then withdrawn. Now the 3.2 mm keratome goes in the same plain. Once it reaches the desired point, the keratome is pushed towards the chamber. At this point of time a dimple is seen at the tip of keratome. Now, gently keratome is forced into the anterior chamber taking care that it does not hit the lens.

CAPSULORHEXIS

Air bubble is injected into the anterior chamber. About 0.2 cc of trypan blue is injected beneath the bubble to stain the anterior capsule. The anterior chamber is first washed with BSS and then viscoelastic is injected at 6 O'clock so that the air bubble goes out of the chamber. A large capsulorhexis is then fashioned. In case it is small, two relaxing cuts are made at its margin at 10 and 2 O'clock.

HYDROPROCEDURE

It is performed to separate the nucleus from its capsular attachments. The anterior capsule is elevated with a 26-G cannula attached to a 2 ml syringe filled with BSS and the fluid is injected slowly and continuously beneath the edge of capsulorhexis to create a fluid wave that passes across the red reflex. The fluid wave is not visible in dense cataracts. In such cases, when hydrodissection is completed, the nucleus appears to move forward following which it must rotate freely inside the capsular bag.

NUCLEAR LUXATION

If the capsulorhexis is 6 mm, the nucleus can be easily luxated into the anterior chamber by injecting the BSS by hydrodissection cannula at 9 O' clock and at the same time slight pressure is applied to lift the nucleus and shift the nucleus towards 3 O' clock. This brings the nucleus out of the rhexis margin. Thereafter little rotatory movement will bring part of the nucleus in anterior chamber. This movement is performed by visco cannula. The viscoelastic is injected between the visible edge of the nucleus and posterior capsule. That helps in further lifting the nucleus. Now the nucleus is rotated clockwise and anti-clockwise. This breaks any attachment with capsule. Then nucleus is rotated in one direction to bring the nucleus out of the bag. If it does not come out of the bag, then more viscoelastic is injected on top of iris with pressure backwards with cannula on iris. Once the margin of nucleus is visible all-round, more viscoelastic is injected behind the nucleus and also on the top of nucleus. These steps helps in pushing the posterior capsule behind and protecting the corneal endothelium. Now lens is ready for fracture and delivery.

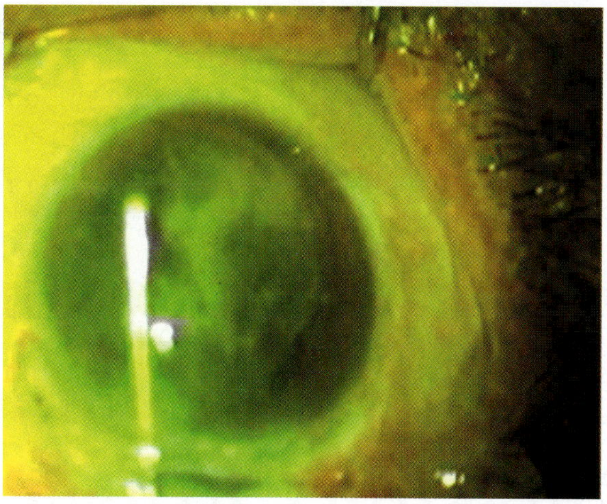

Fig. 26.1: Lens sandwiched between the two instruments

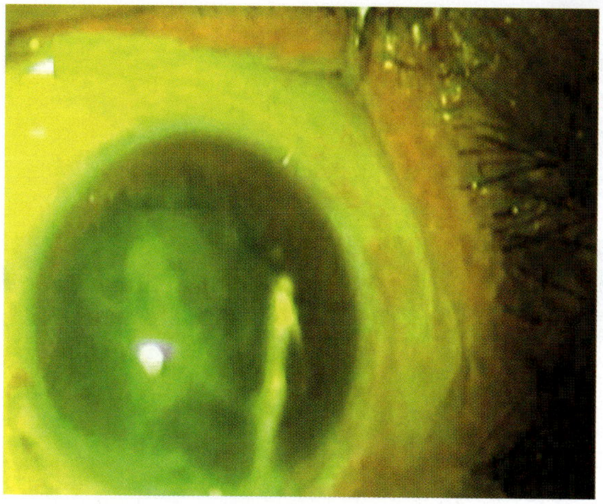

Fig. 26.2: Long axis of the nucleus fragment in verticle meridian

NUCLEUS DELIVERY

I perform the maneuver with the help of an irrigating vectis and Sinskey. My first instrument that enters into anterior chamber is Sinskey. It is kept on the anterior surface of lens. Then irrigating vectis is passed beneath the nucleus. At this point I ensure that the hold of nucleus between the two instruments is strong. With the lens held nicely sandwiched between two instruments (Fig. 26.1). I try to deliver the nucleus out. It usually breaks close to the wound. The upper broken fragment comes out sandwiched between two instruments. Remaining lower part of the nucleus is then pushed back. Its long axis is horizontally placed. This fragment is then moved in such a way that it's long axis becomes vertical (Fig. 26.2). Now, the visco cannula is taken towards 6 O'clock and viscoelastic is injected. At the same time the cannula is slightly pushed backwards on the sclera at the entry site. This will open the wound a little and positive pressure created by the viscoelastic with in the anterior chamber will force the fragment of the nucleus out of the anterior chamber. This maneuver is called viscoexpression. The remaining debris is epinucleus, small pieces of nucleus and cortical matter. Epinucleus and small fragments of nucleus are delivered out of the chamber by viscoexpression. Cortical matter is then aspirated out with two way Simcoe cannula. Once the posterior capsule is clean and free of any debris or cortical fiber the IOL is implanted in the usual fashion.

COMPLICATIONS

Most of the complications are similar as described in the phacosandwich technique. The only difference is in the chances of injury to the corneal endothelium, which may be a little more in this technique of fracturing the nucleus and then taking them out than in the phacosandwich technique, where nucleus comes out in one go.

REFERENCES

1. Blumenthal M, Ashkenazi I, Fogel R, Assia EI. The gliding nucleus. J Cataract Refract Surg 1993;19:435-37.
2. Fry LL. The phacosandwich technique. In: Rozakis GW, Ed, Cataract Surgery; Alternative Small-Incision Techniques. Thorofare, NJ, Slack, 1990;91-110.
3. Kansas PG, Sax R. Small incision cataract extraction and implantation surgery using a manual phacofragmentation technique. J Cataract Refract Surg 1988;14:328-30.
4. Vajpayee RB, Sabharwal S, Sharma N, Angra SK. Phacofracture versus phacoemulsification in eyes with agerelated cataract. J Cataract Refract Surg 1998;24:1252-55
5. Sinha R, Bhartiya P, Vajpayee RB. Manual Phacofracture in Small Incision Cataract Surgery (Manual Phaco) Kamaljeet Singh (Ed) New Delhi, Jaypee Brothers.
6. Singh Kamaljeet The Phacosandwich technique in Small Incision Cataract Surgery (Manual Phaco) Kamaljeet Singh (Ed) New Delhi, Jaypee Brothers.

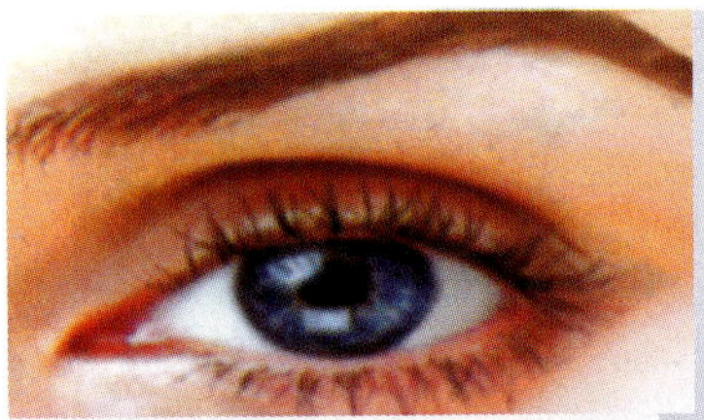

Twenty seven

Manual Multiphacofragmentation (MPF) Allows for Small Incision Cataract Surgery

Francisco J Gutiérrez-Carmona (Spain)

INTRODUCTION

Current surgical techniques used in cataract surgery have two fundamental objectives: (i) to induce the minimum postoperative astigmatism, and (ii) to achieve rapid recuperation of the patient's sight after surgery.

To meet these objectives, it is necessary to perform cataract surgery using a small incision. It has been shown that the smaller the surgical incision, the smaller the residual postoperative astigmatism.

Of all the techniques described for cataract operations, phacoemulsification is the one that allows working with smaller incisions. However, it is a technique which requires a long learning curve, with expensive and complicated instrumentation and equipment.

Our manual multiphacofragmentation (MPF) technique allows cataract surgery through 3.2 mm clear corneal or 3.5 mm scleral tunnel incisions. In this method the nucleus is fragmented into multiple tiny pieces of 2 × 2 mm.

The method enables cataract surgery in soft and hard nuclei. The results obtained in postoperative astigmatism are similar to those obtained with phacoemulsification, but with a shorter learning curve and less financial outlay.

On the other hand, our method is an ideal back-up after discontinuation of emulsification when complications arise in phacosurgery, since with the help of our instrument set, we can conclude the surgery without enlarging the incision.

We designed an instrument set, manufactured by John Weiss and Son Ltd in England, which consist of

- A racquet-shaped nucleotome 8 mm long and 2 mm wide, divided along its short axis by 3 thin transverse bars 2 mm apart, set at 45 degrees to a long straight handle (Fig. 27.1)
- A spatula 8 mm long by 2 mm wide the same shape as the nucleotome, used as a support during the fragmentation (Fig. 27.2)
- Two straight handled manipulators, right and left, used to collect the nuclear fragments (Fig. 27.3).

SURGICALTECHNIQUE

Surgical technique can be carried out with the use of retrobulbar or peribulbar anesthesia, topical or topical + intracameral anesthesia.

To perform MPF it is important to have good pharmacological mydriasis, since the pupil could contract during surgery.

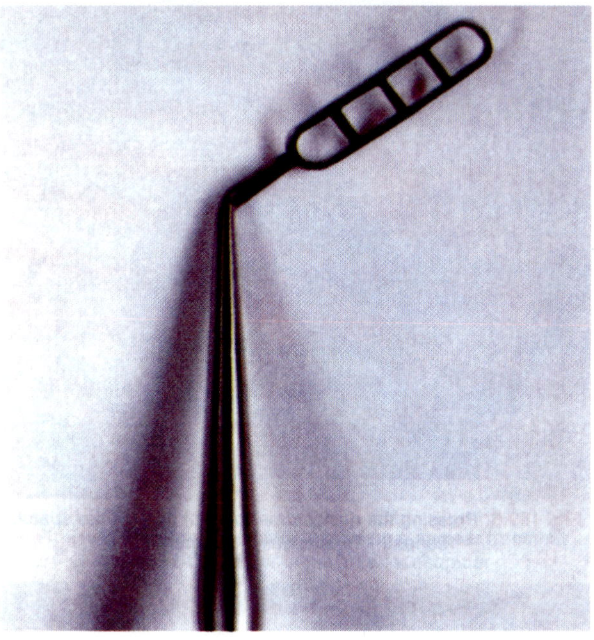

Fig. 27.1: Nucleotome with a racquet-shaped end

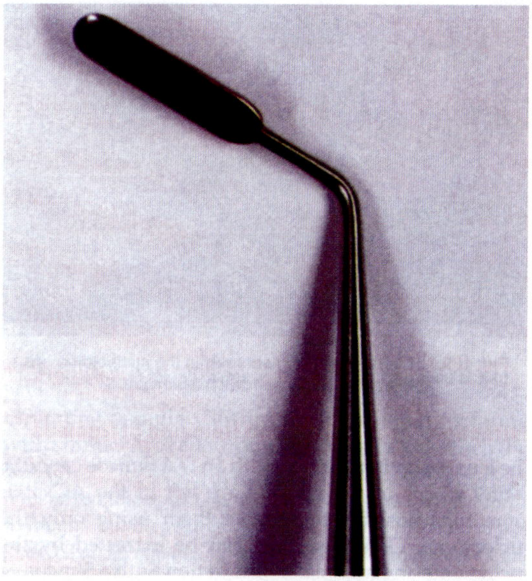

Fig. 27.2: Spatula with an end the same size as the nucleotome

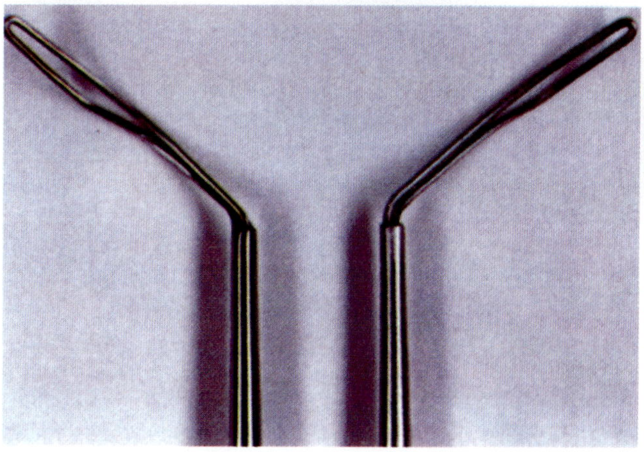

Fig. 27.3: Manipulators, right and left

Anterior Capsulotomy

High density viscoelastic is injected into the anterior chamber (AC) through a superior and temporal paracentesis, and a capsulorhexis is performed with a cystotome. It should be sufficiently wide (6.0-6.5 mm) to allow an easy luxation of the nucleus into the AC.

Incision

The surgery can be performed with a 3.2 mm clear corneal (Fig. 27.4), or 3.5 mm scleral-tunnel incision (Fig. 27.5).

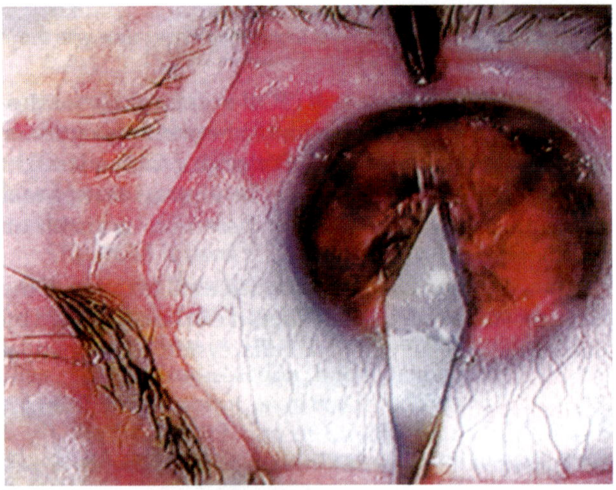

Fig. 27.4: The 3.2 mm clear corneal incision is performed at 12 O'clock

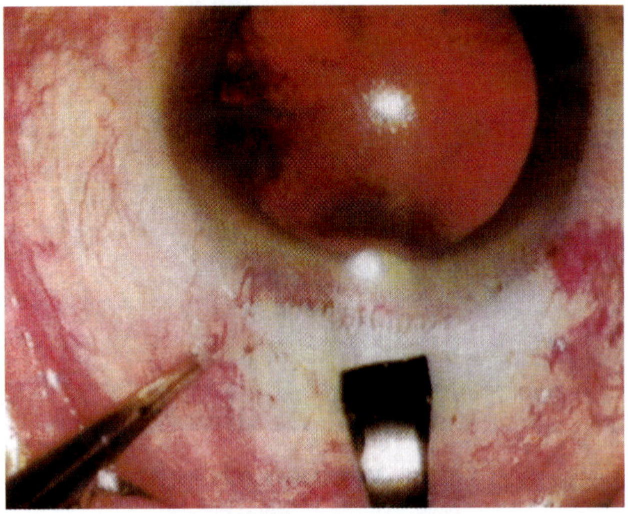

Fig. 27.5: The 3.5 mm scleral tunnel incision is made with the help of a angled crescent knife

The clear corneal incision is performed at 12 O'clock with a 45° stab incision knife and with the help of a disposable angled crescent knife. The scleral-tunnel incision is made after carrying out a fornix-based conjunctival miniflap about 2 mm posterior to the corneal-scleral limbus with the help of a disposable angled crescent knife, without penetrating the AC.

Hydrodissection and Luxation of the Nucleus

After entering the AC with a 3.2 mm phaco knife, balanced salt solution (BSS) is injected through the incision with a Binkhorst cannula between the anterior capsule and the cortex at 12 O'clock, or with a straight Rycroft cannula. The BSS must be injected slowly and continuously until the "wave of dissection" is visible on the posterior capsule.

The injection of BSS is continued until luxation of the nucleus in the AC is partial. Then, it can be completed by rotating the nucleus with a cannula, cystotome or spatula.

Nuclear Fragmentation

Once the nucleus has been luxated into the AC, high-density viscoelastic (Viscoat, Amvisc Plus, etc.) is injected into the surrounding area to fill the AC. The nucleus is then fragmented by placing the spatula beneath and the nucleotome on top of the nucleus (Figs 27.6a and b). Pressure is then created

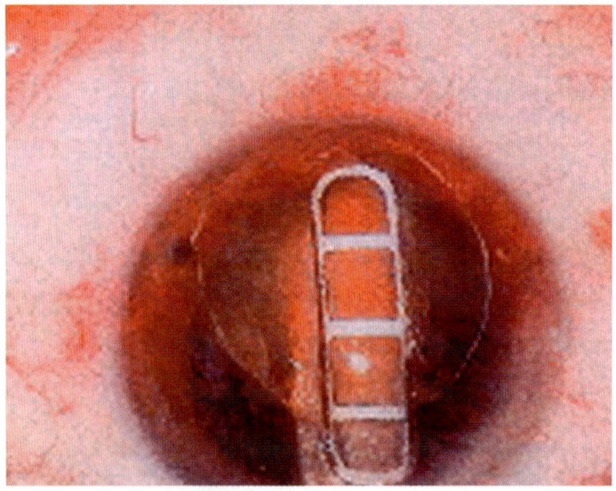

Fig. 27.6a: Pressing the nucleotome (on top) against the spatula.

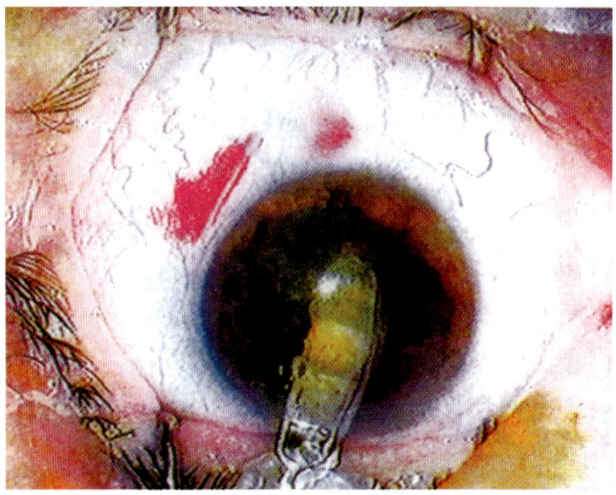

Fig. 27.6b: Pressing the nucleotome (on top) against the spatula (beneath) the nucleus is fragmented

Section 2

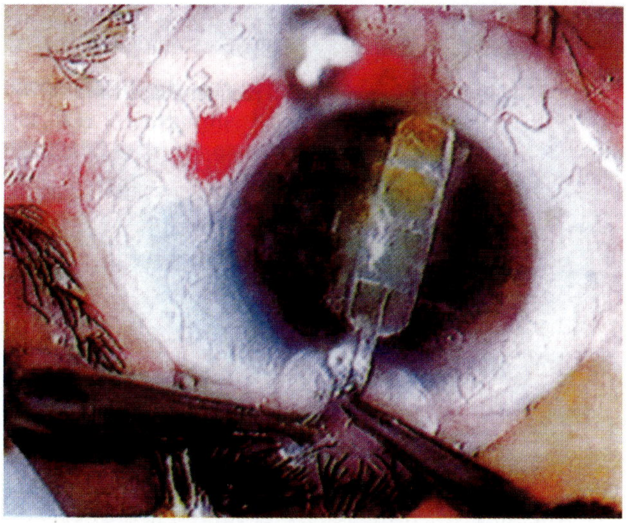

Fig. 27.7: The nuclear fragments within the nucleotome are extracted with a sandwich technique

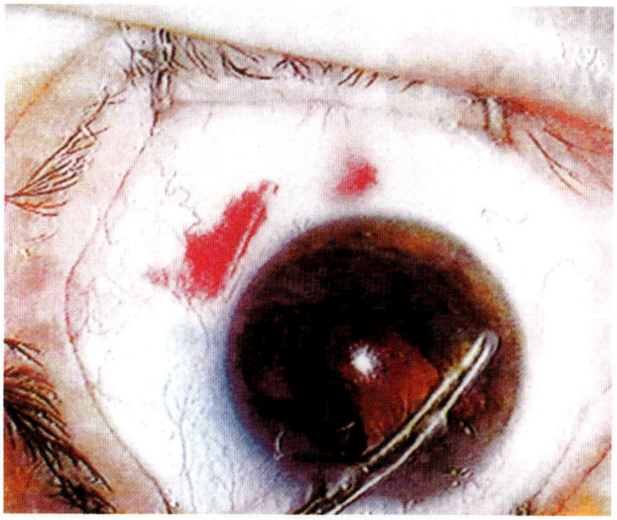

Fig. 27.8: Right manipulator displacing a nuclear fragment toward the center of the anterior chamber

by slowly pressing the nucleotome against the spatula, until this section of the nucleus is fragmented into four pieces which remain within the nucleotome, and which, with the help of the spatula, are extracted from the AC with a "sandwich" technique (Fig. 27.7). This maneuver is repeated until all the nucleus is fragmented.

During nuclear fragmentation, it is important to fill the AC with high-density viscoelastic, as needed, to protect the corneal endothelium and to facilitate safe manipulation during surgery.

Manipulation of Nuclear Fragments

The right and left manipulators are used to displace the remaining fragments of the nucleus to the center of the AC for further fragmentation and extraction (Fig. 27.8).

Extraction of the Cortex and Remains of Nucleus

The lens cortex is aspirated with an I/A Simcoe cannula. If tiny pieces of the nucleus are left in the AC, it is sometimes possible to remove them using only the nucleotome. Otherwise they can be extracted by the nucleotome and spatula, by aspiration with a Simcoe or Charleux cannula, or by gentle irrigation of the AC with BSS using a Rycroft cannula while simultaneously depressing the posterior lip of the incision.

IOL Implantation and Wound Closure

High-density viscoelastic is injected into the capsular bag and a foldable IOL is implanted (Fig. 27.9). The viscoelastic material is then aspirated with an irrigating/aspirating cannula. Closure of the incision is performed with stromal hydration, or with a single cross-stitch (Fig. 27.10).

We recommend to ophthalmologists who are new to this technique that they initially practise it using incisions of more than 3.2 or 3.5 mm and thereafter

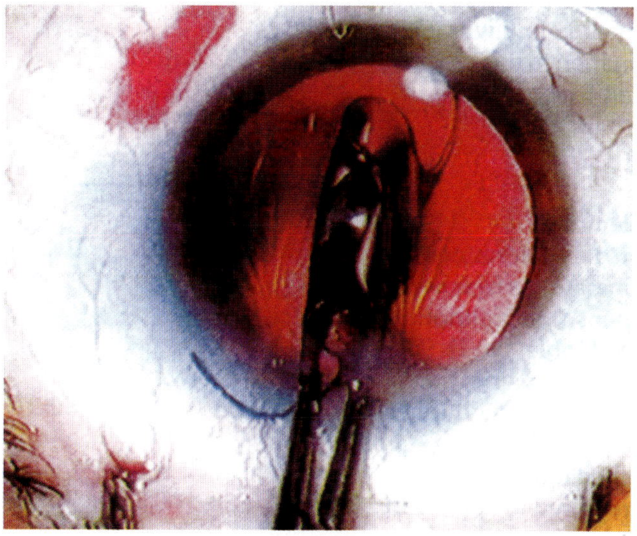

Fig. 27.9: A foldable lens is implanted in the capsular bag

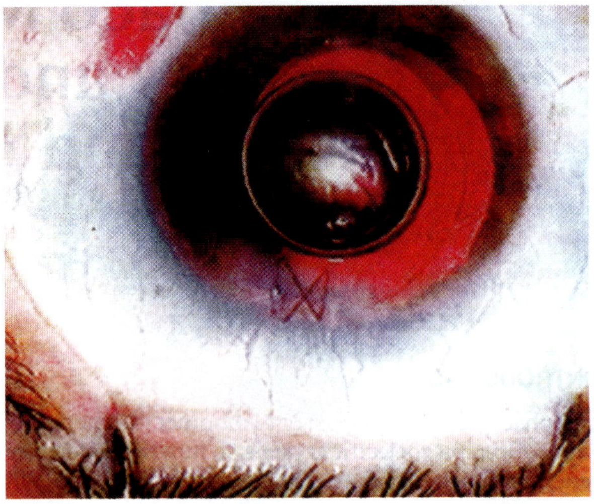

Fig. 27.10: A single cross-stitch is enough to close the wound

reduce the incision size once they have mastered the technique.

Lately I have been performing some steps of my technique with the help of an anterior chamber maintainer (ACM): model Lewicky 20 G from Katena or the ACM 20 G from John Weiss Ref. 0185061.

The ACM works by producing a constant irrigation flow of BSS into the AC. This flow generates a positive intraocular pressure (IOP) that stabilizes the AC depth during some steps of the surgery. On the other hand, with the ACM the quantity of viscoelastic material used persurgery is reduced, diminishing the financial outlay.

The ACM is used

- During the capsulorhexis
- In order to aspirate the anterior cortex and epinucleus in soft and medium hard nuclei before the hydrodissection / hydrodelineation
- For the aspiration of cortical debris
- For the extraction of tiny nuclear fragments, by depressing the posterior incision lip with a straight cannula.

The maneuvers of nuclear multifragmentation and IOL implantation are carried out with the help of high density viscoelastic material.

REFERENCES

1. Uusitalo RJ, Ruusuvaara P, Jarvinen E et al: Early rehabilitation after small incision cataract surgery. Refract Corneal Surg. 1993;9:67-70.
2. Shepherd JR: Induced astigmatism in small incision cataract surgery. J Cataract Refract Surg 1989;15:85-88.
3. Cristobal JA, Minguez E, Ascaso J et al: Size of incision and induced astigmatism in cataract surgery. J Fr Ophthalmol. 1993;16:311-14.
4. Gutiérrez-Carmona FJ: Manual technique allows for small incision cataract surgery. Ocular Surgery News: Surgical Maneuvers. 1997;15(21):14-15.
5. Gutiérrez-Carmona FJ: Manual technique allows for small incision cataract surgery. Ocular Surgery News (International Edition): Surgical Maneuvers. 1998;9(2):10-11.
6. Gutiérrez-Carmona FJ: Nueva técnica e instrumental de facofragmentación manual para incisiones esclerales tunelizadas de 3.5 mm. Arch Soc Esp Oftalmol. 1999; 74:181-86.

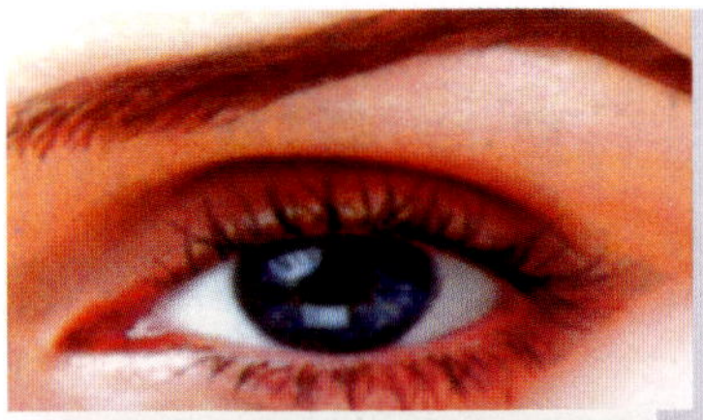

Twenty eight

Closed Chamber Manual Phacofragmentation

Jagannath Boramani
(India)

MANUAL PHACOFRAGMENTATION
ANTERIOR CHAMBER MAINTAINER
CLOSED CHAMBER MANUAL PHACOFRAGMENTATION
BLUMENTHAL'S MINI NUC TECHNIQUE

To say that cataract surgery has advanced expansively during the last decade would be a mere echo of both commonplace perception and conviction. The focus today is on sutureless cataract surgery with minimal surgically induced astigmatism. Manual phacofragmentation is a highly skilled procedure. The various techniques need insertion of large instrument/s through the main incision. As a result, anterior chamber cannot be kept well formed. The corneal endothelium and/or the posterior capsule may get "ravaged" during the excursion. Phacofragmentation can be made safer if it is done in a 'closed and deep anterior chamber'.

The procedure can be performed under the anesthesia of surgeon's choice. I perform it under topical anesthesia. One drop of 0.5% Proparacaine is instilled seven times during 45 minutes prior to surgery. The last drop is instilled after the peritomy. No sedation is used and a constant surgeon-patient communication is maintained. Patients are told to report immediately if they feel pain. If pain is complained, 0.75 cc of 2% Lignocaine is infused through a blunt canula in the subtenon space and if required at any stage of surgery, 0.5 cc of Lignocaine free of preservative is irrigated in the anterior chamber.

An anterior chamber maintainer (ACM) is introduced near lower limbus through a corneal tunnel and the BSS infusion line is kept 'on' to maintain positive pressure in AC. The height of the BSS bottle can be varied as per requirement during the procedure. After preparing a fornix based conjunctival flap and cauterization of bleeders, a 5.5 mm Frown scleral incision is made. A scleral tunnel is prepared extending about 1.5 mm in cornea to prepare a clear corneal valve. The tunnel is funnel shaped and is about 7.5mm wide in clear cornea. The anterior chamber is not entered at this stage through the tunnel. Scleral pocketing is not done. About 5.5mm capsulorhexis is performed using 27G/30G bent needle introduced through a side port incision at 10 O'clock. Conventional hydrodissection and then hydrodelineation are carried out and the nucleus is partially prolapsed out of the capsular bag. If the nucleus is small it is extracted out using Sheet's glide. (Blumenthal's Mini Nuc Technique).

For large nucleus, a 'Closed Chamber Manual Phacofragmentation' is performed. The surgical nucleus is partially prolapsed out of the capsular bag by the technique of surgeon's choice. I generally prolapse the nucleus out by exerting rotational force with hydrodissection canula, at times totally tumbling it and making it upside down. The nucleus should be positioned in such a way that the left (surgeon's) and upper part remain out of

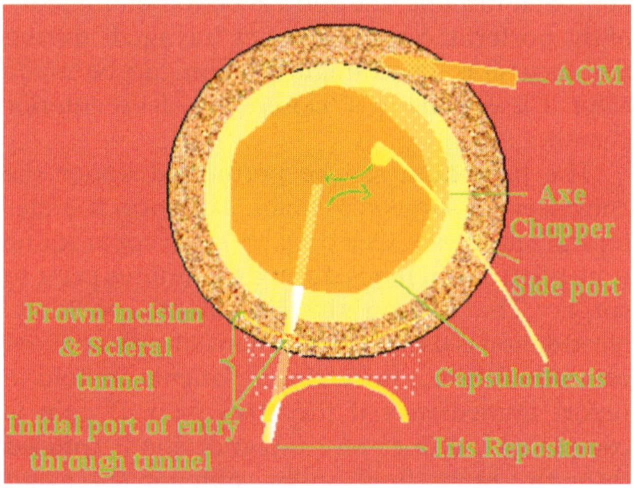

Fig. 28.1: Diagram showing the axe chopper position in front of nucleus and the iris repositor behind the nucleus before phacofragmentation

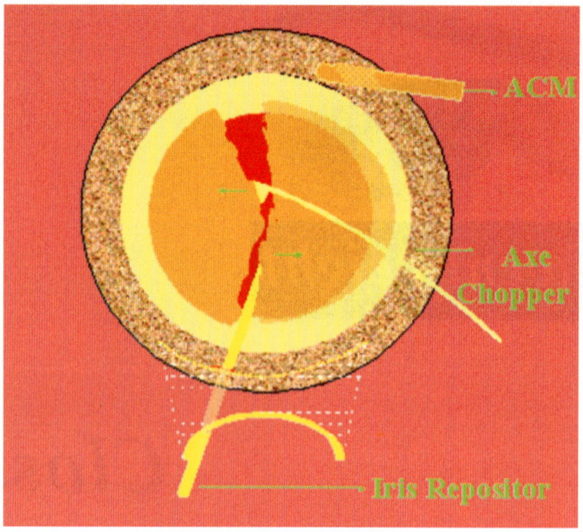

Fig. 28.2: Diagram showing the axe chopper and the iris repositor pushing apart the nuclear fragments

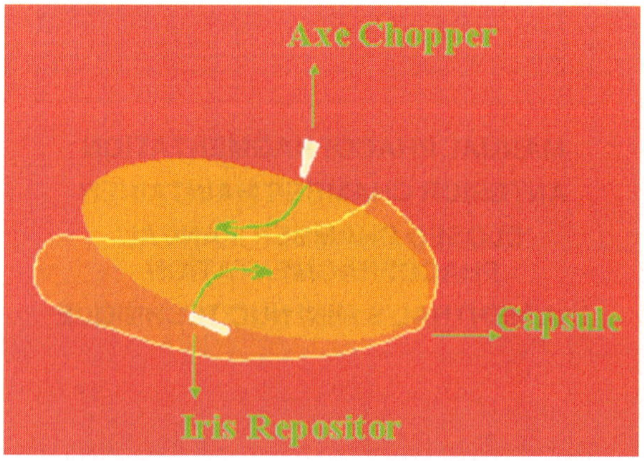

Fig. 28.3: Cross-sectional view of the maneuver (as if viewed from 12 O' clock). The chopper and the repositor should be moved in the direction of the green arrows. Although the movements are continuous curvilinear, the instruments are brought closer to each other initially so as to fragment the nucleus and then moved away from each other to separate the fragments

bag. Instead, the nucleus may be brought totally into the anterior chamber. Using a Stiletto knife a small initial entry (0.9mm) is made into the anterior chamber about 1.5 to 2 mm to the left of midline (Fig. 28.10). An iris repositor is glided under the nucleus a little to the left of the midline. The surgeon gets sufficient space between the nucleus and the posterior capsule due to positive pressure in anterior chamber and the closed chamber maneuvering. Another instrument, 'Boramani's Axe Chopper' is

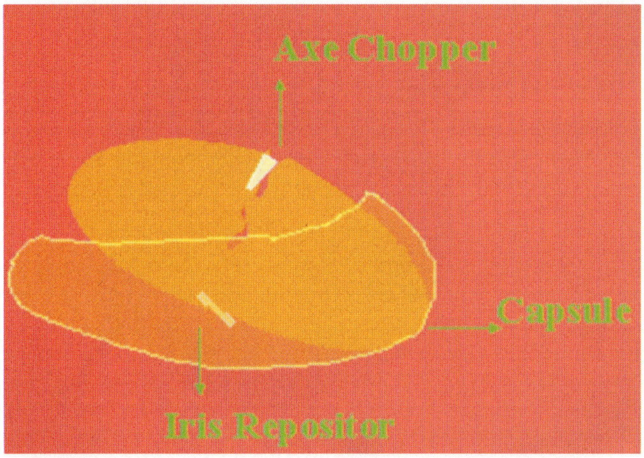

Fig. 28.4: The initial crack when the axe chopper gets buried in the nucleus

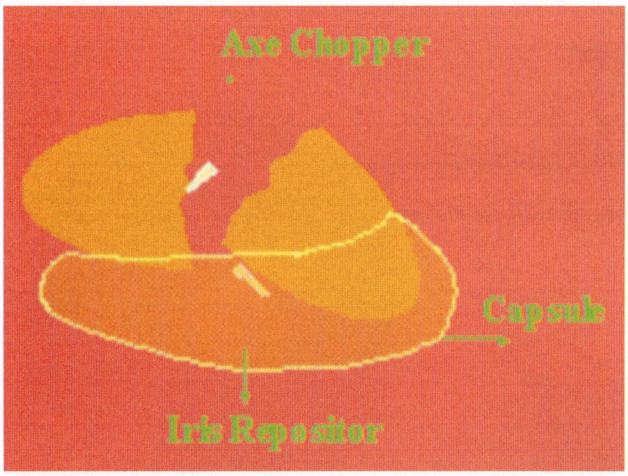

Fig. 28.5: The completion of the phacofragmentation

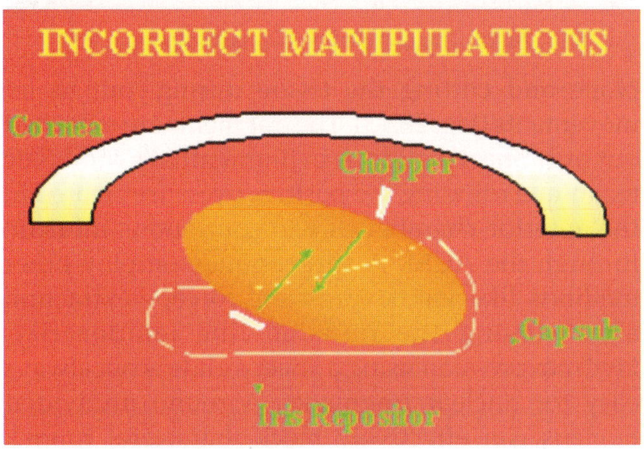

Fig. 28.6: Incorrect manipulations: if the instruments are straightway opposed to each other, a sudden hazardous tumbling of the nucleus can occur

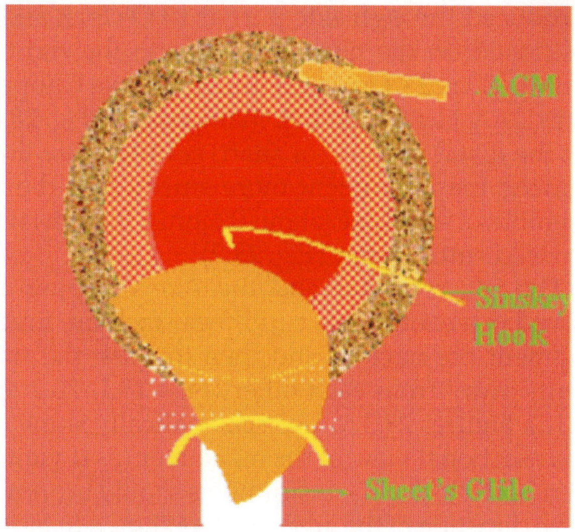

Fig. 28.7: It may be difficult to express out a fragmented nucleus with fluid pressure due to egress of fluid from sides. A Sinskey hook passed through the side port can push the fragment out

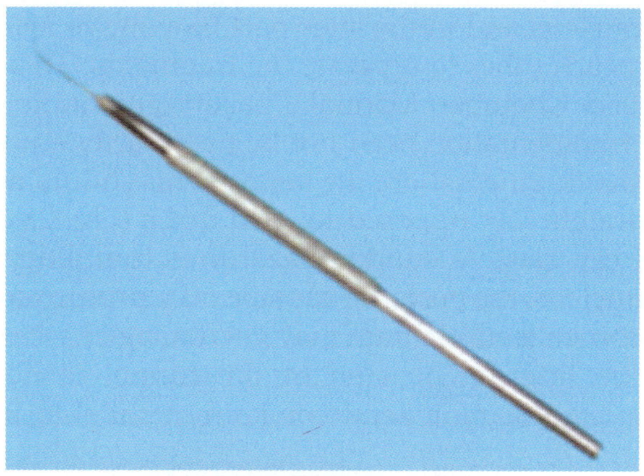

Fig. 28.8: The Axe chopper

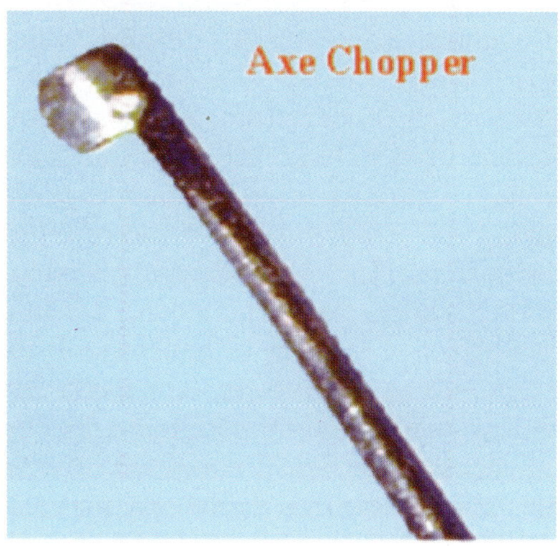

Fig. 28.9: The tip of the axe chopper

introduced through side port at 10 O'clock and is positioned on the nucleus a little to the right of midline (Figs 28.1 to 11). Boramani's Axe Chopper is basically like a lens / IOL manipulator (Fig. 28.8), but the distal portion (or shaft) is little more thick to make the instrument more sturdy and the tip resembles a small axe (about 0.6mm × 0.6mm) with a curved cutting edge (Fig. 28.9).

The iris repositor and the Axe Chopper are moved in a continuous curvilinear fashion, first to fragment the nucleus and then to push the fragments away from each other (Figs 28.1, 28.2 and 28.12). Figures 28.3 to 28.5 schematically show the cross-sectional view of the maneuver (as if viewed from 12 O' clock). The instruments should be moved in the direction of the green arrows shown in Figure 28.3. Please note that although the movements are continuous curvilinear, initially the instruments are brought closer to each other so as to fragment the nucleus and in the later part they move away from each other to separate the fragments. This is 'Closed Chamber Manual Phacofragmentation'. The fragmentation need not be necessarily equal. For the fragmentation, the instruments should not be straightway opposed to each other (Fig. 28.6). This can cause a sudden hazardous tumbling of the nucleus, the posterior capsule may rupture and the corneal endothelium may get damaged.

The internal incision of the tunnel is now completed using a keratome knife parallel to iris

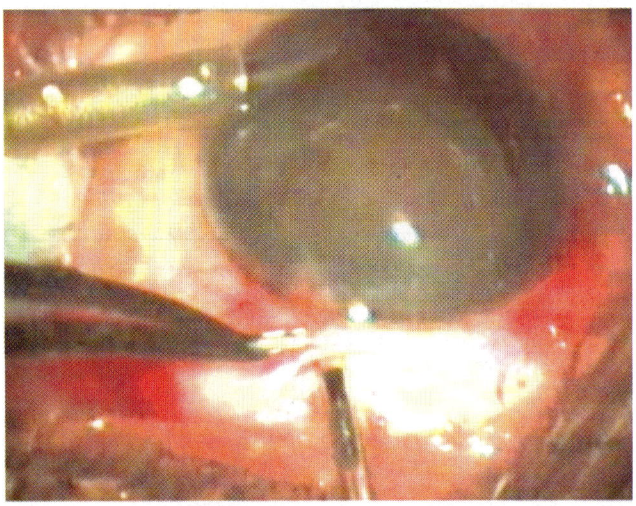

Fig. 28.10: Using a Stiletto knife a small initial entry (0.9 mm) is made into the anterior chamber through the scleral tunnel about 1.5 to 2 mm to the left of midline

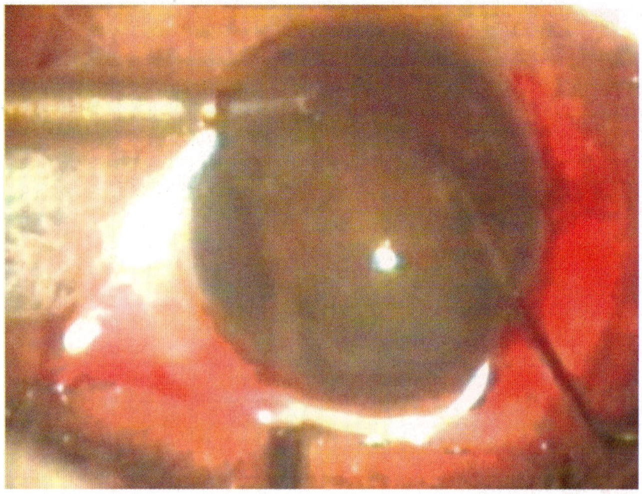

Fig. 28.11: The axe chopper positioned in front of nucleus and the iris repositor behind the nucleus before phacofragmentation

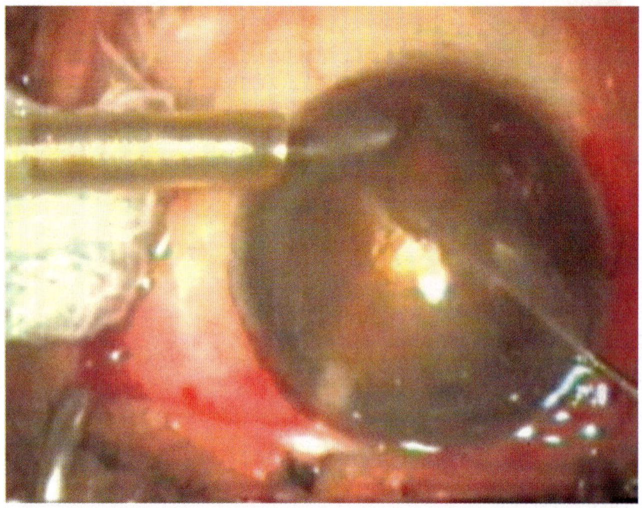

Fig. 28.12: The completion of phacofragmentation

plane and cutting the tissue during 'out to in' movements (Fig. 28.13). The fragments are extracted out over Sheet's glide as in Blumenthal's Mini Nuc technique utilizing the positive pressure created in the anterior chamber due to continuous infusion through the ACM. A surgeon may employ other methods like viscoexpression, forceps extraction after closing the infusion line temporarily. Hydroexpression using a Sheet's glide is not always easy for nuclear fragments. A round undivided nucleus can effectively block the scleral tunnel, allowing build-up of pressure in the anterior chamber to facilitate hydroexpression. A fragmented nucleus can be ineffective, allowing the egress

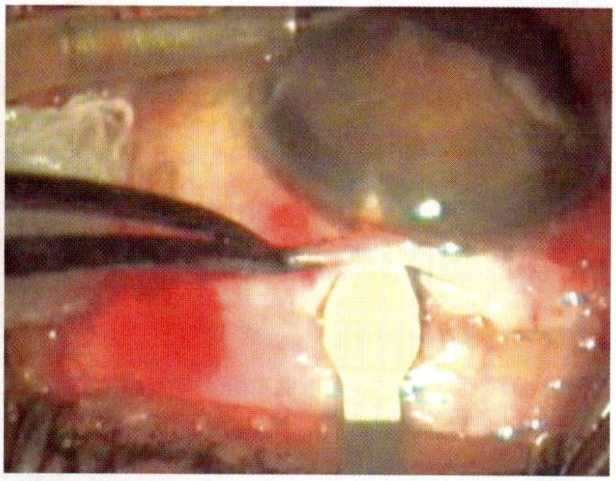

Fig. 28.13: The internal incision is completed with keratome only after phacofragmentation

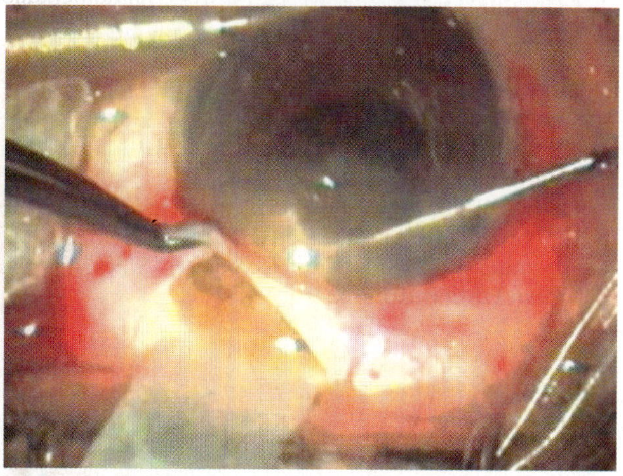

Fig. 28.14: The hydro-expression of the fragment is being assisted with Sinskey hook passed through the side-port

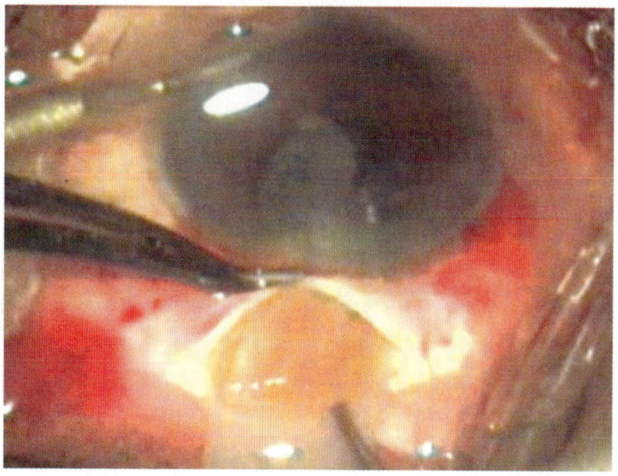

Fig. 28.15: A nuclear fragment being taken out over Sheet's glide

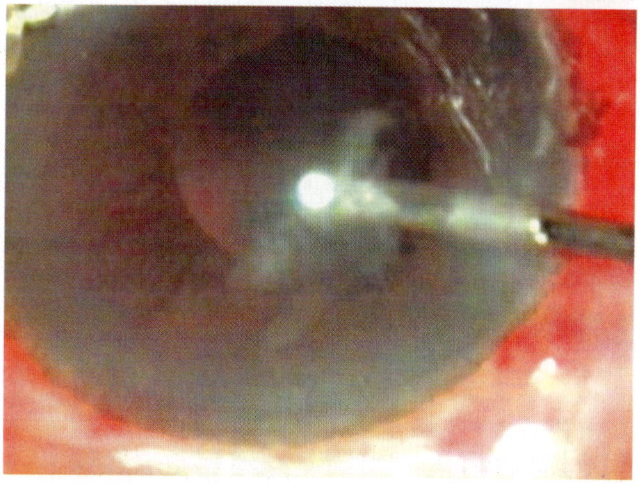

Fig. 28.16: Water jetting of the capsular bag is done through a fine canula passed through the side-port

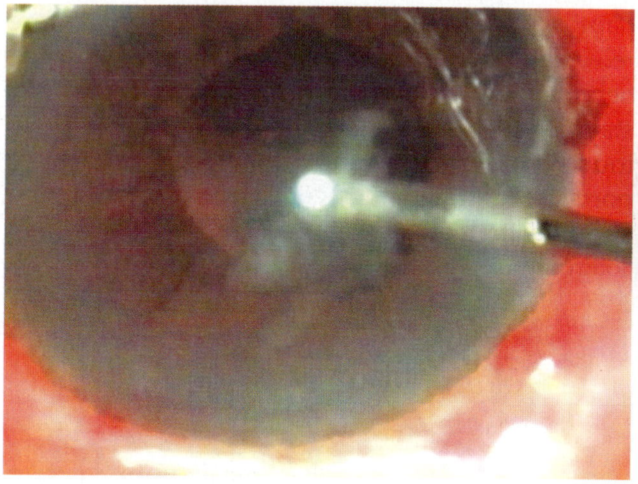

Fig. 28.17: The cortex is aspirated manually using a single port aspiration canula, passed through the side port

of fluid from sides. If such a difficulty is encountered, a Sinskey hook passed through the side port can push the fragment out (Figs 28.7 and 28.14). The epinuclear mass is delivered out using Sheet's glide. Water jetting of the bag is done through a fine canula passed through the side port (Fig. 28.16). The cortex is aspirated manually using a single port aspiration canula, passed through the side port (Fig. 28.17). This canula is attached to a syringe through a silicon tube. An intraocular lens is implanted in the bag (Fig. 28.18). While implanting the lens, once the inferior haptic is placed in the lower bag, it is advisable to support the superior

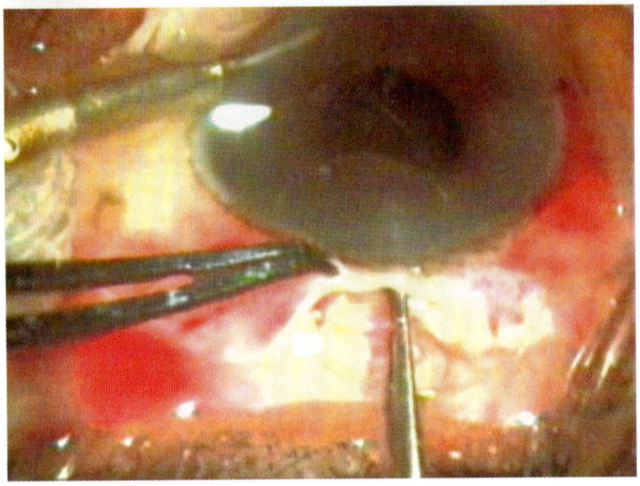

Fig. 28.18: The implantation of an IOL

haptic with the forceps in the left hand before releasing the optic. Otherwise the lens can recede behind due to continuous flow of the BSS, the optic stays in the tunnel and the inferior haptic may touch the corneal endothelium. If necessary the ports are hydrated, the eyeball is pressurized with BSS and the conjunctiva is sealed with wet field coagulator.

The major advantage of this technique is that the phacofragmentation is done in a closed, deep chamber using very fine instruments, thus making it safer.

REFERENCES

1. Blumenthal M. "The modern manual small incision extracapsular with mini-nuc technique". Highlights of Ophthalmology. 2000;28(1).
2. Gutierrez-Carmona FJ. Manual multi-phacofragmentation through a 3.2 mm clear corneal incision. J Cataract Refract Surg 2000;26(10):1523-28.
3. Chawla HB, Adams AD. Use of the anterior chamber maintainer in anterior segment surgery. J Cataract Refract Surg 1996;22(2):172-77.
4. Kansas PG, Sax R. Small incision cataract extraction and implantation surgery using a manual phacofragmentation technique. J Cataract Refract Surg. 1988;14(3):328-30.
5. Bartov E, Isakov I, Rock T. Nucleus fragmentation in a scleral pocket for small incision extracapsular cataract extraction. J Cataract Refract Surg. 1998;24(2):160-65.
6. Blumenthal M, Assia E, Moisseieve Y. Manual ECCE, the present state of the art. Asia-Pacific Journal of Ophthalmology 1995;4:21-24.
7. Keener GT. The Nucleus Division Technique for Small Incision Cataract Extraction. In Cataract surgery Alternative Small Incision Techniques. Slack Inc. First Indian Edition 1995:163-91.

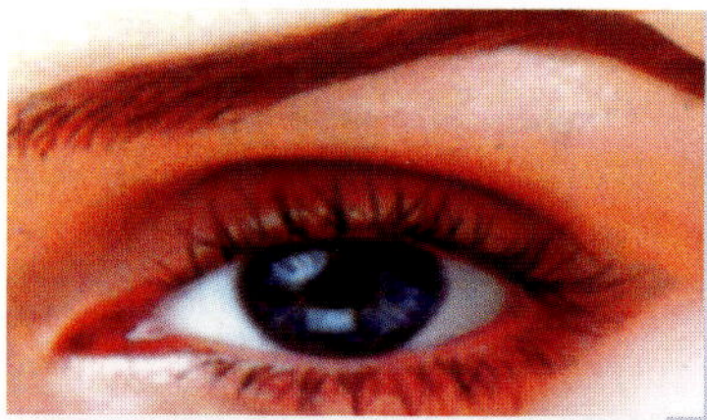

Twenty nine

Phacosection Technique in SICS

MS Ravindra (India)

WHY DID I CHANGE OVER TO SMALL INCISION CATARACT SURGERY?

Modern Tunnel incision cataract surgery (TICS), as it should be called rightly, offers safety, consistency, stability and quick rehabilitation. Small incision cataract surgery is a misnomer, as 'small' is always bigger than 'smaller'! Moreover, the two most important advents in modern cataract surgery is the synthesis of the TUNNEL and CCC. The technique of Cataract surgery has progressed rapidly and would continue to change. Today's technology dependent surgery has its benefits as well as high costs, long learning curve and big list of consumables. At this time it is going through a refinement phase, to further improve the safety features. On the other hand, Surgeons all over the world continue to develop simpler, friendly and elegant surgeries that are cost-effective and yet provide the highest quality results anatomically and functionally. Trend to switch over to sutureless cataract surgery technique has caught on everyone. The advantages are safety, quick rehabilitation, least complications and stable vision.

The Phacoemulsification needs periodic update of the ever-improving expensive equipment. The machines get outdated soon. An experienced assistant is mandatory. There is an increased stress on OR staff. The procedure is highly dependent on equipment and ancillary personnel. I switched over to Phacoemulsification in early 90's. I had one Phaco probe and was not willing to re-use it and the tubings for the next patient. I had to wait till the probe was resterilized. Chemical sterilization is never ever safe. That is time I looked for equally good or better alternatives.

Phacoemulsification was developed in 1960s by Charles Kelman, but the technology has changed a lot since then. Today we are still in search of perfect machine and a perfect, belmishless procedure. May be few years later we will have robots doing this procedure. The complications with phacoemulsiflcation are less forgiving. Much of the over-enthusiasm in Phacoemulsification is generated by the Industry. In our country only a fraction of Surgeons can afford the expensive instrumentation and recurring expenditure. Manual small incision cataract surgery, with all its benefits, is the perfect answer to many of the problems. It elegantly suits high volume cataract operations, is perfect for every type of cataract, from immature to Morgagnians, posterior capsular to rocky hards and from pseudo-exfoliation to subluxated cataracts. Last few years have seen an upsurge to re-discover various manual techniques, within the arena of Phacoemulsification and outside it.

In early 1993 I started switching over from Phacoemulsification to Phacosection. I never had to look back at any point of time! The advantages were just too many, hard nucleus, a low endothelial cell count, the malfunctioning machine, etc. but the biggest advantage was when the OR list was long, as each of the charity camps would have 60 to 100 surgeries to be finished in one day. Don't believe if somebody says the learning curve is shorter, it is as much longer and painful as with Phacoemulsification. The problem is compounded as the industry and trade take great interest in systematically teaching you the machine surgery, but if you need to learn SICS, you are left on the lurch, on your own, searching for an appropriate guru!

PATIENT SELECTION, PREPARATION AND ANESTHESIA

There is really nothing very special, very different or restrictive as regard to preoperative planning. There is no need to be choosy about the patient, as any cataract could be handled safely and comfortably. I don't any more grade my nuclei, as all are one and the same for Phacosection. There is no need to worry about Pseudoexfoliations, posterior polar cataracts, super hard nueclei, subluxations, weak zonules, endothelial disease, miotic pupils etc. as all can be handled very elegantly with least trauma to the eye. The surgery becomes safe as the hydrodynamics, intra-ocular pressures and turbulence are at the lowest. However in the above situations and in eyes with corneal opacities, shallow anterior chamber, post glaucoma surgery, bleeding disorders, etc. the beginners may revert to the technique that they are more familiar with.

Perform a complete ocular examination including assessing the cornea, measuring the intraocular pressure etc. Look for obvious evidences of endothelial disease, guttata, past inflammation, trauma, pupillary rigidity, posterior capsular involvement, pseudoexfoliation etc. They are certainly not contraindications, but you would be cautious to anticipate need for deviations in the surgical technique. Ask for any sudden loss of sight and check if the extent of cataract is in commensuration with the amount of vision loss.

Patient Preparation

The preoperative instructions are similar to any cataract surgery. Broad-spectrum antibiotic eye drops are instilled 3 hourly for a day prior to surgery. A well-dilated pupil will make the surgical procedure comfortable. Tropicamide and Phenylephrine eye drops are used at 20 min. Intervals for 1 hour prior to surgery. Non-steroid anti-inflammatory eye drops can be started preoperatively. There is no role for Acetazolamide, Glycerine or Mannitol.

Anesthesia and Akinesia

You can chose topical, intracameral or parabulbar anesthesia. For the beginners and for those who desire akinesia as well as consistency and peaceful surgery, a single site infero-temporal retrobulbar or parabulbar injection is useful. I use the following anesthesia in apprehensive patients.

1. Add 1 ml of Sodium Bicarbonate into 30 ml vial of 2 percent Xylocaine and Adrenaline (1:200000). Draw 2.5 ml of this mixture in a 5 ml syringe with 23 G, 1 inch needle.
2. Add 1 vial of Hyaluronidase into 20 ml vial of Bupivacaine 0.5 percent. Draw 1 ml of this into the same syringe.

Rub antiseptic on lateral aspect of lower lid. The subcutaneous vessels get slightly dilated and avoid pricking them. Identify the injection site just above the inferior orbital margin, at the junction of middle and lateral 1/3rd. Pass half the length of the needle perpendicularly. Then tilt the syringe so that the tip of the needle is directed toward the apex of the orbit. As you inject the anesthetic into the orbit, note that there is a progressive, subtle, supratarsal fullness, as the orbital septum raises up. This is an excellent sign and indicates that you have achieved a true intraconal block, and you would have an excellent sensory block as well as akinesia. If this does not happen but the inferior lid fills up, than you have achieved a peribulbar block, and would have a good sensory block but poor motor block. A 1-inch needle would never hit the optig nerve or its sheath! I have never seen a globe puncture with my technique and had retrobulbar hemorrhage only once.

Why this mixture? I realised few years ago that the needle does not 'sting' the patient, but the medicine as it gets into the tissues is very painful. This I realised is because of the pH of Xylocaine, which is 4.2 and that of Bupivacaine which is 5.8! With Hyaluronidase the pH of the mixture is 3.0! The stinging pain was eliminated when I added Sodium Bicarbonate, which also enhances the potency of the mixture.

Inducing hypotony continues to be important in my technique where several steps are performed in an open chamber situation. Keep a 200 gms 'weight' over the eye for about 15 minutes before giving the block and about 15 minutes after the block. The 'weight' is home made by filling a circular bag of diameter about 2 inches, made of cloth or Rexin, with tiny steel bearing balls and than sealing the mouth. It is like stitching a round pillow of diameter about 2 inches, in the shape of a bun, but having steel balls instead of foam! It is than covered with several layers of cellophane tape, so that it does not split over when it falls down. The tape is replaced periodically. When in use, the 'weight' rests not only on the eye but also on the orbital margins, and increases the IOP to about 30 mm Hg, which does not obstruct either venous or arterial blood flow to the retina and optic nerve head. Most of other techniques of inducing hypotony have no control on the amount of IOP raised and some of the unexplained subnormal post operative vision and pallor of ONH could be due to a compromised ONH and retinal perfusion by undesirably high IOP. This is particularly true when ONH is already compromised, like in glaucoma and diabetes.

INSTRUMENTATION

Insist on the best microsurgical instruments. Do not compromise on their quality. Indeed you would need very few of them. Ensure that you have following instruments in your routine cataract set in superb condition. They are to be autoclaved, and do not use anything that is kept in chemical lotions and formaline chambers! The only alternative is to ethylene oxide sterilisation, and this works well only for spare instruments for emergency use.

1. *Scleral tunnel blades*
   a. To create the sclerocorneal tunnel the double bevel 'spoon' blade is used, made of stainless steel. While the front bevel blade tends to dissect deeper, the back bevel blade tends to dissect superficially. Double bevel blade is the sharpest, and dissects tissue in a uniplanar direction. It is 2mm wide and 2.5mm long and bent to give the best ergonomic comfort. Because of its circular (slightly oval) design, it can be used to cut in both forward and backward directions. If double bevel is not available, the next best is the front bevel blade, which takes the dissection deeper. At the worst, you will have a premature anterior chamber entry with this blade, and never an anterior wall perforation.
   b. The slit blade or Keratome has a sharp tip. It has a width of 5.0 mm and is used for entering the anterior chamber. This is also be used to

further widen the internal opening of the tunnel, to 6 mm or even larger for handling supra-hard nuclei.

2. *Cystitomes*

A 26 G half inch hypodermic needle is bent at 90 degrees at its tip, in a direction away from the bevel. This is best done by

a. Keep the bevel (not the tip) of the needle pressed against a flat hard surface, like the flat handle of an instrument. Rotate the two instruments in the opposite directions, so that the bevel is bent by the hard surface, without damaging the tip. This is done in a circular motion. The handle and the needle would be initially positioned like the two limbs of an 'A' and than you open up the two limbs in such a way that the bevel is bent. Alternatively, you could use the needle holder to create the 90 degree bend, but the earlier described technique gives consistently excellent cystitomes.

b. The second bend is at the shaft's junction with the hub, in the opposite direction to the first bend. On an average this is about 45 degrees. For deep-set eyes, you bend it lesser, the angle now will be less acute in deep set eyes. For prominent eyes you bend little more, so that the shaft of the needle is more or less perpendicular to the direction of syringe. See that the tip of the needle do not touch any hard surface, and do not reuse the cystitome.

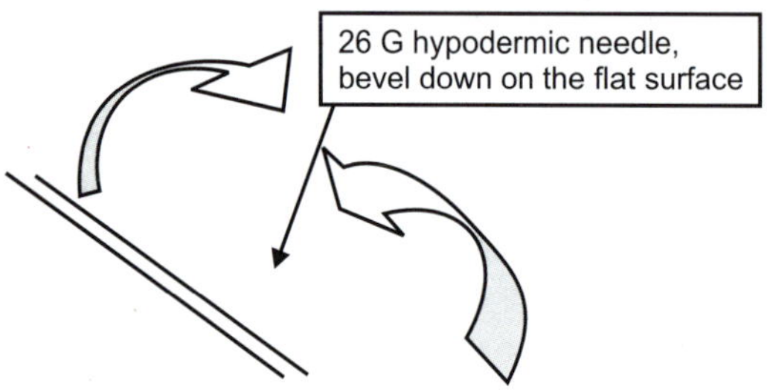

Making a cystitome

3. *Cannulas*

a. The hydrodissection cum nucleus management cannula is 'home made' from 26 G half inch hypodermic needles. The tip is rubbed off against an abrasive oilstone, (available with hardware stores) till it becomes smooth and rounded. The shaft is bent to 45 degrees at the hub. For hydrodissection this cannula is attached to 2 ml syringe containing BSS. For nucleus management it is attached to a syringe filled with Methylceullose (HPMC). Any other type of cannula would not work for nucleus management! You need about 4 cannulas in each set, and they can be reused. Flush them immediately after use so that they do not get blocked.

b. 19 G cannula for quick injection of HPMC viscous.

c. Cortical aspiration is by a bimanual 23 G Simcoe cannula with a 0.3 mm aspiration port on its left side. The gentle concave anterior shape of the cannula is ideal to work through the main tunnel, and is excellent especially for small deepset eyes. The Simcoe cannula is mounted on to a Silicone bulb containing BSS. I have modified Simcoe cannula so that is has a smooth bulbous base, instead of a Luer lock type of base. This easily slips into the bulb, and avoids the need for the connecting piece, which lengthens the cannula and also gives unstability to the whole system. Two bulbs in each set are desirable, as the assistant can fill one bulb when the other one is in use.

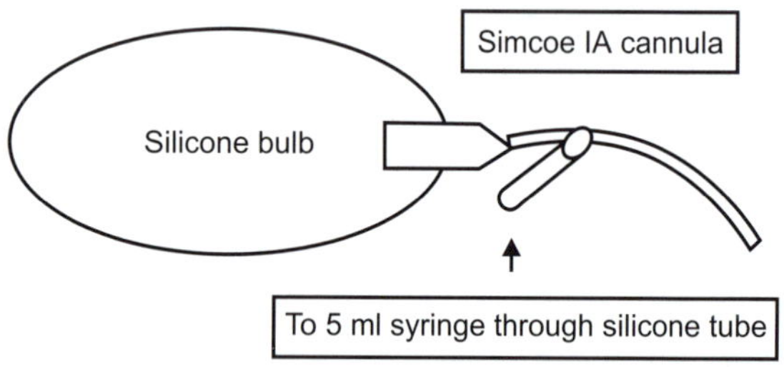

d. The sub-incisional cortex is aspirated through the main tunnel, using right and left J shaped 12 O'clock aspiratoin-irrigation cannulas of Simcoe design. The aspiration port is 0.3 mm and on the left side.

4. *The Sinskey hook* is used for nuclear rotation and for prolapsing it into the anterior chamber. It is also used for nuclear division in very hard cataracts. At the end it is used to dial the IOL into the bag.

5. *Wire Vectis* Gives support to the nucleus while dividing it and sandwiches the nucleus half while it is being extracted.
6. *6 mm marker*, built on the rear side of the wire vectis handle, is used to mark the ends of initial scleral incision.
7. Straight 0.1 mm 1:2 fixation forceps, preferably made of Titanium should be of excellent quality.
8. *Methylcellulose* (HPMC) visco is essential. Do not attempt this surgery without it!
   e. *Irrigating fluid is BSS* and is to be chilled in the refrigerator (not forzen!). Buy the bottles from reputed companies and do not autoclave it. Plastic bottles are better, they collapse as they get emptied and outside air would not enter through the fluid. This always happens with glass bottles, when you vent the bottle through the bung. The coldness of the fluid will reduce the release of prostaglandin and stabilizes the Blood-Aqueous barrier. It also prevents miosis and constricts the iris blood vessels. Always load the Silicone bulbs directly from the bottle, through an IV dripset. Never take the irrigating fluid in an open Galley pot to refill the Silicone bulb. The particles in the air settle down by gravity, and within no time they will contaminate the BSS in the Galley pot. Although Ringer lactate can be used as the quantities of fluid utilised is small and surgery is extremely quick, it is best to use BSS as it creates the best micro-environment for the sensitive cells lining the anterior segment.

At this stage, let me add a note on cleaning and sterilisation of these instruments. Special attention must be taken in the meticulous cleaning of every surface, part, joint and crevice of each instrument, immediately after the surgery is over. Flush the cannulas immediately after use, and once again at the end of surgery, with distilled water. Ultrasound cleaning of all instruments after each surgery is paramount. Instruments are to be kept separated from each other to prevent damage and interlocking. This is done best by the silicone mat. Avoid using the steel boxes and bins. One or two mats kept one over the other, containing the instruments, is double packed directly and tightly in a cotton packing cloth and autoclaved. Load these directly into the autoclave, and avoid surgical bins for this purpose. The moist heat autoclaving is the most efficient method of sterilisation. The extra instruments can be ethylene oxide gas sterilised and for use when needed. Avoid all other chemical sterilisations at any cost.

ENTRY INTO THE EYE

Preperation: On patient's arrival to the surgery, dilate the pupil well with tropicamide and phenylephrine. Avoid the latter in hypertensives. The eye needs to be moderatly hypotonic. This is achieved by keeping the 'weight' (see inducing hypotony) on the eye for about 20 to 30 minutes before the surgery. The IOP increases to about 25 to 30 mmHg and unlike many other techniques of inducing hypotony which are very quick, this technique of inducing hypotony is slow. But it does not compromise either arteriolar or venous circulation in ciliary, retinal and optic nerve vasculature. Hypotony is important, as many steps of the phacosection surgery are done at atmospheric pressures.

Instil a drop of aqueous 5 percent povidone-iodine into the conjunctival sac along with topical anesthetics. Paint the area with 5 percent aqueous povidone-iodine and wash the conjunctival sac with 0.5 percent povidone-iodine. Apply a sterile drape with a side pouch. See that the eyelashes are well tucked under the drape, by the non-touch techniques. The lid margins, which include the eyelashes and lid glands, should not be exposed to the conjunctival sac, and this is achieved by a good draping technique.

Separation of Eyelids An ideal exposure is obtained with a thin wire speculum, with a medium amount of tension in the wire. The speculum is made out of one single wire and should not have any welded elements. Most important consideration is that it should not have the usual bridge wire on the top of the blades. The speculum can be rotated and positioned at any angle, and does not have to be exactly holding the middle of lower and upper lids! e.g. when you are operating at the upper temporal quadrant of the right eye, initially position the speculum the way you normally do it, and than rotate the entire speculum anti-clockwise, so that the 'blades' of the speculum now hold the lateral half of upper lid and medial half of the lower lid.

Your entire surgery can now be performed within the width of the upper blade, and you will never have a surprise slippage of a surgical instrument from the top of speculum blade.

Add on Anesthesia What ever may be the anesthesia you give or don't give, the following simple procedure discovered by me few years ago would go a very very long way to achieve superb patient comfort and relaxation. I can say that this is the secret for good surgery. As your assistant is adjusting the microscope, keep a small piece of cotton on the presumed surgical site and soak it with few drops of Inj. Xyloacine 2 percent. Keep it there for few minutes. The conjunctiva and sclera locally becomes deeply numb, and the patient will be really thankful for that. Patient is now totally relaxed, which helps you to smoothly perform the surgery.

Superior rectus Never take a superior rectus bridle suture, and you are getting rid of all the complications that go with it, including ptosis and vertical phorias and tropias. Many unhappy patients inspite of excellent cataract surgery are due to vertical phorias induced by a superior rectus sutures or induced by pulling the globe down against a contracting superior rectus muscle of reflex Bells phenomenon to counter the discomfort. Hence negating the pain and discomfort factor is the critical issue in safe and successful cataract surgery.

Peritomy Select an area, which is devoid of perforating anterior ciliary vessels. These are relatively large vessels, which branch out from the rectus muscular arteries, proceed anteriorly and dip into sclera about 2 to 5 mm away from the limbus. It is better to avoid their zones completely, as damage to these vessels not only cause much bleeding, but more than that, would compromise blood circulation to the anterior segment. A fornix based 7 mm wide conjunctiva-Tenons-episcleral (CTE) peritomy is made, preferably in the upper temporal limbus. Don't try to separate these three layers. Make the first nick through this CTE, parallel to and about 2 mm away from limbus. Dissect upto sclera. Than sweep one blade of the scissors between the CTE and sclera for about 7 mm. Snuggly nudge the blade toward the limbus, and that cut the entire CTE, at the limbus. You would notice that while the conjuncitva is continuous with the limbal and corneal epithelium, the tenons is inserted into the sclera about a mm or two away from the limbus. If you try to make the nick initially at limbus, than you would not be able to get CTE in one layer. Cauterise bleeding vessels, if any, with thermal cautery. You would need only a very minimal cauterisation.

Do only 'point cautery' of the actual bleeding vessels. The 4-steps are, irrigate the bleeding area

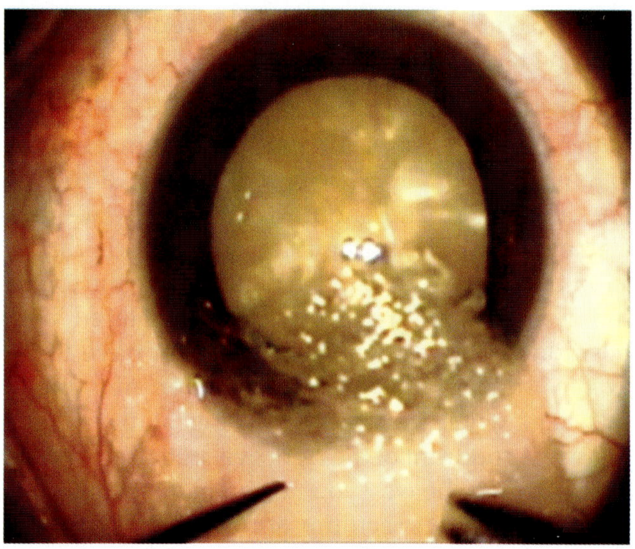

Fig. 29.1: Lignocaine soaked cotton

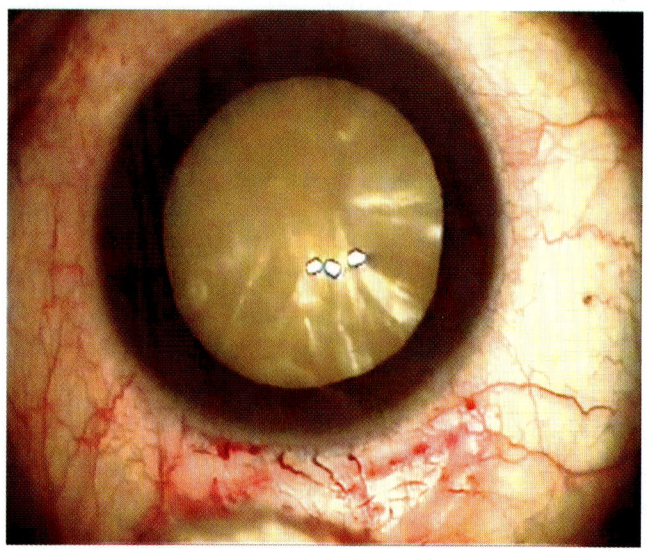

Fig. 29.2: Conjunctival bleeders

with BSS, identify the actual bleeder, and than dry the area and hold it down pressed with a swabstick, and finally apply the cautery exactly on the actual bleeder, quickly, as you remove the swabstick. If you try to do this otherwise, in a pool of blood, you will be unnecessarily cauterising a large area of sclera. Quickly wipe the cautery tip with a cotton swab, so that you don't carry carbon soot to the surgical site. Thermal cautery is ideal and its temperature can be controlled by how long you keep it in the flame. You don't need a cable, electrical supply and a person moving around giving the connections of a diathermy, and you will never encounter a loose connection! There are no electrical waves passing through the patient, and hence it is safe even for those who have a pacemaker!

Tunnel Incision

The sclero-corneal tunnel incision was described over a decade ago by Richard Kratz. It is one of the biggest inventions in the history of cataract surgery and continues to remain the best way to have a small, stable and secure incision.

I have learnt over a decade now that it is not the size or design of the incision that controls the surgically induced astigmatism (SIA). In my series, where I keep the integrity of tunnel intact, without stretching, cooking or tearing, it does not matter whether I made a frown or a straight incision, whether it is a 6 mm long incision or smaller. It did not matter whether I did it superonasal or superotemporal. The latter position is adapted as a routine for the sake of comfort. I don't have to turn the microscope, chair and tables, like a merry go round, as in temporal incisions. It did not matter if I did the incision on the steep axis, flat axis or in between! By making good sclerocorneal tunnels and by not spoiling them, you can easily achieve ZERO SIA.

The initial incision is about 1.5 mm behind the limbus, half scleral depth, and 6 mm long. An arc like 6 mm caliper, designed by me at the back end wire Vectis, is used to mark the 6 mm. The incision is made with a blade fragment to half the scleral thickness. The proximal lip of the incision (not toward the corneal side but toward the surgeon) is grasped with a 0.1 mm 1:2 toothed Titanium forceps. The tunnel is dissected past limbus, to 1.5mm of the clear cornea, at half corneal thickness, with the double bevel spoon blade. How do you know it is half thickness? You could use an expensive 350 micron pre-calibrated blade. Better alternative is to gain experience. Get the feedback on the next day as to how deep you have gone by comparing the thickness of the superficial lamina to the deeper lamina of the corneal portion of the tunnel on your slit lamp. When you start dissecting, remember that you not only go radial toward the center of cornea, but also upward, toward the dome of the cornea. Remember that you are working on the surface of a spherical object. Start at one end of the incision, make the full-depth dissection and then go laterally to cover the entire 6 mm width. This forms a uni-planar tunnel. Always be watching the cutting edge of the blade. Have a dry field so that you recognise a premature passage of the blade tip into the anterior chamber. In case you end up very superficial or very deep, start another tunnel in the right plane from the opposite end of the same surgical site, and than complete it all over. You would have two tunnels, the right one is the second one. Ignore the first one. If the tunnel roof is lacerated, it usually does not need any repair in most of the cases. Recognize the premature entry early. Ignore it and start another tunnel in s superficial plane and continue the surgery. You may need to put a horizontal suture at the end of surgery to minimize the inevitable astigmatism. If bleeding occurs with in the tunnel, direct cautery will help, if it is close to the outer incision. If it is deep inside, cauterize the feeder vessel on the surface of sclera, outside the tunnel. It is not necessary to cauterise small bleeders, which do not bleed into the anterior chamber. They can be left alone and allowed to bleed externally until they spontaneously stop. Bleeding within the tunnel is usually a sign of having gone too deep during the dissection or working close to penetrating anterior ciliary vessels, which can branch out within sclera. The floor of the tunnel must be uniform without tags so that there is free passage of instruments.

The edges of the tunnel are parallel and the internal opening, which is not made at this time, is also 6 mm wide. There are no side pockets, and

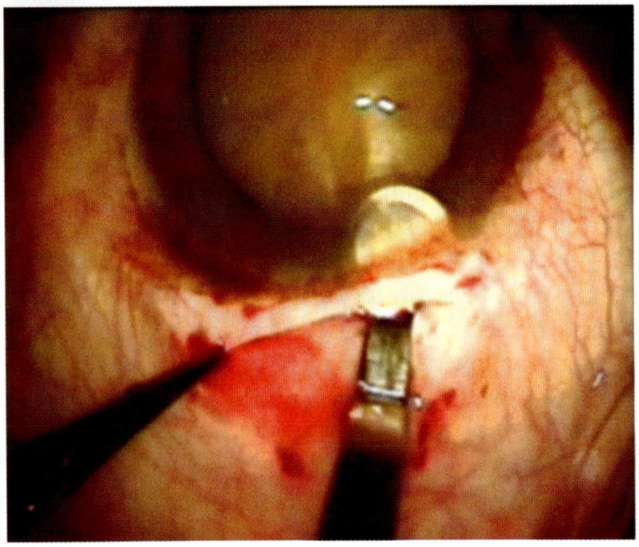

Fig. 29.3: Tunnel making

there is no widening of internal opening, as the nucleus is always taken out bisected.

Structural principles Tunnel making is the secret of success, and is most important from the point of safety and stability. There are actually two openings in a tunnel; the external and internal incisions. The external incision is the groove on the sclera and entry into the tunnel. The internal incision is the actual entry into the anterior chamber. Both of them must work in harmony in order for the tunnel to serve its full function. It is the internal incision that could change the shape of the cornea and contributes to the astigmatism. The outer incisional gape is contributed by the natural elasticity of the sclera and the changes induced by cautery and subsequent healing. This incisional gape does not affect the corneal astigmatism.

Surgically induced astigmatism is the end result of sliding between the two lamina of the tunnel. If the sliding is more, than the SIA is more. The straight lateral edges, unlike a funnel shaped incision, minimize the sliding. When the IOP increases, pressure is exerted at each point of sclera in an outward direction, so as to expand the globe. This force can be divided into vectors, in the plane of sclera. These vector forces extend in all directions, and not only in the direction of tunnel length! The forces in line with the tunnel tend to separate the two-scleral lamina, but the straight parallel sides of the tunnel counter this. A stretched, destructed or torned tunnel would not resist this vector force, and the scleral lamina would slide. In addition, the vector forces that are perpendicular to the first also tend to minimize this slide.

Astigmatic neutral zone is described as a funnel shaped area at 12'oclock limbus. As the eye is a globe, if you think 3 dimensionally, it exists everywhere around the limbus. Geometrically, the actual measurements of this zone is dependent upon just too many factors, including the size of the globe and diameter of the cornea. Incision placed with in this "astigmatic funnel " induces least amount of SIA. The phacosection incision, is always well within this zone.

The upper temporal incisions are supposed to be even more astigmatically neutral then other incisions. The reasons are:

1. The collagen fibres are reported to be circumferentially configured here as compared to

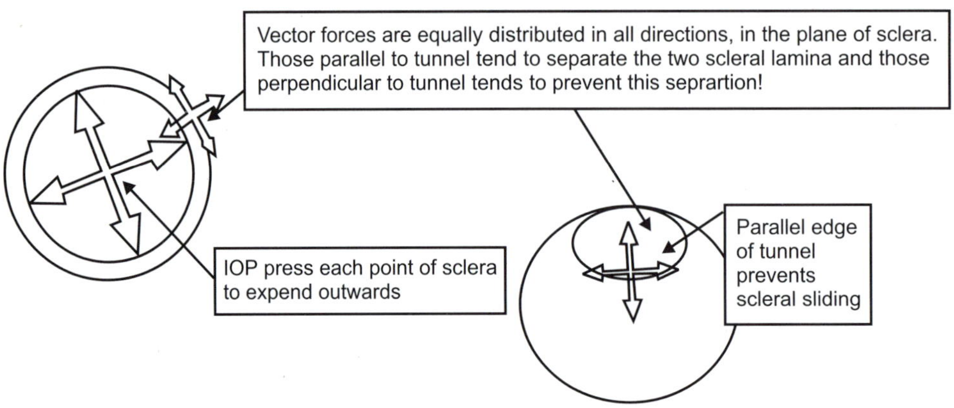

radial configuration at 12 O'clock. So the fibres are not cut across their length, and hence the pull by healing collagen fibres is minimal.

2. The action of rectus muscles tend to separate the two lamina. The action is direct and maximal at 12, 9 and 3 O'clocks. The upper temporal tunnel has least amount of direct pull. However, the vector forces still act on the inner lamina of sclera, at whatever position the tunnel is. As a large portion of our ocular movements is horizontal, the temporal incisions are subjected to this force maximally.

FLUIDICS AND OPEN AND CLOSED CHAMBER CONCEPTS

Phacosection gives the freedom to play around between two important hydrostatic environments in the eye, open and closed chamber situations. The classic example of open chamber is the direct incision extracapsular technique of olden days, where the pressure inside the eye comes down to atmospheric levels (e.g. 16 to 0 mmHg) as soon as the incision is made, and remains so till suturing is done. Any negative or positive pressure attempted is immediately nullified by its direct connection to the atmosphere. It is like a tennis ball, which is torn, or a hole is cut out. The classic example of closed chamber technique is the Blumenthal's technique, where the situation is similar to a football with the valve holding pressurised air inside. Here the intraocular pressure can be controlled and is determined by pressures of inflow and outflow, and quantum of inflow and outflow. The hydrostatic pressure influences the intraoperative IOP. An infusion bottle height of one meter gives an IOP of 80 mmHg (what happens to the venous and arterial flows!). Phacoemulsification can work safely only in a closed chamber, but it seriously lacks the basic element of continuous perfusion, like in a Blumenthal or 3 port vitrectomy. Hence, pressure fluctuations are very high. Initially, if you look at the historic development of phacoemulsification over several decades, the high pressure and a closed eye were created, so as to deepen emulsification process occurs far away from the endothelium, within the inflated capsular bag. The ultrasound of phacoemulsification, in its initial phases of development, literally destroyed the endothelium! To solve this, CCC and endocapsular emulsification techniques were developed. They work best in a closed eye, where intraocular pressures can be kept high, without leakage or any fluid. So, tight and small incisions were developed with valvular configuration, which wouldn't leak fluid. Further, to clean up the mess that is created in AC, machines were modified to have increased fluid exchanges, and this was also aimed at reducing the ultrasonic impact on tissues. This necessitated maintenance of a high pressure in anterior segment. The very high rate and volume of fluid turnover dissipates the heat and sonic energy waves generated within the eye by the phaco-probe during the process of lens emulsification. The temperature of the tunnel goes upto 80 degrees if the fluid flow through the sleeve stops even for a short while! Now the new problem was to meticulously balance the large inflow to the outflow so as to avoid sudden increase or decrease in IOP, so called surges, which can be disastrous. All the current machine developments are aiming at fine tuning the balance between pressures and flows at inlet and outlet of the eye so as to maintain a high-flow, high-pressure low surges and to at minimise the role of ultrasound. Today every emulsifying surgeon aspires to use ultrasound as little as possible and prefer to perform most of the steps manually by one or other way. The pumps in the machine became stronger to give better suction and better hold. Inspite of this the older compulsion of high fluidics and high-pressures is somehow retained as a vestige. Why not we go ahead and get rid of these sidekicks of emulsification era? Now that manual chopping techniques have largely invaded the so Called phacoemulsification, the need for the older concepts of high-pressure and high fluidics appears to be logically superfluous.

In phacoemulsificatoin, more than half the time of surgery, there is no perfusion into the eye to maintain a closed chamber, while all the ports have become leaky and fish mouthed by mechanical pushing of larger sized probes e.g. to insert a 2.8 mm diameter phacoprobe a 2.8 mm slit incision is made. The phacoprobe does not have a slit configuration, but has a cylindrical configuration! It needs a slit of half of its circumference to atraumatically get in. A 2.8 mm cylinder has a circumference of Pie X diameter, that is 22/7 X 2.8 = 8.8 mm. That means the slit needed is 4.4 mm! So when you create a slit of 2.8 mm and introduce a 2.8 mm phacoprobe, you are tearing the tunnel width from 2.8 mm to 4.4 mm, that is by a 157 percent. As the cornea is nonelastic, this tearing would fish-mouth the tunnel, so you need a stromal hydration to close the tunel. It will heal by scarring and so produce changes in the corneal topography. Phacosection scores abundant marks on every one of these fronts.

Phacosection has the best fluidics. The pressure fluctuations and turbulence in AC are the lowest. IOP is maintained at level between 0 to 20 mm Hg unlike 30 to 40 mmHg in Blumenthal and 0 to 80 mmHg in phacoemulsification. At no point in phacosection does the ONH and retinal circulation is compromised. This is particularly important in glaucoma and diabetic retinopathy. The flow rates and the total amount of fluid used in phacosection are lowest. In majority of cases, it is only from 30 to 50 ml. In phacoemulsification, if 300 ml of BSS is used over a 10 minutes surgery, (half the time there is no flow) there would be a flow of 60 ml per minute through the AC when the phacoprobe or IA is being used! This is a very high velocity, giving rise to great velocities, eddies and turbulence within that tiny little anterior chamber! In the newer sleeveless probe phacoemulsification, where the infusion sleeve is removed from the phacoprobe to make the incision smaller, lot more fluids go through the AC and tubings to cool the direct heating of tunnel. Yes, most of the phacosection is performed under hypotonic environment. I have never seen choroidal engorgement, detachment or hemorrhages caused by a few minutes of hypotony! CME is exceptionally rare as it is produced by inflammation and not by hypotony! I have heard people talk of higher pressure in AC and the fluids flowing only from within to out of eye, taking the blood and contaminants out. In phacosection, the bleeding is almost nil due to limited dissection. And as fluidics is minimal, the chance for any outside particles being taken in is miniscule. Any aspiration in the AC is well balanced by simultaneous infusion by Simcoe IA cannula.

ANTERIOR CAPSULOTOMY

The capsulorhexis or continuous curvilinear capsulotomy (CCC) as first proposed separately by Gimbel and Neuhann involves controlled tearing of the anterior capsule to produce a smooth, strong, round and regular opening. The capsulorhexis can be quite difficult to learn. Trying all other techniques, I have designed an easy way to consistently perform CCC in every situation. The concepts are:

i. Done in a closed chamber so that AC can be maintained deep. Iris lens diaphragm is pushed backward so that the anterior capsule-zonule complex is loose. There are least centrifugal forces to pull the-rhexis away from its path. If the AC becomes shallow, the lens iris diaphragm moves anteriorly, and the anterior capsule is put on a stretch due to its zonular attachments, and than there will be a greater tendency for the rhexis margin to run off to the periphery.

ii. Aqueous-air exchange is performed so that the AC is fully filled with Air. The large surface tension of the air keeps the capsular flap nicely folded down. It also enhances the visibility by giving better reflections from various surfaces.

1. *Aqueous-air exchange*: Mount the 26 G cystitome on a 2 ml syringe filled with air. Pass the cystitome into the tunnel upto the limbus. Rotate the syringe so that the 90 degrees bent needle tip is downwards. Puncture the floor of the tunnel *at the limbus* so that you are inside the AC. Don't enter the AC at the corneal end of the tunnel as this would distort the cornea, reducing visibility, when you start doing CCC. Also, remain in the middle 1/3 rd of the tunnel. If you enter the AC near the side of the tunnel, you would end up orelocking, when the shaft of the cystitome hits the side of the tunnel. Now rotate it by 90 degrees so that the tip does not catch the peripheral iris. Proceed to the center of the chamber. If the eye is soft, inject a small air bubble into the eye. Next is to make way for the exit for Aqueous. A 30-G disposable needle is passed throughthe clear cornea at 3 O'clock, just inside the limbus, obliquely so as flows into AC, withdraw the 30 G needle. Now you have a deep air filled, transparent anterior chamber

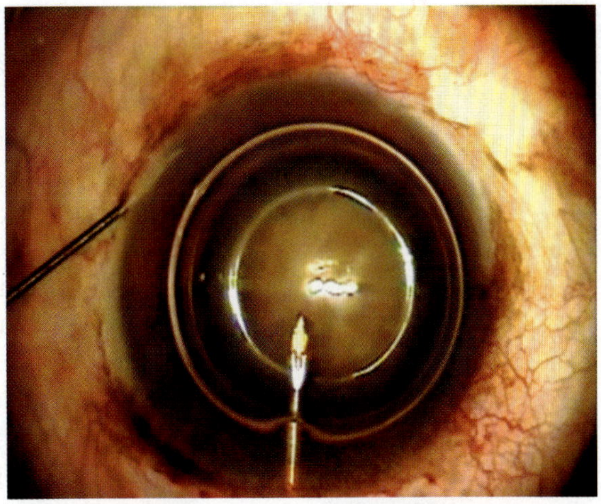

Fig. 29.4: Aqueous air exchange

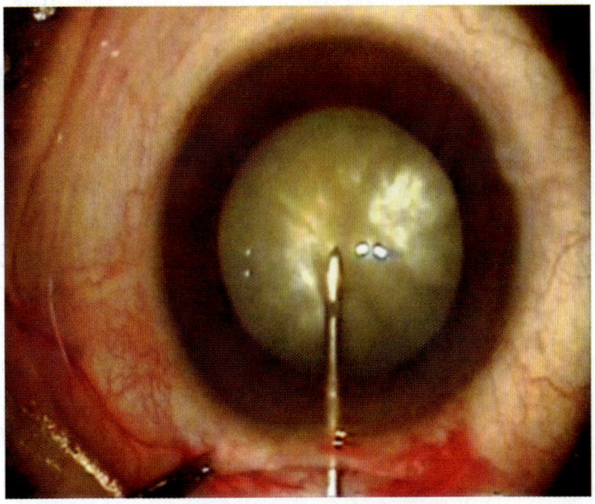

Fig. 29.5: Milking of HMSC

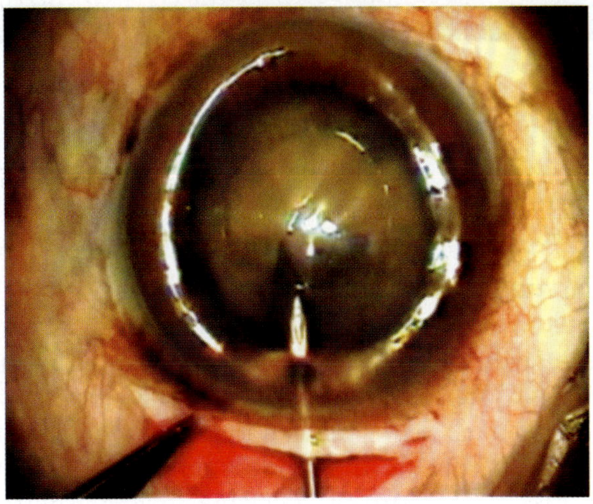

Fig. 29.6: CCC and trypan blue

with lax and retro-pushed anterior capsule, in a closed eye and this is the key to a successful CCC. The large surface tension of the air bubble will hold the capsule tightly back and the flap nicely folded. For hypermature and intumescent cataracts, Than puncture the center of the anterior capsule with the cystitome before injecting air into AC. The milk slowly flows into the AC. It than gets extruded out of AC through the 30 G needle during the aqueous air exchange. Put a drop of Trypan blue on the anterior capsule now, the dry capsule in an air filled AC stains blue instantaneously!

2. *Capsulorhexis*: I perform the rhexis with a 26 G capsulotomy needle as it is easier, simple and economical. The anterior capsule is taut due to air in the anterior chamber. No visco is used. It is important to begin the rhexis at the center of the anterior capsule. After making few can opening incisions to the right of the center, a small triangular flap of anterior capsule is raised. The bent needle is placed near the edge of this flap and the tear continued in an anticlock direction to create a circular tear of the desired size. It is ideal to create a CCC of diameter about 5 mm so that the entire edge of the anterior capsule is physically separated from the posterior capsule.
3. *In small pupils:* The rhexis can be done under the iris. The reflections from the iris surface is seen so vividly under air, that you could identify the tearing capsule through the iris.

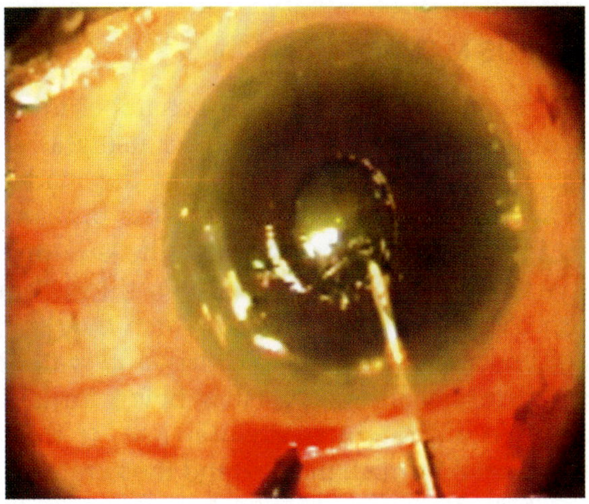

Fig. 29.7: CCC in small pupil

No matter how carefully you perform CCC, an occasional difficulty could be encountered. CCC can tend to run off toward the equator. Stop the procedure, push in some more air to deepen AC and to relax the zonules and than continue the rhexis. When the end point is nearer, ensure that the tear joins the circle from the outside. This ensures that there are no weak points in the rhexis margin. If the tear runs off to the periphery, a long blade Vannas scissors or the cysitome can be used to make a fresh nick in the border of the capsulotomy. Start a new rhexis to go and join the old. A beginner should not hesitate to convert it into a can-open type of capsulotomy.

Why do CCC? Some of the advantages of this technique are:

A. In the bag placement of the IOL is possible. This promotes long-term centration of the IOL, which is all the more important in bifocal, multifocal and higher order aberration corrected IOLs.
B. In the bag IOL insertion is safe. It secludes the IOL, avoids uveal tissue contact with the IOL and reduces the incidence of iritis.
C. The structural rigidity and integrity of the bag are near normal.
D. If an inadvertent posterior capsular tear occurs and insertion of PC IOL in the bag is not feasible, it can now be placed safely in front of the anterior capsule.
E The aspiration of the cortical matter is entirely wlth in the bag, prevents iris pigment release.
F. Less chances of iris being caught during I/A.

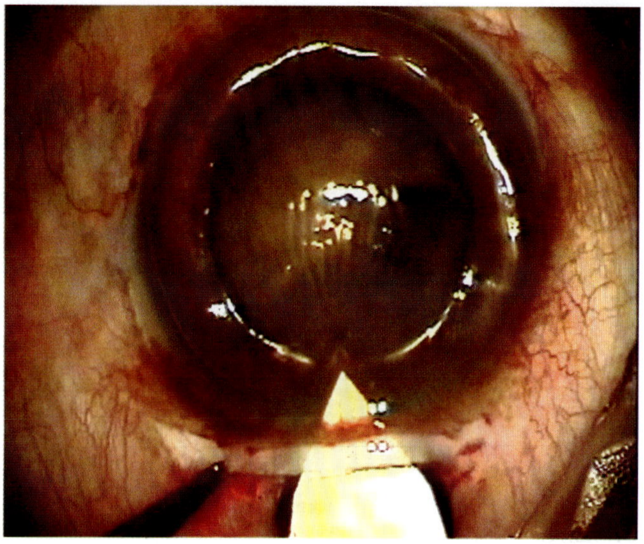

Fig. 29.8: Keratome entry after CCC

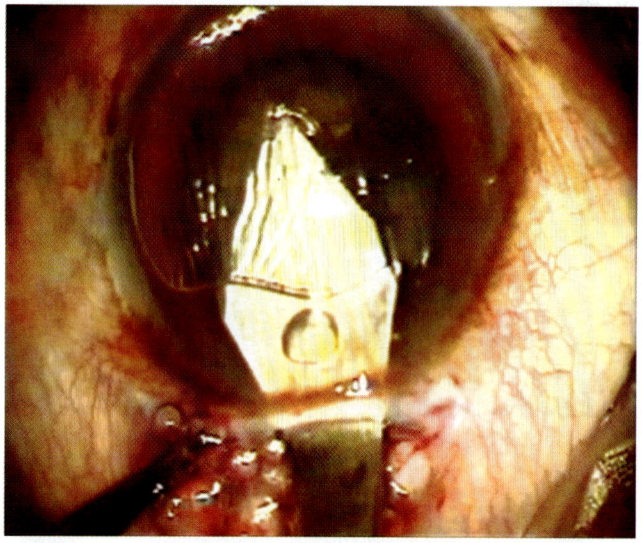

Fig. 29.9: Keratome with sharp tip entry

NUCLEUS MANAGEMENT

At this stage I enter the anterior chamber through the tunnel that was created earlier using a 5-mm sharp keratome or slit blade. Dip the blade tip downward at the anterior end of the tunnel and enter into the AC. Then straighten the keratome to be parallel to the iris and go down till the entire width of the incision is made. Watch the tip as it should not touch the cornea or iris, and watch the internal tunnel incision as it is being formed, it should be a straight horizontal line. If the AC remains well formed, than extend the keratome on either side by a small amount so that you have about 6.0 mm of internal opening. If you are implanting a 6 mm PMMA IOL, depending upon its thickness, you could make the incision to about 6.5 mm wide. The anterior capsular flap and the air in AC are removed with Simcoe cannula.

Hydroprocedures Perform only hydrodissection, to cleavage the plane between the cortex and capsule, so that cortical removal at a later stage becomes an easy job. Hydroprocedure in my technique has *nothing to do* with nucleus management, which is done entirely by mechanical movements. Avoid hydrodelination (separation of cortex from epinucleus) and hydrodelamination (separation of epinucleus and nucleus, and then separation of different layers of nucleus itself) as they would leave behind variable amounts of cortex and epinucleus, which needs to be managed with fluidics at the end.

This is an *open chamber* procedure The 26 G cannula is passed under the anterior capsule, without disturbing the cortex. Than following the curve of the anterior capsule, proceed laterally and posteriorly toward the equator of the lens. Than lift the shaft of the cannula upward toward the iris, tenting up the anterior capsule. Start meeting BSS continuously and watch out for any of the following happenings:

a. Fluid pass across the red reflex
b. Lifting up of the nucleus at 9 O'clock
c. Prolapse of the nucleus into AC
d. Shallowing of AC.

See that the fluid freely flows out of the capsular bag and out through the open tunnel. Open chamber ensures that you don't have to limit the amount of fluid being injected and ensures that the posterior capsule would never give way, which is very important in posterior subcapsular cataract. YES, you could do a hydrodissection in posterior subcapsular cataract, just ensure that it is an open chamber and that there is no viscoelastic in the anterior chamber to hinder the free exit of BSS and the pressure in the capsular bag remains low.

The fluid that dissects capsule from cortex does not produce a golden ring. It is the hydrodelineation that produces a golden ring, because of the total internal reflection from the prism like accumulation of fluid at the genu of fluid sheet as it takes a U turn from the front of the lens to the back of the lens. Hence do not aim to achieve a golden ring and if your technique is yielding golden ring, than find the proper plane in your next case.

The anterior chamber is filled with a viscoelastic only after hydrodissection. Start from 6 O'clock and see that entire AC is filled with visco. This technique coats the endothelium well and protects it throughout out the following procedures. A dispersive visco is better than a cohesive viscoelastic. The former gives a better coat to the endothelium, and would not go away easily with the BSS turbulence. Well, until now the steps were

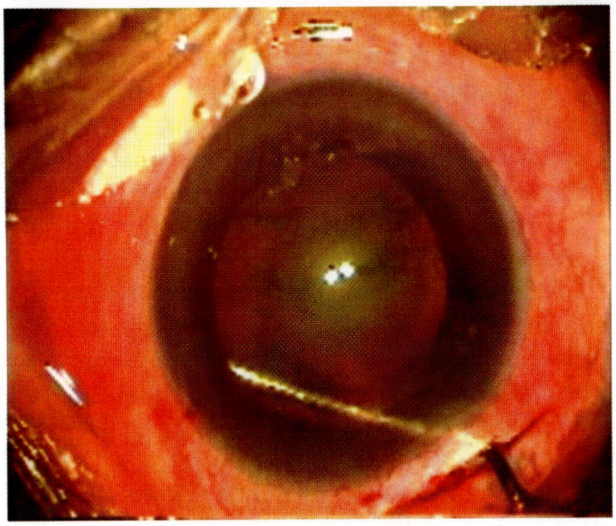

Fig. 29.10: Hydrodissection

conceptually similar to that of phacoemulsifaction. Following are the maneuvers that differentiate the two.

The contents within the capsular bag are in three layers and the relative sizes and texture depends upon the patients' age and status of cataract. In the very young there is no hard central 'nucleus'. In older patients more and more cortex becomes hardened and incorporated into the nucleus. Surrounding the nucleus is the gelatinous, pliable epinucleus which is the transitional material between cortex and nucleus. Indeed epinucleus was never described, either surgically or histologically before the phacoemulsification era! It gained importance because it is too soft to be handled like nucleus arid too hard to be aspirated like cortex!

Based on the nucleus management, there are several different types of doing manual SICS. They can be classified as under:

1. The nucleus is delivered in its wholesome. The tunnel is created like a funnel and the nucleus is pushed out with hydro/visco/mechanical forces. As the circumference of nucleus is bigger than the circumference of tunnel, the tunnel gets stretched during the delivery. You need to create a larger tunnel.
2. Minification of nucleus so that it is stripped of epinucleus, and than its removal. This leaves a large amount of epinucleus and cortex behind. The tunnel is again made like a funnel, with a

larger internal opening and a smaller external opening. The tunnel is still stretches in majority of cataracts as the nucleus is pushed out. Only those nuclei which can be squeezed into a cylinder of diameter 3.80 mm can come out through a 6 mm tunnel, without stretching it! All others tear the tunnel although they are created larger.

3. Division of nuclei and making them into smaller cylindrical pieces, 2 or 3, is logically the most elegant and appropriate technique, which aim at retaining the integrity of the tunnel.

For 1 and 2 you need a larger tunnel. Scleral dissection is extensive, with side pockets. To find such a large area without major scleral vessels is difficult, and so bleeding is more common. You need more cautery which could affect scleral architecture. However, big the tunnel is the nucleus does stretch the tunnel.

In Phacosection, the Aim is

1. To remove as much of lens matter as possible along with nucleus. It includes the entire epinucleus and majority of cortex.
2. To avoid stretching of the tunnel, so that the collagen fibers of cornea (which are non elastic) and the sclera (which are very minimally elastic) are not broken.
3. To give maximum protection to the endothelium.

To achieve these, don't disrupt the integrity of hard nucleus, epinucleus and cortex! This is the exact reason why I insisted to avoid hydrodelineation procedure. Let me use the word nucleus to represent all the three structures in the following description!

To deliver the nucleus into the AC, use the following maneuvers:

a. Right hand holds 26 G cannula mounted on a 2 ml syringe filled with visco. Left eye holds Sinskey hook.
b. Rotate the nucleus within the capsule in an anticlock direction, like you rotate the steering wheel of a car. Imagine that there is a steering column, which holds the center of the nucleus in one position. This maneuvers separates the peripheral cortex from inner cortex. What is being rotated is exactly what you are going to remove. What is left behind is aspirated later.
c. Push the nucleus to its left with Sinskey hook. Pass the tip of the cannula under the right edge of the nucleus and hold it slightly lifted up, in a plane slightly in front of the capsular bag. Now rotate the nucleus anticlockwise, bimanually. As the right edge of the nucleus has been lifted up to the front of the capsule, rest of the nucleus gets rotated out of bag, as though a screw is coming out of a bolt. You actually walk on the equator of the nucleus with the two instruments, with a slight lifting pressure, and the nucleus gets rotated out of the capsular bag. This is a bimanual procedure and hence minimizes lateral shifting of the nucleus. Any lateral movement of the lens will exert an undesirable stretch on the opposite zonules. This zonular stretch is undesirable in myopes, mature cataracts, brown cataracts, pseudoexfoliation, subluxations, etc. Rarely does the epinucleus get separated from the nucleus during these maneuvers.
d. In very soft nuclei, like in posterior capsular or subcapsular cataracts, pass the cannula right into the center of the nucleus, like the stick inside a lollypop, and nudge and maneuver the entire nucleus into the AC. It is easy.
e. Endothelial protection is paramount. This is done by continuous injection of dispersive

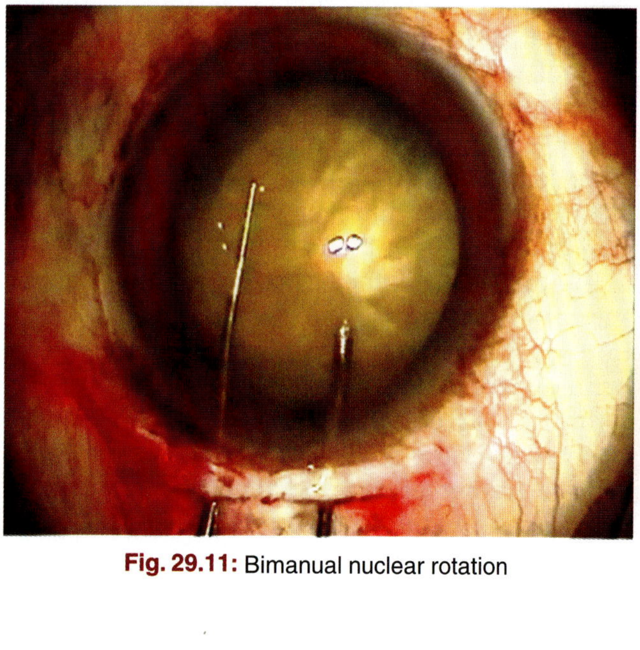

Fig. 29.11: Bimanual nuclear rotation

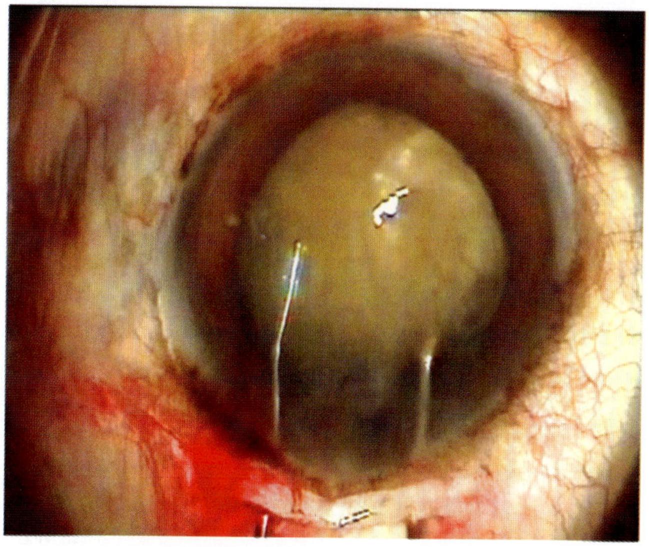

Fig. 29.12: Nuclear prolapse into AC

visco throughout the next few steps. This keeps refilling the space between the nucleus and cornea.

f. Change the left hand instrument to wire vectis. The right hand holds the syringe in a position so that the thumb is on the piston and it is ready to continuously inject visco.
g. Tip the 12 O'clock nucleus anteriorly and pass the wire vectis under the nucleus. Remember that the nucleus is biconvex, and your movement should be in conformity with this. Otherwise you would be hitting the bulge of

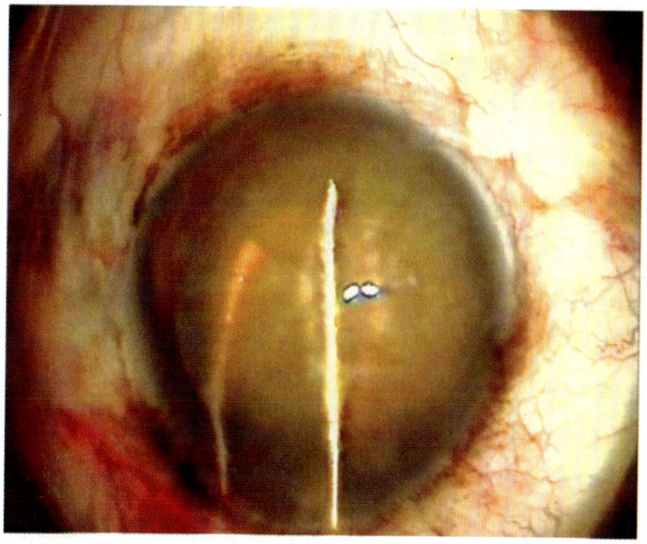

Fig. 29.13: Nuclear bisection

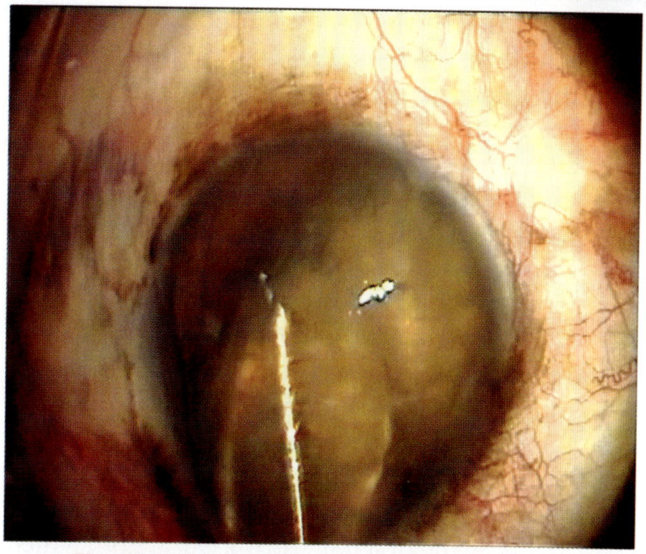

Fig. 29.14: Viscosandwich of first half of nucleus

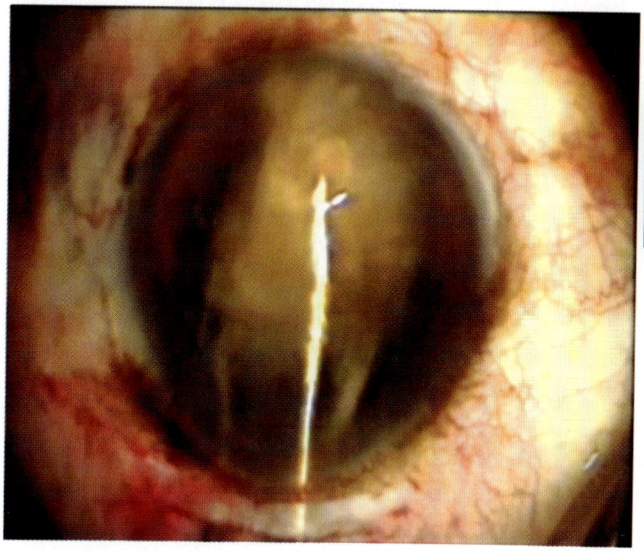

Fig. 29.15: Viscosandwich of 2nd half of nucleus

the nucleus with wire vectis, and the nucleus will move downward! See that nucleus does not move at all when you are inserting the wire vectis. Check, if the lower end of the vectis has gone under the iris, and catch inferior iris between it and nucleus. The shiny vectis is visible through all types of nuclei!

h. Pass the 26g half-inch cannula in front of the nucleus. You could pass it through cortex, if you like so. Continuously inject visco through out these procedures.

i. Hold the vectis steady, supporting the exact middle of nucleus. Press the cannula towards the vectis so that the shaft of the cannula bisects the nucleus. This motion should be slow and steady. You will be surprised to see that the shaft can bisect any nucleus, however hard it may be! Continuously inject visco through out! For very hard nucleus, use the Sinskey hook instead of the cannula. Than you will not be injecting the visco.

j. Inject more visco between two halves of nucleus and confirm that they are fully separated. If any connections are remaining, nudge them with visco injecting cannula so that they get separated. Otherwise, the 2nd half tends to follow the first half during extraction, which is not desirable.

k. Now slide the vectis under the left half of nucleus. The cannula is positioned on the front surface of the nucleus. This sandwich containing vectis behind, nucleus in between and cannula in front are removed from the AC through the tunnel, slowly Don't change the direction of the movement; which should be in line with the tunnel, till the end of the nucleus is out of tunnel! Tip the upper end of the nucleus anteriorly and depress the posterior lip of the tunnel incision as the nucleus slides out of AC, so that the scleral valve does not engage the upper pole. The visco is continuously injected through out, and this prevents AC from collapsing, in addition to maximally protecting the endothelium.

l. Now inject visco in front of the right half of nucleus. It is than moved to the center of AC, in-line with the tunnel. It is similarly sandwiched between the wire vectis and visco injecting cannula and gently taken out of eye in a similar movement.

If the nucleus fails to prolapse into the anterior chamber it is because you have not given enough lift to the right edge before rotating it. If the technique is correct, usually the size of capsulorhexis and nucleus do not affect this, as capsule is quite elastic. However in the initial stages, if the rhexis is grossly undersized, don't try to force the nucleus out, you will break zonules or capsule and loose vitreous. Perform a single relaxing incision at 10 O'clock and then proceed. You just need to nick the edge of rhexis with your cystitome and the nucleus maneuver will tear it to the amount it needs! Usually the tear extends till equator, and never extends to posterior capsule, unless you are very clumsy. In this situation, do not initiate hydrodissection around the relaxing cut. Remove posterior cortex here only at the end and till than it will be holding the fort, preventing the tear from extending'to posterior capsule. When you implant the IOL, a modified C loop is better than J loop, see that the one of the loop is across the relaxing incision. If the tear has extended to posterior capsule, than place the loops of the IOL perpendicular to the position of the relaxing incision.

At times the nuclear fragment can break off in the tunnel at this stage. Push the fragment back into the anterior chamber with visco. Align is such a way that its long axis is in line with the tunnel and remove it with wire vectis. If any resistance is met during extraction of the nuclear fragment, do not persist with the extraction. Check, if the upper pole of nucleus has gone under the scleral valve, through the hole the vectis. If so realign it again into the tunnel. If the nucleus is extra big and hard, don't hesitate to enlarge the tunnel.

CORTICAL ASPIRATION

Very little cortex is left behind. It is easily aspirated using straight and right and left 12 O'clock Simcoe cannulas. The beauty of this open chamber technique is that you don't have to critically match the inflow of fluid to outflow of fluid, drop by drop, as in a closed eye situation! Hence there are no major pressure fluctuations, no turbulence and most importantly there are no surges! You don't need to have the expensive microprocessors and gadgets to monitor the pressures and flows inside the eye, and motors to quickly respond to the calls! Life becomes so easy and comfortable.

Position the aspirating port just under the edge of anterior cortex and suck it into the port. While you start aspirating the anterior leaf into the port, give a gentle centripetal movement to the cannula, and a pie shaped segment of the cortex, like a pizza slice, gets stripped off. A deep anterior chamber

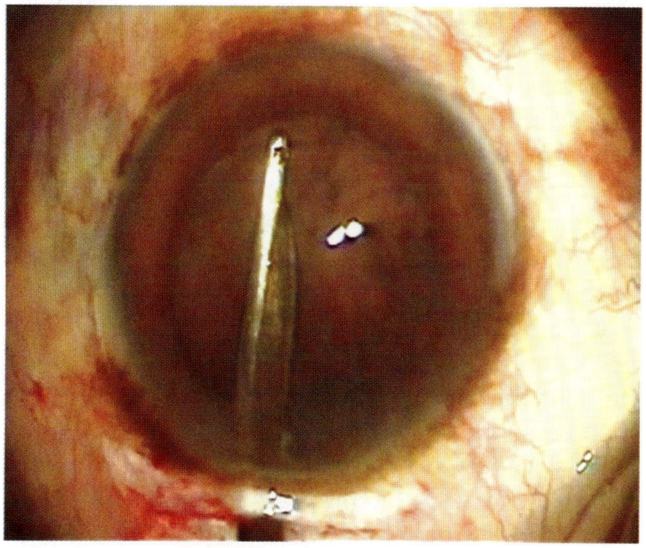

Fig 29.16: Cortical aspiration

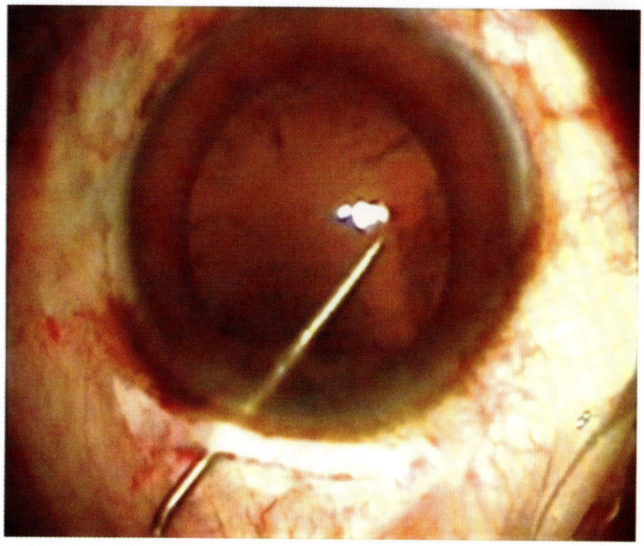

Fig 29.18: Hydroplanning

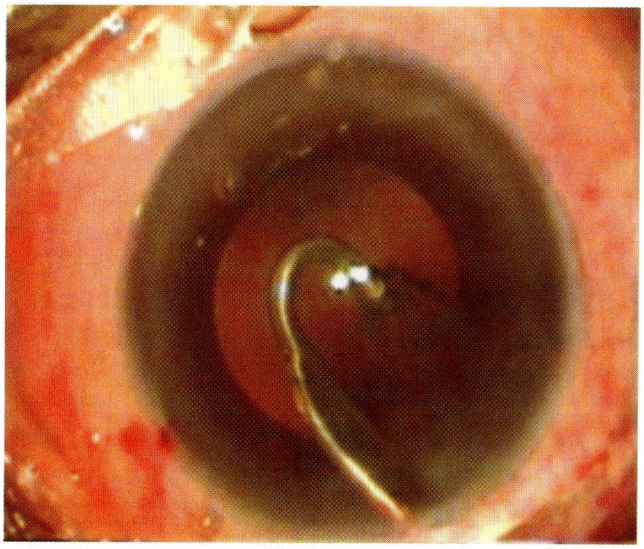

Fig 29.17: Subincisional cortex

facilitates this stripping. When AC is shallow, the posterior capsule strangles the cortex against the anterior capsule, and aspiration can become extremely difficult. In such extreme situations, fill the AC with visco so that the capsular bag remains wide open. Now without injecting BSS, go and hold the anterior cortical leaf and drag into the center. Visco holds the AC deep as long as you don't inject BSS and push it out of chamber! No problems if you have done it, just refill the AC with visco and proceed. It is vital to remove every bit of cortical matter to reduce the incidence of postoperative inflammation as well as after-cataract and capsular fibrosis.

Very rarely, if the hydrodissection is in the wrong plane, the epinuclear bowl is left behind and than it becomes extremely difficult to aspirate it, even with a large port Simcoe cannula. The best is to nudge the epinucleus towards the center, from all directions, using the tip of 26 G cannula. Once the majority of it is in the middle, go under the eninucleus and inject visco. Now the epinucleus can be lifted into AC and removed using the wire vectis and viscoexpression.

Once cortical aspiration is completed, the posterior capsule should be inspected and residual opacities if any are removed by careful polishing with the back of Simcoe cannula with continued aspiration. I do hydroplanning to remove stubborn debris from posterior capsule. Keep the tunnel open, and inject a fine jet of BSS with moderate force, using 26 G cannula, in a direction almost parallel to the posterior capsule. The fluid jet clears away the opacities and debris on the posterior capsule. There will not be any sudden increase in the IOP, as it is an open chamber technique, nor there will be any damage to posterior capsule. This is an excellent technique to get rid of posterior capsular tags, cells, fibers, clumps and opacities. The Simcoe cannula is than used to aspirate the anterior capsular epithelial cells, by gently scrubbing and aspirating them using all the three cannulas. Note that there are no side ports in phacosection.

Few General Principal of Cortical Removal

A. This part of phacosection is an open chamber technique. Preoperative hypotony is of great use here, as it minimizes the vitreous upthrust and keeps the AC deeper. It could be converted into a pseudo-closed chamber with visco or a true-closed chamber if additional side ports are created for I A. Deep AC and deep capsular bag facilitate engagement of the peripheral cortex for aspiration and stripping.

B. The aspiration port must always face the cornea. However, it can be turned in any direction to catch the anterior leaf of cortex, but never toward the capsule.

C. The superior cortex is aspirated with separate right and left 12 O'clock cannulas, through the main tunnel. The aspirating cannula here is curved to a U shape. It also can be used to retract the iris to visualize left over cortex. It is important to remove every piece of superior cortex as it can later get hydrated and gravitate downward, to settle behind the IOL, affecting the vision.

Cortex removal in event of PC tear:

1. Identify and assess the extent and margin of the tear
2. Minimize the extension of the tear by stopping infusion
3. Release all the pressures on the eye, if any
4. Check if hyaloidal face is broken and if vitreous has herneated. If no, form the AC with Visco.
5. Attempt dry aspiration, where there is no infusion and the aspiration is minimal to avoid vitreous fibers getting into the port. Fill the AC with visco. Without irrigating, take the Simcoe cannula right upto the cortex, aspirate and also strip the cortex away from the capsule. Once the cortex gets engaged into the port, vitreous and fluid cannot enter and hence you can strip the cortex out. If AC collapses, refill with visco. If Vitreous fibers get into the port, as evidenced by the movement of iris and posterior capsule, you have no other option but to do a vitrectomy procedure.
6. The cortex should be aspirated from the intact capsule toward the margins of the tear, taking care not to enlarge the tear.

On rare occasions you find the loose cortex sticking on to the corneal endothelium and may obscure visualization for cortical cleanup in the bag. Reverse flushing with the Simcoe cannula will flood the cortex out. Reverse flushing (aspirated fluid in the syringe is pushed back into the AC, through the aspiration port) unlike in phaco-emulsification, do not bring in unsterile fluid into the eye. The other technique is to inject visco on to the endothelium, which will sweep all the material out of the eye. If adherent cortex does not obstruct visualization then leave it alone.

IMPLANTATION OF INTRAOCULAR LENS

The IOL of choice is a full optic 6 mm dia IOL with 12 mm overall diameter, with no dialing holes or optically disturbing optic haptic junctions. It is desirable to have a single piece modified 'C' loop PMMA IOL or a Foldable IOL. The AC and capsular bag is filled with visco. The IOL optic is grasped with the Mcphersen's forceps. Flush the IOL with BSS and coat with Visco. Apply lots of visco over the sclera around the section. Nudge the leading haptic into to the tunnel, and push it gently into the AC. Without releasing the optic, position the lower loop into the capsular bag and push the entire optic of the IOL into the AC. Now release the optic but immediately hold the superior optic with another straight forceps. Otherwise the pressure in the AC and the bend in the IOL haptics that you have created (Note that the tunnel is directed uphill and you then need to go downhill to reach the inferior cul de sac) will push the IOL outward, and the lower loop will come out of the the sac! So don't release the superior optic. Next the upper haptic is dialed into the capsular bag using a dialer or Sinskey hook. Position the IOL in such a way that the folds it creates in the posterior capsule are horizontal. In case the IOL of your choice has optical defects like optic-haptic junctions, holes, etc. position the IOL such that these aberrations are situated in the vertical meridian. If they are situated temporally, they may give rise to intractable visual aberrations like glare, tails, wisps, etc. especially in dim light like while night driving. Phacosection is compatible to any type of IOL. You don't have to limit the choice of IOL to those which have to be squeezed through folders and injectors. You do not have to punish a good foldable IOL, sometimes deforming and even tearing it, by squeezing it through instruments. Economically viable PMMA IOL, which is the gold standards even now, are no problem for the 6 mm tunnel. Please do not compromize the size of the IOL to-less than 6 mm, as it would hamper the mesopic vision, when the pupil dilates.

As you have not distructed or stretched the tunnel, it would be watertight. There is no need for stromal hydration or to check for the integrity of the tunnel. Check the IOP by a gentle tap on the limbus and watch for indentation. Don't press the corneal dome to check the IOP! Draw the conjunctiva over the wound and patch the eye.

The postoperative instructions are very few. The patient can resume all the activities. He can wash his face and also have a shower right from the 1st postoperative day. Spectacle of residual refractive errors can be done in the first week itself, as the refraction is going to be stable. You would be surprised to see that whatever corneal astigmatism

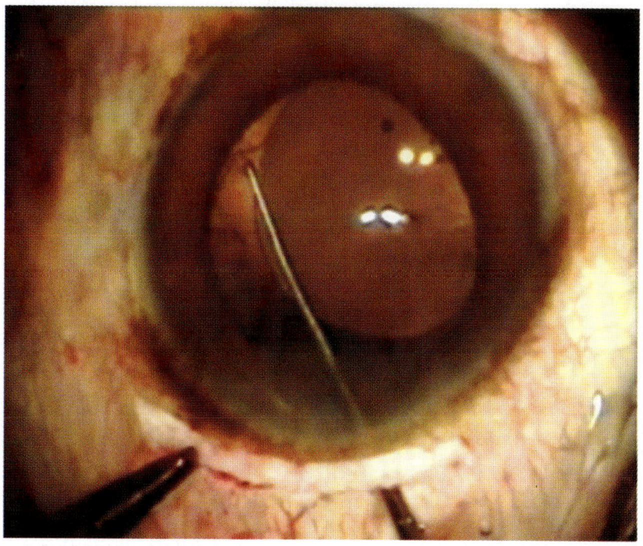

Fig. 29.19: PMMA IOL dialing of upper loop

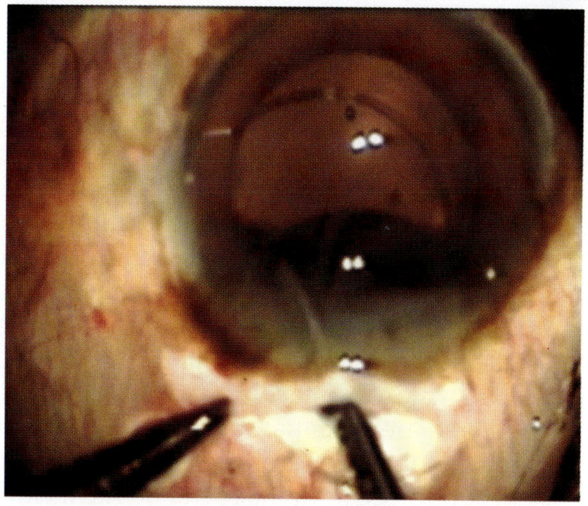

Fig. 29.20: PMMA IOL lower loop into bag

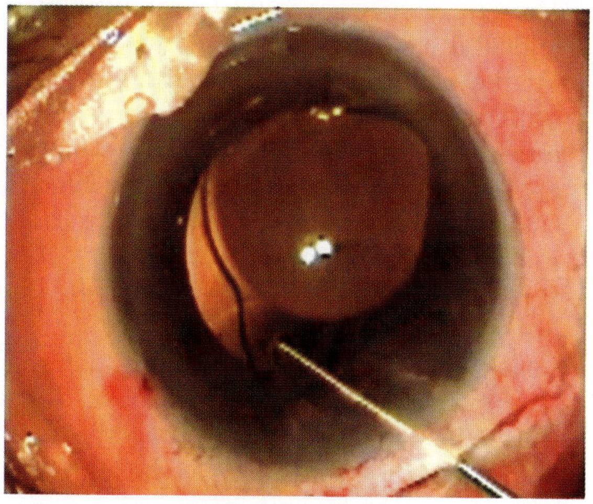

Fig. 29.21: Acrylic IOL

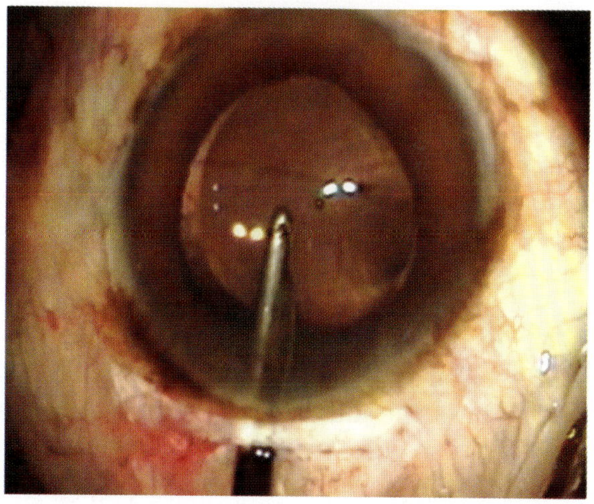

Fig. 29.22: PC folds indicating within the bag positioning of IOL

the patient had preoperatively, and would continue to remain the same for ever. SIA in an unpunished tunnel, even if it is 6 mm wide, is negligible. On the first postoperative day. on Rio-microscopy, the Corneas are crystal clear. The Incidence ot complications in this technique is extremely low.

The obvious advantages of this technique are:

1. Complete asepsis is possible in phacosection. This is almost impossible with machine techniques, with its tubing coming in and out of sterile field and with the refluxes. The tubings that go inside the machine can never be sterilized, and are potential sources of infection.
2. Ultrasound time is Zero! There is no possibility of heat damage or damage due to ultrasound probe to the tunnel or to the anterior segment.
3. The entire surgery is performed in physiological intraocular pressures, very important in all eyes, but especially in those where the optic nerve or retinal circulation is compromized, like in glaucoma, diabetic retinopathy, etc. I have never seen a choroidal bleeding, CME or postoperative inflammation due the intraoperative hypotony.
4. It is a low cost because no expensive gadgets are needed.
5. Least wound trauma and least of astigmatic change as the wound is not stretched, destructed or heated. No need to keep the wound watertight during surgery, as the ambience is physiological pressures.
6. Turbulence is minimized because very little BSS is used, less than 50 ml per surgery, at very low pressures and flow rates.
7. The option of using a 6-mm diameter PMMA lens is open! PMMA lenses create least changes in higher order aberrations, are available with heparin coated optics and are also available in Diffraction Bifocal design, unlike Foldable lOLs. They are also available in long C loop design, which are the best for the capsule.
8. The option of using a foldable lens is always there. The indication may be the material, its stickiness, the square edge, higher order aberration correction or reduced PCO. You don't need to fold the lens or squeeze it through an injector, to put into the capsular bag.

Disadvantages

- There is a very definite learning curve. The technique looks very simple, but needs to be slowly acquainted before mastering it.

GUIDELINES FOR BEGINNERS

The technique and instrumentation in cataract surgery is changing rapidly. It is important to initially try out as many different methods as you can, under proper guidance and training. Learn phacoemulsification fully, as there are many training programs promoted by the industry. It will give you good foundations, particularly in fluidics and nuclear management. Write down the difficulties you had with each surgery and if possible video record when ever you change a step. Don't let go even a small trouble you had at any stage. Watch it later, you would get so much of feedback. Read books on SICS, observe experienced surgeons doing this wonderful procedure and watch videocassettes of Masters. When you visit somebody, record their surgeries, and watch it repeatedly at home.

Once you have begun to implement the change, do it one step at a time. Make small modifications in your extracapsular or phacoemulsification technique. From ECCE the best route would be to master the CCC, nuclear bisection, visco-sandwich and cortical aspiration and than move on to creating smaller incisions and last is to try with shorter and later longer tunnels. Doing a small CCC is easy and later you can do a relaxing incision in the anterior capsule before expressing the nucleus. Avoid using the technique, initially, in very soft and very hard cataracts. Visit an accomplished surgeon before starting, and after doing about 25 cases. The best learning is by video recording your surgery, and to critically analyze them. Donot hesitate to take them to your mentor, and discuss specific difficulties and problems. Attend all cataract update workshops, whether it is SICS or phacoemulsification. There will be plenty of newer developments to learn about and implement.

The beauty of the scleral tunnel is that you can simply withdraw all instruments at any stage of the surgery, and it is a water tight wound now. Nothing can get in and nothing can come out.

If you can do a good extracapsular cataract extraction or good phacoemulsification sugery, you can perform a good phacosection. The learning curves are similar, but the concepts are different. With phacosection, you have the absolute control on the situation, at every single, step and moment, and you remain the master. There are no surprises, no accidents and no gadgets. Everything happens as you dictate. All you need to do is set your mind on it! Enjoy the surgery!

REFERENCES

1. Norman S Jaffe. Cataract Surgery and its Complications (4th edition) CV Mosby company: St Louis, USA.
2. Paul S Koch. Converting to Phacoemulsification, JP brothers publications, 1992.
3. Richard C Troatman, Kurt A Buzard: Etiology, Prevention and Management. CV Mosby company, 1992.
4. Keneith P. Wolf, Lewiston Maine. Phacosection, A small Incision Alternative.

Journals

1. Steve Arshinoff. Mechanics of Capsulorhexis Journal of Cataract and Refractive Surgery 1992;18.
2. Susanne Krag, Kirster Thim, Leif Corydon. Strength of the lens capsule during hydro-expression of the nucleus. J Cataract Refractive Surgery 1993;19.
3. Milind Pande. Continuous curvilinear (circular) capsulorhexis and planned ECCE are they compatable? BJO 1993;77:152-57.
4. Samuel Masket. Yes you can use small incision in problem eyes. Review of Ophthalmology 1995.
5. Luther L Fry. How to do small incision planned extracapsular extraction. Review of Ophthalmology 1995.
6. Chistopher S Connor: Temporal incision. Review of Ophthalmology 1995.
7. Instrumentation guide; Ocular surgery news. Slack incorporated, New Jercey, USA 1995;6(11):44-53.
8. Morgan Chanda. IOP after peribulbar anestheisa, is the Honan balloon necessary? BJO 1995;79:46-49.
9. Ana Matheu et al. Manual nucleofragmentation and endothelial cell loss. J Cataract Refract Surg 1997;23:995-97.
10. Clemens Vass et al. Conreal topographic changes after frown and straight sclerocorneal incisions. J cataract Refract Surg 1997;23:913-21.

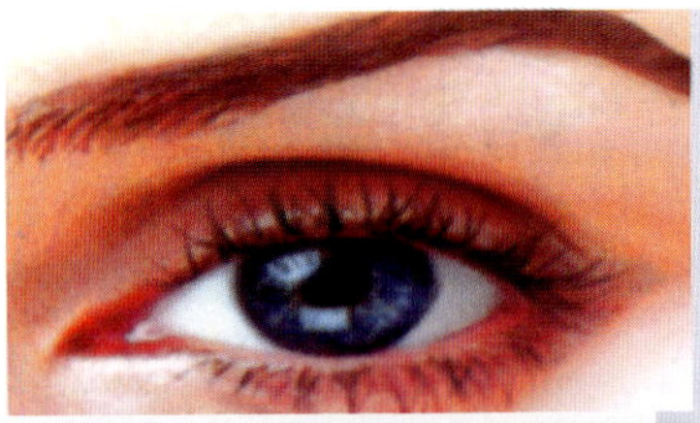

Thirty

Manual Small Incision Cataract Surgery Using Irrigating Vectis

RD Ravindran
K Thiruvenkata Krishnan (India)

INTRODUCTION

Hydroexpression with an irrigating vectis is a simple technique of Manual SICS using a combination of mechanical and hydrostatic forces to express out the nucleus.[1] A simple irrigating vectis is all that is needed to perform the procedure. The technique is specially suited for softer cataracts, which will easily mould through smaller incisions; even harder cataracts can be tackled just by increasing the size of the scleral tunnel. The surgery can be performed either through a superior or temporal scleral tunnel incision. With temporal approach, even with larger incisions the amount of resultant astigmatism will be less and consequently the uncorrected vision will be better.

SURGICAL PROCEDURE

Peritomy

The conjunctiva and the Tenon's layer are dissected separately. This helps to minimize the amount of cautery applied, as there are no tags of Tenon's left, which may cover the bleeders requiring excessive cautery. If the surface is smooth without any episcleral tissue then the scleral dissection also becomes easier. The amount of conjunctival dissection should be minimal and preferably 8 to 10 mm.

Scleral Tunnel and Side Port Incision

It consists of a 6 mm scleral incision placed 1.5 mm to 2 mm from the limbus either superiorly or temporally. The incision may be straight or frown shaped. The scleral tunnel is constructed by carrying forward the scleral dissection using a bevel up crescent blade. A side port entry is made at 9 O′ clock (75 to 90 degrees to the right side of the tunnel) and preferably it should be 1 mm in size. Viscoelastic is injected into the anterior chamber through the sideport incision to make the eye firm. This is to facilitate entry of the main wound with the keratome for creation of the corneal valve and completion of the internal wound in one stretch. The sideport entry also helps to form the anterior chamber at the end of the procedure as well as for the removal of subincisional cortex.

The entry into the anterior chamber is made with a sharp 3.2 mm bevel down keratome taking care to create a corneal valve of atleast 1.5 mm, which provides the self-sealing valve. A broader corneal valve of 2mm is even acceptable as the maneuver performed through the wound is limited and the chance of distortion of corneal dome is minimal. The internal wound is then enlarged to 6 or 6.5 mm using a 5.2 mm blunt tipped bevel down blade. The internal opening should be slightly larger than the external incision to facilitate the delivery of nucleus.

Capsulotomy

Additional viscoelastic is injected and the capsulotomy is performed. Capsulorhexis is preferred except in advanced nuclear cataracts and in patients with small pupil associated with hard cataracts.

Flipping the Nucleus into Anterior Chamber

With a rhexis, a forceful hydrodissection is done until a part of the nucleus prolapses into the anterior chamber. Then with the help of a Sinskey hook or lens dialler or the cannula itself, the nucleus is rotated either clockwise or anticlockwise and delivered into the anterior chamber.

Following can opener capsulotomy, with Sinskey hook engage the superior pole of the nucleus and tip the pole up into the iris pupillary plane. Then the nucleus is rotated with the same instrument in clockwise or anticlock wise direction. until it is completely in the AC, so that it is clearly loosened from its attachments to the equatorial and posterior cortex.

In cases with small pupil, can opener capsulotomy is preferred. Iris and anterior capsule is retracted with Sinskey hook towards 12 o′ clock, superior pole of the nucleus is tipped up. Partially prolapse the nucleus through the pupil, such that iris will support the superior pole of the nucleus. Place the viscoelastic between the nucleus and the iris, and manipulate the iris with the viscoelastic or iris spatula, until the iris is entirely behind the nucleus.

If the capsulorhexis is too small, or the nucleus too large, it may be necessary to make more than two relaxing incisions in the capsulorhexis rim to tip-up the nucleus to distribute the forces present during the tip-up manoeuvre and thus minimize the risk of tearing past zonules. (Refer chapter of prolapse)

Nucleus Removal

Prior to nucleus removal, it is necessary to make sure that the whole nucleus lies in front of the iris. The nucleus can be removed using an irrigating vectis. This technique basically uses a combination of mechanical and hydrostatic forces to express out the nucleus. The irrigating vectis is available in various shapes and sizes.[2] We prefer a 5 mm wide vectis, with one to three 0.3 mm forward irrigating ports with a gentle superior concavity. This vectis is attached to a 5 cc syringe containing Ringer lactate when in use (Fig. 30.1).

After prolapsing the nucleus into the anterior chamber viscoelastics are liberally injected both above and below the nucleus. The upper layer shields the endothelium while the lower layer pushes the posterior capsule and iris diaphragm posteriorly. This creates space for the atraumatic insertion of the vectis. A proper superior rectus bridle suture, which helps in fixating the globe, is

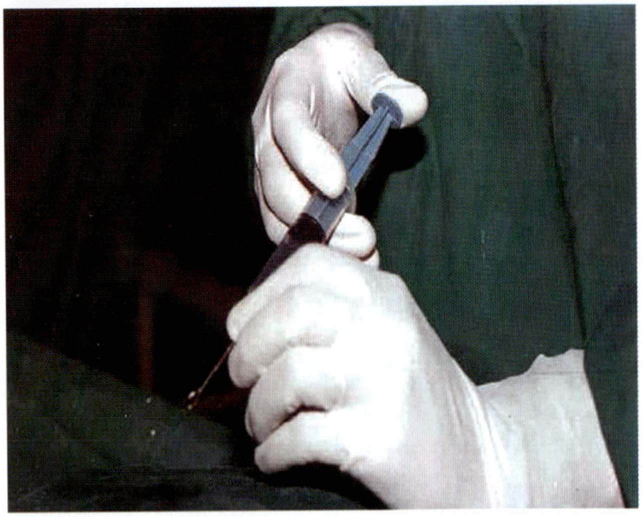

Fig. 30.1: Irrigating vectis connected to a 5 ml syringe

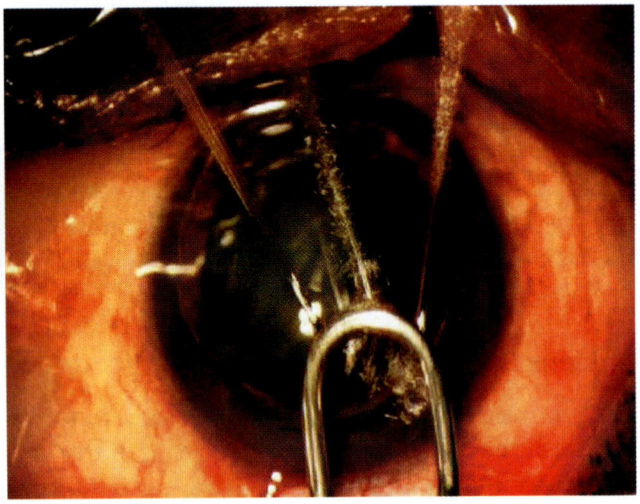

Fig. 30.2: Checking the patency of three port vectis

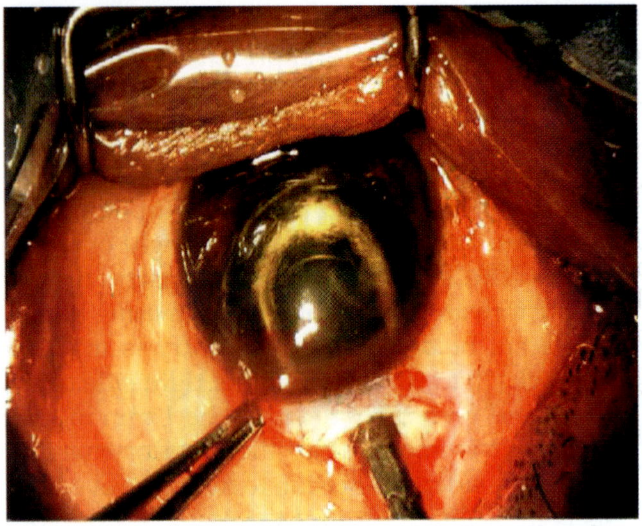

Fig. 30.3: Nucleus engaged with the irrigating vectis

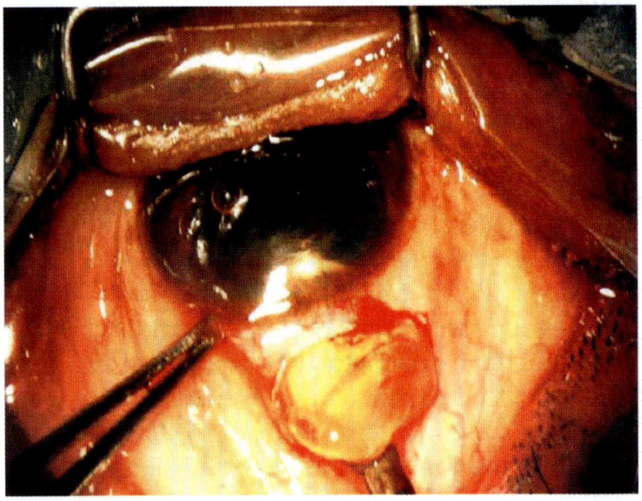

Fig. 30.4: Nucleus moulding out through the tunnel

crucial for the success of this step. The superior rectus suture is loosely held in the left hand or the assistant is asked to hold it. The vectis is now tested outside for the patency of the ports (Fig. 30.2). After confirming the patency the vectis is insinuated, concave side up, under the nucleus. Try to see the margins of the vectis through the nucleus to avoid pinching of the iris and consequent iridodialysis. It is possible to visualize the vectis border in most cataracts except in very white and black nuclei (Fig. 30.3). Now the following movements should occur in synchrony. The irrigating vectis is withdrawn out slowly without irrigating till the superior pole of the nucleus is engaged in the tunnel. At this point the superior rectus is pulled tight and with the globe thus fixed, the irrigating fluid is injected slowly to build up the hydrostatic pressure inside the chamber and the vectis is slowly pulled out while pressing down on the scleral lip. These steps are crucial in protecting the endothelium. The irrigation keeps the anterior chamber well formed, whereas, the downward pressure helps to open up the wound and prevent the nucleus rubbing on the endothelium. The nucleus moulds through the tunnel and comes out (Fig. 30.4).

The irrigation has to be reduced when the maximal diameter of the nucleus just clears the tunnel. This step prevents the nucleus being thrown out forcefully with a consequent sudden decompression and shallowing of the anterior chamber.

Management of Hard Cataracts

By increasing the incision size to 7.0 mm, one can probably manage any size of nucleus. Brunescent nuclei can be removed through a smaller wound by purposely breaking the nucleus into two pieces, if it gets locked in the wound during the removal process **(Fragmentation at the scleral pocket)**.[3] There are two techniques for doing this. The first technique involves lifting the heel of the vectis when the nucleus gets locked in the tunnel. This usually breaks off the superior 1/3 to ½ of the lens nucleus. Alternatively one can remove the vectis as the nucleus gets locked in the wound and chop off a part of the nucleus outside the tunnel with a Sinskey hook. The remainder can be pushed back into the anterior chamber with the longitudinal axis oriented towards 6 – 12 o'clock position and removed using the vectis. These techniques offer the surgeon the opportunity to reduce the size of most, if not all cataract incisions.

Irrigation-aspiration of the Cortex

It is done using the Simcoe cannula. If there is problem in the removal of subincisional cortex, then it can be approached through the sideport using the same cannula. The IOL is implanted preferably in the bag. Injecting fluid through the side-port incision forms the anterior chamber. The wound is checked for any leak. Normally no sutures are required, as the tunnel is self-sealing.

To conclude it is a time-tested technique and practiced by most surgeons in our institute with excellent results. It is safe and probably the best method to start learning Manual SICS. Only a single instrument is used inside the anterior chamber and with a good cover of viscoelastics, the procedure is very safe to the endothelium. With the use of irrigation the anterior chamber remains formed throughout the procedure. With adequate sized wound and capsulotomy, any cataract can be safely managed without any complications.

Unlike instrumental phacoemulsification, manual SICS using an irrigating vectis is universally applicable to nearly all cataract extraction procedures. It can also be performed following RD surgery or vitrectomy, patients with colobomas and even traumatic cataracts more safely than phacoemulsification.

REFERENCES

1. Manual small incision cataract surgery – an alternative technique to instrumental phacoemulsification. Aravind publications, 2000;25–32.
2. Akura J, Kaneda S, Hatta S, Matsuura K. Manual sutureless cataract surgery using a claw vectis. J Cataract Refract Surg 2000;26:491-96.
3. Barrov E, Isakov I, Rock T. Nucleus fragmentation in a scleral pocket for small incision extracapsular cataract extraction. J Cataract Refract Surg 1998;24:160-65.

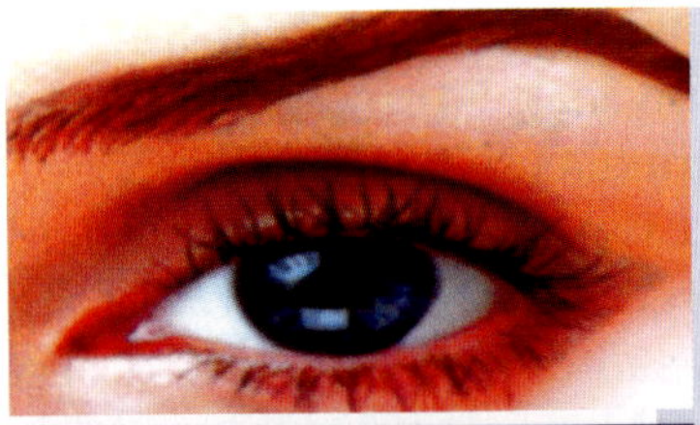

Thirty one

SICS Surgery in Difficult Situations

Arun Kshetrapal
Ramesh Kshetrapal
(India)

INTRODUCTION

Certain difficult situations coexisting with visually significant cataract warrants special techniques and special considerations during cataract extraction surgery. If appropriate technique and precautions are taken up, the result of surgery can be excellent even in these difficult situations. Some of the difficult situations that may be encountered during cataract extraction are:

1. Small pupil
2. White cataract
3. Hard black cataract
4. Subluxated cataract
5. Cataract with pseudoexfoliation
6. Cataract with existing filtration bleb

The significance of a systematic preoperative evaluation is to be emphasized in every case of cataract surgery. A good preoperative evaluation of a case is very important to foresee certain difficulties or problems that may crop up during the surgery. If the surgeon and the assistant are aware and geared up before-hand for the difficult situations that could be encountered during the surgery, then it can be dealt in an efficient way. The surgeon must be well trained and competent enough to deal with such situations and should be aware of all the complications of the technique used to deal with the difficult situations.

SMALL PUPIL

It is preferred to have a widely dilating pupil throughout the surgery especially when performing capsulorhexis, nucleus prolapse and cortical cleanup. Small pupil is the most common problem encountered by most of the surgeons during cataract extraction surgery. Some of the causes of non-dilating pupil are

a. Chronic use of miotics
b. Diabetes
c. Posterior synechiae
d. Previous intraocular surgery
e. Intraoperative trauma
f. Idiopathic
g. Pseudoexfoliation

The management of non-dilating small pupil starts preoperatively. A good preoperative examination can give an idea if the particular pupil is going to dilate or not. Presence of posterior synechiae or presence of amorphous deposition of flakes on the pupillary margin should make the surgeon cautious and a preoperative trial of pupillary dilatation should be given to know the extent of pupillary dilatation and various surgical options should be considered. If the patient is on chronic miotic therapy then it should be stopped before surgery and IOP controlled with alternative drugs.

Cycloplegics and mydriatics along with non steroidal antiinflammatory drugs (NSAIDs) should be used to dilate the pupil and for maintaining pupillary dilatation during surgery. Use of topical ketorolac 0.5 percent has been found to have effective inhibition of surgically induced miosis and it provides a more stable mydriatic effect during surgery.[1, 2]

Managing intraoperative miosis Prolapsing out nucleus into the anterior chamber and the maneuvers to prolapse the nucleus out through the tunnel can lead to surgical trauma to the iris if the surgeon is not careful. This surgical trauma can lead to miosis of the pupil. A pupil which was dilated at the start of surgery but has now become small due to surgical trauma is best managed with intracameral adrenaline. A 0.5 ml of injection Adrenaline 1:10,000 without preservative is used and is diluted in 4.5 ml of ringer lactate. The anterior chamber is then flushed with 0.1 to 0.2 ml of this fluid. The pupillary dilatation starts immediately after flushing the anterior chamber with this fluid and the pupillary dilatation is well maintained after dilatation with adrenaline. Intracameral adrenaline should be used with caution especially in hypertensive patients and patients with cardiac problem. A permission of the anesthetist should be asked for prior to injecting intracameral adrenaline.

Managing non-dilating pupil Non-dilating pupil is a relative term. The extent of pupillary dilatation should be assessed keeping in mind the experience of the surgeon, the type and hardness of the cataract. Even if after maximal dilatation with pharmacological agents the surgeon feels that the pupil is not dilated enough for smooth and uncomplicated completion of surgery then the surgeon should consider surgical methods of pupillary dilatation. Surgical methods of pupillary dilatation are to be achieved depending on the cause of non-dilatation of the pupil. If the pupil is not dilating due to posterior synechiae or if a pupillary membrane is restricting the pupil to dilate, then releasing posterior synechiae or performing membrenectomy will dilate the pupil.

If the pupil is not dilating due to restriction at the sphincter pupillae then sphincter needs to be tackled. The sphincter can be stretched either by using two instruments which can engage the pupillary margins such as Lester lens manipulator or by using special instruments such as Keuch small pupil dilator.

Technique of stretching small pupil Bimanual stretching of the pupil is the easiest method of achieving pupillary dilatation.[3,4] The pupil is stretched right in the beginning of the surgery. Once the anterior chamber has been entered it is filled with viscoelastic to create enough space. Two Lester manipulators are introduced either through the main tunnel or through the side ports and the pupil is stretched in two opposite direction. Both the manipulators are pushed gently fully across the chamber without damaging the anterior chamber structures. Gentle stretching of pupil will cause multiple tiny partial tears in the sphincter which do not have any detrimental effect on the shape of the pupil. Pupil can be stretched in two or many meridians as required. If the pupil is being stretched in the vertical meridian that is at 12 and 6 o'clock position then one manipulator is pushed towards 6 o'clock and the other manipulator is pulled towards 12 o'clock position (Fig. 31.1). If the pupil is being stretched in horizontal meridian that is at 3 and 9 o'clock then both the manipulators are pushed in opposite direction with cross over action (Fig. 31.2). Pulling, instead of pushing the pupillary margin in this meridian will not result in good stretching.

Instead of stretching the pupil, multiple small fine sphincterectomies can be made with the help of Vannas scissors. These small fine sphincterectomies usually do not interfere with normal functioning of the pupil.

Iris hooks can also be used to dilate the pupil, but they are really not required during small incision non-phacoemulsification cataract surgery and most of the cases can be managed by pupil stretching. They add to the cost and time of the surgery.

The Graether pupil expander, a device for mechanically dilating the pupil is also available. It is a soft silicone ring grooved to engage the iris sphincter and maintains pupil dilation during cataract surgery and intraocular lens implantation.[5]

If proper technique is employed to stretch the pupil a reasonable pupillary dilatation can be achieved and the complications due to small pupil can be avoided, however, the techniques of pupillary stretching themselves require some practice before they can be performed smoothly.

WHITE CATARACT

In the developing countries the problem of mature and hypermature white cataracts still exist in a large section of population. Managing white cataracts requires certain alterations in the technique of the surgery as white cataract has certain peculiarities. The capsule is more fragile in cases of white cataract and poses a problem of visibility during capsulorhexis. The intralenticular pressure is more and there are more chances of capsulorhexis extending into the periphery. In cases of hypermature white cataracts the zonules may be compromised. The problem of capsulorhexis is managed to a greater extent by the use of dyes such as trypan blue[6] or indocyanine green.[7, 8]

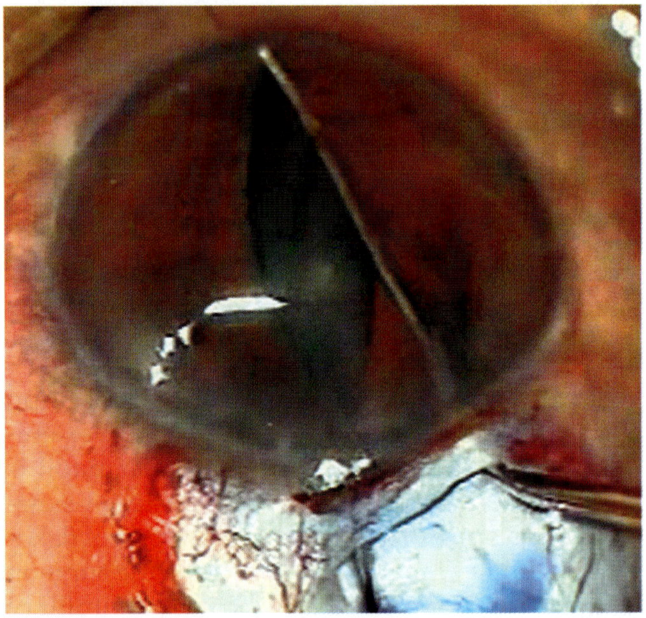

Fig. 31.1: Pupil being stretched by pull and push of lens manipulator

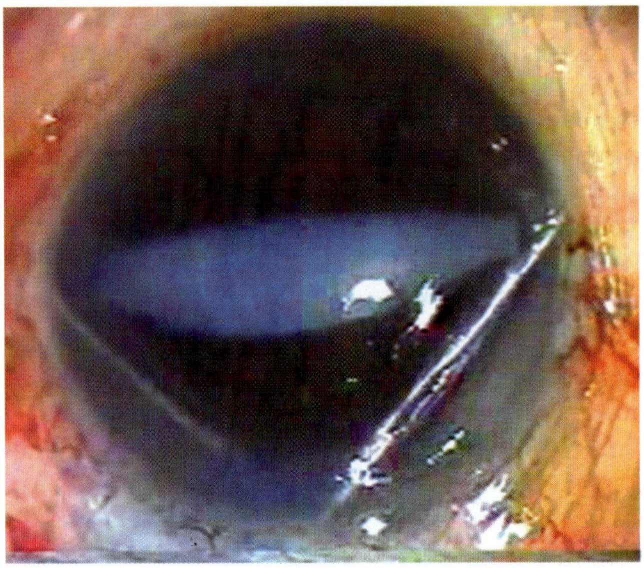

Fig. 31.2: Pupil being stretched by pushing lens manipulators with cross over action

Section 2

Trypan blue is used to stain the capsule. First of all, the aqueous in the anterior chamber is replaced with an air bubble. Now a few drops of trypan blue are placed on to the anterior lens capsule under the air bubble. Due to capillary action the dye spreads over the capsule, if it does not spread then it can be painted over the anterior capsule with the help of cannula. The dye stains the capsule immediately; however it can be left over the capsule for 10 seconds to get a better contrast. Once the dye has been injected it can be washed out with BSS and can be replaced with viscoelastic.

Performing capsulorhexis in case of white cataract requires great skill. The problem of non-visualization of the anterior capsule is taken care of by staining the capsule as just mentioned. This is eases the procedure of capsulorhexis. However there is one more glitch in performing capsulorhexis and that is the raised intralenticular pressure. The anterior capsule is flattened with a good amount of viscoelastic, preferably with sodium hyaluronate 2.3 percent and the capsulorhexis is performed through a side port to prevent leakage. Frequent replenishing of the viscoelastic should be done if there is leakage of viscoelastic. The capsulorhexis should be of adequate size to let out the nucleus out without much of a struggle.

In cases of hypermature Morgagnian type of cataract a small nick in the anterior capsule will let the milky fluid come out, thereby decreasing the intralenticular pressure, but it should be performed in a very controlled manner as sudden expulsion of milky fluid from the lens can extend the capsular opening to the periphery.

In cases of white cataract even though the size of the lens is large but the size of the nucleus is usually small. The large size of the lens is due to the hydrated lens fibers so in most of the cases the capsulorhexis need not be very large.

In cases of white cataracts the posterior pole is not visible and hence any preexisting rent in the posterior pole cannot be appreciated before prolapse of nucleus. In all cases of white cataract, hydrodissection should be carried out with great caution and with minimum of fluid. If possible it is best to avoid hydrodissection, if the nucleus can be made mobile by just rotating it with the help of Sinskey's hook.

White cataracts are most often associated with white plaques adherent to the posterior capsule. The plaques present in the visual axis should be gently peeled off from the posterior capsule with the help of bent 30 G needle and/or with the help of Utrata forceps under high magnification. These plaques generally come out very easily.

If proper technique is used and proper precautions are followed an excellent visual results can be obtained in cases of white cataract.

HARD BLACK CATARACT

The hard brown to black cataracts are more common in the developing countries. They pose a problem because their nucleus is very big in size and they are hard and non-mouldable. Hard cataracts can be easily recognized preoperatively on slit lamp examination. The surgeon should be ready to make some alterations in the surgical steps to deal with hard cataracts.

If the surgeon is planning to take out whole of the nucleus through the tunnel, then a wide tunnel depending on the size of the nucleus should be made. A 6.5 to 7 mm wide tunnel will still be self sealing if it is well constructed. A large capsulorhexis should be made to facilitate easy prolapse of nucleus into the anterior chamber. Since the nucleus is hard and non-mouldable, prolapsing out the nucleus through a small capsulorhexis can result in either zonulodialysis or accidental intra capsular cataract extraction. Once the nucleus is in the anterior chamber then it can be prolapsed out through the tunnel by any of the preferred technique of the surgeon.

Our preferred technique of nucleus expulsion through the tunnel in cases of hard cataract is by hydroexpulsion. Anterior chamber maintainer is not used in our technique. Once the nucleus is in the anterior chamber, viscoelastic is injected all around the nucleus. A Sheet's glide is introduced under the nucleus to guide it towards the tunnel and to avoid malengagement of the nucleus into the anterior chamber angle.[9] Now a paracentesis is made with the help of 26 G bent needle, mounted on a 2 cc syringe which is filled with BSS. When the needle is inside the anterior chamber, BSS is injected through the 26 G needle as a result the nucleus is pushed towards the tunnel. Once the nucleus has been engaged in the tunnel more fluid is injected to raise the pressure inside the anterior chamber and simultaneously posterior lip of the tunnel is pressed backwards. With the increasing pressure of the fluid inside the anterior chamber, the nucleus is pushed out through the tunnel in a very controlled manner. The advantage of this procedure is that it gives the surgeon full control of the situation and the surgeon can actually control the pressure inside the anterior chamber.

The hard nucleuses are slightly difficult to crack inside the anterior chamber. Trying to divide them inside the anterior chamber by an inexperienced surgeon can lead to anterior chamber trauma.

Alternatively they can be chipped off to reduce the size of the nucleus before taking out. The nucleus is prolapsed into the tunnel and a part of the nucleus is projected out of tunnel, the part of the nucleus which is projecting out of the tunnel is chipped off and the nucleus is then pushed back into the anterior chamber and rotated so that the adjacent site of the nucleus presents out of tunnel for chipping. In this way the size of the nucleus is reduced until it can come out through the tunnel comfortably.

Once the nucleus is out the rest of the surgery can be completed in the usual manner.

If at the end of surgery the surgeon feels the self-sealing nature of the tunnel has been compromised or the tunnel is slipping then one should apply a suture to make the tunnel more stable.

Cases with hard brown to black nucleus are slightly difficult to manage but with proper technique good results can be obtained even in cases of hard nucleus with small incision non-phacoemulsification cataract extraction technique.

SUBLUXATED CATARACTS

Small incision non-phacoemulsification surgery can safely be performed in cases of subluxated cataracts. Subluxated cataracts are to be dealt very cautiously and the general principles which apply to subluxated cataract surgery apply to this technique also. The decision to perform a small incision non- phacoemulsification cataract extraction along with intraocular lens implantation depends upon the amount of subluxation of the lens and the surgical skills of the surgeon. The decision on the technique to be used should be taken on merits of individual case.

The anterior chamber is gently entered with keratome to avoid sudden collapse of the anterior chamber. Sudden collapse of anterior chamber can lead to further subluxation of the lens. A capsulorhexis should always be aimed at in all cases of subluxated cataract and an endocapsular ring should be inserted into the capsular bag as soon as possible. Once the endocapsular tension ring is secure in its place then the management becomes relatively easy. In cases of greater degree of subluxation, Cionni's ring can be used to anchor the capsular bag to the sclera.[10] One has to be very gentle in all the maneuvers when dealing with a case of subluxated cataract.

CATARACTS WITH PSEUDOEXFOLIATION

Cataracts with pseudoexfoliation pose a problem because of weak zonules and non-dilating pupil and they are associated with statistically significant increased risk of intraoperative complications during cataract surgery.[11] Non-dilating pupil can be dealt with as mentioned previously by stretching the pupil. The capsulorhexis opening should be sufficient enough to allow the nucleus to pass out without any stress on the capsule as the slightest stress on the capsule can lead to zonulodialysis and subluxation. The weak zonules can be managed with the help of endocapsular tension ring. Stripping of cortical matter from the capsule should be done in a tangential way rather than in a radial fashion in order to preserve the integrity of the zonules. The surgeon should be prepared for alternative methods of IOL implantation in case the capsular bag cannot be secured.

CATARACTS WITH EXISTING FILTRATION BLEBS

Selected patients who have already been operated for trabeculectomy and who have now developed visually significant cataract can be operated with the technique of small incision non-phacoemulsification cataract surgery. A patient having well dilating pupil with soft cataract and intact zonules can be safely operated with this technique. Presence of posterior synechiae leading to small pupil, hard cataracts or cataracts with subluxation in the presence of filtering bleb should be operated very cautiously. A temporal incision is to be made as most of the time a trabeculectomy has been performed at 12 o'clock position.

CONCLUSION

Performing cataract surgery using small incision non-phacoemulsification technique in difficult situations requires the understanding of the basic principles of the technique along with the complications of the technique employed. Approaching these difficult situations in a systematic manner will help the surgeon to surmount over these situations.

REFERENCES

1. Stewart R, Grosserode R, Cheetham JK, Rosenthal A: Efficacy and safety profile of ketorolac 0.5% ophthalmic solution in the prevention of surgically induced miosis during cataract surgery. Clin Ther. 1999;21(4):723-32.
2. Srinivasan R, Madhavaranga: Topical ketorolac tromethamine 0.5% versus diclofenac sodium 0.1% to inhibit miosis during cataract surgery. J Cataract Refract Surg. 2002;28(3):517-20.
3. Shepherd DM: The pupil stretch technique for miotic pupils in cataract surgery. Ophthalmic Surg 1993;24(12): 851-52.
4. Dinsmore SC: Modified stretch technique for small pupil phacoemulsification with topical anesthesia. J Cataract Refract Surg 1996;22(1):27-30.
5. Graether JM: Graether pupil expander for managing the small pupil during surgery. J Cataract Refract Surg 1996;22(5):530-35.
6. Jacob S, Agarwal A, Agarwal A, Agarwal S, Chowdhary S, Chowdhary R, Bagmar AA: Trypan blue as an adjunct for safe phacoemulsification in eyes with white cataract. J Cataract Refract Surg 2002;28(10):1819-25.
7. Horiguchi M, Miyake K, Ohta I, Ito Y: Staining of the lens capsule for circular continuous capsulorhexis in eyes with white cataract. Arch Ophthalmol. 1998;116(4):535-37.
8. Pandey SK, Werner L, Escobar-Gomez M, Roig-Melo EA, Apple DJ: Dye-enhanced cataract surgery. Part 1: anterior capsule staining for capsulorhexis in advanced/white cataract. J Cataract Refract Surg 2000;26(7):1052-59.
9. Blumenthal M, Ashkenazi I, Fogel R, Assia EI: The gliding nucleus. J Cataract Refract Surg 1993;19(3):435-37.
10. Moreno-Montanes J, Sainz C, Maldonado MJ: Intraoperative and postoperative complications of Cionni endocapsular ring implantation. J Cataract Refract Surg. 2003;29(3):492-97.
11. Scorolli L, Scorolli L, Campos EC, Bassein L, Meduri RA: Pseudoexfoliation syndrome: A cohort study on intraoperative complications in cataract surgery. Ophthalmologica. 1998;212(4):278-80.

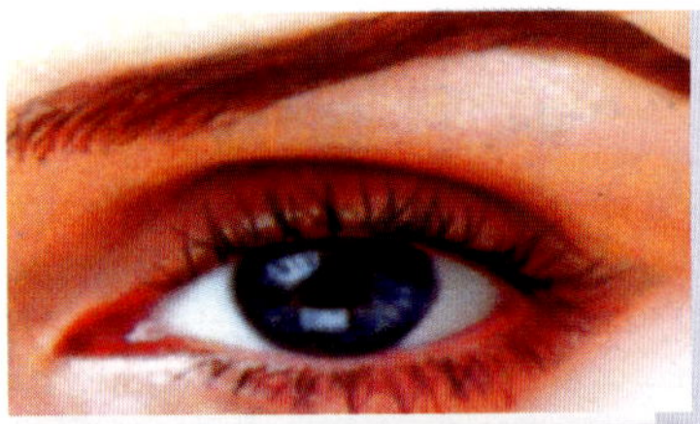

Thirty two

Small Incision Sutureless Temporal Approach Extracapsular Cataract Surgery

Geoffery Tabin (USA)
Sanduk Ruit (Nepal)

Cataracts are currently the leading cause of blindness worldwide with the majority of cases in developing nations. Of the 38 million cases of blindness (visual acuity less than 20/400), an estimated 16 million are caused by age-related cataracts. Moreover, in Nepal alone the percentage of curable blindness resulting from cataracts is more than 80 percent. Estimates for Tibet suggest that the problem is just as critical there. A 1987 Tibet eye study revealed that debilitating cataracts were present in 11.8 percent of the population older than 40 years of age and in more than 50 percent older than 70 years of age.

Because of increasing population age, the incidence of cataract blindness in developing nations is on the rise. In India, 3.8 million people become blind each year from cataracts. With no improvement in current practices, the World Health Organization estimates a doubling of the world's blindness by the year 2020. Most underserved countries today are simply unable to cope with new cases, let alone the rapidly growing backlog. Projections show that to eliminate the backlog within the next 25 years, the recent number of 7 million cataracts operated on, would have to be increased to 32 million by the year 2020. There is a pressing need for faster, less expensive, and more effective ways to deliver high quality cataract surgery. This chapter will explain our method of delivering high quality, low cost, high volume, cataract surgery as well as our surgical technique. We will take a stepwise approach starting with our sutured, large incision extracapsular cataract surgery with a posterior chamber intraocular lens implant technique and progress to how we currently perform small incision, sutureless, temporal extracapsular cataract surgery.

Prior to embarking on our small incision cataract surgery technique, it is important to master the steps involved in our technique while using a large incision. Our method of cataract surgery uses only fluidics to remove the lens from the eye. A modified capsulotomy technique allows smooth nucleus delivery and facilitates placement of the posterior chamber intraocular lens into the capsular bag. Our delivery technique relies on a team approach that involves nurses and ophthalmic assistants, as well as the operating surgeon. It is an efficient team approach that allows us to perform high volume surgery in a minimum of time and ensure excellent results.

In remote areas, we involve the entire community, performing first a complete epidemiologic survey of the region. We arrange for village organizers to ensure that every person in a region with ocular problems is brought to a central screening area. We then have our patients initially screened by well-trained ophthalmic technicians. These technicians are able to prescribe glasses to patients with refractive errors, antibiotics and other medications for common infections and take care of most minor ocular problems. They screen the patients in need of cataract surgery or more sophisticated ophthalmic care. The ophthalmologist then only examines the patients that have been pre-screened to have pathology.

Once the patients have been selected for cataract surgery we have a systematic approach to reduce the chance of infection and deliver high-quality, high-volume care. This is an integral part of our cataract surgery, and will be discussed prior to the details of our actual surgical technique. We will then take a step-wise approach to how we perform our small incision surgery. Our cataract technique has been developed to be one that is applicable for all types of cataracts. It is extremely safe for even most difficult cases with the hardest and largest nucleus, as well as traumatic, pediatric, and uveitic and virtually all other cataract cases. The nucleus delivery involves only fluidics and water pressure to remove the lens from the eye. It is very safe both for preserving the posterior capsule, and the corneal endothelium. Finally, it is a technique that is easily replicable and can be performed with a minimum amount of time without any expensive extra equipment.

PREOPERATIVE MANAGEMENT

As stated above, our preoperative management begins with the surgeon examining the patients who have been pre-screened by ophthalmic assistants. A large majority of our cases have mature cataracts with no view of the posterior segment, even with indirect ophthalmoscopy. The ophthalmic assistants carefully check for a relative afferent pupillary defect to obtain a gross assessment of the retinal and optic nerve function. At our larger eye centers, all patients undergo analysis with a B-scan ultrasound at the time of their biometry where axial length is measured by A-scan ultrasound and keratometry is performed.

The evening before surgery, the patients have their faces washed vigorously with soap and clean water. Antibiotic drops and ointment are instilled the night before surgery. Prior to surgery the ophthalmic assistants cut the eyelashes closely, apply antibiotic ointment over the eyelashes and instill fluoroquinolone eye-drops into the eye. The patients receive another dose of fluoroquinolone antibiotic and at the time of instillation of dilating drops. The ophthalmic assistants now place a local anesthetic in the fornix, and the eye is washed and prepped with Betadine. Trained ophthalmic technicians then perform a peribulbar and a 7th nerve block. After the anesthesia, the eyes again receive a full prep with Betadine scrub and pressure is held over the eye with a Betadine soaked gauze. This preoperative cleaning and sterilization regimen allows a rapid turnover time between cases while maintaining a very low infection rate.

At the conclusion of one case, a new patient is brought onto the operating table from one side as the operated patient is helped off the table from the other side. The surgeon performs a final Betadine prep and then instills a small amount of 5 percent povidone iodine into the fornix of the eye prior to surgery. While the surgeon is prepping and draping the eye, the scrub nurse will have completed arranging a new instrument set which has been brought out for the new patient. Surgery is able to continue with a typical delay between cases of less than 3 minutes.

SURGICALTECHNIQUE FOR CONVENTIONAL CATARACT SURGERY

Our standard surgical technique begins with the eye being opened with a lid speculum. A 4-0 silk suture placed in the superior rectus muscle tendon for traction. Next, a superior limbal peritomy is performed followed by gentle electrocautery to the limbal vasculature. A blade breaker is used to create a sharp razor blade, which then makes a 10 mm half-scleral thickness limbal groove parallel to the limbus. A straight 26-gauge needle is next inserted through the groove and turned so that it is beveled to the side. A V-shaped cut is made in the anterior capsule with the side of the needle so that the apex of the V is connected at the 12 o'clock position. This capsular incision is possible to complete easily and completely even with a hypermature lens or difficult capsular visualization on a white or black capsule. The needle is attached to a syringe with balanced salt solution. If liquid cortex obscures the view, this can be easily irrigated away using a small amount of pressure through the syringe.

Once the V-shaped incision is completed in the anterior capsule, the anterior chamber is entered with a razor blade and a 10 mm incision is completed in a two-plane fashion along the limbus with corneal scissors. Next, a manual irrigation aspiration Simcoe cannula is used to hydrodissect and irrigate under the capsular flap. A fluid wave circles around the lens and the capsular opening fishmouths superiorly. Irrigation floats the lens gently out of the capsular bag and into the anterior chamber. The lens is then easily irrigated out of the eye. No vitreous pressure is used to express the lens. There are no extracapsular tags. The expression of the lens from the eye is always atraumatic with no stress on either the capsular bag posteriorly or the corneal endothelium superiorly.

Once the nucleus has been irrigated from the eye, any residual cortex is removed with the Simcoe cannula. When all of the cortex has been removed an air bubble is instilled to reform the anterior chamber. A posterior chamber intraocular lens is then inserted into the capsular bag under air. The edge of the corneal incision flips inward as the lens is inserted to trap the air bubble and protect the corneal endothelium during placement of the lens. The anterior flap of the capsulotomy floats upward with the air insuring that the leading haptic of the intraocular lens automatically goes under this capsular flap. The trailing haptic is then easily placed or dialed into the capsular bag.

Once this has been completed, the Simcoe cannula is used to irrigate the air from the eye and the anterior chamber is reformed with balanced salt solution.

Keeping the anterior chamber inflated with fluids from the Simcoe cannula, a curved Vannas scissors is brought in with the other hand and slid over the top of the implant to the edge of the anterior triangular capsular flap. A small cutis then made at the base of the V-flap. This torn edge is grasped with suction from the Simcoe cannula and a smooth capsular tear is made, completing a capsulorrhexis with the V superiorly and a smooth curved capsular tear at the base. The lens now sits completely within the capsular bag with a V-opening toward the apex and a smooth tear to the 6 o'clock position, completing what we call the Himalayan capsulorrhexis.

A new air bubble is then instilled into the anterior chamber. The limbal incision is closed with a running 10-0 nylon suture starting within the wound and running to the far end of the wound and back again to tie securely with the knot buried within the wound. At the conclusion of the operation the anterior chamber is refilled with balanced salt solution. The superior conjunctiva is injected with dexamethasone and gentamicin that balloons it up over the corneoscleral wound. The eye is then dressed with ciprofloxacin and dexamethasone and patched. Postoperatively, the patients receive combined steroid and antibiotic drops every 2 hours for the first 3 postoperative days, then 4 times per day for the next 2 weeks, with steroid and antibiotic ointment at bedtime.

This extracapsular technique is highly reproducible with a minimal amount of intraoperative and / or postoperative complications. The operative time for the technique decreases with the increasing experience of the surgeon. Experienced doctors typically complete four uncomplicated cases per hour. It is essential to master this large incision extracapsular technique prior to attempting our small incision surgery. The critical steps to be mastered that are unique to our method include; irrigating the lens out of the capsular bag and into the anterior chamber, completing the Himalayan capsulorrhexis by cutting the base of the triangle and creating a smooth tear holding the capsule with the Simcoe cannula, and placing the intraocular lens easily into the capsular bag. Once this has been accomplished, we then slowly transition to our small incision sutureless technique.

SMALL INCISION SUTURELESS CATARACT SURGERY

Our sutureless, small incision, cataract surgery relies on the same use of fluidics that we use for our conventional extracapsular surgery, except that the lens is delivered through a small, self-sealing tunnel incision. We do not require any expensive viscoelastics or complex maneuvers to break the nucleus within the anterior chamber. The key steps to this surgery are mastering the gentle irrigation of the nucleus into the anterior chamber through the use of fluidics, and irrigating the lens out of the eye through a well-constructed, self-sealing tunnel incision. Our technique involves a self-sealing scleral tunnel. We construct a wound that has a larger internal opening than the external scleral incision. The section must have a properly constructed architecture so that intraocular pressure seals the internal wound. We then gently irrigate the lens into the anterior chamber as with our large incision surgery. We then use the same fluid dynamics that were originally described by Dr. Michael Blumenthal to help the lens flow into the funnel of our incision and irrigate the nucleus out of the eye. However, we differ from Dr Blumenthal in that we do not require an anterior chamber maintainer to provide fluid pressure behind the lens. We rely on the Simcoe cannula and positioning of the eye to irrigate the lens from the eye.

It is best to begin learning our small incision sutureless surgery with the approach the surgeon is most familiar. We generally advocate beginning surgeons start with a superior approach, utilizing a superior rectus bridle suture. This allows easy positioning of the eye throughout the case. Moreover, this superior approach is preferred for the novice because of the occasional need to convert to a sutured extracapsular cataract extraction. It is also easier to perform high volume superior approach surgery on one standard operating table. As will be discussed later we modify our table for temporal surgery.

A fornix based conjunctival flap is created utilizing a peritomy from approximately the 10 o'clock to the 2 o'clock position down to bare sclera. Light cautery is used to blanche the scleral incision area. Next, an initial partial-thickness 30-50 percent scleral depth 6-7 mm scleral incision is made tangential to the limbus. At its midpoint, the incision should be approximately 1.5-2 mm posterior to the limbus. This incision can be made with a razor blade fragment or commercial sharp rounded blade. The former helps with cost containment. Next, a scleral corneal tunnel is fashioned with an angled beveled up crescent blade or similar. From the initial incision, the tissue is dissected in a single plane forward through sclera and limbus approximately 1-1.5 mm into the clear cornea. The plane should be parallel with the ocular surface. The dissected pocket should extend nasally and temporally to the limbus so that its transverse extent is much greater in the cornea than at the scleral opening. This results in a purse or funnel shape to the yet-to-be completed tunnel. It is important to exaggerate this internal flaring of the tunnel, particularly during the initial transition stage.

Next, the same triangular capsulotomy used in our large incision surgery is performed with the apex at 12 o'clock. Again this is made using a straight 26-gauge needle attached to a 1 ml syringe filled with anterior chamber irrigation fluid. The needle is passed into the anterior chamber through the recess of the scleral corneal pocket at about its midpoint. Using a beveled tip of the needle, the linear cut in the capsule is again made from the 4 o'clock to the 12 o'clock position and another then cut from 8 o'clock to 12 o'clock so that the two join at 12 o'clock. The apex of the capsulotomy can then be lifted with the tip of the needle and peeled towards 6 o'clock. This confirms that the capsular cuts are complete and frees any anterior capsule cortex adhesions. If the anterior capsular chamber shallows during these maneuvers or if the view is obscured by liquefied lens material, a small amount of anterior chamber irrigation fluid can be injected through the needle to deepen the chamber or clear the view.

With this accomplished, a sharp pointed keratome or slit knife is used to open the inner aspect of the scleral corneal tunnel into the anterior chamber. The sides of the blade are then used to open the corneal end of the tunnel along its full extent to the limbus nasally and temporally. The purpose of this internal flaring of the tunnel is to allow and encourage the nucleus to engage in the tunnel at the time of expression. It is essential that the internal opening to the tunnel is widely opened. The eventual size of the internal and external openings of the tunnel can and should be varied according to the anticipated size and hardness of the nucleus.

The next step may be varied, depending on the maturity of the cataract. For the less advanced cataract, a Rycroft cannula is used to inject anterior chamber irrigation fluid into the lens to delaminate the lens components and separate the nucleus and epinucleus from the cortex. The whole of the nucleus or one of its poles may prolapse from the capsular bag into the anterior chamber. Hydrodissection is not required with the more advanced cataracts. In these cases, and where the less mature cataract has been mobilized with hydrodissection, the process of subluxating the lens nucleus into the anterior chamber can be initiated or completed by using a flowing Simcoe irrigation-aspiration cannula. The nucleus is gently rotated and tilted. In-flowing fluid is directed behind the nucleus and irrigation is performed under the capsular flap. The nucleus is delivered into the anterior chamber using fluidics and hydrostatic forces to gently rise into the anterior chamber. This maneuver takes a small amount of practice to master. Because the anterior chamber is closed, if difficulty occurs while hydro-expressing the nucleus into the anterior chamber, it is wise to convert at this stage to a large incision extracapsular cataract extraction to be certain not to traumatize the cornea or posterior capsule. During the learning curve, it is important to remain slow and gentle, and convert when needed. Soon it will be very natural to bring the lens above the iris using only fluid dynamics.

At this point, a combination of mechanical and hydrostatic forces can be used to deliver the nucleus from the anterior chamber into the tunnel incision, and then irrigate the lens out of the eye. Once the nucleus has been irrigated above the iris into the anterior chamber, there are several ways one can remove the nucleus. We do not suggest sectioning or fragmentation of the nucleus in the anterior chamber. However, whichever method is chosen it is important to confirm the adequacy of wound size for the observed size and consistency of the nucleus.

One method of nucleus delivery begins by rotating the eye downward. We use toothed forceps to grasp the lip of the incision at one end and rotate the eye downward slightly. Next, we pass a vigorously flowing Simcoe cannula into the anterior chamber around the side of the nucleus then gently underneath it until the tip is beyond the 6 o'clock pole of the nucleus and clearly visible. The accumulating irrigational fluid from the cannula in this position tends to push the nucleus so that it engages the internal mouth of the corneoscleral tunnel. A combination of hydrostatic pressure and a gentle lifting action with the tip of the Simcoe, rather like the action of a spoon, forces the nucleus further into the tunnel. The external foramen of the tunnel can be opened using downward pressure of the heel of the Simcoe. As the nucleus moves into the tunnel, epinucleus may strip off or the nucleus may fragment. However, the whole nucleus should usually be delivered from the eye in one motion. This is our standard and preferred method of nucleus delivery and yields clear corneas postoperative day one.

A second method utilizes an irrigating vectis that is passed into the anterior chamber and under the dislocated nucleus. The bulk of the nucleus can then be lifted and drawn into and through the corneoscleral tunnel using irrigation to add a hydrostatic push to the pull of the vectis. This technique allows rapid delivery of the nucleus and may allow an inexperienced surgeon to more easily deliver the nucleus until full comfort with simple hydrostatic forces has been acquired through experience. It must be cautioned not to lift up too vigorously on the nucleus as this may engage the corneal endothelium and result in an edematous cornea on postoperative day one.

The Simcoe cannula is then used as usual to remove epinuclear and cortical debris from the anterior chamber, posterior capsule, and recesses of the capsular bag. Next, the Rycroft cannula is used to inject air into the anterior chamber. Finally, a polymethylmethacrylate intraocular lens is passed into the eye. The wound construction is such that the air is usually retained in the anterior chamber during this maneuver. However, if this is not the case, the leading haptic intraocular lens can be used to then fold the anterior lip of the incision to prevent escape of the air. The leading haptic is passed into the capsular bag behind the triangular flap of anterior capsule, indicating correct placement within the bag. Using straight or angled tying forceps, the upper loop is placed into the bag behind the straight cut edge of the anterior capsule. Fine positioning is done with a Simcoe cannula or a lens-positioning hook if required. With a Simcoe cannula in moderate flow, the anterior chamber air is removed and replaced with irrigation fluid. The flowing Simcoe cannula continues to maintain the anterior chamber as a fine blade Vannas scissors is introduced. The scissors are used to make a small cut at either the nasal or temporal base of the triangular capsular flap. Next we again use the Simcoe cannula to engage with the edge of the triangular flap on the apical side of the cut in the same manner as with our large incision technique. The capsular flap is gently torn away from the base with a circumferential motion. Care must be taken to ensure the tear does not extend radially toward the equator. With continuing single cannulation aspiration, the freed anterior capsular triangle remains engaged in the cannula port and both the cannula and capsule are removed from the anterior chamber. The Simcoe cannula is used to ensure the anterior chamber is reformed to a satisfactory depth and ocular tension. Avoid the temptation to overpressurize the eye.

The wound, being a 3-planed shelled incision, should self-seal. This may be confirmed by pressing on the globe with an instrument while observing the wound for leakage. If there is leakage, we recommend suturing the wound. With experience, we find that less than 1 percent of our small incision cataract surgeries require any sutures. Subconjunctival injection of antibiotic and steroid is then given just above the cut edge of the conjunctiva. This will balloon the conjunctiva and move it toward the limbus, covering the scleral wound. Caution should be taken to ensure there is not so much pressure on the posterior portion of the wound that there is a wound leak. The lids are closed and a dressing is applied in the usual way. The postoperative course is similar to that for our standard extracapsular technique.

Our results have shown in both the hospital and eye camp settings, a very low complication rate and excellent visual recovery for both our sutured and sutureless techniques. However, the sutured technique leads to considerably more postoperative astigmatism and a lower level of uncorrected visual acuity. 92 percent of our patients obtained 20/40 or better corrected visual acuity with the sutured technique, however, only approximately 50 percent obtained 20/40 or better visual acuity uncorrected. For our sutureless technique, 65 percent of the patients had uncorrected visual acuity of 20/40 or better at 8 weeks postoperatively. The mean corneal astigmatism induced was 0.93 diopters. The sutureless small incision surgery also has advantages with regards to speed and cost savings. Sutureless surgery also has less late postoperative wound or suture complications.

TEMPORAL SMALL INCISION EXTRACAPSULAR SURGERY WITH POSTERIOR CHAMBER INTRAOCULAR LENS

Although the results of our superior small incision sutureless cataract surgery are very good, the superior incision does induce a small amount of with the rule astigmatism that can affect uncorrected visual acuity. We found approximately 0.61 Diopters of induced astigamatism at three months that drifts to approximately 0.93 Diopters at one year. Postoperative astigmatism is a concern in extracapsular cataract extraction and one of the most significant contributors to postoperative visual acuity. Minimizing postoperative astigmatism in order to provide the best possible visual outcomes is essential, particularly in developing nations where limited postoperative eye care is available.

Numerous factors have been hypothesized to affect postoperative astigmatism in cataract surgery. Intraoperative factors such as the length and location of incision and the type and placement of suture have received the most attention in the literature. The majority of studies have examined phacoemulsification surgery, which showed that smaller scleral incisions and sutureless incisions tend to induce less astigmatism. The use of temporal incisions in phacoemulsification has also been investigated.

Only a few studies have directly addressed the astigmatic effects of alternate incisional meridia in extracapsular surgery. The results of one series found, that a lateral approach produced significantly less astigmatism with prolonged astigmatic stabilization when compared to a superior incision. The visual outcomes of the temporal incision surgery in this study were not statistically different from phacoemulsification surgery. These results were not supported by an Australian series that used Holladay-Cravy-Koch's method to measure the magnitude and direction of astigmatic change. In this study, the temporal incision group had high astigmatism while the superior incision group had low astigmatism, however visual acuities were the same in the two groups. Another study found that a lateral incision technique was useful in reducing astigmatism.

We find less induced astigmatism when the same small incision extracapsular surgery is performed from a temporal approach, yielding improved uncorrected visual acuity. We have now switched our standard procedure to a temporal incision in all cases except where a high level of existing with-the-rule astigmatism is present preoperatively. When we perform a high-volume of small incision cataract surgery from a temporal approach, we utilize a long table with the surgeon seated in the middle with easy access to his foot control pedals. Patients are brought to the operating table such that patients with left eye cataracts will have their feet extended to the surgeon's left, and those who will have surgery on their right eye have their feet extended to the surgeon's right. In this manner, we are able to perform high-volume surgery with the same rapid turnaround time as with our superior incision technique.

The surgeon must be experienced and comfortable with small incision cataract surgery before switching to the temporal approach, as it is more difficult to extend the wound and convert to a sutured surgery if a complication arises. Otherwise, the surgical technique is exactly the same. A tunnel incision beginning with a half-thickness scleral groove approximately 1.5 mm behind the limbus that flares out to create a funnel with a wider opening into the anterior chamber. The V-capsulotomy is again performed with the apex towards the surgeon at either the 3 of 9 o'clock position. The lens is hydrodissected and fluid gently moves the lens to the anterior chamber. The eye is then rotated nasally with Simcoe cannula placed beneath the lens such that fluidics brings the lens into the tunnel incision and the nucleus is hydroexpressed. Completion of the case is then exactly the same as for ours superior incision cataract surgery with the one of exception that a single absorbable suture is used to close the conjunctiva over a scleral wound, as we found that some cases left the wound exposed. This added step of a single suture to close the conjunctiva does not significantly alter the surgical time or cause problems for the patient.

In order to quantify the advantages of the temporal approach we conducted a prospective randomized trial where 100 consecutive patients had one eye receive a superior incision and the fellow eye a temporal small incision, sutureless, extracapsular cataract surgery. We conducted this study to examine whether a temporal incision in conjunction with a sutureless closure will decrease postoperative astigmatism in extracapsular cataract extraction, thereby maximizing uncorrected postoperative visual acuity. The temporal approach does produce less induced postoperative astigmatism and improved uncorrected acuity over the superior incision.

Methods

A randomized prospective clinical trial was conducted in which 100 bilateral cataract patients (53 F/47 M, Mean age 61.9 + 10.6 years) had one eye assigned to a superior incision extracapsular cataract extraction with posterior chamber intraocular lens implantation and the other eye assigned to an identical surgery with a temporal incision approach. Both the temporal and superior incision approach surgeries were performed by the same two surgeons at Tilganga Eye Center (Kathmandu, Nepal) in December 2002.

The extracapsular cataract extraction with posterior chamber intraocular lens surgery was performed as described previously. In brief, with the patient under retrobulbar anesthesia, a 6-7-mm limbal half-scleral thickness limbal groove was made, followed by a scleral tunnel extending to 10-mm at the corneal entrance, and a V-shaped capsulotomy created using a straight 26-G needle. The vertex of the "V" is at 12 o'clock in the superior incision cases and at 3 o'clock (OS) or 9 o'clock (OD) in the temporal incision cases. The internal width of the scleral tunnel was then enlarged. After manual irrigation with a Simcoe cannula, the lens was floated out of the capsular bag and fluid pressure was used to bring the nucleus into and through the tunnel, residual cortex was aspirated, and a posterior chamber intraocular lens was inserted. The power of the IOL was determined preoperatively based on keratometry measurements and axial length. After creating a cut with a curved Vannas scissors, the capsulorrhexis was completed. Air and viscoelastic were removed from the anterior chamber, which was reformed with a balanced salt solution. Dexamethasone and gentamicin were injected into the conjunctiva, and the eye was patched overnight.

Outcomes

Keratometry measurements were made at 1st day, 1st week, 1st month, and 3rd months postoperatively. At each of these points, the absolute value of the simple subtracted astigmatism [k1-k2], absolute value of the simple subtracted change in astigmatism from preoperative values [(Post-op k1-k2) - (Pre-op k1-k2)], and the astigmatic change were recorded. Refraction and corrected visual acuity were measured at 1st and 3rd months postoperatively. To assess corneal astigmatism, the Holladay-Cravy-Koch spherocylinder method of Surgically Induced Refractive Change (SIRC) was used at 1st and 3rd months.

ASTIGMATIC CHANGE

Preoperatively, there was no significant difference in mean absolute astigmatism between the temporal incision (0.581 + 0.50 D) and superior incision (0.718 +0.65 D, p = 0.06) eyes. One week postoperatively, the patients in the superior incision group had a higher absolute astigmatism (1.67 + 1.3 D) than the temporal incision group (0.79 + 0.7 D). Eyes that underwent the superior incision surgery also showed a larger absolute astigmatic change from preoperative measurements (1.60 + 1.3 D) than those that underwent the temporal incision surgery (0.8 + 0.8 D, p = 0.006). (See Figures 1 and 2)

A comparison of the Surgically Induced Refractive Change (SIRC) as measured by Holladay-Cravy-Koch's method at 1st month showed greater magnitude of induced cylindrical change among the superior incision group (1.437 + 0.9 D, n=57), when compared to the temporal incision group (0.892 + 0.84, n=58) (p=0.001). In addition, the superior section showed greater against-the-rule (ATR) change (0.662 + 1.57 D) when compared to the temporal incision group, which manifested a smaller degree of with-the-rule (WTR) change (-0.163 + 0.81 D, n=58, p=0.002). At 3 months postoperatively, these results persisted, with the superior incision showing a larger ATR astigmatic change (0.61 + 1.65 D, n=68) while the temporal incision showed a smaller WTR change (-0.23 + 0.95 D, n=47) (p=5.9E-5).

At 1 month postoperatively, there was a significantly higher percentage of superior incision patients (75%) who had ATR astigmatism, as opposed to temporal incision patients (38%: Z=4.36). This difference also held true for ATR astigmatic change (65% among SS vs. 38% among TS: Z=-3.09). Conversely, a significantly higher percentage of temporal section patients manifested WTR astigmatism when compared to superior section patients (58% vs. 19% : Z=4.53) and also WTR astigmatic change (55% vs. 23% : Z=3.69). (See Table 1) An identical pattern was also found at 3 months after surgery.

REFRACTION AND VISUAL ACUITY

At 1 month postoperatively, patients in the temporal incision group required a lower cylindrical correction (-0.91 + 0.71 D) than the patients in the superior incision group (-1.47 + 1.09 D) (p<0.001). This pattern persisted at 3 months after surgery (temporal incision -0.99 + 0.76 D, superior incision -1.68 + 0.88 D). There was no difference in corrected visual acuity between the two groups at 1 month after surgery (p=0.52, 0.07). 91.4% (n=93) of temporal section patients and 92.0 percent (n=88) of superior section patients had acuities of 20/40 or better one month postoperatively. Only one patient (1.1%) in the temporal section group and two patients (2.3%) in the superior section group had corrected visual acuities of 20/80 or worse. These patients had pre-existing macular problems that were not picked up by B scan ultrasonography and were hidden behind mature cataracts. There was no difference in the magnitude of spherical correction between the two groups.

Complications

There were no cases of posterior capsular rupture and no cases of vitreous loss. There were no other visually significant complications in this study. Ten percent of patients in both groups developed transient corneal edema, which resolved by one week postoperatively.

CONCLUSION

In many developing nations, extracapsular cataract extraction is still the most widely used and available cataract surgery. In rural areas and in eye camp settings, phacoemulsification is too expensive and bulky to be an effective surgical option. Therefore, given the reality of extracapsular surgery with intraocular lens implantation in these settings, minimizing postoperative refraction is of paramount importance.

Our results clearly suggest that sutureless temporal incisions produce less postoperative corneal astigmatism than superior incisions in extracapsular cataract extraction with posterior chamber intraocular lens implantation. The degree of astigmatic change induced by the temporal incision ECCE/PCIOL surgery compares favorably with published data on extracapsular cataract surgery and scleral tunnel approach phacoemulsification. Our results support the claim that a superior incision induces a higher magnitude ATR astigmatism, while the temporal incision induces a lower magnitude WTR astigmatism. While the exact difference in cylindrical power between the two groups varies based on the method of analysis, most of our measures show a difference of 0.5-0.7 D of cylindrical refraction at 1 and 3 months after surgery. While definitive studies are yet to be done, there is general consensus that this amount of astigmatic change is likely to be visually significant. ATR astigmatism is thought to be more visually significant than WTR astigmatism, and the surgically induced astigmatic change might be compounded over time by the ATR change that many people develop with age of 7.

All of the patients in this study were operated on at Tilganga Eye Centre in Kathmandu, where excellent refractive services are available. This could explain the fact that the corrected visual acuities in the temporal and superior incision groups were identical despite the difference in astigmatic cylinder. However, the vast majority of people blind from cataracts in Nepal live in rural areas. For many of them, cataract extraction surgeries done at 'eye camps' may be the only eye care they receive. Such patients are often unlikely to seek regular refraction after surgery due to financial barriers and a dearth of optical shops. The optical shops these patients may have access to often lack a wide range of cylindrical corrective lenses. Rigid contact lenses are rarely available outside of the large cities and impractical for use in most rural settings.

The excellent visual outcomes and the low complication rates confirm those of the initial studies introducing this sutureless extracapsular cataract surgery with posterior chamber intraocular lens surgery as an efficacious surgical technique to address the backlog of cataracts in developing nations. A temporal incision can reduce postoperative astigmatism among patients often lost to follow-up, allowing them to maximize their long-term visual function.

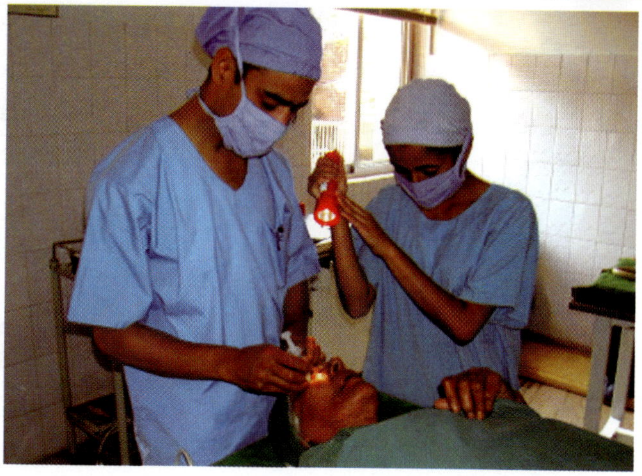

Fig. 32.3: Trained ophthalmic technicians give peribulbar anesthesia

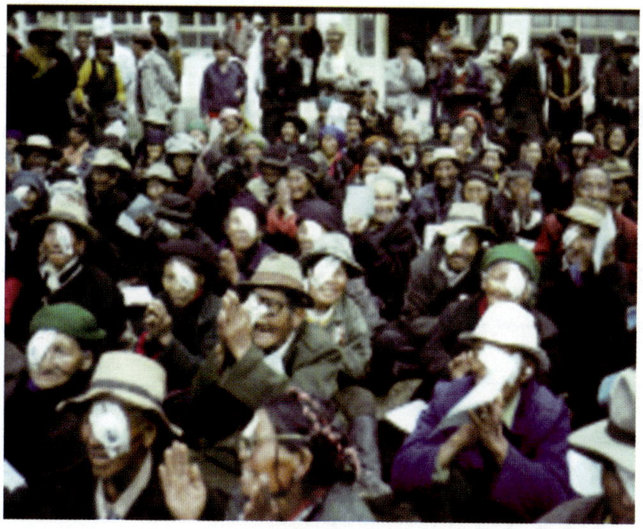

Fig. 32.1

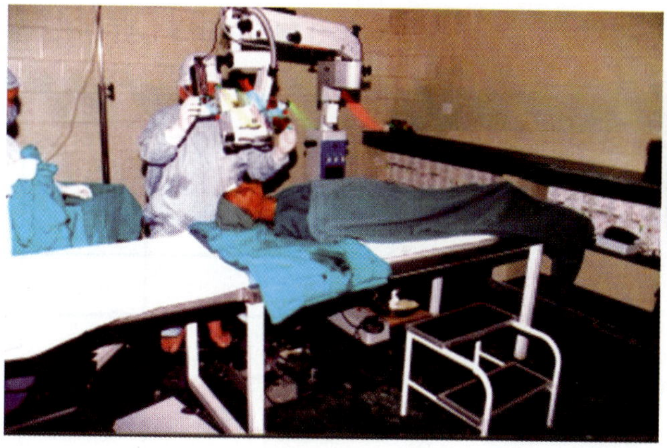

Fig. 32.4

Quality is the best driver of demand

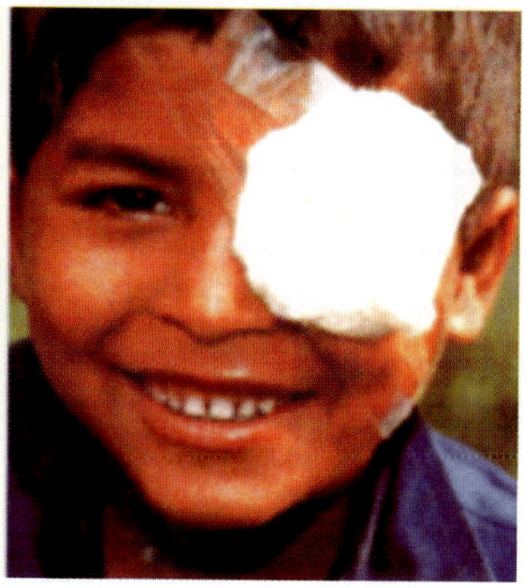

Fig. 32.2

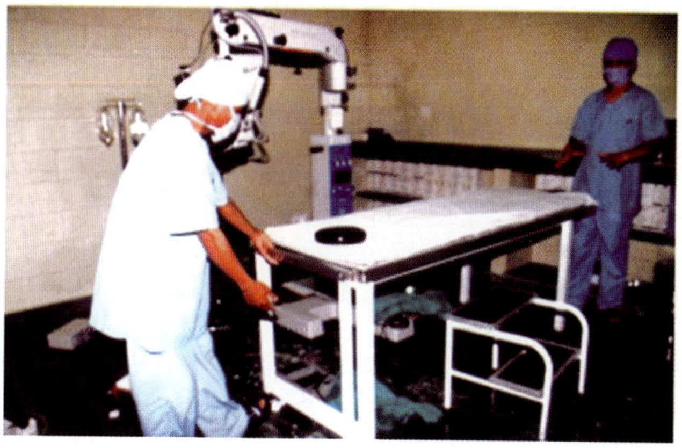

Fig. 32.5

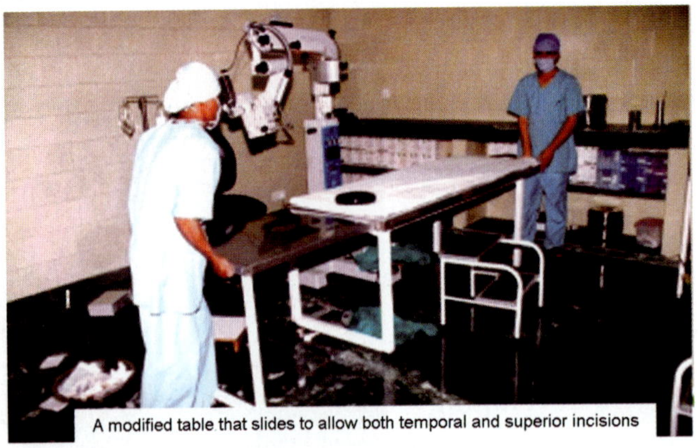

Fig. 32.6: A modified table that slides to allow both temporal and superior incisions

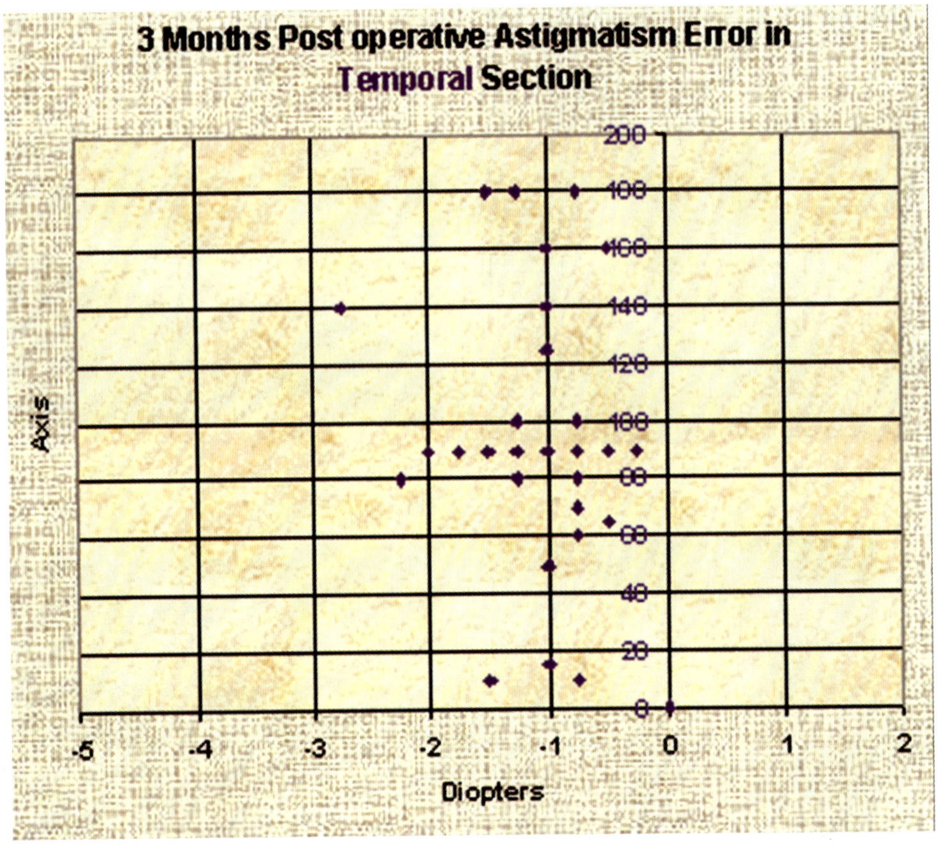

Fig. 32.7: Results of Temporal & Superior Section

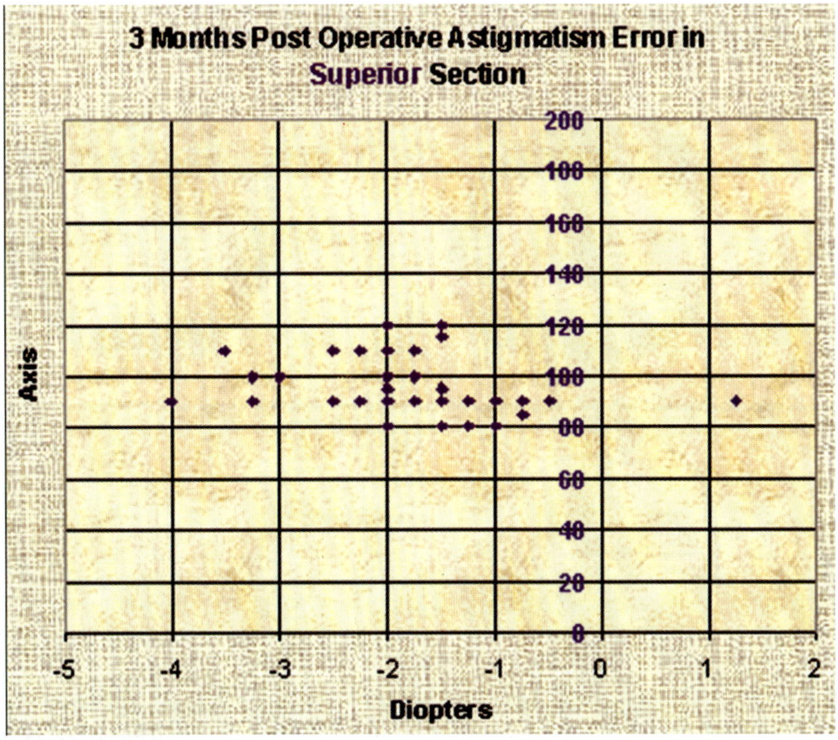

Fig. 32.8

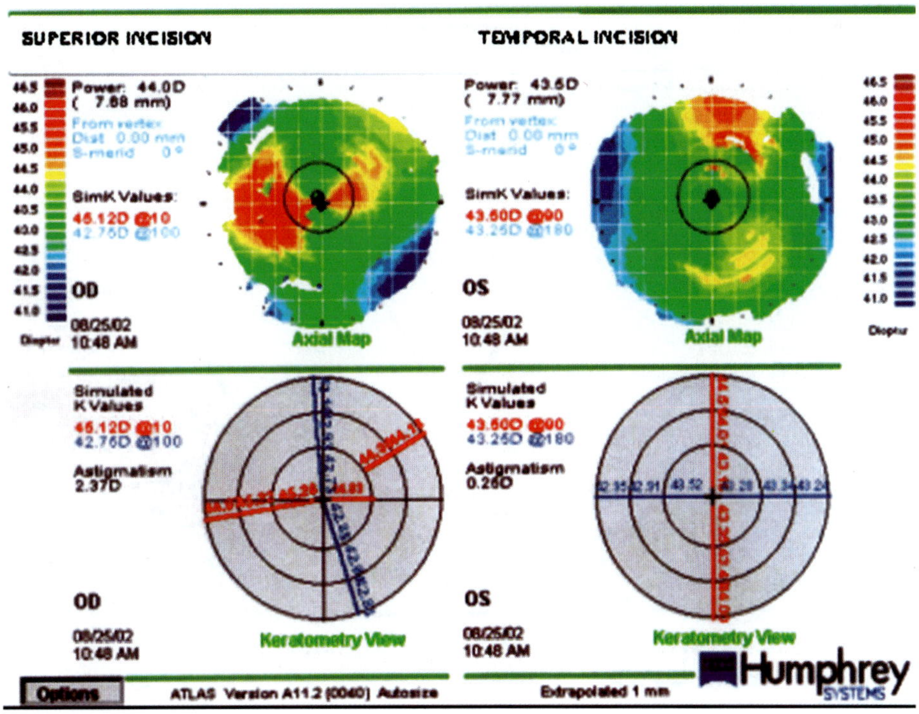

Fig. 32.9

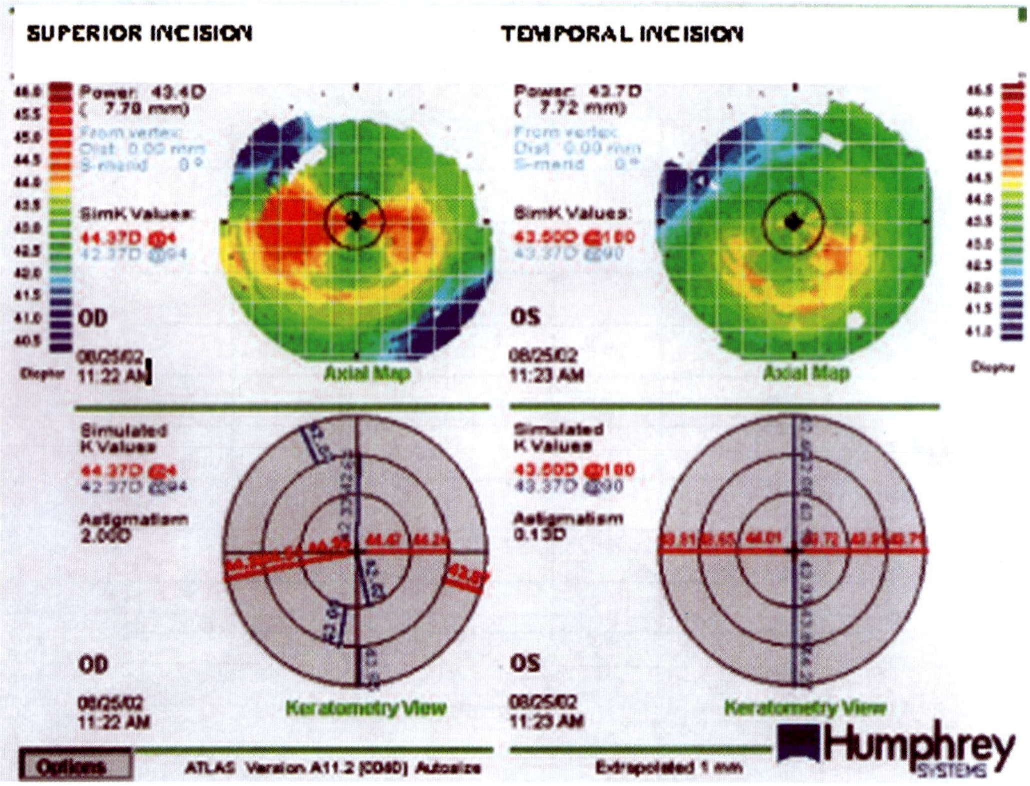

Fig. 32.10

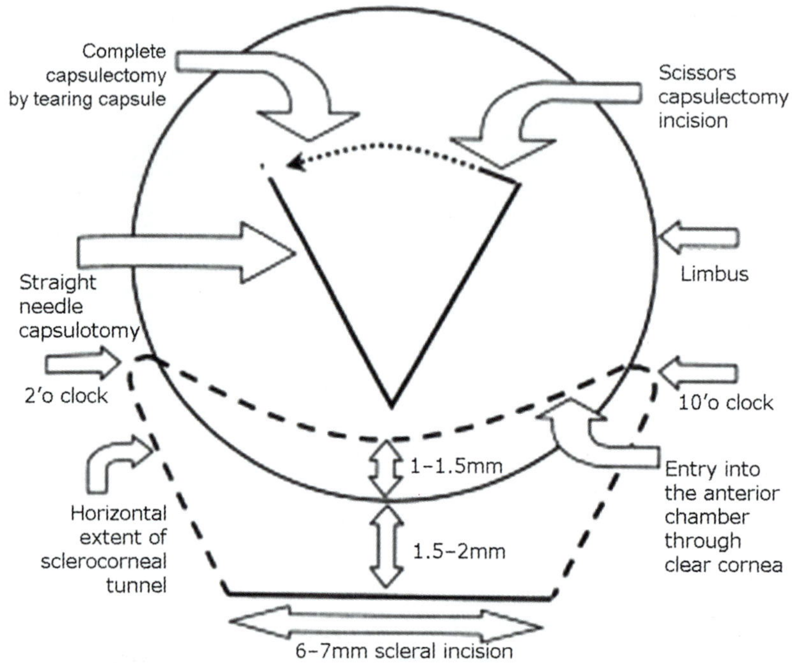

Fig. 32.11: Diagram of our sutureless ECCE/IOL techniques sclerocorneal tunnel and capsulotomy from the surgeon's perspective

REFERENCES

1. WHO Fact Sheet No 213. Global Initiative for the Elimination of Avoidable Blindness. 2000.
2. Thylefors B. A global initiative for the elimination of avoidable blindness [editorial]. Am J Ophthalmol 1998;125:90-93.
3. Ruit S, Tabin GC, Nissman SA, et al. Low-cost high-volume extracapsular cataract extraction with posterior chamber intraocular lens implantation in Nepal. Ophthalmology 1999;106(10):1887-92.
4. Ruit S, Paudyal G, Gurung R, et al. An innovation in developing world cataract surgery: sutureless extracapsular cataract extraction with intraocular lens implantation. Clinical and Experimental Ophthalmology 2000;28:274-79.
5. Chitkara DK, Smerdon DL. Risk factors, complications, and results in extracapsular cataract extraction. J Cataract Refract Surg 1997;23:570-74.
6. Cockerman GC, Hettinger ME, Azar DT. Astigmatism and Cataract Surgery. In: Albert DM, Jakobiec FA, Eds. Principles and Practice of Ophthalmology, 2nd ed. Philadelphia: Saunders, 2000:1538-50.
7. Flaxel JT, Swan KC. Limbal wound healing after cataract surgery: A histologic study. Arch Ophthalmol 1969;81:653-59.
8. Stainer GA, Binder PS, Parker WT, Perl T. Modulation of post cataract astigmatism by suturing techniques. Int Opthalmol Clin 1983;23:57-67.
9. Steinert RF, Brint SF, White SM, Fine IH. Astigmatism after small incision cataract surgery. Opthalmology 1991; 98:417-24.
10. Neumann AC, McCarty GR, Sanders DR, Raanan MG. Small incisions to control astigmatism during cataract surgery. J Cataract Refract Surg 1989;15:78-84.
11. Oshika T, Tsuboi S. Astigmatic and refractive stabilization after cataract surgery. Ophthalmic Surg 1995;26:309-15.
12. Gills JP, Sanders DR. Use of small incisions to control induced astigmatism and inflammation following cataract surgery. J Cataract Refract Surg 1991;17(Suppl):740-44.
13. Azar DT, Stark WJ, Dodick J, et al. Prospective, randomized, vector analysis of astigmatism after three, one, and no-suture phacoemulsification. J Cataract Refract Surg 1997;23:1164-73.
14. Levy JH, Pisacano AM, Chadwick K. Astigmatic changes after cataract surgery with 5.1 and 3.5 mm sutureless incisions. J Cataract Refract Surg 1994;20:630-33.
15. Gimbel HV, Sun R. Postoperative astigmatism following phacoemulsification with sutured versus unsutured wounds. Can J Ophthalmol 1993;28:259-62.
16. Mueller-Jensen K, Barlinn B. Long-term astigmatic changes after clear corneal cataract surgery. J Cataract Refract Surg 1997;23:354-57.
17. Long DA, Monica ML. A prospective evaluation of corneal curvature changes with 3.0 to 3.5 mm corneal tunnel phacoemulsification. Ophthalmology 1996;103:226-232.
18. Anders N, Pahm DT, Antoni HJ, Wollensak J. Postoperative astigmatism and relative strength of tunnel incisions: A prospective clinical trial. J Cataract Refract Surg 1997;23:332-36.
19. Oshima Y, Tsujikawa K, Oh A, Harino S. Comparative study of intraocular lens implantation through 3.0 mm temporal clear corneal and superior scleral tunnel self-sealing incisions. J Cataract Refract Surg 1997;23:347-53.
20. Gross RH, Miller KM. Corneal astigmatism after phacoemulsification and lens implantation through unsutured scleral and corneal tunnel incisions. Am J Ophthalmol 1996;121:57-64.
21. Cravy TV. Routine use of a lateral approach to cataract extraction to achieve rapid and sustained stabilization of postoperative astigmatism. J Cataract Refract Surg 1991;17:415-23.
22. Wong HC, Davis G, Della N. Corneal astigmatism induced by superior vs. temporal corneal incisions for extracapsular cataract extraction. Australian and New Zealand J of Ophthalmology 1994;22(4):237-41.
23. Axt JC, McCaffery JM. <outbind://3/das/journal/view/29716525/O/2403719?sid=192075220&source=MI> Reduction of postoperative against-the-rule astigmatism by lateral incision technique. J Cataract Refract Surg 1993;19(3):380-86.

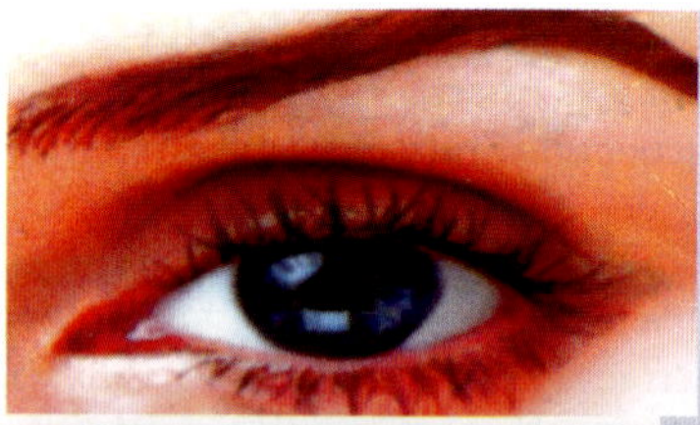

Thirty three

Phaco Sandwich Technique in SICS

Kamaljeet Singh
(India)

INTRODUCTION

Fry is a credited with the phaco sandwich technique. This technique is simple, allows removal of lens through a sutureless 6.0 – 6.5 mm self sealing scleral tunnel incision and produces much less astigmatism compared to extra-capsular cataract surgery. The author has adopted this technique for over 5 years and results have been gratifying.

INSTRUMENTATION

Essentially the instruments required are similar to what an ECCE surgeon requires. Additional instruments are.

- Crescent knife
- 3.2 mm angled Keratome
- 5.2 mm Keratome
- Irrigating vectis
- Sinskey type dialer, iris repositor

PREOPERATIVE PREPARATION

The essential thing in this surgery is wide dilatation of pupil, which allows easy prolapse of the nucleus in anterior chamber, prevents iris entrapment during delivery of nucleus. Pupil dilatation and its maintenance in dilated status is achieved by instilling tropicamide and phenylephrine combination + flurbiprofen eye drops. These are instilled 1 hour before the surgery. Author suggests a conventional ECCE if the pupil is less than 5 mm in diameter, at least in initial 50 cases. Acetazolamide one tablet is given 2 hours prior to surgery.

Anesthesia

A peribulbar anesthesia with a cocktail of 3 ml of Xylocaine with adrenaline and 3 ml sensosrcaine mixed with hylase is used. Superpinky ball or ocular massage for long is not recommended as it produces hypotony.

SURGICALTECHNIQUE

Wound Construction

After applying speculum and holding superior rectus a fornix based conjunctival flap is fashioned. Bipolar cautery should be carried out carefully. It gives a bloodless field to operate and there is no inadvertent bleeding during the making of scleral tunnel, but its excessive use should be avoided as it causes postoperative astigmatism. 6 mm to 6.5mm partial thickness scleral tunnel incision is made 1.5 mm behind limbus (Fig. 33.1). Harder the nucleus longer is the incision. In initial 25 patients longer incision is recommended to avoid nucleus touch to the corneal endothelium. The scleral pocket is made with crescent knife (Fig. 33.2). Disposable crescent blades are the best. Their reuse might lead to a poor tunnel. This is the single most important step in this surgery. Therefore, no compromise should

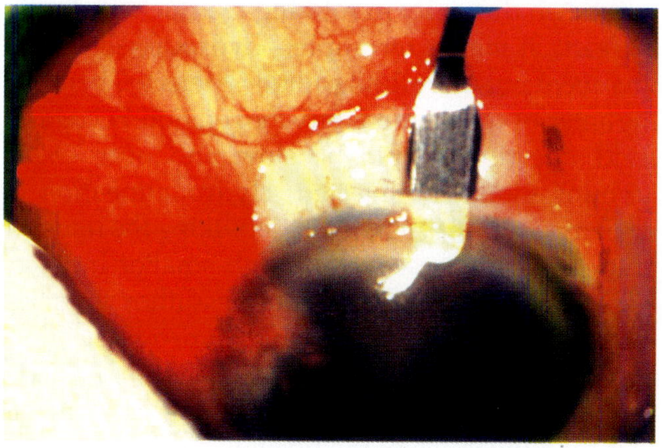

Fig. 33.1: Scleral tunnell being made

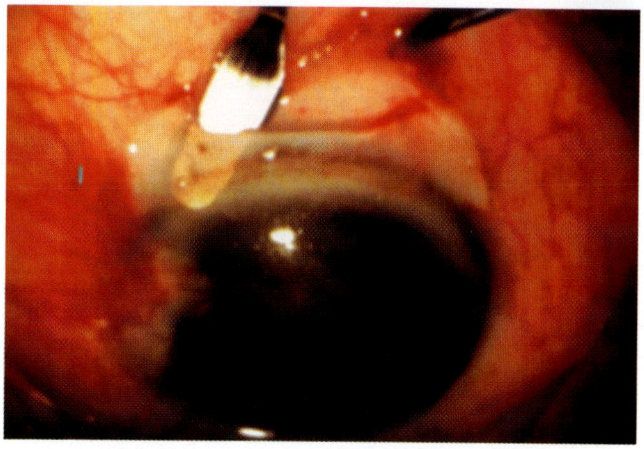

Fig. 33.2: Scleral pocket being fashioned

be accepted. Scleral pocket is extended in the corneal stroma. While making scleral tunnel, sclera induces greater resistance than the cornea. Therefore when the surgeon reaches close to limbus his movement should be very gentle. Otherwise, it may lead to early entry into the anterior chamber causing formation of a leaky corneal valve. The corneal tunnel should extend up to 1.5 mm from the limbus and the corneal incision should be 2 mm wider than the scleral incision. Entry into the anterior chamber is made with a 3.2 mm angled keratome. It should be sharp–blunt Keratome leads to Descemet's detachment. A dimple on the anterior surface of cornea is seen when pressure of the keratome is applied towards the anterior chamber (Fig. 33.3). Then entry into the anterior chamber is made (Fig. 33.4). This movement should be well controlled otherwise it may hit the anterior capsule causing rupture of the anterior capsule, which may jeopardizes the fashioning of capsulorhexis.

Capsulotomy

Viscoelastic is injected into the anterior chamber. Here, the care should be taken to slightly press the scleral side so that the aqueous leaks out and the viscoelastic takes it place. It will make the anterior chamber deep and capsulotomy becomes easier. Any type of capsulotomy can be fashioned in SICS —can-opener, envelope or capsulorhexis, all are useful. In fact author suggests can-opener and envelope technique in initial few cases, because the prolapse of the nucleus in AC is much easier

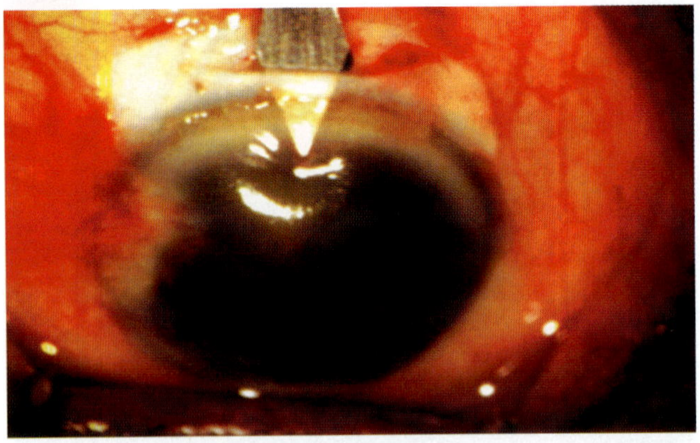
Fig. 33.3: Dimple at the cornea before entry into anterior chamber

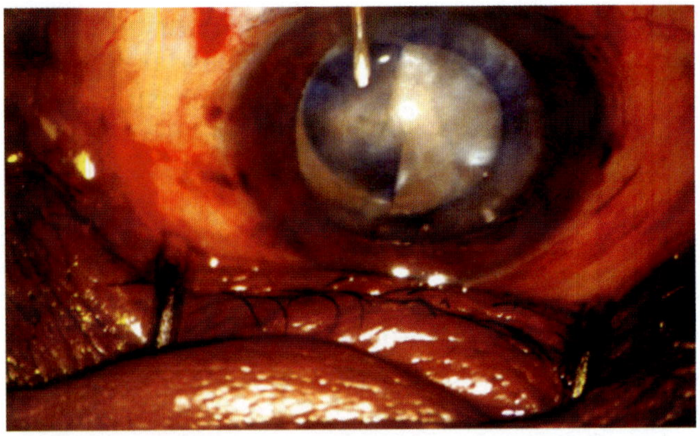
Fig. 33.5: Capsulorhexis in progress

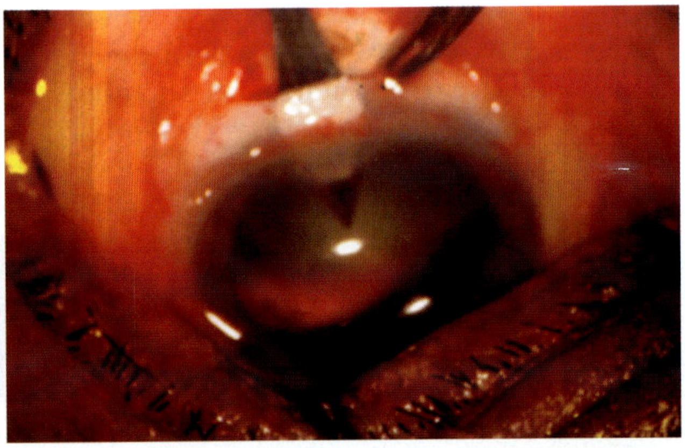
Fig. 33.4: Entry into anterior chamber with 3.2 keratome

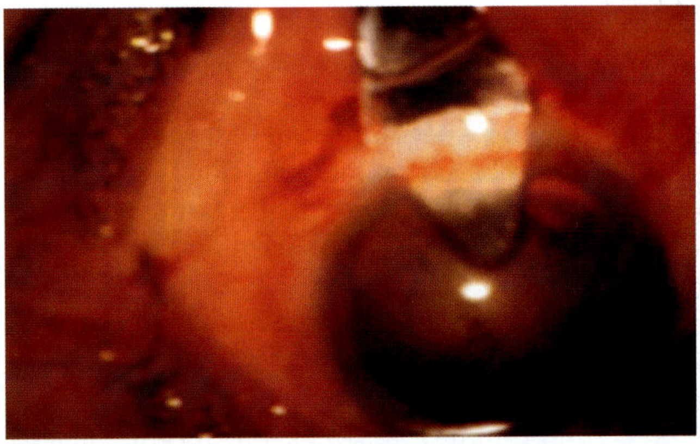
Fig. 33.6: Extension of incision

than when a capsulorhexis has been fashioned. Size is important in case one prefers to make capsulorhexis (Fig. 33.5). It should be not less than 6.5 mm and slightly eccentric on the upper side. Both these things will help in prolapse of the nucleus in the AC. In case the capsulorhexis is small, whole nucleus with capsular bag may come in the AC. Then it would be intra-capsular rather than extra-capsular surgery. In this case two relaxing incisions on the edge of capsulorhexis at 11 and 2 o'clock may facilitate the prolapse of nucleus in anterior chamber. Once the rhexis ix complete the incision is extended to desired size of 6-6.5mm (Fig. 33.6).

Hydrodissection-Hydrodelineation

Aim of hydrodissection is to break all the adhesions between cortex and capsule. This results in a freely rotating nucleus within the bag. The technique of hydrodissection has been described elsewhere. Two points need to be mentioned here. Don't try to strain the zonules by pushing your rotating instrument too hard. If hydrodissection is complete there will be no difficulty in rotating the nucleus. If it is difficult, it means incomplete hydrodissection. In this event put more fluid should be injected beneath the anterior capsule and retry the rotation. Secondly, fluid injection should be slow and only small amount should be injected. Hydrodelineation is not a must in SICS. It helps in debulking the nucleus and delivery of nucleus through smaller incision becomes easier. But presently, the author does the expression of nucleus without hydrodelineation because the epinucleus is a soft structure. Its accidental touch to the endothelium causes less damage to it than the touch of the nucleus.

Nuclear Luxation

This is single important step in a successful SICS. Nuclear luxation or prolapse in anterior chamber is easier, if the pupil is widely dilated and a good rotation of the nucleus is achieved after hydrodissection. In initial few cases, prolapsing the nucleus in anterior chamber is easy if can-opener or envelope type of capsulotomy has been performed. The nucleus is prolapsed by rotating the nucleus after filling the chamber with viscoelastic. The moment, rim of nucleus is visualized, the cannula is brought below the rim of nucleus; and again viscoelastic is injected in between the nucleus and capsule. The upper pole of nucleus will prolapse in the AC (Fig. 33. 7). In small pupils one can depress the nucleus at 5 O'clock with the cannula. The upper pole tilts anteriorly at 11 O'clock. Now the nucleus is rotated toward 12 O'clock. Thus achieving the aim of prolapse of upper pole of nucleus. Once you are sure about prolapse of nucleus in AC, inject more viscoelastic between the cornea and anterior surface of nucleus and also behind the nucleus. This maneuver requires copious use of viscoelastic to prevent injury to the corneal endothelial cells. Once this is achieved the nucleus is now ready for delivery.

Nuclear Delivery

The author uses irrigating vectis and a Sinskey type of dialer but the difference here is that it is like a hammer at the end and much thicker than the dialer. Thus it has blunt end, which prevents injury to posterior capsule. The author calls it a dumbbell. Fluid flow through the vectis is checked. First thing is to enter anterior chamber through the incision with the dumbbell in your left hand. This is kept at the center of nucleus (Fig. 33.8). No pressure is applied. Then the irrigating vectis is passed behind the nucleus in such a way that the nucleus is sandwiched between these two instruments (Fig. 33.9). Now pressure is applied from below the nucleus and also on the anterior surface of lens. Pressure should be more from the top than from beneath. Once you are sure about the hold, the sandwiched nucleus is brought out of the wound taking care that the sandwiched nucleus does not touch the corneal endothelium. In this process two things may result. If the lens is soft, it will come out in one go. If it is hard, it may break into several pieces. A part of that will come out sandwiched between two instruments. Remaining pieces of nucleus are taken out by either viscoexpression.

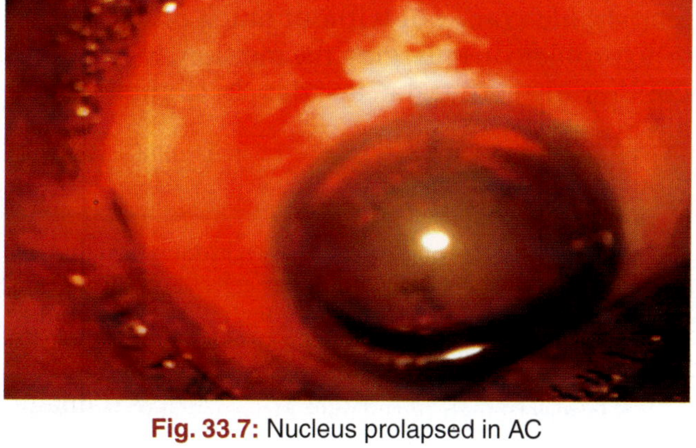

Fig. 33.7: Nucleus prolapsed in AC

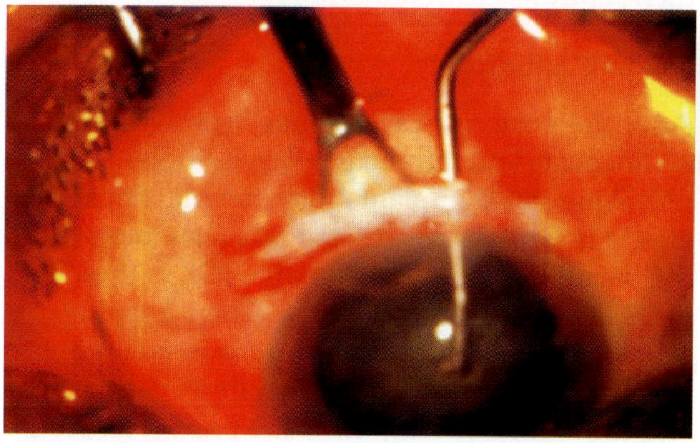

Fig. 33.8: The Sinskey or dumbbell goes first in the anterior chamber; the vectis follows afterwards

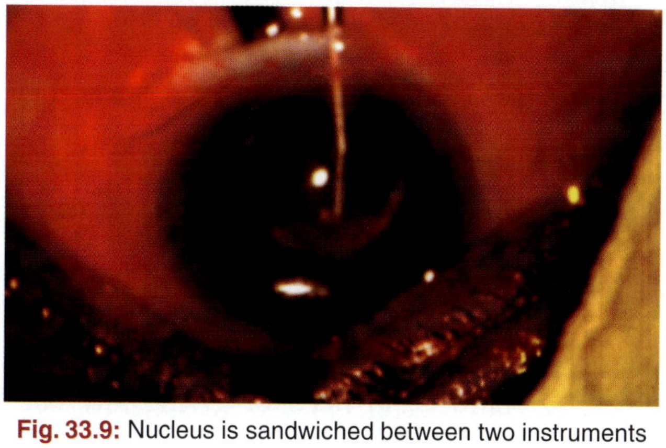

Fig. 33.9: Nucleus is sandwiched between two instruments

One needs to be very cautious here. The anterior surface of nucleus or its pieces should always have viscoelastic in front of them. In case one finds difficulty in delivering out the nucleus, the incision length should be increased. This problem is normally encountered in brown hard cataracts. Rarely in very big nucleus the tunnel has to be abandoned and a routine ECCE is performed.

Cortical Cleanup

Remaining debris is perinucleus and cortical matter. This is removed by two way Simcoe cannula, which is attached to a bottle. Cannula is opened with full flow. Take this free flowing cannula to 6 O'clock and slight pressure with the cannula on tunnel will cause perinucleus to come out. Remaining material is cortex. A part of this will come out with perinucleus by hydro-expression. Cortical fibers are then aspirated with the cannula.

IOL Implantation

After the posterior capsule has been washed and no fibers are left, intraocular lens is implanted. The technique of IOL implantation is simple. First viscoelastic is injected in the anterior chamber within the bag. All PMMA nonfoldable IOL is then held with the IOL holder forceps. Then keeping the direction of haptic downwards it is pushed into the lower capsular bag. The optic goes in the anterior chamber with the same push (Fig. 33.10). Now the trailing haptic is inserted in the bag by dialing it with the Sinskey hook if IOL has holes, or with the Y shaped dialer, if there is no hole in the IOL.

Wound Closure

Conjunctiva is reposited back by holding the conjunctiva with two forceps. Cautery is then applied at two ends. Sutures are usually not applied in the section. They are needed only when the valve is compromised. A figure of eight suture usually suffices in that case. Then gentamycin and dexamethasone injection is instilled on the top of conjunctiva. There is no need of giving any subconjunctival injection.

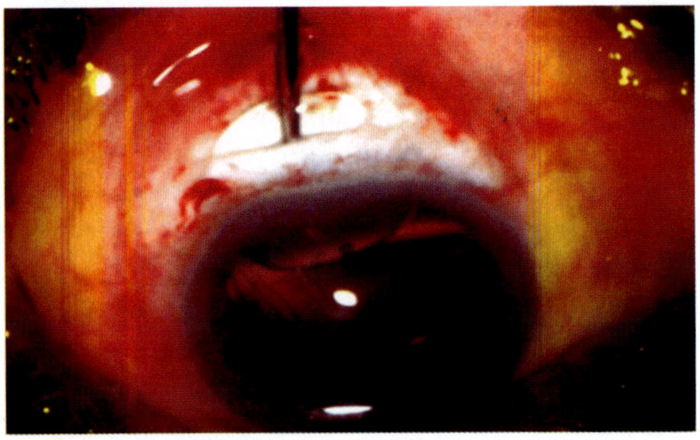

Fig. 33.10: IOL is implanted after thorough wash

Complications

The complications of phaco sandwich technique per se are few. Intraoperative complications include damage to corneal endothelium, iridodialysis, and posterior capsule rupture postoperatively transient corneal edema may be frequent, if too much handling has been done with in the chamber.

Recommendation

Before contemplating the manual small incision cataract surgery by the phaco sandwich technique the surgeon should thoroughly examine the cataract for its hardness. Initially one should not try this technique in very hard cataracts. This surgery is fine for up to grade 3 and 4 hardness. The wound should be enlarged to 6.5 mm. 1 mm larger than this is recommended for harder nuclei. The nuclear luxation into the anterior chamber, at least of the upper pole is must. Before sandwiching the nucleus copious amount of viscoelastic has to be used on the top of nucleus and behind the nucleus. The lens should come out without much of fuss. There is no problem in enlarging the incision, which gives you shining cornea the next day. In slightest doubt always apply suture.

REFERENCES

1. Fry, Luther. The phacosandwich technique in George W Rozakis et al (Ed); Cataract Surgery: Alternative Small Incision Techniques. Thorofare Inc. 71-110; 1995 Indian edn.
2. Singh, Kamaljeet. The Phacosandwich technique in Kamaljeet Singh (Ed). Small Incision Cataract Surgery (Manual Phaco). Jaypee Brothers, India 2002;101-07.

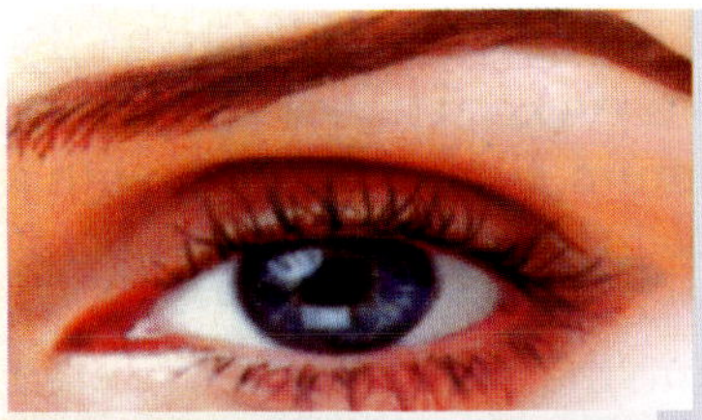

Thirty four

Sutureless Cataract Surgery with Nucleus Extraction—Fishhook Technique

Albrecht Hennig
(Nepal)

BACKGROUND

In 1997, I met Prof Michael Blumenthal during a conference in Nepal and learnt about his mini-nuc technique, which I introduced in our Lahan Eye Hospital in southeast Nepal. Being a busy eye hospital with often 300-350 cataract surgeries per day, performed by four surgeons, there was need for a different, more simplified technique. Instead of anterior chamber maintainer and hydroexpression of the nucleus, we use a small hook for nucleus extraction. From 1998 till August 2003, more than 160,000 sutureless cataract operations with nucleus extraction have been performed at Lahan. In the meantime, this technique has spread to many Asian and African countries and even some surgeons in Germany use it when phacoemulsification is not appropriate. It is named "Lahan Technique", "Hennig Technique" or more often "Fishhook Technique". In 2000, a video of this technique was honoured with a Special Award during the Annual Meeting of German Ophthalmic Surgeons (DOC).

THE HOOK

The hook is made of a 30G ½ inch needle, bending it with fine pliers or a needle holder. There are two bends:

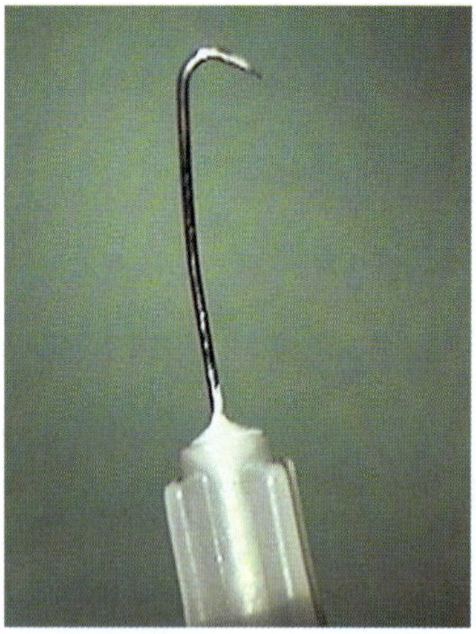

Fig. 34.1: "Fishhook", showing the bent tip of the 30G ½ inch needle

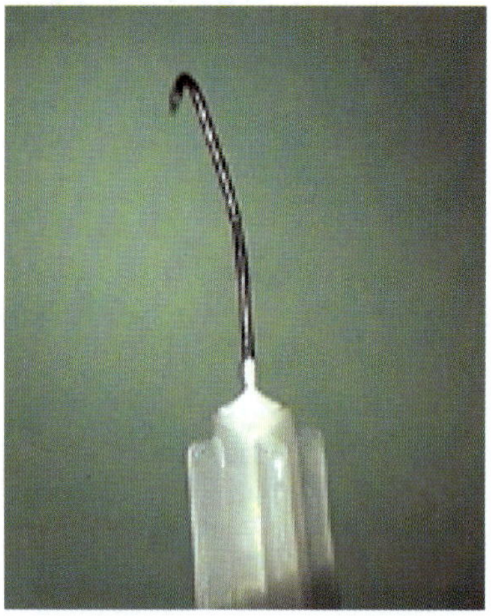

Fig. 34.2: "Fishhook", side view

1. The tip of the needle (Fig. 34.1), which will insert into the central nucleus.
2. A slight bend between the tip and the plastic mount (Fig. 34.2) to assure an easy insertion between the lower part of the nucleus and the posterior capsule.

   The hook is mounted on a 1 ml tuberculine syringe and can be re-autoclaved and used for hundreds of nucleus extractions.

THETECHNIQUE

Tunnel Construction

After fornix-based conjunctival preparation and scleral cauterization, the sclero-corneal tunnel can be done at 12 o'clock or temporal, ideally at the steepest corneal meridian to keep the postoperative astigmatism at a minimum. Scleral fixation with a good catching forceps, e.g. Pierse or Paufique, helps to perform a controlled corneo-scleral tunnel with a minimum of 1 mm into the clear cornea. We start with a scleral Frown incision (Fig. 34.3) with a central distance of at least 2 mm behind the limbus (Fig. 34.4). The width of the tunnel depends on the age of the patient and the size of the nucleus. Very big brown nuclei may require an inner opening to the anterior chamber of at least 8 mm (Fig. 34.5).

For beginners we recommend conventional tunnel instruments. Experienced surgeons may use a diamond knife (double lancet with sharp sides), which enables them to perform the three tunnel steps as well as a linear capsulotomy with the same instrument.

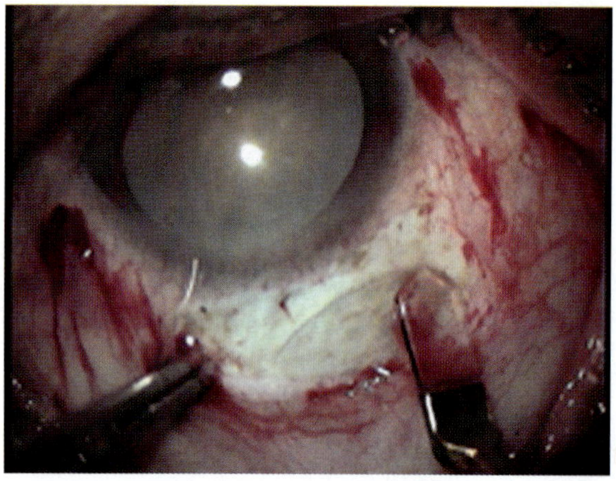

Fig. 34.3: Frown incision

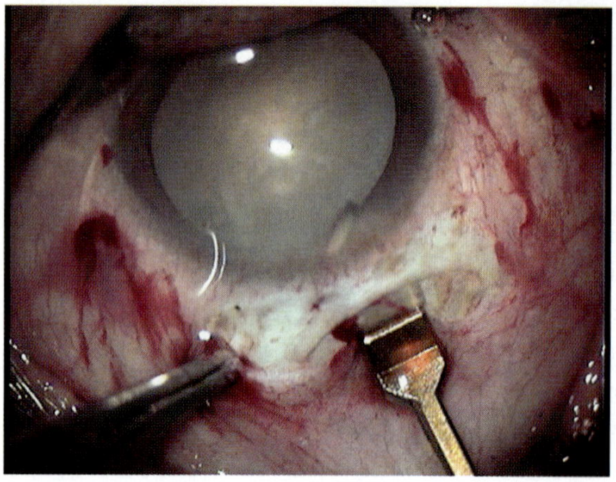

Fig. 34.4: Sclero-corneal tunnel

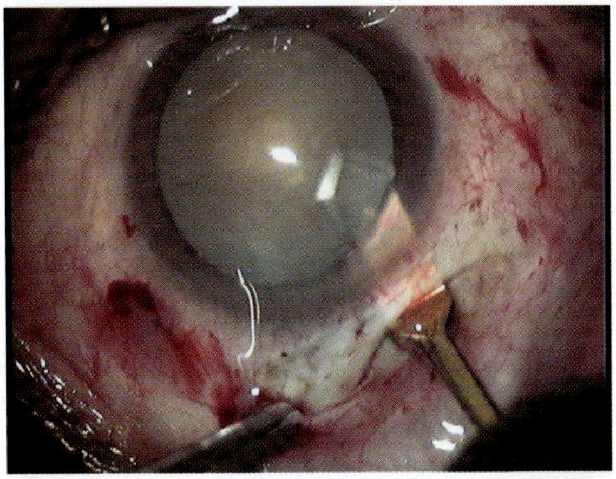

Fig. 34.5: Opening of the anterior chamber

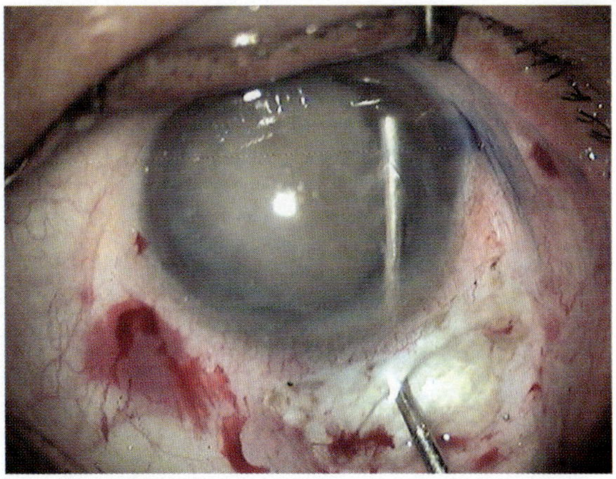

Fig. 34.7: Hydrodissection and nucleus mobilization

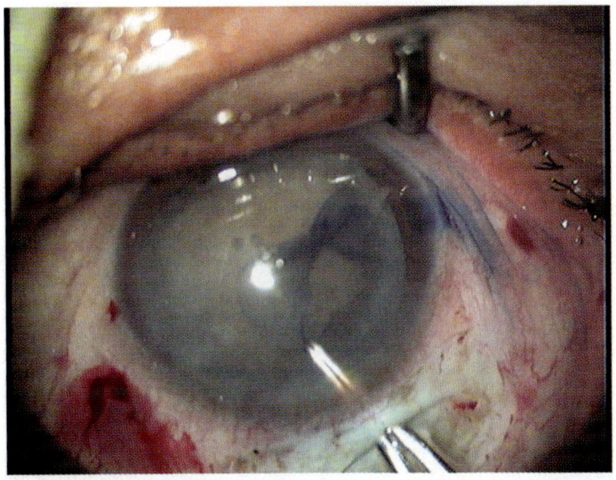

Fig. 34.6: Continuous curvilinear capsulorhexis

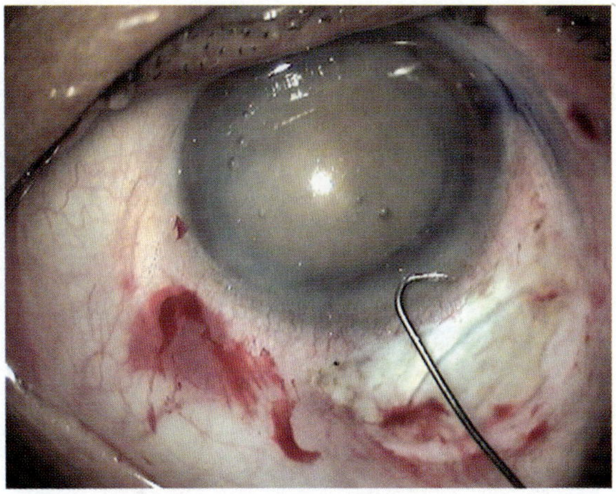

Fig. 34.8: The hook before insertion

Capsular Opening

A linear capsulotomy is either done with the keratome after preparing the inner corneal opening, or with a diamond knife. Preferred is a continuous curvilinear capsulorhexis (CCC) of 6-7 mm diameter (Fig. 34.6). However, CCC may be difficult in various advanced cataracts.

Hydrodissection and Nucleus Mobilization

After linear capsulotomy a forceful hydrodissection separates the capsule from the rest of the crystalline lens. Using the same irrigating cannula, the nucleus plus cortex is mobilized and slightly lifted up at the tunnel opening site.

In case of CCC, a careful hydrodissection is done on one side. If the CCC is large enough the cortex plus nucleus will tilt and partly prolapse mostly contralateral to the hydrodissection side. Then the elevated cortex-nucleus part is rotated towards the tunnel opening position (Fig. 34.7).

Nucleus Hook Extraction

After placing some viscoelastics between nucleus and posterior capsule and into the anterior chamber, the bent 30G needle hook (Fig. 34.8) is inserted between nucleus and posterior capsule with the sharp needle tip pointing to the right side. Then the hook is turned and slightly pulled back, so that the needle tip is engaged into the central lower portion of the nucleus (Fig. 34.9).

Without lifting, the nucleus is pulled out of the capsular bag and through the tunnel (Fig. 34.10).

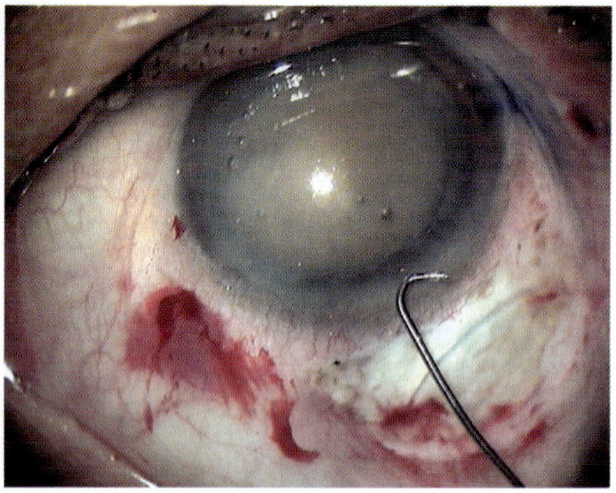

Fig. 34.9: Insertion of the hook between nucleus and posterior capsule

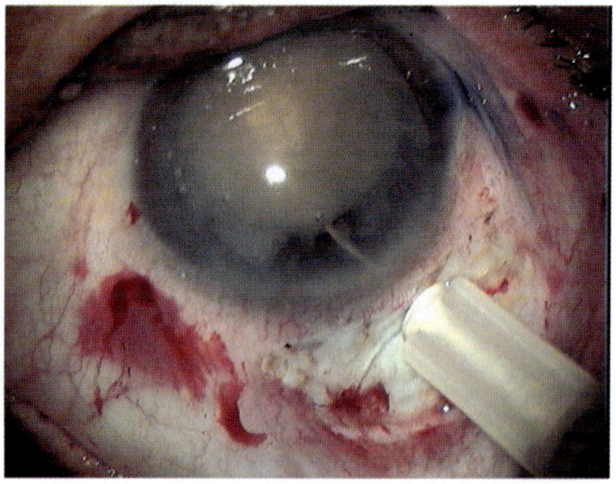

Fig. 34.10: Hook extraction of the nucleus out of the capsular bag

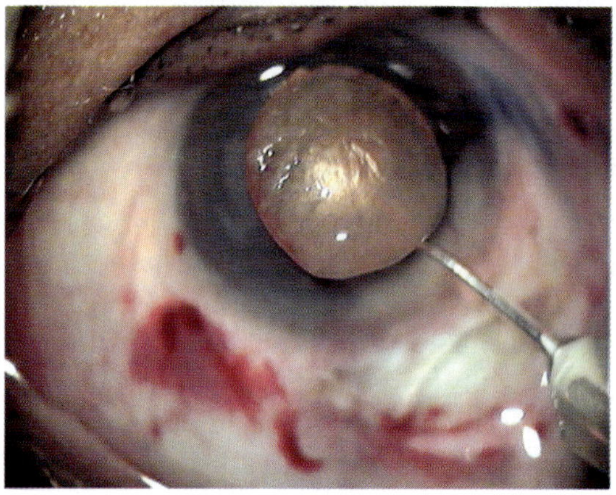

Fig. 34.11: Extracted nucleus, top view

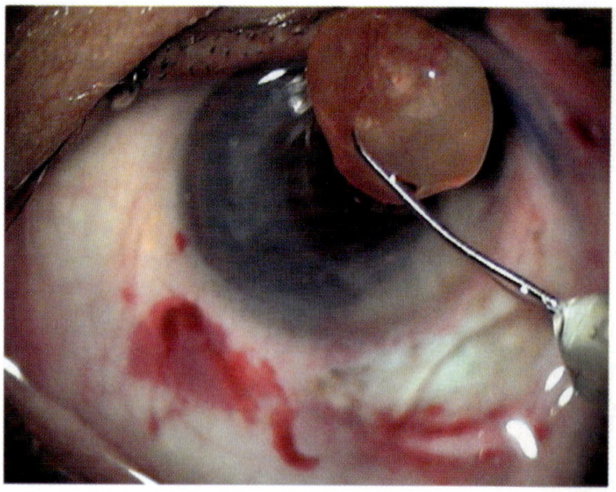

Fig. 34.12: Extracted nucleus, side view

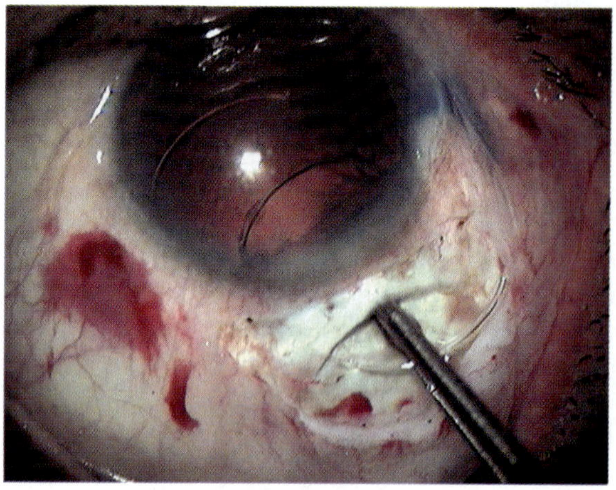

Fig. 34.13: Insertion of IOL

Cortex remains in the anterior chamber, acts as a cushion and thus protects the endothelium from any contact with the nucleus.

Once the tip of the hook is correctly inserted into the nucleus, there is no risk to damage any part of the eye, nor does the nucleus rotate or tilt while being extracted (Figs 34.11 and 34.12).

Completing the Surgery

After hydroexpression of remaining cortex and removal with a Simcoe cannula, a 6 mm optic PMMA IOL is inserted into the capsular bag (Figs 34.13 and 34.14).

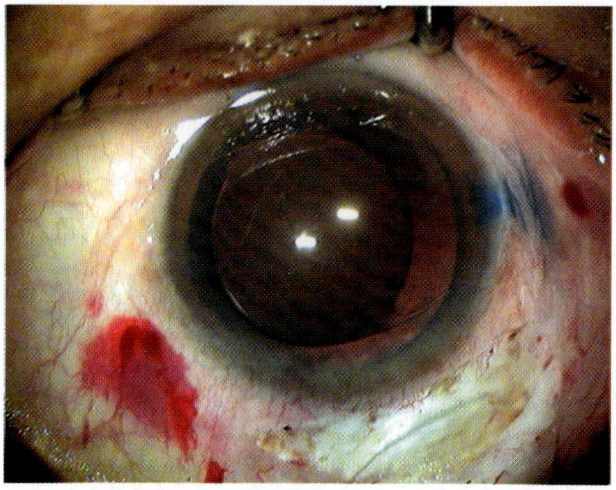

Fig. 34.14: IOL placed in capsular bag

In case of linear capsulotomy, two small cuts are done with fine scissors on both sides of the anterior capsule, and the anterior capsule removed.

OUTCOME

In the hands of experienced surgeons sutureless cataract surgery with nucleus hook extraction has a very low surgical complication rate and provides excellent immediate uncorrected postoperative visual acuity.[1]

This is underlined by another outcome study on high volume surgery where six surgeons performed 2,111 sutureless cataract surgeries within six days.[2]

LEARNING CURVE

Sutureless tunnel surgery is more difficult to learn than ab-externo ECCE/PC IOL with sutures. Ophthalmologists without surgical experience may start with sutured ab-externo ECCE/PC IOL. Once they achieve consistent good results with a low surgical complication rate, a step-wise conversion to sutureless surgery is advised.

There is a much shorter learning curve for experienced phaco surgeons. They just need to learn the preparation of a larger tunnel and have to get familiar with the nucleus hook extraction. Once this technique is mastered, experienced eye surgeons at our hospital are able to perform 15-20 sutureless cataract operations per hour.

SPECIAL HIGHLIGHTS

The sutureless cataract surgery with nucleus hook extraction is a safe, fast and inexpensive technique, which provides immediate good visual outcome.

The only additional instrument needed is a 30G needle, bent to a hook.

Among all other sutureless cataract surgical techniques, our technique is the only one where the nucleus is extracted straight from the capsular bag through the tunnel, avoiding corneal endothelium touch.

Nucleus extraction requires a smaller tunnel size than nucleus removal by hydroexpression.

With more than 160,000 sutureless cataract surgeries performed in Lahan and many more in other eye centers around the world, the nucleus hook extraction is one of the techniques most often used in sutureless non-phaco cataract surgery.

Acknowledgements

I thank Dr. Jan Tynovsky, who in 1998 played an important role in the development of the hook extraction technique.

Special thanks goes to my German colleague Dr. Bernd Schroeder, who reviewed the text and produced the photographs.

I am grateful to all my colleagues and hospital staff members. Due to their dedicated and hard work, every year thousands of blind cataract patients get their sight restored with the help of our surgical technique.

REFERENCES

1. Hennig A, Kumar J, Yorston D, Foster A: Sutureless cataract surgery with nucleus extraction: Outcome of a prospective study in Nepal. Br J Ophthalmol 2003; 87(3):266-70
2. Hennig A, Kumar J, Singh AK, Singh S, Gurung R, Foster A: World Sight Day and cataract blindness. BrJ Ophthalmol 2002;86:830-31.

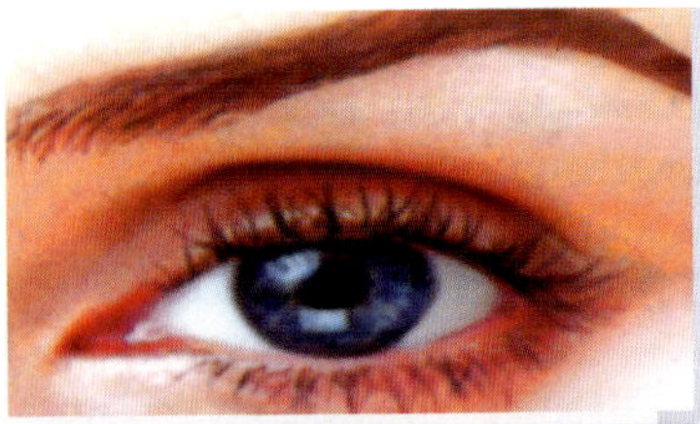

Thirty five

The Jaws Slider Pincer Technique for Small Incision Non-phaco Cataract Surgery

Keiki Mehta
Cyres Mehta (India)

Small incision, non-phaco techniques are very important to achieve consistent success in cataract surgery. There are many techniques available which permit it to be done with a high level of accuracy and competency. However all techniques at present are dependent on the lens lying flat with the hard nucleus being sheared off , or chopped off, with the nucleus lying horizontally, flat abutting the posterior capsule. The risk factors with this techniques is that the dome of the cornea may be damaged with endothelial cell loss leading to corneal decompensation, or damage may occur to the iris if entrapped between the choppers or splitters, or the incision may be damaged leading to an non occluding incision requiring sutures which enhance the astigmatism, or the posterior capsule is likely to be damaged often irretrievably with the result that a implant cannot be inserted and the with the added possibility of nuclear drop, either partial or total.

The obvious answer to prevent any possibility of damage is to handle the lens vertically. In an effort to analyze the technique in two consecutive eye camps, all cases were selected , to be done with the slider pincer technique only.

THE INSTRUMENTS

The "Jaws" slider pincer is a specially designed instrument to cut even the hardest cataract into longitudinal slices. It has its tip designed as a beak of a bird and properly rounded to permit its easy entry into the eye . The jaws of the slider pincer literally slide open thus placing no stress whatsoever on the 3.2 mm incision. The jaws are made of hardened tungsten steel to prevent any whiplash on handling hard cataracts. The tips of the pincer forceps are designed with the part placed at 12 o'clock being blunt with roughened edges to prevent slippage , while the 6 o'clock placement pincer is made curved and sharp to permit easy slicing through the substance of the lens (Figs 35.1 to 35.5).

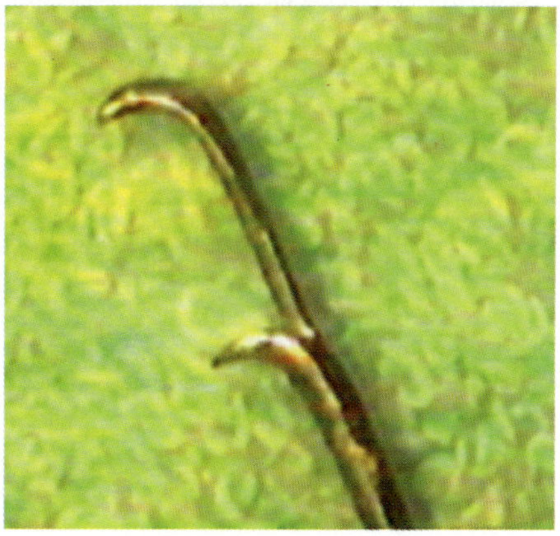

Fig. 35.1: The Slider pincer instrument. Note the inner part of the upper slider is sharp while the lower part is flat to prevent it slipping off the nucleus when held

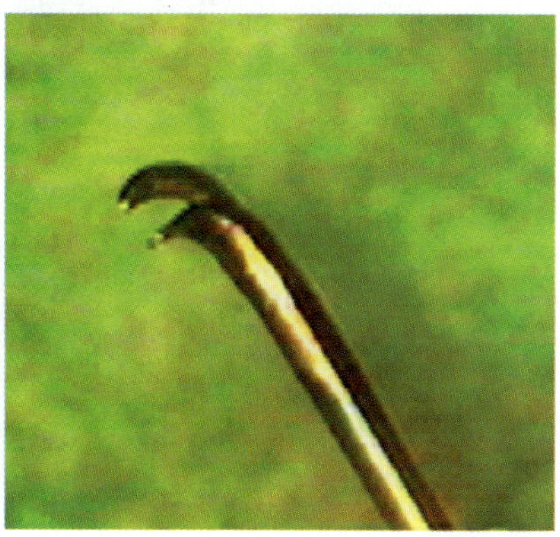

Fig. 35.2: The slider pincer now being closed . Note the close approximation

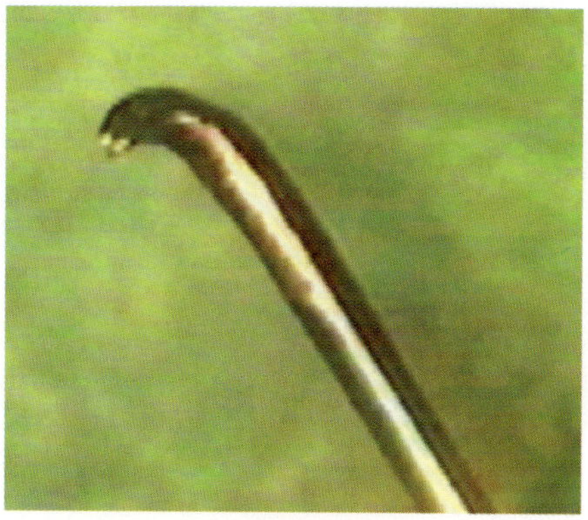

Fig. 35.3

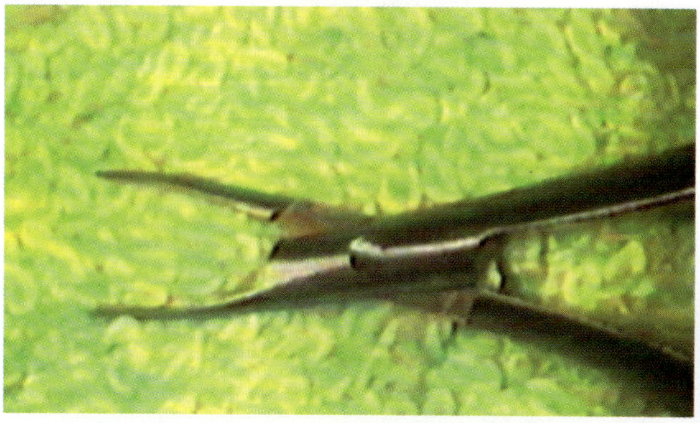

Fig. 35.4

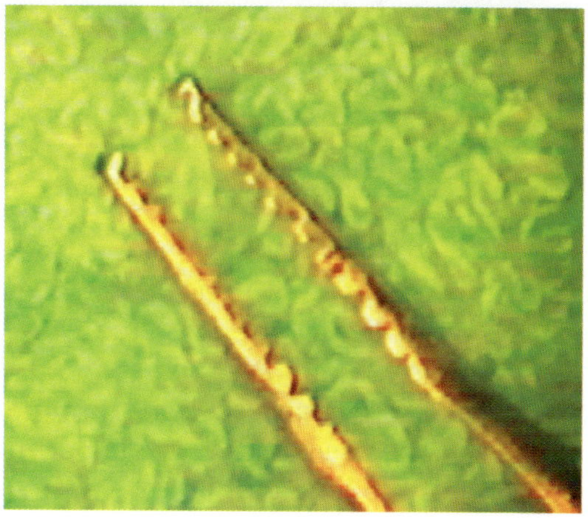

Fig. 35.5

THETECHNIQUE

The standard technique utilized was to do a corneal tunnel entry with a 3.2 mm diamond knife (Fig. 35.6), a good capsullorhexis (Fig. 35.7) followed by hydrodissection which is done in two parts. The first part is carried out using either BSS or Ringer-

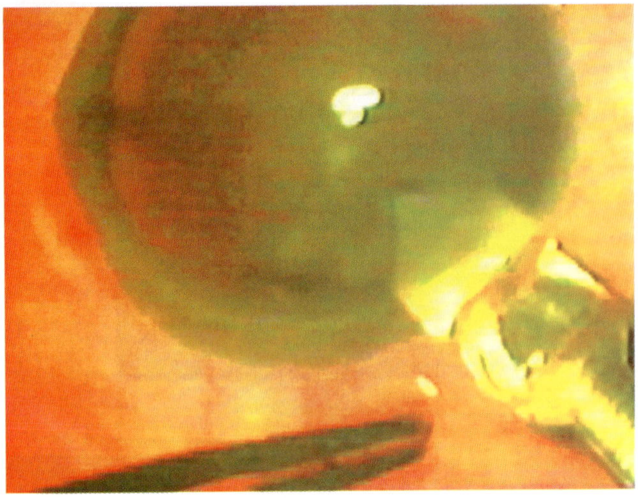

Fig. 35.6

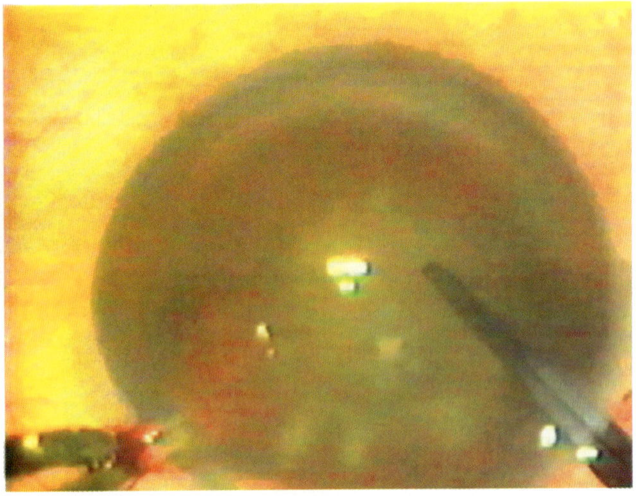

Fig. 35.7

lactate. The moment it is noticed that the fluid wave has spread below the lens, the cannula is removed and a specially designed cannula which is three port attached to a viscoelastic cannula (Figs 35.8 and 35.9). The use of this cannula permits the easy rotation of the lens with no pressure on the posterior capsule.

Once the lens is made to rotate out of the capsular bag, the specially designed pincer forceps is introduced via the incision. Since it is curved, it manages to easily enter the eye with no stress on the incision (Fig. 35.10). It is introduced in its closed form, sideways and then gradually opened up to encompass the width of the nucleus (Fig. 35.11). Once it is properly positioned the jaws are closed

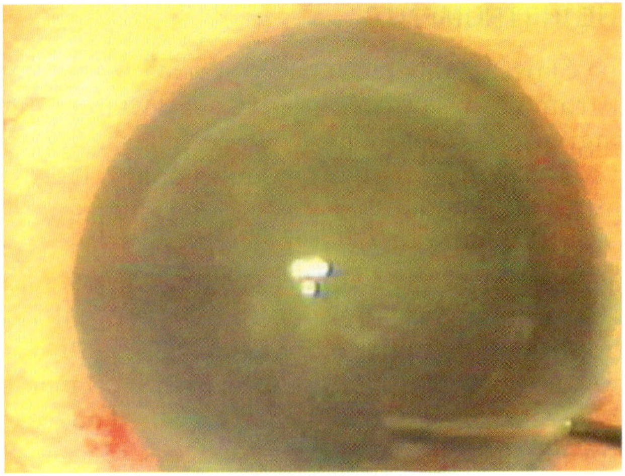

Fig. 35.8

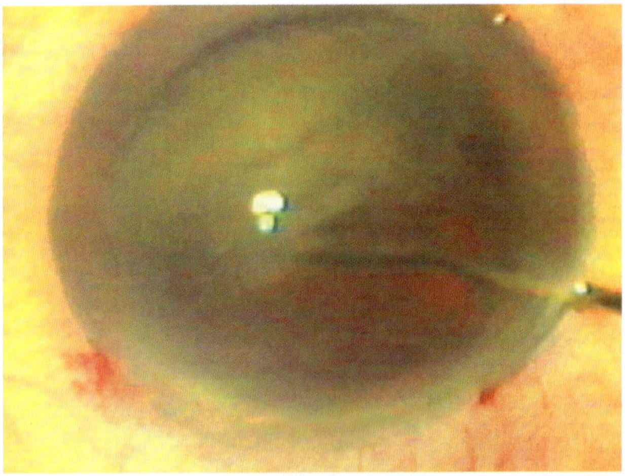

Fig. 35.9

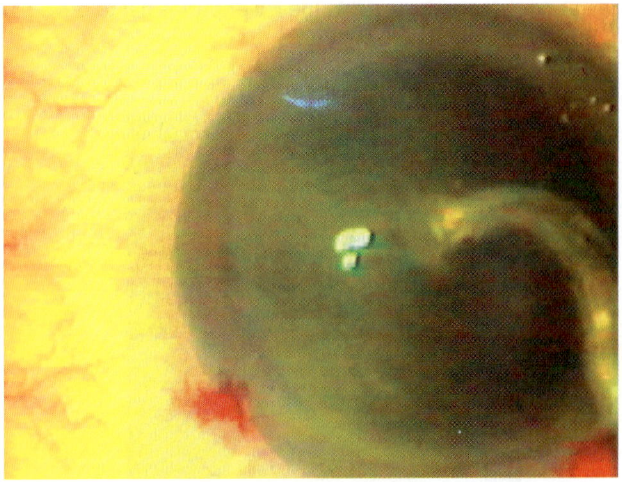

Fig. 35.10: Once the nucleus is in the anterior chamber, the 'jaws' is inserted via the 3.2 mm incision on the surface of the nucleus

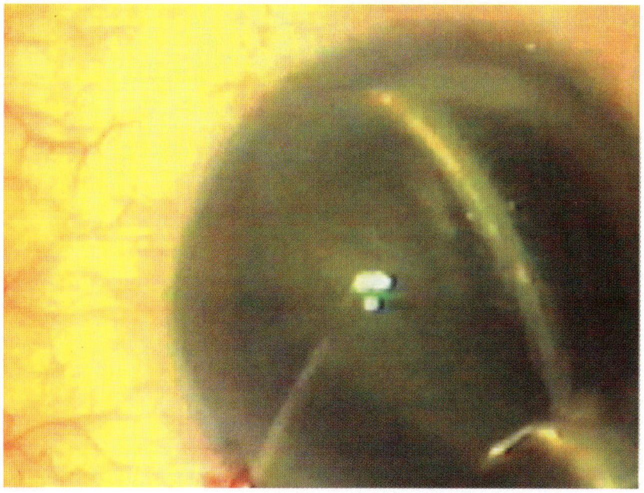

Fig. 35.11: The Jaws is opened up fully until it encompasses the nucles. A repositor from the side may be used to properly position the lens

which automatically sections the nucleus into two parts (Fig. 35.12). On an average, +2 or +3 density cataract , two pieces are adequate, as the pieces will compress when held with a forceps and come out easily enough from a 3.2 mm opening. However if the density is higher, especially if it is Grade +5 or over (suprahard) cataract it may be necessary to cut the cataract into three or even four slices. Thus the initial slice will be from 1 o'clock to 5 o'clock, while the middle piece will cut at 12 o'clock to 6 o'clock , while the last piece will be from 11 o'clock

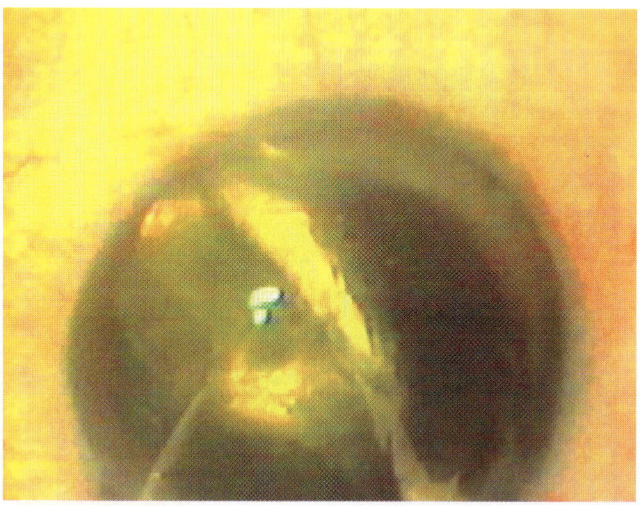

Fig. 35.12: As the slider is approximated, it immediately slices through the nucleus. Literally with this instrument no resistance is noted even with the hardest nucleus

to 7 o'clock position. Thus these hard pieces will be easy to remove. Always remember to cut the pieces longitudinally as cross cutting a piece has no advantage and makes it more troublesome to remove.

Utilizing the specially designed non-apposing curved forceps the pieces can be easily removed in their entirety (Figs 35.13 to 35.15). The tips of the forceps do not appose and thus can never grasp iris accidentally. One of the biggest advantages of this procedure over the "sandwich" technique of

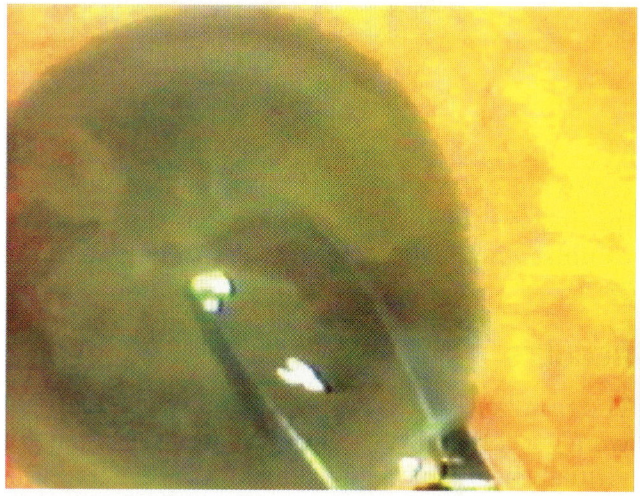

Fig. 35.13: Using the special delivery forceps literally shaped like the obstetrical forces and the tips do not meet to prevent accidental grasp age of the iris. . The inner edges of the forceps blade are grooved to prevent slippage which prevent the fragment from slipping out

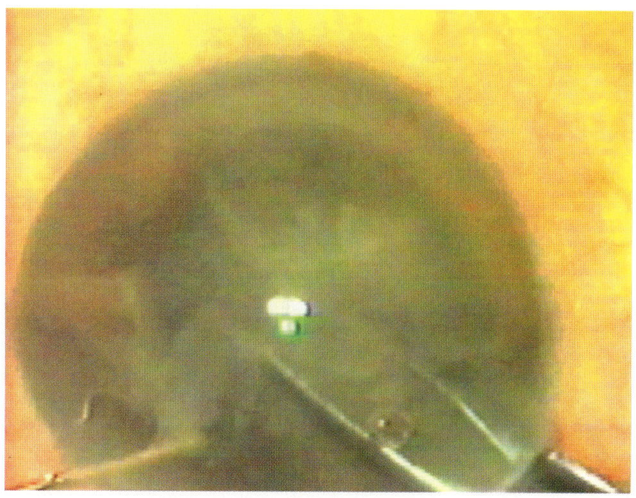

Fig. 35.14: Individual pieces are grasped with the special forceps.

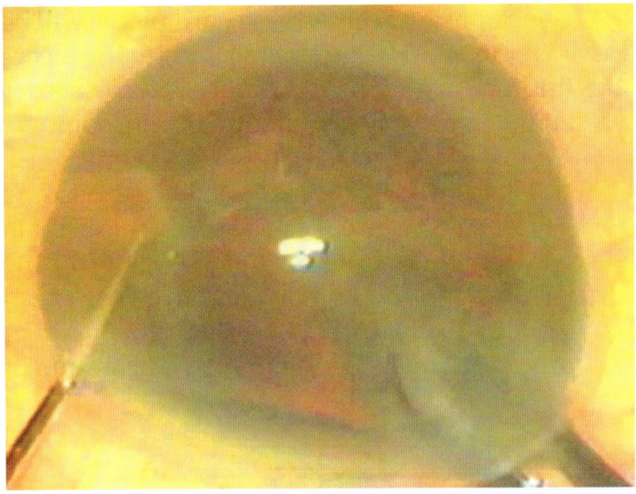

Fig. 35.15

removing the nucleus is that there is no stress on the incision which does not shear and lead to troublesome irregular astigmatism (Figs 35.16 to 35.20).

RESULTS

The results from the 200 cases done consecutively were exceptionally good. The complications were virtually negligible and well within the usual results as compared to phacoemulsification. On the other hand if the results were compared to phaco done in Grade+5 or suprahard cataracts (+6 or more) the results were significantly better. Even in the hardest

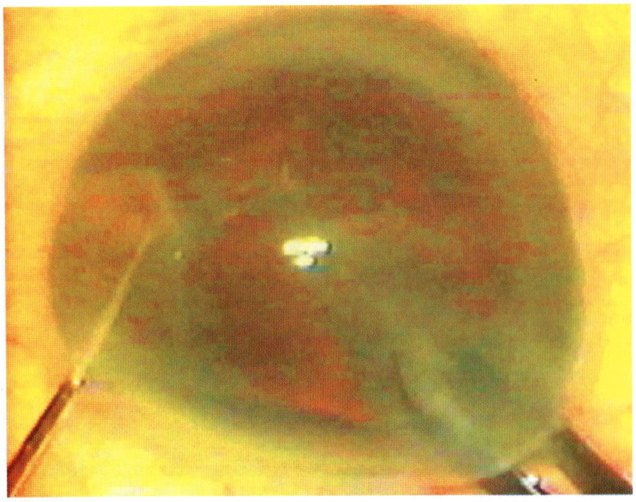

Fig. 35.16: An simple I/A completes the procedure

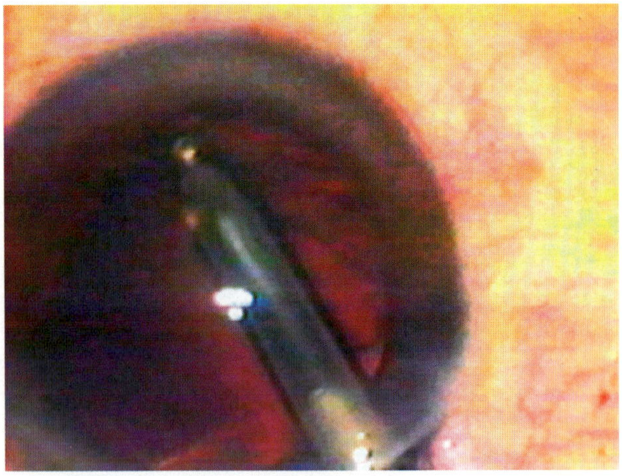

Fig. 35.17: I/A completed, final fragments of the cortex aspirated out

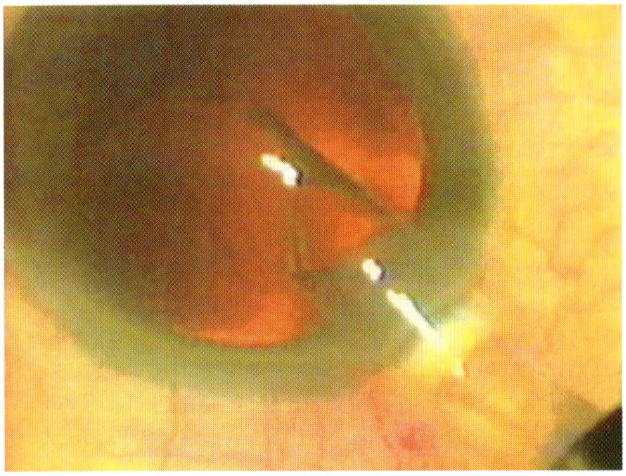

Fig. 35.18: A foldable IOL is inserted via the small 3.2 incision

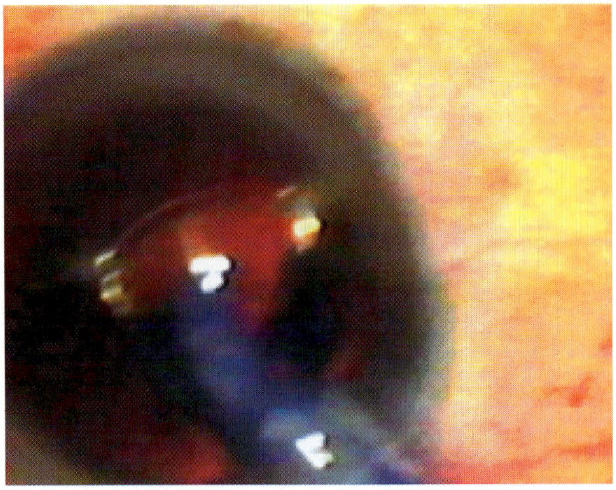

Fig. 35.19: Foldable silicone Allergan IOL (SI40) is injected in

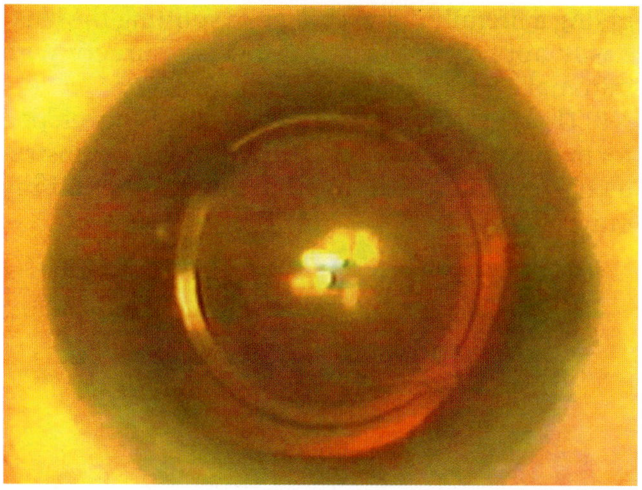

Fig. 35.20: IOL in the eye. Notice how quiet the eye is. Notice that the 3.2 mm tunneled openings always seal themselves. The final appearance, completely undistinguishable from a true phaco by anyone

cataracts in no case was the posterior capsule compromised.

In an effort to analyze the cases further, endothelial cell studies were carried out. The results once again show that the results with the pincer forceps was measurably better than with phaco and the results were far superior if the very hard cataracts were selected where the ultrasound energy compromised the endothelium still further.

In addition 50 cases were done using the sandwich technique. Surprisingly the endothelial cell loss with the sandwich is quite high and more, so if the cell count is done with the eye measured at 15 degree deflection. As compared to the pincer forceps it would seem virtually mandatory that if small incision non phaco be considered then the pincer forceps is the answer to the problem and the "sandwich" technique should be relegated to posterity.

Variations

In a very hard cataract the split may not go through and through the nucleus. Spin the nucleus on its vertical axis and do it from the other side to complete the chop.

In thin hard cataracts typically associated with white hyper mature cataract, spear the lens with a sharp instrument to support it against the splitter.

Complications n=254

Complications	No	%
Corneal striae	14	5.5
Capsular break	4	15
Mild Zonular disinsert	5	1.9
Lens flop	21	8.3
Iris tear	4	15
Iris dialysis	1	0.4
Hyphema	9	3.5
Iritis >5 days	4	1.5

Perhaps the greatest advantage of the pincer slider technique is that it prevents the development of extensive endothelial cell loss which is, unfortunately, a common problem of the Non-phaco sandwich technique, or the vectis slide, in the hands of novices. Though per se, it is a very nice technique when done by a master, however when a novice tries the same techniques, especially in a Grade 3+ in an effort to do it rapidly and with the fear that the nucleus may not come it or slip to the side, the novice tries to pull too hard and then abrades the cornea.

Why do these problems occur with the sandwich technique

1. The corneal dome has inadequate space for gymnastics.
2. The perception of depth is often inadequate unless exceptional microscopes are used.
3. Multiple entry in and out of the eye will invariably lead to inadvertent corneal touch with grave results.
4. A panicky surgeon leads to a lost eye. Nothing panics a surgeon as much as a uncooperative lens in a small incision, non-phaco surgery.
5. Subsequent often flat chambers due to traumatized wound entries lead to a further exacerbation of the problem

All these problems are completely obviated using the 'Jaws' slider pincer technique with the lens in the 'lens salute' mode. It is a far safer technique and needs to be a part of the armamentarium of not only small incision non-phaco surgeon but also with the phaco surgeon for he can now do every had cataract with minimal energy and be assured of splitting the hard nucleus every time without any problems.

IN SUMMARY

A simple effective technique which can be done easily, under direct vision, with minimal risks, giving a literally 100% chance of splitting the lens . Easily applicable even to eye camp surgery with minimal complications .

NB: This Jaws instrument was originally developed for me by Mr Malkeet Singh of Indo-German Instruments Company, Mumbai, to whom I extend my grateful thanks.

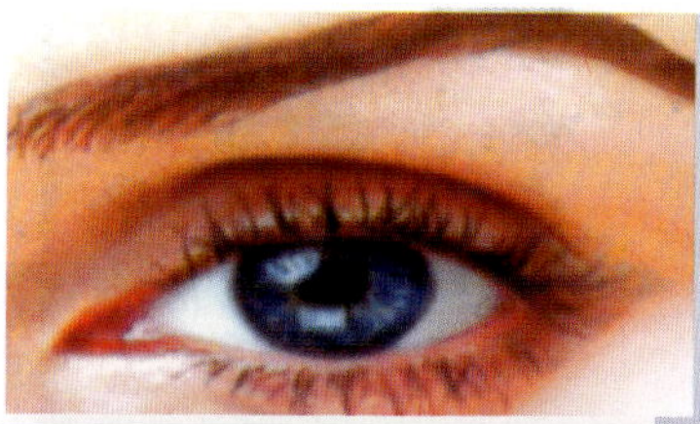

Thirty six

The Double Wire Snare Splitter Technique for Small Incision, Non-phaco Cataract Surgery

Keiki Mehta
Cyres Mehta (India)

There are many techniques which are available for doing effective small incision cataract surgery. Many splitting techniques have been devised to guillotine a nucleus. Single strands of wire, or nylon or polypropylene have been in use for some time as has the single strand, tonsil type, snare.

The problem is that using a single looped snare does not work as holding the lens eccentrically leads invariably to the nucleus being irregularly cut. Naturally if one is to hold an oval object it has to be held at its equator. At any other place it is bound to slip, or will excentrically leaving a small and a large fragment of the nucleus.. The question was also how to split a lens into three parts, preferably equally . This is important as only then the nuclear fragments could be removed through a 4.00 mm incision without stressing the edges of the incision

WHAT IS THE MYSTIQUE OF 4.00MM

It has always been the dream of any small incision surgeon to take a nucleus out of a 'foldable IOL" incision without widening it. Astigmatism is always negligible through a small incision, and a 4.00 mm incision always seals by itself if the tunnel is made well. In addition once can use the Sclero-corneal tunnel incision which leaves the eye the next day , literally looking as if it is unoperated (Figs 36.5 and 36.6).

The answer to the problem is obvious . Have a dual splitter which would work simultaneously, leaving three fragments , each of which is smaller than 4.00 mm. The techniques in doing this procedure ranged from using choppers, splitters, both single sided and double sided, as well is using a wire.

In an effort to have a really functional unit, a disposable splitter was designed using two strands of wire and a disposable needle . However the ability to use a double wire to split the lens into its component parts as not yet been explored to its full potential. In India, hard cataracts are the norm rather than the exception. Splitting a lens into two will not permit to the fragments of a hard nucleus to be removed easily through a 4.00 mm incision. It is for this reason that the concept of splitting a lens into three parts rather than two makes sense.

DOUBLE WIRE SNARE .THE TRISECTOR : MANNER OF CONSTRUCTION (Fig. 36.1)

A 20 gauge needle is cut off at the tip and the edges of rounded but maintaining a slight bevel as it permits easier entry into the eye.It is made by using two strands of 28 gauge flexible stainless steel wire threaded though a 20 gauge blunted disposable needle. Of the two loops of wire, one leg of each is entwined around the other. Thus the two loops which should be four strands are now converted to three strands. The end of the three strands is now threaded through the 20 G needle and the excess wire is looped around in the form of round loop so that it can be held easily in one hand while supporting the blunt needle with the other hand (Figs 36.2 to 36.4).

No viscoelastic is used in the needle as it did lead to the wire locking and not moving smoothly in the bore of the needle. It is important that the loops of the wire should be uniform and equal. The wire selected is a stainless steel wire which has a quantum of tensile strength and is the one which is normally utilised by the orthopaedic surgeons as a fine wire gauge. Since it costs virtually nothing to make, a fresh unit of can be made just prior surgery, and discarded following its use.

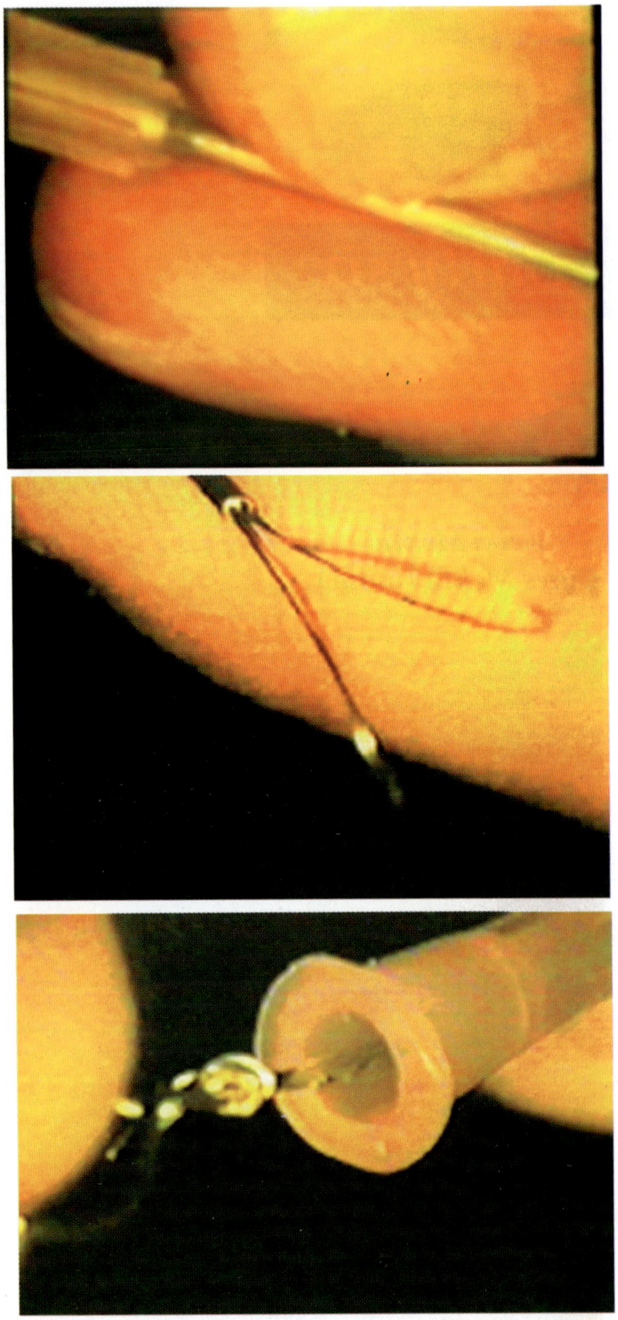

Figs 36.1A to C: Dual splitter: Manner of construction: (A) Standard 20 gauge, 1" length disposable needle selected (B) Loops extended. Note divergence (C) The four wires are knotted together and made into a small loop

SURGICAL TECHNIQUE

The surgeon has the option of utilizing either topical anesthesia if his level of skill and competence

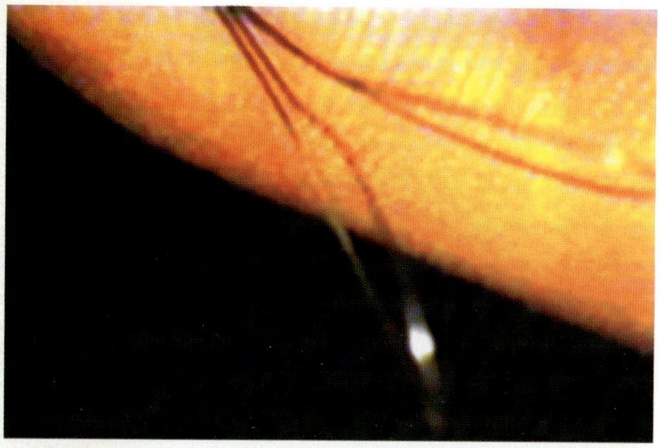

Fig. 36.2: The four wires constitute two loops. Make them spread outwards

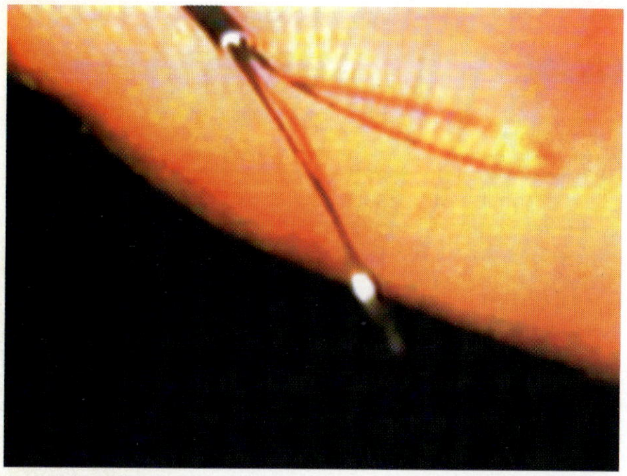

Fig. 36.3: Loops extended. Note divergence

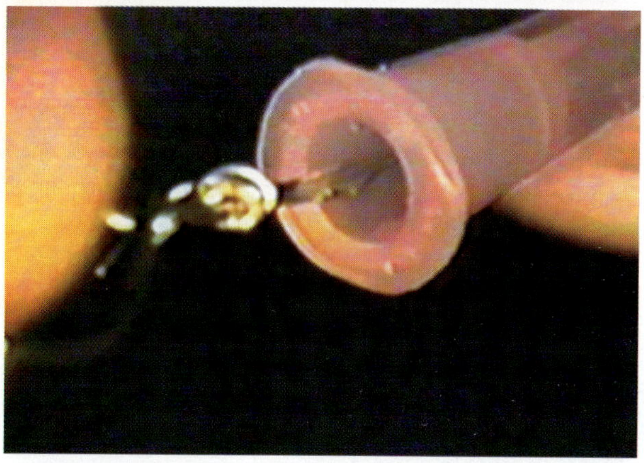

Fig. 36.4: The four wires are knotted together and made into a small loop

permits him to do so, or alternatively he can utilize a standard retrobulbar or a peribulbar block. The conjunctiva needs to be excised at the corneo-scleral

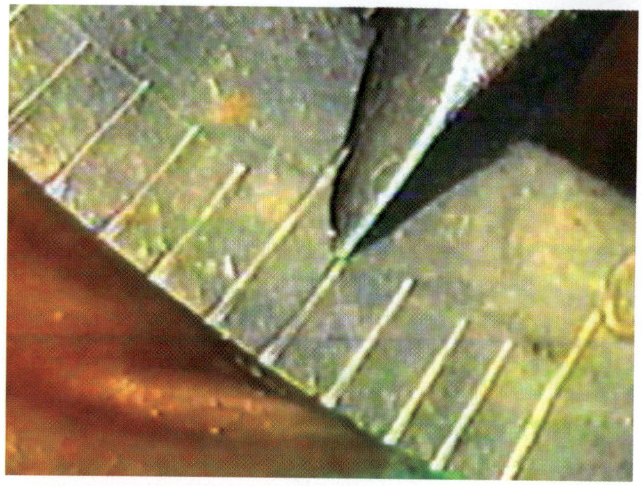

Fig. 36.5: 4.00 mm incision is adequate. Measure it and mark it to achieve consistant results

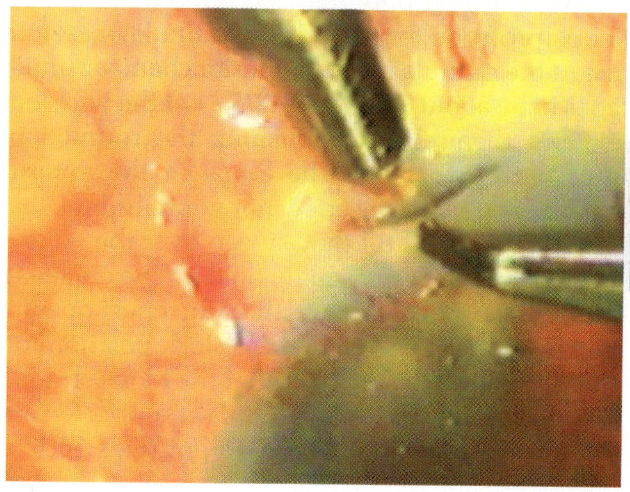

Fig. 36.6: A 4.00 mm sclero-corneal tunnel made

junction, simple cautery to control the bleeding is carried out. Care must be taken that the cautery setting is not so high as to leave grey marks on the sclera. The incision is made in a semi arcuate fashion in the sclera and the dissection carried forwards till it enters the clear cornea. Making the incision in this manner permits a virtual zero astigmatism to be induced by this "smiling" incision.

An adequate sized tunnel length is essential so that the wound subsequently self-seals itself. The anterior chamber is filled with viscoelastic. The ideal viscoelastic to use is Healon which can maintain the chamber depth ,which is so essential in this procedure. A good sized capsullorhexis is essential (Fig. 36.8). The minimum size is usually seven mm. Following the rhexis, a good hydro dissection is carried out the in such a manner that the edge of the nucleus tips forward. This tipping of the nucleus forward is also known as the 'lens salute'.

The viscoelastic is again placed in the anterior chamber and a blunt rotator is placed on the opposite pole of the slightly prolapsed nucleus and swept around in a manner that the nucleus literally rolls over on itself into the anterior chamber. As a final maneuver, the lens is rotated using a blunt IOL rotator to be sure that it lies the anterior to the capsule (Figs 36.9 and 36.10).

The next step is the insertion of the wire loops, into the anterior chamber. Retract the loops in the cannula so that only the 2.00 mm of the narrow loops protrude forward of the cannula. Carefully insert the cannula into the anterior chamber until it goes in by about 3 mm (Fig. 36.7). Let the wire loop expand themselves by pushing the round loop holder from behind. The loops in the anterior chamber are first inserted horizontally and then gradually turned till they sweep over the edge of the nucleus and then snugly hold it. The nucleus is gradually rotated utilizing the side report opening which we had remained at 2 o'clock position into the loops in such a manner that the loops straddle the nucleus equally . The cannula is supported and the wire loops smoothly pulled out (Figs 36.11 to 36.14).

Following the trisection of the nucleus , usually the middle part often simply slips out at the time of the wire loop removal. If it does not, it is of no consequence. Viscoelastic is re-injected and an iris repositor is introduced to separate the fragments apart making sure the fragments always remained vertical aligned to the incision (Figs 36.16 to 36.19).

A specially designed forceps which has special recurved tracks grooved into its substance of the jaws, with short square grooves virtually along the lines of a tank tracks. The force of fixing comfortably through a 4.0 mm incision and the individual fragments are held the and simply removed. The harder to the nucleus they easier it is to hold. In the advantage of the tracks is that once it is grasped

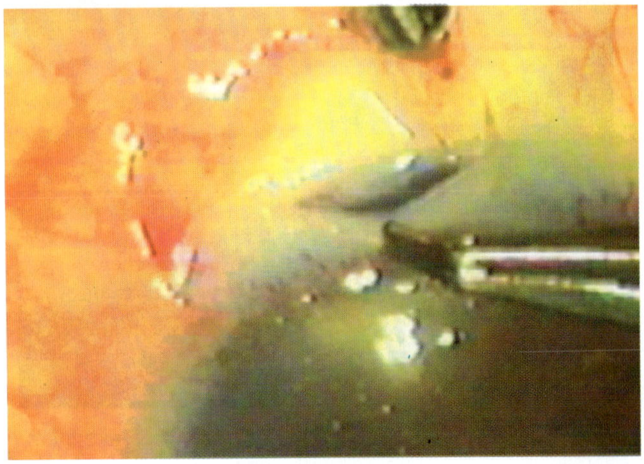

Fig. 36.7: Tunnel dissected till it extends almost 3.00 mm into the cornea

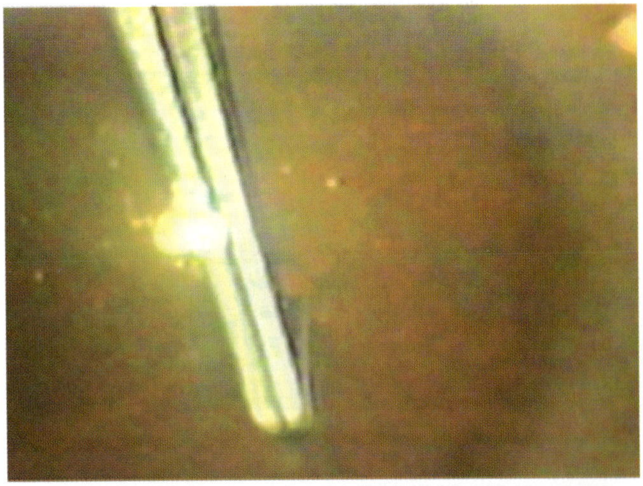

Fig. 36.8: Rhexis carried out. Minimum size 6.00 mm

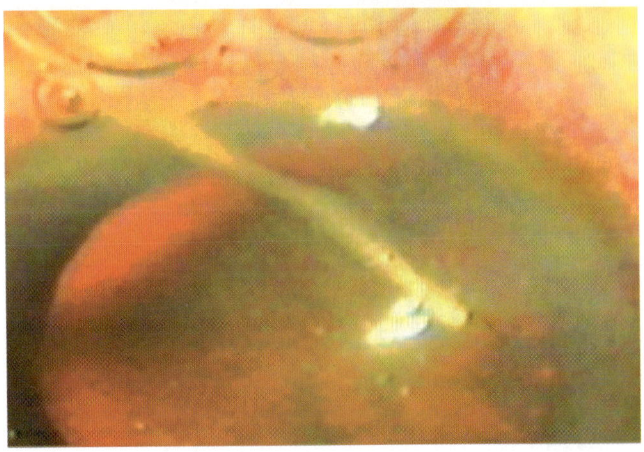

Fig. 36.9: Induced a lens tilt by oblique hydrodissection

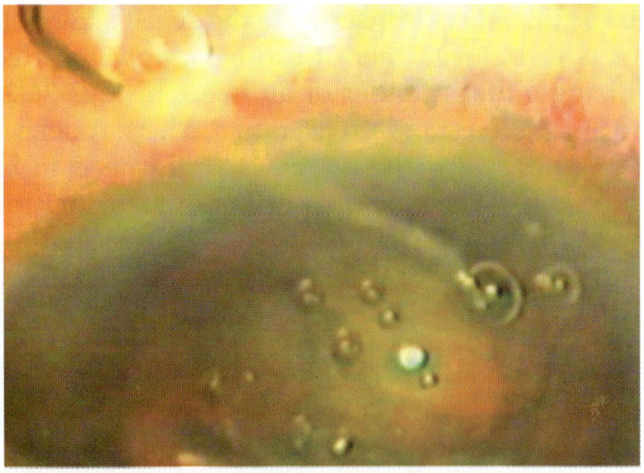

Fig. 36.10: Rotate the lens out of the bag. Simply turn it over with a blunt rotator

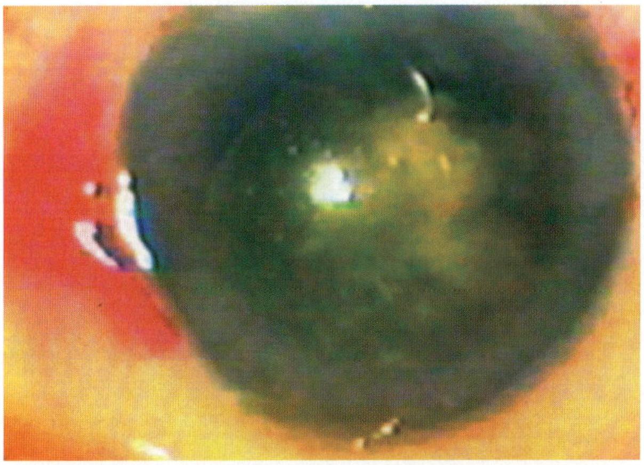

Fig. 36.11: Nucleus lies out of the bag, in the A/C

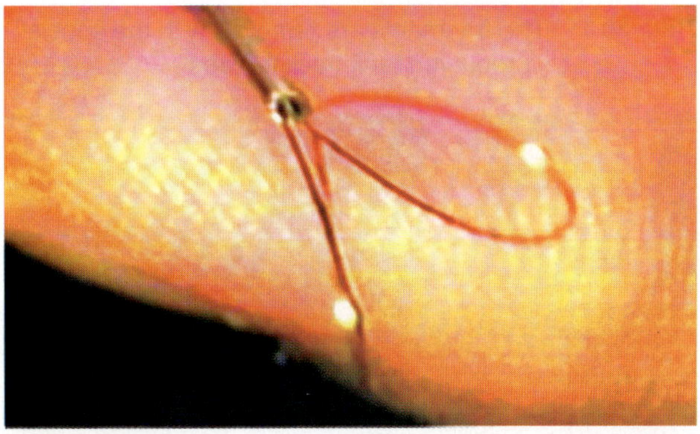

Fig. 36.12: Check the wire double splitter for proper action

the fragments come out in the single stroke (Figs 36.19 to 36.21).

A good cortical cleanout is done in and subsequently after polishing the capsule, in the

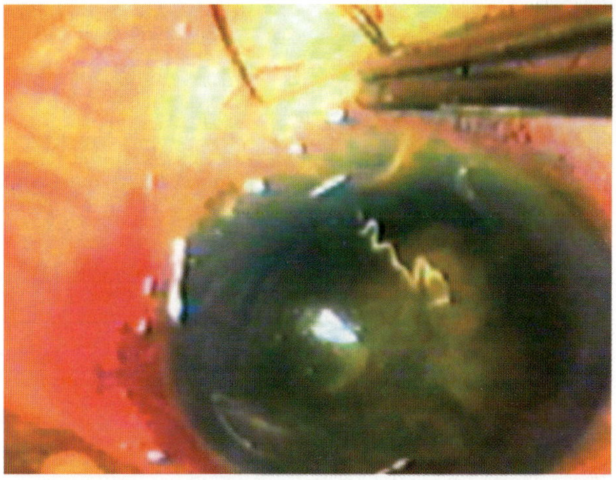

Fig. 36.13: Wire loops inserted in the semi retracted position to easily navigate the 4.00 mm opening

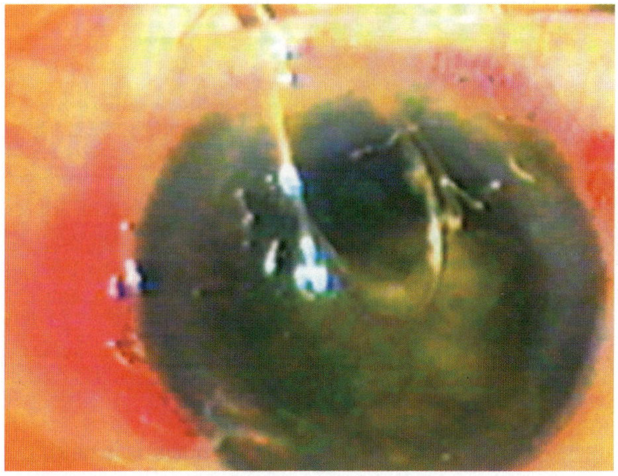

Fig. 36.14: The wire loops are allowed to circumambulate the nucleus. Note the loops are horizontal

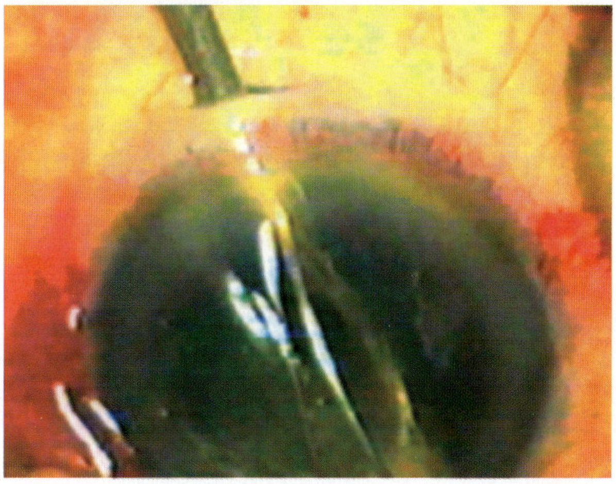

Fig. 36.15: Gradually swung around till the loops now lie vertical

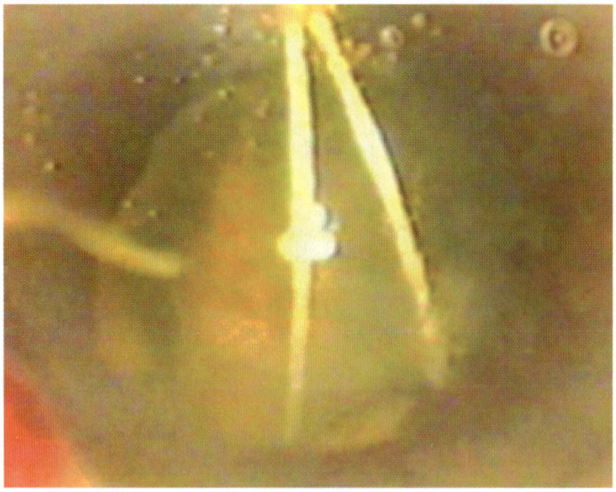

Fig. 36.16: Pull the loops snug to hold the nucleus. Note the spread of the wire loops

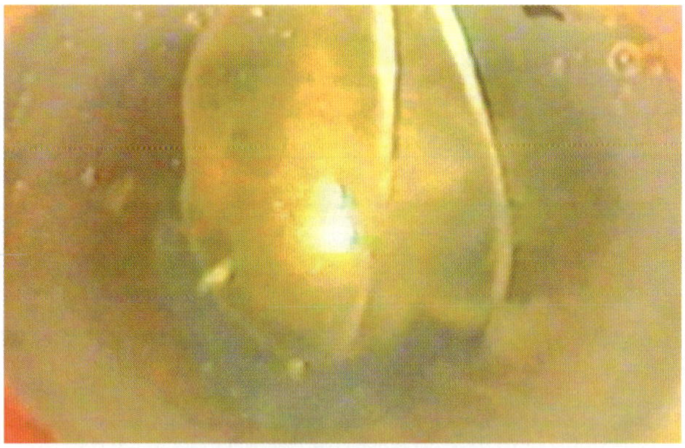

Fig. 36.17: Note how snuggly the nucleus is held. It remains immobile

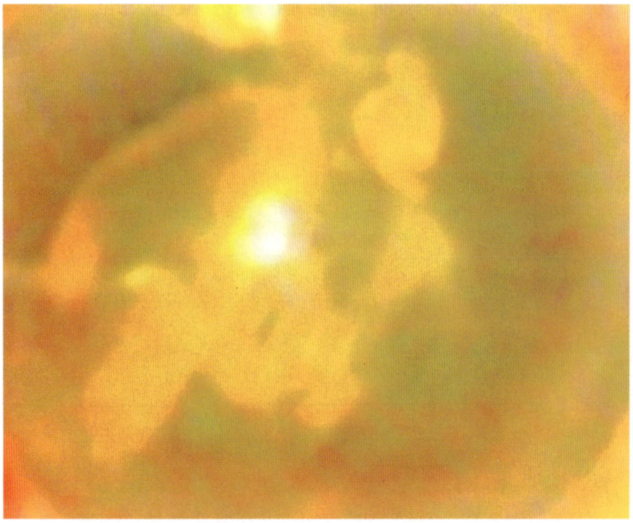

Fig. 36.18: The nucleus is sliced into three parts

intraocular lenses is inserted in the eye. If a foldable lens is to be used then it can be simply inserted utilizing either a folder or an injected (Figs 36.22 and 36.23). If a standard 5.5 mm P. M. M. A. lens is to be utilized for the opening would need to be widened by 1.5mm. Utilizing and arcuate incision makes the opening self-sealing . The edges of the cut conjunctiva can be apposed utilizing a coaptation forceps. The viscoelastic to his washout, chamber is reformed.

IN SUMMARY

The eye is exceptionally quieter. Ironically, the harder to the nucleus the easier the trisector works and the hall mark of the procedure. It is an

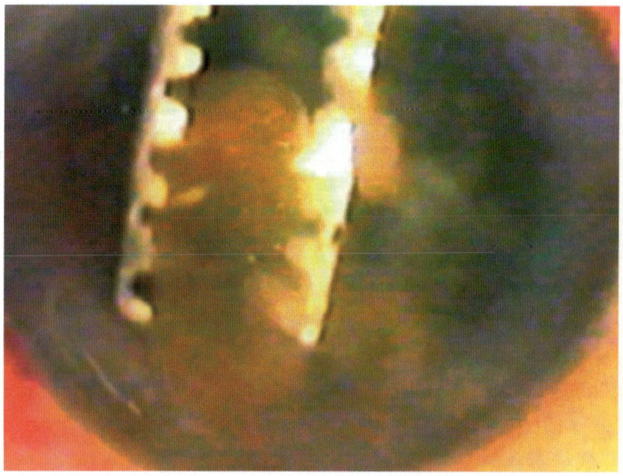

Fig. 36.19: The fragments are removed with the special recurved tank track forceps

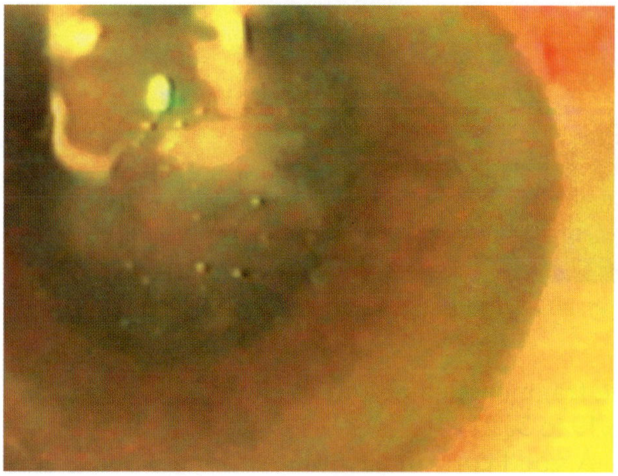

Fig. 36.20: Final fragment lifted out

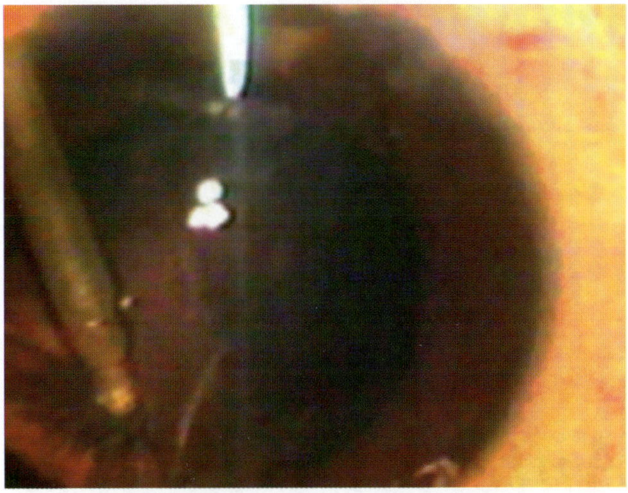

Fig. 36.21: I/A carried out

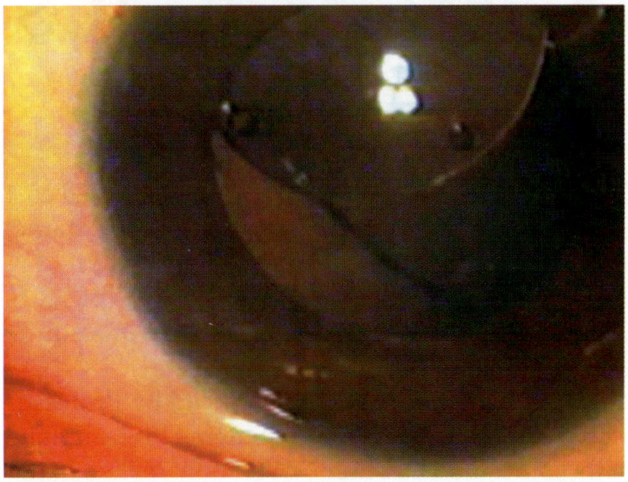

Fig. 36.22: IOL inserted. Here a silicone Storz IOL is injected in

exceptional technique which is of great use, not only for one who does small incision non-phaco techniques, but also for the phaco surgeon ,who is often faced with a hard cataracts usually coupled with the compromised endothelium, and for whom this would prove to be an ideal choice.

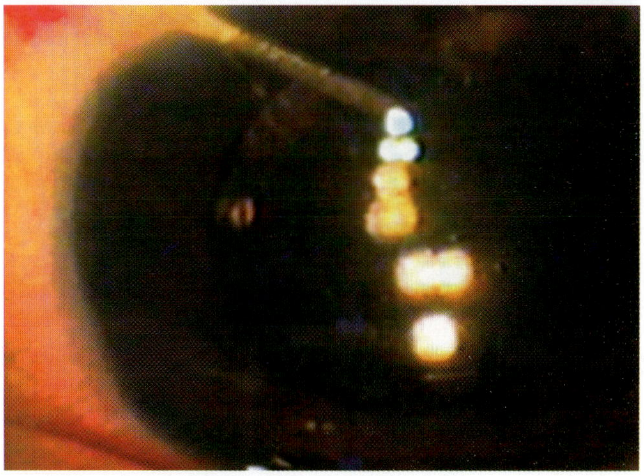

Fig. 36.23: Final picture

This technique is also very useful when the nucleus is hard, especially in the deep brown incompressible cataracts where trying to do a sandwich method causes undue stress on the corneal edges leading to sheer which will lead to an unstable astigmatism. The advantage of splitting the nucleus into three parts permits easier removal of the smaller fragments.

The other alternative methods utilize a back stop or a flat back blade , inserted under the nucleus and a vertical splitter designed , like a bread board, so that it cuts the nucleus into two or into three fragments. But in both these techniques it presupposes that the chamber depth is adequate. Indian cornea have smaller, steeper cornea's and a shallower anterior chamber depth where , utilizing the back stop and cutter there is always the likelihood of corneal. Simply rotating the nucleus into the loops of the wire is a simpler, safer technique. As with all new techniques a certain element of practice is required to gain facility with this method. But the learning curve is short, and the results are gratifying.

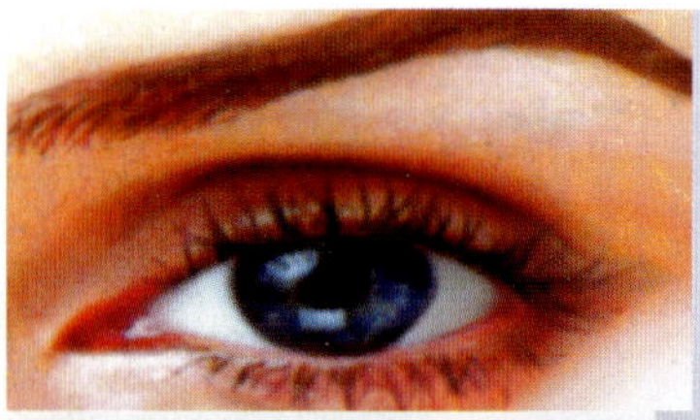

Thirty seven

Versatility of Anterior Chamber Maintainer in SICS

KPS Malik
Ruchi Goel (India)

The simplicity, safety, wider applicability and cost effectiveness of non phaco Small Incision Cataract Surgery (SICS) has inundated the present day cataract surgeon with various techniques of SICS. Every innovation is aimed at achieving a procedure, which is bereft of complications.

SICS, using ACM was introduced by Professor M. Blumenthal. We started practicing his technique with some modifications. We soon realized that the property of ACM to maintain a deep anterior chamber could be utilized in phacosection and phacosandwich techniques also. Both the methods involve greater instrumentation inside the chamber endangering the corneal endothelium. ACM can also be used in phacoemulsification whenever a higher vacuum is required. It prevents chamber collapse and allows emulsification of hard nuclei with considerable ease. Recently, we have started using ACM in mini-incisional surgery through a 1.5 mm clear corneal section. We shall now describe how ACM plays a pivotal role in each of these procedures.

MODIFIED BLUMENTHALTECHNIQUE

Professor M Blumenthal, performs all the maneuvers under fluid without using viscoelastics.

We have modified his technique and advocate copious use of viscoelastics to safeguard the corneal endothelium.

We prefer to use a frown shaped external incision of 5.5 to 6.5 mm length. A self-sealing corneo-scleral tunnel is dissected using crescent knife. The inner wound diameter should be approximately 8 mm long with well made side pockets. The details of tunnel making have been described in other chapters. Prior to entry with a slit knife two side ports are made at 10 O'clock and 6 O'clock for capsulorhexis and ACM entry respectively.

Insertion of ACM

For making the 6 O'clock opening a 20 G MVR blade is held tangential to the 6 O'clock limbus and is entered from the temporal side, away from the vascular arcade, creating a valvular opening for insertion of ACM. The blade should be held in such a manner that its widest portion is parallel to the surface of iris. The opening should be of adequate size to snugly fit the ACM. Too small an opening results in struggle during insertion. If it becomes larger than the required size, there can be repeated slipping of the ACM, which will prevent building up of sufficient hydropressure to push the nucleus out.

The ACM is a hollow steel tube with 0.9 mm outer diameter and 0.65 mm inner diameter. While inserting, it is held firmly from the steel portion with the thumb and the index finger and entered with bevel up and then turned 180 degrees so that the bevel faces the iris. If part of the bevel remains in the corneal stroma, corneal haziness can occur due to stromal hydration. Prior to insertion, it should be flushed with BSS not only to check its patency but also to remove any air column in the tubing. The tube of ACM is attached to the BSS bottle suspended 50-60 cm above the patient's eye.

The capsulotomy is performed through the opening at 10 O'clock position. Without going into the details, we would like to emphasize that the capsular opening which is preferably but not necessarily a capsulorhexis should be more than 6 mm in size and the capsular rim at 12 o'clock area should be narrow to facilitate passage of Sinskey's hook behind the upper pole during nuclear prolapse from the bag. It also assists in aspiration of the 12 o'clock cortex. If the size of CCC is small, relaxing cuts at 7 and 11 o'clock should be given. Nuclear prolapse if attempted through a small capsular opening can result in zonular dialysis.

In hypermature milky white cataracts, flow from ACM clears the chamber of the milky fluid released by the puncture of the anterior capsule. After the capsulotomy, the anterior chamber is entered with a slit knife. Hydroprocedures are then performed to reduce the size of the nucleus and free the nucleus from the capsular bag. Once the nucleus starts rotating freely within the bag, the chamber is filled with viscoelastics and the nucleus is prolapsed out of its bag with the help of Sinskey's hook. Free nucleus in deep AC is then ready for being propelled out by the hydropresure generated by the ACM.

Principle of the Technique

- Engage the nucleus into the sclerocorneal pocket tunnel with the help of a lens glide/ iris repositor
- Push the nucleus out by hydropressure
- Pull the nucleus out by a needle if required

For engaging the nucleus into the corneoscleral tunnel, after injecting viscoelastic both in front and behind the nucleus, a lens glide/ iris repositor is passed behind the nucleus one-third or half the nucleus width distance. Once the iris repositor is in position, ACM is opened and slight pressure is applied on the scleral side. Intermittent pressure, engages more and more nucleus out of the tunnel's mouth. Subsequent taps enable the epinucleus and cortex to flow out of the anterior chamber.

At times, a free nucleus fails to engage in the section. This could be due to the following reasons:

- Small internal wound diameter
- Irregular/ incompletely dissected tunnel
- Leaking anterior chamber
- Premature entry into anterior chamber
- Vitreous in anterior chamber

The tunnel should be revisited with the slit knife. If the nucleus still fails to engage and there is no vitreous in anterior chamber, ACM is disconnected from the BSS and attached to a syringe containing viscoelastics. Viscoelastic is then injected through the ACM by the assistant while the surgeon keeps

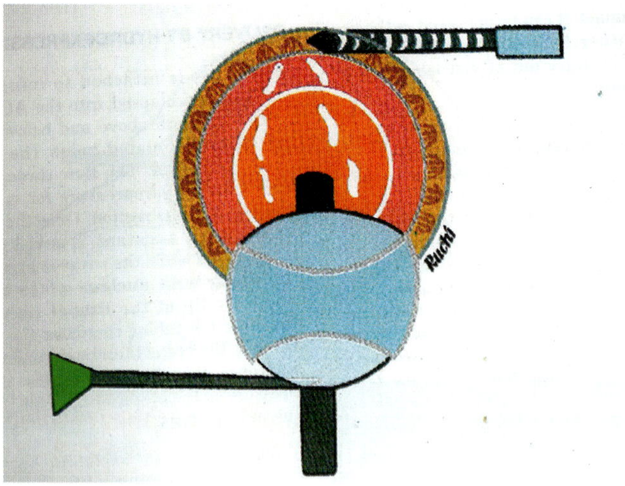

Fig. 37.1: Assisted delivery in Modified Blumenthal technique

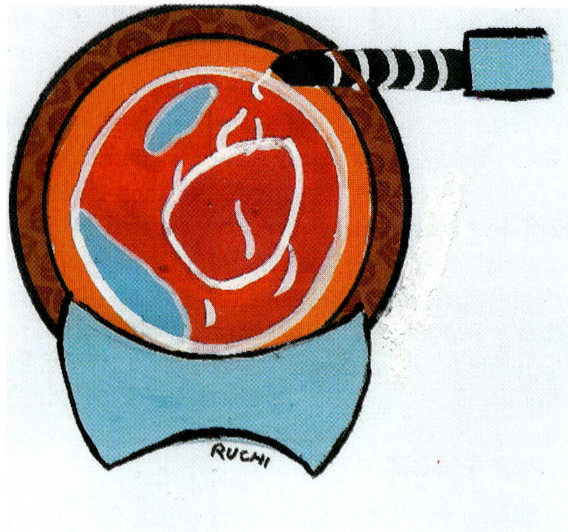

Fig. 37.2: Flow through ACM pushes the vitreous back in case of posterior capsular tear during cortical wash

a watch on the progress of the nucleus and the intraocular tension. The pressure created by the viscoelastic pushes the nucleus towards the section. Once the nucleus is engaged, the ACM is reconnected to the BSS bottle and the nucleus is delivered in the usual manner. At times, if the nucleus is engaged but fails to deliver due to hypotony, the bottle height may be increased.

Assisted Delivery

If a small portion of the nucleus shows out of the section but further progress is stalled even with full flow of ACM, nuclear delivery can be assisted by 23 G needle held in the other hand. The nucleus is engaged at right angle to its axis with a 23 G needle and while the ACM generated hydropressure pushes it out, the needle assists by pulling it and intermittent pressure on the iris repositor guides the nucleus out (Fig. 37.1).

If the nucleus is very large and hard, a bit of it may be sheared off, remaining nucleus is pushed back into the anterior chamber and the smaller diameter may be allowed to flow out.

A bimanual irrigation aspiration is carried out using an olive tipped cannula and ACM. In case of inadvertent posterior capsular rupture, flow through ACM pushes the vitreous back and facilitates cortical aspiration (Fig. 37.2). Cortical clean up is followed by placement of posterior chamber intraocular lens in the bag and hydration of the side ports.

PHACOFRACTURE AND PHACOSECTION

In both these techniques, the construction of corneoscleral differs from the previous method. Here, the size of the internal and the external incision are equal and the side pockets are not dissected. The incision size in phacofracture varies from 4.5 to 5.5 mm whereas, in phacosandwich it is kept from 6-7 mm. After dissecting the tunnel, two side ports are created as described in the previous section. Capsulotomy, fixing the ACM, hydroprocedures and nuclear prolapse are performed in the usual manner. After suspending the nucleus in an ocean of viscoelastic, an irrigating wire vectis is insinuated behind the nucleus and a Sinskey's hook is placed on the top.

In phacosandwich technique, the nucleus is delivered sandwiched between the two instruments while the assistant injects viscoelastics through the ACM, maintaining a deep anterior chamber through out (Fig. 37.3).

In phacofracture technique, the two instruments are approximated toward each other to crush the nucleus into two halves, while the assistant injects the viscoelastic through the ACM. The two halves are separated and each half is brought out

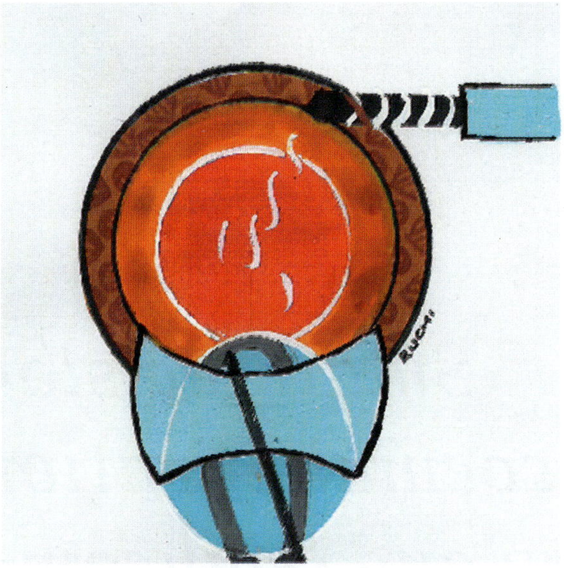

Fig. 37.3: Phacosandwich technique using ACM

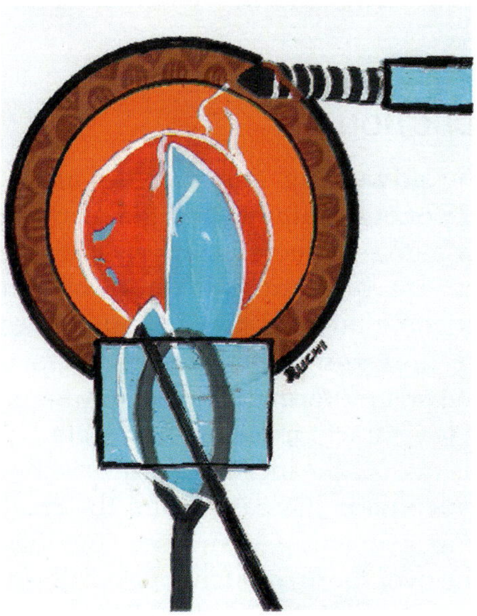

Fig. 37.4: Phacofracture technique using ACM

sandwiched between the microvectis and the Sinskey's hook (Fig. 37.4).

ACM IN PHACOEMULSIFICATION

We advocate use of ACM in all grades of cataracts during the learning phase. It is especially useful in grade 4/5 nuclei where higher vacuum is required to prevent chamber collapse. After the trenching is complete, the vacuum is increased to 200 mm of

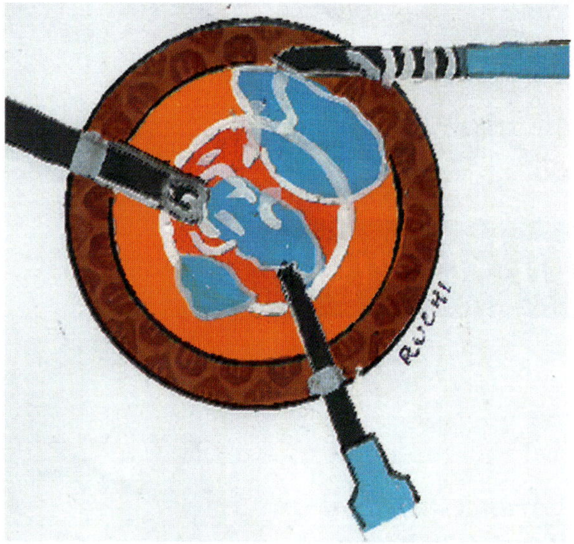

Fig. 37.5: Microincisional surgery using ACM

Hg and ACM flow is put on. The nuclear pieces are then engulfed without the danger of chamber collapse.

Mini-incisional Surgery

In mini-incisional surgery, a clear corneal tunnel 1.5 mm in length is created. 3 side ports are made at 10 O'clock, 3 O'clock and 6 O'clock positions for performing capsulorhexis, inserting the blunt tipped 18 G needle and inserting the ACM respectively.

A 30 degrees phacotip with a shortened sleeve is used. The shortened sleeve reduces the temperature created by phacotip vibrations, preventing corneal burn. The tip of the 18 G needle is blunted and is fashioned in the form of irrigating chopper and attached to BSS bottle. ACM is attached to another BSS bottle. Trenching is performed keeping the machine parameters as usual (Flow: 25cc/mt, Vacuum: 20 mm of Hg and Power: 50 to 80%.

ACM is put on during the trenching itself. After the trenching is complete, vacuum is increased depending upon the hardness of the cataract and the nucleus is emulsified (Fig. 37.5).

In conclusion, ACM is an inexpensive, useful instrument, which can be employed in various techniques for maintaining a deep anterior chamber and thereby preventing endothelial damage, a dreaded complication of cataract surgery.

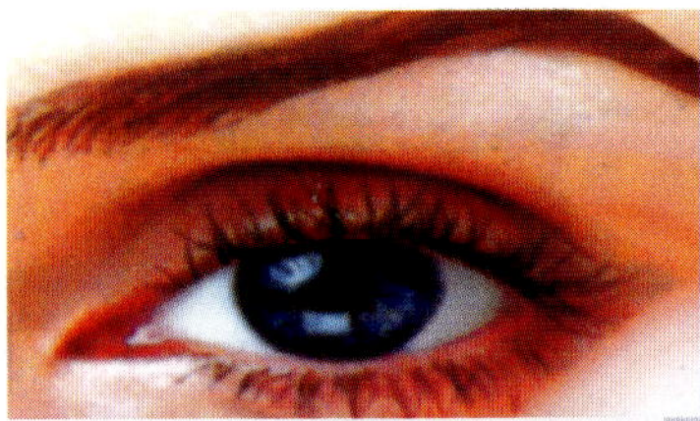

Thirty eight

Small Incision Non-phacoemulsification Surgery and Glaucoma

Arun Kshetrapal
Ramesh Kshetrapal
(India)

INTRODUCTION

With the advancing age there is an increased incidence of both cataract and glaucoma and both of them cause a decrease in vision. Both these diseases are preventable cause of blindness. Cataract and glaucoma may be found to coexist in one eye and sometimes cataract can lead to glaucoma or long-term miotic therapy for glaucoma can lead to cataract formation. As the life expectancy is increasing so is the incidence of coexisting cataract with glaucoma is increasing and the challenge of managing coexisting glaucoma and cataract is becoming ever more frequent.[1] Beside the difficulty in diagnosis of glaucoma in the presence of cataract there are many other problems to be considered in the surgical management of glaucoma such as compliance of the patient, side effects and cost, etc.

DIAGNOSIS OF GLAUCOMA

The diagnosis of glaucoma in the presence of cataract is slightly difficult as out of the three cardinal points in diagnosis of glaucoma, that is raised IOP, optic disc cupping and visual field defect; it becomes difficult to evaluate the latter two. The problem can be overcome by looking at the past records of the patient and evaluating the other eye.

DECISION

The decision as to how to operate and when to operate on a case of coexisting visually significant cataract and glaucoma lies entirely on the merits of individual case. There are various options available for surgical management of coexisting cataract and glaucoma. The surgeon can either go in for a sequential approach; that is to perform trabeculectomy before proceeding for cataract extraction with IOL implantation at a later date or can opt for combined cataract extraction and IOL implantation with trabeculectomy in a single sitting.

COMBINED SURGERY

Combined trabeculectomy with small incision (< 6 mm) cataract extraction often succeeds in reducing IOP[2] and the results are promising.[3] The combined surgery can control IOP effectively and can improve visual acuity rapidly.[4] There is strong evidence for better long-term control of IOP with combined glaucoma and cataract operations compared with cataract surgery alone.[5] Combined surgery has the advantages for the patient with visually significant cataract and uncontrolled glaucoma. When the two procedures are performed together in a single sitting it becomes very convenient for the patient as he has to undergo the mental trauma of a surgical procedure only once. The patient saves lot of time in terms of rehabilitation and cost. The visual rehabilitation is faster. The most important advantage of combined procedure is the prevention of postoperative spike of IOP seen after cataract surgery alone. This postoperative spike of IOP can be detrimental in a case of glaucoma.

Having decided to perform surgery in a single sitting the surgeon has two options, either to perform trabeculectomy and cataract extraction at two different sites or to perform both the procedures at a single site. In this chapter we will discuss about single site technique of combined trabeculectomy and cataract extraction through a small incision without the use of phacoemulsification.

INDICATIONS

The main indication for performing combined trabeculectomy with cataract extraction is when the patient is having both a visually significant cataract that requires extraction and IOL implantation along with uncontrolled glaucoma. It seems justified to extend the indication for combined surgery in cataract patients with coexisting open angle glaucoma in case of poor compliance, inability of sufficient medical care, or unacceptable medication.[6]

PREOPERATIVE EVALUATION

Evaluating a case preoperatively not only gives us a chance to confirm the diagnosis but also to uncover the problems that may arise during the surgery. A detailed history along with a good clinical examination should be performed using a slit lamp.

The condition of cornea is to be taken into consideration during preoperative evaluation. The cornea could be very hazy and edematous especially in cases of lens induced glaucoma. Operating upon such a case with corneal haze or edema can lead to difficulty in visualization of capsule and cortical material during surgery. Lowering of IOP with oral acetazolamide or with intravenous mannitol can help in clearing up the corneal haze and edema which will facilitate visualization of cortex and capsule per operatively. Administration of glycerin drop can also facilitate clearing of corneal edema.

Sometimes, especially in cases of lens induced glaucoma there could be cells and aqueous flare in the anterior chamber. This should be taken care of with steroids preoperatively for few days till the cells disappear from the anterior chamber. This will also help in reducing postoperative inflammation.

The status of the pupil and the extent of pupillary dilatation should be assessed preoperatively. Presences of any amorphous deposits on the pupillary margin are suggestive of pseudoexfoliation. If patient is on miotic therapy then they should preferably be stopped at least a week before surgery and oral acetazolamide can be added to control the IOP.

Fundus examination if possible should be carried to determine the status of the optic nerve head.

The surgeon should also determine as to what proportion of visual loss is due to cataract and what proportion of visual loss is due to glaucoma. This should be brought into the patient's knowledge before operating and to inform him or her about the vision likely to be gained after the surgery.

THETECHNIQUE

Many techniques have been described in the literature for performing combined trabeculectomy and cataract extraction through a small self-sealing tunnel without the use of phacoemulsification. The basic principle in all the procedures is to achieve sclerectomy of the posterior lip of the sclerocorneal tunnel which is covered by anterior lip of the tunnel. This can be achieved either with the help of a blade knife or a scleral punch.

Anesthesia: This surgery is most safely performed under a peribulbar anesthesia. The technique of anesthesia is the same as given for any other ocular surgery. A mixture of 2.5 ml of lignocaine 2 percent and 1.5 ml of bupivicaine 0.5 percent along with hyaluronidase is used and is injected in the peribulbar space along the inferior orbital rim at the junction of lateral one-third and medial two-third. Addition of sodium bicarbonate instead of hyaluronidase in lignocaine can make this procedure painless. Topical 2 percent lidocaine hydrochloride jelly without systemic sedation may be a safe and effective alternative anesthetic method in combined surgery.[7]

Conjunctival flap: The conjunctival flap can either be a limbus or a fornix based. The use of either flap in combined surgery achieves the same IOP lowering.[8] A fornix based conjunctival flap is preferred when considering a combined surgery as it has the advantage of better exposure of the surgical site. Conjunctiva is lifted up in the superior quadrant with the help of a non traumatizing forceps about 1 to 1.5 mm away from the limbus and a radial nick is given with the help of a Wescot's scissors (Fig. 38.1). The conjunctiva along with tenon is under-

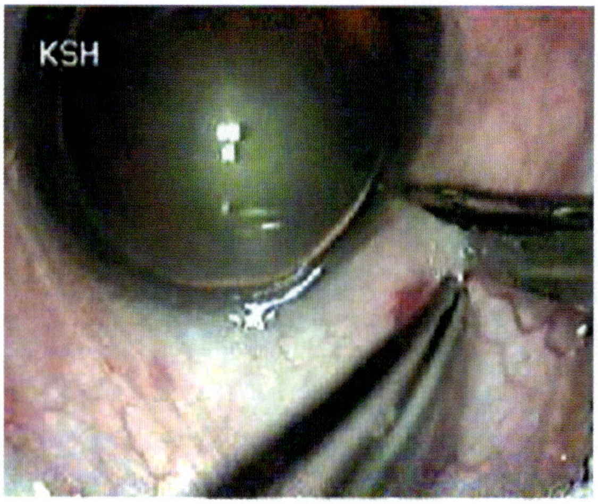

Fig. 38.1: Radial nick is given in conjunctiva

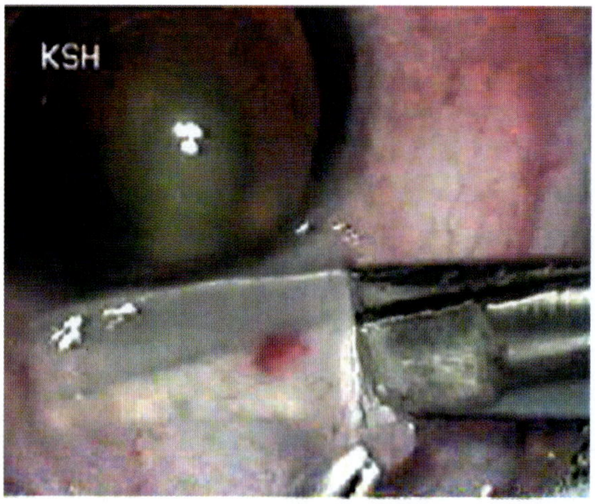

Fig. 38.2: Conjunctiva is undermined

mined (Fig. 38.2) and cut along the limbus (Fig. 38.3) to give a fornix based triangular conjunctival flap. A rim of 1 mm of conjunctiva can be left at the limbus so as to facilitate suturing if the surgeon desires. The exposed sclera is then scrapped clean for the remnants of tenons capsule if present with the help of BP blade and if required minimum cauterization of the scleral site is done to achieve hemostasis. Excess cauterization is avoided as it makes the sclera stiff and later on it can lead to excess fibrosis which can be detrimental for the surgery.

Scleral Tunnel: The three plane scleral tunnel is constructed very meticulously when performing a combined surgery. A 5.5 mm or 6 mm wide partial

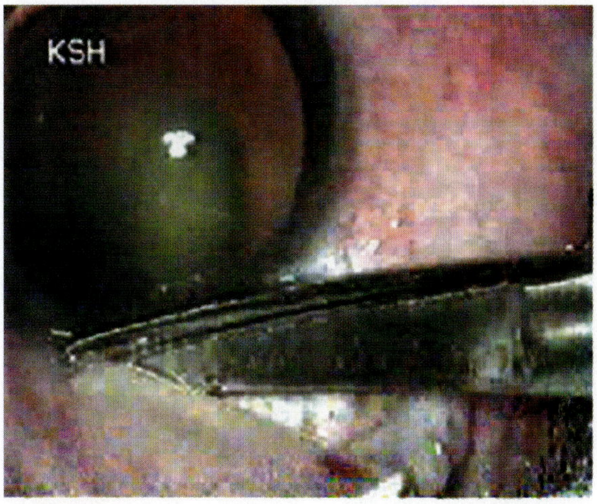

Fig. 38.3: Conjunctiva is cut along the limbus

thickness frown scleral incision is made with the help of blade knife or with the help of depth-preset knife (300 microns). The center of the frown incision is placed about 2.5 to 3 mm posterior to the limbus which 0.5 to 1 mm more posterior to the usual incision when performing cataract extraction alone. The scleral tunnel is constructed with the help of a crescent blade. It is of utmost importance to enter at correct depth and to maintain the same depth throughout the tunnel. The scleral tunnel is carried forward for about 1.5 to 2 mm into the cornea. The dissection at the corneal end of the tunnel has to be 2 mm wider then the scleral end. Now anterior chamber is entered with a suitable sized keratome. Once the anterior chamber is entered it should be reformed with the viscoelastic and then the sides of the tunnel is enlarged to make it funnel shaped.

Capsulorhexis: Every attempt should be made to achieve a continuous curvilinear capsulorhexis however, in certain cases of lens, induced glaucoma it becomes very difficult to perform a capsulorhexis. Adequate amount of viscoelastic should be used in such cases to counter balance the intralenticular up thrust. Staining of capsule with trypan blue dye is a very good tool when performing capsulorhexis in mature and hypermature cataracts. An appropriate sized capsulorhexis should be made keeping the size of nucleus in mind so that the nucleus can be prolapsed easily into the AC. In cases of lens-induced glaucoma the nucleus in most of the cases is not very big, it is the hydration of the cortex which has caused the lens to swell up and increase in size. In cases when the pupil is not dilating which is frequently seen in cases with long standing miotic therapy, the capsulorhexis can be made under the iris, even without visualization of the capsulorhexis margin if the surgeon has sufficient amount of proficiency. Alternatively the pupil can be enlarged with various techniques as described elsewhere in this book. In cases of pseudoexfoliation, when combined surgery is being performed the size of capsulorhexis should be adequate as slightest pressure on the capsulorhexis margin during proplapse of the nucleus into the anterior chamber can lead to zonulodialysis.

Hydrodissection: The technique of hydrodissection does not differ significantly in a case where a combined surgery is being performed. It is performed in the usual way except in cases where the posterior capsule is not visible. When the posterior capsule is not visible the hydrodissection has to be very slow and minimal fluid is to be used. In cases of mature and hypermature cataract, hydrodissection can be avoided and the nucleus can be easily mobilized by engaging it with the help of Sinskey's hook.

Nucleus Management: The prolapse of the nucleus from the bag into the anterior chamber and then through the tunnel out the anterior chamber is on the same principles as is done for cataract extraction alone. The nucleus can be prolapsed into the anterior chamber by any of the preferred techniques of the surgeon and then the nucleus is prolapsed out through the tunnel with a technique with which the surgeon is most comfortable. Once the nucleus is removed, a careful cortical clean up is done and the capsule is well polished and an IOL is implanted after filling the anterior chamber with viscoelastic.

Sclerectomy: Sclerectomy is done after the IOL has been implanted and before the viscoelastic is removed. Various techniques of performing sclerectomy are available. Here in this chapter we will discuss one technique of performing posterior lip sclerectomy using a scleral punch and one technique without the use of scleral punch.

Scleral Punch Technique: A Holth scleral punch (Fig. 38.4) is used in this technique to perform

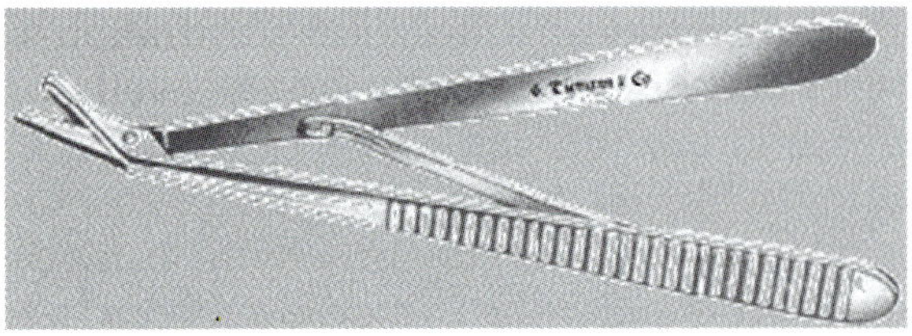

Fig. 38.4: Holth scleral punch

sclerectomy of the posterior lip of the scleral tunnel. After the IOL has been implanted, the anterior chamber is replenished with viscoelastic which has escaped during IOL implantation.

The posterior lip of the scleral tunnel is held at the corneal end with the help of a Pierse Hoskins forceps and it is pulled out beyond the posterior margin of the anterior lip (Fig. 38.5). To hold the corneal end of posterior lip, lift up the anterior lip with Pierse Hoskins forceps held in right hand and with another Pierse Hoskins forceps held in the left hand reach for the anterior end of the posterior lip. Press lightly with one limb of the forceps at the corneal end of the lip so that the lip becomes slightly everted which can now be easily grasped with the forceps in the left hand.

Once the posterior lip has been grasped by the forceps in left hand, the sclera is engaged between the limbs of scleral punch held in right hand

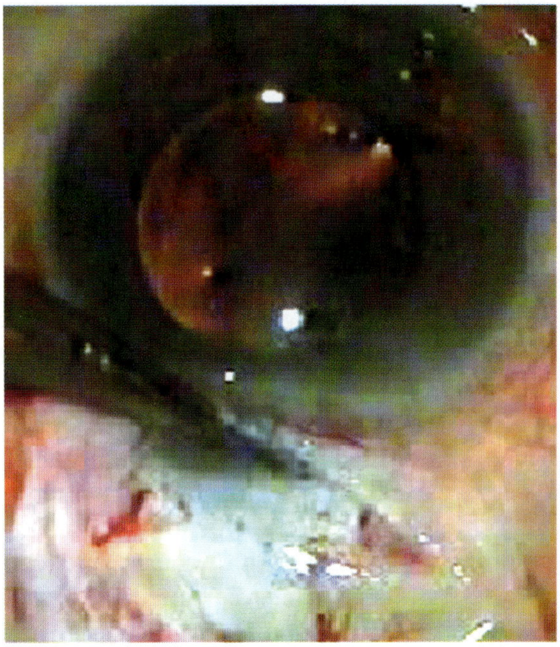

Fig. 38.5: Inner lip of tunnel is held with a forceps

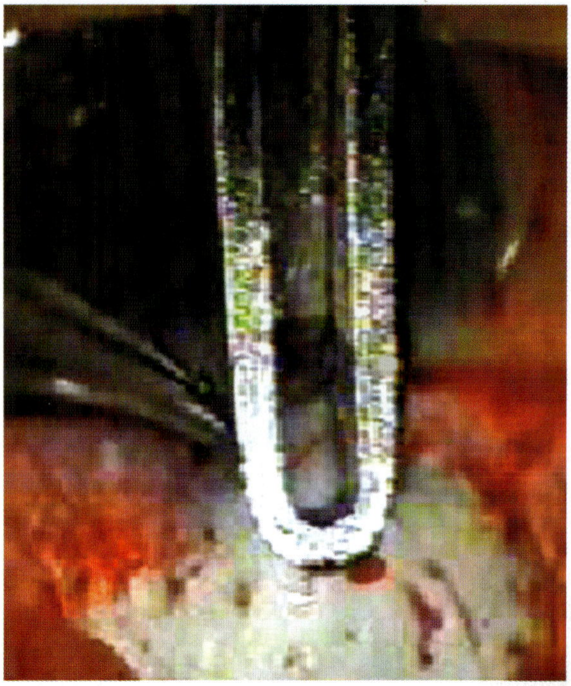

Fig. 38.6: Sclera is punched out wiht Holth punch

(Fig. 38.6) and a portion of the sclera is punched out by closing the punch and the piece of the sclera is removed (Fig. 38.7). The extent of the sclera to be punched out should be continuously monitored through the punch from where the surgeon can visualize the area being punched out. It should not cross the line of incision, as the punched out area will be more then what the anterior lip can cover.

An iridectomy is performed in the area of sclerectomy to complete the procedure. Care should be taken while punching the sclera. Sometimes if the surgeon is not careful enough, the iris can be caught in between the punch which then will be punched out along with the sclera. The area of the punched out sclera should be barely enough so that it is covered by the anterior lip of the tunnel.

Sclerectomy without the help of scleral punch: Various techniques of performing sclerectomy of the posterior lip without the use of scleral punch have been described. The posterior lip of the scleral tunnel is held with the help of a forceps as described earlier or the lip is exposed by pulling on to the anterior lip towards the cornea by an assistant. The surgeon then with the help of a blade breaker knife makes two radial incisions, parallel to each other

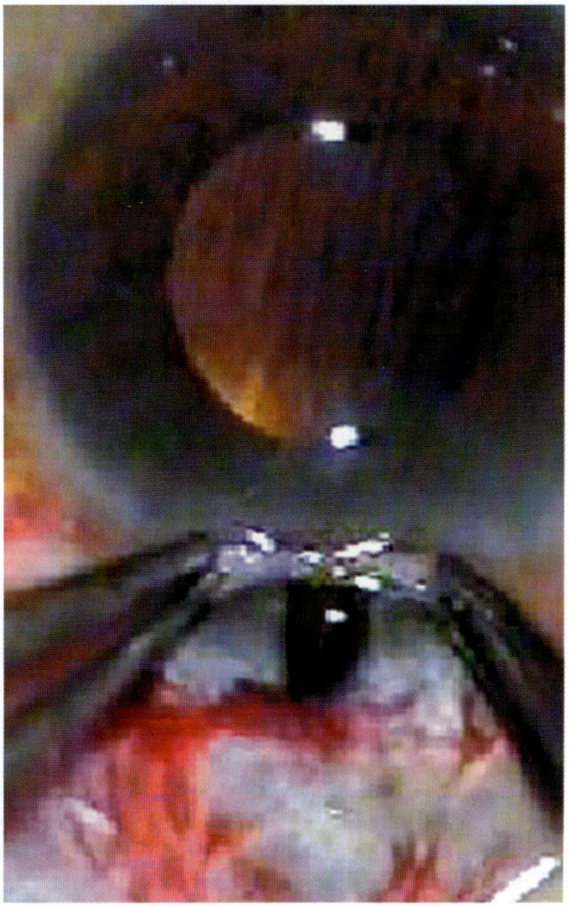

Fig. 38.7: Punched out posterior lip of tunnel

and about 1.5 mm apart extending about 2 mm from the corneolimbal junction towards the sclera. A third incision is made at the corneolimbal junction that is parallel to the limbus and connects the two radial incisions. Once these two radial incisions and corneolimbal incision have been made, a hinged flap of the corneosclera is obtained which is excised horizontally with the help of vannas scissors. In this manner, a portion of sclera is removed from the posterior lip.

After completion of sclerectomy, if the self sealing nature and the integrity of the scleral tunnel are in doubt, then the tunnel should be sutured to prevent any complication.

Once the sclerectomy has been performed, the viscoelastic is removed and anterior chamber is formed with ringer lactate or if needed then it can be filled with air.

Conjunctival Closure: The conjunctival flap is sutured at one or both ends to the limbus with 8-0 or 10-0 nylon sutures to obtain tight limbal closure. If the conjunctival flap had been initially fashioned leaving a 1 mm rim of conjunctiva at the limbus then the conjunctiva to conjunctiva can be sutured by a running 10-0 nylon suture. Alternatively the conjunctiva can be cauterized back to cover the incision site and it works equally well.

ANTIMETABOLITES

Antimetabolites such as 5-fluorouracil (5-FU) or mitomycin-C when used in conjunction with combined surgery can be beneficial. The antimetabolites are indicated for intractable glaucoma and high risk patients where the chances of failure are more. Application of 3 mg/ml of mitomycin-C for 2 minutes on the sclera, at the site of scleral tunnel has been found to be beneficial in combined surgery. After application the excess drug has to be washed out with copious amount of fluid to prevent complications such as scleral melting, bleb leak and hypotony. Contact of mitomycin-C to the conjunctiva should be avoided as it may cause conjunctival necrosis.

Combined surgery augmented with mitomycin-C achieves a lower IOP then combined surgery alone without the use of mitomycin –C. The use of 5-fluorouracil is not as effective as mitomycin-C and has a variable influence on the results.[9]

COMPLICATIONS

Besides the usual complications of small incision non-phacoemulsification cataract extraction certain specific complications are seen with combined surgery.

Intraoperative complications: The most dreaded intraoperative complication is making of an oversized sclerectomy which cannot be covered by the anterior lip of the scleral tunnel. Once an oversized sclerectomy is made then every attempt should be made to suture the incision as watertight as possible without pulling on to the lips of the scleral tunnel and closing the conjunctiva with sutures and making it as watertight as possible. The other common complication could be intraoperative hyphema. The bleeding vessel should be identified and if possible should be cauterized. If the bleeding vessel cannot be seen or is at a location where the cautery cannot be performed then the surgeon should wait for the bleeding to stop on its own and then wash out all the blood from the anterior chamber and then the conjunctiva is closed. Alternatively adrenaline can be used to achieve hemostasis if the patient is having normal blood pressure and there is no contraindication to its use.

Postoperative complications: The most common complication seen postoperatively is severe fibrinous reaction with or without hyphema. The anterior chamber reaction along with exduates clears in 2 to 3 days time after frequent use of topical steroids. Postoperative shallow anterior chamber is seen in cases when the anterior chamber was not well formed on the table. If the anterior chamber is shallow along with low IOP, over filtration should be suspected and the patient should either be pad and bandaged until the anterior chamber deepens or the patient should be taken into operating room and anterior chamber reformed with the help of air and the incision closed watertight with sutures.

If the anterior chamber is shallow along with raised IOP then a pupillary block should be suspected and instillation of topical mydriatics can relieve the pupillary block.

CONCLUSION

Each case of coexistent visually significant cataract and glaucoma has to be managed on its own merits. The surgeon should decide the course of management of a case on the surgical capability of the surgeon and no generalization should be made. The techniques described in this chapter should only serve as guide for individual surgeon's preferences in management of cataract and glaucoma. However, if the combined surgery is performed with appropriate technique, excellent results can be expected with high rate of success.

REFERENCES

1. Heffelfinger BL, Berman MN, Krupin T, Rosenberg LF, Ruderman JM: Surgical management of coexisting glaucoma and cataract. Ophthalmol Clin North Am. 2000;13(3):545-52. Review.
2. Lyle WA, Jin C: Comparison of 3- and 6-mm incision in combined Phacoemulsification and trabeculectomy. Am J Ophthalmol 111:189, 1991.
3. Kubota T, Touguri I, Onizuka N, Matsuura T: Phacoemulsification and intraocular lens implantation combined with trabeculotomy for open-angle glaucoma and coexisting cataract. Ophthalmologica. 2003;217(3): 204-07.
4. Chen H, Ge J, Liu X, Lu F: The clinical analysis of 260 combined surgery of glaucoma and cataract. Yan Ke Xue Bao. 2000;16(2):102-05.
5. Friedman DS, Jampel HD, Lubomski LH, Kempen JH, Quigley H, Congdon N, Levkovitch-Verbin H, Robinson KA, Bass EB: Surgical strategies for coexisting glaucoma and cataract: An evidence-based update. Ophthalmology. 2002;109(10):1902-13. Review.
6. Storr-Paulsen A, Perriard A, Vangsted P: Indications and efficacy of combined trabeculectomy and extracapsular cataract extraction with intraocular lens implantation in cataract patients with coexisting open angle glaucoma. Acta Ophthalmol Scand. 1995;73(3):273-76.
7. Lai JS, Tham CC, Lam DS: Topical anesthesia in phacotrabeculectomy. J Glaucoma 2002;11(3):271-74.
8. Simmons ST, Litoff D, Nicholas DA, et al: Extracapsular cataract extraction and posterior chamber intraocular lens implantation combined with trabeculectomy in patients with glaucoma. Am J Ophthalmol 1987;104:465.
9. Casson RJ, Salmon JF: Combined surgery in the treatment of patients with cataract and primary open-angle glaucoma. J Cataract Refract Surg. 2001;27(11):1854-63. Review.

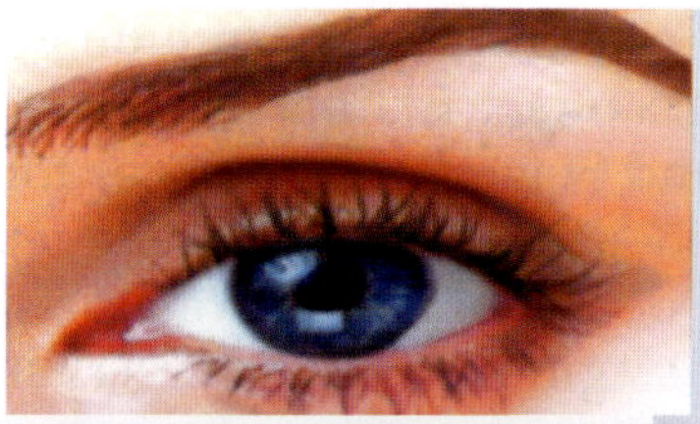

Thirty nine

SICS in Pediatric Cataracts

MS Ravindra (India)

WHY SICS AND IOL IN A CHILD?
SURGICAL PROCEDURE
TUNNEL INCISIONS
VISCOELASTICS
ANTERIOR CAPSULECTOMY
REMOVAL OF LENS MATTER
PRIMARY IOL IMPLANTATION
MANAGEMENT OF POSTERIOR CAPSULE
SELECTION OF IOL POWER
POSTOPERATIVE MEDICATIONS
FOLLOW-UPS

Surgical management of pediatric cataracts has always been challenging. After Sceie's paper on 'Aspiration of congenital and soft cataract', pediatric cataract surgery has evolved through various techniques including iridectomy, discission, linear extraction, curette evacuation, extracapsular extraction, intracapsular extraction, aspiration, etc. Until recently the preferred method of choice has been Pars plana Lensectomy with anterior vitrectomy, followed by postoperative correction of aphakia.

Today the method of choice for pediatric cataract is SICS, with or without PCIOL implantation. Although the age at which an IOL is implanted as a primary procedure is yet to be decided, majorities of surgeons today implant an IOL for one-year age and above. Visual results are greatly dependent on the time of uni/bilaterality, initial presentation, the time of surgery and the methods of optical and visual rehabilitation. Newer surgical techniques have certainly made the rehabilitation easier and have contributed significantly for better results. Pediatric cataract disrupts the development of the visual pathways and its surgical correction, in a way, is a part of overall management of amblyopia. I implant a PCIOL at all ages, the youngest I have implanted is a 20-day-old child with unilateral cataract.

WHY SICS AND IOL IN A CHILD?

Pars plana in a child is very small, and is almost non-existent. Pars plana Lensectomy surgery is associated with increased risk of retinal tears, as majority of the time the entry will be through pars plicata or peripheral retina. Also the posterior capsular support is removed irregularly and the posterior chamber IOL implantation either as a primary procedure or as a secondary procedure later becomes a difficult issue. Placing the IOL in the sulcus with retention of anterior capsule necessitates another limbal incision and more over the IOL centration is going to be difficult.

A direct limbal incision needs to be adequately sutured. Children being less manageable and difficult to follow up, suture related problems, including infection, could be more prevalent. Also limbal sutures for a direct incision need more frequent follow-ups, which obviously needs anesthesia. A direct incision, as against a tunnel incision, results in an unstable cornea, with perpetual alterations in the corneal astigmatism, initially with the rule, and ending up with a large against-the-rule in the later stages of life.

Amblyopia, even in a child with surgically well managed cataract is not a rare entity. Uncorrected aphakia is as good a stimulus to amblyopia as the cataract itself! Visual rehabilitation has to be meticulous. The role of an early IOL needs to be re-emphasized.

Fitting and maintenance of aphakik contact lenses in children is difficult, they get decentred or lost. Allergy and infections are common. Parents may loose compliance leading to uncorrected aphakia and Amblyopia.

SURGICAL PROCEDURE

The child's eye is not a miniaturised adult eye. Operating on it is a totally different plan altogether. Not only the spaces are smaller and the texture and feel of tissues is different, the way tissues respond to surgical trauma is also different. Do not be surprised by a vehement postoperative inflammation, which now is much lesser with the introduction of Vitrectomy as part of the procedure. Why so, no body seems to know!

The right time for cataract surgery in a dense **unilateral** congenital cataract is from birth to 6 weeks of age (Birch and Stager[1]). The chances for good visual acuity, better than 6/24, is lesser after this age. In bilateral dense congenital cataracts, permanent sensory nystagmus occurs if surgery is delayed beyond 3 to 4 months of age. In partial cataracts and acquired cataracts after infancy, several issues need to be considered about the timing of surgery. When a child presents after infancy with dense central cataract, surgery needs to be done at the earliest, within weeks. Partial cataracts can be managed with trial patching, if the level of visual loss is proportionate to the density and size of cataract. Mydriasis may be helpful. Surgery in partial cataract is indicated when the cataract reduces the visual acuity to 6/18. However, individual judgments are needed.

Surgery

The complications like secondary cataract, glaucoma, corneal decompensation, IOL decentrations, deprivation amblyopia, etc. were so high in the past that cataract surgery in a child by and large was disappointing. The advent of vitrectomy in mid-1970s revolutionized pediatric cataract surgery. In 1976, Parks et al introduced removal of central posterior capsule and anterior vitreous during the cataract procedure.[2,3] The second major revolution is the introduction of the IOLs. Although Choyce implanted an IOL in the eye of a child with traumatic cataract as early as 1956,[4] IOL did not become a routine in a child until the 1990s.[5] Currently, IOLs are widely used for children beyond one year of age. Studies in unilateral congenital cataracts indicate that IOL implanted in the first 6 months of life may produce better visual acuity but there is a higher risk of complications.[6]

Many adult cataract surgery techniques, such as clear corneal incisions, hydrodissection, foldable IOLs, and manual curvilinear anterior and posterior capsulorhexis, can be adapted in older children. But younger children need special techniques.

Anesthesia

Once you have decided to operate, the child is taken under general anesthesia. Surgery under

Ketamine is not recommended. Ensure that the pupil is well dilated. A small piece of cotton soaked with topical mydriatics, kept in the lower fornix, would quickly dilate the pupil even after the induction. A bridle suture for the superior rectus is avoided for the fear of postoperative vertical phorias and tropias. Intraoperative Bells phenomenon in lighter plane anesthesia is avoided by supplementing with topical anesthesia. Just before the surgery, keep a small piece of sterile cotton soaked in Xylocaine 2 percent on the proposed area of surgery for few minutes, although the surgery is done under GA. This reduces the sensory pain inputs to the CNS, and so minimises the need for a deeper plane anesthesia as well as the total dose of muscle relaxants. The topical anesthesia reduces the reflex contraction of superior rectus during the surgery, and the extraocular muscles remain relaxed, thus reducing the vitreous upthrust. The Keratometry and Biometry are performed prior to surgery under GA, if they are not done earlier and then a library of IOLs are to be kept ready. Valsalva maneuvers and coughing are common during the recovery from general anesthesia, and hence secure suturing of wounds is important in children.

TUNNEL INCISIONS

Self-sealing tunnels of adult design although are universally used in children now, will often leak because of thinner and less rigid sclero-cornea. Synthetic, absorbable 10-0 sutures, like Vicryl, are always used at the end of surgery to close all incisions, although they may appear secure and non-leaking. A sclero-corneal tunnel incision is generally opted in children with a superior or superotemporal approach. Place the incision so as to avoid perforating anterior scleral vessels. Temporal corneal incisions are avoided in children, as they are less secure, do not heal well and also they produce visible corneal scarring. The superior orbital margin as well as the Bell's phenomenon protects the superior incision against injuries.

Avoid any stay suture on the muscle. A pull on the muscle, against its contraction, will induce post-operative vertical phorias/tropias. A fornix based conjunctiva-Tenons flap is raised. To avoid separating the two layers, make the first nick 2 mm away and parallel to limbus, and dissect till you reach sclera. Pass one blade of the scissors between sclera and the dissected tissue, sweep down to the limbus and then cut the two layers from the limbus. About 5 to 7 mm wide conjunctival incision is adequate. Avoid the zone where there are perforating anterior ciliary vessels.

A sclerocorneal incision is ideal. A half thickness, frown or straight scleral incision measuring 4.5 mm or 6.5 mm (depending on the IOL chosen) is made 2 mm behind the supero-temporal limbus. Take the dissection into the cornea, for about 1.5 mm, but **at this time do not enter the AC.** The dissection through the sclerocorneae may be tricky, as the sclera is thin and fibers are more elastic and compact. A double bevel, very sharp spoon blade is my instrument of choice. A Fleiringa ring is desirable as it provides an external skeleton for the less rigid sclera and minmises the tendency for scleral collapse.

As there will be no nucleus in a child, the size of incision depends upon the IOL chosen. For a PMMA 6 mm. optic IOL, a 6.5 mm scleral incision is made. For an atraumatic introduction of a foldable IOL through a 2.8 mm injector, you need a 4.4 mm long incision. A 2.8 mm diameter injector has a circumference of 8.8 mm and so would need a 4.4 mm slit to enter. Make the incision adequate, and never squeeze a larger object through a tight tunnel. You would tear scleral lamellae, and result in a leaking wound that ultimately would scarify badly. This is particularly important in children, as the scleral rigidity is lower.

VISCOELASTICS

A high viscosity cohesive Viscoelastics is essential for pediatric cataract surgery to facilitate maintenance of anterior chamber stability, to counter the low scleral rigidity and increased vitreous upthrust. In special situations like with a compromised endothelium, it is helpful to use initially a low viscosity Dispersive agent like HPMC followed by Cohesive viscoelastic, like a soft shell. Cohesive viscoelastics are also needed for secondary IOL implantation in aphakic children, as it dilates the pupil and reduce the trauma of releasing posterior synechiae.

ANTERIOR CAPSULECTOMY

CCC is highly desirable in a child, to minimises extensive capsular fibrosis. It is also needed if there is an inadequate posterior capsular support, so as to resort to sulcus fixation. The anterior capsule is very elastic in child and poses great challenges. Perform an anterior capsulotomy with a 26 G cystitome, the tip of which is bent away from the bevel to 90 degrees. Mount it on a 2 ml syringe filled with air. Enter the AC with the cystitome, through the bed of the tunnel, at the limbus, not at the anterior end of the tunnel you have just created. Exchange the aqueous with air. This is done by slowly injecting air into AC and letting the aqueous escape through a 30 G needle, introduced obliquely at the left limbus. Anterior capsule is highly elastic in children and so aim for a small CCC. Remember that the Zonular fibers extend centrally to cover a very large area of the anterior capsule and resist a circular capsular tear, especially if the CCC is aimed to be big. As a closed chamber is essential, if air tends to escape, then fill the AC with a viscoelastic and complete the tear.

Manual continuous curvilinear capsulorhexis is difficult to perform. More force is required when pulling the capsular flap before tearing begins. Control of the capsulectomy and prevention of 'runaway rhexis' can be extremely difficult. In difficult cases, fill the AC with a high viscosity Viscoelastic. This flattens and slackens the anterior capsule and assists easier tearing in a controlled fashion. If the capsule is very resistant to tear, use a Utrata forceps to complete the CCC, under viscoelastic. You need to enlarge the entry to introduce the Utratas. You can actually generate an enormous amount of traction with this forceps! Utrata's capsulorhexis forceps performs better that a needle cystitome in these cases (Fig. 39.1). Regrasp the capsulorhexis edge frequently. Begin with a capsulotomy smaller than desired. When tearing, force is directed towards the center of the pupil (Fig. 39.2). The elasticity of the capsule makes the opening larger. Achieve about 5 mm dia CCC.

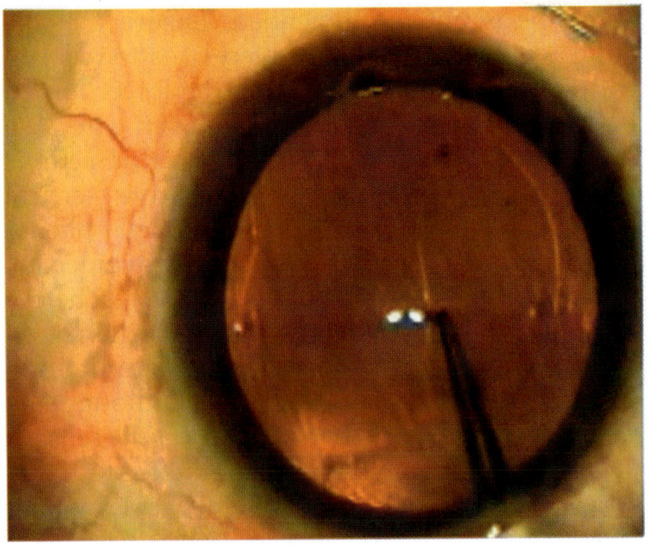

Fig. 39.1: Tenting up post capsule with utrata

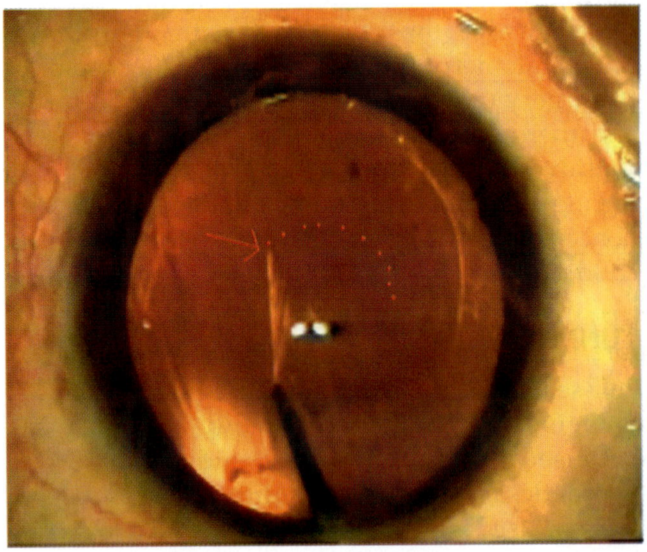

Fig. 39.2: PCCC continuing tear

Ultimately, if the capsule begins to extend peripherally, stop before the edge runs away under the iris (Fig. 39.3). Convert into one of the techniques described below. CCC is difficult in children. Vasavada and Chauhan failed to create an intact CCC using manual techniques in 80 percent of infants on whom this technique was attempted.[7] Alternative methods are:

A Vitrectomy probe can be used to create anterior capsulectomy. A Venturi pump system works better than a Peristaltic pump system. The vitrectomy probe is introduced into the closed eye

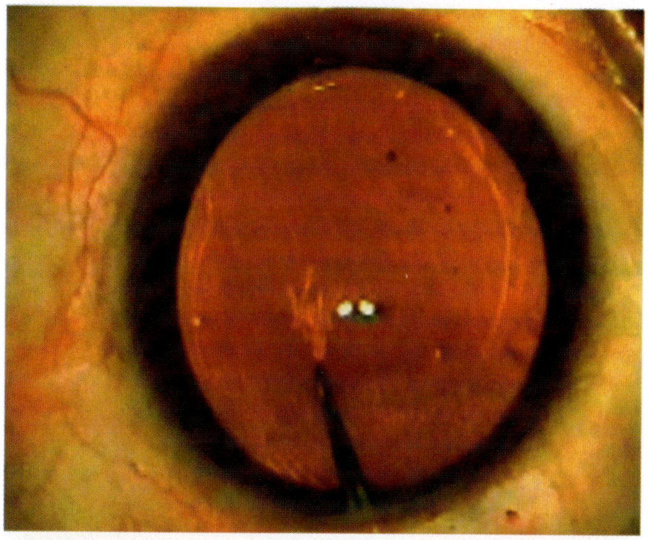

Fig. 39.3: PCCC removing posterior capsule

through a tight tunnel stab incision made at the limbus with an MVR blade. Irrigation is through a Blumenthal infusion cannula through a tunnel stab incision at 6 0′ clock. With a cutting rate of about 300 cycles per minute and the port oriented posteriorly, the center of the anterior capsule is aspirated up into the cutting port to create an initial opening. Enlarge the capsular opening using the cutter in a circular fashion. Keep the cutter just in front of the capsular edge and aspirate the capsule into the port rather than working in the plane of the capsule and chopping it directly. Any lens matter that exits is aspirated simultaneously. This technique can be easily performed even in white cataracts. A smooth, round capsulectomy can be produced, which resists radial tearing. The more elastic the anterior capsule, the smoother the edge of the rhexis and works best in young patients in whom the manual CCC is difficult. This technique is less ideal in older children because the capsule elasticity begins to approach that of an adult capsule. The capsular edge appears more scalloped and tears easily.

A third option for creating an anterior capsulotomy in a child is through the use of Radio frequency diathermy. I use Ellman Surgitron unit in difficult situations of anterior capsulectomy, with its special hypodermic needle mount attachment. A high frequency, low energy current in its purest form is used, so as to optimise the cutting energy and minimise the heat. The steel cystitome is mounted on the handpiece and the tip is placed in contact with the anterior capsule, under viscoelastic. The footswitch is then activated and the capsulectomy size and shape are controlled as it is moved along a circular path. Gas bubbles are formed but do not usually interfere with visualization. The cut edge of the capsule rolls up slightly and a larger capsulectomy results than that is initially aimed at. Corneal endothelial cells are not damaged. RF diathermy capsulectomy edge is less elastic when compared to that of manual CCC. Kloti's dedicated endodiathermy and Fugo blade can also be used for RF anterior capsulectomy.[8]

REMOVAL OF LENS MATTER

Now enlarge the cystitome entry at the base of the tunnel, at the level of limbus, with a MVR blade. Use a Simcoe cannula through this port to simultaneously irrigate BSS and aspirate cataractous lens. Hydrodissection and delineation can be attempted but a classical dissection of layers is difficult in a child. However, the hydroprocedures will loosen the lens matter, and assist in its aspiration. Instead of a continuous injection, small bursts of fluid injection at different levels and clock hours aid the cortical separation. The lens matter does not have the layered anatomy of an adult cataract. Neither it has the fibrous continuity, that if you engage one end of the lens matter into the port, the entire segment could be aspirated. The lens matter comes out in irregular clumps, like putty and has a gummy consistency. Complete cortical aspiration is mandatory to minimise postoperative inflammation even if a primary posterior capsulectomy is done. Pupil would tend to constrict, and this can be minimised with preoperative topical NSAIDs. Use a drop of preservative free Adrenaline in the irrigating fluid in difficult situations. Rarely there could be mild inflammatory fibrinous exudation intra-operatively, and this can be minimised by adding Inj. Heparin into the irrigating solution. An AC maintainer introduced at 6 0′ clock will be of use, as it keeps the AC deep and pressurized, and keeps the pupil dilated. Indeed AC maintainer is of great help if used throughout the surgery. Phacoemulsification is not only useless to extract the lens but also as the anterior chamber is unstable,

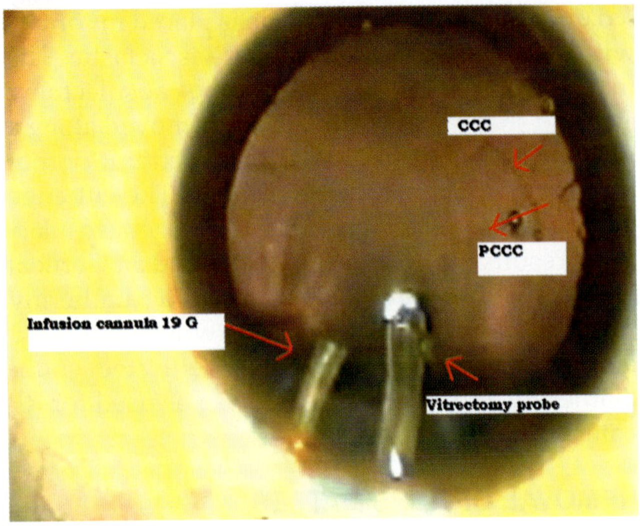

Fig. 39.4: Anterior vitrectomy

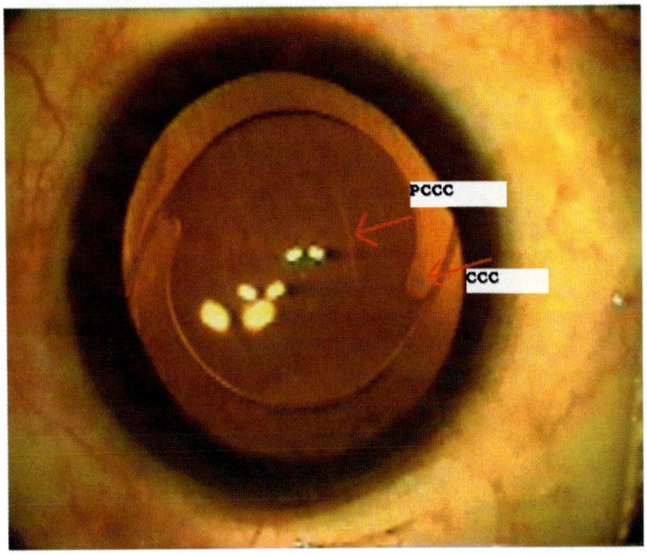

Fig. 39.5: PMMA IOL after PCCC and vitrectomy

could be hazardous. However, the Vitrectomy handpiece can be used with active suction (Fig. 39.4). Bursts of cutting can be used intermittently to facilitate the aspiration of the resistant lens matter. Despite meticulous removal of equatorial lens epithelium, a Soemmering's ring will form in most children.

PRIMARY IOL IMPLANTATION

The consensus is to implant an IOL in all children older than 2 years.[9,10] The majority of axial growth occurs during the first 2 years of life.[11] This makes selection of an IOL power for an infant difficult. Low scleral rigidity make IOL implantation technically more challenging in infants. Despite these complexities, IOLs are being implanted in infants with increasing frequency.

IOL in children has to be implanted within the bag. Avoid fixating one haptic in the bag and the other in the sulcus, as it leads to IOL decentration. Dialing the IOL into the capsular bag is difficult in children. So implant it into the bag, in the first attempt itself. When it is needed to dial the IOL into the bag, you may need to do it bimanually, in a deep AC, under Viscoelastic. Acrylic and PMMA IOLs are preferred in children because of their proven track record. Recent studies have recommended the heparin surface modified variety of PMMA IOLs to reduce the incidence of posterior synechiae and lens deposits (Fig. 39.5). While silicone IOLs are not recommended in children, the second-generation silicone material appears to be an acceptable alternative for older children.[12] When capsular fixation is not possible, sulcus placement of both the haptics of an IOL in a child can be done. Rigid PMMA IOLs are preferred for sulcus fixation, as it minimises the decentration.

For secondary IOL implantation, under the protection of a Viscoelastic, meticulously dissect the synechiae between the iris and the residual capsule, all along the periphery. Many a time, a Soemmering's ring keeps the anterior and posterior capsules separated. Reopen this peripheral capsular bag all round and aspirate the material. Insert the PMMA or Acrylic IOL within the peripheral capsular bag (Fig. 39.6). If this is not possible, a heparin surface modified PMMA IOL is inserted into the sulcus. An optic capture is done posteriorly through the capsule, to ensure long-term centration.

When capsular support is inadequate, do not implant IOL unless the child cannot tolerate contact lenses or spectacles. In these very rare situations, consider Kelman quadriflex AC IOLs. All though their long-term safety is yet to be established, they seem to be well tolerated in children with normal anterior segments if properly implanted without iris tucks or mal-sizing. Transscleral fixation of posterior chamber IOL can be considered, but pupillary capture, suture erosion, lens tilt and displacements are seen more often in children.

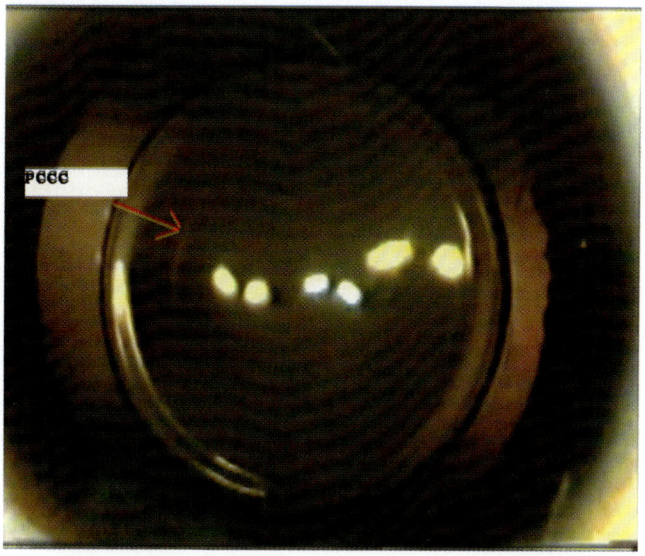

Fig. 39.6: Acrylic IOL after PCCC and vitrectomy

MANAGEMENT OF POSTERIOR CAPSULE

As the incidence of PCO is 100 percent in pediatric cataract surgery, a posterior capsular CCC and anterior Vitrectomy is mandatory, atleast till the age of 5 years. This is done under a viscoelastic, in a deep AC, with a Utratas capsulectomy forceps. I do the initial central nick with a 23 G needle. I hold the edge of the nick with Utrata, and complete the CCC. The Hyaloidal face is not disturbed at all. Again aim for a very small rhexis, smaller than the anterior rhexis. Aim for about 2 to 3 mm size, and it will end up larger. Now excise anterior hyaloid face and anterior vitreous with a Vitrectomy probe. I prefer low aspiration and a cutting rate of 600, and the eye needs to be continuously infused during the procedure. A closed chamberVitrectomy is preferred and hence use the port at the base of the tunnel to enter the probe, and not the main tunnel itself. Working with the Vitrector probe through the main tunnel also distorts the cornea, limiting the visibility.

The advent of primary posterior capsulorhexis and anterior vitrectomy in young children has dramatically improved the success rates and minimised the need for secondary surgery. Complications like retinal detachment and cystoid macular edema are reported to be exceedingly rare after pediatric cataract surgery with or without primary Capsulectomy and Vitrectomy. Nd-YAG Laser posterior capsulotomies is needed almost in every child if posterior capsulectomy is not primarily performed, and this also carries a greater risk of retinal detachment and cystoid macular edema. In addition, as pediatric capsules undergo intense fibrosis, larger amounts of Laser energy are often needed as compared with adults, and the posterior capsule opening may close down, requiring repeated laser treatments or a secondary pars plana membranectomy.

Studies have shown that a posterior capsulectomy without a central vitrectomy would be unlikely to prevent the development of a secondary membrane.[18] In fact, the opacification rate was not significantly decreased by a posterior capsulectomy alone. Only when an anterior vitrectomy was added did the opacification rate fall. In a prospective and randomized study, Vasavada and Trevidi[19] showed that visual axis obscuration across the anterior vitreous face occurred in 70 percent of those eyes in which vitrectomy was not performed after posterior CCC in children 5 to 12 years of age. No eye developed visual axis obscuration when a posterior CCC was combined with an anterior vitrectomy. Once an anterior vitrectomy is performed, an IOL optic capture is no longer necessary.

SELECTION OF IOL POWER

The choice of IOL differs with the surgeon. I prefer a Heparin coated PMMA IOL of diameter 6 mm. The long C loops, which confirm to the shape of the capsular fornix are more desirable than the J like loops of most of the IOLs. A foldable IOL of Acrylic make can be chosen, but the enormous fibrotic capsular contraction forces would surely distort the IOL to some extent, resulting in higher order visual aberrations. As a large number of IOLs do decenter marginally, avoid IOLs smaller than 6 mm. IOL should have full 6 mm optic (many IOLs have an edge which is non-optical), be made of one piece and shall have no holes. Their mesopic pupil size is going to be bigger than in an adult eye and any of the anomalies in the peripheral lens optic will show up in the quality of vision in the night, when the pupil is dilated. Remember that the child has to go through decades of active life, and needs the best-designed IOL.

To introduce the IOL, the AC is entered with a microkeratome, at the anterior end of the tunnel that was previously made. It is either a 4 mm or a 6 mm opening, depending on the IOL chosen. The AC is filled with Visoelastic and the IOL is inserted straight into the capsular bag. Care is taken that the lower haptic gets into the capsular bag and neither into the vitreous cavity through the PCCC nor into the ciliary sulcus. The rest of the IOL can be rotated into the bag using a Sinskey hook. If there is an AC maintainer, switch it of during this procedure. Reinject Viscoelastic again and again to keep the AC deep. A Dispersive Viscous like Methylcellulose is better at this stage than a Cohesive Viscoelastic, as the former protect the endothelium better and also maintain spaces adequately.

Selecting the IOL power in a child is challenging. Gordon and Donzis[13] have documented the axial growth pattern in normal eyes, but controversy exists about whether the pseudophakic eye grows predictably along the same curve. In the normal phakic child, there is little change in refraction (0.9 D from birth through adulthood on average) because the power of the natural lens decreases dramatically as the eye grows axially. We know that on Atropinisation a child's eye is often hypermetropic, the very strong accommodative effort makes the eye 'emmetropic'. However, an IOL in a child's eye does not change its power like this to match the growth of the eye. So, an IOL aiming emmetropia in early childhood would leave the patient highly myopic in older age.

Dahan et al [14] reported that younger the child at the time of implantation, the greater the myopic shift over time. They suggested that a child under age of 1 year should receive 80 percent of the IOL power needed for emmetropia. Between 1 to 2 years, implant an IOL with 90 percent of the power needed for emmetropia. There would be initial hyperopia, which needs to be corrected with glasses immediately after the surgery, till they move on to emmetropia or slight myopia in adulthood.

Knight-Nanan et al [15] suggested for less than 1 year of age, an IOL of power lesser by 6 D than emmetropic to compensate for the myopic shift. Awner et al[17] suggested aiming for a postoperative refraction of 4 D for children younger than 2 years of age, 3 D for children 2 to 4 years of age, 2 D for children 4 to 6 years of age, 1 D for children 6 to 8 years of age, and emmetropia for children older than 8 years of age at the time of implantation. For children between 2 and 8 years of age, you can select an IOL power that will leave mild to moderate hyperopia, milder with increasing age.[16] Some suggest aiming for emmetropia regardless of age when in children above 2 years of age. This approach aims at avoiding hyperopic amblyopia but is likely to result in significant myopia at a later date. To calculate the power of IOL, modern theoretical IOL formulas like Sanders-Retzlaff-Kraff (SRK) II, SRK-T, Holladay and Hoeffer Q formulas are preferred.

The Viscoelastic has to be completely removed from the AC, from behind the IOL and from the capsular bag. Gently flush the back of the cornea to remove its coating that is stuck to it. Most of the eyes need a suture or two to close the tunnel. 10-0 Vicryl could be used so that the child does not need to be taken into OR for suture removal. If an AC maintainer is used, one stitch would be needed to close the port. Bury the knots so that they do not irritate and the child can open the eyes and use it instantaneously.

Phacoemulsification has no role in a pediatric eye. The ultrasound energy is bad for the child's eye, and moreover there is no hardness in a child's cataract to emulsify.

POSTOPERATIVE MEDICATIONS

A drop of Povidone-iodine 5 percent is instilled and antibiotic, steroid and atropine ointments are placed in the eye. The eyes are patched and a shield applied for one day. Topical atropine (0.5% in children younger than 1 year of age, and 1% thereafter) is instilled once per day for 2 to 4 weeks. Prednisolone acetate is used topically, and the frequency is titrated according to the clinical picture. Generally 3 hourly medication is advised for 2 weeks during the day and then three times per day for an additional 2 to 6 weeks. An antibiotic drop is used for 1 week. Residual hyperopia is corrected for **NEAR** after 1 week. Separate glasses for near and distance are given in school going age. Postoperatively, the child needs very frequent topical steroids. Short acting cycloplegics may be of use for few days, to reduce the inflammatory response. If there is a hyperinflammatory reaction, children are prone for this, increase the topical steroids and a short-term systemic steroid regimen can be considered in consultation with the pediatrician.

In bilateral cataracts I perform simultaneous bilateral surgeries. Intraoperatively, the two eyes are totally isolated, and operation theater procedures are as though they are performed on two different individuals. The gowning, gloving, painting, draping, instruments, etc. are separate for the two eyes. No instruments cross over from one eye to the other. Simultaneous surgery prevents two GA inductions and also minimizes the risk of Amblyopia in the second operated eye.

FOLLOW-UPS

The use of protective glasses during the day and a shield at night is recommended for at least 2 weeks postoperatively. The child is seen after every week for one month and later at 3 months and 6 months postoperatively. The follow-ups later are based on amblyopia management. Yearly examinations under GA is essential in order to monitor intraocular pressure, peripheral retina, retinoscopy, A scan ultrasound, assessment of anterior segment and the IOL, and detect any PCO. Monitor any other ocular or systemic abnormalities. Aphakic or pseudophakic glaucoma is an important concern if the eye is microphthalmic. An unexpected myopic shift is an indication of glaucoma in a child. Amblyopia treatment is paramount during the follow-ups.

The surgical management of cataracts in children is challenging. Decreased scleral rigidity and increased vitreous upthrust make it more difficult. The anterior chamber is unstable, the capsular management needs caution and the eye is likely to react with severe postoperative inflammation. Selection of an IOL power is tricky. Compliance with postoperative instructions is difficult for the parents. The long expected life spans of children make the issues more challenging. These special patients are uniquely challenging. The child deserves best surgical techniques for optimal rehabilitation. Visual results are very satisfactory. Prescribe glasses to correct for the near vision initially, and later, in the school age, correct the left over hypermetropia for both near and distance. You may need to modify the spectacle powers once in 6 months. Squint and Amblyopia, if any, needs to be addressed meticulously. Clear corneae, briskly reacting pupils, clear media, absence of inflammatory sequelae, absence of synechiae, well centred IOL, and a smiling face and what more you want!

REFERENCES

1. Birch EE, Stager DR. The critical period for surgical treatment of dense, congenital, unilateral cataracts. Invest Ophthalmol Vis Sci. 1996;37:1532-38.
2. Parks MM. Posterior lens capsulectomy during primary cataract surgery in children. Ophthalmology. 1983;90:344-45.
3. Taylor D. Choice of surgical technique in the management of congenital cataract. Trans Ophthalmol Soc UK. 1981;101:114-117. Vasavada AR, Trivedi RH, Singh R. Necessity of vitrectomy when optic capture is performed in children older than 5 years. J Cataract Refract Surg. 2001;27:1185-93.
4. Choyce DP. Correction of uniocular aphakia by means of anterior chamber acrylic implants. Trans Ophthalmol Society UK. 1958;78:459-70.
5. Wilson ME. Intraocular lens implantation: Has it become the standard of care for children? Ophthalmology. 1996;103:1719-20.
6. Lambert SR, Buckley EG, Plager DA, Medow NB, Wilson ME. Unilateral intraocular lens implantation during the first six months of life. J AAPOS. 1999;3:344-49.
7. Vasavada A, Chauhan H. Intraocular lens implantation in infants with congenital cataracts. J Cataract Refract Surg. 1994;20:592-98.
8. Fugo RJ, Coccio D, McGrann D, Becht L, DelCampo D. The Fugo Blade. The next step after capsulorhexis. Presented at the American Society of Cataract and Refractive Surgery symposium on cataract, IOL and refractive surgery, Congress on Ophthalmic Practice Management, Boston, Massachusetts, 2001.
9. Taylor D. The Doyne lecture: Congenital cataract: The history, the nature, and the practice. Eye. 1998;12:9-36.
10. Lambert SR, Drack AV. Infantile cataracts. Surv Ophthalmol. 1996;40:427-58.
11. Gordon RA, Donzis PB. Refractive development of the human eye. Arch Ophthalmol. 1985;103:785-89.
12. Pavlovic S, Jacobi FK, Graef M, Jacobi KW. Silicone intraocular lens implantation in children: Preliminary results. J Cataract and Refract Surg. 2000;26:88-95.
13. Gordon RA, Donzis PB. Refractive development of the human eye. Arch Ophthalmol. 1985;103:785-89.

14. Dahan E, Drusedau MUH. Choice of lens and dioptric power in pediatric pseudophakia. J Cataract Refract Surg. 1997;23:618-23.
15. Knight-Nanan et al. Intraocular lenses in children with cataract. J Cataract Refract Surg. 1996;2:730-36.
16 Crouch Jr ER, Pressman SH, Crouch ER. Posterior chamber intraocular lenses: Long-term results in pediatric cataract patients. J Cataract Refract Surg. 1995; 32:210-18.
17. Awner S, Buckley EG, DeVaro JM et al. Unilateral pseudophakia in children under 4 years. J Pediatr Ophthalmol Strabismus. 1996;32:230-36.
18. Metge P, Cohen H, Chemila JF. Intercapsular implantation in children. Cur J Cataract Refract Surg 1990;2:319-23.
19. Vasavada AR, Trivedi RH, Singh R. Necessity of vitrectomy when optic capture is performed in children older than 5 years. J Cataract Refract Surg. 2001;27:1185-93.

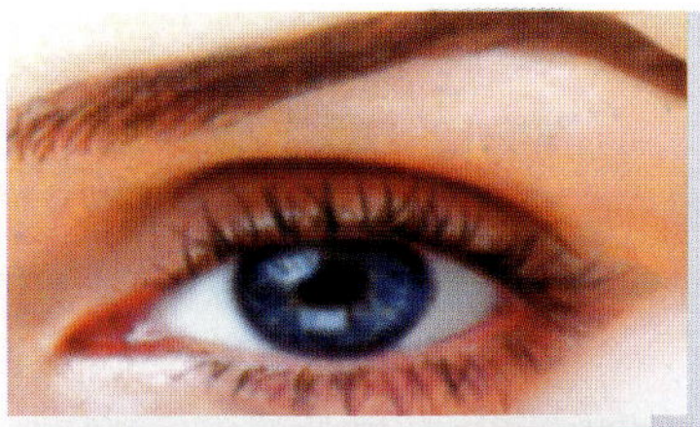

Forty

Mini Nuc Cataract Surgery Under Topical Anesthesia

RM Shanbhag (India)

TECHNIQUES OF OPHTHALMIC ANESTHESIA

The techniques of ophthalmic anesthesia have changed over the years. In the eighteenth century couching was done under cocaine topical anesthesia. Then came facial and retrobulbar anaesthesia techniques followed by peribulbar anesthesia technique. Of late subtenons and topical anesthesia have evolved.

OCULAR COMPLICATIONS OF RETRO/ PERIBULBAR ANESTHESIA

The most common complication is retrobulbar hemorrhage due to which the surgery has to be postponed for few days.

Other complications are:

- Globe perforation
- Optic nerve injury
- Central retinal artery occlusion
- Intra arterial injection

Optic nerve sheath injury all of which can lead to permanent damage in vision. The systemic toxicity of anaphylaxis due to injection in the vessel is another serious complication.

WHY IS TOPICAL ANESTHESIA POSSIBLE TODAY

This is due to self sealing incision which causes a closed globe without iris prolapse and other serious attendant complications. The anterior maintainer keeps the pupil well dilated and the intraocular structures in there normal positions with constant intraocular pressure in all stages of surgery which helps to minimise pain.

THE DISADVANTAGES OF TOPICAL ANESTHESIA

The eye is mobile eye with less profound anesthesia which is not necessary in cooperative patients. Eye lids and peri orbital area is not anesthetized which again makes little differences to a cooperative patients. Discomfort from microscope light is felt by few patients compared to injection anesthesia. Potential epithelial toxicity can occur due to which it is advisable to put anesthetic two minutes before surgery.

ADVANTAGES OF TOPICAL ANESTHESIA

The advantages of topical anesthesia is manifold as there is no risk from needle injection with the complications already mentioned. No bridal suture is required to be taken which reduces the risk of superior rectus palsy and also reduces the risk of iris prolapse during delivery of lens. The return of vision is rapid and almost immediate compared to retrobulbar injection which numbs the optic nerve. The rapid return of vision contributes a lot to mental healing of the patients. The eye following topical anesthesia need not be patched contributing to greater postoperative comfort.

CASE SELECTION FOR TOPICAL ANESTHESIA

It is preferable to have the following patients for this procedure:

- Patients with uncomplicated cataracts.
- Patients with well dilated pupils
- Patients which are best avoided are anxious patients
- Patients with hearing problems
- Patients who are mentally handicapped

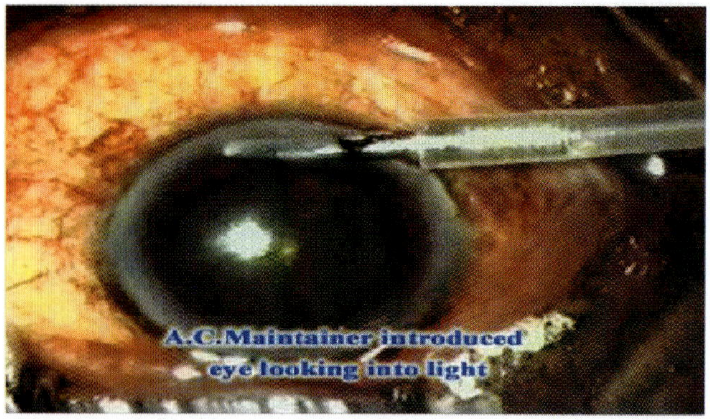

Fig. 40.1

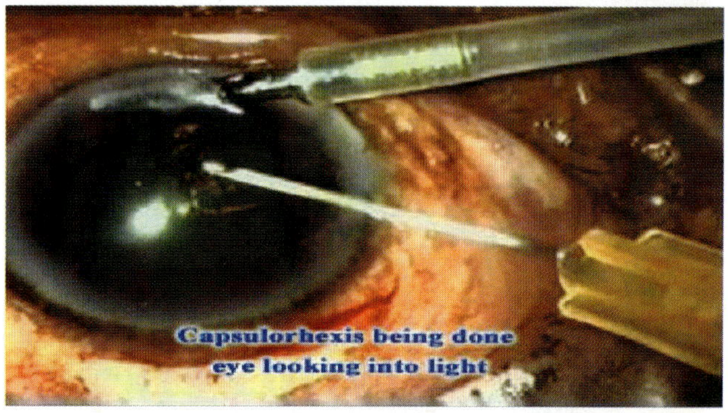

Fig. 40.2

TECHNIQUE OF MINI NUC CATARACT SURGERY UNDER TOPICAL ANESTHESIA

First of all the surgeon should be well versed and should have done many surgeries with block anesthesia before venturing into topical anesthesia since the eye is mobile. The patient should be instructed pre operatively to keep both eyes open and carry out the two movements, i.e. looking in the light of microscope and looking down without movement of head. Four percent lignocaine drops are instilled in the eye, two to five minutes before surgery after eye is prepared aseptically and after cutting of conjunctiva when patient is looking down (Fig. 40.1) and applying cautery on the sclera sponges dipped in four percent lignocaine may be applied to the sclera in case of discomfort. The side ports (Fig. 40.2) and introduction of anterior chamber maintainer and capsulorhexis (Fig. 40.3) and hydrodisection (Fig. 40.4) of the lens is performed while the patient is looking into the microscope light. Then the patient is again asked

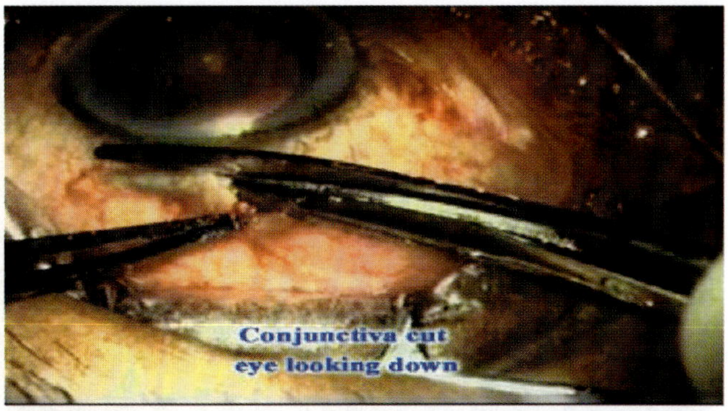

Fig. 40.3

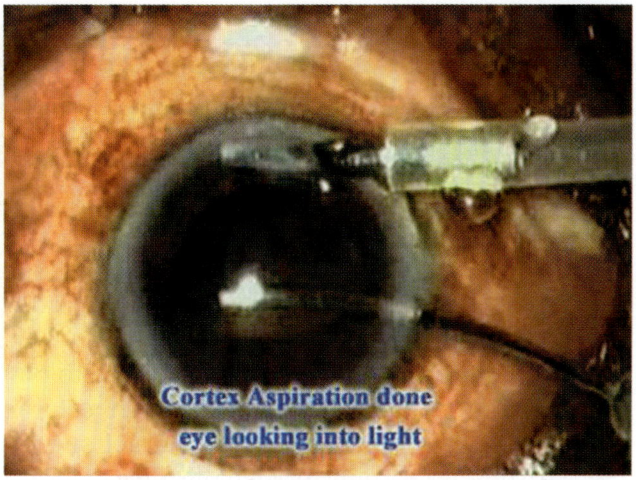

Fig. 40.4

to look down during the introduction of glide (Fig. 40.5) and pressure on the glide during delivery of the hard core nucleus and epinucleus. The patient then looks into the microscope light while aspirating the cortex through the side ports (Fig. 40.6).

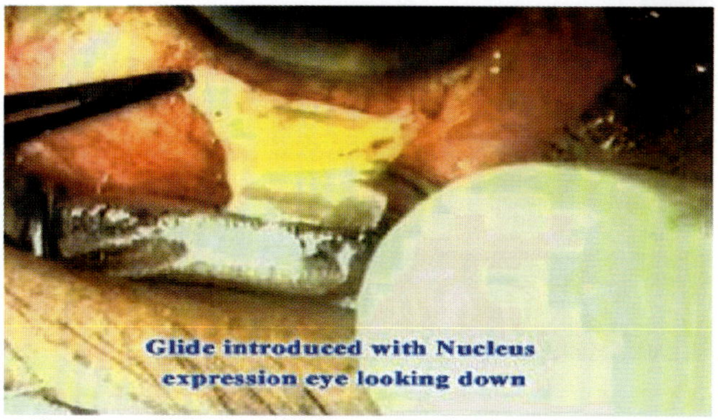

Fig. 40.5

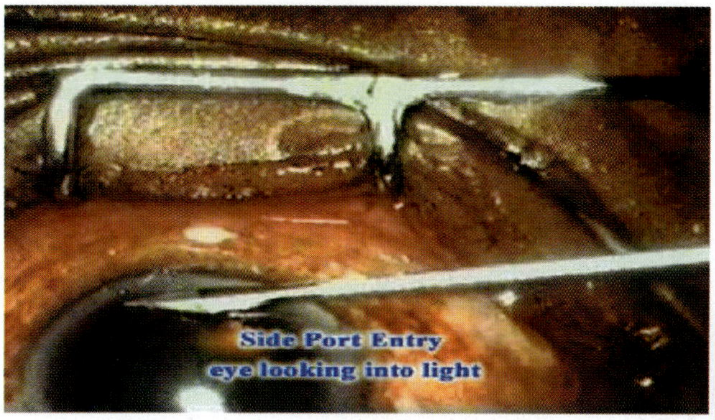

Fig. 40.6

The intraocular lens is then inserted in the bag and conjunctiva glued with cautery.

REFERENCES

1. Surgical rehabilitation of vision—Michael Blumenthal et al.
2. Anesthesia in Cataract surgery—Highlights of ophthalmology, Benjamin F Boyd.
3. Textbook of Ocular Pharmacology—Zimmerman.

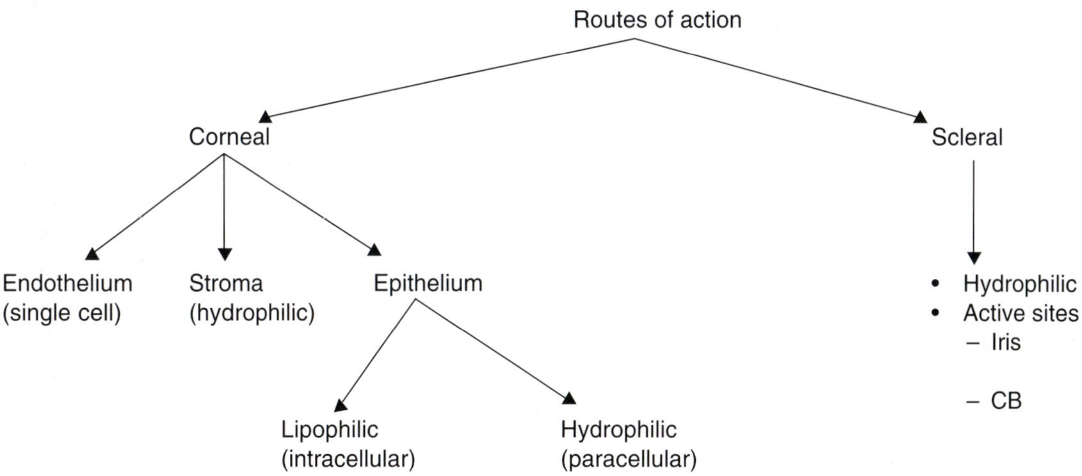

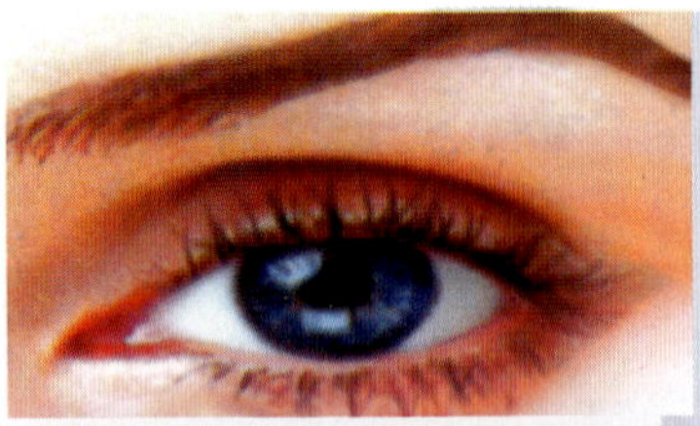

Forty one

Ocular Pharmacokinetics in Manual Small Incision Cataract Surgery

Ashok Garg (India)

INTRODUCTION

Ocular therapeutics have a significant role to play in any type of intraocular surgery. In cataract surgery specially small incision cataract surgery (SICS) drugs are administered in the form of topical eye drops, systemic administration, eye ointments, injections or infusion forms. The aim of drug administration in SICS is to:

- Prepare bacteria free sterile environment for safe surgery (preoperatively).
- To assist in surgical steps for safe surgery (Perioperative)
- To bolster the compromised defence mechanisms of surgically traumatized eye (Postoperatively) to achieve complications free post surgical phase to obtain best visual results.

Use of different forms of medications may vary from surgeon to surgeon and from place to place. Here, I shall describe a commonly accepted protocol for ocular pharmacokinetics being practiced worldwide with little modifications.

The various ocular medications being used in preoperative, perioperative and postoperative phases of the small incision cataract surgery are broadly classified into following groups.

I. Antibiotics
II. Povidone Iodine (Halogens)
III. Mydriatics and cycloplegics
IV. Miotics
V. Irrigating solutions and Viscosurgical devices.
VI. Anti-inflammatory drugs
- Steroidal group
- Non-steroidal group (NSAID).

ANTIBIOTICS

Antibiotics are chemical substances produced by microorganisms that have the capacity to inhibit growth of or even destroy bacteria and other microorganisms in dilute solution.

Antibiotics are most commonly used in preoperative phase of SICS for prophylaxis against and for treatment of ocular infections. Organisms that may otherwise be considered normal flora such as *Staph epidermidis* are potential pathogens to eye for intraocular surgery. The use of pre-operative topical antibiotics may decrease or eliminate bacterial flora from the conjunctiva that their use will not prevent intraoperative contamination of wound or anterior chamber. The goal of achieving high antibiotic concentration. In anterior segment can be achieved by frequent topical instillation of antibiotics drops into the conjunctival sac. However in severe infections of eye or in systemic infection, systemic antibiotic therapy is also indicated for 48 hours before surgery. Generally broad spectrum topical antibiotic drops are frequently instilled intensively started 24 hours preoperatively and bactericidal antibiotics are used postoperatively in combination with topical steroids.

Although, a large number of antibiotics of different groups are available commercially but following group antibiotics are most commonly prescribed.

a. Fluoroquinolone group.
b. Aminoglycosides
c. Cephalosporins
d. Polypeptides including polymixin B, Bacitracin.

Fluoroquinolone Group

So far the most significant and most commonly used latest antibiotics in ophthalmic surgery belongs to Fluoroquinolone group.

Antibiotics (systemic or topical) of Fluoroquinolone group are generally prescribed because of their broad spectrum of activity against groam +ve and gram -ve pathogens as well as good aqueous humour concentration in both routes.

Various drugs of this group used in SICS in preoperative and Postoperative phases include :-

Topical Ciprofloxacin - 0.3 percent
Topical Ofloxacin - 0.3 percent
Topical Lomefloxacin - 0.3 percent
Topical Levofloxain - 0.5 percent
Topical Moxifloxacin - 0.5 percent
Topical Gatifloxacin - 0.3 percent

For systemic use generally ciprofloxacin (500 mg twice a day) or gatifloxacin (400 mg twice a day) or levofloxacin (500mg twice day) for 48 hours prior to the surgery are recommended

Aminoglycosides

Among aminoglycosides gentamicin was previously commonly used for preoperative phase. Now tobramycin with broad spectrum activity is most commonly prescribed after Fluroquinolones for topical instillation commonly. It is available as 0.3 percent topical ophthalmic solution.

Cephalosporins

Second and third generation systemic and injected forms of Cephalosporins are used in postoperative phase of SICS specially in desperate cases with high order infections.

Polypeptides including Polymixin B and Bactracin

Polypeptides including Polymixin B and Bactracin are preferred by some ophthalmologist for preoperative phase of SICS. Topical preparation consists of Polymixin B 10000 units/ml and Bacitracin 500 units/ml.

Generally during perioperative phase of SICS no antibiotics in any forms are given in the eye to prevent the risk of intraocular infection or contamination. However many ophthalmologists prefer to instill subconjunctival antibiotic injection at the end of the intraocular surgery to produce a constant and prolonged depot of medication supplying effective concentration in the anterior segment. The main route for subconjunctival antibiotic injection is through the tear film and cornea.

In uneventful postoperative phase, only broad spectrum high order antibiotics are prescribed along with topical steroids for 2-4 weeks depending upon the postsurgical ophthalmic status.

In situations confronted with postoperative infections, treatment should be given with the use of a narrow spectrum antibiotic active against the infective organism identified by culture. The choice of route of administratioin of the antibiotic will depend on the site and severity of the infection and the degree of ocular iatrogenic inflammation.

So the best pre-requisite for the correct choice of an antimicrobial which at the same time will be fully active, safe and well tolerated, is an exact clinical and bacteriological diagnosis.

When more than one antibiotics are used in such situation, apart from spectrum of the individual antibiotics, synergism and antigonism must be kept in mind. Generally, they achieve their effects by disturbing the metabolic activities of the bacteria. The details of various antibiotics with their dosage and various routes of administrations specially intravitreal injections have been discussed in details in separate chapter on Management of Postoperative Endophthalmitis.

Povidone Iodine (Halogens)

Iodine is aqueous and alcoholic solution and is an active bactericidal agent. Commercially, it is available as 5 percent sterile ophthalmic prep. Solution. It contains Povidone Iodine (0.5% available iodine) stabilized by glycerin.

It is indicated in the eye for prepping of the periocular region (Lids, brow and cheek) and irrigation of the ocular surfaces (cornea, conjunctiva and palpebral fornics) prior to SICS.

This topical solution is an isotonically balanced pre-operative microbicidal solution that can be safely used directly on the cornea and conjunctival cul-de-sac as well as on periocular region. This solution is strictly used for external use only. It is contraindicated for intraocular injection or irrigation.

Topical Povidone-Iodine is commonly used in preoperative phase of SICS worldwide. Salient features of this topical solution are:

- Assure asepsis in less than 30 seconds and stained skin is virtually impossible to reinfect for atleast one hour enough to complete the surgery.
- It is non toxic, has excellant skin tolerance and does not burn the skin.
- It has broad spectrum of action sporicidal, bactericidal, antimycotic, viricidal and protozocidal.
- It decreases the incidence of post-operative endophthalmitis.

So Topical Povidone Iodine preparation should be commonly used in SICS.

MYDRIATICS AND CYCLOPLEGICS

This Mydriatics and cycloplegics are two classes of drugs which are used preoperatively in combination to produce maximal mydriasis prior to SICS when surgical control is made through the pupil. A well dilated pupil makes the SICS much easier with lesser perioperative complications. Topical Phenylephrine (5%) and tropicamide (0.8%) combination is commonly used in preoperative phase for faster action. The major advantage of this combination is that it produces quick mydriasis and mydriatic effect persists to facililate SICS. Generally 1-2 drops of the topical combination are instilled into the operating eye every 15-20 minutes starting one hour before the surgery, however frequency may vary as per choice of the ophthalmic surgeon.

MIOTICS

Miotics have important role to play during perioperative stage of SICS generaly cholinergic agents like Acetylcholine, Carbachol and pilocarpine are used in ophthalmic surgery.

These agents produce miosis by the direct stimulation of the spherical pupillae. Acetylcholine cannot be used topically as it is rapidly destroyed by the cholinesterase, so it is used directly into the anterior chamber (Intra cameral). As acetylcholine is unstable in solution, so it supplied as dry powder and fresh ophthalmic solution (1:100 acetylcholine chloride) is prepared before the use usually 0.5-2 ml of this solution is required to produce satisfactory miosis. Solution need not to be flushed from the anterior chamber after intracameral injection when adequate miosis is produced.

Acetylcholine has short duration of action (10-20 minutes) and only fresh solution is used before use.

Carbachol and Pilocarpine are effective both in topical and intracameral form. Generally Topical 1% and 2% Pilocarpine is used for ophthalmic surgery.

For intracameral administration Topical carbachol is available in the concentration of 0.01 percent in 1.5 ml disposable ampoules. Gently instill not more than 0.5 ml of carbachol into the anterior chamber during SICS. Miosis is achieved within 2-5 minutes after application.

An Intracameral preparation of cholinergic agents for intraoperative use during SICS induces miosis and inhibits post-operative pressure rise. These cholinergic agents are most helpful in constricting the pupil before closing the corneoscleral wound.

Irrigating Solutions and Ophthalmic Viscosurgical Devices

Irrigating solutions are used during SICS:

- Preoperatively to cleanse the conjunctiva and periocular skin.
- During surgery to remove intraocular debris and to replace intraocular volume.
- Irrigating solutions are aqueous solutions used to cleanse and to maintain moisture of ocular tissues.

Intraocular irrigating solution: (Balanced Salt Solution BSS or BSS plus) are used during ocular surgery to protect the lens and cornea. Balanced salt solutions provide magnesium and calcium ions as cellular nutrients. These nutrients are required for intercellular and intracellular function during prolonged ocular surgery. Calcium, bicarbonate, glucose and glutathione present in BSS help to maintain a deturgesced or thin cornea by avoiding corneal clouding. BSS plus solution is iso-osmotic with intraocular tissues and provides uncompromised endothelial nourishment. The details have been discussed in separate chapter on ophthalmic viscosurgical devices and other ocular surgical adjuncts in this book.

Extreme care should be taken while selecting intraocular irrigating solution for SICS. One should be careful about the quality and sterility of the product. Any compromise in the sterility or quality of irrigating solution can lead to Fluminating post-operative infections leading to complete loss of vision.

OPHTHALMICVISCOSURGICAL DEVICES (VISCOELASTIC SUBSTANCES)

When the eye is entered during SICS anatomical relations are disturbed and tissues may be in contact allowing no room for manipulation. Viscoelastic substances are used to restore the anatomy and to temponade the tissues. The anterior chamber proving not only the apposition, but also preventing iris contact and adhesion.

Viscoelastics are used in Intraocular surgery to:

- Protect corneal endothelium from mechanical trauma.
- To maintain an anatomical situation created by surgeon and maintenance of anterior chamber.
- Separate tissue planes.
- Prevents capillary bleeding.
- Forms a temporary blockade.
- To protect and isolate newly created or restored tissue surfaces.
- To prevent the formation of undesirable fibrin coagulum.
- To provide coating ability to implants, instruments and corneal epithelial surface.

Two groups of viscoelastic agents are used for intraocular surgery.

Sodium Hyaluronate

It is a large polysaccharide molecule. One percent Sodium Hyaluronate is true viscoelastic agent. It is highly viscous, elastic and pseudoplastic of very high molecular weight.

It is available as preloaded syringe with 27 G or 30 G cannula containing sodium hyaluronate 10 mg/ ml or 14 mg/ml strength (in 0.25, 0.50, 0.80, 2 ml and 4ml syringes).

During SICS, as soon as sodium hyaluronate is entered anterior chamber, the role of viscoelastic begins. It fills, maintains and cushions the anterior chamber. During anterior capsulotomy it prevents scrolling up of margins. Hydraulic separation of nucleus and cortex can be easily done with sodium hyaluronate. Sodium hyaluronate can be easily distinguished from vitreous.

Its use is limited as it is very expensive and every patient cannot afford the cost specially in developing countries.

Methylcellulose

It is an artificial compound somewhat viscous, low cost but not truly viscoelastic substance. It is water soluble, non toxic to the endothelium, transparent and nonpyrogenic. It is basically used as lubricant and maintain anterior chamber. Commercially 2 percent of hydroxymethyl cellulose is used for SICS. It is highly purified Hydroxy propyl and methyl groups, increases the hydrophilicity of the compound.

Injection of methyl cellulose serves to support a deep anterior chamber during SICS and allows through manipulation with less trauma to corneal endothelium and other surrounding tissues. It impedes vitreous leakage into the anterior chamber. thereby decreasing the chances of postoperative flat chamber. Care should be taken to remove as much possible of methyl cellulose by irrigation/ aspiration at the close of surgery for preventing corneal endothelial cell loss as a result of performed procedure.

It is available as 2 percent HPMC solution in 2ml vials or prefilled sterilised disposable syrings with sterile 27 G cannula.

Rest of details is discussed in separate chapter on ophthalmic visco surgical devices earlier.

ANTIINFLAMMATORY DRUGS

Postoperative therapy is decided individually. The operated eye must be protected from exogenous infections as well as iatrogenic inflammatory responses specially in uvea. Before selecting anti-inflammatory drug ophthalmic surgeon should keep in mind the type of AID to be used, duration and potential adverse side effects specially in wound healing, aggravating herpetic infections and the induction of glaucoma in susceptible patient.

Two types of anti-inflammatory drugs can be used in postoperative phase following SICS.

a. Corticosteroids :
b. Non-steroidal anti-inflammatory drugs.

Corticosteroids

Topical corticosteroids are indicated in post-operative phase to control iatrogenic inflammation of the eye.

Steroids have powerful anti-inflammatory action. It is shown to be potentiation of epinephrine vasoconstriction, stabilization of lysosomal membranes, retardation of macrophage movement, inhibition of prostaglandin synthesis and inhibits fibroblastic proliferation and vascularisation.

Steroids may be administered locally in the form of eye drops, ointments or injections in post-operative phase to control iatrogenic inflammation.

A number of topical steroid-antibiotic combinations are commercially available for use. The most common combinations prescribed are:

- Dexamethasone (0.1%) with Tobramycin (0.3%) suspension or ointment.
- Dexamethasone (0.1%) with Lomefloxacin (0.3%) in soln and oint.
- Dexamethasone (0.1%) with Ofloxacin (0.3%) in soln.
- Fluorometholone (0.1%) with Tobramycin (0.3%) in soln.
- Loteprednol (0.5%) with Ciprofloxacin (0.3%) in soln.
- Rimexolone (1%) with Ciprofloxacin (0.3%) in soln.

Topical steroid-antibiotic combination provides a greater patient compliance and convenience. In such combinations steroids provide powerful anti-inflammatory effect while associated antibiotics provide broad spectrum bactericidal effect. Even pus, exudates and bacteria growth products cannot inactivate the antibiotic in such combinations.

Patient is advised to put 1-2 drops in the conjunctival sac 2-4 times daily for 3-4 weeks depending upon the assessment of condition by ophthalmologist. Care should be taken not to discontinue the treatment prematurely and abruptly.

Non-steriodal Anti-inflmmatory Drugs (NSAIDs)

NSAIDs act mainly as anti-inflammatory agents by inhibiting cyclo-oxygenase and lipo-oxygenase enzymes which lead to inhibiton of products—like prostaglandins, thromboxane and leukotriens which induce inflammation.

Need of NSAIDs in ocular inflammation was felt due to severe complications associated with more established steroid therapy. Although a overlap between the mechanisms of action of both NSAIDs and steroids exists yet the use of NSAIDs in ophthalmology is safer than the use of steroids.

Topical NSAIDs drops are potentially useful for adequate pupillary dilation specially its maintenance during intraocular surgery undergoing ECCE or SICS. Endogenous factors other than prostaglandins and surgical techniques have been responsible for this condition. NSAIDs use can cause pharmacological effect on the pupil lessening intraoperative miosis.

NSAIDs that are commonly used for this indication include:

Fluribiprofen — 0.03 percent
Suprofen — 1 percent
Indomethacin — 1 percent suspension.

Topical Fluribiprofen and Indomethacin maintains pupillary dilatation in statistically significant higher number of patients undergoing SICS.

Topical NSAIDs drops are potentially useful in managing postoperative inflammation following SICS. Flurophotometric analysis offers a quantitative means of studying anterior chamber inflammation.

Several clinical studies have shown the efficacy of topical NSAIDs in controlling iatrogenic inflammation specially indomethacin (1 percent), fluribiprofen (0.03 percent), ketorolac (0.5 percent) and diclofenac (0.1 percent).

Fluorophotometry studies conducted by the author have shown that topical NSAIDs achieve better inflammation control than the steroids in double masked randomised studies. Topical diclofenac (0.1 percent), indomethacin (1 percent suspension) or 0.1 percent ophthalmic solution have been proved to be better in controlling inflammation following SICS. Latest studies have strongly advocated the use of topical diclofenac 0.1 percent four times daily starting 24 hours after cataract surgery to control postoperative inflammation. It is possible practically to prescribe a topical NSAID for a topical corticosteroids to control iatrogenic inflammation specially in eyes with significant steroid responsive glaucoma. Some research studies have even advocated the use of topical diclofenac (0.1 percent) in preoperative phase (starting 24 hours prior to the surgery) to control iatrogenic inflammation of the eye.

REFERENCES

1. Garg Ashok. Text Book of Ocular Therapeutics, 2nd ed, New Delhi, Jaypee Brothers, 2002.
2. Garg Ashok. Advances in Ophthalmology, 1st ed., New Delhi, Jaypee Brothers, 2003.
3. Zimmerman. Text Book of Ocular Pharmacology; Lippincot and Williams and Wilkins, 1997.
4. Kershner. Ophthalmic Medications and Pharmacology; Slack Inc, 1994.
5. Kanski. Clinical Ophthalmology, 4th ed: Butterworth–Heineman, 1999.
6. Fechner. Ocular Therapeutics; Slack Inc, 1998.
7. Duvalle. Ophthalmic medications and Pharmacology, 7th ed. C.V. Mosby, 1985.
8. Bartlett JD. Clinical Ocular Pharmacology, 4th ed, Boston, Butterworth – Heineman, 2001.
9. Seal. Ocular Infection Management and Treatment; Martin-Dunitz, 1998.
10. Steven Podos: Text Book of Ophthalmology, New Delhi, Jaypee Brothers, 2001.

Section Three

Complications and Their Management

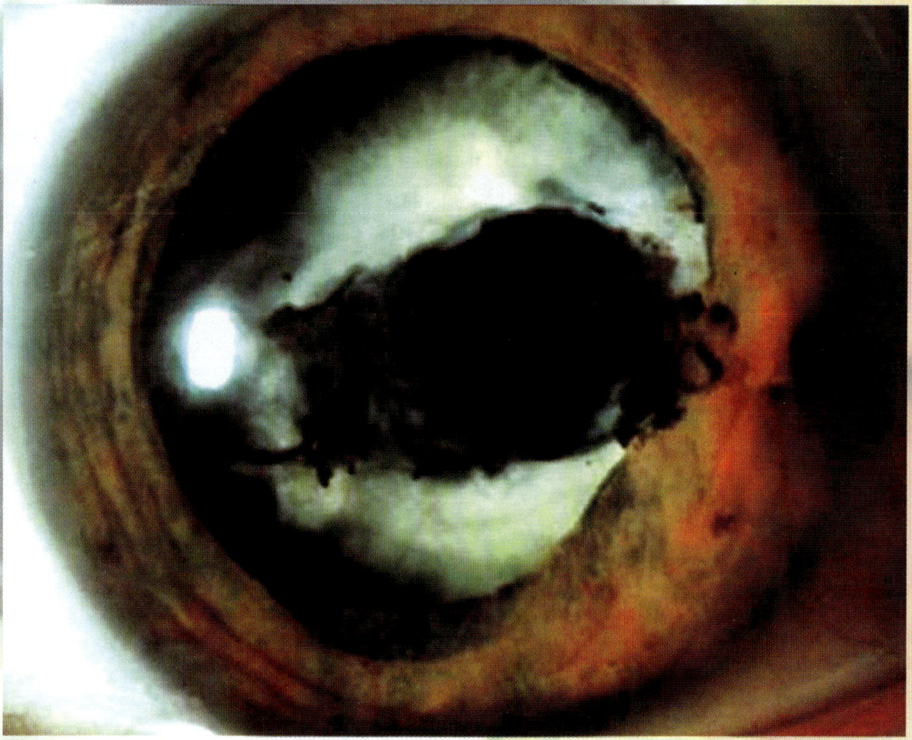

- Management of Anterior Segment Complications in SICS
- Posterior Segment Complications in SICS and Management
- Management of Astigmatism in SICS
- Complications and their Avoidance in Manual Small Incision Cataract Surgery
- Postsurgical Cystoid Macular Edema
- Favit—A New Method to Remove Dropped Nuclei
- Management of Nucleus Prolapse in Manual Small Incision Cataract Surgery
- Management of Dislocated Lens and Lens Fragments by Vitreoretinal Approach
- Management of Dislocated Implants by Vitreoretinal Approach
- Posterior Dislocation of Lens Material During Cataract Surgery
- Management of Postoperative Endophthalmitis
- Update on Posterior Capsule Opacification: Etiopathogenesis, Clinical Manifestations, Pharmacological and Surgical Prevention
- Update on Delayed Postoperative Opacification of Rigid and Foldable Intraocular Lenses

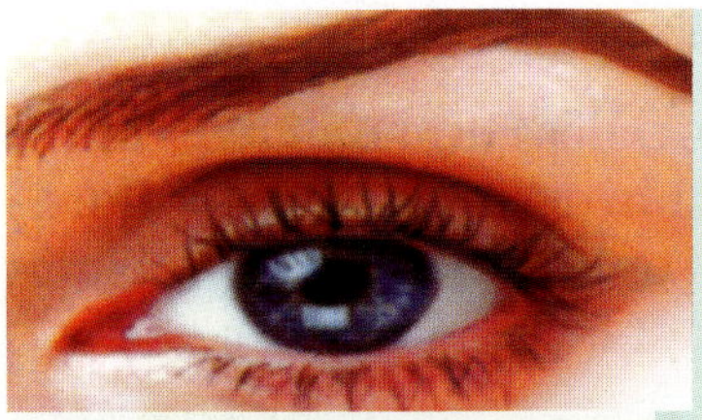

Forty two

Management of Anterior Segment Complications in SICS

Arif Adenwala
S Natarajan (India)

Complications are the important part of any surgery. Due to recent advances in cataract surgery the number of complication have reduced.

Thorough preoperative evaluation, immaculate operative technique and good postoperative care can minimize the rate of both intraoperative and postoperative complications.

Intraoperative complications: These include complications related to different steps of surgery.

ANESTHETIC COMPLICATIONS[7]

Anesthetic complications are mainly related to the type of anesthesia used. They are less common in topical and subtenon anesthesia and common in retrobulbar and peribulbar anesthesia.

The complications seen are:

a. *Retrobulbar hemorrhage:* This can be seen by both retrobulbar or peribulbar injection. It is recognized by:
   - Proptosis
   - Tensed eyeball, and
   - Difficulty in separating the eyelid

   Treatment: Immediate digital massage for 15-20 minutes. This allows the bleeding to stop. Then check the IOP digitally and then continue with the surgery. The intraocular pressure is also eased by lateral canthotomy. If IOP is not under control, then postpone the surgery and give antiglaucoma agents.

b. *Globe Perforation:* It is common complication seen during/with retrobulbar injections. Also occasionally optic nerve damage is also seen. To avoid this complication – peribulbar anesthesia with short needle is used. Early diagnosis of globe perforation is very important. It is diagnosed by sudden hypotomy.
   Treatment: It includes complete evaluation of eye to find the site of perforation. The site of perforation is accordingly sealed with cryotherapy. Evaluate the periphery to check the retinal status. If there is retinal break or detachment then treat accordingly.
c. *Subconjunctival hemorrhage:* This is commonly seen during or with peribulbar, subtenons anesthesia and retrobulbar injection. It is differentiated from retrobulbar hemorrhage by its fresh red color and normal intraocular pressure.
d. *Chemosis:* This is treated by making incision or conjunctiva and draining the fluid out of swelling.

WOUND RELATED COMPLICATIONS[5]

An adequate and properly constructed wound is important prerequisite for SICS (Fig. 42.1). The complication related to wound depends on:

1. Depth of incision.
2. Length of incision.
3. Width of incision
4. Shape of incision.

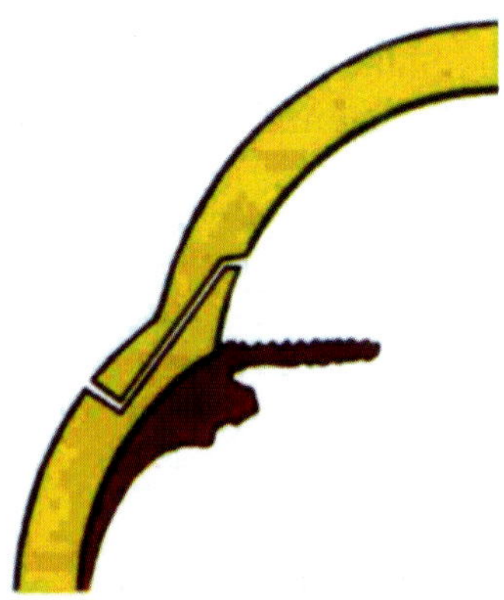

Fig. 42.1: Correct incision (*Courtesy :* Dr KPS Malik and Dr Ruchi Goel, New Delhi)

Depth of the Incision[5]

Depth refers to the thickness of the flap. External incision should be 0.3 mm deep or about one third–one half the thickness of the sclera. The problems associated with depth of incision may be:

Superficial Incision

If the incision is superficial – then it leads to buttonholing of anterior wall of tunnel. This buttonholing may also result from improper direction of blade or forward dissection (Fig. 42.2).

Management

a. Proper placement of crescent knife – angle the crescent knife downwards to increase the dissection of sclera.
b. Abandon the present tunnel and reenter at a deeper plane from another site of internal incision.

Button holing can also be prevented by making scleral pockets at medial and lateral end of tunnel and then joining both the pockets.

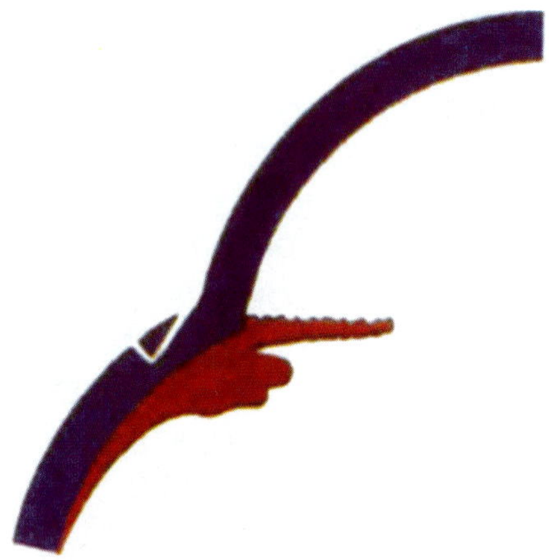

Fig. 42.2: Shallow incision leading to buttonholing of roof of the tunnel (*Courtesy :* Dr KPS Malik and Dr Ruchi Goel, New Delhi)

Deep incision: Deep tunnel wound leads to:

A. *Premature entry onto AC[5]:* This would lead to prolapse of iris tissue out of the wound (Fig. 42.3).
   Management: Reposit the iris tissue back into AC. Inject viscoelastic both in front and behind the nucleus to keep iris back. Place lens glide or iris

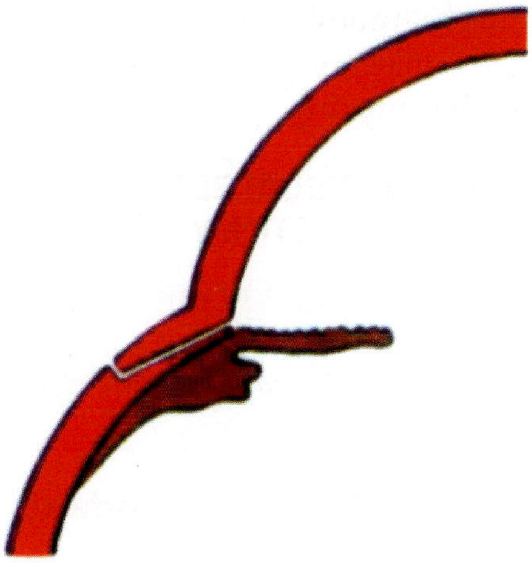

Fig. 42.3: Premature entry
(*Courtesy:* Dr KPS Malik and Dr Ruchi Goel, New Delhi)

repositor behind the nucleus and try to deliver the nucleus. Wire vectis can also be used. Since it is wider, pushes back the iris more firmly. But if prolapse is large one should suture the wound and abandon the site and make new entry at another place.

B. *Scleral disinsertion:* The floor of the tunnel is formed by posterior half of the sclera. Deep incision would cut through the floor of tunnel – thus resulting in disinsertion of inferior sclera. This may lead to large shift of wound downwards and flattening of vertical meridian of cornea. This will cause large against the rule astigmatism, which would continue to increase postoperatively (Fig. 42.4).
Management: The tunnel is sutured with radial bites so that the two edges of floor are connected or joined.

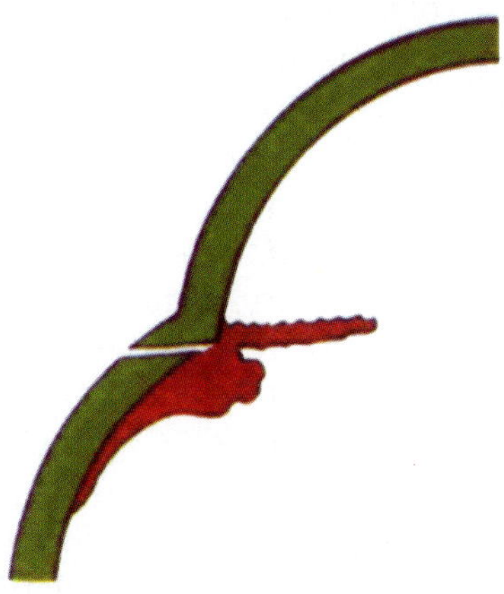

Fig. 42.4: Deep incision leading to scleral disinsertion
(*Courtesy:* Dr KPS Malik and Dr Ruchi Goel, New Delhi)

C. *Detachment of Descemets's membrane*[5]*:* The descement's membrane may be injured or detached either while making entry into AC with keratome or while entering the AC with rough edge cannula.
Management: Descemet's membrane must be uncurled and kept in this position so that corneal stoma is protected from aqueous. Inject viscoelastic/air into anterior chamber. This has tamponade effect on Descemet's membrane. The detached part settles down fast if placed under pressure for few hours.

The other option is Descemetopexy[11], a surgical technique of reattachment of stripped Descemet's membrane.

Reopening of the central portion[12] of the wound and unrolling the Descemet's membrane with iris repositor.

Suturing of Descemet membrane if it is seen in the incisional area.

1. *Width of wound*[5]*:* The distance between external incision and internal entry into the AC is the width of the incision. For production of astigmatic neutral incision, the external incision should be as far as posterior as possible.
The main complications seen are increase incidence of bleeding.
Management: Proper cauterization of episcleral vessels before starting with the incision is very important. If the width is small, then valvular effect of wound is reduced and the section is no longer self-sealing. There is also increase incidence of iris prolapse.
Treatment: Close the incision with suture and make incision at longer distance than previous one.
2. *Length of the incision*[5]*:* It is very important part of the incision. If the incision is smaller than the size of nucleus then there is difficulty in removal of the nucleus. This may lead to further complications of damage to corneal endothelium, corneal edema and uveitis. If the length is large then there is increase in postoperative astigmatism. There is also increase incidence of postoperative shallow AC, wound gaping and iris prolapse.

Thus, the length of the incision should be around 5-6 mm. If cataract is very hard you can increase the length to 7 mm or use any of the method of nuclear delivery in which we divide the nucleus into smaller pieces.

Iris prolapse: This is one of the important complications seen in SICS. This may be due to: -

a. *Improperly structured wound:* due to increase in size, incision very close to the limbus and deep incision.
b. Increase positive pressure in the eye.

Management: The main principles followed are:

a. Ensure that the eyeball is soft before the surgery. This can be done by applying digital pressure after the peribulbar block.
   Use of thin wire speculum is important in ensuring minimal external pressure.
   If superior rectus is taken then it should be released to reduce the pressure.
b. The wound should be properly constructed with adequate size.
   If length is more then proper suturing should be done to reduce the length of the wound. A small iridectomy may also help in reducing iris prolapse. Iris repositor is used to reposition the iris. Viscoelastic can also be used. Lens glide or wire vectis – may be used for delivery of nucleus in presence of iris prolapse.

3. *Side port entry:* Side port is created by lance tip MVR blade (19G/20G). This opening is used mainly for:
   a. Anterior capsulotomy
   b. Cortex aspiration
   c. Injection of visco/air into AC.

Complications related to it are:

a. Bleeding if made in vascular area.
b. If opening is large–it may lead to increase leaking and shallow AC
c. Descemet's detachment.
d. Injury to the iris.
e. Injury to the lens.

There can be prevented by using sharp instruments–inserting at avascular area. The direction should be towards center of area.

If the incision is large, it can be sutured with 10/0 nylon suture. Hydration of side ports should always be done to prevent any leak through side ports.

Descemet's membrane detachment can be managed by injection of air bubble in anterior chamber or by suturing.

COMPLICATIONS RELATEDTO ANTERIOR CAPSULOTOMY

There are two basic types of capsulotomy used for cataract surgery.

- Continuous curvilinear capsulorhexis.
- Can opener capsulotomy.

Continuous Curvilinear Capsulorhexis[5]

The commonest type of capsulotomy done in SICS is continuous curvilinear capsulotomy (CCC). The ideal size of CCC should be about 0.25 mm less than that of optics of IOL. The complication related to the rhexis depends on its size, shape and position.

- *Small rhexis:* A small rigid rhexis can result in: -
  1. Increase in zonular stress while prolapsing the nucleus into the anterior chambers. This can lead to zonular dehiscence and avulsion of bag into AC.
  2. Increase incidence of PC tears and nuclear drop during hydroprocedure because of capsular blockage syndrome.

Management: Enlargement of small sized rhexis by continuation of the spiral tears.

If the CCC is small then it is converted to can opened capsulotomy by giving 1-2 relaxing cuts at rhexis margins. The cuts should not be extended away from the equator. After nucleus delivery, second rhexis can be done in order to insert the IOLs in the bags. They can be done by taking small nick with 26 no. needle and then CCC is completed with utrata forceps for 26 no. needle. Dyes such as tryptan blue are used for better visualization of the capsule.

- *Large rhexis*[7]*:* If CCC is large then it may result in premature delivery of nucleus into the AC. It may also cause difficulties in placing the IOL in the bag.
- *Peripheral extension of CCC:* The CCC may extend into the periphery towards the equator or posterior capsule. The most common complication associated is advertent perpendicular capsule tear extending to the peripheral zonules underneath the iris. This is more common when the

anterior chamber is shallow mainly when there is positive pressure on the globe.

Management:

a. The capsulorhexis is stopped when the tear develop a peripheral heading.
b. Refill the anterior chamber with viscoelastic.
c. The direction of vector force at the edge of capsular flap is changed to resume the circular tear. The following measures can be taken:
  - Cut the outgoing flap of the capsule and then proceed with rhexis on the remaining capsular area.
  - Use of utrata/capsular forceps to bring the capsular extension inside in path of rhexis.
  - Initiate the rhexis at starting point and more in opposite directions.
  - Another option is to convert the rhexis into can opener capsulotomy with multiple perforations.
  — *Eccentric rhexis:* There is chance of IOL decentration at later stage. This is prevented by making continuous circular rhexis and in the bag lens implantation.

- *Can opener Capsulotomy:* It is a technique of capsulotomy in which you make multiple perforations in anterior capsule. The most common complication associated with the procedure is creation of unequal capsular flaps. The flaps may be aspirated into the irrigation aspiration cannula. This can cause an inadvertent capsular tear towards the zonlues.

If left unrecognized it could lead to large posterior capsular rent or some times nuclear bag may be aspirated.

Management

a. Multiple fine punctures should be created, thus eliminating large capsular flaps.
b. Continuous curvilinear rhexis should be done thus avoiding the creation of capsular tag.
c. Use of trypan blue helps in visualization of anterior capsular flaps.

COMPLICATIONS DURING HYDROPROCEDURES[5]

Hydroprocedures are techniques, which are used to free the nucleus and epinucleus from the capsular bag so that nucleus could move or rotate freely in the bag. It also helps in reducing the size of nucleus, so that it could be delivered easily through the small incision. Minimum amount of fluid should be used for the procedure.

Complications

If large amount of irrigating fluid is injected vigorously there it can lead to peripheral extension of small radial tears and zonule ruptures, thus leading to rupture of posterior capsules that will lead to vitreous loss and posterior dislocation of lens.

There is high incidence of these complications in case of hard nuclear cataract in which there is minimal cortical matter and the posterior capsule in thin. In case of posterior polar cataract, hydrodissection is avoided and only hydrodelineation is done. This prevents the posterior capsular tear.

Management The following steps should be taken to prevent the complication:

a. Inject small amount of fluid beneath the capsule. About 0.1-0.2 ml is sufficient.
b. Inject the fluid by just lifting the anterior capsule. We could see fluid wave coming out of the wound if you are in proper plane.

After injecting the fluid one should tap the anterior surface of the nucleus to release the fluid out of the bag. If this is not done, then it will cause more pressure on the posterior capsule leading to rupture. One should perform hydrodissection first and then hydrodelineation so that cortical matter does not hamper the visualization. Do not inject more fluid in case of hard nucleus cataract. All there procedures can prevent the complication related to hydroprocedures.

COMPLICATIONS DURING NUCLEUS DELIVERY

All the methods of SICS except few require the delivery of nucleus into the anterior chamber. This is one of the important steps of small incision cataract surgery. The inability to prolapse the nucleus may be due to following reason:

Small CCC

The size of the rhexis should be adequate to deliver the nucleus out of the bag. In case of hard cataract one should make larger rhexis. Smaller rhexis can be managed by making another rhexis that should be of larger size. One can also give extension cuts at 2-3 sites, which help in reducing the tension on capsular bag and helps in delivery of nucleus into the anterior chamber.

Incomplete Rotation of Nucleus in the Bag

This is usually due to improper hydrodissection. This can be managed by repeating hydrodissection in a correct plane.

Small Pupil or Miosis

Miotic pupil not dilating with mydriatic may be due to presence of posterior synechiae. The synechiae makes the delivery of nucleus difficult, if one tries to rotate the nucleus – it can lead to increase in zonular stress leading to zonular dehiscence or lens displacement. It can also lead to damage of iris sphincter and bleeding.

Prevention

This can be prevented by breaking the posterior synechiae. Inject the viscoelastic into the[8] AC and pass the synechiatome under the iris to break the synechiae. One can also pass the iris repositor to separate posterior surface of iris and anterior capsule. Pupils can also be enlarged by using iris hooks. Stretching of pupil cause microsphinctrotomy which help in enlargement of pupil. Vannas scissor can also be used to make sphincterotomy by taking small nicks so that shape of pupil is maintained. These patients usually do not dilate with adrenaline injections. Pupils can become smaller during the surgery also. This is usually seen with increase iris handling or when the surgical time required is more. This can be managed by:

a. Use of adrenaline either in the irrigating fluid or directly into anterior chamber. It has to be diluted before giving intracamerally.
b. High molecular weight viscoelastic can also be used to dilate the small pupil.
c. Avoid damage to iris during AC maneuvers.
d. If pupil is not dilating then sphincterotomy or radial iris cuts can be made.

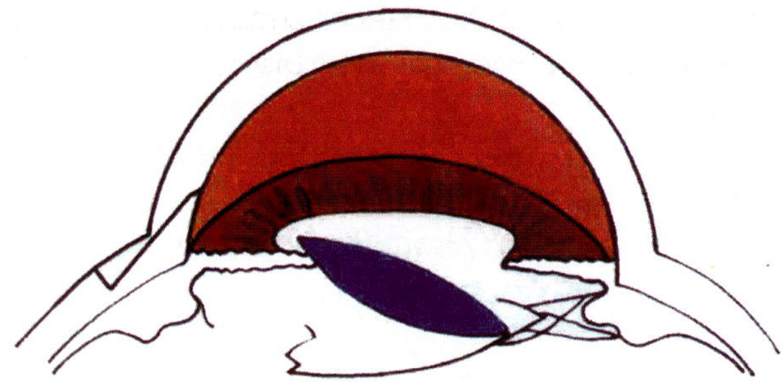

Fig. 42.5: Dehiscence of superior zonules of lens (*Courtesy:* Dr KPS Malik and Dr Ruchi Goel, New Delhi)

Zonular Dehiscence[5]

It is one of important complication seen while delivering the nucleus into the anterior chamber. Dehiscence usually occurs as result of increase stress on zonules when nucleus is rotated out of the bag. This is commonly seen in cases of hard nuclear cataract, in cases of small pupil, improper technique of rotation of the nucleus and in cases of small rhexis. This is commonly seen in beginners who start learning the basic steps of the surgery. Increase application of pressure while rotating over the nucleus forcibly can lead to zonular dialysis or delivery of whole nuclear bag (Fig. 42.5).

Management In case of small rhexis opening, try to make second larger rhexis or take relaxing cuts at 2-3 places. Then after injecting viscoelastic try to deliver the nucleus out of the bag. While rotating nucleus with Sinskey hook pressure should not be applied posteriorly but it should be more anteriorly in the clockwise or anticlockwise direction. This would decrease zonular stress, thus preventing zonular dehiscence and dislocation of nucleus.

Detection of zonular dehiscence: Nucleus is freely rotating in the bag but does not prolapse into the anterior chamber. It shifts towards the left side or downward. This may be associated with vitreous loss. The management depends on vitreous loss in AC.

A. If there is no vitreous loss / no vitreous in AC First see the size of rhexis. If size is small then give relaxation cuts or convert into can opener (multiple perforation) capsulotomy. Check the size of tunnel. Inject viscoelastic above the nucleus. Try to rotate the nucleus and delivery it into anterior chamber without increasing the area of zonular dehiscence.

Now deliver the nucleus out of the wound. Aspiration of cortex should be done with little irrigation, as increase flow of irrigation can increase the area of zonular dehiscence. There should be minimal manipulation while inserting the IOL.

B. If there is vitreous in AC In this case complete automated vitrectomy is done. Then nucleus delivery and IOL implantation is proceeded. Special precaution should be taken so that there is no increase in vitreous loss.

C. If the amount of zonular dehiscence is large In this case any attempt for nuclear rotation and delivery into the anterior chamber can lead to total dislocation of nucleus into the vitreous.

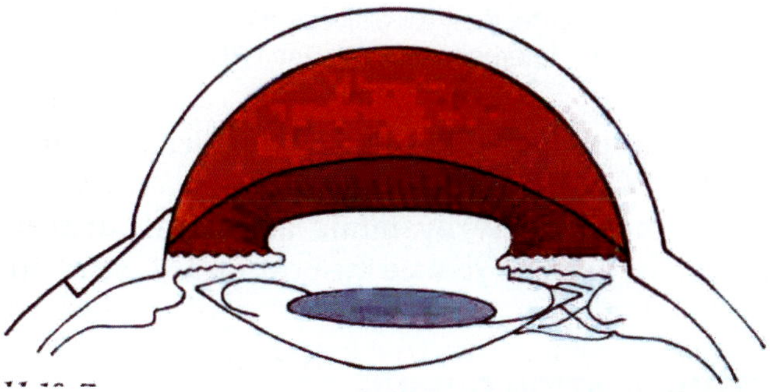

Fig. 42.6: Management of Zonular Dehiscence (Capsular Bag stretched by IOL Haptics) (*Courtesy:* Dr KPS Malik and Dr Ruchi Goel, New Delhi)

Treatment

Initial step is to increase the size of tunnel. Take relaxation cuts on rhexis or convert it into can opener capsulotomy. Deliver the nucleus out of wound with the help of plain wire vectis. Cortical aspiration is done under minimal or dry aspiration. IOL is implanted into the sulcus away from area of zonular dehiscence (Fig. 42.6).

The other option is to convert into manual or conventional extracapsular cataract extraction. Either end of the tunnel is cut down radially to limbus and then limbal section enlarged by corneal scissors.

Damage to Corneal Endothelium[6]

This is one important complication seen during nucleus delivery. Endothelial touch or damage to endothelium is more common in case of hard nuclear cataract. If while rotating the hard cataract into anterior chamber in presence of small tunnel there is increase chance of endothelial damage. Endothelial touch is also common when instruments are inserted through the scleral tunnel.

Management Damage to the endothelium is prevented by using large amount of viscoelastics. It should be inserted above the nucleus so that nucleus does not touch the corneal endothelium. The size of incision should also be large enough so that there is enough space for maneuvering of the instruments. If preoperative evaluation show early decompensation or corneal guttata then high viscosity agent is used so that if stays inside the AC and gives adequate support / cushion like effect to the endothelium.

Dropped Nucleus

This is one of an important complication of cataract surgery (Fig. 42.7). It is commonly seen in Phacoemulsification. The common predisposing factors are:

a. Hard nuclear cataract
b. Small pupil
c. Pseudoexfoliation due to weak zonules
d. Beginners who have started doing phacoemulsification.

Dropping the part or whole nucleus in vitreous cavity is feared complication of phacoemulsification.

Protocol that should be followed in management of retained nuclear fragment.

a. Initial observation – in cases of small retained nuclear fragment and / or mild inflammation.
b. Continuous local steroid eyedrops.
c. *Vitrectomy is indicated:* If size of fragment is more than 25 percent of actual size of nuclear. If inflammation is not controlled
d. We can delay vitrectomy so that corneal edema reduces and ocular inflammation reduces.
e. Perform adequate core vitrectomy and then proceed for phaco fragmentation.
f. Implant secondary IOL if not done before.
g. Examine the periphery to look for retinal breaks or retinal detachment.

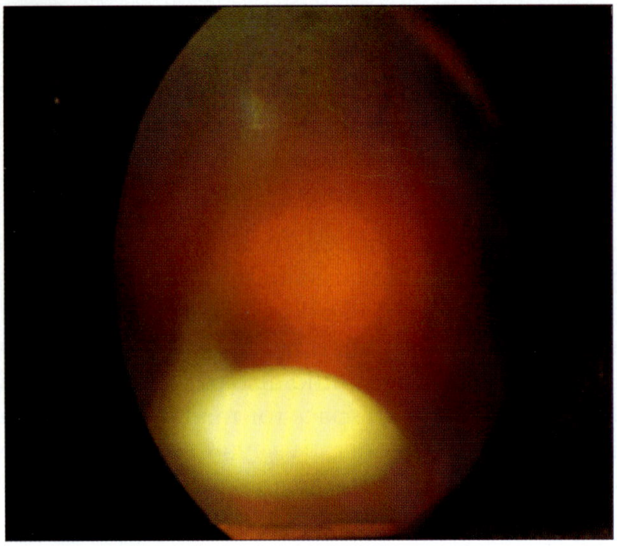

Fig. 42.7: Dropped nucleus

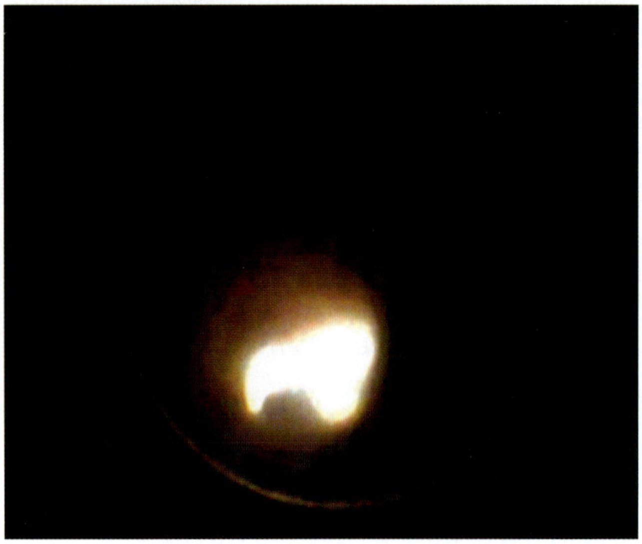

Fig. 42.8: Vitrectomy for dislocated nucleus + VH + laterogenic GRT + Total RD

Management Initial steps depend on grade of the nuclear and size of dropped nuclear fragment. In manual SICS–usually the whole nucleus drops into the vitreous cavity. A proper and complete automated vitrectomy is very important. Any lens material and vitreous in anterior chamber should also be removed. A 3 part pars plana approach is used (Fig. 42.8).

If the nucleus is soft then the fragment can be brought to the center of vitreous cavity and eaten up with vitreous cutter.

But if the Nucleus is hard then, use perfluorocarbon liquid to float the nucleus and then by using fragmatome – break the nucleus into small pieces and then remove the actual fragmentation of the nucleus should be performed in the midvitreous cavity and not on or near the retinal surface.

If there is coexisting RD also then encircling scleral buckle is recommended. After nuclear is removed then endolaser is applied around retinal breaks. Then silicone oil may be injected for tamponading effect.

If nucleus is present in anterior vitreous, we can bring the nucleus in the anterior chamber and deliver it through cataract section.

After removal of dropped nucleus, one should evaluate the status of retina. The next step is implantation of IOL. The variety of IOL to be implanted depends on integrity of posterior capsule. The *IOL* may be implanted in the bag in the sulcus or scleral fixated PCIOL or ACIOL may be used.

Postoperatively systemic and local steroids should be given to reduce the postoperative inflammation that may occur.

COMPLICATION DURING CORTICAL ASPIRATION

The main complications seen are:

a. Retained lens matter.
b. Posterior capsular tears or rupture.

Retained Lens Matter[19]

Lens matter such as anterior capsule, cortical matter or nuclear fragments may be left behind in eye. Nuclear or cortical fragments of about 25 percent usually tend to absorb spontaneously without any sequelae or complications. But large amount of cortical lens matter can result in –

a. Uveitis.
b. Corneal edema.
c. Secondary glaucoma.
d. Cystoid macular edema
e. Posterior capsular opacification
f. Retinal detachment

Residual lens matter is usually left behind in following cases:

a. Small pupil.
b. Posterior capsular tears with or without vitreous in AC
c. Small rhexis.
d. Subincisional cortex.

Management In cases of small pupil, inject adrenaline into irrigation fluid or in the anterior chamber. Lens fragments in anterior chamber should be removed preserving as much capsular bag as possible. If vitreous is seen in anterior chamber first do automated vitrectomy. This would prevent traction on the vitreous. Then corneal matter is removed with dry irrigation. Try to removal the entire cortical fragment without increasing the capsular tear. The central visual pupillary area should be clear of cortical matter.

If capsular tear is small then lens is implanted in the bag over the tear and if tear is large then lens is implanted in the sulcus or scleral fixating lens is used. Large size optics lens is used for in the bag implantation.

If the tear is large and the large cortical fragments cannot be removed then whole capsular bag is removed and anterior chamber lens or scleral fixated lens are used.

In case of small rhexis and small pupil if we try to aspirate blindly there is high chance of posterior capsular tear. The cortical matter left behind can be removed by phenomenon of water jetting in which irrigating saline is flushed. It is better to leave piece of cortical matter that is not in pupillary area rather than increase the chance of posterior capsular tear.

Adequate hydroprocedures also loosens the cortical matter and these small bits of residual cortex can get absorbed within 3-4 weeks if left behind.

In presence of posterior capsular tear, cortical matter away from area of rent is aspirated first so that the size of tear is not increased.

Posterior Capsular Rupture

Posterior capsule is very important as it provides support for posterior chamber IOL implantation. The commonest step in which posterior capsular tear occur is during cortical matter aspiration.

The other stages being :
a. Hydroprocedures
b. Delivery of nucleus.
c. IOL implantation.

Posterior capsular tear may occur as:
a. Posterior tear without vitreous loss[7], i.e. with intact hyaloid face.
b. Posterior tear with vitreous loss
c. Large tear with vitreous in anterior chamber.
d. Loss of Capsular bag

Prevention

Extra precautions are taken in cases in which posterior capsular tear is suspected or cases in which posterior capsule are thin.

In case of posterior polar cataract, hydrodissection is not carried out by hydrodelineation is done.

Another important aspect is that minimal quantity of fluid is used for hydrodissection thus decreasing the pressure in the bag.

Management

If posterior capsular tear occur during cortical removal Initial step is to do a good automated vitrectomy is done. Then cortex is aspirated with dry irrigation. Try to aspirate the cortex away form the capsular tear site. Also try to remove the cortex under the cover of viscoelastics.

Inject high molecular viscoelastic. Implant the lens in bag or in the sulcus depending on size of tear. Scleral fixating lens may also be used.

Site of IOL implantation in presence of capsular tear This is very important step in case of PC tear. One should always try to implant posterior chamber lens in almost all cases. The site of implantation will depend on:
a. size of PC tear
b. size of capsule.

If the size of PC tear is small then one should implant PC IOL over the PC rent, i.e. in the bag. After implantation confirm that IOL is well placed in situ. This is done by tap test. This is done by tapping the IOL in the center and then to see for the stability of the lens. If IOL is in situ after tapping it remains stable. But if tear is not well placed after tapping it shifts its position and starts telling

If the size of PC tear is large then assess the size of rhexis. Inject viscoelastic over the out capsule. Insert IOL over the CCC in the sulcus one should see that IOL does not increase the size of PC tear and is not placed in the bag.

If the size of tear is large and the rhexis size is not sufficient – then the other alternative is of scleral fixative lens.

Anterior chamber lens can also be used. But before implanting one should remove the nuclear bag completely. We should not forget to do peripheral iridectomy, as secondary angle closure glaucoma is common after anterior chamber lens implantation.

Position of PCIOL on case of posterior capsular tears If posterior chamber lens is implanted in the bag then direction of is very important. The position of the haptic should be such that it should not

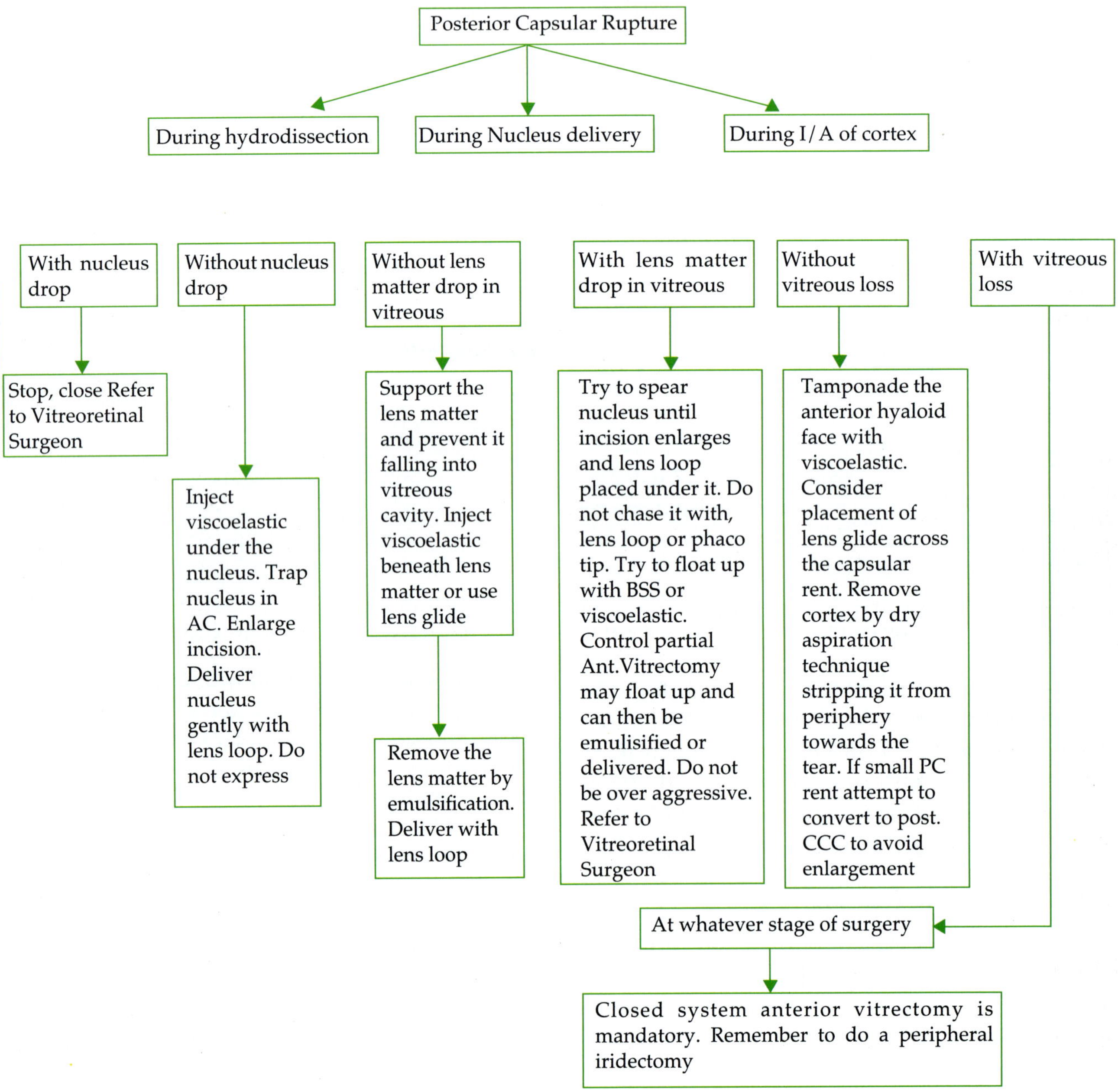

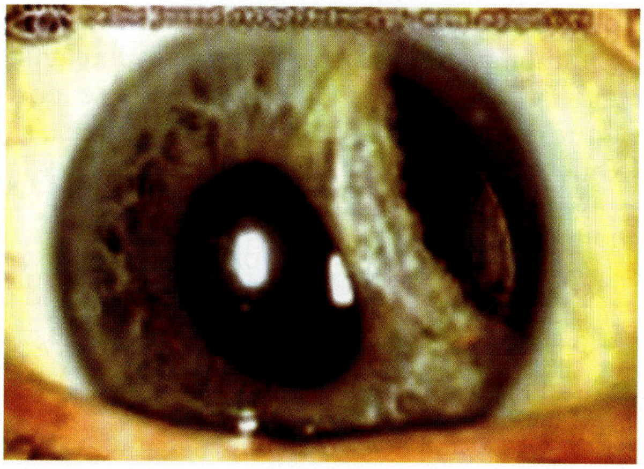

Fig. 42.9: Postoperative iridodialysis (*Courtesy:* Online Journal of Ophthalmology–Author: Carsten Meyer, M.D., Marburg, Germany)

increase the size of capsular tear. The Lens implantation can be done at some setting or one can also go for lens implantation after 6-8 weeks after the inflammation of the eye subsides. If it is done at the same sitting will lead to increase postoperative inflammation.

Management of Posterior Capsular Rupture

Iridodialysis

This is another common intraoperative complication seen after manual small incision surgery. When deep scleral tunnel is made, the chance of iris getting damaged at 12 o'clock position is common. Iridodialysis can also occur while removing the nucleus with the plain wire vectus. The site of dialysis is usually is 6 o'clock position (Fig. 42.9).

Prevention Iridodialysis can be prevented by proper wound construction. When the wire vectus is insinuated under the nucleus, the iris at 6 o'clock should not be caught in vectus, otherwise it will lead to iridodialysis.

Treatment In cases of small iridodialysis no treatment is required. But in cases of large iridodialysis suturing with 10/0 prolene is done.

SHALLOW ANTERIOR CHAMBER

This is another common complication, which is seen intraoperatively. It can occur at any stage of the operation and is associated with increase in intraocular pressure and subsequent iris prolapse.

High intraocular pressure is seen in Malignant glaucoma.

Low intraocular pressure is seen in wound leak and in Choroidal detachment.

The complication related to this may be more severe in open wound surgery like cataract but it is less in closed chamber surgery like SICS / Phaco.

It can be due to:

- Tensed eyeball preoperatively due to improper digital massage.
- Tight superior rectus sutures.
- Stout wire speculum
- Squeezing of eyes by uncooperative patient. This is commonly seen in topical anesthesia.
- Suprachoroidal hemorrhage.

Always check the intraocular pressure before starting the surgery. This will prevent many intraoperative and postoperative complication.

Management Release the superior rectus sutures and remove wire speculum. Iris reposition is done or one can do iridectomy. Inject viscoelastics to increase the depth of anterior chamber.

If the anterior chamber is shallow then give IV Mannitol and then wait for 10-15 minutes and then proceed with the surgery. Do not proceed the surgery with shallow chamber as posterior capsule is pushed forwards and this will increase incidence of capsular tears. In case of cortical wash first clear the central pupillary area free of cortex and then implant the lens. After implantation one can proceed with peripheral cortical removal.

COMPLICATIONS RELATEDTO INTRAOCULAR LENS[4]

The commonest lens used in cataract surgery nowadays is the Posterior Chamber IOL. The posterior chamber lens may be implanted at three sited mainly

- In the Bag,
- In the Sulcus, and
- Scleral fixated lens.

The complications related to its positioning are:

Pupillary Capture

This complication occurs when part of IOL or whole optic moves anterior to iris surface to get entrapped in the pupil. This is commonly seen.

a. When IOL is implanted in sulcus
b. In presence of PC tear with vitreous loss.

It is associated with secondary postoperative uveitis and pigment dispersion. Lenses with angulated loops reduce the incidence of pupillary capture.

Treatment

- Initial treatment includes pupillary dilatation. This causes the part of IOL or optic to move backwards.
- Pupil is then constricted after IOL is well placed in the bag.
- Redialing of IOL may also be required.
- Laser Iridotomy may be done to prevent late complications of pupillary capture like pupillary glaucoma.

Decentred IOL

This includes the following syndromes:

a. Sunrise syndrome
b. Sunset syndrome
c. East-West syndrome

The variety of syndrome will depend on position at which IOL is subluxated.

This decentration occurs mainly:

a. When one haptic is in bag and other is in sulcus.
b. When PCIOL is implanted in presence of PC tear with vitreous loss
c. Due to zonular dialysis or capsular fibrosis.

Treatment

- Initial treatment involves evaluation of degree of decentration of *IOL*.
- If the amount of aphakic part is minimal then there is no need of any intervention. (The lens covers visual areas).
- Also if the patient is asymptomatic then no treatment is required.

Surgical treatment

1. Redialing of IOL to its proper position. Care should be taken that the IOL does not get dislocated posteriorly. This complication is common in case of large posterior capsular tear.
2. If patient complains of diplopia due to exposed aphakic part then–iridoplasty is done. This causes closure of aphakic part thus visual axis is covered by the lens only.
3. If there is large subluxation then IOL is removed and replaced/exchanged with scleral fixated IOL or Anterior Chamber IOL is implanted.

Windshield Wiper Syndrome

It is complication in which the IOL moves from side to side with head movement. This usually occurs when the diameter of implant is too small for the eye. It is seen mainly in (a) myopic eyes or (b) when the loops are placed in the sulcus and (c) When there is failure of adhesion of superior loop to posterior capsule.

Treatment Fixating the loop of lens with McCannel suture. This prevents the movement of IOL.

Posterior Dislocation of IOL

This complication is mainly seen intraoperatively or immediate or early postoperatively. But in some cases it can occur in later period also.

Posterior Iris Shafing Syndrome

These are associated with Shafing of the posterior surface of iris by sulcus-fixated lens. It is rubbing of the iris surface with lens loop. It is referred as white out syndromes.

Erosion and Perforation of Ciliary Body

This is also seen in scleral fixated lens.

UGH Syndrome

This complication of Uveitis Glaucoma and Hyphaema syndrome is seen in cases of anterior chamber lens.

POSTOPERATIVE COMPLICATIONS[6]

Manual small incision cataract surgery has minimized the rate of postoperative complication, which was seen before in conventional Extra Capsular Cataract Extraction.

It can be divided into:

Early	Late
• Wound leak	Pseudophakic bullous keratopathy
• Striate keratopathy	Irregular pupil
• Corneal edema	Delayed postoperative uveitis
• Iritis	Decenterd IOL
• Hyphema	Pupillary capture
• Iris prolapse	Retinal detachment
• Decentered IOL	Endophthalmitis
• Raised IOP	Posterior dislocation of IOL
• Hypotony	Posterior capsular opacification.
• Choroidal detachment	Secondary glaucoma.
• Endophthalmitis.	
• Macular edema	

Wound Leak

It is common complication seen if there is no proper wound construction.

This can occur in following cases

- *Irregular dissection of the tunnel:* If scleral tunnel is split into layers then self sealing action is lost. It is mainly seen in case of blunt instruments and also when beginners start learning small incision surgery. It can be prevented by using sharp instruments for all the cases as far as possible. Intraocular button holing of the tunnel can also increase the incidence of postoperative wound leak.
  Treatment is suturing of the wound.
- *Size of wound is large:* The proper self sealing action of the wound to lost. In these cases wound leak is prevented by taking single suture after the surgery is over.
- *Side port entry*: The size of opening becomes more. This will increase the leakage of aqueous through the port and thus leading to wound leak. This can be prevented by using sharp blade with proper technique. It can be treated be taking single suture if leaking is seen postoperatively.
  Hydration of side port and main wound also ensures self sealing action of wound and reduce incidence of postoperative wound leak.
  Intraocular pressure of about 20 should be present at end of surgery for tight closure of scleral tunnel.

Shallow AC

Common cause of shallow AC

a. *Wound leak:* They may occur through the main wound usually and sometimes through side port. The management of wound leak has already been discussed above.
b. *Choroidal Detachment:* It is another important cause of shallow anterior chambers. It can lead to reduce intraocular pressure.

   Management Initial treatment includes pressure pad and bandage, which is given for 24 hrs. This can lead to formation of anterior chamber and then settling of choroids back into its normal site. Medical treatment—includes systemic steroids and local mydriatic eyedrops. Inspite of the above management the chamber remains shallow then surgical management is required. This includes drainage of suprachoroidal space. After drainage air bubble is kept into anterior chamber.

Iris Prolapse[2]

This is another important complication seen postoperatively (Fig. 42.10). This may be due to:

- Wound gaping- Secondary to improper wound construction of the wound and in cases of large size tunnel.
- Sudden increase in intraocular pressure in patients with chronic cough and bronchial ashthma.

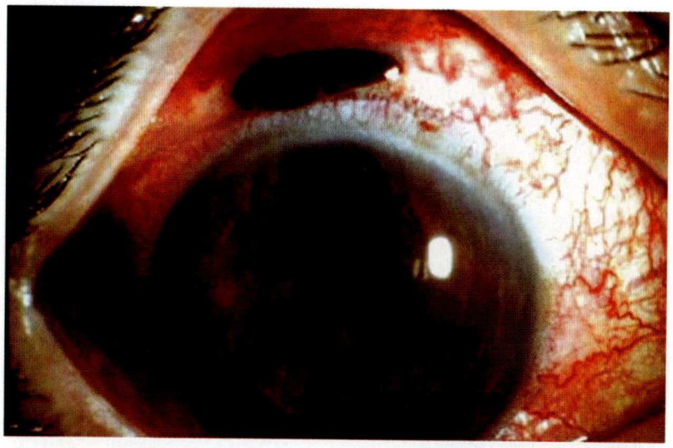

Fig. 42.10: Iris prolapse. (*Courtesy :* Online Journal of Ophthalmology - Author: Prof. J. Wollensak, Berlin, Germany)

- Postoperative blunt trauma.
  Early treatment is very important to prevent the complications such as endophthalmitis.

  Management Immediate iris prolapse is treated by iris reposition and formation of anterior chamber with viscoelastics and resuturing of scleral tunnel.

  a. If iris is epithelized then iris abscission is done.
  b. The scleral tunnel should be free of any uveal tissue. A single suture is taken to form the anterior chamber. Iris prolapse usually cause shift in position of the lens. The lens is dialed properly so that it is well placed.

Corneal Complications

This is one of most important vision threatening complication seen postoperatively. This includes:

a. *Striate keratopathy*: this is characterized by folds in decrement membrane (Fig. 42.11).
b. *Corneal edema:* Important cause – for corneal edema includes:

a. Preoperative corneal degeneration – which includes corneal guttata or from low endothelium count.
b. Hard nuclear cataract.
c. Endothelial touch with the instrument- this is usually seen in small tunnel and hard cataract
d. Diabetes
e. Increase in intraocular pressure

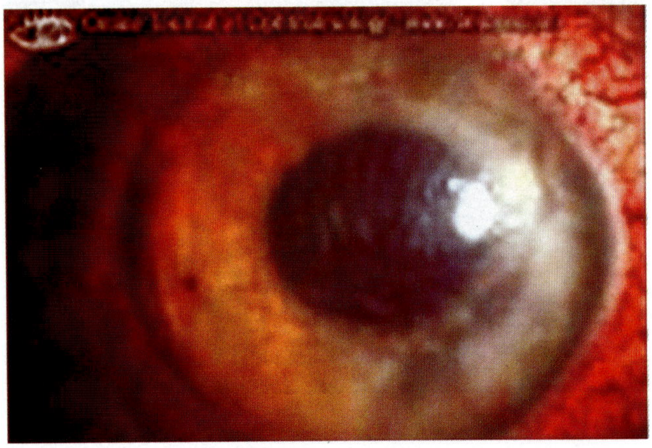

Fig. 42.11: Striate keratopahy

Management Corneal complication arising from endothelial damage can be prevented by using high molecular weight viscoelastics. The chamber should be always deep. Viscoelastics acts as support for the endothelium and prevents if from getting damage from hard cataract.

Immediate management includes:

- Frequent instillation of local steroids.
- Topical mydriatics
  Mild corned edema usually gets cleared with this management within 7-10 days. Initial one week of management is very important in treatment of corneal edema.
  In case of severe corneal edema-local instillation of 5 percent sodium chloride is very important. It is available in eyedrop and ointment forms. Corneal endothelial cells recover function and regain its clarity very soon. But these eyedrops should not be used for more than one month.
  Topical antiglaucoma agents can be instilled in order to reduce intraocular pressure, which may be increased in cases of severe corneal edema.
  Very severe corneal edema usually does not respond to this management. This will eventually lead to corneal decompensation. These patients usually require–Penetrating Keratoplasty.

Iritis

Inflammation of uveal tissue commonly occurs:

a. Secondary to increase handling. The handling of uveal tissue – seen in cases of hard cataracts, small rigid pupils, small tunnel and due to instrumental trauma.
a. Viscoelastics in AC can also cause iris reaction.
b. If cortical wash is incomplete.
c. In case of PC tear with vitreous loss if not managed properly.

Prevention

a. Decrease handling of uveal tissue
b. Wash away all viscoelastics from AC
c. Try to remove as much cortex as possible.
d. Do a good automated vitrectomy.

Management

a. *Local steroids:* Eyedrops like Prednisolone eyedrops or Hydrocortisone eyedrops are used.

These are instilled at a frequent interval initially. The frequency is gradually reduced as inflammation reduces.

b. *Local mydriatics:* Atropine or Atropine substitutes like Homatropine can be used. These drops cause breaking of posterior synechiae and gives rest to eyeball.
c. Systemic Steroids like Prednisolone 1 mg/kg can be used in cases of severe reactions.

Hyphema

Common source of blood in anterior chamber includes:

a. Bleeding from scleral tunnel
b. Trauma to iris
c. Expulsion hemorrhage

Improper cauterization of episcleral blood vessels can lead to blood clots in anterior chamber. These can be present intraoperatively also. If scleral tunnel is not self-sealing, blood can flow into the anterior chamber from the conjunctival vessels.

Intraoperative increase handling of iris or instrumental trauma of uveal tissue can lead to hyphema postoperatively.

Prevention

a. Proper cauterization of episcleral blood vessels
b. Good wound construction.
c. Decrease uveal tissue handling

Management The absorption of hyphema occurs through two routes. Main route is canal of Schlemm and other route is iris vessels.

a. Propped up position.
b. If IOP is high – start antiglaucoma agents which mainly include local β-blockers
c. Topical steroids and oral steroids–are also started
d. Cycloplegic eyedrops
e. Systemic Vitamin C

Hyphema may take 5-7 days to clear. But if there is severe hyphema then paracentesis with drainage of anterior chamber can be done Irrigation of the anterior chamber with BSS with or without fibrinolysin is performed.

Decentred IOL

The common condition in which decentration of IOLs are seen:

a. Implantation of IOL in presence of PC tear and vitreous loss due to large tear–IOL may slide downwards or sideward, leading to decentration.
b. In case of can opener capsulotomy – haptic of IOL may get entangled in capsular flap – leading to decentration of IOL
c. IOLs with small optics
d. Improper implantation of IOLs.
e. Implantation of lens in sulcus.

Prevention Proper implantation of lens in the bag is very important. In large PC tear in many cases scleral fixated lens are used. Proper dialing of IOL is also important. IOL tap test should always be done.

Management This will depend on:

a. Degree of decentration
b. Complaint of patient

If degree of decentration is minimal and without any complaints. No intervention is carried out. If there is obvious decentration – then redialing of IOLs should be done. In presence of PC tear and vitreous loss, lens implantation is a very important step and should be done with minimal handling. There are chances of IOL getting displaced into vitreous. One can also remove the IOL and replace it or fix the IOL transclerally. Try to construct the pupil and then examine the amount of aphakic part of pupil. If there is large aphakic area then intervention is required.

Distorted or Irregular Pupil

In many cases only pupillary dilatation can correct pupillary capturem i.e. cases in which optics get entangles in iris tissues. If vitreous gets incarcerated then Nd: YAG Laser can be used to cut the tractional bands or in case of thick fibrosis bands, Vitrectomy is done.

This change in shape of pupil is caused by:

a. Presence of posterior synechiae – formed due to iris handling.
b. Decentred IOL – leading to pupillary capture. This is seen mainly in case of large PC tear with vitreous loss.
c. Incarceration of vitreous in pupillary area–causes tractional forces leading to distortion of pupil.

Management Includes – treatment of associated iritis/iridocyclitis. Local and systemic steroids are given. Local mydriatics are very important to dilate the pupil.

Raised Intraocular Pressure/Secondary Glaucoma

Immediate rise in IOP postoperatively may due to

a. Presence of viscoelastic material.
b. Air bubble in anterior chamber.
c. Pupillary block glaucoma due to vitreous
d. Uveitis secondary to retained cortical matter
e. Suprachoroidal hemorrhage with shallow AC.
f. Malignant glaucoma.

Prevention

a. Complete cleaning of viscoelastic material from the anterior chamber.
b. Size of air bubble kept in AC should be small. After injecting air bubble in AC, always flush irrigating saline through side port behind the air bubble. This will reduce the size of bubble and will help in its absorption.

Treatment

a. Local/systemic steroids given to reduce the tissues reaction seen due to retained cortical matter.
b. If cortical matter is more, then AC wash is done to remove the cortical matter. If it is seen in vitreous then pars plana removal of cortical matter is done.
c. Vitreous incarceration will require surgical vitrectomy
d. Peripheral iridectomy and antiglaucoma medication may need to be started
e. Treatment of suprachoroidal hemorrhage includes drainage of suprachoroidal fluid.

Hypotony

Important causes leading to decrease in intraocular pressure are

a. Wound leak.
b. Choroidal detachment
c. Retinal detachment

Management of wound leak has already been covered and treatment of retinal and choroidal detachment is dealt in other Chapter.

Pseudophakic Bullous Keratopathy

It is one of the important cause of decrease visual acuity after SICS. Long standing corneal edema not responding to medical management can lead to Bullous keratopathy. This occurs secondary to endothelial damage or extensive descemet's detachment intraoperatively.

Treatment includes

a. Antiglaucoma agent to reduce the IOP
b. Local and systemic steroids.
c. 5 percent NaCl Eye ointment is also beneficial

These agents can be used for 2 to 3 months and the response is seen. Usually long standing Bullous keratopathy fails to respond to the therapy and these are the cases, which will respond best to penetrating Keratopathy.

Conjunctival Flap Retraction[6]

When large conjunctival flap is taken with excess of cauterization, the conjunctival flap fails to cover the scleral funnel properly. Use of excess of topical steroids also causes non-healing of conjunctival flap.

This complication can be prevented by avoiding excessive cauterization, use of adequate conjunctival flap and covering the tunnel by cauterization of conjunctiva with forceps. This helps in covering the scleral wound adequately.

Pupillary Capture of IOL[6]

Common causes of pupillary capture includes

a. Placement of IOL in sulcus.
b. Implantation of IOL in presence of large PC tear with vitreos loss
c. Presence of vitreous in AC can cause traction leading to pupillary capture.

Management Long standing pupillary capture can lead to adhesion between iris and lens. This adhesion may cause disturbance in stability of the lens leading to pupillary capture. Inject Viscoelastics and try to break the synechiae and release the adhesion. This can reduce the pupillary capture of IOL. If the patient is asymptomatic with good visual acuity then the pupillary capture is left behind. The incidence of uveal reaction is more after rehandling of the lens.

Posterior Capsular Opacification

This is most common cause of decrease visual acuity after cataract surgery. Commonest causes are:

a. In almost all paediatric cataract.
b. Patients in which cortical matter is left behind
c. Patients with large posterior capsular tear with vitreous loss some amount of retained cortical matter can cause capsular opacification.
d. High incidence in surgical aphakics (ECCE).

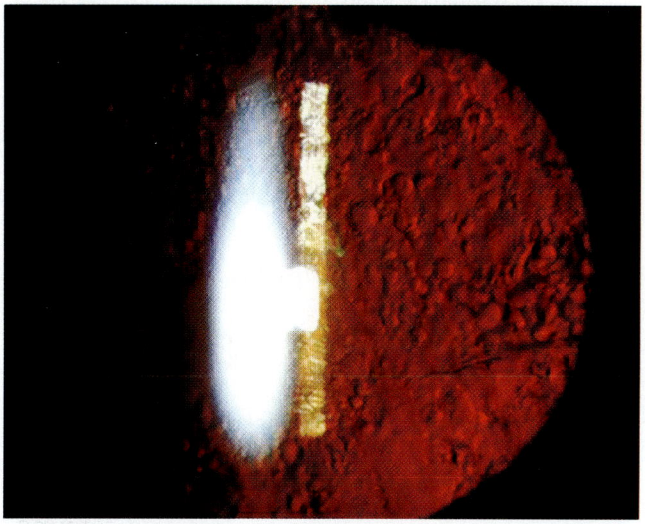

Fig. 42.12: Elschnigs Pearl
(*Courtesy:* Eye Atlas, the Online Atlas of Ophthalmology)

Management Includes mainly slit lamp examination to confirm the diagnosis and evaluate the thickness of PCO. In case of surgical aphakia the PCO is of fibrous variety (Fig. 42.12).

Treatment

A. *Nd: YAG Laser Capsulotomy:* It is many times OPD procedure. In this case capsulotomy is done with No. 26 needle. This treatment requires accurate focusing and use of minimum amount of energy to puncture the capsule. The wave length used is 532 μ. In Q Switched laser the power setting is between 1 and 2.5 mj/pulse and with mode locked laser it is between 3 and 5 mj/ pulse (Fig. 42.13).

Antiglaucoma agent is instilled prior to laser therapy to prevent rise in intraocular pressure. While performing YAG capsulotomy, it is important not to damage the *IOL*. An opening of 3 mm is usually sufficient to improve the visual acuity. The opening should be made in the visual axis.

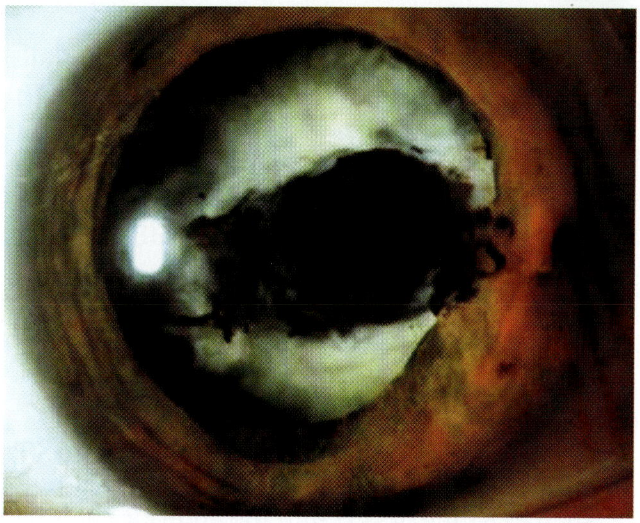

Fig. 42.13: Nd: YAG Laser Capsulotomy. (*Courtesy:* Online Journal of Ophthalmology - Author: Prof. J. Wollensak, Berlin, Germany)

A. *Surgical Capsulotomy* This is mainly indicated in cases of thick capsular opacification, which is not breaking with YAG Laser. It is also used for pediatric cases and in mentally retarded patients who have difficulty in focusing for laser treatment. This is done by using No. 26 needle or with the help of IOL dealer. In cases of thick fibrous PCO – vannas scissor can be used to cut the fibrous band.

Expulsive Hemorrhage[4]

It is one of the most dreaded complications of cataract surgery. The incidence in open chamber surgery is more than closed chamber operation, like Manual Small Incision Surgery and Phacoemulsification. The first report of expulsive hemorrhage associated with cataract surgery is attributed to de Wenzel who described it in 1786.

Types: Hemorrhage may be limited or massive (explusive).

Expulsive hemorrhage may occur:

a. On the table.
b. Postoperatively.

Prevention

a. Always check the intraocular pressure digitally before starting the surgery.
b. Avoid open chamber surgery.
c. Try to go for phacoemulsification or manual small incision surgery.
d. Check the blood pressure preoperatively.

Treatment

a. Immediately close the wound. This ensures no exit area for the contents to move. Take multiple sutures for firm closure of wound,
b. Immediate posterior sclerotomy to release the suprachoroidal blood. Forced injection of fluid such as saline or BSS into the anterior chamber helps in pushing the retina and choroids backward. This also promotes evacuation of sub choroidal haemorrhage.
c. After bleeding has stopped, reopen the wound and do good anterior vitrectomy. This is done to prevent the fibroplastic reaction caused due to disturbed vitreous and blood within the eye. Then the anterior chamber is formed and resuturing is done.

Pars plana vitrectomy is indicated in case of severe intraocular hemorrhage. Evaluation of peripheral retina is also important. If there is associated retinal detachment then it is managed accordingly.

Postoperative Management

Main aim is to reduce the inflammation. Corticosteroids are used. They are given both systemically and topically. Mydriatics are also given to give rest to eyeball. Systemic Nonsteroidal antiinflammatory agents are used to reduce the pain.

REFERENCES

1. Gholam A Payman, Donald R, Sanders, Morton F. Goldberg. The lens cataract and its management, principle and practice of ophthalmology 580-618.
2. Jack J. Kanski Disorders of the lens. Clinical Ophtalmology, 286-309.
3. Howard Fine, Mark Packer, Richard S. Hoffman. Small Incision Cataract Surgery 349-56.
4. Norman S. Jaffe, Mark S. Jaffe, Gary F. Jaffe. Cataract Surgery and its Complications
5. KPS Malik, Ruchi Goel. Intraoperative complications of SICS – Manual of Small Incision Cataract Surgery 77-85.
6. KPS Malik, Ruchi Goel. Postoperative complications of SICS, Manual of Small Incision Cataract Surgery. 89-96
7. KR Murthy. Phaco Surgery and Foldable IOLs. Complications during phacoemulsification. 11.1-11.2.
8. Colman R. Kraff and Manus C. Kraff. Cataract Surgery. Complications in Ophthalmic Surgery. 4.2-4.22.
9. Mary Abraham. Complications of Phacoemulsifications . Modern Ophthalmology.
10. Jaffe NS: Results of intraocular lens Implantation surgery. Third Binkhorst Medal Lecture. Am. J Ophthalm 1978;85;13-23.
11. Sparks GM: Descemetopexy; Surgical reattachment of stripped Descemet membrane. Arch Ophthalmology 1967;78:31-34.
12. Sugar HS. Prognosis in stripping of the Descemet's membrane in cataract extraction. Am Journal of Ophthalm 1967;63;140-43.
13. Christensen L: Postoperative Flat Chamber. In Symposium in Cataract. New Orleans Acad of Ophthalm. 1965 The CV Mosby Co.
14. Leipmann ME: Intermittent visual "White Out" a new intraocular lens implantation. Ophthalmology 1982;89: 109-112.
15. Apple DJ, Reidy JJ, Olson RJ et al. The Comparison of Ciliary Sulcus and capsular bag fixation of the IOL. J Am Intraocular Implant Society. 1985;11:44-63.
16. Bloom SM. Wyszynski RE. Brucker AJ. Scelral fixation suture for dislocated posterior chamber IOL. Ophthalmology 1990;21:851-54.
17. Girad Lj, mino N. Wesson M et al. Scleral fixation of Subluxated postchamber lens. Journal of cataract and Refractive Surgery 1998;14:326-27.
18. Clinical Practice in Opthalmology 230-33.

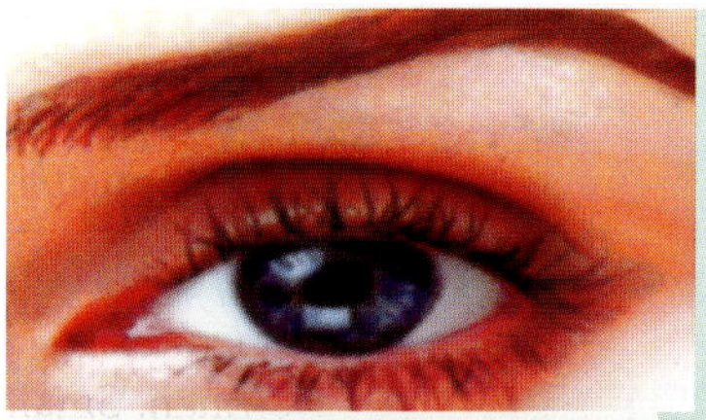

Forty three

Posterior Segment Complications in SICS and Management

S Natarajan
Arif Adenwala (India)

Cataract Surgery can lead to various posterior segment complications. The complications seen are:

1. Cystoid macular edema.
2. Vitreous hemorrhage.
3. Dislocated IOLs.
4. Suprachoroidal hemorrhage.
5. Endophthalmitis.
6. Retinal detachment.
7. Choroidal detachment.
8. Vitritis.

CYSTOID MACULAR EDEMA

It represents one of the most common cause of poor visual acuity after cataract surgery (Figs 43.1, 43.2A and 43.2B). The various theories put forward to explain the pathogenesis are:

a. *Vitreous traction on macula*: If there is posterior rupture with vitreous loss there is capsular traction caused on macula from the vitreous. In cataract extraction there is high incidence of vitreomacular traction syndrome leading to cystoid macular edema.
b. *Vitreous incarceration in wound*[20]: Vitreous gets incarcerated in case when complete vitrectomy is not done. The incidence is quite less nowadays due to use of automated vitrectomy.

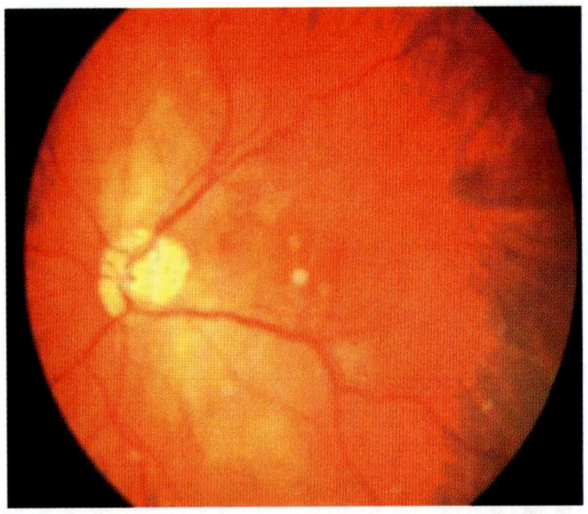

Fig. 43.1: Fundus photograph
CYSTOID MACULAR EDEMA

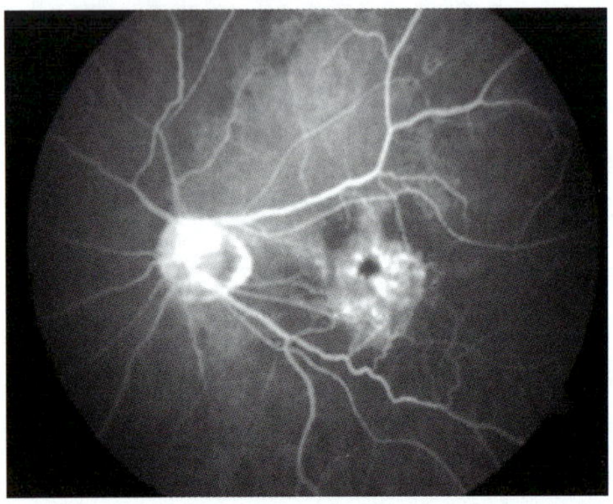

Fig. 43.2A: Fundus fluoroscien angiography
CYSTOID MACULAR EDEMA

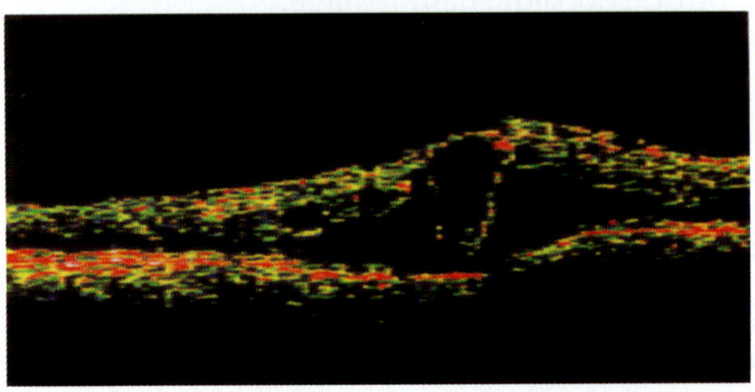

Fig. 43.2B: Optical coherence tomography
CYSTOID MACULAR EDEMA

c. *Secondary inflammation:* This can cause of breakdown of blood aqueous barriers and lead to formation of cystoid macular edema.
d. Inflammatory mediators like prostaglandin can also cause formation of cystoid macular edema.

Management

Main aim of management is to compare the visual acuity after decreasing the macular edema.

Treatment includes:
a. Medical
b. Surgical

MEDICAL

Therapeutic agents need for treatment of CME includes :
1. Corticosteroids preparations
2. Non-inflammatory agents steroidal anti
3. Carbon anhydrase inhibitor agents
1. *Corticosteroids:* Steroids decrease the release of arachidonic acid from the cell membrane thereby reduces the level of prostaglandin. This will help in treatment of cystoid macular edema. Various preparations available are:
   a. *Topical:* Prednisinone. Acetate eyedrops 1% Dexamethasone eyedrops
   b. *Peribulbar:* Triamcinolone 20 mg. This is injected in Subtenons space.
   c. *Oral/Systemic:* Predn. Tablets 1 mg/kg.

   The long-term improvement in CME is not well seen and so steroids are not a main line of management.
2. *Non-steroidal anti-inflammatory agents:* These drops block the cyclooxygenase enzyme and thus reduce the level of prostaglandins. These drugs are very useful in decreasing the macular edema.

Preparations available are:
1. *Systemic:* Indomethacin is the best drug available for the treatment of CME.[10] It is also available in sustained release form. Indomethacin 25 mg QID is given for 4-6 weeks to reduce the edema.
2. *Topical:* Flurbiprofen eyedrops (0.3%)
   Diclofenac eyedrops (0.3%)
   Ketorolac eyedrops

These agents have to be given for at least 4 to 6 weeks to show its response.

Carbon anhydrase inhibitor: These agents have shown to reduce the level of macular edema if given postoperatively. They help in pumping the edema fluid out.

Preparations

i. Acetazolamide 250 mg. Tab.
ii. Methazolamide

Long-terms are of these agents are not indicated due to its adverse side effects.

SURGICAL

It includes:

a. YAG Laser Vitreolysis, and
b. Vitrectomy

Nd: YAG Laser Vitreolysis: Patients with CME and vitreous incarceration responds slowly to management than individual without vitreous. Thus, presence of vitreous increases the time of resolution of CME.

Therefore, Nd: YAG Laser vitreolysis breaks down the vitreous strands, which get absorbed and reduces macular edema. Fibrosed vitreous strands are difficult to break. This will require vitrectomy.

VITRECTOMY

The main role of vitrectomy is:

1. Removal of vitreous adhesions
2. Removal of inflammatory mediator in vitreous.

Vitrectomy is usually delayed till CME is stable. Vitrectomy is beneficial in cases of aphakia chronic cystoid macular edema. Indications[19] for vitrectomy based on randomized controlled study on chronic aphakic macular edema.

A. Vitrectomy should not be considered until the visual acuity has been stable for 2-3 months.
B. Vitrectomy should be considered if visual acuity is 20/80 or worse.
C. Vitrectomy can be performed by pars plana or limbal route.
D. Hypertension is regarded as bad prognostic factor.

- **Main line of management of CME**: It includes:

Topical corticosteroids + Topical NSAIDs for about 4 to 6 weeks.
↓
If no response
↓
Peribulbar or Subtenon depot injections can be given
↓
If no response
↓
Start on carbonic anhydrase inhibitor
↓
Last step is the surgical management

- Nd: YAG laser vitreolysis
- Vitrectomy.

Prognosis

The prognosis for full restoration of visual acuity is generally good. The macula regains its normal appearance after edema subsides.

Last step is surgical treatment:

a. YAG Laser Vitreolysis
b. Vitrectomy

Photocoagulation may be tried but it is not quite successful.

Vitreous Hemorrhage

Vitreous hemorrhage[7] is defined as the presence of extravasated blood with the space outlined by internal limiting membrane posteriorly and laterally, the non-pigment epithelium of ciliary body anterolaterally and the lens zonules and postero lens capsule anteriorly.

The occurrence of massive vitreous hemorrhage to impair the vision seriously after cataract surgery is uncommon. But mild variety of hemorrhage is common.

Blood from vitreous can gain entrance into anterior chamber and vice versa via rent in anterior hyaloid membrane. Most intravitreal hemorrhages are caused by rupture of diseased blood vessels. Massive intravitreal hemorrhage results from rupture of short posterior ciliary artery, long posterior ciliary artery or choroidal artery (Fig. 43.3).

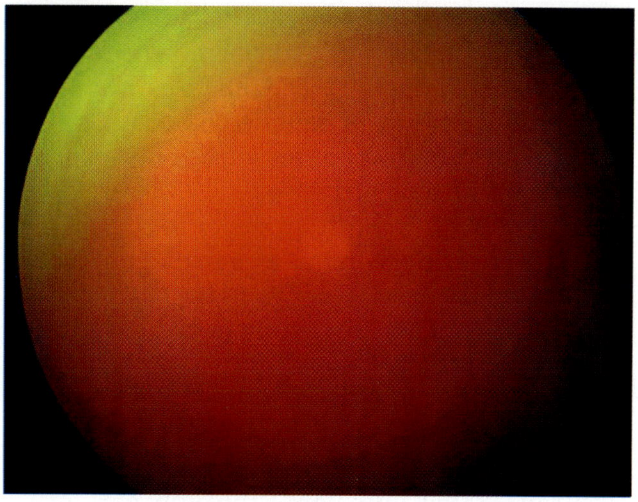

Fig. 43.3: Vitreous hemorrhage

Fate of Blood within the Vitreous[1]

a. Blood may undergo absorption resulting in no or little damage.
b. Hemorrhage within the vitreous may organize rapidly and form fibrous bands.

Treatment: The choice of treatment depends on several factors.[1] They include:

1. The patient's age
2. The duration of disease
3. Visual acuity
4. Intraocular pressure
5. Amount of hemorrhage
6. Status of retina
7. Neovascularization of iris
8. Associated conditions like diabetes and hypertension

The treatment options available are[7]*:*

1. Observation
2. Laser photocoagulation.
3. Anterior retinal cryotherapy.
4. Vitrectomy

1. *Observation:* Fresh vitreous hemorrhage often clears in days to weeks, and therefore, critical observation is very important. Reevaluation of retina is very important if absorption does not take place, we should proceed to next step.
   Eyes suitable for treatment are those with:
   - Poor visual acuity
   - No improvement in vitreous transparency has occurred
   - Anterior segment is healthy
2. *Anterior retinal cryotherapy (ARC)*[7]: It is indicated in eyes with fresh vitreous hemorrhage. ARC causes breakdown of blood retinal barrier, which leads to clearance of liquefied blood.
3. *Vitrectomy:* Indications for vitrectomy are:
   - Eyes with attached retina
   - Good PVD
   - Non-clearing vitreous hemorrhage over 2-3 months.
     These patients are best managed by vitreous surgery.
   - Eyes with advanced proliferative retinopathy with vitreous hemorrhage not clearing in 6-8 weeks also require early vitrectomy.
     Automated vitrectomy through pars plana approach is performed. Organized vitreous hemorrhage can lead to tractional retinal detachment. Vitrectomy with retinal detachment surgery is performed.
4. *Intravitreal urokinase*[11]*:* Urokinase is a plasminogen activator and the conversion to plasmin-results in lysis of fluid clot within few minutes. This promotes absorption of vitreous hemorrhage.
   Future trends in treatment: The treatment including vitreolysis with hyaluronidase, autologous plasmin enzyme is being tried. The chance that these agents will reduce the frequency of vitrectomy and will facilitate as adjuvants in vitreous surgery is unclear.
5. *Laser photocoagulation:* It is indicated in cases of proliferative vasculopathies.

ENDOPHTHALMITIS

Postsurgical endophthalmitis is a catastrophic complication of cataract surgery. The incidence following surgery is around 0.072 percent.[17]

Types: Postsurgical Endophthalmitis[17] (Fig. 43.4).

1. Fulminant (within 4 days)
   Gram-negative bacteria
   Streptococci
   Staph aureus
2. Acute (5-7 days)
   Staph epidermides
3. Chronic (more than 4 weeks)

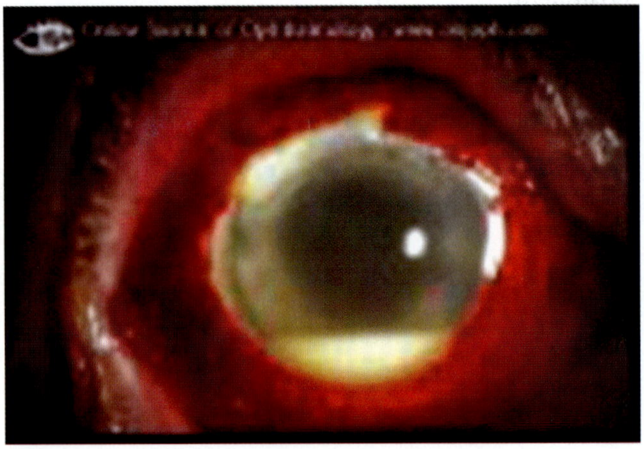

Fig. 43.4: Coagulase negative cocci POSTOPERATIVE ENDOPHTHALMITIS (*Courtesy* Atlas of Ophthalmology by Dr Robert Machemer and George Michelson)

Propionibacterium acne
Fungi – Aspergillus, Fusarium
Staph epidermides

Management: This mainly includes:

I. *Identification of organisms*[18]: Samples taken to identify the organisms are mainly from aqueous and vitreous.
   a. *Aqueous (AC) tap:* About 0.1 ml of aqueous is aspirated with 25-gauge needle attached to tuberculin syringe.
   b. *Vitreous tap:* About 0.1 ml of vitreous is removed from mid vitreous. Tuberculin syringe is used. The samples are inoculated in various culture media and sent for culture sensitivity.

II. *To find the source of infection:* The materials used during operation are sent for microbiological diagnosis.

Prophylaxis[18]

- Preoperative treatment of the preexisting infection of the lid conjunctiva and cornea.
- Use of preoperative antibiotics.
- Povidone – iodine 5 percent prepared by diluting 10% Betadine with 1:1 BSS.
- Postoperative use of local antibiotics.
- Meticulous attention to aseptic surgical procedure with isolation of lashes and lid margin from the operative area.

Treatment: This includes

Medical: Broad-spectrum antibiotic covering both gram positive and gram-negative organisms is used till the culture reports are available.

Antibiotics: are given in various preparations:

A. Intravitreal antibiotics are main line of treatment.[17] The combinations commonly used are:

Vancomycin 1000 mg in 0.1 ml + Cefazolin 2.25 mg in 0.1 ml
OR
Vancomycin 1000 mg in 0.1 ml + Amikacin 400 mg in 0.1 ml.

There combinations cover both gram positive and gram-negative organism. Antifungal agent, which is given intravitrealy, is Amphotericin 5-10 µgm in 0.1 ml.

B. *Topical* Fortified preparation are made and instilled topically.
   Fortified Gentamicin 15 mg 1 ml and Vancomycin 50 mg 1 ml.
   These drops have to be instilled very frequently initially till the infection subsides.

C. *Periocular injection* This includes anterior subtenon route or subconjunctivally.

D. *Systemic* Usually different antibiotics are given through different routes.

Steroids Corticosteroids reduce the postoperative inflammations. These agents can be given systemically, topically and intravitreal. But the role of steroids is very controversial.

Surgical: Surgical management includes Vitrectomy.

Role of Vitrectomy in Endophthalmitis

Vitrectomy plays an important role in management of endophthalmitis. The advantages are:

- It decreases the infectious load and inflammatory material.
- It provides vitreous sample for culture study.
- It helps in giving intravitreal injections.
- It removes the media opacities (exudates).

Thus, Vitrectomy helps in a more rapid visual recovery.

The endophthalmitis vitrectomy study (EVS) was done to determine the role of PPV in comparison to intravitreal injections. According to this study, vitrectomy is indicated

- When visual acuity reduces to perception of light
- When vitreous haze precludes a view of the fundus.

Technique 3 Port vitrectomy is done. In pseudophakic eyes, vitrectomy can be safely placed behind the IOL allowing safe vitreous cutting.

The important principles to be taken in account are:

- Maximum cutting rate is used
- Minimum suction is used
- Do not induce PVD if it is not already present.

After vitrectomy is completed, intravitreal injections are given. Lighted infusion cannula is used to visualize the tip of vitrector when view is poorer.

DISLOCATED IOLs

Dislocation of IOL can occur Intraoperatively or postoperatively.

Intraoperatively when PC IOL is implanted over the large PC tear. There is a chance lens getting dislocated posteriorly. Dislocation of IOL can be seen at a later stage also.

Dislocation of AC lens is very rare.

Management[4] A dislocated PCIOL may be left undisturbed in the eye without any surgical intervention. But it is best to remove the IOL to prevent retinal injury at a later stage. There are various methods available for removal of dislocated IOLs.

Main steps included are detailed examination to find the exact location of the dislocated IOL. There are four kinds of options available:

a. Observation
b. IOL removal
c. IOL exchange
d. IOL repositioning

Surgery may be deferred in cases[6]:

a. If refractive correction is visually satisfactory and convenient to patients
b. If patient is not willing for the surgery
c. If medical problem or ocular conditions prohibit further surgery. However, substantial intraocular inflammatory retinal detachment and cystoid macular edema are relative indication for the surgery.

Techniques available for removal of IOL are:

Surgical approach: Surgical removal of dislocated IOL can be removed via limbal or pars plana approach.

IOL holding forceps: After partial vitrectomy, 25 G needle is inserted through scleral groove posterior to limbus.

Then 25 G IOL forceps holding a slip knot on 10/0 suture is then inserted through the scleral incision for engaging the IOL haptic. After looping the haptic, the forceps are released from the suture, to grasp the end of haptic, thus preventing the suture from slipping. Then the IOL is repositioned in citiary sulcus. The same procedure is done with other haptic.

The scleral incision is closed with 10/0 nylon suture.

Use of perfluorocarbon liquid[4] This liquid is used to float the dislocated IOL anteriorly while keeping the retina posteriorly. Then 9/0 polypropylene suture is passed through scleral tunnel to engage the haptic of IOL. The IOL is then anchored in citiary suture. The perfluorocarbon liquid is not used in large amount as it will induce and cause the floated IOL to move towards the peripheral retina or vitreous

The Grieshabes snare[4] The Grieshabes snare consists of 20 G litre and handle with a moveable spring loaded finger slide for adjusting the amount of polypropylene suture loop. The suture loop is inserted posteriorly to engage a dislocated rupture in the vitreous cavity. Then the external portion of the loop is cut free and guided through 30 G needle for anchoring by anterior sclerotomy.

Temporary haptic externalization[4] The main features include the temporary haptic externalization for suture placement after pars plana vitrectomy. This is followed by reinternalization of rupture bed with 10/0 polypropylene sutures for anchoring by anterior sclerotomies.

Silicone lens reposition IOL exchange may be considered in certain cases of silicone IOLs. Silicone IOLs are usually slippery and more difficult to grasp than PMMA IOLs. A serrated forceps are used to grasp the IOLs but these forceps should not damage the optics of IOL. But these silicone IOLs can be repositioned on sulcus over the anterior capsular rhexis.

IOL replacement Distortion of IOL usually occurs secondary to posterior capsular tear. After removal of IOL, the placement of AC IOL or scleral finalised PC IOL may be performed. But due to disadvantage of anterior chamber IOLs, scleral fixated PC IOLs are usually professed.

Posterior chamber IOLs can be repositioned by following way:

1. Repositioning in the suture or in bag – depending on the size of capsular remnants available
2. Iris suture finalisation
3. Scleral suture finalisation

Thus, recognization of adequate capsular support is very important.

The anterior segment surgeon encountering the PC IOL dislocation intraoperatively should perform good vitrectomy to reduce the vitreous incarceration in the wound. Then postoperatively, topical and systematic steroids should be given with antiglaucoma agents. Then either observe the patient for some days or in some cases immediately refer the patient to VR surgeon.

CHOROIDAL DETACHMENT

Postoperative choroidal detachment can occur at three stages[2]:

- Immediately after surgery
- 7–21 days after surgery
- Months – year after surgery

Immediate choroidal detachment are very common after cataract surgery. It is usually associated with shallow anterior chamber. The detachment is usually anterior to equator.

Treatment: Most postoperative choroidal detachments subside within 3 weeks and so no treatment is required.

Medical

a. Cycloplegic agents:
   These agents cause relaxation of ciliary muscle and thus tension on uvea is minimized.
b. IV Mannitol:
   This is hyperosmotic agent, which deepens the anterior chamber and permits aqueous to be directed into anterior chamber.

Surgical

The surgical steps include:

a. Perform a suprachoroidal tap[2]
b. Form the anterior chamber with air
c. Resuturing of wound to repair the leak.
d. Laser or surgical iridectomy or incision of the anterior hyaloid face–helps in treatment of pupillary block, which is seen with choroidal detachment.

RETINAL DETACHMENT

The incidence of postoperative retinal detachment is less in SICS than in intracapsular cataract surgery.

Postoperative retinal detachment is common in aphakics then in pseudophakics.[13] The rate is 1.7[10] percent and the percentage of aphakics in retinal detachment cases is 53 percent[11] (Fig. 43.5).

The association between vitreous loss and subsequent detachment has been demonstrated.[14] The percentage without vitreous is 1-2 percent and with vitreous loss is 70 percent.

The predisposing factors causing retinal detachment are:

a. Presence of vitreous loss intraoperatively
b. Patient of high myopia with predisposing retinal degeneration like with lattice degeneration
c. Retinal break / tear in fellow eye
d. Retention of lens fragment
e. Dislocation of IOL
f. YAG Laser capsulotomy

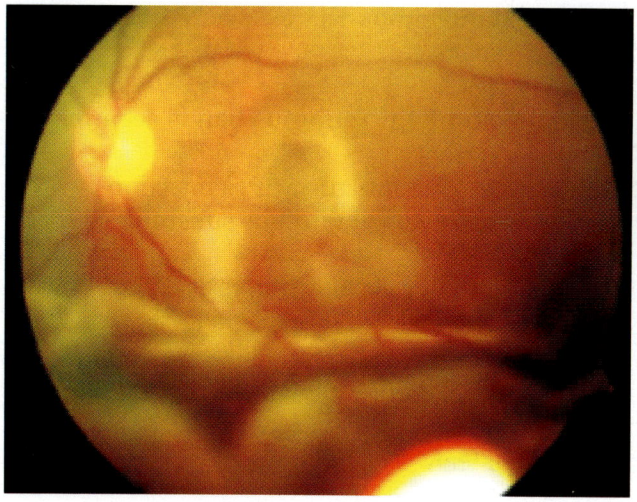

Fig. 43.5: Postoperative retinal detachment

The incidence of RD in aphakia is more. Also the incidence increases with vitreous loss.

Type of retinal detachment seen postoperatively are:

A. *Rhegmatogenous R.D:* Seen in patients with lattice degeneration or other predisposing retinal degeneration
B. *Tractional RD:* Seen secondary to vitreous traction caused to vitreous loss intraoperatively. Intraoperative vitreous loss may get organized into fibrous band. These bands lead to formation of tractional retinal detachment

Treatment

1. Scleral buckling: Is very effective in treatment of uncomplicated RD Radial or circumferential implants are used. Silicon materials can also be used
2. *Pneumatic retinopexy:*
   - Includes are of gas bubble to seal the retinal break and reattach the retina.
   - In this you treat the break by cryotherapy and then inject the gas bubble to seal the break.
3. *Pars plana vitrectomy:* It is microsurgical procedure in which you insert the instrument like cutter, cannula through small opening in pars plana.

   Indications of Pars plana vitrectomy are:

   a. Tractional RD.

   Vitrectomy helps in removal of vitreous bands, which form the tractional RD.

   b. Rhegmatogenous RD associated with very large breaks.

   c. Severe PVR:

   To break the thick fibrous bands seen in the vitreous cavity
4. Intravitreal vitreous substitutes injections:

   The commonly used vitreous substitutes are:

   i. Acts

   ii. Expanding gases like SF6/C3F8

   iii. Silicon oil

   iv. Perfluorocarbon liquid

Silicon oil is commonly used vitreous substitutes. They are usually in cases of severe PVR and grant retinal tear.

VITRITIS

Inflammation of the vitreous is usually associated with anterior chamber reaction.[22]

Severe vitritis is seen in cases with posterior capsular tear and in presence of vitreous loss. It is also seen in cases of retained cortical matter leading to inflammatory reaction in the vitreous. If the reaction is more then it leads to obscuration of the fundus visualization.

Management Most important step is the prevention of posterior capsular tear and vitreous loss.

In the presence of vitreous loss, cortical matter is removed with dry aspiration. The cortical matter can also be aspirated under the cover of a viscoelastics. Care should be taken that cortical matter does not get mixed with vitreous.

Medical treatment includes the use of corticosteroids. Posterior subtenon depot steroids are usually used.

REFERENCES

1. Morman S Jaffe, Mark S Jaffe, Gary F Jaffe. Vitreous Haemorrhage. Cataract Surgery and its complications. 21:487-505.
2. Morman S Jaffe, Mark S Jaffe, Gary F Jaffe. Choroidal Detachment. Cataract Surgery and its complications. 14:376-83.
3. Spraul CW, Grossncklous HE. Vitreous haemorrahge. Surv. Ophthalmology 1997;42:3-39.
4. Clement K. Chan, Gerald RS Schultz. Management of Dislocated Implants by Vitreoretinal Approach. Advances in Ophthalmology 109-18.
5. Hary W Flynn. Jr William E Smiddy. Removal of retained lens fragments. Vitreo Retinal Surgical Techniques. 231-39.
6. Surgical Technique for the management of dislocated posterior chamber intraocular lens. 239-49.
7. Sandeep saxena, Lalit Verma, Subhadra Jalali, Avinash PAthengay. Management of vitreous hamorrhage. Indian Journal of Ophthalmology 2003;51:189-96.
8. de Wenzel MJB; Traite de la cataracte, Paris 1786.P-J Duplain.
9. Gass JDM, Norton EWD. Follow up study of cystoid macular edema following cataract extraction. Trans Am Acad Ophthalm 1969;73:665-82.
10. Klein RM, Kalzin HM, Yannuzzi LA. The effect of indomethacin pretreatment on aphakic CME. Am. J Ophthal 1979;87:487-89.
11. Dugmore WN, Raichand M. Intravitreal Urokinase in the treatment of Vitreous Haemorrage. Am J Ophthalm 1973;75:779-81.
12. Mcpherson Ar, O Malley RE, Bravo J: Retinal detachment following late postcapsulotomy. Am J Ophthal 1983;95: 593-97.
13. Norton EWD. Retinal detachment in aphakia.Trans Am Ophthalm Soc 1963;61:770-89.
14. Kratz RP. Aphakia and retinal Detachment. In: Emery J. (Ed). Current Concepts in Cataract Surgery, The CV Mosby Co, 340.
15. Surgical management of posteriorly dislocated silicone plate intraocular lens (Johnson W, Schneiderman TE). Current Opinion Ophthalmol 1998;9;11-15.
16. Campo RU, Chung KD, Oyakawa Ry, Pars plana vitrectomy in management of dislocated posterior chamber lenses. Am J Ophthalmol 1989;18:529-34

17. Dr. Lalit Verma, Dr. Pradeep Venkatesh and Dr. HK Tewari; Management of Endophthalmitis. CME Series (No. 4)
18. Jack J. Kanski Disorders of the lens. Clinical Ophthalmology 286-309.
19. Fung WE. Vitrectomy for Chronic Aphakic Cystoid Macular Oedema. Ophthalmology 1985;92/81: 102-11.
20. McDonnell PJ. Jenarda C, Green WR. Vitreous incarcenation complicating cataract surgery. Ophthalmology 1986;93:247-53.
21. Norman S. Jaffe, Mark S. Jaffe Gary F. Jaffe. Cystoid macular edema. Cataract surgery and its complications, 434-49.
22. KPS Malik, Ruchi Goel. Postoperative complications of SICS. Manual of Small Incision Cataract Surgery 89-96.

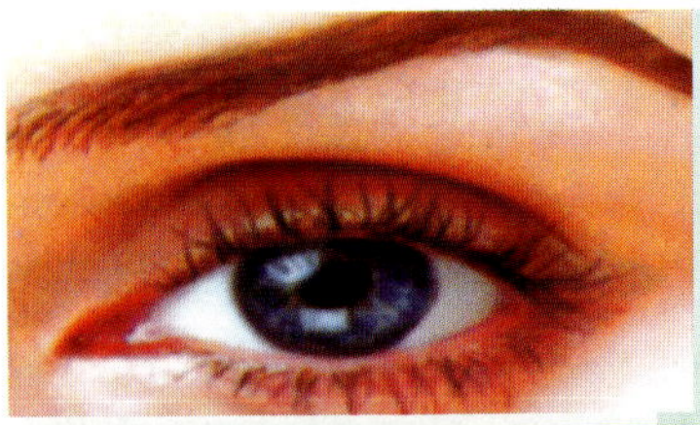

Forty four

Management of Astigmatism in SICS

Kamaljeet Singh
(India)

WITH THE RULE AND AGAINST THE RULE ASTIGMATISM
THE EFFECT OF SURGERY
INCISION TYPE
LENGTH OF THE INCISION
ASTIGMATICALLY NEUTRAL FUNNEL
DISTANCE FROM CORNEA
THE ENTRY POINT AT CORNEA
MANAGING PREEXISTING ASTIGMATISM

Any kind of ammetropia- myopia, hypermetropia or astigmatism present after the surgery gives rise to doubts in the mind of patient. In present age patients desire for a postoperative result that can give them a vision without glasses, not only for near but for distance also. Therefore, our endeavour should be to examine the patient thoroughly before the patient is taken to the operation theater. The surgeon should know the preoperative keratometry and his precataract refractive status. Postoperative astigmatism is annoying to the patient, especially if the astigmatism is more than 2.5 D. Because astigmatism of this order, even when fully corrected, causes blurring of the image, leads to field distortion and produces monoocular diplopia. All these problems cause asthenopia, and the patient remains unsatisfied.

Therefore, it should be very clear in our mind as to what we wish to achieve after the surgery. Our goal is customer's full satisfaction. He wants and deserves-vision for both near and distance. In order to achieve this, we must aim for a postoperative refraction of –1.5D cylinder at 180 degrees. This gives two point foci rather than one point focus. He can easily read 6/12 for distance and N6 for near. Patients are happiest with this kind of result, because they can do their routine activity without glasses. They can watch TV in their room and can also read the newspaper.

WITH THE RULE AND AGAINST THE RULE ASTIGMATISM

The rule is that cornea is more curved in vertical meridian than in the horizontal meridian. So far as our discussion is concerned there are two kinds of astigmatism— with-the-rule (WTR) and against-the-rule (ATR).

WTR astigmatism is said to be present, when on keratometry the cornea is more curved vertically than horizontally. In contrast, ATR astigmatism is said to be present, when cornea is less curved vertically than horizontally. This can be understood by the following example.

Suppose, on keratometry, vertical K reading is 48D and horizontal K reading is 43D. This means that the vertical meridian of cornea is more curved, or steeper. This is, therefore, an example of WTR astigmatism. On the other hand, if vertical K reading is 43D and horizontal K reading is 48D ATR astigmatism, which means cornea is steeper in horizontal meridian, is said to be there.

THE EFFECT OF SURGERY

In a study conducted by Merriam change on the horizontal and vertical meridians of the cornea after cataract surgery was observed in 5 different incisions for cataract: extracapsular cataract extraction (ECCE), 6 mm superior scleral tunnel (6 Sup), 3 mm superior scleral tunnel (3 Sup), 3 mm temporal scleral tunnel (3 Temp), and 3 mm temporal corneal incision (3 Cor). After each superior incision, the steepness and length of the transition from the initial to final plateau for each meridian depend on incision length. Considering the uncertainty of measuring K, the corneal meridians stabilized 4.5 months after ECCE, 1.2 months after 6 Sup, and 0.3 months after 3 Sup. No significant change was detected on the horizontal and vertical meridians after 3 Temp and 3 Cor.

In another study conducted by Huang to compare the corneal astigmatic changes induced by clear corneal incisions with those induced by scleral tunnel frown incisions, both from a temporal approach, in sutureless cataract surgery. Corneal stability was achieved with minimal astigmatic change 1 week after scleral frown incisions, while clear corneal incisions induced greater WTR astigmatism with delayed stabilization 1 to 3 months postoperatively.

In a study conducted by Zheng, the change in induced astigmatism was calculated for 8 years after ECCE (n = 144), for 3 years after 6 mm superior incisions (6 Sup) (n = 93), for 2 years after 3 mm superior incisions (3 Sup) (n = 120), and for 18 months after 3 mm temporal incisions (3 Temp) (n = 65). Two weeks after ECCE the mean induced cylinder was +3.47 D, which decayed to about -1.25 D after 6 months. Induced cylinder increased gradually to about -1.6 D after 8 years, although this further change was not significantly different than that at 6 months after surgery. For the phako groups, the net induced cylinder on the first post-operative day was +1.23 D (6 Sup), +0.49 D (3 Sup), and -0.19 D (3 Temp). After 6 Sup the wound was astigmatically stable after approximately 3 months, and 3 years after surgery net induced cylinder was -0.66 D; after 3 Sup the wound was astigmatically stable after about 6 weeks, and after 18 months net induced cylinder was -0.35 D. Maximum visual acuity was reached after a mean of approximately 6 weeks after ECCE, 2 weeks after 6 Sup, and between 1 day and 1 week after 3 Sup and 3 Temp.

In SICS we make basically 3 kind of incisions-parallel to limbus, straight and frown. The post-operative astigmatism depends upon the type of incision made, whether the incision has been made within the astigmatically neutral funnel, the length of incision and the distance from the cornea. Here, we have to understand that the frown incision gives minimum astigmatism. If the incision is with in the astigmatically neutral funnel, the astigmatism is least, smaller the incision less is the astigmatism and finally farther is the distance from cornea smaller is the astigmatism.

INCISION TYPE

When the incision is made parallel to limbus, the inferior edge of the incision may fall back, which flattens the cornea in this meridian. If the incision is made at 12 O'clock this incision flattens the vertical meridian of the cornea, causing against the rule astigmatism. When straight incision is fashioned, there are no chances of inferior edge falling back. Whatever astigmatism is produced by the straight incision is because of the instability of the central portion of the wound, which is much less than the smile incision. Least astigmatism is produced by the frown incision, because the edges of this incision are further away from the cornea. These edges become stable much earlier. Therefore, this incision produces minimum possible astigmatism.

LENGTH OF THE INCISION

Many studies have documented beyond doubt that the longer the incision more is the astigmatism. Usually, the incision size in SICS is between 6 and 7 mm. This causes astigmatism up to 1.0 D. If the incision is larger than this, the induced astigmatism may increase to 3D, because the approximation of the wound is not good causing sagging of inferior edge of the wound. These edges must be sutured in order to get less astigmatism.

ASTIGMATICALLY NEUTRAL FUNNEL

The concept of astigmatic funnel arose from two mathematical relationships; firstly, that corneal astigmatism is directly proportional to the cube of the length of the incision and the second, that, it is inversely related to the distance from the limbus. Incisions made within this funnel will be for all practical purposes, astigmatism equivalent. Curvilinear limbus parallel incisions fall outside this funnel and are hence unstable. Therefore, any incision within this funnel causes almost negligible astigmatism.

DISTANCE FROM CORNEA

More is the distance from cornea less are the chances of astigmatism because the wound at the sclera has little effect on the corneal curvature.

THE ENTRY POINT AT CORNEA

The wound of entry in SICS is much larger than the external scleral wound. This also results in considerable astigmatism. Opening in the anterior chamber, the edges of which are straight cause much less astigmatism than the ragged edges of the corneal wound.

MANAGING PREEXISTING ASTIGMATISM

We make an incision at 12O'clock if the preoperative keratometry shows with-the-rule astigmatism. In presence of against-the-rule astigmatism the incision is made on the temporal site. If the astigmatism is high, the incision goes close to the limbus, becomes paralimbal and long. If no or small degree of astigmatism is present, the small, frown and away from the limbus is fashioned. There are many other ways and means like keratotomy and LASIK for which reader is referred to appropriate book on the subject.

REFERENCES

1. Huang FC, Tseng SH. Comparison of surgically induced astigmatism after sutureless temporal clear corneal and scleral frown incisions. J Cataract Refract Surg. 1998; 24(4):477-81
2. Merriam JC, Zheng L, Urbanowicz J, Zaider M. Change on the horizontal and vertical meridians of the cornea after cataract surgery Trans Am Ophthalmol Soc. 1997;95:387-410; discussion 410-15.
3. Zheng L, Merriam JC, Zaider M. Astigmatism and visual recovery after 'large incision' extracapsular cataract surgery and 'small' incisions for phakoemulsification. Trans Am Ophthalmol Soc. 2001;99:187-95; discussion 195-97.
4. Sachdev Mahipal, Mishra P, Thanikachalam S. The manual small incision: Surgical aspects-I in Small Incision Cataract Surgery (manual Phaco) Kamaljeet Singh (ed) Jaypee Brothers: New Delhi, India 2002;75-83.
5. Percival P, Thornton S. The plan for ametropia and astigmatism in A Colour Atlas of Lens Implantation Percival Piers (Ed). Wolfe Publishing Ltd: England 1991;164-67.

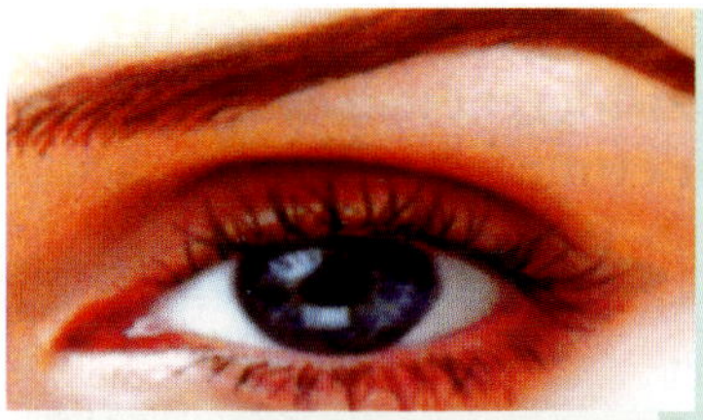

Forty five

Complications and their Avoidance in Manual Small Incision Cataract Surgery

Francisco J Gutiérrez-Carmona (Spain)

No surgical technique is exempt from complications which can occur at any step in the surgical procedure. Obviously, surgical skill is a very important factor in avoiding such complications, but equally important is the surgeon's experience in dealing with these complications which only comes after performing a significant number of cataract surgeries.

One important factor in the frequency of complications is dependent on surgical preparation and the clinical status of the patient. From the point of view of a patient's preparation, it is important that the type of surgical procedure to be performed, and the type of anesthesia to be used be explained to him thoroughly before the operation.

This psychological preparation will serve to increase the patient's collaboration during the surgery whether with local or topical anesthesia.

On the other hand, before and during surgery, we need to maintain the patient in optimum condition with regard to blood pressure, heart rate, etc. as with any other patient pathologies (diabetes, hypertension, etc.).

Concerning the eye to be operated on, it is important to do a meticulous study of the anterior and posterior segment and intraocular pressure before surgery.

This will help in planning the surgery and diminish the frequency of complications.

INTRAOPERATIVE COMPLICATIONS AND THEIR AVOIDANCE

Wound Construction

The clear corneal tunnel incision or scleral tunnel incision both present the distinct advantage of allowing cataract surgery in a closed system. The location and construction of the wound are factors in avoiding later complications during surgery. The location of the scleral tunnel incision should be between approximately 1.5 and 2.0 mm away from the limbus and the clear corneal incision should be made inside the limbus with an intrastromal tunnel between 1.0 and 1.5 mm. This will avoid a premature entrance into the anterior chamber and the iris prolapse during hydrodissection, capsulorhexis, etc., at the same time reducing the risk of Descemet's membrane detachment.

In the scleral tunnel incision a frequent complication is during undermining, a buttonhole may occur in the scleral flap. This may be caused by a groove that is too shallow, either throughout or only in some areas. If the dissection is too deep this can produce scleral disinsertion. To avoid this it is necessary to make a tunnel of 0.30 mm thickness (Fig. 45.1).

Bleeding from the incision into the anterior chamber is more frequent with scleral tunnel incision. Davis B. Davis, MD has pointed out that the most important consideration in the prevention of hyphemas is to undermine well into a vascular, clear corneal limbus before entering the anterior chamber. Bleeding can be managed by means of careful bipolar cautery.

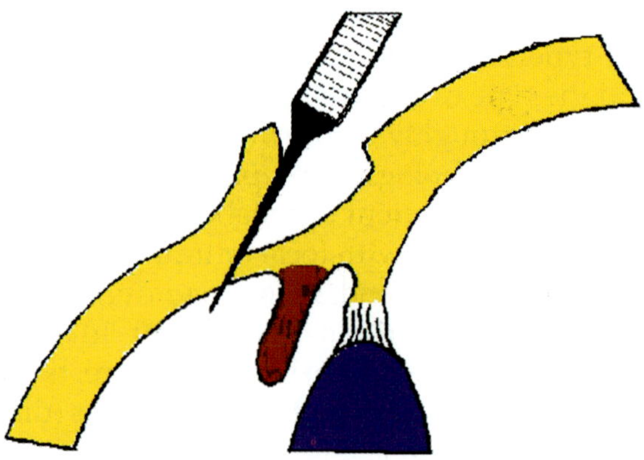

Fig. 45.1: When underminig the wound the dissection should be carried into clear cornea at least half-way into the blue zone, within 0.5 mm or less of the conjunctival attachment line

Capsulotomy

The capsulorhexis should be sufficiently wide not less than 6 mm to allow an easy luxation of the nucleus into the anterior chamber. If the capsulorhexis is small we will encounter great difficulties in the luxation of the nucleus into the anterior chamber resulting in a zonular rupture. As such, we should enlarge the capsulorhexis by means of making various cuts on its margins with capsulotomy scissors and forceps or with the help of a cystitome (Fig. 45.2).

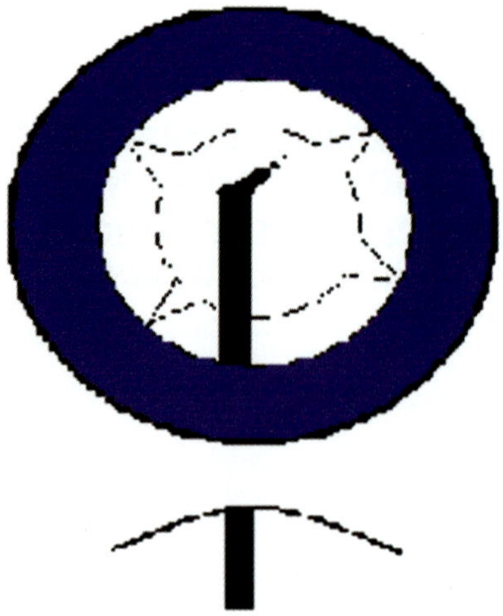

Fig. 45.2: In a small capsulorhexis several cuts should be made with a cystotome on the margin in order to facilitate an easier luxation of the nucleus

Nuclear Luxation

Difficulty in nuclear luxation occurs primarily under two circumstances; when the pupil is small and when the nucleus is soft. Before surgery any pupil must be examined with respect to its size and rigidity. If the pupil is small and fibrotic, it is best to simply perform sphincterotomies (Fig. 45.3), sector iridectomy or to stretch the pupil with two Kuglin hooks.

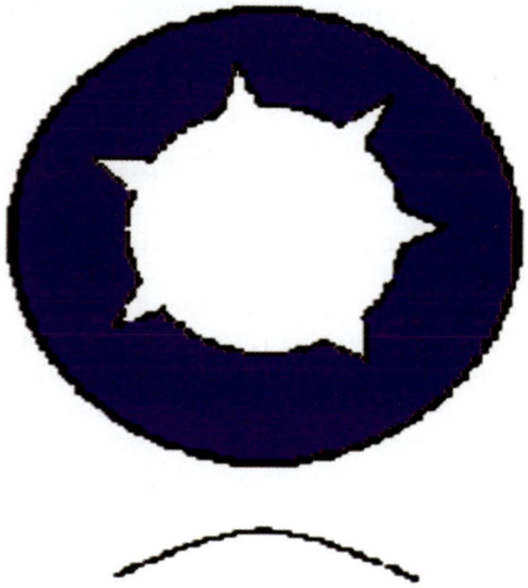

Fig. 45.3: When the pupil is small and fibrotic several sphincterotomies should be made with capsulotomy scissors to allow an easy luxation of the nucleus

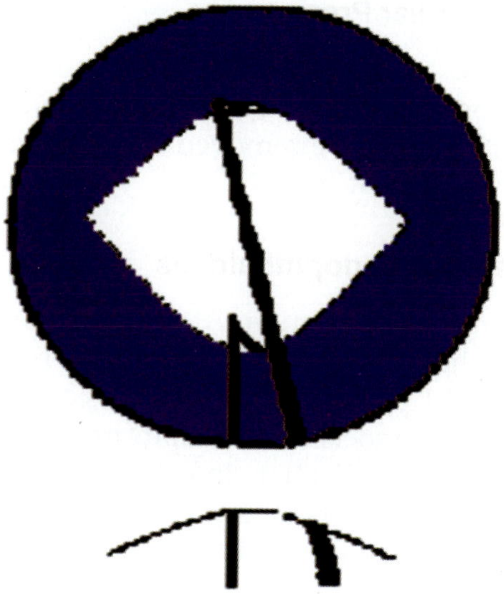

Fig. 45.4: In very small pupils a mechanical enlargement of the pupil should be made with two Kuglin hooks to avoid the dialysis of the posterior capsule

Soft nuclei may also present a problem with luxation. For the very soft ones, simple aspiration can be used. However, there are some nuclei that tend to fracture when an attempt is made to luxate them. In this case, hydrodissection and the subnucleus injection of viscoelastic material will facilitate luxation.

Dialysis or Rupture of the Posterior Capsule

Dialysis of the posterior capsule can occur in an effort to luxate the nucleus. The use of viscoelastic material as an aid in luxating the nucleus will avoid this problem in the case of medium-dilated pupils; in the case of very small pupils, it is avoided by sphincterotomies, sector iridectomy or mechanical enlargement of the pupil with two Kuglin hooks (Fig. 45.4).

Rupture of the posterior capsule may occur during hydrodissection or nuclear fragmentation while trying to push the spatula or vectis between the nucleus and posterior capsule. It can be avoided by hydroexpressing the nucleus out of the capsular bag and then pushing the posterior capsule away from the nucleus by the injection of viscoelastic material.

Iris Trauma

It may occur if the superior leaf of the iris is captured on the spatula or vectis and the nucleus. It can be avoided by the injection of viscoelastic material at 12 o'clock out of the plane of insertion of the spatula or vectis to retrodisplace the iris prior to introducing the instruments.

POSTOPERATIVE COMPLICATIONS AND THEIR AVOIDANCE

Corneal Edema

Transient corneal edema can appear in the postoperative period. This edema quickly resolves and is not clinically significant. Avoiding cornea touch will prevent corneal edema. The use of high density viscoelastic material during nuclear fragmentation will prevent the endothelial cell loss and corneal edema.

Shallow Anterior Chamber

This complication is usually due to the closure of the incision. This can be managed by applying a suture.

High Intraocular Pressure

This is due to the large amount of viscoelastic material used during surgery. To prevent it the viscoelastic should be removed from the anterior chamber with great care.

Postoperative Endophthalmitis

This is a rare complication. Although its reported incidence has decreased significantly from 1 to about 0.05-0.1 percent, it still remains a source of dread for all eye specialists. Despite improvements in asepsia and sterilization, infectious endophthalmitis continues to persist as one of the most important sight-threatening condition.

REFERENCES

1. Gutiérrez-Carmona FJ. Manual technique allows for small incision cataract surgery . Ocular Surgery News: Surgical Maneuvers:1997;14-15.
2. Gutiérrez-Carmona FJ: Nueva técnica e instrumental de facofragmentación manual para incisiones esclárales tunelizadas de 3.5 mm ArchSoc Esp Oftalmol 1999;74:181-86.
3. Gutiérrez-Carmona FJ: Manual multi-phacofragmentation through a 3.2 mm clear corneal incisión. J Cataract Refract Surg 2000;26:1523-28.
4. Keener GT (Jr): The nucleus division technique for small incisión cataract extraction. In: Rozakis GW, (Ed) Cataract Surgery; Alternative Small-Incision Techniques. Thorofare, NJ Slack, 1990;6:163-91.
5. Kansas PG. Small incision cataract extraction and implantation surgery using a manual phacofragmentation technique. J Cataract Refract Surg 1998;14:328-30
6. Quintana M: Implantación de LIO plegable con facosección manual y pequeña incisión. Microcirugía ocular 1998;6(1):37-44.
7. Blumenthal M. Manual ECCE, the present state of the art. Klin Monatsbl Augenheilkd 1994;205:266-70
8. Koch PS: Structural analysis of cataract incision construction. J Cataract Refract Surg 1991;17 (Suppl.): 661-67.
9. Boyd BF, et al. Complicaciones Transoperatorias de la Facoemulsificación. En: El Arte y la Ciencia en la Cirugía de la Catarata; Highlights of Ophthalmology Int'l , edición en español 2001;11:249-68.
10. Davis DB. Scleral Incisions With Cataract Surgery. American Intra-Ocular Implant Society Journal, Spring. 1983;9:192.

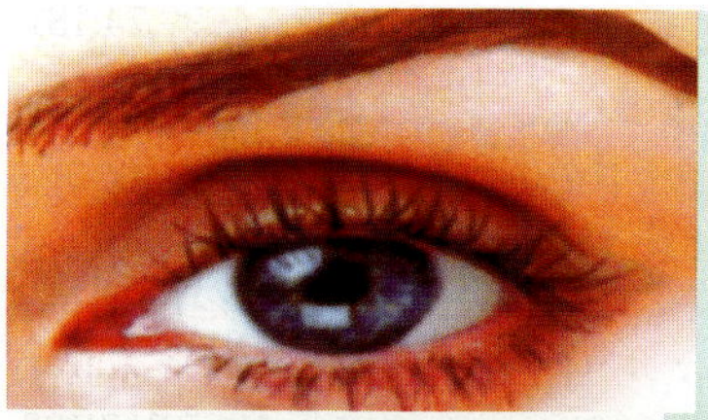

Forty six

Postsurgical Cystoid Macular Edema

PN Nagpal
Kamal Nagpal
Manish Nagpal (India)

INTRODUCTION

Ocular tissues, like those of other organs, exhibit well-defined morphological reactions to local trauma and insult in the form of hyperemia, vasodilatation, increased permeability of blood vessels and edema. Cystoid macular edema (CME) following cataract surgery is one such manifestation, and it can result in either temporary and rarely a permanent reduction of visual acuity. Although its etiology remains obscure, its relationship to the details of the surgical procedures and their complications are becoming clearer. Likewise, more insight into the phenomenon is also being imparted by the agents being used in the preventive or curative line of management in CME.

This entity was first referred to by Vogt in 1918 and in 1953 was defined by Dr. SR Irvine as "a newly defined vitreous syndrome following cataract surgery".[1] Gass and Norton[2] demonstrated this entity on fluorescein angiogram as intraretinal cysts arranged like flower-petals and was subsequently given the name of "Irvine-Gass" syndrome.[3]

PATHOPHYSIOLOGY

Macula has certain distinguishing features which predispose it to CME. These are:

- Thick Henle's layer with a greater capacity of absorbing fluid
- The avascularity of the foveal avascular zone (FAZ) leading to decreased drainage of inflammatory or toxic metabolites from this region
- The internal limiting membrane is the thinnest at the macula
- It is the most functionally and metabolically active area of the retina
- Adhesion of the cortical vitreous to the macula.

CME is the final common pathway of several intraocular and systemic diseases. Successful primate models of CME have been experimentally made[4] with the help of the following presumed causative factors:

- Disruption of blood-retinal barrier at the retinal vasculature and retinal pigment epithelium
- Ischemic injury to the retina
- Intraocular events related to surgery—inflammation, hypotony and vitreous traction
- Systemic disorders such as diabetes and systemic hypertension

CME is essentially a disease of increased capillary permeability in the perifoveal capillaries and the capillaries of the disk as demonstrated angiographically. Endogenously produced mediators such as prostaglandins and others liberated after surgery can produce such a response and are considered contributory to its development.[5]

Stimulation of prostaglandin release takes place presumably at the anterior uvea. Simultaneously, there is an inhibition of the active transport—the Bito's pump which is responsible for their removal from intraocular fluids.[6] At these two areas—the disk and macula, the internal limiting membrane is the thinnest. This might explain their susceptibility to the inflammatory products from the anterior segment which travel through the vitreous to the retinal surface postoperatively, resulting in the barrier breakdown.

Localization of the site of the breakdown has been attempted, using horseradish peroxide and immunohistochemical[7] methods. It has been found to occur primarily at the inner bloodretinal-barrier (retinal vasculature) although leakage is also encountered at the outer barrier (pigment epithelium).

A role of mechanical stress[8] in the pathogenesis of CME has been suggested. Vitreous adhesions are present anteriorly at the lens and the vitreous base and posteriorly at the major vessels, optic disc and macula. At all these sites, the inner limiting membrane is thin, and there are firm fibrous vitreous attachments to the Muller cells. A chronic traction to the Muller cells, therefore, results in their chronic irritation. This may cause a local release of a variety of mediators facilitating vascular leakage. A complete vitreomacular separation, though rare can allow resolution of cystoid changes and improvement of visual acuity.[9]

Hypertension and diabetes with their own vascular and rheological consequences also work in conjunction with the inflammatory mediators to increase the leakage from the perifoveal capillaries. Thus, such patients have a greater tendency to develop aphakic or pseudophakic CME.

SURGICAL FACTORS

Over the years as the trends and practices of cataract surgery have evolved, various associations and risk factors related to the surgical procedure have been condemned for their role in the development of CME. Here, we summarize these in brief.

- Type of cataract surgery—ICCE Vs ECCE Vs phacoemulsification
- IOL—manufacture and quality, site of placement and its contact with the uvea
- Status of the posterior capsule
- Vitreous disturbance during surgery and its incarceration to the surgical wound or adhesion to iris
- Postoperative hypotony
- Postoperative inflammation
- Endodonesis and pseudophakodonesis
- History of CME in the other eye
- Retinal phototoxicity from the operating microscope
- Hylase in the retrobulbar block
- Patient factors such as age (young patients)[10] blue iris, hypertensive or diabetic patients
- History of postoperative CME in the other eye

In order to understand better the etiology of CME, numerous insights into the surgical factors have been made. Some of the earliest studies which were performed on ICCE cases without lens implants took into consideration angiographic CME at different intervals from the time of surgery, helping us to understand the natural history of the disease (Table 46.1).

Type of surgery Various authors reported the incidence of clinically significant CME following ICCE with IOL to range from 3.4 to 20 percent. The same surgeons reported a 0 to 4.4 percent incidence in ECCE with IOL (Table 46.2).

Quentin, *et al*[22] compared CME and vision in patients of ICCE and Choyce anterior chamber lenses with those of ECCE and posterior chamber lenses in the fellow eyes of 65 patients. On discharge, there was an angiographic CME in 23 percent of the ICCE group and 7.6 percent of the ECCE group. After 6 months, an incidence of 1.5 percent of clinical CME was seen in both the groups while, angiographic CME was observed in 22 percent of the ICCE group and 12 percent of the ECCE group.

Taylor[23] reviewed 1808 of his own cataract patients and found an incidence of clinical CME of 2 percent in ICCE patients without IOL, 9.9 percent in ICCE with iris-supported IOL and 1.2 percent in ECCE with PC IOL. Others have also found that iris-fixated IOLs are associated with an incidence of CME ranging from 3.4 to 6.1.[10,20,21,24]

As far as phacoemulsification is concerned, the "cataract research outcome team"[25] declared that the pooled results of postoperative vision and most postoperative complications including CME did not differ much for surgeries performed either by phacoemulsification or standard ECCE. The incidence of angiographic CME between these two procedures has also been reported to be comparable.[26,27]

POSTERIOR CAPSULE STATUS AND VITREOUS DISTURBANCE

Improved microsurgical skills and a good dealing with the disturbed vitreous seem to have reduced the incidence of CME. Nikica[28] compared the incidence of CME in three groups of patients that had undergone different types of surgical procedures. The first group comprised of patients of ECCE with PC IOL, the second group of ECCE with anterior vitrectomy with AC IOL due to posterior capsular rupture and the third group of ICCE with AC IOL. The incidence of CME as diagnosed on FA was 1.5 percent, 35.7 percent and 9 percent respectively in the first, second and third groups. The difference in the second and third group patients was, therefore, presumed to depend upon vitreous loss.

Table 46.1: Studies on ICCE cases without lens implants taking into consideration angiographic CME at different intervals from the time of surgery

Study	*No. of eyes*	*Time interval after surgery*	*CME (angiographic) (Percentage)*
Klein and Yannuzzi—1976[11]	75	2-7 days	5
Meredith, *et al*—1976[12]	44	2 weeks	60
Hitchings, *et al*—1975[13]	71	6 weeks	51
Irvine, *et al*—1971[14]	100	4-16 weeks	40
Miami study group—1979[15]	113	4 months	14
Miami study group—1979[15]	87	8 months	15
Miami study group—1979[15]	94	6-24 months	9
Hitchings — 1977[16]	57	24 months	12

Table 46.2: Percentage incidence in ECCE with IOL

Study	*CME (percentage) ICCE with IOL*	*CME (percentage) ECCE with IOL*
Moses—1978[17]	8.5	4.4
Stark, *et al*—1982[18]	10–20	2
Binkhorst—1977[19]	3.8	1.2
Worst, *et al*—1977[20]	4.1	1.0
Jaffe, *et al*—1982[21]	3.4	0

Alpar[29] found a significant difference in the incidence of CME in patients with on-the-table posterior capsulotomy with and without 1 percent healon, injected between the posterior capsule and vitreous prior to completion of the capsulotomy. In those who did not receive the injection, the incidence of angiographic CME was 26 percent and clinical CME 10.5 percent, while in those who got the injection, there was a 2.8 percent incidence of angiographic CME. This indicated that by maintaining space between the posterior capsule and anterior hyaloid membrane, healon prevented the development of CME. This supported the theory that the anterior hyaloid membrane protects the posterior segment.

Winslow[30] reported an incidence of 7 percent in ECCE cases and 38 percent in ECCE with primary capsulotomy, while Binkhorst[19] found that in 328 eyes with ECCE with IOL with intact capsule, there was no clinical CME and in 172 eyes with ECCE with IOL with PC defect there was a 3.5 percent incidence. Wright *et al*[31] found an incidence of angiographic CME in 24 percent of cases with a primary capsulotomy and in 16 percent with intact capsules in ECCE with PC IOLs. Bergman[32] reported a 12.5 percent incidence of clinically significant CME in those ECCE cases that were complicated by vitreous disturbance.

Spaide[33] on logistic regression of 141 patients who had clinically significant CME following cataract surgery found that of all the systemic and ocular factors studied, the best predictors of vision {(20/200, 6/60) or worse} were the presence of iris in the wounds and an FA of grade 4 (see below). Integrity of the posterior capsule, iritis, vitreous in the wound or type of IOL did not predict the visual status.

Kraff *et al*[34] summarized the factors connected to pseudophakic CME by evaluating the following in their relation to early postoperative angiographic CME.

- UV filter in the operating microscope—no statistically significant difference
- UV light filtering IOL—statistically significant difference noted
- Primary capsulotomy during ECCE—higher rate as compared to capsule intact group
- Hylase in the retrobulbar block—no significant difference
- Prophylactic indomethacin drops—statistically significant lowering in the incidence

A higher incidence of CME has been noticed in patients receiving secondary implants, which depends upon vitreous disturbance in the second surgery and smaller (<1year) interval between the two surgeries.[35]

DIAGNOSIS AND NATURAL COURSE

Clinical assessment of macular edema is often not fruitful in all cases because its often very slight and subtle and its incidence varies at different post-operative periods. Therefore, CME can be considered as being clinically significant, which has an incidence of about 1.5 percent[25] in extracapsular surgeries and is symptomatic, or *angiographic*. Angiographic CME is much more common—in up to 60 percent following ICCE and about 20 percent following ECCE. Vision is generally not affected, and the condition is mild and innocuous. It usually subsides spontaneously in a few days and can only be diagnosed on fluorescein angiography (FA). However, a functional deficit in the form of abnormal ERG (focal and pattern),[36] fall in contrast sensitivity[37,38] and an abnormal photostress test[39] have been noted.

Irvine-Gass syndrome occurs following cataract extraction in eyes with initially improved postoperative visual acuity. Symptoms may appear between one month to three months following surgery, as a result of leakage into the macula. Most commonly the symptoms appear within the first six months, although they may be delayed for several years.

Symptoms

Symptoms are mainly in the form of a fall in visual acuity, and rarely redness, pain and photophobia.

Signs

Signs of complicated anterior segment surgery may be present in the form of ruptured posterior capsule, displaced lens, retained lens matter, vitreous in anterior chamber, with adherence to the wound or the iris, iris incarceration in the wound or distortion by the IOL. Subtle signs of an active inflammation such as mild flare, cells and ciliary injection may be detected. There may be an evidence of mild anterior vitritis.

Fundus examination reveals loss of foveal reflex. Slit-lamp biomicroscopy reveals macular thickening with cystoid concentric spaces arranged in a petaloid pattern around the fovea. They may appear like a honey-comb. The central cysts are larger in size with smaller cysts peripherally. Small perifoveal splinter hemorrhages may be present. Papilledema with peripapillary hemorrhages may appear.

Fluorescein Angiography (Figs 46.1A to C)

Early diffuse leakage through out the macula is seen in the perifoveal capillaries in the form of pin point spots 10 to 15 minutes after the injection. These coalesce to form a characteristic appearance of fluorescein in the cystoid spaces, filling them up in classical stellate perifoveal configuration like a flower petal. This can appear in the late phase, therefore, it is important to wait till 30 minutes after the injection. Late staining of the disk may also be seen, which worsens the prognosis.

FA rating of CME is as follows.

0—no leak
1—edema < perifoveal region
2—perifoveal edema
3—moderate edema—1 DD in size
4—severe perifoveal edema > 1 DD
+— confluent foveal cysts

The relation between macular thickening and visual acuity has been studied with the help of stereoscopic fluorescein angiograms.[40] It was found that there was a significant relationship between mean macular thickness and vision recorded at the time of the angiogram. However, the existing visual acuity had no relationship with the amount of dye leakage.

Menzo,[41] upon studying the iris and retinal angiograms in implanted eyes found a correlation between the presence of CME and iris leakage. A satisfactory diagnosis of CME can also be made upon fluorography following oral fluorescein ingestion.[42]

Quantitative assessment of macular edema can accurately be obtained by optical coherence *tomography*.[43] These tomograms correspond closely to the known histopathological characteristics and therefore may be useful in an objective monitoring of the edema.

Chronic CME

It is defined as clinically significant CME persisting for more than 6 months. Ruiz *et al*[44] found that chronicity developed in 36 percent of the clinical CME cases. Of these, majority (71%) were those with vitreous loss and an AC IOL. Of the chronic cases, only 29 percent had a final vision of 20/40 or better.

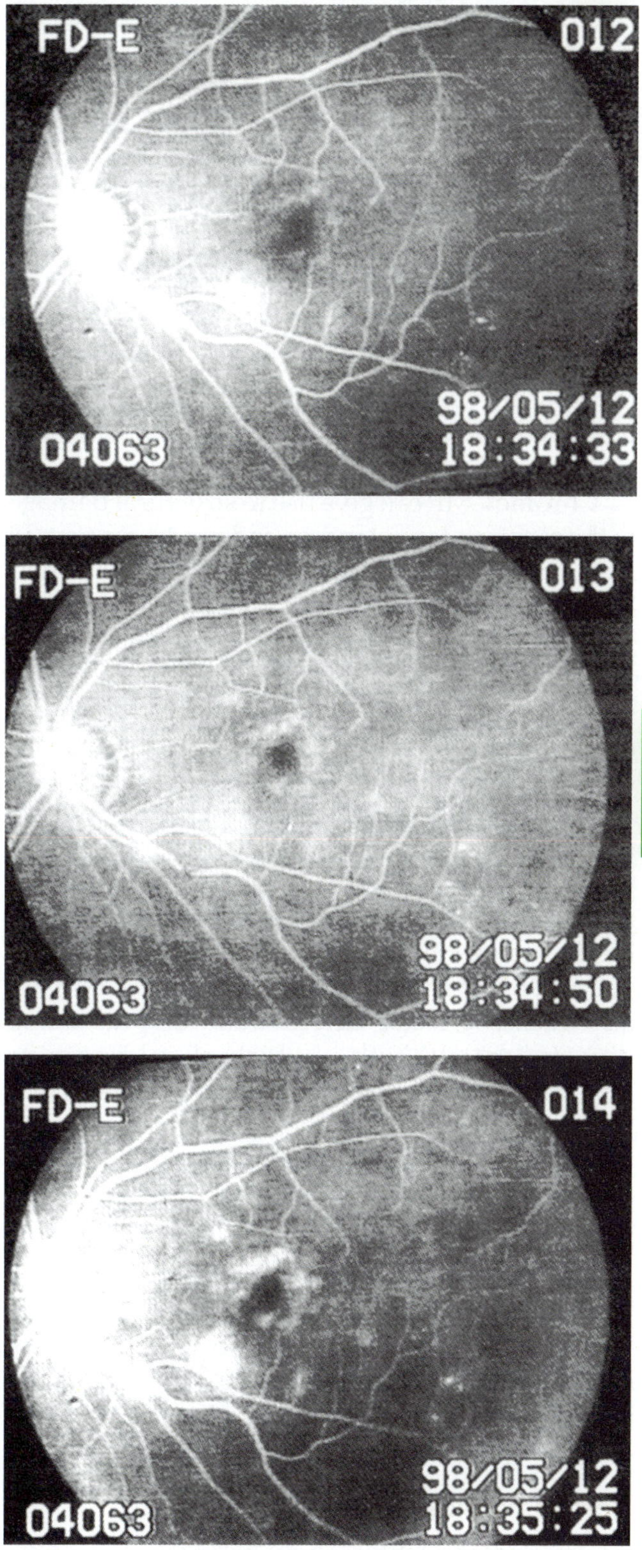

Figs 46.1A to C: Fluorescein angiogram of cystoid macular edema (CME)—increasing perifoveal leakage to form classical flower petal pattern

Acute CME usually develops within the first 3 months following surgery. It responds well to topical nonsteroidal antiinflammatory drugs (NSAIDs) and steroids. Chronic CME develops later, even years after surgery and typically persists for more than 6 months despite treatment. It seems to be less responsive to topical antiinflammatory agents. If detected early, the prognosis can be better, however, the final vision is often less than that in the acute disease. Gass and Norton[3] studied the resolution time of CME and found that improvement—both visual and angiographic occurred within 6 months in 50 percent cases and within 36 months in 72 percent of cases.

Chronic CME can give rise to structural damage to the retina on long standing and produce a cystoid maculopathy. Other complications include macular hole and premacular membrane.

DIABETES AND CME

There is a higher incidence of angiographic as well as clinical CME in diabetics due to the already compromised blood ocular barrier.[45] On FA, it is about 32 percent in those without a preoperative retinopathy and 81 percent in patients who have retinopathy at the time of surgery. The prognosis is poorer in the presence of retinopathy in terms of a higher rate of clinical CME, its longer course and a poorer final visual outcome. A cataract surgery also causes a faster deterioration of preexisting diabetic maculopathy, which should receive treatment prior to or immediately after the surgery.

TREATMENT

Treatment modalities that have been used can be either medical or surgical.

Medical line alone forms the mainstay of treatment in majority of cases. For maximum visual benefit, the treatment should be early and aggressive once the diagnosis has been established because a late and half-hearted attempt often has disappointing results.

Corticosteroids

Corticosteroids act by inhibiting arachidonic acid release from the cell membrane, which is a precursor of prostaglandins and leukotrienes. They may be dispensed from topical, sub-tenon's or systemic routes.

Topical steroids such as 0.1 percent dexamethasone or 1 percent prednisolone drops are used 4 times in a day. Their IOP raising properties should, however, be kept in mind in the steroid responder group of patients. Newer steroids such as rimexolone 1 percent have demonstrated significant antiinflammatory properties with a minimal potential to elevate the IOP,[49] thereby, making it a promising drug.

Peribulbar or sub-Tenon's injections of steroids such as triamcinolone (20 mg) or methylprednisolone (20 mg) every 30 days has an advantage of placing the drug closer to the macula. However, these are associated with greater potential complications such as a persistent rise in IOP and a risk of globe perforation.

Systemic steroids—1 mg / kg / day prednisolone are also accompanied with significant side effects on prolonged therapy such as gastric ulcers, hypertension and hyperglycemia. Recurrence of this condition is frequent after stopping the steroid treatment. Therefore, a maintenance steroid therapy is recommended after the condition subsides.[10]

Nonsteroidal Antiinflammatory Drugs (NSAIDs)

NSAIDs (discussed below) are at least as effective as steroids in the treatment of established cases of CME by inhibiting the blood-aqueous barrier breakdown.[50] They block the cyclooxygenase pathway which is responsible for converting arachidonic acid to prostaglandins.

Carbonic Anhydrase Inhibitors

Acetazolamide has clinical effects on the retinal pigment epithelium (RPE) via the membrane-bound carbonic anhydrase activity in the RPE, causing an increase in the rate of subretinal fluid absorption.[51] Oral route for administration of the drug has been studied with promising results. The recommended dose is 500 mg twice a day, for three weeks.

Hyperbaric Oxygen

Instituted at 2.2 atmosphere for 1.5 hours two times daily, for 7 days and then 2 hours daily for next 14 days has been shown to help in resolution of CME and improvement of vision.

Nd: YAG Laser Vitreolysis

The Nd: YAG laser can be employed to lyze off the strands of vitreous that are adherent to the anterior segment structures or incarcerated to the corneoscleral wound. This line of management has successfully been attempted both in CME patients and prophylactically in those who were prone to it.[52] There was an improvement of vision. However, the complications encountered include retinal detachment and an IOP rise. It can be considered as the first line of management of those cases with obvious vitreous adhesions.

Argon Laser Photocoagulation

Argon laser photocoagulation of cases having chronic clinical CME not responding to medical line of treatment has been attempted.[53] It has been reported to have a 50 percent success rate.

Pars Plana Vitrectomy

It is reserved for cases that have failed to show any improvement in vision despite prolonged medical line of treatment and have vitreous adhesions to anterior segment structures.[54–58] Vitrectomy aims at mechanically removing all the vitreous adhesions, and also releasing the traction over the retina. This reduces the formation of mediating agents. The results are promising, in the form of improvement of vision and subsidence of edema. Pars plana approach is recommended because adhesions to the posterior surface of the iris can also be tackled. If indicated, it can be supplemented with an IOL removal, exchange or repositioning, in order to remove chronic uveal insult by a malpositioned IOL in cases of chronic CME not responding to medical treatment.

PROPHYLAXIS

A large amount of clinical data[37, 46–48] has proven beyond doubt the benefit of prophylactic management of this condition. This is becoming possible with the increasing number of topical NSAIDs that are being made available today. Topical drugs useful for this purpose include 0.1 percent diclofenac sodium, 1 percent indomethacin, 0.03 percent flurbiprofane and 0.5 percent ketorolac (ketorolac is relatively more effective than the others). There is a lowering in the incidence of CME—both clinical and angiographic, earlier recovery from the disease, better visual outcome and better functional visual status such as greater contrast sensitivity. In prone cases—with history of CME in the other eye—these agents are given from 2 to 3 days prior to the surgery till 3 to 6 months postoperative. They have very few side effects and the potential side effects of the steroids are absent. They are also well-tolerated topically.

REFERENCES

1. Irvine SR. A newly defined vitreous syndrome following cataract surgery. Am J Ophthalmol 1953;36:599-19.
2. Gass JDM, Norton EWD. CME and papilledema following cataract extraction. Arch Ophthalmol 1966;76:646-61.
3. Gass JDM, Norton EWD. Follow up study of CME following cataract extraction. Trans Am Acad Ophthal Otolaryngol 1969;73:665-82.
4. Tso MO. Animal modelling of CME. Surv Ophthalmol 1984;28:512-19.
5. Sears ML. Aphakic CME—the pharmacology of ocular trauma. Surv Ophthalmol 1984;28:526-34.
6. Miyake et al. Active transport system of prostaglandins—clinical implications and considerations. J Cataract Refract Surg 1992;18:100-05.
7. Vinores SA et al. Immunohistochemical localization of BRB breakdown sites associated with post surgical CME. Histochem J 1994;26:655-65.
8. Schubert HD. CME—the apparent role of mechanical factors. Prog Clin Biol Res 1989;312:277-91.
9. Hikichi T et al. Course of vitreomacular traction syndrome. Am J Ophthalmol 1995;119:55-61.
10. Stern AL et al. Pseudophakic CME—a study of 50 cases. Ophthalmol 1981;88:942-46.
11. Klien EM et al. CME in the first week after cataract extraction. Am J Ophthalmol 1976;81:614-15.
12. Meredith TA et al: Perifoveal vascular leakage and macular edema after ICCE. Br J Ophthalmol 1976;60:765-69.
13. Hitchings RA et al: Aphakic macular edema—incidence and pathogenesis. Invest Ophthalmol 1975;14:68-72.
14. Irvine AR et al: Macular edema after cataract extraction. Ann Ophthalmol 1970;3:1234-40.
15. The Miami Study Group: CME and pseudophakic eyes. Am J Ophthalmol 88: 45-48, 1979.

16. Hitchings RA. Aphakic macular edema—a two year follow up study. Br J Ophthalmol 1977;61:628-30.
17. Moses L. Incidence of CME following cataract extraction and pseudophakos implantation—ICCE Vs ECCE Vs phacoemulsification. J Am Intraoc Implant Soc 1978;4:17.
18. Stark WJ et al. Intraocular lenses—experience at the Wilmer Institute. Ophthalmol 89: 104-08, 1982.
19. Binkhorst CD. 500 planned ECCE with iridocapsular lens implantation. Ophthalmic Surg 8: 37-44, 1977.
20. Worst JGF et al. The artificial lens—experience with 2000 lens implantations. J Am Intraocu Implant Soc 3: 14-19, 1977.
21. Jaffe NS et al. CME after ICCE and ECCE with and without IOL. Ophthalmol 89: 25-29, 1982.
22. Quentin CD et al. CME and visual acuity after ICCE and Choyce AC lens Vs ECCE and PC lens in the partner eye. Ophthalmologe 90(4): 364-66, 1993.
23. Taylor DM et al. Aphakic CME—long term clinical observations. Surv Ophthalmol 28: 437-41, 1984.
24. Kraff MC et al. The medallion suture lens—management of complications. Ophthalmol 86: 643-54, 1979.
25. Powe NR et al. Cataract patient outcome research team. Arch Ophthalmol 112: 239-52, 1994.
26. Colin J. Comparision of phacoemulsification and ECCE. Ophthalmologie 3: 233-34, 1989.
27. Kraff MC et al: Prophylaxis of pseudophakic CME with topical indomethacin. Ophthalmol 1982;89:885-90.
28. Nikica G et al: CME in AC IOL implantation following PC rupture. Doc Ophthalmol 1992;81:309-15.
29. Alpar JJ: On the table posterior capsulotomy and 1% sodium hyaluronate. J Cataract Refract Surg 1986;12:391-93.
30. Winslow RL et al: One year follow up of CME following IOL implantation. Ophthalmol 1978;85:190-96.
31. Wright PL et al: Angiographic CME after PC IOL implantation. Arch Ophthalmol 1988;106:740-44.
32. Bergman M: CME after complicated cataract surgery and implantation of AC IOL. Acta Ophthalmol Copenh 1994;72:178-80.
33. Spaide RF et al: Chronic CME and predictors of visual acuity. Ophthal Surg 1993;24:262-67.
34. Kraff MC et al: Factors affecting pseudophakic CME—five randomized trials. J Am Impl Soc 1985;11:380-85.
35. Shammas HJ: CME following secondary lens implantation. J Am Intraoc Impl Soc 1981;7:40-42.
36. Salzman J et al: Electrophysiological assessment of aphakic CME. Br J Ophthalmol 1986;70:819-24.
37. Ginsburg AP et al: Effects of flurbiprofen and indomethacin on acute CME—functional vision and contrast sensitivity. J Cataract Refract Surg 1995;21:82-92.
38. Ibanez HE et al: Prospective evaluation of the effect of CME on contrast sensitivity. Arch Ophthalmol 1993;111:1635-39.
39. Severin SL: Qualitative photostress testing for the diagnosis of CME. J Am Intraoc Impl Soc 1980;6:25-27.
40. Nussenblat RB et al: Macular thickening and visual acuity—measurement in patients with CME. Ophthalmol 1987;94:1134-39.
41. Menezo JL et al: Iris and macular angiography in intraocular implants. J Am Intraoc Impl Soc 1984;10:25-28.
42. Noble MJ et al: Oral fluorescein and CME. Br J Ophthalmol 1984;68:221-24.
43. Hee MR et al: Quantitative assessment of macular edema with OCT. Arch Ophthalmol 1995;113:1019-29.
44. Ruiz RS et al: Visual outcome in pseudophakic eyes with clinical CME. Ophthal Surg 1991;22:190-93.
45. Pollack A et al: CME following cataract extraction in patients with diabetes. Br J Ophthalmol 1992;76:221-24.
46. Rossetti L et al: Effectiveness of diclofenac eyedrops in reducing inflammation and the incidence of CME after cataract surgery. J Cataract Refract Surg 1996;22:794-99.
47. Solomon LD: Efficacy of topical flurbiprofen and indomethacin in preventing pseudophakic CME. J Cataract Refract Surg 1995;21:73-81.
48. Flach AJ et al: Prophylaxis of aphakic CME without corticosteroids. Ophthalmol 1990;97:1253-58.
49. Assil KK et al: Control of ocular inflammation after cataract extraction with rimexolone 1% ophthalmic suspension. J Cataract Refract Surg 1997;23:750-57.
50. Miyake K: Indomethacin in the treatment of postoperative CME. Surv Ophthalmol 1984;28:554-68.
51. Wolfensberger TJ et al: Membrane bound carbonic anhydrase in human RPE. Invest Ophthal Vis Sci 1994;35: 3401-07.
52. Tchah H et al: Lysis of vitreous strands with neodymium: YAG laser. Korean J Ophthalmol 1990;4:34-39.
53. Perez R et al: Argon laser photocoagulation in chronic clinical CME. P R Health Sci J 1993;12:109-13.
54. Harbour JW et al: Pars plana vitrectomy for chronic pseudophakic CME. Am J Ophthalmol 1995;120:302-07.
55. Dugel PU et al: Pars plana vitrectomy for intraocular inflammation related CME unresponsive to steroids. Ophthalmol 1992;99:1535-41.
56. Mackool RJ: Closed vitrectomy and the IOL. Ophthalmol 1981;88:414-24.
57. Federman JL et al: Vitrectomy and CME. Ophthalmol 1980;87: 622-28.
58. Fung WE: Anterior vitrectomy for chronic aphakic CME. Ophthalmol 1980;87:189-93.

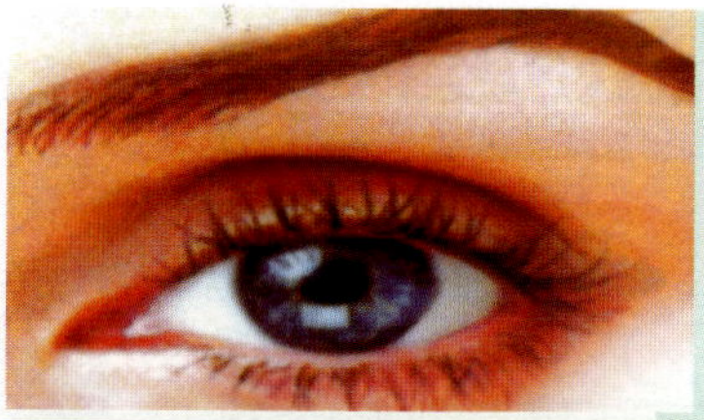

Forty seven

Favit—A New Method to Remove Dropped Nuclei

Amar Agarwal
Athiya Agarwal
Ashok Garg
Azimuddin Siraj
(India)

INTRODUCTION

Various techniques have been used to remove dropped lenses like the usage of perfluorocarbon liquids or the use of a needle. We have removed dropped nuclei by all these techniques. We have then devised our own technique of removing dropped nuclei which is a totally new concept. We have named this technique as Favit.

BASICS

Today, with phacoemulsification surgeries on the rise, the number of dropped nuclei are also on the rise. We have devised a new technique to remove these nuclei. Before we move into the technique, let us remember that phaco should not be done in the presence of vitreous. The reason is that if the vitreous fibrils get sucked into the phaco probe, it will also tug on the retina which can lead to a tear in the retina and retinal detachment.

PERISTALTIC VS VENTURI PUMP

Normally, when we perform three-port vitrectomy for macular holes or any other vitreoretinal pathology, we use the vitrectomy machine which has a venturi pump. In this, one hand holds the endoilluminator and the other the vitrectomy probe. This vitrectomy probe can do two functions: (i) of cutting, and (ii) of aspiration. The third port has an infusion cannula through which BSS (fluid) flows continuously.

If we use the same technique when we are managing dropped nuclei we have a problem. We have to make another port—in other words a third port for the fluid to pass through with the infusion cannula. The problem is that we perform clear corneal incisions under topical anesthesia. These cases will have to undergo a conjunctival cut and a sclerotomy to fix the infusion cannula. All this will have to be done under a peribulbar block.

To solve this problem, we decided to use the peristaltic pump in our Favit technique. In this, the advantage is that the vitrectomy probe has three functions: (i) cutting, (ii) aspiration, and (iii) of infusion. In other words, there is an infusion sleeve present which allows fluid to pass through. Another advantage is that every phaco machine (e.g. Alcon) also has a vitrectomy set up. If one is an anterior segment surgeon, he or she does not have to buy a separate vitrectomy machine. A peristaltic vitrectomy machine comes with the phaco machine.

The disadvantage of the peristaltic pump while performing vitrectomy is that if you take your foot of the pedal while aspirating it will still aspirate for some time. Whereas in a venturi system, the moment you take your foot of the pedal the suction immediately stops. The point is that if you are doing vitrectomy, with the peristaltic pump you should be careful that you do not create a retinotomy.

In the Storz machine, both vitrectomy and phaco are in the venturi system so there is no problem.

FAVIT TECHNIQUE

Let us now look at the technique of Favit. If you are doing phacoemulsification, you are either doing a clear corneal incision or a scleral incision. In the left hand, you have a chopper or a straight rod. If during surgery, there is a posterior capsular rupture and the nucleus drops into the vitreous, this nucleus will generally go and lie on the retina over the disk and macula (Fig. 47.1).

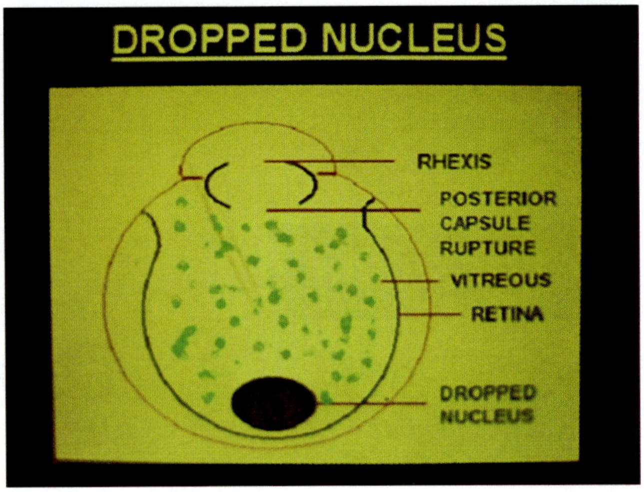

Fig. 47.1: Dropped nucleus—nucleus lying on the retina due to a posterior capsular rupture

First of all, go in with an irrigating aspirating probe and remove the cortex. Do this first, otherwise when you perform vitrectomy your visualization will get hampered with the cortex.

Then immediately convert to a vitrectomy setup. Ask the assistant to fix the vitrectomy probe to your phaco machine set up. In other words you will be using a vitrectomy probe with a peristaltic pump.

Now, pass the vitrectomy probe through the clear corneal incision or through the scleral tunnel incision you had made. This probe will pass into the anterior chamber and then pass through the posterior capsular rupture into the vitreous cavity. In the other hand, hold an endoilluminator and pass it through the side port opening. This will also go through the posterior capsular rupture into the vitreous cavity (Fig. 47.2).

Start the anterior vitrectomy. This can be done with the aid of the operating microscope light. Once the anterior vitrectomy is done, move downwards to perform a midvitrectomy. For this, off the microscope light and use the light of the endoilluminator. At this time, ask your assistant to place a contact lens on the cornea. Any contact lens can be used which is normally used for three-port vitrectomy. The assistant should be careful while holding the lens because the vitrectomy is being done through a clear corneal approach. The problem is

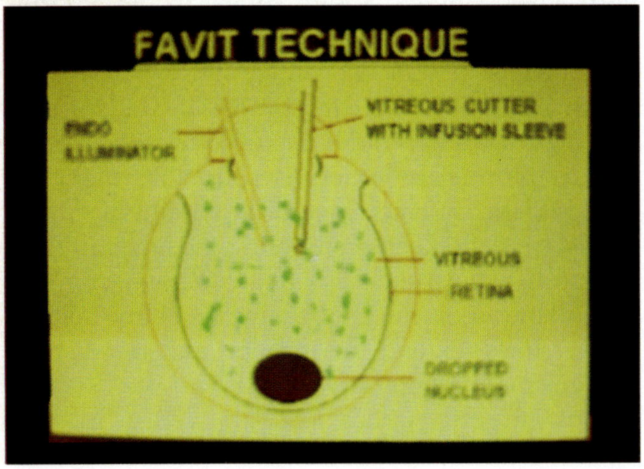

Fig. 47.2: Favit technique—note the endoilluminator and the vitrectomy probe with infusion sleeve are passed through the corneal incisions into the vitreous cavity through the posterior capsular rupture

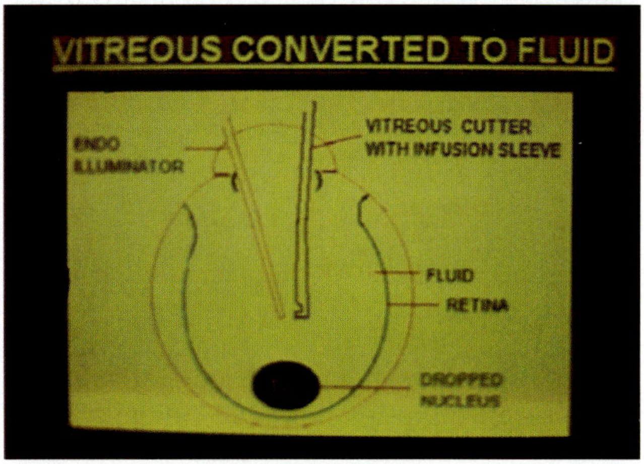

Fig. 47.3: Vitrectomy is done so that the vitreous is converted to fluid (BSS). Vitrectomy contact lens is placed on the cornea

that your vitrectomy and endoilluminator will be occupying a little bit of space of the cornea. So the assistant should push against your hands otherwise the visualization will be very bad

Once a midvitrectomy has been done, proceed to do a posterior vitrectomy. Clear all the vitreous fibrils around the nucleus. Watch the nucleus. There should be no vitreous fibrils around it. Another point one should note is to check the movement of the nucleus. When vitreous is around it the nucleus will not move much. When the vitreous gets cleared, the nucleus will start moving around a lot. This indicates that the nucleus is free of vitreous attachments (Fig. 47.3).

Once the nucleus is free of vitreous attachments, bring the vitrectomy probe out. Then shift to a phaco probe (Fig. 47.4). Once again in a phaco probe fluid will also pass through it. So, pass the phaco probe through the clear corneal incision and pass the endoilluminator through the side port. Keep the settings as 50 percent phaco power, 50 mm Hg suction and 18 ml/minute flow rate.

Once the phaco probe is over the nucleus apply only suction. The nucleus will then come towards the phaco tip. At that stage, when the nucleus touches the phaco tip apply a very small burst of phaco power which will embed the nucleus into the phaco tip (Fig. 47.5). This is just akin to doing a

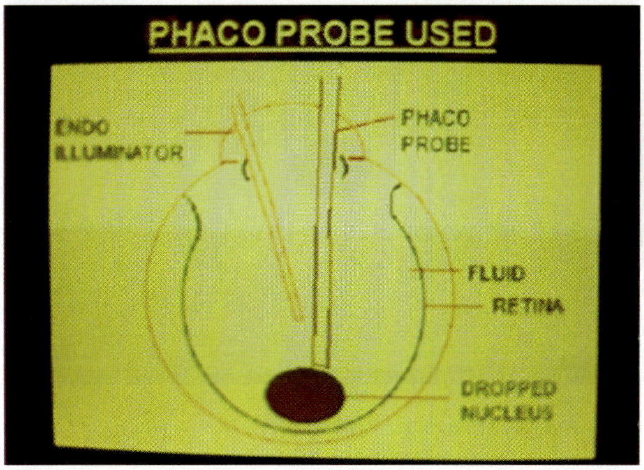

Fig. 47.4: Phaco probe is now passed into the eye

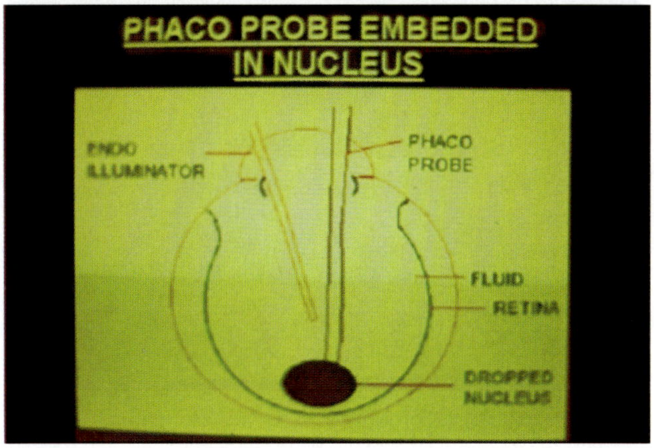

Fig. 47.5: Phaco tip embeds the nucleus

phaco chop when you embed the nucleus in the phaco tip. Once the nucleus gets embedded, it has been impaled. Lift the phaco probe anteriorly. The nucleus will also get lifted (Fig. 47.6). Bring the nucleus anteriorly above the iris. The nucleus will not fall back as it has been impaled in the phaco tip. All this time, keep your foot pedal in position 2. Position 3 is used only at one time for a fraction of a second when you are impaling the phaco tip into the nucleus.

When the nucleus is brought anteriorly, use the left hand with the endoilluminator to guide the nucleus above the iris (Fig. 47.7). At this stage, check the status of the nucleus. If the nucleus is not very hard, remove it with phaco in the anterior chamber. Do not use pulse mode, and do not chop the nucleus. If you use pulse mode the nucleus might fall back as there is a time in the pulse mode when ultrasound is not being used. Do not chop or divide the nucleus otherwise one-half might fall back into the vitreous cavity. Use continuous mode ultrasound and keep on nibbling the nucleus like a rat eating a piece of cheese. Start nibbling from one side till the whole nucleus is removed. If the nucleus is very hard, extend the incision and remove the nucleus manually.

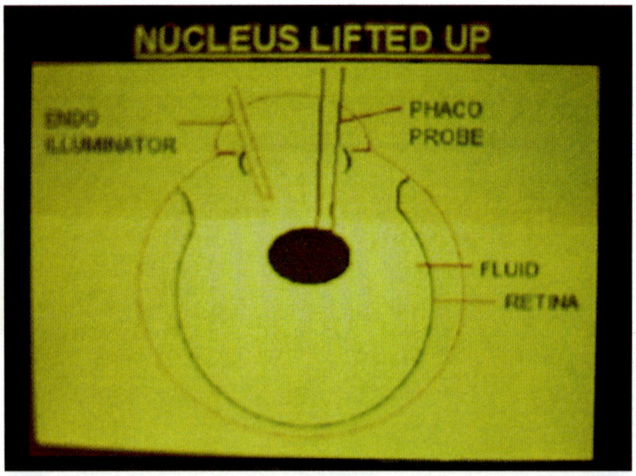

Fig. 47.6: Nucleus is lifted up by the phaco probe

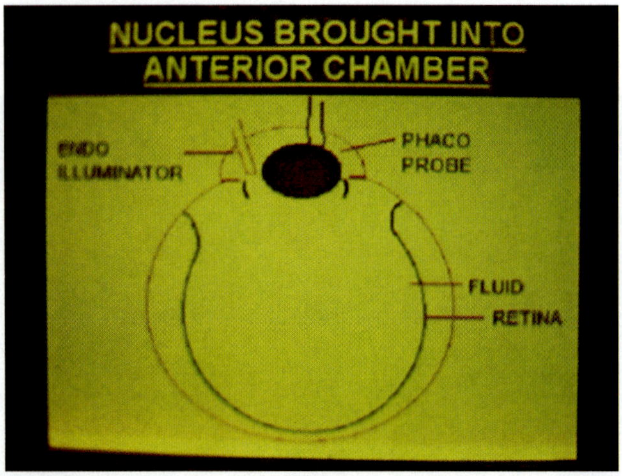

Fig. 47.7: Nucleus is brought into the anterior chamber. It can be removed manually (if a hard cataract) or by phacoemulsification (if a soft cataract)

Once the nucleus has been removed, go in again for a vitrectomy to see if any cortex or small fragment is left behind. If it has been left behind, remove it. Perform an iridectomy with the vitrectomy probe. Then inject viscoelastics, and implant a 6.5 mm nonfoldable PCIOL in front of the rhexis. Apply suitable sutures.

ANESTHESIA

If you have done your phaco under peribulbar, there is no problem, the case can just be continued and the nucleus retrieved. If you have done the case under topical, one can perform the Favit technique under topical anesthesia also. If you are not very confident, one can do a parabulbar anesthesia. In this just make a nick in the conjunctiva in the superotemporal quadrant. Take a syringe with xylocaine and a cannula. The cannula can be the one you are using for injecting viscoelastics. This cannula is then passed on the side of the globe till it reaches near the optic nerve. Inject one ml of xylocaine. Wait for a couple of minutes and then start the vitrectomy. The patient will not have any pain.

RESULTS

Phacoemulsification surgery is gaining immense popularity among ophthalmic surgeons, but unfortunately for those in their learning curve, is wrought with complications. The most dreaded of them all, is the dropped nucleus.[9] A variety of options are available to retrieve the dislocated lens from the vitreous. Notable are anterior floatation of the nucleus using perfluorocarbon liquids,[1,2,11,12] using

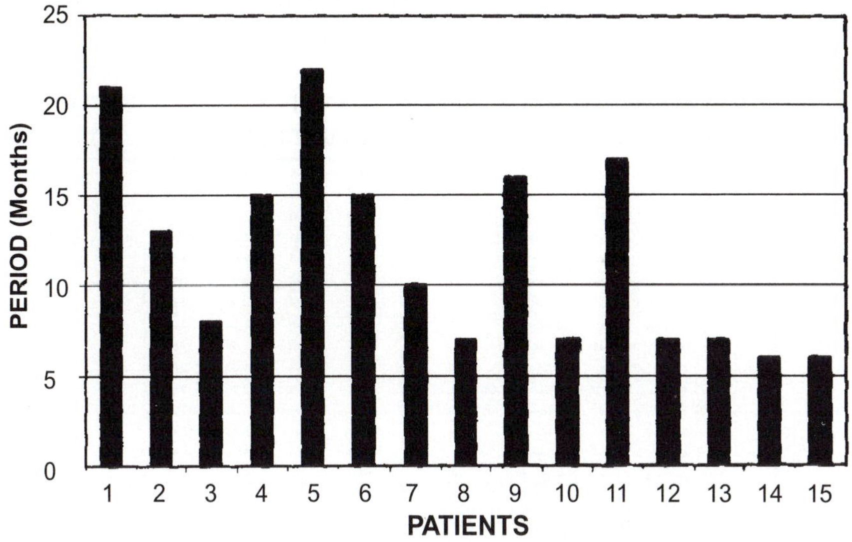

Fig. 47.8: Follow-up period

a vitrector,[3,5,8,10] three-port vitrectomy combined with midvitreous phacofragmentation,[7,9,13] and fragmatome dissolution of the lens.[6] We have designed and used a new technique called Favit-(PHAco combined VITrectomy) in the management of dropped nucleus which we have found safe and effective in our hands. We analyzed 15 of our consecutive eyes that underwent this technique over the last two years and are submitting our results in terms of best corrected visual acuity and complication rate.

The charts of 15 patients (Ten male and five female) who consecutively underwent the FAVIT technique of phaco dropped nucleus retrieval at our center were retrospectively analyzed. The patients were aged between 56 and 75 years (mean age 65.2 years). All the FAVIT surgeries were performed by a single surgeon (AA). Eleven of the eyes had undergone the FAVIT procedure in the same sitting as the primary phaco procedure and four of them had this done as a separate procedure though all were done on the same day. The mean age of the study group (Table 47.1) was 65 years (range 56-75 years). The average follow-up period (Fig. 47.8) was 11.8 months (range 6-22 months). The intraocular pressure did not rise more than 18 mm Hg in any of the eyes. Fourteen (93.33%) eyes had a BCVA of $\geq$ 20/100 (Fig. 47.9). Of the 14, 10 (66.66%) had a BCVA of $\geq$ 20/40. Two eyes (13.33%) went in for late corneal decompensation (one had a visual acuity of 20/200 and the other 20/100). One eye (6.66%) developed cystoid macular edema (CME) with a BCVA of 20/40 (Fig. 47.10). None of the 5 intraocular lenses decentered, and there were no late retinal complications like proliferative vitreoretinopathy or detachments.

DISCUSSION

Nucleus drop is a common complication occurring when surgeons learn phacoemulsification.[9] The nucleus cannot be left in the vitreous cavity because it incites a chronic inflammatory reaction, glaucoma and subsequent drop in final visual acuity.[3,4, 8-10] Popular among the treatment modalities presently done is anterior floatation of the nucleus using perfluorocarbon liquids,[1,2,11,12] especially in the management of hard nuclei. After a vitrectomy, perfluorocarbon liquids float the nucleus anteriorly because of their high specific gravity, and retinal damage is minimal.[2,12] Apart from the high cost, it necessitates a third port for infusion during vitrectomy and needs to be completely removed from the vitreous after the procedure, because it risks toxic effects on the retina, corneal decompensation and glaucoma.

Table 47.1: Retrospective study of Favit technique

TABLE - 1

S.No.	AGE	SEX	EYE	NUCLEUS GRADE	SURGERY DATE	COMPLICATION	IOL IMPLANTED	IOL DECEN-TRATION	IOP		FOLLOW UP PERIOD (MONTHS)	VISUAL ACUITY	
									PRE OP	LAST FOLLOW UP		PRE OP	LATE
1	65	F	RE	3+	12-Sep-96	CORNEAL EDEMA	PMMA	NIL	14.60	15.60	21	20/200	20/200
2	58	M	RE	2+ psc+	15-May-97	NIL	NIL	NIL	16.80	16.50	13	20/200	20/40
3	62	F	RE	2+psc+	19-Oct-97	CMO	PMMA	NIL	17.40	17.30	8	20/200	20/40
4	60	F	RE	2+	17-Mar-97	NIL	NIL	NIL	15.00	14.90	15	20/200	20/60
5	63	M	LE	2+	26-Aug-96	NIL	NIL	NIL	13.40	14.00	22	20/100	20/40
6	72	M	LE	4+	13-Mar-97	NIL	NIL	NIL	10.00	12.00	15	20/200	20/40
7	63	M	RE	3+	30-Aug-97	NIL	NIL	NIL	17.30	16.40	10	20/200	20/80
8	61	M	RE	2+	26-Nov-97	NIL	NIL	NIL	12.20	12.20	7	20/100	20/60
9	56	M	RE	4+psc+	04-Feb-97	NIL	NIL	NIL	17.30	17.00	16	20/200	20/40
10	75	M	RE	3+	19-Nov-97	NIL	NIL	NIL	11.60	12.00	7	20/40	20/30
11	70	M	LE	3+psc	17-Jan-97	CORNEAL EDEMA	NIL	NIL	12.30	13.10	17	20/200	20/100
12	74	F	RE	3+	14-Nov-97	NIL	NIL	NIL	17.30	17.50	7	20/200	20/40
13	68	M	LE	2+	29-Nov-97	NIL	PMMA	NIL	16.80	17.40	7	20/100	20/40
14	72	M	RE	3+	03-Dec-97	NIL	PMMA	NIL	17.10	17.60	6	20/200	20/40
15	59	F	LE	3+	12-Dec-97	NIL	PMMA	NIL	16.90	17.20	6	20/200	20/20

psc postenor sub-capsular cataract
CMO Cystoid macular edema
PMMA Poly methyl methacrylate intraocular lens
IOP Intra-ocular pressure

Section 3

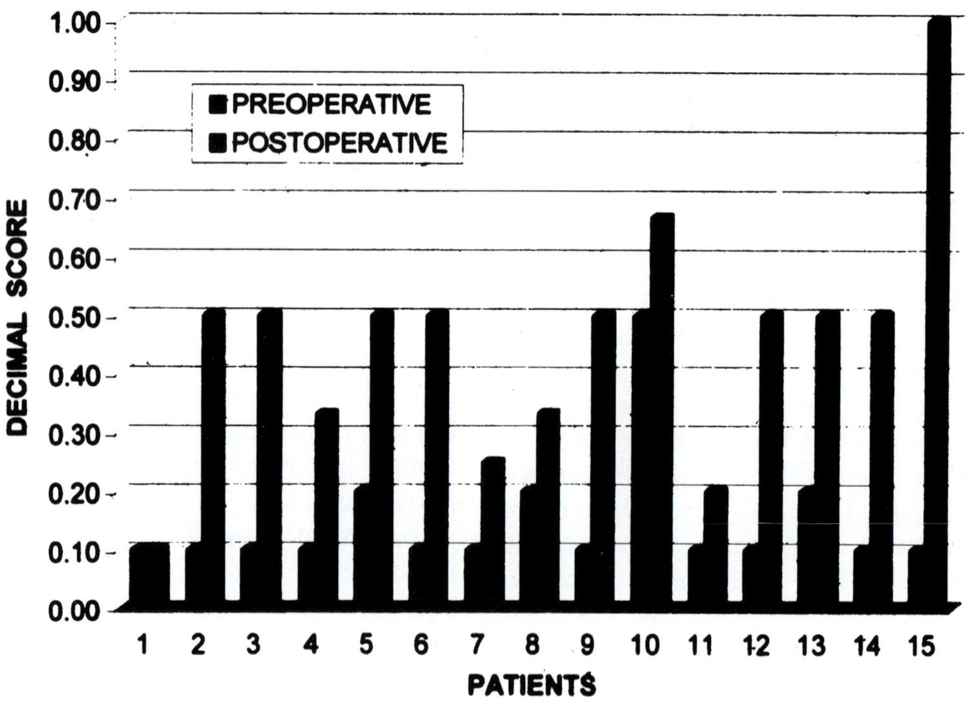

Fig. 47.9: Visual acuity

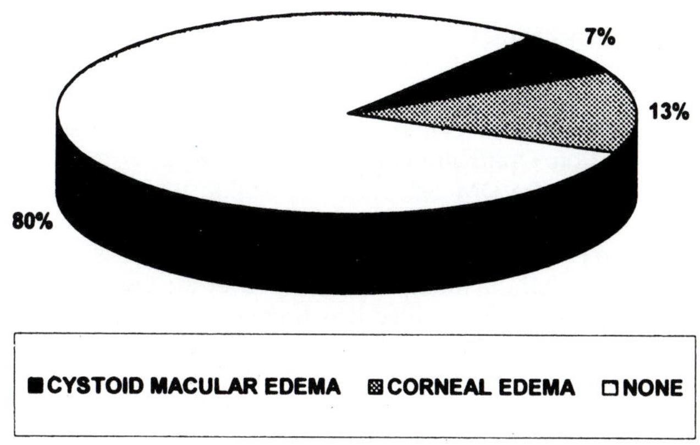

Fig. 47.10: Complications

A vitrector[3,5,8,10] is an effective method of removal of retained lens matter and is helpful in resolving chronic lens fragment induced persistent uveitis and glaucoma. This necessitates three ports of entry and is difficult in cases of hard nuclei and risks retinotomy.[5] Fragmatome dissolution,[6] another popular technique also requires three ports of entry and risks retinotomy, especially in cases of dense nuclear sclerosis.

A three-port vitrectomy combined with midvitreous phacoemulsification,[7,9,13] though safe to the cornea, risks ultrasound induced CME retinal damage,[12] and surgical time is prolonged due to repeated nucleus fall back during the procedure.[2,13]

We believe FAVIT provides several advantages over currently used techniques. All the above mentioned techniques use a three-port vitrectomy through the pars plana. Ours is a two-port cover vitrectomy using the existing ports (corneal / scleral tunnel and chopper side-port) of the primary phaco procedure. So, in FAVIT, there is no separate conjunctival incision, sclerotomy and its complications like choroidal effusion. In addition, the surgery can be continued after the nucleus drop as the change over time is short.

We could perform a two-port vitrectomy because our vitrectomy probe was connected to a peristaltic pump. This probe served three functions—infusion (through the infusion sleeve around it), cutting and aspiration. Normally, when vitrectomy is performed, a vitrectomy machine with venturi pump will be used. In this, one hand holds the endoilluminator and the other, the vitrectomy probe. This vitrectomy probe with the venturi unit does only two functions—cutting and aspiration. A third port for an infusion cannula is needed.

As phacoemulsification cannot normally be done in the vitreous cavity because of risk of vitreous incarceration,[4,6] we first converted the vitreous gel into fluid by performing the two-port core vitrectomy. While impaling the nucleus with phaco, it was brought up to the port by suction, and there was no thrust on the retina as it now was in a fluid filled cavity. The chances of an accidental retinotomy was minimal because of the cushioning effect of the nucleus. As it was elevated *in toto*, there is no retinal risk associated with scattered nuclear fragments as in a fragmatome. The lens was brought anterior to the iris and was stabilized by the endoilluminator providing better control during subsequent phacoemulsification. This technique is fast even in dense nuclear sclerosis, as the nucleus is elevated first *in toto* and subsequently taken out by enlarging the entry incision of the primary phacoemulsification procedure, minimizing the phaco energy used within the eye. Further, since most phacoemulsification machines are provided with a peristaltic pump, the change over is easy, and the need for a separate venturi unit is not there. This technique is cheap, and does risk any toxicity as in perfluorocarbon liquids.

We find this technique safe and effective in our hands. The complication rate is extremely low and the postoperative vision is good. Only one of the eyes developed CME and the final best corrected visual acuity (BCVA) was 20/40. The cornea decompensated in two eyes. The primary procedure in these cases was performed by a surgeon in his or her phacoemulsification learning curve, and hence, the decompensation could not be directly attributable to the FAVIT procedure.

SUMMARY

Whenever one discusses whether one can do phaco in the vitreous cavity, the answer is an absolute no. The reason is that the vitreous fibrils get entangled in the phaco probe and as they are connected to the retina they pull on the retina producing a rhegmatogenous retinal detachment.

What we are doing is different. We are first of all performing a vitrectomy. We have now converted the vitreous into saline or BSS (balanced salt solution) depending on the irrigating fluid being used. The nucleus is now lying on the retina surrounded by fluid. In other words, the retina is akin to the posterior capsule. It is just like the nucleus lying on the posterior capsule surrounded by aqueous humor or fluid.

Now, what we are doing is just taking of the nucleus like we would do it in the anterior chamber. We are using suction and then very little phaco power to embed the nucleus. The nucleus is brought anteriorly and then removed. The chances of tears occurring in the retina are not there because we have first converted the vitreous into fluid.

Another point to note is since we are doing a two-port vitrectomy, we need not make the third port which makes things more messy. This is the reason why we use the peristaltic pump of the phaco machine and not a separate venturi vitrectomy machine.

REFERENCES

1. Shapiro MJ, Resnik KI, Kim SH et al: Management of the dislocated crystalline lens with a perfluorocarbon liquid. Am J Ophthalmol 1991;112: 401-05.
2. Lewis H, Blumenkranz S, Chang S: Treatment of dislocated crystalline lens and retinal detachment with perfluorocarbon liquids. Retina 1992;12:299-304.
3. Magherio RR, Magherio AR, Pendergast Scott D et al: Vitrectomy for retained lens fragments after phacoemulsification. Ophthalmology 1997;104:1426-32,
4. Fastenburg DM, Schwartz PL, Shakin JL: Management of dislocated nuclear fragments after phacoemulsification. Am J Ophthalmol 1991;112:535-39.
5. Borne MJ, Tasman W, Regillo C et al: Outcomes of vitrectomy for retained lens fragments. Ophthalmology 1996;103:971-76.
6. Lambrou FH (Jr), Stewart MW: Management of dislocated lens fragments during phacoemulsification. Ophthalmology 1992;99:1260-62.
7. Kapsuta MA, Chen JC, Wai-Ching Lam: Outcomes of dropped nucleus during phacoemulsification. Ophthalmology 1996;103:1184-87.
8. Gilland GD, Hutton WL, Fuller DG: Retained intravitreal lens fragments after cataract surgery. Ophthalmology 1992;99:1263-69.
9. Topping TM: Retained intravitreal lens fragments after cataract surgery. Ophthalmology 1992;99:1268.
10. Blodi BA, Flynn HW (Jr), Blodi CF et al: Retained nuclei after cataract surgery. Ophthalmology 1992;99:41-44.
11. Rowson NJ, Bacon AS, Rosen PH: Perfluorocarbon heavy liquids in the management of posterior dislocation of the lens nucleus during phakoemulsification. Am J Ophthalmology 1992;76:169-70.
12. Movshovich A, Berrocal M, Chang S: The protective properties of liquid perfluorocarbons in phacofragmentation of dislocated. Retina 1994;14:457-62.
13. Charles S: Vitreous Microsurgery (2nd edn) Williams and Wilkins: Baltimore, 1987;48-51.

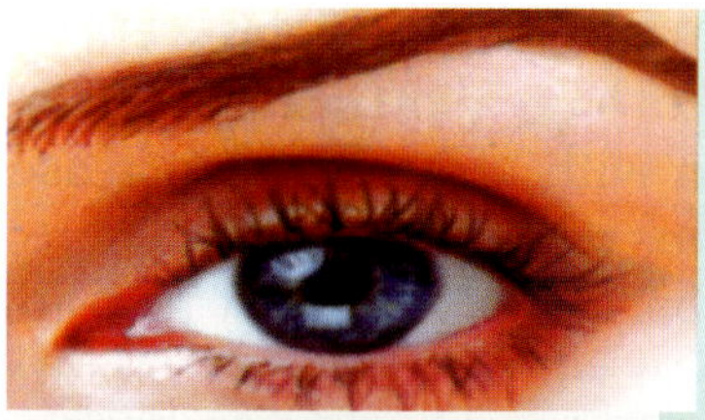

Forty eight

Management of Nucleus Prolapse in Manual Small Incision Cataract Surgery

Venkatesh Rengaraj
RD Ravindran (India)

Manual SICS involves the manual removal of nucleus through a scleral tunnel.[1,2] To achieve this one has to safely prolapse the nucleus from the capsular bag into the anterior chamber. As is the case with most surgical techniques, this looks simple when one observes an experienced surgeon performing the prolapse. But there are few hurdles for the beginners; this does not imply that it is a difficult step. It is just a matter of learning few techniques and of course lot of practice.

The technique of nucleus prolapse into the anterior chamber depends on the type of capsulotomy done. Either a canopener or a capsulorhexis can be performed to prolapse the nucleus. As there are more advantages of having an intraocular lens in the bag it is preferable to prolapse the nucleus from the capsular bag through a capsulorhexis with an intact rim.

NUCLEUS PROLAPSETHROUGH CANOPENER CAPSULOTOMY

With can opener capsulotomy the nucleus can be prolapsed mechanically without any of the hydro procedures. The simple Sinskey hook or the lens dialer is used for performing this step. The hook is placed at the edge of the equator or slightly posterior to it at the 12 o'clock position by retracting the pupillary border of the iris. The nucleus is then pushed down towards 6 o'clock till the superior equator of the nucleus clears the pupillary margin. At this point the nucleus is lifted up using the shaft of the hook and rotated so that the superior pole of the nucleus gets prolapsed over the iris. Once one part of the nucleus is out, it is engaged and rotated either in a clockwise or anti-clockwise direction, until the whole nucleus is in the anterior chamber.

Some surgeons find it easier to engage the nucleus at the 9'oclock position to perform the step described above. In patients with white cataracts, the loose and fluffy superficial cortex is aspirated exposing the firm nucleus underneath, before prolapsing it mechanically with the Sinskey hook.

This technique is ideal for surgeons converting from ECCE with sutures to Manual SICS, who are yet to master capsulorhexis. With canopener capsulotomy we loose the advantages of having intraocular lens in an intact bag. In addition with the manipulation of nucleus and subsequent contact with the iris tissue during prolapse we often find the pupil constricted resulting in difficulty during aspiration of the lens matter.

NUCLEUS PROLAPSETHROUGH CAPSULORHEXIS

Prolapsing the nucleus into anterior chamber after capsulorhexis using fluid (**Hydroprolapsing method)** is a crucial step. Normally hydrodissection or fluid injection underneath the capsule breaks the adhesions between cortex and capsule.[3,4] Here, we use the same step for creating hydrostatic pressure within the bag without putting any stress on the zonules to prolapse the nucleus.[5]

First prerequisite is an adequate sized rhexis. The margin of the rhexis is highly elastic and can allow safe expression of nucleus, which is larger than the opening.[6-10] Hydroprolapsing method is safe when the diameter of the rhexis is 5 mm or more.[11,12] Getting a right sized capsulorhexis is crucial and its significance in small incision cataract surgery cannot be overemphasized. With smaller or incomplete rhexis, it is safer to make a few relaxing cuts and proceed as described under canopener capsulotomy. If one is experienced and skill permits, one can go in for a double rhexis. Second prerequisite is to have a soft eye. Overfilling the anterior chamber with viscoelastic increases the resistance to nucleus prolapse. Partially emptying the anterior chamber of viscoelastic by pressing the floor of the incision with shaft of the cannula will permit the nucleus to easily prolapse.

Partial Hydroprolapse and Wheeling

Hydrodissection is usually done at 9 or 3 O' clock position and the fluid injection is continued without decompressing the bag as in phacoemulsification, until one part of the equator of nucleus is forced out of the rhexis. The purpose of continued injection of fluid is to increase the hydrostatic pressure within the bag to pop out the nucleus. This maneuver is safe, as the posterior capsule can withstand a pressure of 59+/- 10 mm Hg without rupturing.[12] Once part of the equator is out, hydroprolapse is stopped (Fig. 48.1). Viscoelastic is injected beneath the exposed equatorial region. Then using a Sinskey hook the nucleus is wheeled either clockwise or anticlockwise to bring the whole nucleus into the anterior chamber (Fig. 48.2).

Intracapsular Flip

In this technique of intracapsular flip, hydrodelineation or fluid injection between the hard nucleus and epinucleus is performed prior to hydro-

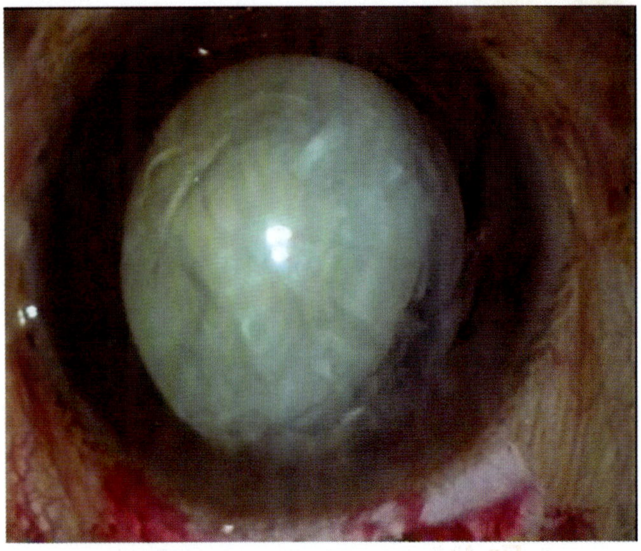

Fig. 48.1: Partial prolapse of the nucleus over the iris

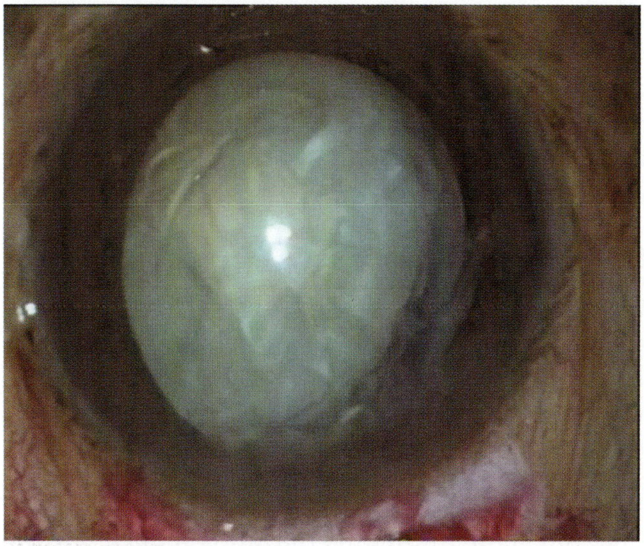

Fig. 48.2: Completion of the prolapse using a Sinskey hook

prolapse. It helps in minimizing the size of the nucleus facilitating easy maneuverability of the nucleus and also creates a soft epinuclear shell protecting the posterior capsule during the flipping procedure. Here again the hydroprocedures are continued until one part of the equator of the nucleus is forced out of the bag. Then by using the same hydrodissection cannula, the part of the equator opposite to the prolapsed area is rotated towards the posterior capsule (Fig. 48.3). The maneuver is continued through 180 degrees within the

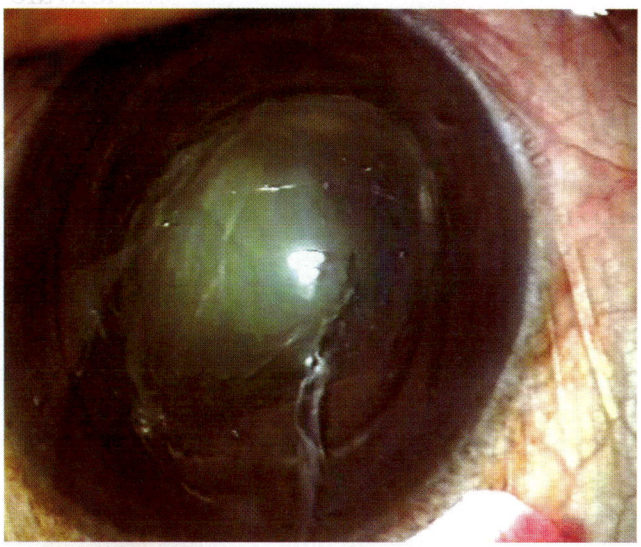

Fig. 48.3: Intracapsular flip in progress

capsular bag (flipping of the nucleus), till it comes out of the bag, into the anterior chamber. The use of hydrodissection cannula to flip the nucleus within the capsular bag is safe as only the shaft of the cannula comes in contact with the epinucleus.

The manipulation of nucleus during intracapsular flip has minimal contact with uveal tissue. Hence, if one masters this technique, it will be possible to prolapse the nucleus without altering the size of the pupil, thereby epinucleus and cortex can be swiftly removed. In addition the whole process of nucleus prolapse is achieved using a single instrument, resulting in lesser surgical time. This technique is not safe in eyes with very hard cataracts or poor zonular support.

TECHNIQUES FOR SPECIFIC TYPE OF CATARACTS

Mature Cortical Cataracts

White cataracts can be managed by doing a capsulorhexis after staining the capsule with 0.1ml of 0.06% trypan blue dye.[13] Nucleus can be levered out of the bag using a sinskey hook even without hydroprocedures, if the cortical attachment is loose with the nucleus. It will be also worthwhile to debulk the cortical matter using a simcoe cannula before prolapsing the nucleus. The staining here not only helps for the rhexis but also for the safe prolapse of the nucleus without damaging the zonules (Fig. 48.5).

Hypermature Cataracts

Here again after staining the capsule, a small trap door is created in the anterior capsule. Through this trap door the liquid cortex is aspirated using a Simcoe cannula. The capsular bag with the nucleus is inflated with viscoelastics and then a capsulorhexis is completed. As described earlier the nucleus can be safely prolapsed using a Sinskey hook or even a Simcoe cannula by flipping, if the nucleus is small as seen in Morgagnian cataracts.

Hard brown/black Cataracts

In these cases the safest technique will be to perform a canopener capsulotomy and prolapse as described

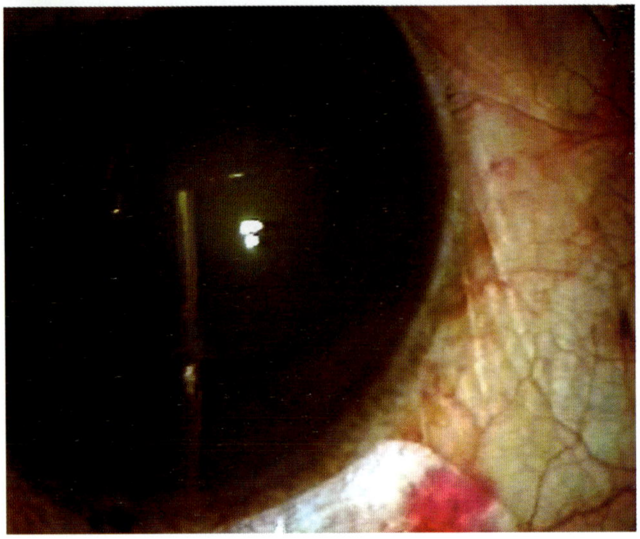

Fig. 48.4: Nucleus lying in the anterior chamber

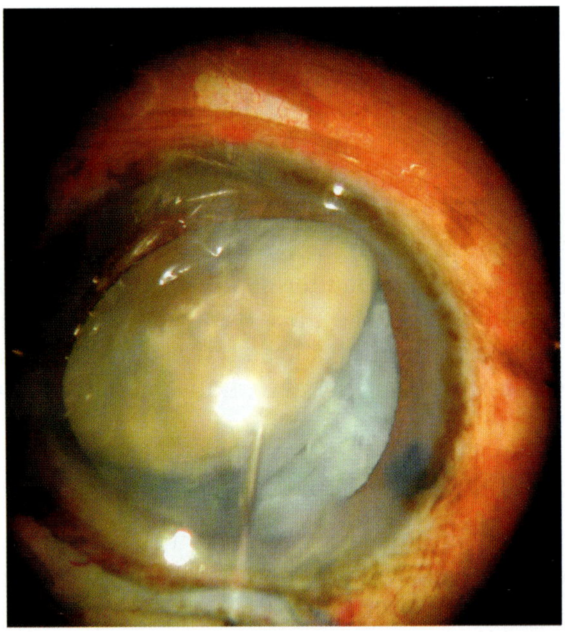

Fig. 48.5: Trypan blue assisted nucleus prolapse in white cataract

earlier. If the surgeon is keen to perform a capsulorhexis, it will be safe to stain the capsule and perform a larger capsulorhexis (6.0 - 6.5mm) followed by less forceful hydrodissection. As the capsule is stained, it will be easy to retract the capsule and lever out a part of the nucleus with a sinskey hook. Then gently wheel the nucleus out, watching the movement of the capsular bag throughout the procedure. If the capsular bag seems to be compromised few relaxing incisions in the capsule can avoid intracapsular extraction of nucleus. Alternatively a bimanual technique can be tried which is described under the small pupil approach.

Small Pupil Approach

One can resort to procedures like stretch pupilloplasty with Kuglen's hooks or sphincterotomies. In certain high-risk cases like pseudoexfoliation with a small rigid pupil and an associated hard nucleus it would be prudent to go in for a small sector iridectomy or a key hole iridectomy. In case it is a pliable small pupil and one's aesthetic sense does not allow mutilating the pupil, there is still an alternative technique, namely what we have termed *the bimanual technique.* This technique is useful if one has failed to prolapse the nucleus by the mechanical method or in case of a small pupil with hard cataracts.

Bimanual Technique

Normally a canopener capsulotomy is prefered and two instruments are used for bimanual prolapse. One is a Sinskey hook in the right hand and the other a cyclodialysis spatula in the left. As described before, with the Sinskey hook the nucleus is pushed towards 6 O' clock. Once the superior part of the nucleus is visualized the cyclodialysis spatula is inserted under it, either through the main wound or through the paracentesis. The exposed part of the nucleus is then tipped up with the spatula. The role of the spatula is not only to tip out the superior pole but also to act as a fulcrum over which the nucleus is rotated out. The nucleus is dialed out by repeatedly engaging the equator with the Sinskey hook till the nucleus cmpletely prolapses into the anterior chamber.

Subluxated Cataracts

Manual SICS can be done in selected cases of subluxated cataracts where in the pupil is well dilated and nucleus is not very hard.[14] Here again staining the capsule with trypan blue stain will facilitate in capsulorhexis as well as in implanting the CTR and in safely prolapsing the nucleus.

Technique

After assessing the extent of subluxation and density of nucleus, the capsule is stained, capsulorhexis is followed by cortical cleaving hydrodissection, and CTR is inserted manually through the paracentesis. The nucleus is then hydrodelineated and irrigation continued until one pole of the nucleus prolapses out of the capsular bag. Rest of the nucleus is wheeled into the anterior chamber using a Sinskey hook.

SUMMARY

To summarize the technique of nucleus prolapse requires only simple instrumentation, namely a Sinskey hook and a 2 ml syringe with a 26 G cannula. During the learning process one can perform the canopener capsulotomy and prolapse the nucleus mechanically. For reasons discussed earlier, capsulorhexis with hydroprolapse or intracapsular flip is ideal as the surgeon masters the technique. Moreover, the management of white and brown cataracts has become easier with the availability of cost-effective capsular stains, which can be effectively used, and the whole procedure made safe.

REFERENCES

1. Bayramlar H, Cekic O, Totan Y. Manual tunnel incision extracapsular cataract extraction using the sandwich technique. J Cataract Refract Surg 1999; 25:312-315.
2. Akura J, Kaneda S, Hatta S, Matsuura K. Manual sutureless cataract surgery using a claw vectis. J Cataract Refract Surg 2000;26:491-96.
3. Thim K, Krag S, Corydon L. Capsulorhexis and nucleus expression. Eur J Implant Ref Surg 1990; 2:37-41.
4. Fine IH. Cortical cleaving hydrodissection. J Cataract Refract Surg 1992;18:508-12.
5. Assia E, Blumenthal M, Apple DJ. Hydrodissection and viscoextraction of the nucleus in planned extracapsular cataract extraction. Eur J Implant Ref Surg 1992;4:3-8.
6. Krag S, Thim K, Corydon L. The stretching capacity of capsulorhexis. An experimental study on animal cadaver eyes. Eur J Implant Ref Surg 1990;2:43-45.
7. Thim K, Krag S, Corydon Leif. Stretching capacity of capsulorhexis and nucleus delivery. J Cataract Refract Surg 1991;17:27-31.
8. Assia EI, Apple DJ, Tsai JC, Lim ES. The elastic properties of the lens capsule in capsulorhexis. Am J Ophthalmol 1991;111:628-32.
9. Assia EI, Apple DJ, Morgan RC, Legler UFC et al. The relationship between the stretching capability of the anterior capsule and zonules. Invest Ophthalmol Vis Sci 1991;32:2835-39.
10. Tana P, Belmonte J. Elasticity of the capsulorhexis and delivery of the nucleus. Eur J Implant Ref Surg 1993;5:103-08.
11. Vasavada A, Desai J. Capsulorhexis: Its safe limits. Indian J Ophthalmol 1995;44:185-90.
12. Krag S, Thim K, Corydon L. Strength of the lens capsule during hydroexpression of the nucleus. J Cataract Refract Surg 1993;19:205-08.
13. Melles GRJ, de Waard PWT, Pameyer JH, Beekhuis wh. Trypan blue capsule staining to visualize the capsulorhexis in cataract surgery. J cataract Refract Surg 2000; 26:1052-59.
14. Venkatesh R. Use of Capsular Tension Ring in Phacoemulsification. Indications and Technique (Letter). Indian J Ophthalmol 2003;51:197.

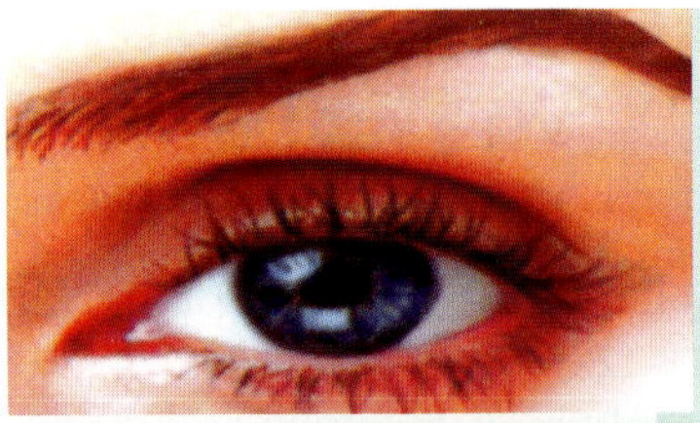

Forty nine

Management of Dislocated Lens and Lens Fragments by Vitreoretinal Approach

Clemant K Chan
Steven G Lin (USA)

INTACT LENS

The dislocation of the entire lens with an intact lens capsule is a rare occurrence. It is encountered in certain ocular conditions, such as Marfan's syndrome, homocystinuria, hyperlysinemia, Ehlers-Danlos syndrome, Weill-Marchesani syndrome, scleroderma, and trauma, etc. The lens subluxation is usually in an upward and temporal direction in Marfan's syndrome and Weill-Marchesani syndrome, while it is often downward in homocystinuria.[1] The intact dislocated lens rarely causes much intraocular inflammation, and the resulting refractive error can often be corrected with an aphakic contact lens without any surgical intervention. However, sometimes the ectopic lens may be associated with intraocular inflammation, glaucoma, retinal breaks, or a retinal detachment. Even in the absence of a sight-threatening intraocular problem, the movement of the ectopic lens with a change in body position may induce bothersome visual symptoms. In such a situation, the removal of the dislocated lens may be warranted.

LENS FRAGMENTS

The dislocation of partial lens fragments resulting from a mishap during phacoemulsification for cataract extraction is an uncommon but potentially serious complication in the clinical setting. When the lens fragments are minimal and are mostly of lenticular cortical material with minimal inflammation, the fragments may gradually resolve with conservative medical management (topical anti-inflammatory and sometimes hypotensive therapy with or without systemic therapy) without the need for surgical intervention. However, when the lens fragments are substantial, particularly with a major portion consisting of nuclear material, further surgical intervention is usually necessary.[2] In that situation, the persistence of the lens fragments may induce marked intraocular inflammation and ocular hypertension. The phacocytic response due to the released lens proteins may induce a type of phacolytic glaucoma (lens particle glaucoma). Either the free proteins or the protein-filled macrophages may block the trabecular meshwork outflow.[3,4] Increasing anterior segment and vitreous opacification may also occur. In an extreme situation, a phacotoxic or phacoanaphylactic reaction may occur, since the exposed lens proteins may be viewed by the body's immune system as foreign antigens.[5-7] If not treated, severe ocular complications such as the following may develop: persistent glaucoma induced by peripheral anterior synechiae, dense pupillary membranes, cystoid macular edema (CME), retinal detachments or injury, etc.[2-4] Thus most cases of dislocated lens fragments in the vitreous cavity after a cataract surgery require surgical intervention.[2,8-10]

TIMING OF SURGERY

Although a few studies advocate immediate surgery after the dislocation,[11,12] most reports indicate that the visual prognosis is not affected by a brief delay in surgery after the dislocation of the lens fragments.[13,14] Blodi reported that those patients undergoing surgery within 7 days experienced a significantly lower chance of long-term glaucoma.[12] However, most studies demonstrated that the timing of the surgery for removing the posterior lens fragments has little influence on the final visual outcome. Gilliland *et al* showed no statistical significance in the visual outcome and the incidence of glaucoma when the vitrectomy was performed at 0 to 7 days, versus 7 to 30 days, or more than 30 days after the dis-location of the fragments.[13] Kim *et al* also found no statistical differences in achieving a final visual acuity of 20/40 or better, when the lens fragments were removed within 7 days (70%), between 1 and 4 weeks (60%), and after 4 weeks (70%) following the dislocation.[14] Prompt intervention may allow the completion of all of the surgery at one time, while the cataract patient is still lying on the operating table. However, an appropriate informed consent may or may not be possible in that situation. The prompt removal of the lens fragments allows earlier visual rehabilitation and quicker resolution of the glaucoma and the intraocular inflammation.[11,12,14]

SURGICALTECHNIQUES

When there is posterior migration of a significant amount of lens fragments during cataract surgery, the anterior segment surgeon may proceed with the clean–up of the anterior cortical material.[11-15] If there is vitreous loss, an anterior vitrectomy may also be performed. Schechter previously described a technique of retinal visualization for the anterior segment surgeon by the placement of a glass slide on the cornea, before the removal of the lens fragments.[16] However, this approach is not comparable to the superior visualization and control provided by a standard 3-port pars plana vitrectomy.[11] Thus the best method for the removal of the dislocated lens or lens fragments is the vitreoretinal approach. The ophthalmic surgeon should be familiar with vitreoretinal techniques, and avoid "blindly" passing instruments into the vitreous cavity to retrieve the posterior lens fragments. Any attempt to irrigate the lens fragments out of the eye,[17] or to engage the lens fragments with sharp instruments from an anterior approach without a clear view of the posterior segment, may induce vitreoretinal traction leading to an intraocular injury. The insertion of a posterior chamber IOL (PCIOL) into the remaining capsular bag of the opened capsule should usually be avoided, since a subsequent IOL dislocation is likely. If it is safe to do so, a PCIOL designed for the sulcus fixation may be inserted, or an ACIOL may be placed, during the primary surgery. The placement of the IOL during the primary surgery obviates the need for the secondary IOL insertion at a later date. Previous studies showed that properly inserted IOLs during the primary operation do not adversely affect the visual outcome.[13-15] If there is a posterior dislocation of a large and rock-hard nuclear fragment, which may require its subsequent removal with a cryoprobe or perfluorocarbon liquids through a limbal incision, then the placement of an IOL should be avoided.[15]

Pars Plana Vitrectomy and Phacofragmentation

Proper vitreoretinal techniques with clear visualization of the posterior segment of the eye are required for the safe and consistent removal of the posteriorly dislocated lens fragments. A standard 3-port pars plana vitrectomy is performed. The cataract wound should first be inspected, as wound reinforcement with additional sutures may be necessary.[15] Any fluffy cortical lens material or hemorrhage in the anterior chamber, as well as adjacent to the implant and the iris is removed by the vitrectomy probe with caution, in order to avoid the inadvertent dislocation of the recently inserted implant.[2,15] Any fibrin membranes on the IOL surface may be peeled with a small needle with a bent tip, a microsurgical hook or forceps. Any herniated vitreous through the capsulotomy or pupil should also be removed with the vitrectomy probe. Posterior capsular remnants may be removed from eyes with pre-existing ACIOLs. If necessary, viscoelastic substances (VESs) may be injected into the anterior chamber to coat the corneal endothelium for the reduction of the striate keratopathy and the enhancement of the view through the cornea. Topical or subconjunctival mydriatics and cycloplegics, or intracameral epinephrine may be administered to prevent miosis.[2] A partial core vitrectomy is then performed to eliminate the formed vitreous, anterior to and surrounding the lens fragments, otherwise formed vitreous may plug up the phaco tip and induce vitreoretinal traction during the emulsification process.[2,8-15] The layer of vitreous under the fragments may be initially left in place to serve as a cushion for the fragments.

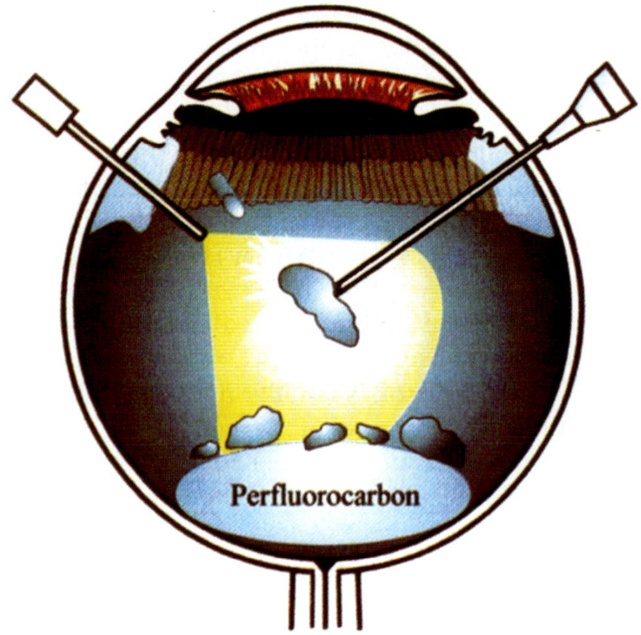

Fig. 49.1: The "aspiration-only" mode is activated on the phacofragmentation handpiece to engage the lens fragments for emulsification in the midvitreous cavity. A small amount of perfluorocarbon liquid protects the posterior retina from any injury by the lens fragments

Next, a phacofragmentation handpiece may be introduced through a pars plana sclerotomy to engage the lens fragments (Fig. 49.1). First the suction-only mode is activated on the handpiece to bring the fragments to the midvitreous cavity.[15,18] Soft lens fragments may be directly aspirated into the handpiece, while hard lens fragments require substantial ultrasonic emulsification before their aspiration.[13-15,18] The hard lens fragments may bounce from the tip of the handpiece and bombard the retina during the emulsification process. To protect the retina, a layer of perfluorocarbon liquid may be placed on the posterior retinal surface. Care must be taken to avoid placing a large amount of perfluorocarbon liquid, because it creates a convex meniscus, which tends to displace the lens fragments toward the peripheral retina or the vitreous base. Placing a layer of viscoelastic on top of the perfluorocarbon liquid neutralizes the convexity of the meniscus (Fig. 49.2).[19] One maneuver to stabilize the lens fragments is the use of a fiberoptic light pipe with a hook or pick to

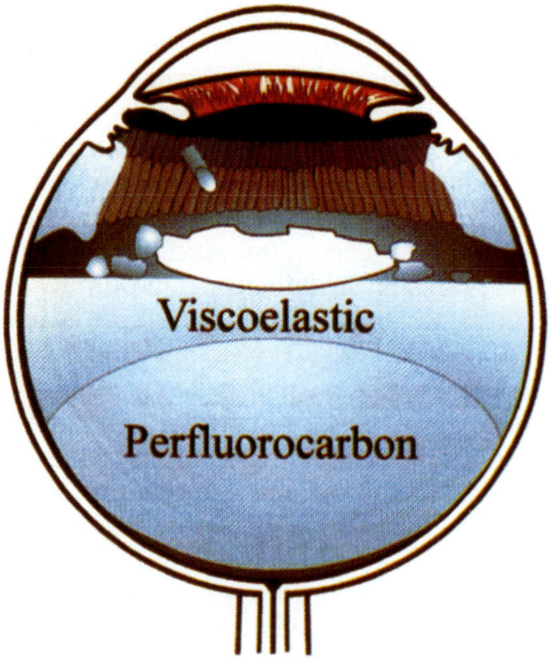

Fig. 49.2: A layer of viscoelastic is placed on top of the perfluorocarbon liquid to eliminate the convex meniscus of the perfluorocarbon liquid, thus recentering the lens fragments toward the visual axis (*Adapted from* Elizalde J [Poster] The Vitreous Society 17th Annual Meeting Rome)

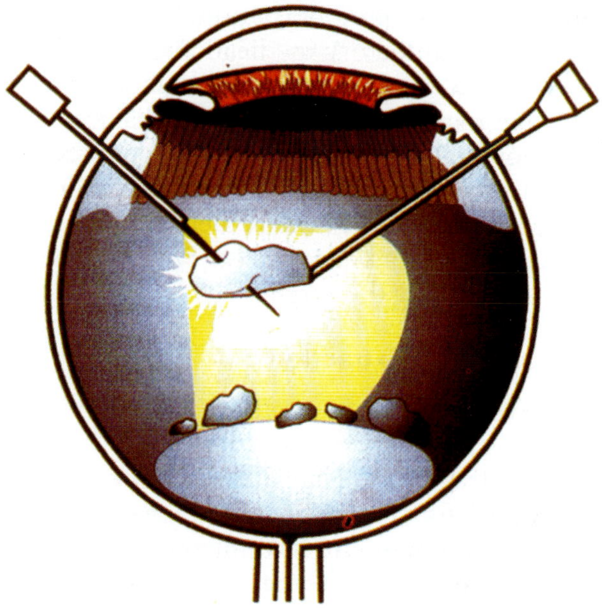

Fig. 49.3: A large lens fragment may be stabilized in the midvitreous cavity for emulsification by spearing it with a lighted pick

spear a large fragment, while the surgeon emulsifies the fragment with the handpiece held by his or her other hand (Fig. 49.3).[11] Employing a low level of ultrasonic power during the emulsification process decreases the tendency of blowing the lens fragments from the phaco tip.[15] The more advanced phacofragmentation units (e.g. Accurus) with proportional phacofragmentation capability also tend to reduce the erratic movement of the lens fragments on the tip of the handpiece. Another maneuver that allows the "controlled" removal of the lens fragments is the bimanual "chopstick" or "crush" method. With this technique, the surgeon gently crushes each lens fragment engaged on the tip of the phaco handpiece with the tip of the fiberoptic light pipe held with his or her other hand. The crushed fragment is easily aspirated, without falling from the handpiece (Fig. 49.4).[2,18]

Once, all of the loose lens fragments are removed, a more complete vitrectomy may be performed. Any residual lens fragments caught at the vitreous base may also be removed at this time.

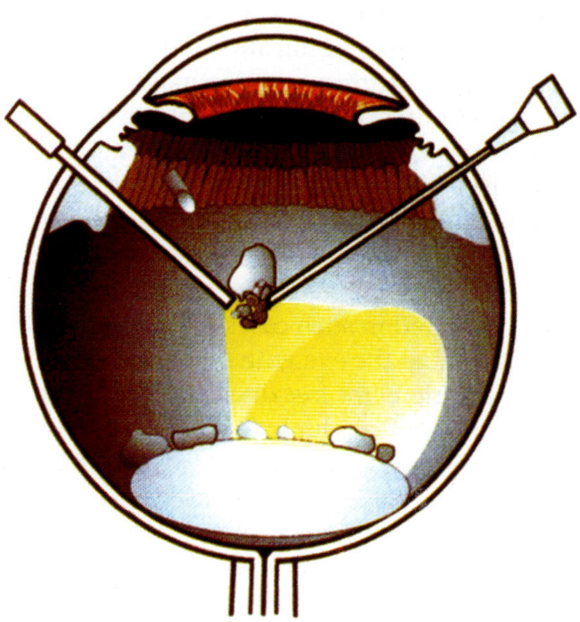

Fig. 49.4: The "chopstick" or "crush" technique involves crushing the engaged lens fragment with the tip of the light pipe against the phaco tip to facilitate the removal of the fragment without dropping it

Before closure, the entire retina including the periphery should be carefully inspected. Any retinal breaks or detachment must be properly treated.

During the postoperative period, topical antibiotic and antiinflammatory medications are applied to the operated eye. Utilizing the techniques described above in removing the retained or dislocated lens fragments, favorable visual outcome can be obtained in a large percentage of cases. Previous reports indicated the achievement of a final visual acuity of 20/40 or better in 52 to 87.5 percent of the eyes undergoing the surgery.[11,13,14,20]

Posterior Cryoextraction

The cryoprobe can be used for the removal of an intact dislocated lens or a large and rock-hard nuclear fragment. **This approach involves the insertion of a cryoprobe to engage the lens or a hard lens fragment for its removal through a large limbal incision, after a relatively complete vitrectomy and fluid-air exchange.[18,21,22]** However, this method can be hazardous. The required excellent visibility for monitoring the position of the cryoprobe and the associated ice ball to avoid complications may be difficult to achieve in an air-filled eye. The proper application of the cryoprobe to engage the lens sitting on the retinal surface, and avoiding the contact between the enlarging ice ball and the surrounding tissues, while bringing the engaged lens toward the corneoscleral limbus are often challenging tasks. The already poor visibility associated with the corneal haze due to prior excessive anterior segment surgical manipulation often encountered in such cases may become even worse after filling the eye with air.[22] In the process of engaging the lens, the freezing from the cryoprobe may spread to the residual vitreous fluid, and the adjacent soft tissues including the iris, retina, and choroid, resulting in a potential intraocular injury. Under certain circumstances, severe retinal necrosis, vitreous hemorrhage, and even choroidal or expulsive hemorrhage may occur.

Removal by Perfluorocarbon Liquid

Although the vitrectomy probe, microforceps, and phacofragmentation handpiece can be safely used to remove soft or moderately hard lens fragments,[8,9,15,18] they do not work well for removing large and rock-hard lenticular nuclear fragments. Ultrasonic fragmentation may be both difficult and unsafe due to the hardness of such lens nuclei and the often poor view through the hazy cornea and media associated with such cases.[22] Besides the posterior cryoextraction,[15,18,21,22] several other techniques for removing the hard nucleus have been reported.[22-24] They include the double-needle trapping of the nucleus after placing the patient in a prone position,[23] and injecting sodium hyaluronate under the nucleus to buoy it up toward the anterior chamber.[24] The needle-trapping technique is difficult to apply and may be hazardous.[22,23] The sodium hyaluronate technique requires clear visibility, and it may induce postoperative glaucoma.[22] Hypotony and miosis may also occur, as the fluid infusion must be turned off during the injection of the sodium hyaluronate.[22,24] In 1991, Shapiro *et al* reported the use of perfluoro-n-octane in the removal of hard lenses.[22] The details of this technique include an initial anterior cortical and capsular clean-up with the vitrectomy probe, followed by a vitrectomy, before the infusion of the perfluorocarbon liquid to float the hard lens fragment anteriorly. The hard lens fragment is allowed to be temporarily lodged between the anterior surface of the perfluorocarbon globule and the ciliary body or the iris. A soft-tipped cannula is then introduced through the sclerotomy to manipulate the lens fragment centrally behind the pupil. (Fig. 49.5A) After floating the recentered hard lens nucleus into the anterior chamber with gentle infusion pressure from the balanced salt solution (BSS), the lens nucleus is manually extracted from the eye with a lens loop via a limbal incision (Fig. 49.5B). The direct expulsion of the hard lens nucleus into the anterior chamber and out of the eye by filling the perfluorocarbon globule into the anterior chamber is not attempted, in order to avoid the mechanical abrasion of the corneal endothelium by the perfluorocarbon liquid and the hard lens nucleus. After the closure of the limbal wound, the perfluorocarbon liquid can be easily aspirated with a small-gauge cannula, due to its low viscosity and its tendency to pool posteriorly.[22] Since Shapiro's paper, several other authors also have reported on the successful removal of hard lens nuclei with various types of perfluorocarbon heavy liquids.[25,26]

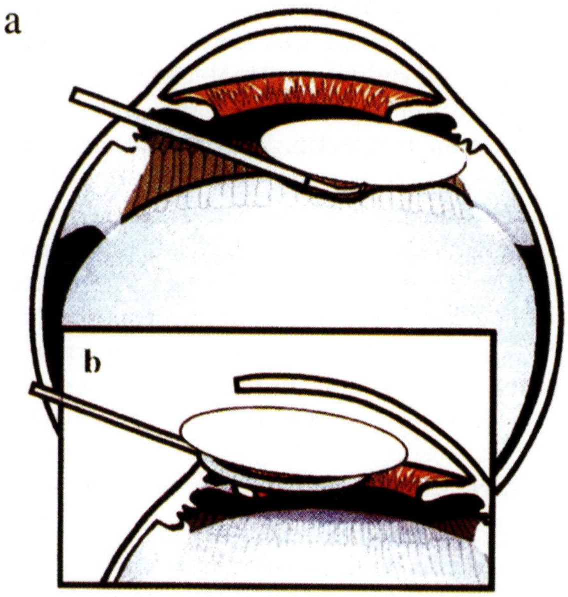

Figs 49.5A and B: (A) The hard lens or lens fragment lodged between the meniscus of the perfluorocarbon globule and the ciliary body or iris is brought centrally with a soft tip cannula, and (B) after floating the lens into the anterior chamber with gentle infusion of balanced salt solution, it is extracted from the eye with a lens loop through a limbal incision (Shapiro *et al Am J Ophthalmol* 112:401-05, 1991)

Thus, the main advantage of the perfluorocarbon liquid is that their high density, inert behavior, and low viscosity, allow the safe removal of the hard lens nucleus with minimal instrumentation, even when the visibility is poor.[22,25,26]

Removal by Endoscopy

In the presence of severe corneal densities, marked miosis, prominent iris synechiae, and IOL opacities, the direct visualization of the lens fragments may be difficult to accomplish through the conventional pars plana technology. In such situations, the endoscopic guidance of lens fragment removal provides a distinct advantage. Boscher *et al* reported a consecutive series of 30 eyes with dislocated lens fragments or IOLs, managed with the endoscopic techniques in 1998.[27] An endoscopic probe incorporated with a video monitor, a fiberoptic light source, and a diode laser was used. Under the endoscopic guidance, the dislocated lens fragments were emulsified with a pars plana phacoprobe, or removed through a limbal wound. In the same manner, the dislocated IOLs were either removed or fixated in the ciliary sulcus. The perfluorocarbon liquid was used in some cases.[27] The main advantages of the endoscopic techniques include: quick localization of the lens fragments embedded in the vitreous base, easy detection of small anterior retinal breaks, improved visualization of the anterior retropupillary structures for surgical manipulations (vitreous base, peripheral capsule, ciliary sulcus, etc.), and the lack of requirement of a clear cornea or ocular media. The main disadvantages of this technique include: the absence of stereopsis, the lack of a 3-dimensional "birds-eye" view, as well as a steep learning curve in mastering the manipulation of the endoprobe and the video monitor.[27]

DISLOCATED LENS FRAGMENTS ASSOCIATED WITH RETINAL BREAKS AND DETACHMENTS

The retinal breaks and detachments in eyes with dislocated lens fragments may be due to a direct retinal injury by the hard fragments, vitreoretinal traction induced by the vitreous loss, or excessive surgical manipulations during the primary cataract surgery.[2] The retained lens fragments may also be associated with vitreous hemorrhage and uveitis, factors that may increasingly exacerbate the vitreoretinal traction, inducing subsequent retinal breaks and detachments.[2] Standard vitreoretinal techniques are used to repair the retinal breaks and detachments after the removal of the lens fragments. Peripheral retinal breaks may be treated by laser or cryotherapy, while posterior retinal breaks are more safely treated with laser. When a retinal detachment is present, a scleral buckle may be placed to support the peripheral retinal breaks. Gas tamponade is utilized for a retinal detachment associated with posterior breaks, after a vitrectomy. When a giant retinal tear or an extensive retinal dialysis is present, the perfluorocarbon liquid may be necessary. Lewis *et al* advocated the use of perfluorocarbon liquids in the treatment of the retinal detachment in the presence of dislocated lens fragments, regardless of whether the retinal detachment is simple or complex.[28] In such a situation, the inert perfluorocarbon liquid serves the dual purpose of safely floating up the lens fragments for their removal, and simultaneously reattaching the elevated retina. After extracting the lens fragments and applying laser or cryopexy to the retinal breaks, the perfluorocarbon liquid can be easily removed. A long-acting gas or silicone oil is employed for severe retinal detachments with proliferative vitreoretinopathy. The earlier reports of dislocated lens fragments indicated a relatively high prevalence of associated retinal breaks or detachments (7 to 50%).[11,13] More recent reports showed a much lower prevalence (3 to 5%).[29] The decreased prevalence may be due to better attention by the anterior segment surgeons in minimizing surgical trauma at the time of the lens fragment loss, and/or improved surgical techniques by the vitreoretinal surgeons during the subsequent management.[29]

SUMMARY

A dislocated lens with an intact capsule may or may not require its removal. Surgical intervention is usually necessary for dislocated lens fragments, particularly when marked intraocular inflammation, glaucoma, or medial opacity is present. Lenticular nuclear fragments almost always need to be removed. The standard 3-port pars plana vitrectomy combined with modern phacofragmentation techniques constitute the best method of removing the posterior lens fragments. Spearing the large lens fragments with a lighted pick, crushing the fragments against the phaco tip, and utilizing the proportional fragmentation control facilitate the smooth removal of the lens fragments. Although a large posteriorly dislocated rock-hard lens or lens fragment may be extracted with a cryoprobe, the frequently poor visibility and the hazard of the expanding ice-ball associated with the cryoextraction may complicate the process. The inert behavior and special properties of the perfluorocarbon liquid make it the ideal agent for the safe removal of a hard lens or lens fragments in an atraumatic fashion. Endoscopy may be employed in the presence of marked corneal densities, severe miosis, prominent iris synechiae and implant opacities. It allows a clear view of the anterior retina and the vitreous base. However, the absence of stereopsis, the lack of a 3-dimensional birds eye view, as well as a steep learning curve are important disadvantages associated with the endoscopic techniques. When the dislocated lens fragments are associated with a retinal detachment, the perfluorocarbon liquid allows the simultaneous removal of the fragments and the reattachment of the retina. Utilizing modern vitreoretinal techniques for management, favorable visual prognosis is achieved for the majority of the eyes with retained or dislocated lens fragments. A large proportion of those eyes may recover a visual acuity of 20/40 or better. Although the timing of the surgery may not influence the final visual outcome, prompt surgical intervention allows earlier visual rehabilitation.

REFERENCES

1. Morris DA. Cataracts and systemic disease. In Tasman W, Jaeger EA (Eds): Duane's Clinical Ophthalmology, Lippincott-Raven Philadelphia 1996;5:13-14.
2. Fastenberg DM, Schwartz PL, Shakin JL et al. Management of dislocated nuclear fragments after phacoemulsification. Am J Ophthalmol 1991;112:535-39.
3. Epstein DL. Chandler and Grant's Glaucoma (3rd edn) Lea and Febiger: Philadelphia: 1986;320-31.
4. Epstein DL. Diagnosis and management of lens-induced glaucoma. Ophthalmol 1982;89:227-30.
5. Verhoeff FH, Lemoine AN: Endophthalmitis phacoanalphylactica. Am J Ophthalmol 1982;5:737.
6. Apple DJ, Mamalis N, Steinmetz RL et al. Phacoanalphylactic endophthalmitis associated with extracapsular cataract extraction and posterior chamber intraocular lens. Arch Ophthalmol 1984;102:1528.
7. Smith RE, Weiner P. Unusual presentation of phacoanalphylaxis following phacoemulsification. Ophthalmic Surg 1976;7:65.
8. Michels RG, Shacklett DE. Vitrectomy techniques for removal of retained lens material. Arch Ophthalmol 1977;95:1767-73.
9. Hutton WL, Snyder WB, Vaiser A. Management of surgically dislocated intravitreal lens fragments by pars plana vitrectomy. Ophthalmol 1978;85:176-89.
10. Ross WH. Management of dislocated lens fragments following phacoemulsification surgery. Can J Ophthalmol 1993;28:163-66.
11. Lambrou FH, Stewart MW. Management of dislocated lens fragments during phacoemulsification. Ophthalmol 1992;99:1260-62.
12. Blodi BA, Flynn HW Jr, Blodi CF et al. Retained nuclei after cataract surgery. Ophthalmol 1992;99:41-44.
13. Gilliland GD, Hutton WL, Fuller DG.Retained intravitreal lens fragments after cataract surgery. Ophthalmol 99:1263-67, 1992.
14. Kim JE, Flynn HW Jr, Smiddy WE et al. Retained lens fragments after phacoemulsification. Ophthalmol 1994;101:1827-32.

15. Topping TM. Discussion of Lambrou FH, Stewart MW. Management of dislocated lens fragments during phacoemulsification, and Gilliland GD, Hutton WL, Fuller DG. Retained intravitreal lens fragments after cataract surgery. Ophthalmol 1992;99:1268-69.
16. Schechter RJ. Glass-slide vitrectomy for use by the cataract surgeon [letter]. Am J Ophthalmol 1991;112:100.
17. Verhoeff FH: A simple and safe method for removing a cataract dislocated into fluid vitreous. Am J Ophthalmol 1942;25:725.
18. Charles S. Vitreous Microsurgery (2nd edn). Williams and Wilkins: Baltimore, 1987;48-51.
19. Elizalde J. Combined use of perfluorocarbon liquids and viscoelastics for safer surgical approach to posterior lens luxation. [poster] The Vitreous Society 17th Annual meeting, Rome, Italy, 1999.
20. Ross WH. Management of dislocated lens fragments after phacoemulsification surgery. Can J Ophthalmol 1996; 31:234-40.
21. Barraquer J. Surgery of the dislocated lens. Trans Am Acad Ophthalmol Otolaryngol 1975;76:44.
22. Shapiro MJ, Resnick KI, Kim SH et al. Management of the dislocated crystalline lens with a perfluorocarbon liquid. Am J Ophthalmol 1991;112:401-05.
23. Calhoun FP, Hagler WS. Experience with Jose Barraquer method of extracting a dislocated lens. Am J Ophthalmol 1960;50:701.
24. Haymet BT. Removal of dislocated hypermature lens from the posterior vitreous. Aust NZJ Ophthalmol 1990;18:103.
25. Rowson NJ, Bacon AS, Rosen PH: Perfluorocarbon heavy liquids in the management of posterior dislocation of the lens nucleus during phacoemulsification. Br J Ophthalmol 1992;76:169-70.
26. Greve MD, Peyman GA, Mehta NJ et al. Use of perfluoroperhydrophenanthrene in the management of posteriorly dislocated crystalline and intraocular lenses. Ophthalmic Surg 1993;24:593-97.
27. Boscher C, Lebuisson DA, Lean JS et al. Vitrectomy with endoscopy for management of retained lens fragments and/or posteriorly dislocated intraocular lens. Graefe's Arch Clin Exp Ophthalmol 1998;236:115-21.
28. Lewis H, Blumenkranz MS, Chang S. Treatment of dislocated crystalline lens and retinal detachment with perfluorocarbon liquids. Retina 1992;12:299-304.
29. Smiddy WE, Flynn HW Jr, Kim JE. Retinal detachment in patients with retained lens fragments or dislocated posterior chamber intraocular lenses. Ophthalmic Surg Lasers 1996;27:856-61.

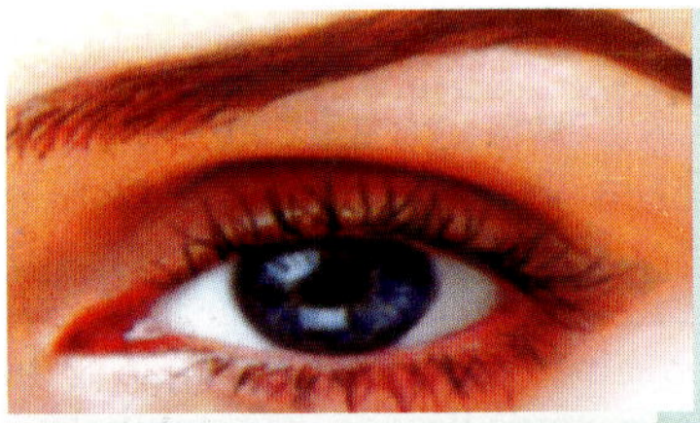

Fifty

Management of Dislocated Implants by Vitreoretinal Approach

Clemant K Chan
Gerald R Schultz (USA)

ANTERIOR CHAMBER INTRAOCULAR LENS (ACIOL)

Dislocation of the ACIOL into the vitreous cavity is relatively infrequent in comparison to the posterior chamber IOL (PCIOL). However, the ACIOL may dislocate during trauma, particularly in the presence of a large sector iridectomy. A subluxated or posteriorly dislocated ACIOL may be simply repositioned into the anterior chamber.[1,2] If the dislocated ACIOL is attached to formed vitreous or is sitting deep in the posterior vitreous cavity, an initial partial vitrectomy to eliminate the vitreoretinal traction is preferred before the repositioning or removal of the ACIOL.[2] If there is any substantial anterior segment injury associated with the dislocation (e.g. marked iridodialysis, large hyphema, excessive angle damage, etc.), it is best to remove the dislocated ACIOL through a limbal incision.

POSTERIOR CHAMBER INTRAOCULAR LENS (PCIOL)

Location of PCIOL Fixation

A dislocated PCIOL may occasionally be left undisturbed without causing a problem.[3] However, it is usually best to remove or reposition a posteriorly dislocated PCIOL to avoid a sight-threatening retinal injury. The removal of the dislocated PCIOL represents a simple and direct approach. Mittra *et al* reported favorable visual results and minimal complications with the removal of the dislocated PCIOL, and the implantation of an open-loop, flexible ACIOL at the same time.[4] Proper PCIOL repositioning provides the best potential for optimal visual rehabilitation. Past reports have described the repositioning of the PCIOL at various intraocular locations. McCannel first introduced the idea of a retrievable suturing technique for anchoring an IOL on the iris in 1976.[5] Stark described the anchoring of the subluxated PCIOL on the iris in 1982,[6] and Sternberg reported the attachment of the posteriorly dislocated PCIOL to the iris with the pars plana technology in 1986.[7] Girard advocated anchoring the PCIOL at the pars plana,[8] or imbricating the haptic loops into the sclerotomies with sutures.[9] Smiddy,[10] Campo,[11] and Anand[12] presented their versions of repositioning the dislocated PCIOL in the ciliary sulcus with a pars plana approach. The repositioning at the ciliary sulcus allows the dislocated PCIOL to be restored to a position most similar to the original state.

Opened Eye or External Approach

This approach involves modifications of various suturing techniques for inserting an external primary or secondary PCIOL—sometimes in association with aphakic penetrating keratoplasty, or with an IOL exchange, in the absence of appropriate capsular or zonular support.[13-23] The suture material can be easily tied to the externally located IOL before its reinsertion. A relatively large limbal incision is required for the externalization and the subsequent reinsertion of the dislocated PCIOL.

Closed Eye or Internal Approach: Pars Plana Techniques

This approach avoids the making of a large surgical incision that may induce undesirable astigmatism or tissue injury. The integrity of the globe is maintained, and the fluctuation of the intraocular pressure (IOP) is minimized throughout the case. However, many of the internal techniques require the passage of sharp instruments or needles into the eye, which sometimes can be associated with the risk of an injury to the intraocular structures. Relatively intricate intraocular maneuvers may also be involved. In recent years, a number of internal techniques for the repositioning of the PCIOL with a pars plana approach have become increasingly popular.[24-36]

Scleral Loop Fixation

In 1991, Maguire and Blumenkranz *et al* described the preparation of a 9-0 or 10-0 polypropylene suture loop by making a simple knot or a series of twists on the suture with a pair of microforceps.[24] The same microforceps are used to grasp the suture adjacent to the suture loop for insertion through an anterior sclerotomy corresponding to the location of the ciliary sulcus, after a partial pars plana vitrectomy to eliminate the vitreoretinal traction. The inserted suture loop is then used to engage one of the dislocated haptics for anchoring at the anterior sclerotomy. The same maneuver is repeated for the opposite haptic (Fig. 50.1).

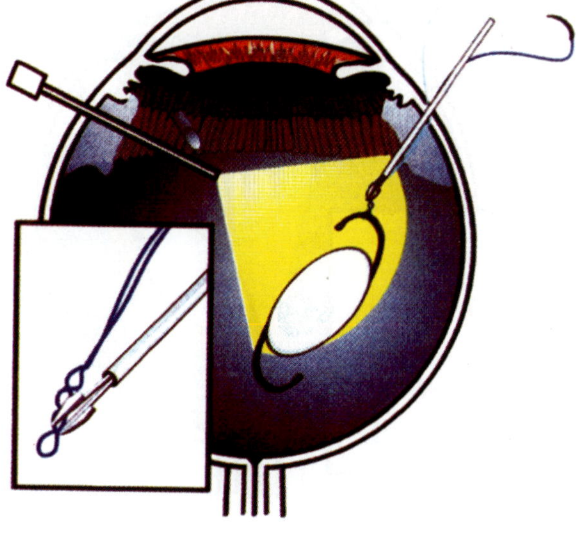

Fig. 50.1: The scleral loop fixation technique involves engaging the haptics of the dislocated PCIOL with a 9-0 or 10-0 polypropylene loop prepared by making a series of twists on the suture with forceps, followed by fixation in the ciliary sulcus (Maguire *et al: Arch Ophthalmol* 109:1754-58,1991)

The Grieshaber Snare

Grieshaber first manufactured a snare designed by Packo in the early 1990s. It consists of a 20 gauge tube and handle with a movable spring-loaded finger slide for adjusting the size of a protruding polypropylene loop. The distal portion of the tube with the polypropylene loop is inserted through an anterior sclerotomy for engaging a dislocated haptic in the vitreous cavity. Once the looped haptic is pulled up against the anterior sclerotomy, the external portion of the polypropylene loop is cut free and guided through a 30 gauge needle for anchoring by the anterior sclerotomy (Fig. 50.2). Little *et al* reported the successful transscleral fixation of the dislocated PCIOL with the snare method in a series of cases in 1993.[27]

Use of Perfluorocarbon Liquid

Various authors reported the removal of the dislocated crystalline lens or the management of the dislocated PCIOL with the aid of perfluorocarbon liquids in the early 1990s.[28-33] In 1993, Lewis and Sanchez described the following maneuver:[33]

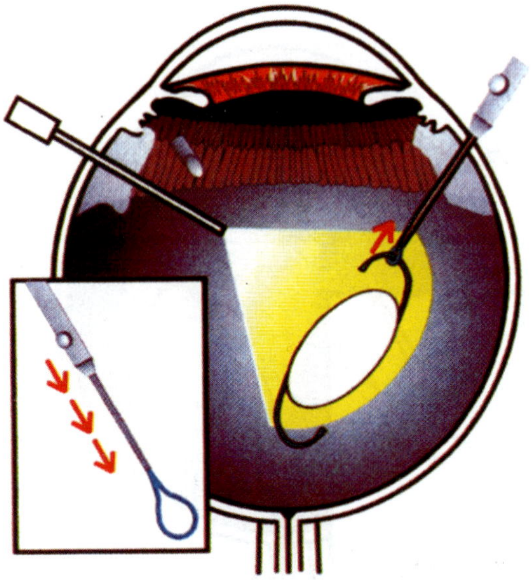

Fig. 50.2: The Grieshaber snare consists of a 20 G tube and handle with a movable spring-loaded finger slide for adjusting the amount of a protruding polypropylene suture loop. The suture loop is inserted posteriorly to engage a dislocated haptic. The external portion of the suture loop is then cut free and guided through a 30 G needle for anchoring at the sclera, after the engaged haptic is pulled up against the anterior sclerotomy

The perfluorocarbon liquid is first used to float the dislocated PCIOL anteriorly; then 9-0 polypropylene sutures are inserted through the horizontal anterior sclerotomies to engage the positioning holes of the optics at 90 degrees from the haptics, which are anchored in the ciliary sulcus along the vertical meridians (Fig. 50.3). This maneuver allows a four-point fixation associated with the proper centering of the IOL. However, not all of the optics have positioning holes. Care must also be taken to avoid infusing a large amount of the perfluorocarbon liquid, which tends to induce a convex meniscus, and can cause the floated IOL to glide toward the peripheral retina or the vitreous base. A layer of viscoelastic may be placed on the surface of the perfluorocarbon liquid to neutralize the convex meniscus, and allow the recentering of the dislocated IOL.[34]

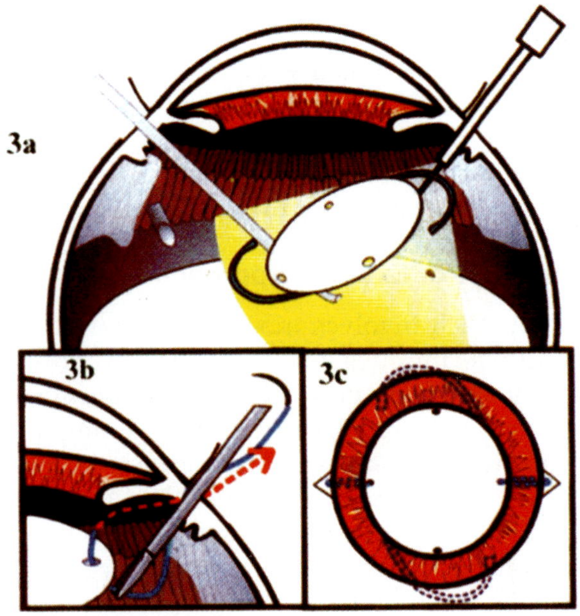

Fig. 50.3: The perfluorocarbon liquid is used to float the dislocated PCIOL anteriorly (A). The haptics are anchored in the ciliary sulcus along the vertical meridians, while the 9-0 polypropylene sutures are inserted through the horizontal anterior sclerotomies to engage the positioning holes of the optic (B); resulting in a stable 4-point fixation (C). (Lewis *et al*: *Ophthalmol* 100:1055-59, 1993)

The 25 gauge IOL forceps

In 1994, Chang introduced the 25 gauge IOL forceps. The passive-action forceps have smooth platforms at the distal end for grasping tissue or holding a suture, and a small groove at the proximal end for gripping a haptic.[35] After a partial vitrectomy, a sharp 25 gauge, 5/8 inch needle is inserted through a scleral groove at 0.8 mm posterior to the corneoscleral limbus, to create a tract for the 25 gauge forceps. The forceps holding a slip knot (lasso) on a 10-0 polypropylene suture is then inserted through the grooved scleral incision into the eye for engaging an IOL haptic. After looping the haptic, the forceps are released from the suture and are used to regrasp the end of the haptic, thus, preventing the suture from slipping off the haptic. After tightening the slip knot, the IOL is repositioned in the ciliary sulcus by anchoring the needle of the 10-0 polypropylene suture within the scleral groove (Fig. 50.4). The same maneuver may be repeated for the opposite haptic, if necessary. The scleral groove is closed with an interrupted 10-0 nylon suture.

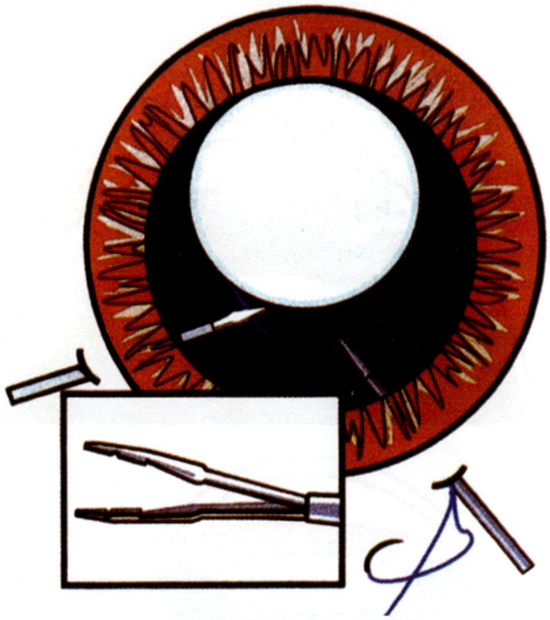

Fig. 50.4: The 25 G Chang passive-action IOL forceps have smooth distal platforms for grasping tissues or sutures, and a proximal groove for gripping a haptic. A slip knot is inserted through a paralimbal scleral groove incision to engage the haptic of the IOL. The forceps are then used to regrasp the distal end of the haptic to prevent the slippage of the suture loop. After tightening the slip knot, the needle of the 10-0 polypropylene suture is anchored within the scleral groove for the implant fixation in the ciliary sulcus. (Chang *et al: Am J Ophthalmol* 119:165-74, 1995)

Temporary Haptic Externalization

Chan first described this method in 1992. Its main features involve the temporary haptic externalization for suture placement after a pars plana vitrectomy, followed by the reinternalization of the haptics tied with 9-0 or 10-0 polypropylene sutures for secured anchoring by the anterior sclerotomies.

Detailed method[36,37]

- A 3-port pars plana vitrectomy is performed for the removal of the anterior and central vitreous adjacent to the dislocated IOL, in order to prevent any vitreoretinal traction during the process of manipulating the IOL.
- Two diametrically opposed limbal-based partial thickness triangular scleral flaps are prepared along the horizontal meridians at 3 and 9 O'clock. Anterior sclerotomies within the beds under the scleral flaps are made at 1 to 1.5 mm from the limbus (Figs 50.5A and B). As an alternative to the scleral flaps, the anterior sclerotomies may be made within the scleral grooves at 1 to 1.5 mm from the horizontal limbus (Fig. 50.5C).
- A fiberoptic light pipe is inserted through one of the posterior sclerotomies, while a pair of fine non-angled positive action forceps (e.g. Grieshaber 50.8) is inserted through the anterior sclerotomy of the opposing quadrant to engage one haptic of the dislocated IOL for the temporary externalization (Fig. 50.6A). A double-armed 9-0 (Ethicon TG 160-8 plus, Somerville NJ) or 10-0 polypropylene suture (Ethicon CS 160-6 Somerville NJ) is tied around the externalized haptic to make a secured knot. The same process is repeated for the other haptic after the surgeon switches the instruments to the opposite hands (Fig. 50.6B).
- The externalized haptics with the tied sutures are reinternalized through the corresponding anterior sclerotomies with the same forceps (Fig. 50.7). The internalized haptics are anchored securely in the ciliary sulcus by taking scleral bites with the external suture needles on the lips of the anterior sclerotomies. By adjusting the tension of the opposing sutures while tying the polypropylene suture knots by the anterior

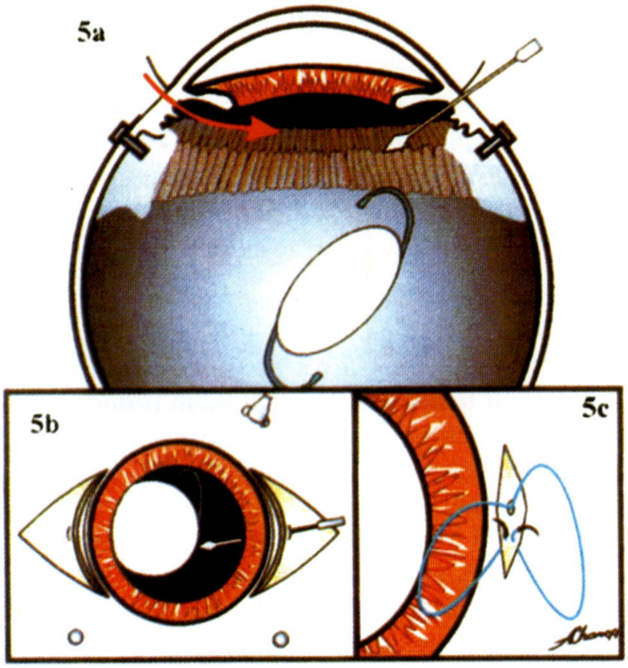

Figs 50.5A to C: Temporary haptic externalization method: (Step 1): Anterior sclerotomies at 1 to 1.5 mm from the horizontal limbus are made under partial thickness scleral flaps (A and B). Instead of scleral flaps, anterior sclerotomies may also be made within scleral grooves (C). (Chan: *Ophthalmol* 99:51-57,1992)

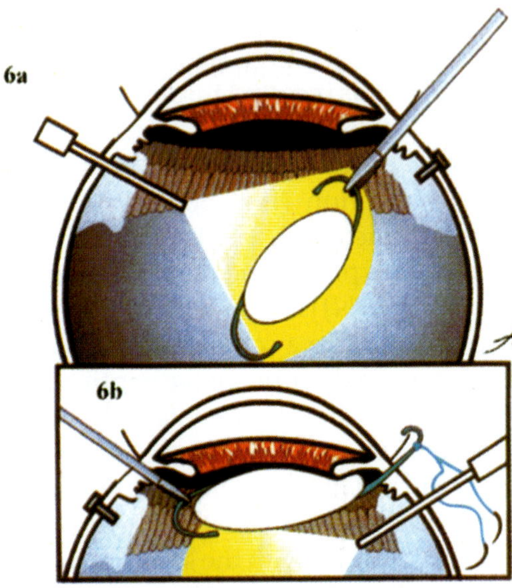

Figs 50.6A and B: Temporary haptic externalization method: (Step 2): After a partial pars plana vitrectomy, a double-armed 9-0 or 10-0 polypropylene suture is tied around the haptic which has been externalized with fine non-angled positive action forceps through one of the two anterior sclerotomies (A). The same process is repeated for the opposite haptic (B) (Chan)

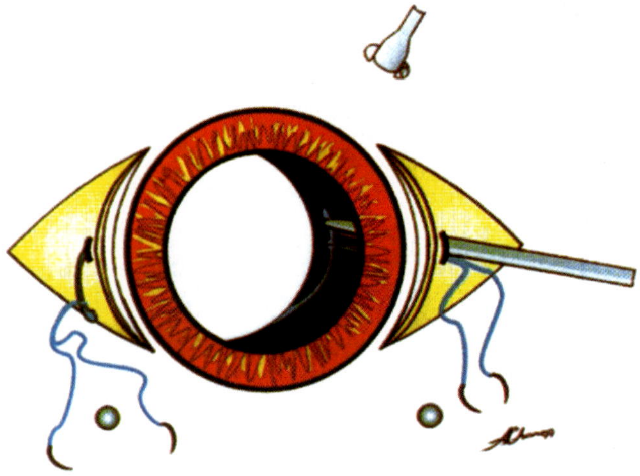

Fig. 50.7: Temporary haptic externalization method (Step 3): The haptics tied with the polypropylene sutures are reinternalized through the corresponding anterior sclerotomies with the same forceps (Chan)

sclerotomies, the optic is centered behind the pupil, and the haptics are anchored in the ciliary sulcus (Figs 50.8A and B).

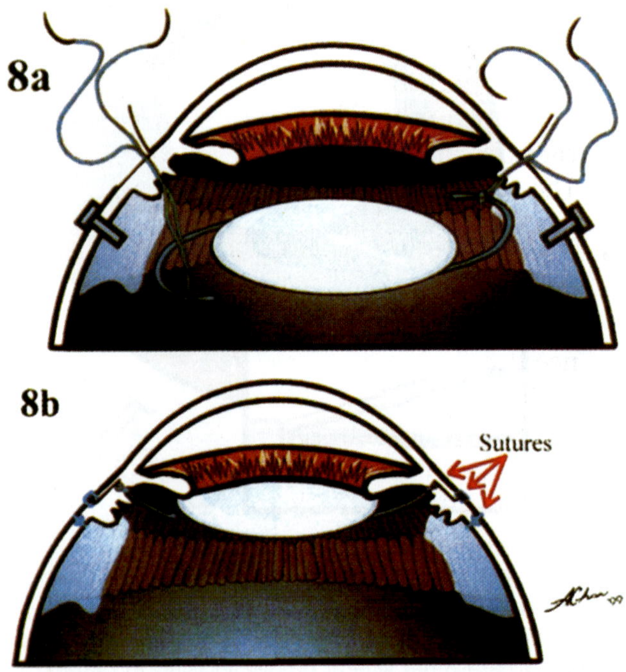

Figs 50.8A and B: Temporary haptic externalization method: After adjusting the tension of the polypropylene sutures tied to the reinternalized haptics (A), the implant is fixated in the ciliary sulcus by anchoring the sutures by the anterior sclerotomies (B) (Chan)

Important features The horizontal meridians are chosen for the location of the anterior sclerotomies for easier manipulation of the forceps, haptics and sutures during the repositioning process. The location of the anterior sclerotomies determines the final position of the IOL. Previous anatomic studies have reported the ciliary sulcus to be between 0.46 to 0.8 mm from the limbus.[38] Thus the distance of 1 to 1.5 mm from the limbus places the anterior sclerotomies close to the external surface of the ciliary sulcus. Making the anterior sclerotomies at less than 1 mm from the limbus increases the risk of injuring the anterior chamber angle or the iris root.

The following steps are taken to ease the passage of the haptics through the anterior sclerotomies and reduce the chance of haptic breakage: (i) The anterior sclerotomies should have adequate size—if necessary, they may be widened before the haptic reinternalization, and (ii) Fine non-angled positive action intraocular forceps are used for the haptic manipulation to give the surgeon the maximal "feel" and "control". Excessive pinching of the haptics is avoided during the passage of the haptics.

Several measures may also be taken to prevent the decentering and tilting of the IOL:

- The anterior sclerotomies are made at 180° from each other.
- The sutures are tied at equal distance from the ends of both haptics.
- A four-point-fixation option—to enhance more stability, two separate polypropylene sutures can be tied on each haptic, and the associated needles are anchored on the two "corners" of each anterior sclerotomy (Fig. 50.9). This results in the stable configuration of a four-point fixation of the IOL.

After the initial report of 12 eyes, additional 22 eyes successfully undergoing this method of repositioning between 1992 and 1999 were presented.[37] Thach *et al* also reported 57 patients undergoing IOL repositioning with this technique at the 1998 AAO meeting in New Orleans.[39] In Chan's series, the average age of the patients was 74. The average follow-up time was 17.5 months. The average preoperative best-corrected visual acuity (BCVA) was 20/400 (range—light perception to 20/30), and

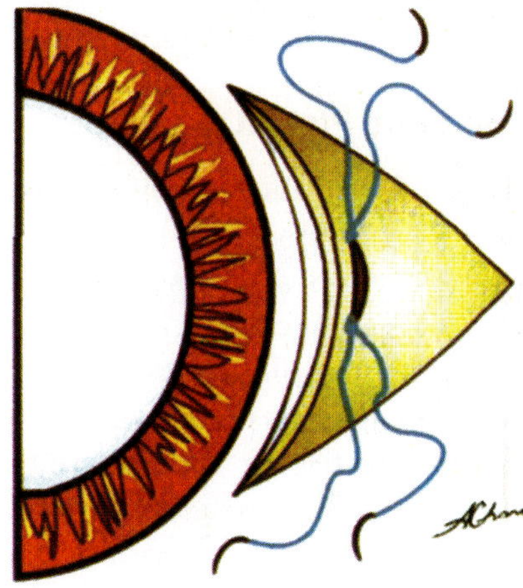

Fig. 50.9: Temporary haptic externalization method: To enhance the centering and prevent the tilting of the IOL, two 9-0 or 10-0 polypropylene sutures are tied on each haptic which has been externalized with fine non-angled forceps, and then anchored on the 2 corners of each anterior sclerotomy after the reinternalization of the haptics. This results in a stable 4-point fixation associated with the appropriate cêntering of the IOL (Chan)

the average postoperative BCVA was 20/50 (range of no light perception to 20/20). There were no major complications, e.g. retinal breaks or detachment, macular pucker, endophthalmitis, ocular ischemia, etc. Despite fixating the scleral sutures along the horizontal meridians, there were no signs of any injury to the ciliary arteries or nerves. The following minor complications were encountered:[37]

- Cystoid macular edema (CME)—20.4 percent (10 eyes); most resolved after topical and/or periocular therapy
- Mild IOL decentration—14.7 percent (5 eyes)—non-sight threatening
- Suture erosion through the conjunctiva—1 eye, no scleral flaps for covering the sutures were made for this eye
- Recurrent IOL dislocation—1 eye, the IOL was too small for the involved eye.

This repositioning technique combines the best features of the external and the internal approaches, while avoiding any intricate and cumbersome intraocular manipulations. With the easy placement of the anchoring sutures in an "opened" environment and the maintenance of the integrity of the globe in a "closed" environment, this technique allows the secured and precise fixation of the dislocated IOL in the ciliary sulcus on a consistent basis.[36,37]

One-piece Silicone Plate IOL

There is a lack of fibrous adhesion between the lens capsule and the one-piece silicone IOL with plate haptics even years after its insertion into the capsular bag.[37-40] The "slippery" surface of the one-piece silicone plate implant makes it relatively mobile, even years after its placement. The silicone plate implant is fixated in the capsular bag by capsular contraction.[37-40] After its implantation, there is fibrotic fusion of the anterior and posterior capsules as well as capsular purse-stringing due to the anterior capsular contraction.[38-41] These effects induce the posterior bowing of the silicone plate implant against the posterior capsule, resulting in the posterior capsular tightening and stretching.[40-44] Thus any dehiscence of the capsular bag outside of the capsulorhexis allows the release of the "built-up" tension, and the expulsion of the implant through the dehiscence.[38-41] Frequently, further capsular contraction after a posterior YAG capsulotomy may then vault the one-piece silicone plate implant through the opening into the vitreous cavity, in a delayed fashion.[38-41]

Previous reports have advocated the repositioning of the dislocated silicone plate implant anterior to the capsular remnants or in the ciliary sulcus. Schneiderman and Johnson, described the technique of picking the slippery silicone plate implant off the retinal surface with a lighted pick.[40,41] The surgeon extends the tip of the pick under the edge of the silicone plate implant to gently elevate it off the retinal surface. The elevated edge is then grasped with the intraocular forceps for the repositioning or removal of the implant. Alternatively, the plate implant may be brought anteriorly by hooking the lighted pick through one of its positioning holes, and then grasped with forceps at the anterior or midvitreous cavity (Fig. 50.10). Another method is to aspirate the plate implant with a soft-tip cannula. The perfluorocarbon liquid may also be used to float the dislocated plate implant. The one-piece silicone plate implant is designed for insertion into the capsular bag.

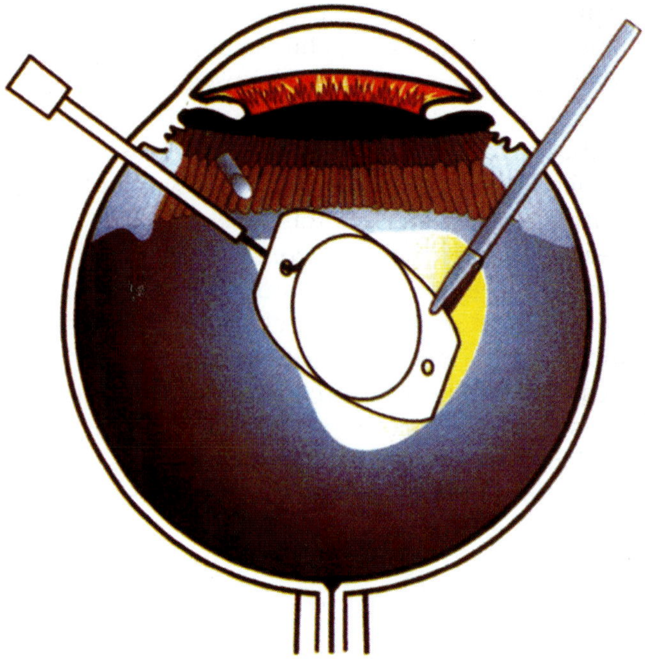

Fig. 50.10: The slippery silicone plate implant may be lifted on its edge or hooked through a positioning hole with a lighted pick, and then grasped with intraocular forceps for its repositioning or removal. (Schneiderman *et al: Am J Ophthalmol* 123: 629-35, 1997)

Thus the silicone plate implant repositioned anterior to the capsular remnants or in the ciliary sulcus tends to be unstable, particularly without the support of sutures. None of the suturing methods (including the temporary haptic externalization technique described in Chapter 49) work well for the one-piece silicone IOL with plate haptics. The temporary externalization of the bulky plate haptics of the silicone plate implant is awkward, and the suture placement through its "floppy" surface tends to result in the "cheese-wiring" of the implant. Frequently, the best approach for managing the dislocated one-piece silicone plate implant is its removal.

Managing Eyes with Two Intraocular Implants

The presence of two intraocular implants complicates the surgical management. This usually occurs when the anterior segment surgeon inserts a second implant (usually an ACIOL) without removing the posteriorly dislocated implant. When the dislocated implant is soft and consists of relatively inert material (e.g. one-piece silicone implant with plate haptics), it may be left alone with a minimal chance of causing a retinal injury, although the movement of the implant may create a visual disturbance. Mobile dislocated implants with hard surfaces and sharp edges may induce an intraocular injury, and therefore should be removed. The association of vitreous hemorrhage, glaucoma, uveitis, retinal breaks, or a retinal detachment with the dislocated implant also requires surgical intervention. The presence of the second intraocular implant eliminates the option of repositioning the dislocated implant, and it also interferes with the removal of the dislocated implant. A number of techniques have been described in the removal of the dislocated implant in the presence of a second implant. The dislocated implant may be treated as an intraocular foreign body, and removed through a pars plana incision with standard vitreoretinal techniques, as reported by Williams *et al.*[42] The dislocated implant may also be removed through a limbal incision with or without the simultaneous removal of the second implant.[42] Wong recently described a technique of temporarily suspending the dislocated implant at the anterior vitreous cavity by passing a 6-0 nylon suture through one of the IOL positioning holes, followed by gently tilting up the edge of the second implant to allow the delivery of the dislocated implant out of the eye through a limbal incision.[43] Another option is the removal of the second implant followed by the repositioning of the dislocated implant. This option may be chosen if there is marked anterior segment pathology associated with the second anterior chamber implant (marked iridodialysis or hyphema, progressive corneal edema, etc.), and the dislocated posterior chamber implant can be safely fixated in the ciliary sulcus. The final option is the removal of both implants, particularly when the presence of any implant may aggravate the ocular condition; such as poorly controlled glaucoma, or an advanced retinal detachment with severe proliferative vitreoretinopathy. Whether there is the removal of one or both implants through a limbal or a pars plana opening, a relatively large incision is required, and complex maneuvers are necessary. This leads to a high chance of ocular morbidities. Thus the placement of a second implant should be avoided in the setting of a posteriorly dislocated implant.

SUMMARY

A dislocated AC or PCIOL may be removed, exchanged, or repositioned. The repositioning of the dislocated PCIOL in the ciliary sulcus with modern vitreoretinal techniques provides an optimal environment for visual recovery. The implant repositioning techniques may be broadly divided into the external and the internal approaches. The former involves modifications of the suturing techniques for a primary or secondary implant in the absence of appropriate capsular or zonular support, while the latter is best accomplished with the pars plana technology. Some of the recent vitreoretinal methods of PCIOL repositioning gaining wide acceptance include the scleral loop fixation, [24] the snare approach,[27] the use of perfluorocarbon,[30,32,33] the 25 gauge implant forceps,[35] and the temporary haptic externalization.[36] The temporary haptic externalization method combines the best features of the external and the internal approaches, avoids difficult maneuvers, and allows the consistent IOL fixation in the ciliary sulcus. Unique features are associated with the silicone plate implants. The capsular contraction after a posterior YAG capsulotomy often leads to a delayed posterior dislocation of the plate implant. Special techniques can be used to pick up the slippery plate implant from the retinal surface for its removal or repositioning. The plate implant repositioned anterior to capsular remnants or in the ciliary sulcus may be unstable, and it is often best to remove the dislocated plate implant. The placement of a second implant in the presence of a dislocated implant is ill advised, as it complicates subsequent surgical management. Surgical options include the removal of the dislocated implant through a pars plana or a limbal incision with special techniques, the repositioning of the dislocated implant after removing the second implant, or the removal of both implants. Surgical maneuvers in the setting of double implants are associated with increased morbidities and complications.

REFERENCES

1. Flynn HW Jr. Pars plana vitrectomy in the management of subluxated and posteriorly dislocated intraocular lenses. Graefe's Arch Clin Exp Ophthalmol 1987;225:169-72.
2. Flynn HW Jr, Buus D, Culbertson WW. Management of subluxated and posteriorly dislocated intraocular lenses using pars plana vitrectomy instrumentation. J Cataract Refract Surg 1990;16:51-56.
3. Jacobi KW, Krey H. Surgical management of intraocular lens dislocation into the vitreous—case report. J Am Intraocul Implant Soc 1983;9:58-59.
4. Mittra RA, Connor TB, Han DP et al. Removal of dislocated intraocular lenses using pars plana vitrectomy with placement of an open-loop, flexible anterior chamber lens. Ophthalmol 1998;105:1011-14.
5. McCannel MA. A retrievable suture idea for anterior uveal problems. Ophthalmic Surg 1998;7(2):98-103.
6. Stark WJ, Bruner WE. Management of posteriorly dislocated intraocular lenses. Ophthalmic Surg 1980; 11:495-97.
7. Sternberg P Jr, Michels RG. Treatment of dislocated posterior chamber intraocular lenses. Arch Ophthalmol 1986;104:1391-93.
8. Girard LJ. Pars plana phacoprosthesis (aphakic intraocular implant—a preliminary report. Ophthalmic Surg 1981;12:19-22.
9. Girard LJ, Nino N, Wesson M et al. Scleral fixation of a subluxated posterior chamber intraocular lens. J Cataract Refract Surg 1988;14:326-27.
10. Smiddy WE. Dislocated posterior chamber intraocular lens. A new technique of management. Arch Ophthalmol 1989;107:1678-80.
11. Campo RV, Chung KD, Oyakawa RT. Pars plana vitrectomy in the management of dislocated posterior chamber lenses. Am J Ophthalmol 1989;108:529-34.
12. Anand R, Bowman RW. Simplified technique for suturing dislocated posterior chamber intraocular lens to the ciliary sulcus [letter]. Arch Ophthalmol 1990;108:1205-06.
13. Stark WJ, Goodman G, Goodman D et al. Posterior chamber intraocular lens implantation in the absence of posterior capsular support. Ophthalmic Surg 1988;19:240-43.
14. Hu BV, Shin DH, Gibbs KA et al. Implantation of posterior chamber lens in the absence of posterior capsular and zonular support. Arch Ophthalmol 1988;106:416-20.
15. Shin DH, Hu BV, Hong YJ et al. Posterior chamber lens implantation in the absence of posterior capsular support [letter]. Ophthalmic Surg 1988;19:606-07.
16. Dahan E. Implantation in the posterior chamber without capsular support. J Cataract Refract Surg 15:339-42, 1989.
17. Pannu JS. A new suturing technique for ciliary sulcus fixation in the absence of posterior capsule. Ophthalmic Surg 1988;19:751-54.
18. Spigelman AV, Lindstrom RL, Nichols BD et al. Implantation of a posterior chamber lens without capsular support during penetrating keratoplasty or as a secondary lens implant. Ophthalmic Surg 1988;19:396-98.
19. Drews RC. Posterior chamber lens implantation during keratoplasty without posterior lens capsule support. Cornea 1987;6:38-40.
20. Wong SK, Stark WJ, Gottsch SD et al. Use of posterior chamber lenses in pseudophakic bullous keratopathy. Arch Ophthalmol 1987;105:856-58.
21. Waring GO III, Stulting RD, Street D. Penetrating keratoplasty for pseudophakic corneal edema with exchange of intraocular lenses. Arch Ophthalmol 105:58-62, 1987.
22. Shin DH. Implantation of a posterior chamber lens without capsular support during penetrating keratoplasty or as a secondary lens [letter]. Ophthalmic Surg 1988;19:755-56.
23. Lindstrom RL, Harris WS, Lyle WA. Secondary and exchange posterior chamber lens implantation. J Am Intraocul Implant Soc 1982;8:353-56.
24. Maguire AM, Blumenkranz MS, Ward TG et al. Scleral loop fixation for posteriorly dislocated intraocular lenses. Operative technique and long-term results. Arch Ophthalmol 1991;109:1754-58.
25. Bloom SM, Wyszynski RE, Brucker AJ. Scleral fixation suture for dislocated posterior chamber intraocular lens. Ophthalmic Surg 1990;21:851-54.
26. Friedberg MA, Pilkerton AR. A new technique for repositioning and fixating a dislocated intraocular lens. Arch Ophthalmol 1992;110:413-15.
27. Little BC, Rosen PH, Orr G. Trans-scleral fixation of dislocated posterior chamber intraocular lenses using a 9-0 microsurgical polypropylene snare. Eye 1993;7:740-43.
28. Lewis H, Blumenkranz MS, Chang S. Treatment of dislocated crystalline lens and retinal detachment with perfluorocarbon liquids. Retina 1992;12:299-304.
29. Shapiro MJ, Resnick KI, Kim SH. Management of the dislocated crystalline lens with a perfluorocarbon liquid. Am J Ophthalmol 1992;112:401-05.
30. Liu K, Peyman GA, Chen M. Use of high density vitreous substitute in the removal of posteriorly dislocated lenses or intraocular lenses. Ophthalmic Surg 1991;22:503-07.
31. Rowson NJ, Bacon AS, Rosen PH. Perfluorocarbon heavy liquids in the management of posterior dislocation of the lens nucleus during phakoemulsification. Br J Ophthalmol 1992;176(3):169-70.
32. Greve MD, Peyman GA, Mehta NJ. Use of perfluoroperhydrophenanthrene in the management of posteriorly dislocated crystalline and intraocular lenses. Ophthalmic Surg 1993;24(9):593-97.
33. Lewis H, Sanchez G. The use of perfluorocarbon liquids in the repositioning of posteriorly dislocated intraocular lenses. Ophthalmol 1993;100:1055-59.

34. Elizalde J. Combined use of perfluorocarbon liquids and viscoelastics aOL by temporary externalization of haptics, [poster #132]. The Vitreous Society 17th Annual Meeting, Rome, 1999.
35. Duffey RJ, Holland EJ, Agapitos PJ et al. Anatomic study of transsclerally sutured intraocular lens implantation. Am J Ophthalmol 1999;108:300-09.
36. Thach AB, Dugel PU, Sipperley JO et al. Outcome of sulcus fixation of dislocated PCIOL's using temporary externalization of the haptics. [paper] AAO Annual Meeting, New Orleans, Louisiana, 1998.
37. Milauskas AT. Posterior capsule opacification after silicone lens implantation and its management. J Cataract Refract Surg 1987;13:644-48.
38. Milauskas AT. Capsular bag fixation of one-piece silicone lenses. J Cataract Refract Surg 1990;16:583-86.
39. Joo CK, Shin JA, Kim JH. Capsular opening contraction after continuous curvilinear capsulorhexis and intraocular lens implantation. J Cataract Refract Surg 1996;22:585-90.
40. Schneiderman TE, Johnson MW, Smiddy WE et al. Surgical management of posteriorly dislocated silicone plate haptic intraocular lenses. Am J Ophthalmol 1997; 123:629-35.
41. Johnson MW, Schneiderman TE. Surgical management of posteriorly dislocated silicone plate intraocular lenses. Curr Opin Ophthalmol 1998;9:11-15.
42. Williams DF, Del Piero EJ, Ferrone PJ et al. Management of complications in eyes containing two intraocular lenses. Ophthalmol 1998;105:2017-22.
43. Wong KL. Simplified technique to remove a posteriorly dislocated PCIOL with a coexistent PCIOL [poster 133]. The Vitreous Society 17th Annual Meeting, Rome, 1999.

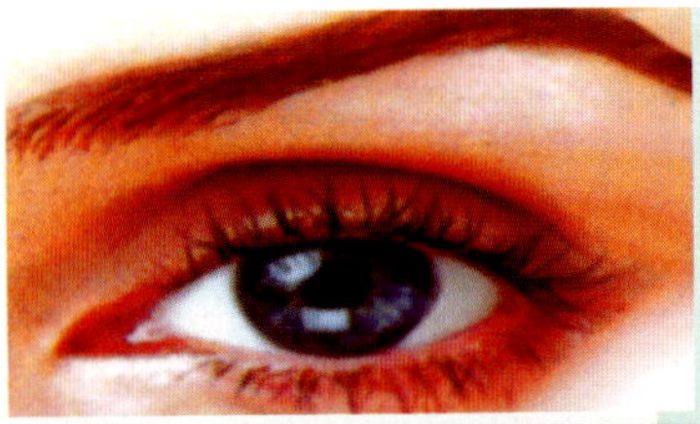

Fifty one

Posterior Dislocation of Lens Material During Cataract Surgery

Steve Charles (USA)

SURGICAL PSYCHODYNAMICS

Cataract surgery has been one of the most frequently performed surgical procedures worldwide for over a century. While inexperience is known to cause a higher complication rate, high volumes and phenomenal success rates can also lead to complacency and judgement errors when complications do occur. Busy schedules, observers, and videography may contribute to faulty decision making when the capsule ruptures. High success rates, outpatient surgery, no stitch, no patch, emmetropia, and topical anesthesia elevate patient expectations unrealistically furthering the problem.

EARLY RECOGNITION AND MANAGEMENT OF DEFECTS INTHE LENS CAPSULE

Optical systems that enhance the red-reflex and the clear corneas achievable with modern cataract surgery assist in early recognition of capsular defects. The surgeon must admit that the defect has occurred rather than rationalize because of the psychological factors described above. When a capsular defect is recognized, the first action should be to construct a barrier between the posterior capsule and the anterior vitreous cortex. Colvard has proposed a plastic barrier that can be deployed in this space, but none are available at this time. High viscosity viscoelastics injected into the defect can serve as a temporary barrier enabling removal of remaining lens material. Many surgeons focus exclusively on prevention or management of posterior dislocation of lens material rather than the more serious matter of reducing vitreoretinal traction and subsequent retinal detachment. Any maneuver designed to prevent posterior dislocation that increases vitreoretinal traction should not be used. Kelman has described use of a needle through the pars plana to prevent lens material from falling posteriorly. This method ignores the pressure that must be placed on the eye to place the needle and the anterior movement of the vitreous that occurs without a barrier. The next section discusses management of vitreous that prolapses through the capsular defect. This discussion intentionally precedes the discussion of the management of lens material because retinal detachment prevention is the most important issue.

VITREOUS LOSS

Use of the phacoemulsifier to remove vitreous is a dangerous step that should never be undertaken. Phaco probes liquefy hyaluronic acid but do not cut collagen fibers. Use of a large bore needle to aspirate "liquid" vitreous should be avoided because of the obligate vitreoretinal traction it creates. The theoretical "pockets" of liquid vitreous are more difficult to locate than the fountain of youth.

Cellulose sponge vitrectomy as reported by Kasner has been an obsolete and dangerous method for two decades in spite of the important role it played at one time. A cellulose sponge causes significant traction on the retina as the sponge is lifted to transect the adherent vitreous. Removal of all vitreous by a vitreous cutter causes virtually no inflammation, while marked inflammation is the rule after sponge vitrectomy. Mechanical damage to the iris caused by contact with the sponge as it swells and is lifted appears to be the cause of this inflammation. The author had also observed cellulose material on the anterior vitreous cortex after sponge vitrectomy had been performed. One can speculate that this retained material causes inflammation in addition to that caused by iris trauma. Testing for vitreous can be accomplished by injecting air into the anterior chamber via the sideport incision and looking for fragmentation of the bubble. Alternatively, a single drop of sterile fluorescein from a newly opened ampoule can be used to stain the vitreous.

Vitrectomy with a high quality vitreous cutter is the preferred method of managing vitreous that presents in the anterior chamber. Alcon builds high quality cutters for use with their phaco systems such as Legacy. These cutters should be operated at the highest possible cutting frequency and very low vacuum. Posterior vitreous surgeons use vacuum settings rather than flow for better control over vitreoretinal traction. The anterior segment machines frequently utilize peristaltic pumps, which cannot be directly controlled for vacuum. The best procedure is to use very low flow rate and vacuum settings to reduce traction on the retina. The cutter should be advanced or held stationary during vitrectomy, never retracted. ***Pulling the cutter back while vacuum is applied dramatically increases vitreoretinal traction.*** Sideport infusion is preferable to "dry" vitrectomy, because it prevents hypotony and therefore reduces the chance of choroidal hemorrhage. Air can be used instead of infusion fluid to keep the vitreous from hydrating. The air helps to delineate the surface of the vitreous and keep it confined by surface tension. Sweeping the wound for vitreous is dangerous because of the vitreoretinal traction it causes.

DISLOCATED LENS MATERIAL

Phacoemulsifiers, lens loops, and saline fluid streams should never be utilized in an attempt to extract lens material from the vitreous cavity (Figs 51.1 to 51.3). If lens material falls posteriorly, there is a natural tendency for the surgeon to chase it with the phaco probe. The phaco probe gives the appearance of vitreous emulsification, but does not sever the collagen fibers. The surgeon must consciously stop, relax, and plan before performing any further maneuvers. The best plan is usually to let

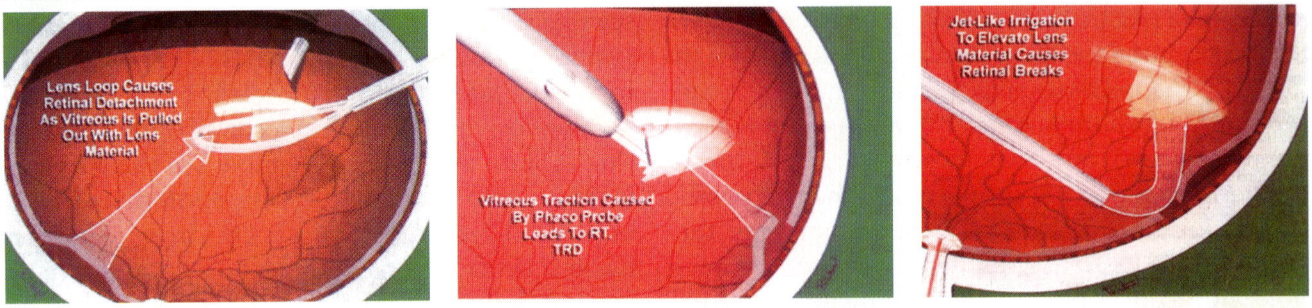

Figs 51.1 to 51.3: Dislocated lens material: What not to do?

the material fall posteriorly and focus on vitreous clean-up and IOL implantation. Lens loops can put significant traction on the retina and cause retinal breaks and detachments. Saline injected under pressure was used by Foulds and later Machemer to create experimental retinal detachments. There is significant risk of retinal breaks if saline is used in an attempt to move the lens material anteriorly.

If the pupil is large, the cornea clear, and the surgeon and available staff are optimum for posterior vitrectomy, immediate intervention may be undertaken. In most instances, it is preferable to perform posterior vitrectomy and removal of lens material at a second procedure (Fig. 51.4). This procedure should be performed when the cornea is clear, the wound is sealed, and the pupil well dilated. The timing can be from several days to weeks later. If there is a moderate amount of cortex, no inflammation, no glaucoma, and no lens-corneal touch, vitrectomy may not be necessary.

Posterior vitrectomy requires the surgeon specifically trained in posterior techniques and a sophisticated vitrectomy system. A suture supported infusion cannula placed through the pars plana is essential. A hand-held, planoconcave fundus contact lens (Machemer) is easier and faster to use than a sewed-on contact lens. Wide-angle visualization systems increase cost, complexity, and the learning curve although they provide an excellent view. A fiberoptic endoilluminator is essential for all cases. Light reflexes from the cornea prevent the surgeon from having an optimal view if coaxial illumination is used. Iris retractors increase inflammation, cost and may cause a distorted pupil after surgery.

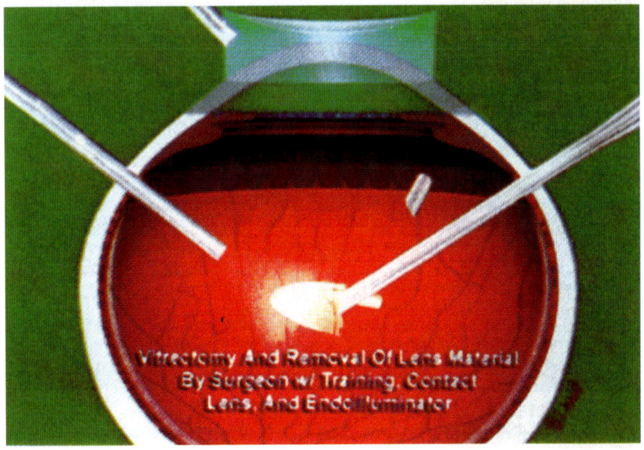

Fig. 51.4: Dislocated lens material: What to do?

All vitreous should be removed before aspirating any dislocated lens material (Figs 51.5 and 51.6). ***Many surgeons function under the false concept that lens material can damage the retina if it falls posteriorly. Inappropriate techniques, not the lens, damage the retina***. It is dangerous and unnecessary to leave a layer of vitreous under the lens material until it is removed. Some cortex may be removed with the vitreous cutter, but nuclear material requires the phacofragmenter. Fragmenters are 20-gauge like vitreous cutters eliminating the need for the larger wounds required for phacoemulsifier probes. The Alcon titanium fragmenter utilizes the same drive electronics and piezo driver as the Legacy phaco probe and is able to handle the majority of nuclear sclerosis cases.

After removal of the vitreous, the fragmenter is introduced with the endoilluminator in the other sclerotomy. The fragmenter is moved to the surface of the lens material and suction applied with the

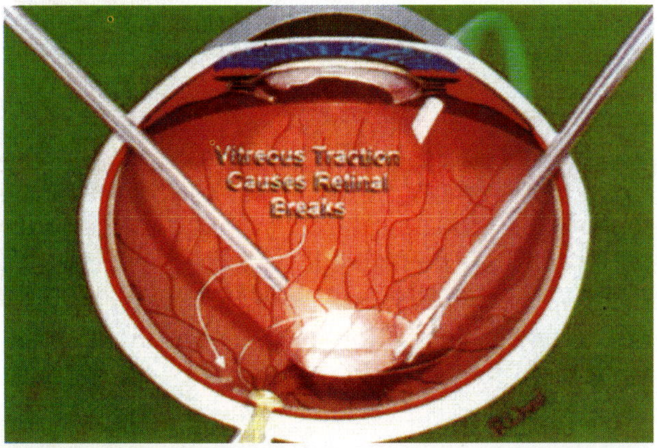

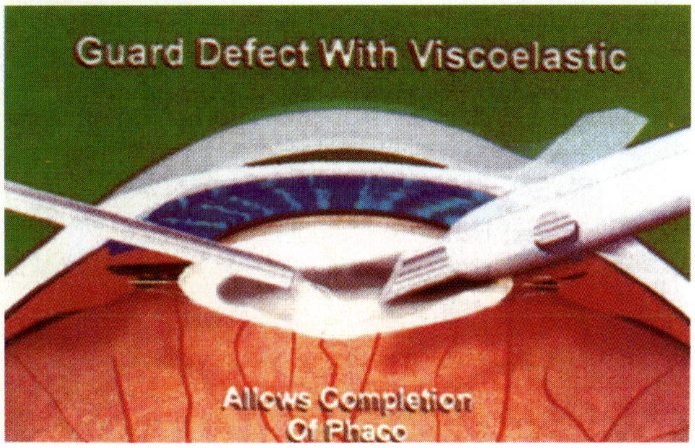

Figs 51.5 and 51.6: Dislocated lens: Precautions

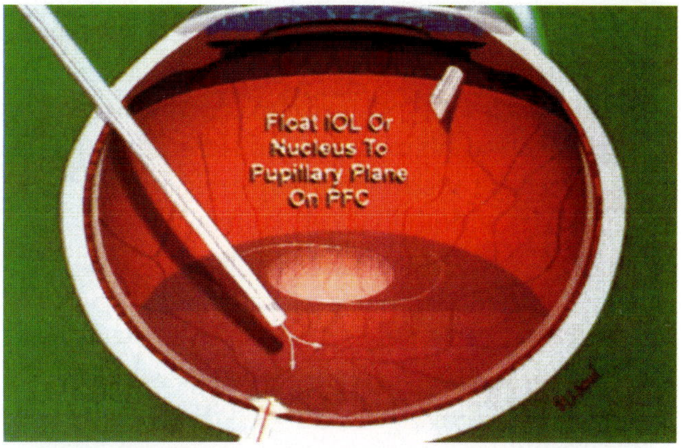

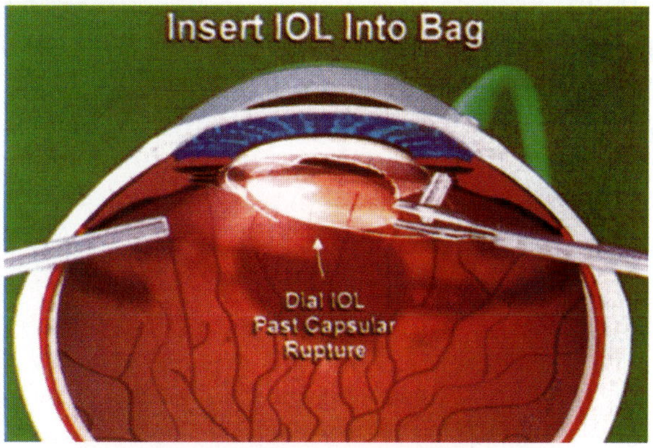

Figs 51.7 and 51.8: Removal of dislocated IOL with perfluorocarbon liquids

linear (proportional) suction. The lens material is moved away from the retina and then the footpedal is used to activate sonification. The fragmenter power is adjusted until sufficient sculpting without bouncing is accomplished.If the fragmenter drills into the lens, the endoilluminator is used to push the fragment off the tip. Alternatively, the endoilluminator can be used to crush and divide the fragment that is speared on the fragmenter tip. This process is continued until all lens fragments are removed.

Perfluorocarbon (PFC) liquids (Chang) were introduced to vitreoretinal surgery for unfolding giant breaks and stabilizing the retina during dissection of epiretinal membranes (Figs 51.7 to 51.9). PFC liquids can also be used to float the lens material away from the retina allowing aspiration-fragmentation to be performed anteriorly. This method increases cost and requires subsequent procedures to remove residual PFC liquids. The PFC liquid method is safe, but unnecessary unless there is extremely dense nuclear sclerosis that should not have been managed with phaco in the first place.

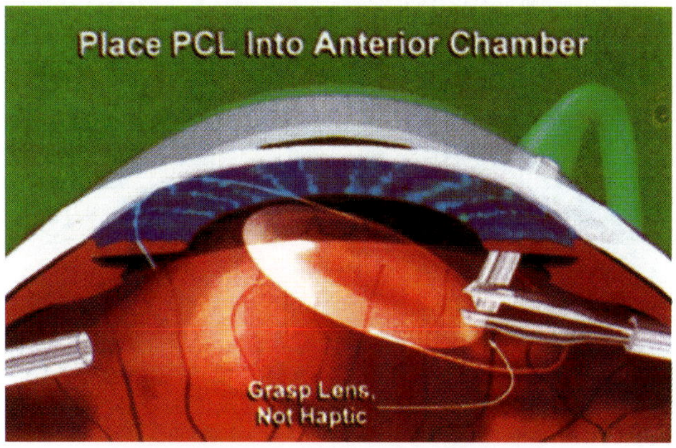

Fig. 51.9: Removal of dislocated IOL with perfluorocarbon liquids

INTRAOCULAR LENS IMPLANTATION

Some retinal surgeons are opposed to lens implantation in cases of posterior dislocation of lens material. The author recommends lens implantation unless there is insufficient capsular support and low corneal endothelial cell counts or significant glaucoma. If the capsule can support an IOL, it can be placed in the bag with the haptics rotated away from the capsular defect. If the posterior capsule will not support an IOL, the IOL can be implanted in the ciliary sulcus anterior to the stronger anterior lens capsule.

If the capsule is not sufficient to support the IOL, an anterior chamber lens can be used. Anterior chamber lenses are contraindicated if there are low endothelial cell counts or open angle glaucoma. Judgement is required to set the level of cell counts and severity of glaucoma that represent contraindications.

SUMMARY

It is essential for the cataract surgeon to mentally rehearse a plan for capsular rupture, vitreous in the anterior chamber, and posterior dislocation of lens material. Simulation of rare complications is similar to that used in flight simulator-based pilot training. Constant attention to prevention of vitreoretinal traction and retinal detachment rather than an obsession with prevention of posterior dislocation of lens material is crucial. Sophisticated mechanical vitrectomy rather than cellulose sponge vitrectomy must become the standard.

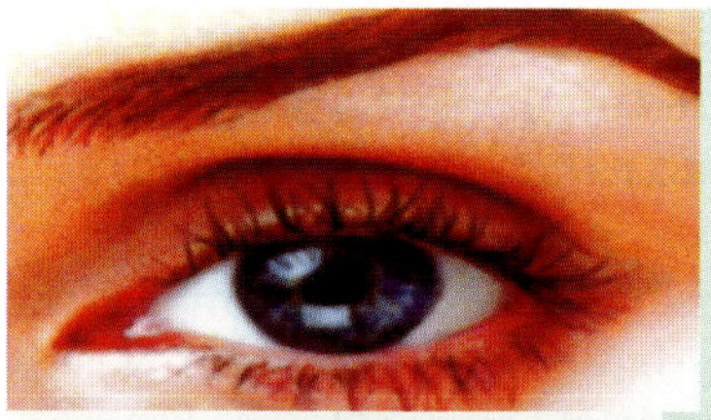

Fifty two

Management of Postoperative Endophthalmitis

Amar Agarwal
Ashok Garg
Sasikanth (India)

INTRODUCTION

Endophthalmitis is any severe intraocular inflammation. Once the sclera gets involved in the infection, it is called panophthalmitis.

ETIOLOGY

Endophthalmitis[1-6] could occur due to an operation, trauma, through a filtering bleb or as a metastatic infection. The etiologic agent could be a normal conjunctival commensal organism. The most common pathogens in acute endophthalmitis are *Staphylococcus epidermidis* and other coagulase-negative staphylococci. Other pathogens which can cause endophthalmitis are: *Staphylococcus aureus, Pseudomonas*, gram-negative microorganisms, fungus, etc. If there is a filtering bleb and endophthalmitis occurs, it could most likely be due to *Streptococcus. Bacillus* species are commonly found in patients having endophthalmitis due to trauma. Late postoperative endophthalmitis could be due to *Propionibacterium acnes* (Table 52.1).

CLINICAL FEATURES

Acute Postoperative Endophthalmitis

Acute postoperative endophthalmitis typically presents with a sudden loss of vision. The patient

Table 52.1: Common etiological agents with their causes

Cause	Microorganism
1. Acute postoperative endophthalmitis	*Staphylococcus epidermidis*
2. Endophthalmitis associated with a filtering bleb	*Streptococcus sp*
3. Endophthalmitis associated with trauma	*Bacillus sp*
4. Late postoperative endophthalmitis	*Propionibacterium acnes*
5. Others	*Staphylococcus aureus Pseudomonas, Fungus,* etc

will complain of pain. There will be circumciliary congestion, loss of the red reflex, hypopyon and the formation of a pupillary membrane (Fig. 52.1). Sometimes, there can be a low-grade infection and so the patient might not have pain. One should be careful that one does not ignore these cases.

Chronic Postoperative Endophthalmitis

One can develop endophthalmitis even several months after surgery. These cases are chronic postoperative endophthalmitis cases. The organism that very commonly implicated is *Propionibacterium acnes*. Other organisms that can produce this sort of infection are *Candida parapsilosis*, diphtheroids, etc.

The *Propionibacterium acnes* organisms grow slowly and are not capable of overwhelming the immunologic defences of the eye. They sequester themselves within the capsular bag out of reach of host defenses so that, they cannot be totally eliminated (Table 52.2). They stimulate an immunologic reaction, i.e. manifest as a persistent inflammation. The time interval for presentation and severity of symptoms usually correlates directly with the virulence of the organisms.

Chronic postoperative endophthalmitis presents differently compared to acute endophthalmitis. In this, vision loss is not very significant. There will be cells in the anterior chamber that respond to topical steroids and return when steroids are tapered off. Other features include keratic precipitates, vitreous reaction or beaded fibrin strands.

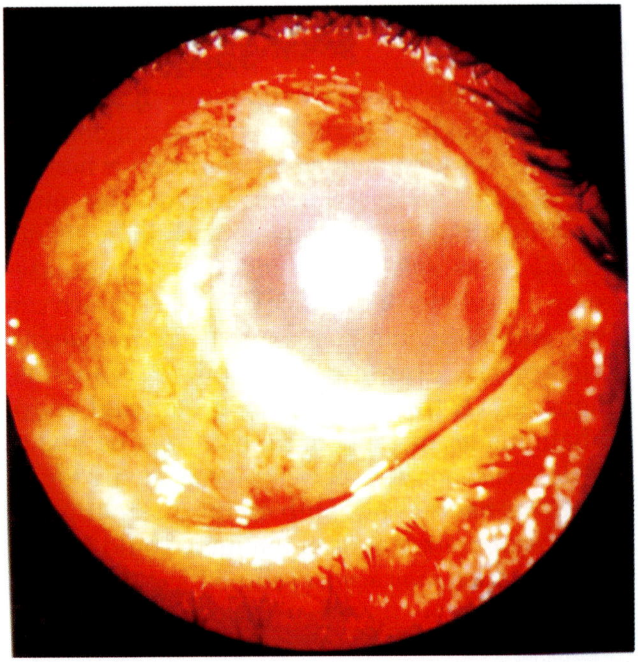

Fig. 52.1: Endophthalmitis—note the circumciliary congestion and the hypopyon (*Courtesy:* Dr. PN Nagpal, Retina Foundation, India)

Table 52.2: Propionibacterium acnes

Propionibacterium Acnes
↓
Organism Grows Slowly
↓
Sequesters in the Capsular Bag
↓
Out of Reach of Host Defenses
↓
Stimulates Immunologic Reaction
↓
Persistent Inflammation

Endogenous Endophthalmitis

Endogenous endophthalmitis is usually associated with a significant systemic illness or intravenous drug usage. One should always search for the cause of the endophthalmitis. Systemic therapy is useful in these cases. Otherwise one has to shift to vitrectomy.

DIAGNOSIS

Anterior Chamber Tap

One can do an anterior chamber tap (Fig. 52.2). In this, a sterile needle with a syringe is passed into the anterior chamber and a little bit of fluid removed and sent for culture sensitivity. The problem here is that in 40 percent of cases in which the vitreous tap is positive the anterior chamber tap is negative.

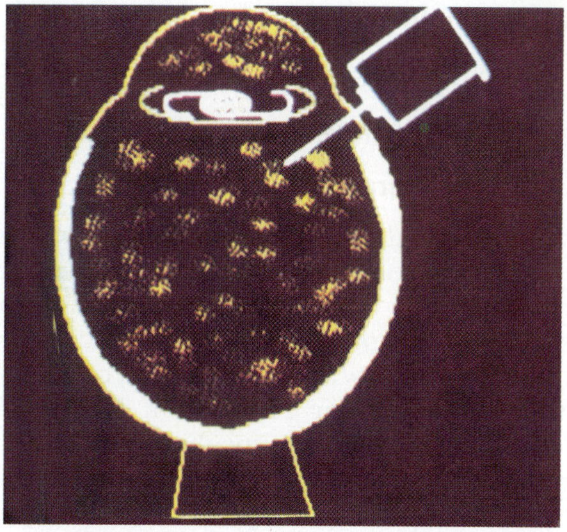

Fig. 52.2: Anterior chamber aqueous tap

Vitreous Tap

The problem in this is that it is dangerous. The method is to use a sterile needle and syringe and pass the needle 3 to 3.5 mm behind the limbus (Fig. 52.3). The problem here is that when we aspirate there can be traction on the vitreous which in turn can lead to a retinal break. It is better to do the vitreous tap just before vitrectomy. In this, the infusion cannula is fixed, then the vitrectomy probe passed into the eye. This probe is connected to a sterile container so that the initial vitreous removed comes into the container, and this is sent for culture and sensitivity (Fig. 52.10). The advantage of this technique is that one does not pull on the vitreous, but the probe cuts the vitreous fibrils and then aspirates, thus it solving the problem of a retinal break.

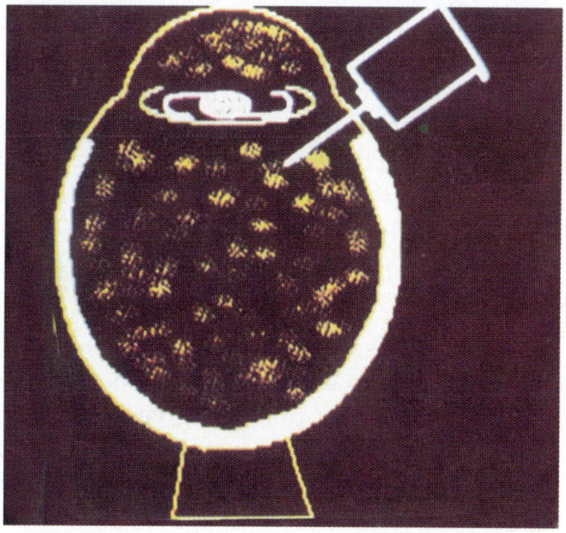

Fig. 52.3: Vitreous tap

MEDICALTREATMENT

Topical Therapy

Vancomycin is the best antimicrobial agent for endophthalmitis. It is mainly effective against gram-positive organisms, but is also active against *Bacillus sp.* and *Propionibacterium acnes*. The mechanism of action is inhibition of the cell wall assembly, damaging protoplasts and inhibiting RNA synthesis. It is given as 25 mg/ml every 2 to 4 hours combined with fortified gentamicin 14 mg/ml. This is also given every 2 to 4 hours and 1 percent prednisolone acetate is given 4 times a day. If vancomycin is not available one can give cephalosporins. The cephalosporins are synthetic penicillins active against the bacterial cell wall. They are very useful against *Pseudomonas*.

Systemic Therapy

For intravenous therapy, the optimal combination is 500 mg IV vancomycin every 6 hours with 2 gm ceftazidime every 8 hours.

Subconjunctival Therapy

Vancomycin 25 mg or gentamicin 20 mg is given.

INTRAVITREAL INJECTIONS

Intravitreal Therapy

For intravitreal injections, the dosage is vancomycin 1.0 mg for acting against the gram-positive organisms. To be effective against the gram-negative organisms, vancomycin should be given in combination with an aminoglycoside like amikacin 200 µg or gentamicin 100 µg. The mechanism of action of aminoglycoside is to inhibit protein synthesis. Ceftazidime, which is a third-generation cephalosporin given in the dosage of 1 mg in 0.1 cc intravitreally, is advantageous because it covers gram-negative organisms including *Pseudomonas* and is not as toxic as the aminoglycosides. When intravitreal injections are given, the drug is loaded in the syringe and the needle passed just as in doing a vitreous tap. The needle should be passed through the pars plana about 3 to 3.5 mm behind the limbus. The needle should be directed towards the midvitreous.

Fungal Case

The drug of choice is amphotericin B. Their mechanism of action is to alter membrane permeability. For systemic therapy one can give ketoconazole 400-600 mg daily. Amphotericin B is given intravitreally as 5 mg. The method of intravitreal drug preparation is shown in Table 52.3.

VITRECTOMY

Timing of Vitrectomy

Vitrectomy is most useful for cases which are between the mild and the advanced. In the mild cases, there is vitritis, but the retina can be seen. In these cases, one can give subconjunctival, systemic antibiotics or intravitreal injections. In the advanced cases, vitrectomy has very poor prognosis as in these cases corneal decompensation has occurred. So, one can only do an open sky vitrectomy in such cases and the visual results are very poor. The best results are in the intermediate cases. In the intermediate cases there would be hypopyon, vitritis with the retina not being seen and the corneal decompensation not started. If the mild cases do not improve, and the retinal view starts getting lost one should contemplate vitrectomy.

Preoperative Evaluation

One should check for perception of light. If the cornea is very bad then one should remember that one cannot do much for visual recovery. One should also check on the duration of onset of the endophthalmitis to give a clue as to the etiologic agent.

Advantages of Vitrectomy

1. Aids in identifying the pathogen.
2. Removes inflammatory mediators and debris from inside the eye thereby clearing the visual axis.
3. Late complications related to cellular proliferation on vitreous matrix are reduced.
4. Reduces the number of organisms.
5. Increases penetration and diffusion of antibiotics.

Theater Set-up

The operating room personnel should be informed about the infected case. At times, it is best to operate in a non-ophthalmic operating room with only the minimal equipment required for the case.

Anesthesia

General anesthesia is vastly superior to local anesthesia in these cases because the inflamed orbit makes retrobulbar block hazardous and ineffective. But most of the cases would be done under local anesthesia, as these are true emergencies. One can supplement the peribulbar block with a pin-point (subcutaneous) anesthesia.

VITRECTOMY: SURGICAL SEQUENCE

Wound Closure

If a cataract wound, surgical wound or ruptured filtering bleb is present, they must be sutured with 8/0 monofilament nylon sutures. If any intraocular foreign body is present, it must be removed.

Table 52.3: Intravitreal drug preparation

Drug	*Step 1*	*Step 2*	*Step 3*	*Step 4*
GENTAMICIN 100 µg in 0.1 ml NaCl for injection USP	One vial is filled with gentamicin 80 mg/2 ml	Withdraw 0.25 ml in syringe 1 (10 mg)	Empty contents of syringe 1 into second 10-ml syringe and add 9.75 ml of 0.9 NaCl for injection (preservative-free) to make up 10 ml solution (1 mg/1 ml)	Withdraw 0.1 ml from syringe 2 into TB syringe. This will contain 100 µg/0.1 ml of gentamicin)
AMIKACIN 200 µg in 0.1 ml NaCl for injection USP	One vial is filled with amikacin 100 mg/2 ml	Withdraw 0.4 ml into TB syringe 1, which will contain 20 mg of amikacin.	Empty contents of syringe 1 into a second 10-ml syringe and add 9.6 ml of 0.9% NaCl for injection (preservative-free) to make up 10 ml solution (2 mg/ml)	Withdraw 0.1 ml from syringe 2 into TB syringe. This will contain 200 µg/0.1 ml of amikacin
VANCOMYCIN 1 mg in 0.1 ml for injection USP	One vial of vancomycin powder, 500 mg, is diluted with 10 ml 0.9% NaCl for injection USP (Preservative-free) (50 mg/ml)	Withdraw 1 ml into syringe 1 (50 mg/ml)	Empty contents of syringe 1 into a second syringe and add 4 ml of 0.9% NaCl for injection (preservative-free) to make up 5 ml solution (10 mg/ml)	Withdraw 0.1 ml from syringe 2 into TB syringe. This will contain 1 mg of vancomycin
CLINDAMYCIN 450 µg in 0.1 ml NaCl for injection USP	Clindamycin is available in vials containing 150 mg/ml	Withdraw 0.3 ml into syringe 1	Empty contents of syringe 1 into a second 10-ml syringe and add 9.7 ml of 0.9 NaCl for injection (preservative-free) to make up 10 ml solution (4.5 mg/ml)	Withdraw 0.1 ml from syringe 2 into TB syringe, which will contain 450 µg of clindamycin
CEFTAZIDIME 1 mg in 0.1 ml NaCl for injection USP	One vial of ceftazidime powder, 500 mg, is diluted with 10 ml 0.9% NaCl for infection USP (preservative-free) (50 mg/ml)	Withdraw 1 ml into syringe 1 (50 mg/ml)	Empty contents of syringe 1 into a second syringe and add 4 ml of 0.9 % NaCl for injection (preservative-free) to make up 5 ml solution (10 mg/ml)	Withdraw 0.1 ml from syringe 2 into TB syringe, which will contain 1 µg of ceftazidime
DEXAMETHASONE 400 µg	Withdraw 0.1 ml in a TB syringe from a vial of dexamethasone containing 4 mg/1 ml and inject intravitreally			
AMPHOTERICIN B 5 mg in 0.1 ml sterile water	One vial of amphotericin B containing 50 mg is diluted with 10 ml sterile water for injection USP (preservative-free) (5 mg/ml)	Withdraw 0.1 ml (500 µg) in a TB syringe	Add contents of TB syringe to a syringe containing 9.9 ml of sterile water for injection USP (50 µg/ml)	Withdraw 0.1 ml in a TB syringe, which will contain 5 µg of amphotericin B and inject intravitreally

Limbal or Pars Plana Approach

The pars plana approach is a better alternative. The limbal approach produces corneal trauma and iris trauma. It also prevents good visualization for vitrectomy. Saying this, the limbal approach can be used by the novice surgeon in a true emergency.

Pupillary Membrane

In many cases, a pupillary membrane is present which obstructs visualization of the vitreous cavity. One should first remove this membrane by entering the anterior chamber through a limbal stab incision using a bent needle or a cystitome (Fig. 52.4). Then, using the needle the distal edge of the membrane is engaged, and the membrane pulled towards the needle entry site (Fig. 52.5) where it could be removed from the anterior chamber (Figs 52.7 and 52.8). One can also use the vitrectomy probe to remove this membrane. Pass the vitrectomy probe through the limbal or clear corneal wound and clear the membrane. Have the infusion of the fluid passing through the vitrectomy probe. In other words use the multi-function probe which has infusion, cutting and aspiration in it.

IOL Removal

One should make a decision about removing the IOL or not. If one feels the causative agent is related in the IOL as in *Propionibacterium acnes* where the organism is in the capsular bag, then one should remove the IOL and the capsule (Fig. 52.8).

Infusion Cannula Versus Infusion Sleeve

In posterior vitrectomies, one always uses a separate infusion cannula (Fig. 52.9). But, in endophthalmitis, there are certain problems. One is that the choroid is thickened and so the cannula tip is not seen. Further the media is very hazy. Second

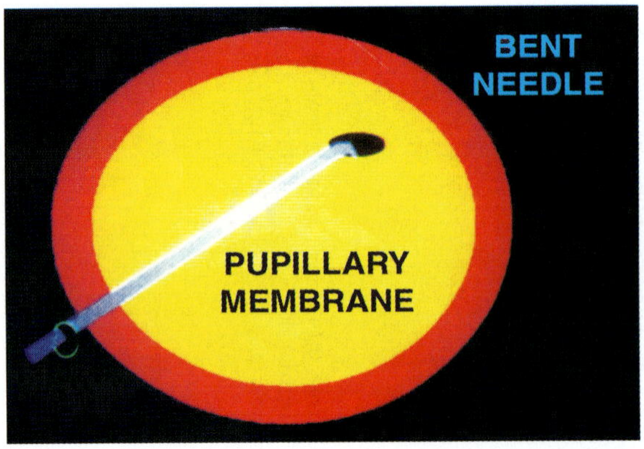

Fig. 52.4: Pupillary membrane being removed with a cystitome

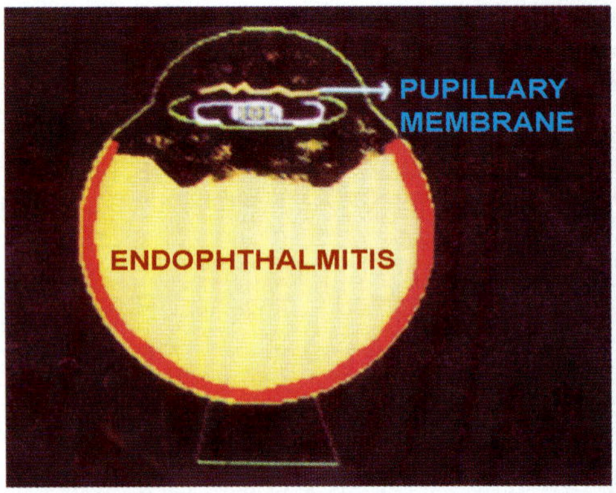

Fig. 52.6: Pupillary membrane present in front of the IOL

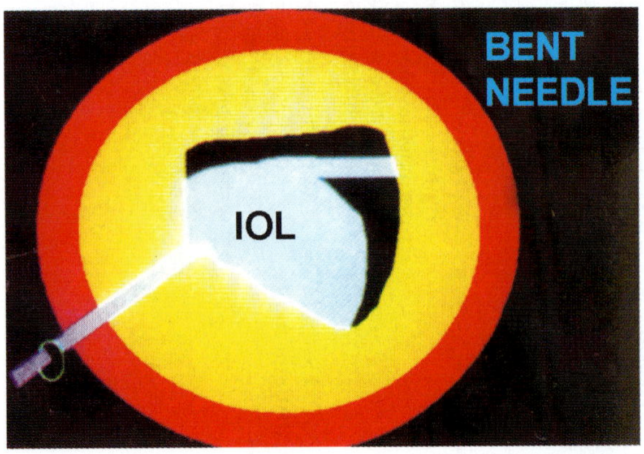

Fig. 52.5: Pupillary membrane removed with cystitome

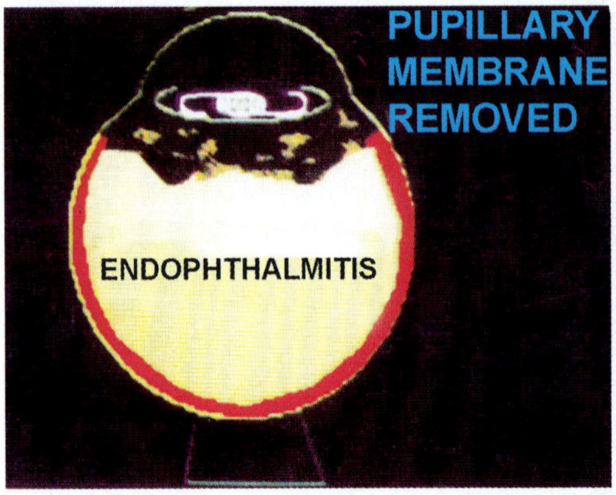

Fig. 52.7: Pupillary membrane removed

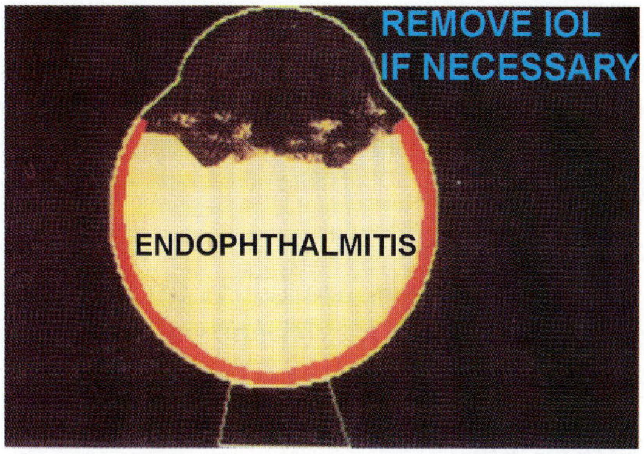

Fig. 52.8: IOL removal done

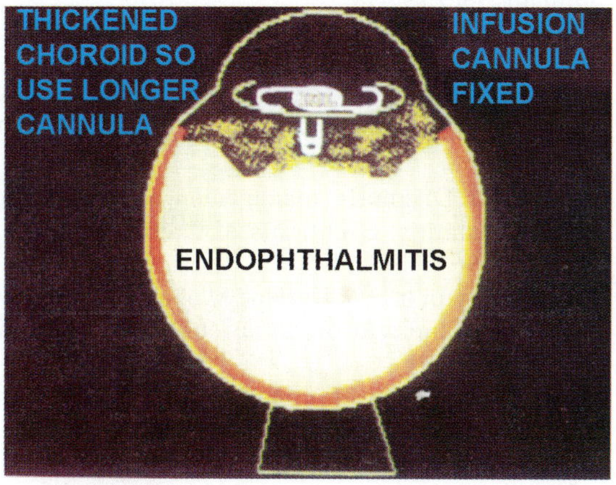

Fig. 52.9: Infusion cannula fixed

problem is that another sclerotomy has to be done which is traumatic. Thirdly, the need for haste might make one not fix an infusion cannula. This is why in endophthalmitis, one might use an infusion sleeve. In this, only a two-port vitrectomy is done in which one port is for the endoilluminator and the other for the vitrectomy probe and aspiration. This probe has an infusion sleeve so that the fluid passes through the same port. We prefer to use a two-port vitrectomy in endophthalmitis cases.

Culture and Sensitivity Testing

Once the infusion cannula is fixed and checked that it is in the vitreous cavity, one should only then make the second sclerotomy for the vitrectomy probe (Fig. 52.10). This probe is first connected to a sterile container so that when cutting is done the

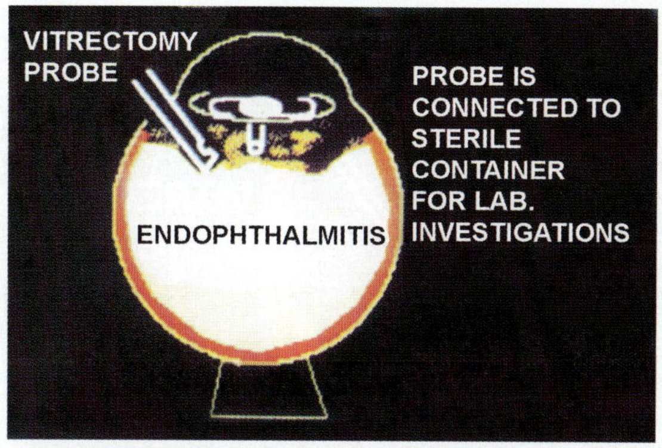

Fig. 52.10: Vitreous tap taken for culture and sensitivity

initial vitreous can be collected and send for culture sensitivity.

Core Vitrectomy

The third sclerotomy is made for the endoilluminator. The vitrectomy is done with low suction force, preferably with linear suction control. The anterior hyaloid face is first removed (Fig. 52.11). One should take care not to damage the iris which can be quite necrotic. If bleeding occurs from the iris, one can use an endodiathermy to control the bleeding.

After the anterior vitreous is removed, a core vitrectomy is done (Fig. 52.12). This avoids traction on the frequently necrotic retina. Vacuum cleaning and membrane peeling should never be done in these cases because of the necrotic retina. These retinas are very prone to retinal breaks. The vitrectomy is done so that the media gets clear, and one starts visualizing the posterior retina.

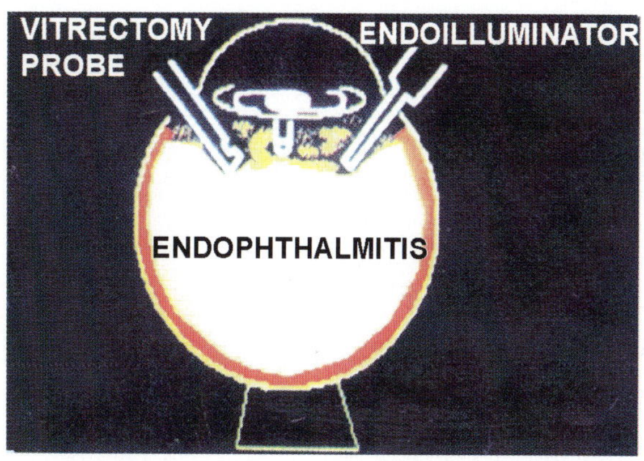

Fig. 52.11: Anterior and midvitrectomy done

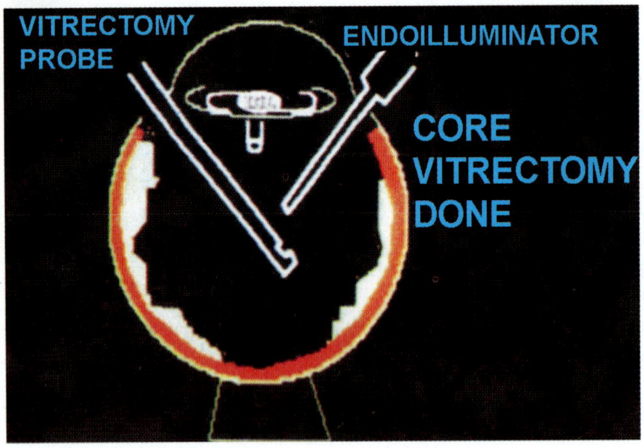

Fig. 52.12: Core vitrectomy done

Antibiotics

Antibiotics diluted in the infusion fluid are not recommended because of the question of toxicity and the difficulty in assessing the total retinal dose. The infusion system should be removed and the 8/0 nylon suture used to close all the sclerotomies except the lower temporal one. Then the antibiotic should be injected in the midvitreous cavity through this sclerotomy taking care of the intravitreal dosage. A 26 gauge needle can be used for this purpose. Then, the sclerotomy is closed with the preplaced 8/0 suture. Finally, at the end of the case subconjunctival injections are also given.

RESULTS

Delay in vitrectomy could lead to a poor visual recovery. If the cases are taken up on time, the prognosis is good. A lot depends also on the etiological agent.

REFERENCES

1. Charles S: Vitreous Microsurgery (2nd ed), Williams and Williams 1987;195-98.
2. Ryan SJ: Retina (2nd ed), CV Mosby: St Louis, 1994;2525-37.
3. Albert DM, Jakobiec FA: Principles and Practise of Ophthalmology WB Saunders: Philadelphia, 1994;1159-69.
4. Speaker M: Diagnosis, management and prevention of endophthalmitis. Highlights of Ophthalmology 1993; 21(11): 89-96.
5. Mao LK, Flynn Jr HW, Darlene M et al: Endophthalmitis caused by Staphylococcus aureus. Am J Ophthalmol 1993;116: 584-89.
6. Kloess PM, Stulting RD, Waring III GO et al: Bacterial and fungal endophthalmitis after penetrating keratoplasty. Am J Ophthalmol 1993;115:309-16.

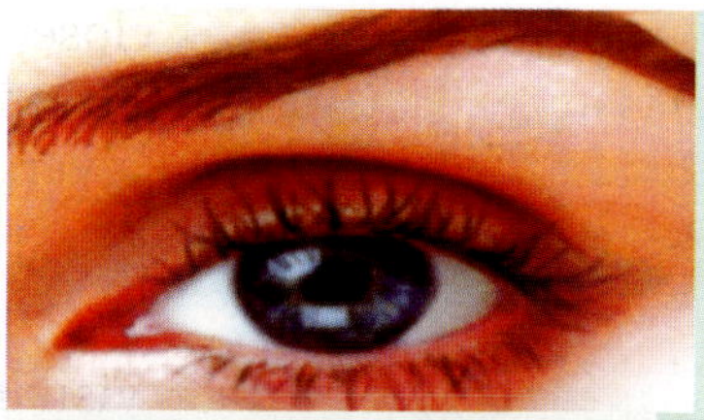

Fifty three

Update on Posterior Capsule Opacification: Etiopathogenesis, Clinical Manifestations, Pharmacological and Surgical Prevention

Suresh K Pandey
Liliana Werner
David J Apple
Andrea M Izak (USA)

INTRODUCTION

Opacification of the posterior capsule caused by postoperative proliferation of cells in the capsular bag remains the most frequent complication of cataract surgery. In addition to classic posterior capsule opacification (PCO), postoperative lens epithelial cell (LEC) proliferation is also involved in the pathogenesis of other entities. These include anterior capsule opacification (ACO) and interlenticular opacification (ILO); a more recently described complication related to piggyback IOLs. Thus, there are three distinct anatomic locations within the capsular bag where clinically significant opacification may occur postoperatively (Fig. 53.1). *In this chapter we will discuss the etiopathogenesis, clinical manifestations, pharmacological, surgical as well implant related factors for prevention of the PCO. Interested readers may consult the published articles for other modalities of capsular bag opacification including ACO and ILO.*[1,10-12,88,89,92,93,95-98,101-104]

POSTERIOR CAPSULE OPACIFICATION (SECONDARY CATARACT)

BACKGROUND AND SIGNIFICANCE

Posterior capsule opacification (PCO, secondary cataract) has been recognized since the origin of extracapsular cataract surgery (ECCE) and was noted by Sir Harold Ridley in his first intraocular lens (IOL) implantations.[3,8] It was particularly common and severe in the early days of IOL surgery when the importance of cortical clean-up was less appreciated. Through the 1980s and early 1990s, the incidence of PCO ranged between 25-53 percent.[7,8]

Improvements in cataract surgical technique have led to a gradual, but steady, decrease in the incidence of this complication. Our data show that through a combination of modern techniques and IOL designs, the incidence of Nd: YAG laser posterior capsulotomy is now decreasing into single digits.[4-6,78-80]

WHY TO ERADICATE PCO?

Although cataract is the most common cause of blindness in the world, after-cataract is an extremely common cause as well. Jan GF Worst, MD stated recently – *"the most meaningful development in intraocular implant research in the next five years will be—effective prevention of secondary cataract formation"* (International Intraocular Implant Club Report, Vol. 1, No. 2, January 1999). Eradication of PCO following ECCE has major medical and financial implications:

A. Nd:YAG laser secondary posterior capsulotomy, can be associated with significant complications. Potential problems including IOL damage, postoperative intraocular pressure elevation, cystoid macular edema, retinal detachment, and IOL subluxation (Fig. 53.2).[36,37,40,41]
B. Dense PCO and/secondary membrane formation particularly common following pediatric IOL implantation.[73] A delay in diagnosis can cause irreparable amblyopia.
C. PCO represents a significant cost to the US healthcare system. Nd:YAG laser treatments of almost one million patients per year have cost upto $250 million annually.
D. A posterior capsulotomy can increase the risk of posterior segment complications in high myopes and patients with uveitis, glaucoma, and diabetic retinopathy.
E. PCO of even a mild degree can decrease near acuity through a multifocal IOL, and may interfere with the function of accommodating IOL designs.
F. Finally, a significant incidence of PCO means that cataract surgery, alone, may not restore lasting sight to the 25 million people worldwide who are blind from cataract.

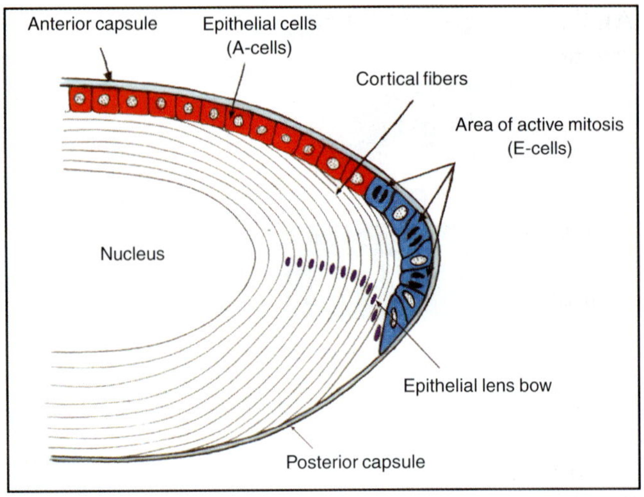

Fig. 53.1: Schematic illustration of the microscopic anatomy of the lens and the capsular bag, showing the "A" cells of the anterior epithelium and the "E" cells, the important germinal epithelial cells of the equatorial lens bow

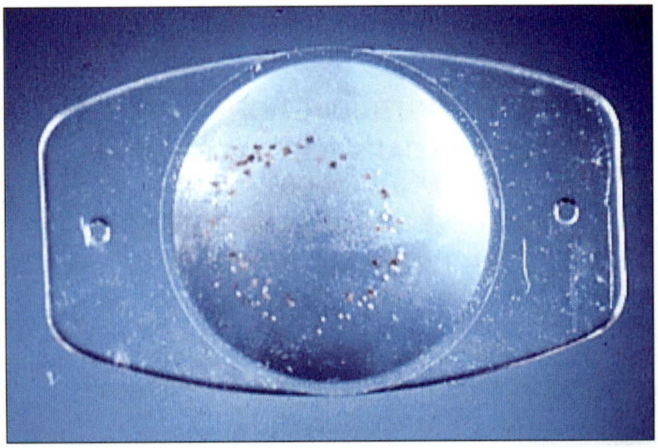

Fig. 53.2: Gross photograph of an explanted foldable posterior chamber intraocular lens (STAAR, 1-piece silicone-plate, small hole) showing multiple Nd: YAG laser lesions on the optical surface

ETIOPATHOGENESIS

Postoperative proliferation of lens epithelial cells in the capsular bag is central to the pathogenesis of PCO. Proliferation of these cells can also lead to

ACO, and ILO.[14,25-29,49,54,70,71] In the normal crystalline lens, the epithelial cells are confined to the anterior surface at the equatorial region and the equatorial lens bow. This single row of cuboidal cells can be divided into two different biological zones (Fig. 53.1):

A. The anterior-central zone (corresponding to the zone of the anterior lens capsule) consists of a monolayer of flat cuboidal, epithelial cells with minimal mitotic activity. In response to a variety of stimuli, the anterior epithelial cells ("A" cells) proliferate and undergo fibrous metaplasia. This has been called "pseudofibrous metaplasia" by Font and Brownstein.[24]
B. The second zone is important in the pathogenesis of "pearl" formation. This layer is a continuation of anterior lens cells around the equator, forming the equatorial lens bow ("E" cells). Unlike within the A-cell layer, cell mitoses, division, and multiplication are quite active in this region. New lens fibers are continuously produced in this zone throughout life.

The majority of clinical PCO is caused by the proliferation of remnant or regenerated lens epithelial cells left in the capsular bag following cataract surgery (Figs 53.3 and 53.4A and B). Although both types of cells (from the anterior central zone and from the equatorial lens bow) have the potential to produce visually significant opacification, most cases of classic PCO are caused by proliferation of the equatorial cells. The term posterior capsule opacification is actually a misnomer. It is not the capsule which opacifies. Rather, an opaque membrane develops as retained cells proliferate and migrate onto the posterior capsular surface.

IOL	Total	Nd:YAG	YAG %
3 PC Acrylic-PMMA (AcrySof)	470	22	4.7%
3 PC Silicone-PMMA	148	18	12.2%
1 PC Silicone Plate, Large Hole	109	22	20.2%
3 PC Silicone-Polyimide	91	20	22.0%
1 PC Silicone Plate, Small Hole	155	36	23.2%
3 PC Silicone-Prolene	409	97	23.7%
3 PC PMMA (Rigid)	3781	1158	30.6%
1 PC All-PMMA (Rigid)	2346	738	31.5%
All Lenses since 1/88	7509	2111	28.1%
Foldable lenses	1382	215	15.6%
Rigid Lenses	6127	1896	30.9%

Fig. 53.3: Gross photograph of a human eye obtained postmortem (Miyake-Apple posterior photographic technique) showing Soemmering's ring formation. The equatorial remnants of a classic Soemmering's ring are composed of cortical material and proliferating E-cells. Although extensive cortical remnants remain forming a massive Soemmering's ring, the central optic region of the visual axis has remained clear in this case, due to the barrier effect provided by the intraocular lens

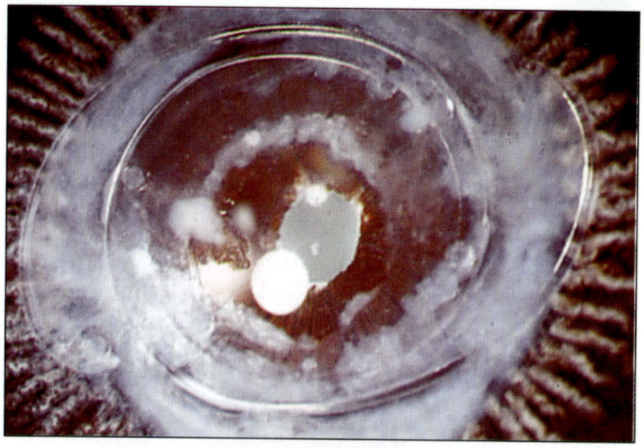

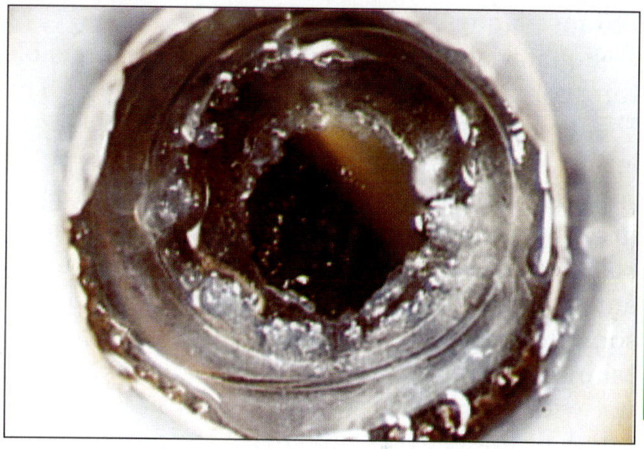

Figs 53.4A and B: Gross photographs of a pseudophakic human globe obtained postmortem implanted with a 1-piece all PMMA lens. Note the presence of a Nd:YAG laser posterior capsulotomy, (A) Posterior view (Miyake-Apple posterior photographic technique), (B) Anterior (surgeon's) view

The opacification usually takes one of two morphologic forms. One form consists of capsular **pearls**, which can consist of clusters of swollen, opacified epithelial "pearls" or clusters of posteriorly migrated equatorial epithelial (E) cells (bladder or Wedl cells). It is probable that both lens epithelial cell types can also contribute to the **fib-**

rous form of opacification. Anterior epithelial (A) cells are probably important in the pathogenesis of fibrosis PCO, since the primary type of response of these cells is to undergo fibrous metaplasia. Although the preferred type of growth of the equatorial epithelial (E) cells is in the direction of bloated, swollen, bullous-like bladder (Wedl) cells, these also may contribute to formation of the fibrous form of PCO by undergoing a fibrous metaplasia. This is a particularly common occurrence in cataracts in third world settings where cataract surgery has been delayed for many years, and where posterior subcapsular cataracts have turned into fibrous plaques.

Equatorial cells (E-cells) are also the responsible for formation of a Soemmering's ring. The Soemmering's ring, a dumb-bell or donut-shaped lesion that often forms following any type of rupture of the anterior capsule, was first described in connection with ocular trauma. The pathogenetic basis of a Soemmering's ring is rupture of the anterior lens capsule with extrusion of nuclear and some central lens material. The extruded cortical remnants then transform into Elschnig pearls. It is not widely appreciated that a Soemmering's ring forms virtually every time that any form of ECCE is done, whether manual, automated or with phacoemulsification (Figs 53.5A to E). This material is derived from proliferation of the epithelial cells (E-cells) of the equatorial lens bow. We have noted that these cells have the capability to proliferate and migrate posteriorly across the visual axis, thereby opacifying the posterior capsular. Because the Soemmering's ring is a direct precursor to PCO, surgeons should strive to prevent its formation.

Cells, types other than lens epithelial cells may be involved in PCO. As extracapsular cataract surgery (ECCE) is always associated with some breakdown of the blood-aqueous barrier, inflammatory cells, erythrocytes, and many other inflammatory mediators may be released into the aqueous humor. The severity of this inflammatory response may be exacerbated by the IOL. This foreign body elicits a three-stage immune response that involves many different cell types, including polymorphonuclear leukocytes, giant cells, and fibroblasts. Collagen deposition onto the IOL and onto the capsule may cause opacities and fine wrinkles to form in the posterior capsule. In most cases, however, this inflammatory response is clinically insignificant. Iris melanocytes also have been shown to adhere to and migrate over the anterior surface of the posterior capsule.

CLINICAL MANIFESTATIONS

The interval between surgery and PCO varies widely, ranging anywhere from three months to four years after the surgery. Although the causes of PCO are multifactorial as reported in the several studies, there is an inverse correlation with age.[7,18,20,23,35] Young age is a significant risk factor for PCO, and its occurrence is a virtual certainty in pediatric patients.[105]

Visual symptoms do not always correlate to the observed amount of PCO. Some patients with significant PCO on slit lamp examination are relatively asymptomatic while others have significant symptoms with mild apparent haze, which is reversed by capsulotomy.[17]

PREVENTION OF POSTERIOR CAPSULE OPACIFICATION

PCO prevention has been an active research interest of ours since 1982. Based on our work, we would review the principles of PCO prevention. These measures can be divided into two categories. One strategy is to minimize the number of retained/regenerate cells and cortex (including the Soemmering's ring) through thorough cortical clean-up. The second strategy is to prevent the remaining cells from migrating posteriorly. The edge of the IOL optic is critical in the formation of such a physical barrier.

We have identified three surgery-related factors and three IOL-related factors that are particularly important in the prevention of PCO (Fig. 53.6).

Three Surgery Related Factors to Reduce PCO

Hydrodissection-enhanced Cortical Clean-up

A very important and underrated factor is the hydrodissection component of the operation (Figs 53.7A to C). Dr. I. Howard Fine perfected and popularized this technique and coined the term

Grade 0

Grade 1

Grade 2

Grade 3

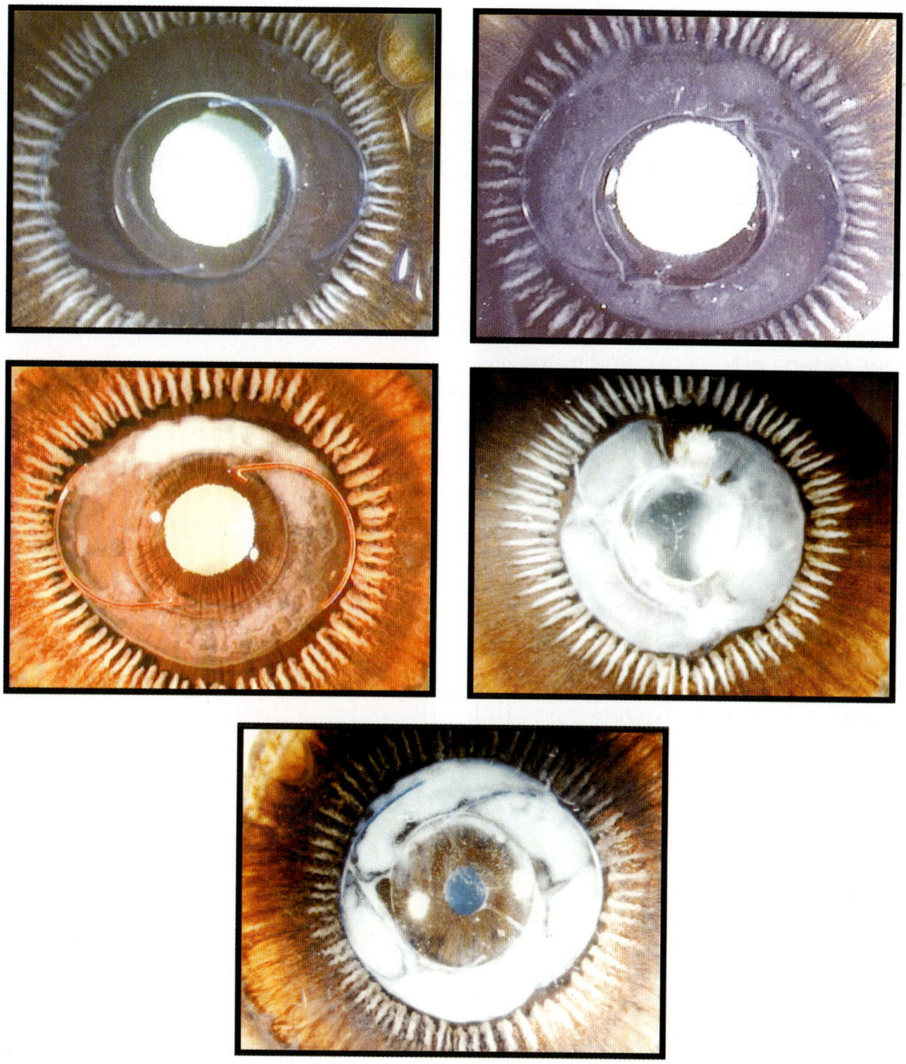

Grade 4

Figs 53.5A to E: Biocompatibility analyses can be obtained by evaluating and scoring peripheral PCO (Soemmering's ring) and central PCO. Using these techniques we have been able to note apparent differences in materials in terms of inhibiting both central and peripheral PCO. Gross photographs from behind (Miyake-Apple posterior photographic technique) of human eyes obtained postmortem showing varying degree of the Soemmering's ring formation: (A) Grade 0 (Alcon AcrySof^{TM} acrylic IOL), (B) Grade 1 (Allergan SI-40 silicone IOL), (C) Grade 2 (Silicone optic/polyimide haptics), (D) Grade 3 (PMMA optic/PMMA haptics), (E) Grade 4 (PMMA optic/prolene haptics)

cortical cleaving hydrodissection.[22] Until fairly recently, many surgeons had a rather fatalistic attitude regarding removal of lens cortex and cells during ECCE, either manual or automated, or with phacoemulsification. The common opinion was that removing all or even most equatorial cells from the bag is impossible. PCO was therefore considered an inevitable complication. This conclusion was partly because PCO occurred in upto 50 percent of cases. We now know from autopsy and experimental studies that good cortical and cellular clean-up can be accomplished in a much more efficient fashion in a majority of cases than had previously been believed. The hydrodissection procedure with special focus on freeing and rotating the lens nucleus facilitates lens substance removal without

6 Factors to Reduce PCO

3 Surgery-Related Factors ("Capsular" Surgery)

1. Hydrodissection-enhanced cortical clean-up.
2. In-the-bag fixation.
3. CCC diameter slightly smaller than that of IOL optic. This places the CCC edge of the anterior surface of the optic and helps sequester the capsular bag, creating a "shrink wrap" of the capsule around the IOL optic

3 IOL-Related Factors ("Ideal" IOL)

1. Biocompatible IOL to reduce stimulation of cellular proliferation.
2. Maximal IOL optic-posterior capsule contact, angulated haptic, "bioadhesive" biomaterial to create a "shrinkwrap."
3. IOL optic geometry: Square, truncated edge.

Fig. 53.6: Factors that significantly influence the formation of PCO. Three factors are related to the type and quality of surgery and three are related to IOL material/design

zonular-capsular rupture. Recently, we have shown an important additional long-term advantage of hydrodissection; namely, a means of more efficient removal of cortex and cells that in turn is essential in reducing PCO. With careful, meticulous hydrodissection, the operation is much easier and faster, cortex and cell removal is much more thorough and formation of an unwanted Soemmering's ring is minimized. A successful performed cortical cleaving hydrodissection provides an easy way to extract the entire lens cortex as well as nucleus, often without the need

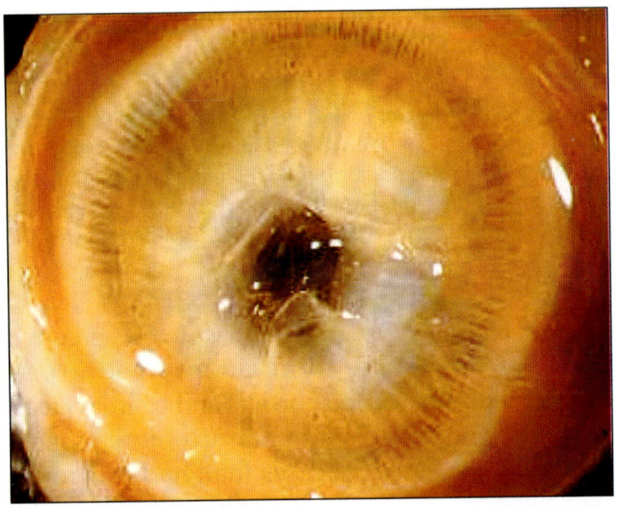

Fig. 53.7A: Control group; Gross photograph obtained from behind (Miyake-Apple posterior view) showing the obscuration of the central visual axis

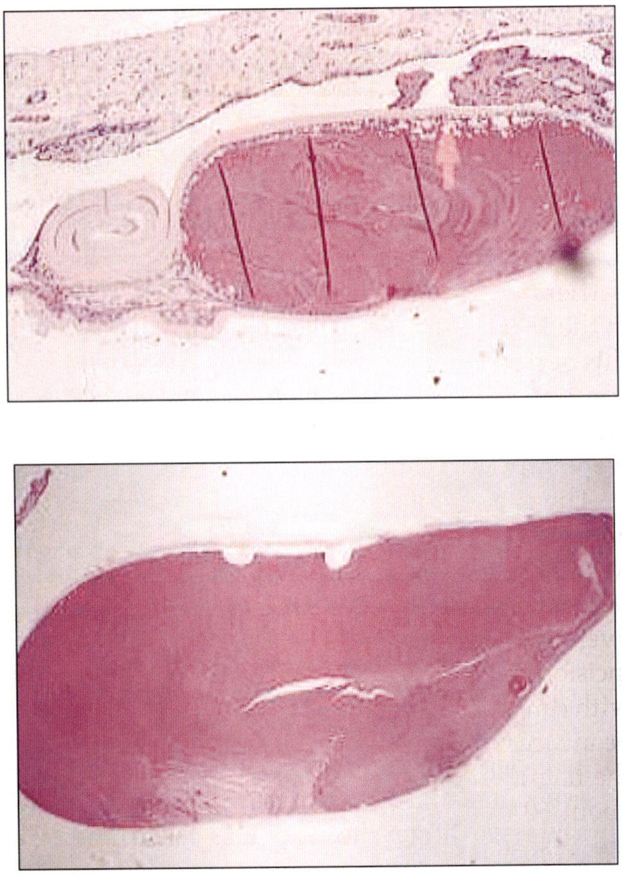

Figs 53.7B and C: Photomicrographs taken from the right and left sides of the capsular bag, respectively. Note the presence of exuberant cortical material and lens epithelial cells (H and E X200, H and E X100 respectively)

for cortical aspiration. The necessary tenting up of the anterior capsule is best achieved by using a cannula with a bend at the tip allowing a flow of fluid toward the capsule to efficiently separate capsule from cortex.

In-the-Bag (Capsular) Fixation

The hallmark of modern cataract surgery is the achievement of consistent and secure in-the-bag (capsular) fixation (Fig. 53.6). The most obvious advantage of in-the-bag fixation is the accomplishment of good optic centration and sequestration of the IOL from adjacent uveal tissues. The numerous other advantages have been described in detail elsewhere. However, it is not often appreciated that this is also extremely important in reducing the amount of PCO.

The primary function of in-the-bag fixation is enhancing the IOL-optic barrier effect, which is functional and maximal when the lens optic is fully in-the-bag with direct contact with the posterior capsule. In case one or both haptics are not placed in the bag, a potential space is created, allowing an avenue for cells to grow posteriorly toward the visual axis. The reader may recall the barrier ridge IOL design devised by Kenneth Hoffer in the 1980s, which did not function sufficiently in this period. The reason was not a problem with the concept or the IOLs themselves, but in that time only about 30 percent of posterior chamber IOLs were implanted in the bag.

The growth of incidence of in-the-bag fixation, although steady and positive, reached what appears to be a limit with non-phaco ECCE of about 60 percent. Apparently, the reason is that many cases over the years had been done with classic large-incision extracapsular surgery with rigid IOLs, often with can-opener anterior capsulotomy. We have to be aware of the fact that secure and permanent in-the-bag fixation only occurred in a maximum of about 60 percent of cases. This rate appears to be the best achievable with these early techniques. However, when considering modern foldable lens implantation, the number rapidly rises to over 90 percent. It is not the foldable IOL itself, or even the small incision in and of itself that provides this positive result, but rather the fact that successful foldable IOL insertion generally requires meticulous surgery, with the necessity of performing a continuous curvilinear capsulorhexis (CCC) and secure implantation of both IOL loops in the bag.

Capsulorhexis Edge on IOL Surface

A less obvious, but significant addition to precise in-the-bag fixation, is creating a CCC diameter slightly smaller than that of the IOL optic. For example, if the IOL optic were 6.0 mm, the capsulorhexis diameter would ideally be slightly smaller, perhaps 5.0 to 5.5 mm. This places the cut anterior capsule edge on the anterior surface of the optic, providing a tight fit (analogous to a "shrink wrap") and helping to sequester the optic in the capsular bag from the surrounding aqueous humor (Fig. 53.6). This mechanism may support protecting the milieu within the capsule from at least some potentially deleterious factors within the aqueous, especially some macromolecules, and some inflammatory mediators. The concept of capsular sequestration based on the CCC size and shape is subtle, but more and more surgeons appear to be applying this principle and seeing its advantages.

Three IOL-related Factors to Reduce PCO

In addition to the three above-mentioned surgery-related factors we will describe briefly the three IOL-related factors, which in our opinion play an important role in the eradication of PCO.

Biocompatibility

Lens material biocompatibility (Figs 53.6, and 53.11 to 53.13) is an often misunderstood term. It may be defined by many criteria, e.g. the ability to inhibit stimulation of epithelial cellular proliferation: the less the cell proliferation the less the chance for secondary cataract formation. The Alcon AcrySof™ IOL scored well with these criteria, with respect to Soemmering's ring formation, PCO and with respect to anterior capsule opacification. In addition, the amount of cell proliferation is greatly influenced by surgical factors, such as copious cortical clean-up. Furthermore, the time factor plays a role, such as the duration of the implant in the eye. Additional long-term studies are required to assess the overall role of "biocompatibility" in the pathogenesis of PCO.

Maximal IOL Optic Posterior Capsule Contact

Other contributing factors in reducing PCO are posterior angulation of the IOL haptic and posterior convexity of the optic (Fig. 53.6). This is due to the creation of a "shrink wrap", a tight fit of the posterior capsule against the back of the IOL optic. The relative "stickiness" of the IOL optic biomaterial probably helps producing an adhesion between the capsule and IOL optic. There is preliminary evidence that the Alcon AcrySof™ IOL biomaterial provides such enhanced adhesion, or "bioadhesion".[46-48,58] This will require further study.

Barrier Effect of the IOL Optic

The IOL optic barrier effect (Fig. 53.6), plays an important role as a second line of defense against PCO, especially in cases where retained cortex and cells remain following ECCE. The concept of the barrier effect goes back to the original Ridley lens. If accurately implanted in the capsular bag, it provided an excellent barrier effect, with almost complete filling of the capsular bag and contact of the posterior IOL optic to the posterior capsule ("no space, no cells"). A lens with one or both haptics "out-of-the-bag" has much less of a chance to produce a barrier effect. Indeed, the IOL optic's barrier function has been one of the main reasons that PC-IOLs implanted after ECCE throughout the decades did not produce an unacceptably high incidence of florid PCO. Actually, the barrier effect has enabled the success of IOL implantation after ECCE during the past decades.

A subtle difference between classic optics with a round tapered edge and optics with a square truncated edge became evident recently (Fig. 53.6). The effect of a square-edge optic design as a barrier was first discussed by Nishi *et al* in the articles related to PCO.[59-69] In a clinicopathological study, our laboratory was the first to confirm this phenomenon in human eyes.[74,75] We reported our results of a large histopathological analysis covering the IOL barrier effect, with special reference to the efficacy of the truncated edge. A truncated, square-edged optic rim appears to be cause a complete blockade of cells at the optic edge, preventing epithelial ingrowth over the posterior capsule.[42,43,50,51,55,56,83,86,87] The enhanced barrier effect provided by this optic geometry probably functions as an "icing on the cake". It seems to provide another reserve factor, in addition to the five abovementioned factors, contributing in diminishing the overall incidence of visually significant PCO.

Our studies upto-date have shown, that the Alcon AcrySof™ IOL best achieves the goals of these three IOL-related factors (Fig. 53.6). Other IOL designers are rapidly moving to provide comparable features, especially a conversion to sharp edges. A major disadvantage of the truncated edge is the possible formation of clinical visual aberration, e.g. glare, halos and crescents. Subtle changes in manufacturing are now helping alleviate these complications. An example of this include introduction of Optic Edge™ IOL manufactured by Allergan. This IOL has squared posterior edge and a round anterior edge. Therefore, it avoids the glare and other disadvantages and on the other hand the squared posterior edge is helpful to prevent/delay development of PCO.

Confirmation of 6 Factors in Clinical Studies

We would like to mention 3 studies that confirm the advantage of applying one or more surgical/IOL related factors to prevent or delay PCO formation. In a large clinical study, Ram, Pandey, Apple, Werner and associates[79] has confirmed previous pathological studies showing the need for mandatory in-the-bag fixation of posterior chamber IOLs (both rigid and foldable) to help reduce the incidence of PCO. This is true for both ECCE and phacoemulsification. This study was performed in Chandigarh, India, and was a combined effort of the Postgraduate Institute of Medical Education and Research (PGIMER), Chandigarh, India, and the Center for Research on Ocular Therapeutics and Biodevices, Storm Eye Institute, Charleston, SC, USA. This study comprised 278 eyes of 263 patients having ECCE and 318 eyes of 297 patients having phacoemulsification with PC IOL implantation. Posterior capsule opacification leading to a decrease in Snellen visual acuity of 2 or more lines was considered visually significant.

The presence of PCO and IOL haptic fixation were evaluated postoperatively using slit lamp biomicroscopy. Haptic position was noted as in-the-bag (B-B), 1 haptic in the bag and 1 in the sulcus (bag-sulcus [B-S]), or both haptics out of the bag (sulcus-sulcus [S-S]). In addition, the rate of visually significant PCO was compared among 3 IOL biomaterials: poly(methyl methacrylate), silicone, and hydrophobic acrylic. Visually significant PCO occurred in 42.45 percent of eyes having ECCE and 19.18 percent of eyes having phacoemulsification ($P < .001$, chi-square test) after a mean follow-up of 2.4 years +/- 0.7 (SD). In both groups, visually significant PCO was significantly less in eyes with B-B fixation than in those with B-S or S-S fixation ($P < .001$). The rate of visually significant PCO in all eyes in the phacoemulsification group with B-B fixation was low (11.90%) and was significantly lower in eyes with a hydrophobic acrylic IOL (2.22%; $P < .05$, chi-square test). The results of this study suggested in-the-bag PC IOL fixation is required to consistently reduce the incidence of PCO. Thorough removal of lens substance, including hydrodissection-assisted cortical clean-up, and in-the-bag PC IOL fixation seem to be the most important factors in reducing PCO, regardless of surgical procedure or IOL type used. Intraocular lens biomaterial and design also help prevent PCO.

Ravalico and associates[81] studied an ideal capsulorhexis size that could able to reduce PCO incidence. These authors retrospectively evaluated 107 patients who had extracapsular cataract extraction with capsulorhexis and capsular bag IOL implantation. The PCO site (central, paracentral, and peripheral) and degree (mild, moderate, and severe) were evaluated in relation to the capsulorhexis edge location relative to the IOL optic. Patients were divided into three groups. Group 1: capsulorhexis free edge located on the IOL optic for 360 degrees; Group 2: capsulorhexis free edge located asymmetrically on and peripherally to the IOL optic; Group 3: capsulorhexis free edge located peripherally to IOL optic for 360 degrees. Each group was divided into two subgroups; one received polyHema IOLs and the second, PMMA IOLs. Results of this study have shown that, in Groups 1 and 2, the capsular transparency was higher than in Group 3 ($P < .04$). Central opacification percentage was lower in Group 1 than in Groups 2 and 3 ($P < .04$). No statistically significant differences between the polyHema and the PMMA subgroups were seen. These authors concluded that capsulorhexis with a slightly smaller diameter than the IOL optic appears to be better than a large-size capsulorhexis in reducing the incidence of PCO.

T. Akahoshi, MD, had reported his experience of AcrySof™ IOL implantation in more than 17,000 human eyes in Japan. The incidence of YAG capsulotomy had been found to be 1.19 percent (207 out of 17,329) after 75 months of the follow-up period. Among the YAG treated cases, 81.2 percent had an eccentric and incomplete coverage of the lens optics by the anterior capsulorhexis margin. In 8.2 percent of the cases, the anterior capsule margin was on the optics edge and 10.6 percent was completely outside. Long-term follow-up revealed that the incidence of after cataract formation in AcrySof™ is extremely low. The size and position of the CCC, however, seems to be one of the most important factors to reduce the YAG capsulotomy rate. (T. Akahoshi, MD Clear corneal cataract surgery and AcrySof™ implantation. Presented in the ASCRS Symposium on Cataract, IOL and Refractive Surgery, Boston, MA, April 28, 2001).

Pharmacological Prevention of PCO

Several experimental studies using intraocular infusion of drugs like colchicine, methotrexate, retinoic acid and 5-fluorouracil (5-FU) had also been performed in animal models to prevent PCO.[19,76,77,82,83,91,92,95]

We designed an intracapsular ring to prevent capsular bag contraction and also to inhibit LECs proliferation and metaplasia by sustained release of 5-FU. We prospectively studied the effects of the intracapsular rings on the prevention of PCO by analyzing the postmortem ocular specimens macroscopically and histologically. We also evaluated the toxic effects of 5-FU on the corneal endothelium, capsular bag and retina of the rabbits.[72] Seventeen rabbits were divided into 3 groups: (i) six rabbits (6 eyes) had phacoemulsification (PE) only (control group); (ii) six rabbits (6 eyes) had PE with implantation of an open loop hydrogel intracapsular ring, (iii) five rabbits (5 eyes) had PE with implantation of ring with sustained release of 0.25 μg/hour of 5-FU for 9 days. All eyes in the 3 groups were followed for 8 weeks before enucleation. Assessment of capsular bag shrinkage, positioning of the intracapsular ring and evaluation of central and peripheral PCO for intensity and area were done by stereomicroscopy from a posterior (Miyake-Apple) view.[2,53] Residual equatorial lens epithelial cells were counted by the same observer in histological sections. Transmission electron microscopy (TEM) of cornea, capsular bag and retina was done to evaluate the toxicity of 5-FU.

No significant difference was seen in the degree of capsular bag shrinkage in the 3 groups. Decentration of the intracapsular ring was seen in 2 eyes (1 each in group 2 and 3 respectively). A statistically significant difference ($p < 0.05$, Student "T" test) was obtained between the control group and eyes with intracapsular ring, concerning the area and intensity of central PCO. No difference was seen between the latter and the group with rings releasing 5-FU. No evidence of toxicity of 5-FU to intraocular structures (cornea, capsular bag and retina) was demonstrated with TEM analysis. Our study revealed that implantation of intracapsular ring may prevent central PCO after cataract surgery by mechanically blocking migration of lens epithelial cells towards the central visual axis. The potential pharmacological effect of 5-FU for PCO prevention was not demonstrated in this experimental study.[72]

The use of intracapsular tension rings to prevent PCO and PCO-related capsular bag shrinkage has recently been reported by several authors.[44,45,52] Kugelberg and co-workers[44] examined after-cataract development and eye growth in lensectomized newborn rabbits implanted with open PMMA capsular tension rings of two different sizes (7 mm and 10 mm). The wet mass of the after-cataract was measured at 3 months after surgery in eyes with and without ring. A significant reduction in the wet mass of the after-cataract was seen in the eye with 10 mm rings in comparison to those with the 7 mm rings or the aphakic eyes.

Nishi and coworkers[62,63] investigated the inhibitory effect of a discontinuous capsular bend created by an IOL with a band-shaped loop or a capsular tension ring on migrating lens epithelial cells. The round form of the open-circular loop of a PMMA IOL was changed to a band-like shape, 1 mm wide and 0.2 mm thick. A capsular tension ring of the same shape with a diameter of 14 mm was also made. They implanted the IOL or the ring into the capsular bag in 5 rabbit eyes after cataract surgery. The same IOL with an unmodified haptic or a conventional capsular tension ring was implanted in the contralateral eye as a control. Gross and histopathological examinations were performed in the enucleated eyes after 8 weeks. LECs accumulation was seen at the equatorial corner outside the IOL haptic or the ring, with inhibition of LEC migration toward the center. In the control eyes, LECs accumulated inside the haptic or ring, forming a Soemmering's ring, showing markedly less inhibition of LECs migration.

Hara and coworkers[30,31] determined the efficacy of an equator ring in maintaining the circular contour of the capsular bag equator and the transparency of the posterior capsule after crystalline lens extraction in 12 rabbit eyes. A flexible silicone ring was implanted in the capsular bag in seven rabbit eyes. A 13.0 mm Sinskey-style posterior chamber IOL was also implanted inside the ring. Three other eyes received only equatorial rings and two eyes received only IOLs. All eyes were followed up for 3.5 months. The authors reported equatorial distortion and severe PCO in 2 eyes that received only the IOL. In nine (90%) of the 10 eyes implanted with the rings, the circular contour of the equator was preserved, and seven (70%) of these 10 eyes had transparent posterior capsules.

Hashizoe *et al*[33] also evaluated the efficacy of a flexible, silicone equator ring in maintaining capsular bag integrity at the equator and transparency of the posterior capsule, but using *cynomolgus* monkeys. The eyes were followed for an average of 5.9 months. The ring effectively maintained the circular contour of the capsular bag and posterior capsule transparency. The authors concluded that the equator ring is a promising device for maintaining capsular bag integrity and minimizing PCO after cataract surgery.

Nagamoto and Bissen-Miyajima[57]designed four prototypes of rings for supporting and preserving the postoperative integrity of the capsular bag, independently of IOL implantation following circular curvilinear capsulorhexis (CCC). An open, PMMA ring, inserted experimentally in cadaver eyes through a 3.5 mm incision, adjusted well to various capsular bag sizes and could be implanted with common IOL types. Although some capsular shrinkage occurred, in general the roundness of the capsular bag equator was preserved. The control specimens with the IOL alone had capsular shrinkage in areas that were not in contact with the haptics, thus the capsular bag was deformed. The untreated controls capsular bag (no ring, no IOL) folded and lost their roundness.

An open-loop intracapsular ring has the advantage of being implanted in the eye through a small incision. We used intracapsular rings manufactured from a hydrogel biomaterial, i.e. copolymer of hydroxy propyl methacrylate (HPMA)-methylmethacrylate (MMA). Recently flexible closed-loop equator rings manufactured from silicone elastomer have also been investigated by some authors.[30,31] No study compared the efficacy of open-loop, intracapsular hydrogel rings and silicone rings in preventing PCO and capsular bag shrinkage.

Intraocular application of pharmacologic agents has also been investigated by several authors as a means to prevent PCO.[15,16,32,34,38,38] The idea is to selectively destroy the LECs and avoid toxic side effects on other intraocular tissues such as the sensitive corneal endothelium. Most of the pharmacologic agents being tested are used for cancer therapy (e.g., antimetabolites as methotraxate, mitomycin, daunomycin, 5-FU, colchicine, and daunorubicin), anti-inflammatory substances, hypo-osmolar drugs, and immunological means have also been investigated.

Published studies concerning the pharmacological prevention of PCO were mostly cell culture and *in vitro* experiments but some animal test results are also available. Hartmann *et al*[32] and Sourdille and Ducournau[93] reported the first clinical studies in patients using an antimetabolite, daunorubicin, for PCO prevention, nevertheless longer follow-up is necessary to evaluate the long-term effect of this drug. Pharmacologic agents in combination with a sustained drug delivery system (SDDS) have been used by some authors.[32,44] The idea is to extend the intraocular delivery time to a longer period and thereby avoid toxic intraocular drug levels by release of a constant therapeutic drug concentration.

Solomon *et al*[92]as shown in a rabbit model that slow release of 5-FU prevents toxic drug levels. The effect of this antimetabolite on PCO reduction was significant in comparison to the controls. Legler *et al*[17] performed a similar study with colchicine. Significant PCO reduction was observed with no toxic side effects in the group with the lowest colchicine concentration. In this study,[44] the SDDS had the shape of a wafer and was inserted in the capsular bag without an IOL.

In our current *in vivo* study, the drug tested was 5-FU and we found that the shrinkage of the capsular bag diameter was less in groups 2 and 3 when compared to group 1. However, this difference was not statistically significant. This can probably be correlated with the degree of peripheral PCO. There was no significant difference in the intensity and area of peripheral PCO among the 3 groups. Also, in our study the eyes were followed up only for 8 weeks. Due to the small numbers of specimens in each group, we could not conclude that the open intracapsular ring was not effective to prevent the shrinkage of the capsular bag.

Gross evaluation of enucleated eyes using the Miyake-Apple posterior view revealed that implantation of an intracapsular ring prevented central PCO when compared to control group (Figs 53.7 to 53.9). This correlates well with the results of Kugelberg and co-workers[44] concerning aftercataract and eye growth in lensectomized newborn rabbits, and with the study by Nishi and coworkers[62,63] investigating the inhibitory effect of a discontinuous capsular bend on migrating lens epithelial cells.

In our aforementioned rabbit study,[72] we also performed the counting of the equatorial LECs in histological sections as reported by Ruiz *et al*[82] We noticed that LECs were significantly less in eyes with an intracapsular ring (groups 2 and 3) when compared to the control group (Figs 53.7 to 53.9). This could be explained by the presence of the ring

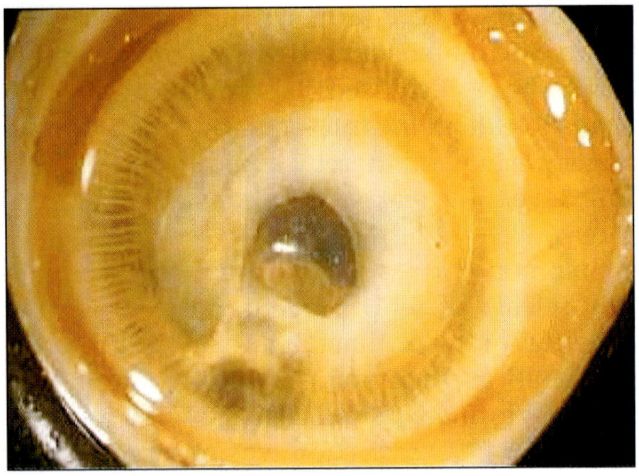

Fig. 53.8A: Intracapsular ring group; Gross photograph obtained from behind (Miyake-Apple posterior view) showing the presence of some lens epithelial cells with relatively clear visual axis

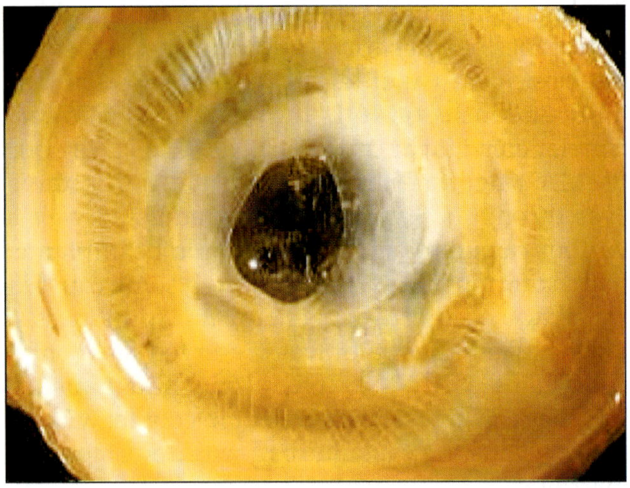

Fig. 53.9A: Intracapsular ring with 5-FU group; Gross photograph obtained from behind (Miyake-Apple posterior view). Note the clear visual axis

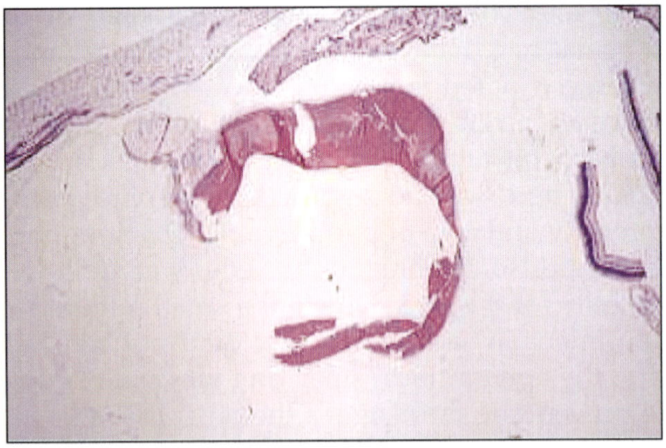

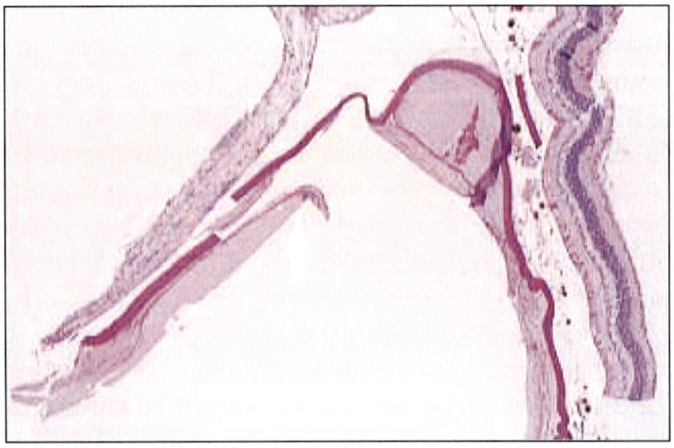

Figs 53.8B and C: Photomicrographs taken from the right and left sides of the capsular bag respectively. Note the mechanical blockage due to the presence of the intracapsular ring (H and E X100)

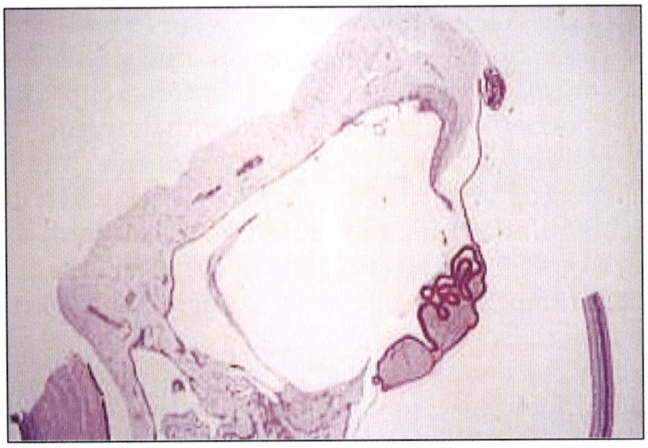

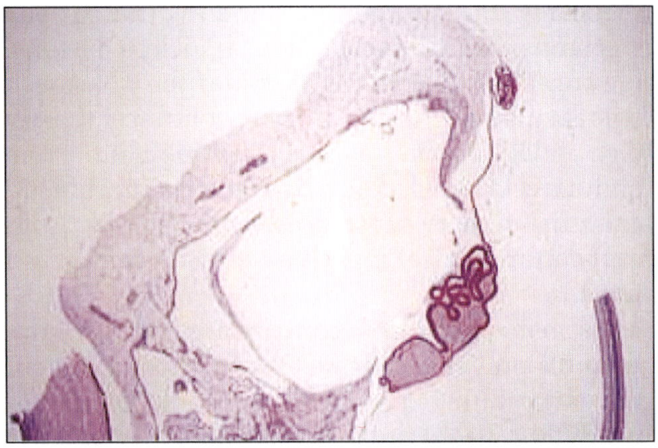

Figs 53.9B and C: Photomicrographs taken from the right and left sides of the capsular bag respectively

Figs 53.7 to 53.9: Assessment of posterior capsule opacification in the 3 groups in our *in vivo* rabbit study[72]

in the capsular bag not allowing the central migration of the LECs, creating a barrier effect (no space-no cell theory). Although in our study the intracapsular ring with a round edge presented a barrier effect, this was not able to completely prevent the central migration of the residual regenerative cortex in some eyes. Figure 53.8 shows an example of migration of regenerative / retained cortex in one of the eyes in group 2 which underwent implantation of the intracapsular ring. Future studies may be helpful to precisely address the effect of squared-edged intracapsular ring on the hindrance of PCO as several recent studies demonstrated that square edged IOL optics offer a better barrier effect, when compared to round edged IOL optics.

The antimetabolite 5-FU specifically acts on mitotic cells by inhibiting the enzyme thymidylate synthetase. Therefore, the postmitotic tissues of the anterior and posterior chambers of the eye should not be affected by the action of this antimetabolite and only the proliferative activity of the LECs of the anterior capsule could be affected by the sustained release of this drug. We could not find any evidence of toxicity of 5-FU to the corneal endothelium or retina with TEM analyses. We are aware that the corneal endothelium in rabbit corneas, in contrast to human, has a tremendous regenerative capacity. As reported by Van Horn and coworkers,[100] even if 50 percent of the central corneal endothelial cells are destroyed by transcorneal freezing, within 10 days sufficient cell division and migration occur to completely repopulate the area of Descemet's membrane denuded of cells, and the corneal thickness returns to normal. Thus, results regarding the toxicity of 5-FU to corneal endothelial cells need to be interpreted with caution. In human eyes, cells that do not rapidly replicate, such as those of corneal endothelium, iris, ciliary body, and retina, are supposed to be less sensitive to the drug. Except for the lens epithelium, all structures within the anterior and posterior chambers are postmitotic.

Our experimental study could not demonstrate an additional effect of 5-FU for prevention of PCO when compared to the mechanical effect provided by the presence of the intracapsular ring. The 5-FU drug delivery properties of the biomaterial were dependent on the hydration of the polymer.[15] The rate of 5-FU release was calculated by the manufacturer (Corneal Laboratories) according to a preliminary (*in vitro*) study[15] and the peak (nontoxic) of 5-FU concentration for the intraocular tissues as studied by Rootman and associates.[82] Based on these studies, 5-FU concentration in the anterior chamber and capsular bag of the rabbits was maintained at 1 μg/ml during 7 days. According to the manufacturer, the ring could be modified to contain larger amounts of 5-FU, with eventually a better effect on prevention of PCO. Nevertheless, additional studies would be necessary to determine the effects of this modification on ocular structures, with regards to 5-FU toxicity.

In summary, according to our macroscopic and histological evaluations, the presence of an intracapsular ring seems to prevent central PCO after cataract surgery by a mechanical effect. An open-loop intracapsular ring can be implanted in the eye through a small incision and offers a barrier effect preventing the central migration of the LECs towards the posterior capsule. Associated release of 5-FU might have an additional impact on the inhibition of PCO, at least on central PCO, although this could not be demonstrated statistically in our study. Concerning the toxicity of the 5-FU release to the corneal endothelium, no definitive conclusion can be drawn from this study, on account of the proliferation capacity of rabbit corneal endothelial cells. This fact raises concerns on the applicability of this concept to the human eye.

ANALYSIS OF ND:YAG POSTERIOR CAPSULOTOMY RATES

Complete analysis of our large series of eyes obtained postmortem has helped us develop the above-mentioned six factors that we believe greatly contributes to the reduction of PCO. Furthermore, an analysis of Nd: YAG laser posterior capsulotomy rates among 8 commonly used intraocular lens models has led us to the optimistic conclusion that the incidence of PCO is rapidly diminishing, especially at least in the industrialized world. Figure 53.10 shows the ranking of the Nd: YAG laser posterior capsulotomy rates (%) for eight lens designs as of December 2000, starting with the lens showing the lowest percentage at the top and the highest rate at the bottom (Fig. 53.10). Note that the

IOL	Total	Nd:YAG	YAG %
3 PC Acrylic-PMMA (AcrySof)	470	22	4.7%
3 PC Silicone-PMMA	148	18	12.2%
1 PC Silicone Plate, Large Hole	109	22	20.2%
3 PC Silicone-Polyimide	91	20	22.0%
1 PC Silicone Plate, Small Hole	155	36	23.2%
3 PC Silicone-Prolene	409	97	23.7%
3 PC PMMA (Rigid)	3781	1158	30.6%
1 PC All-PMMA (Rigid)	2346	738	31.5%
All Lenses since 1/88	7509	2111	28.1%
Foldable lenses	1382	215	15.6%
Rigid Lenses	6127	1896	30.9%

Fig. 53.10: Tabulation of Nd:YAG laser capsulotomy rates on 8 different IOL types between January 1988 upto 2001. These are listed with the highest capsulotomy rates below. Note that the 2 rigid optic designs had the highest rates

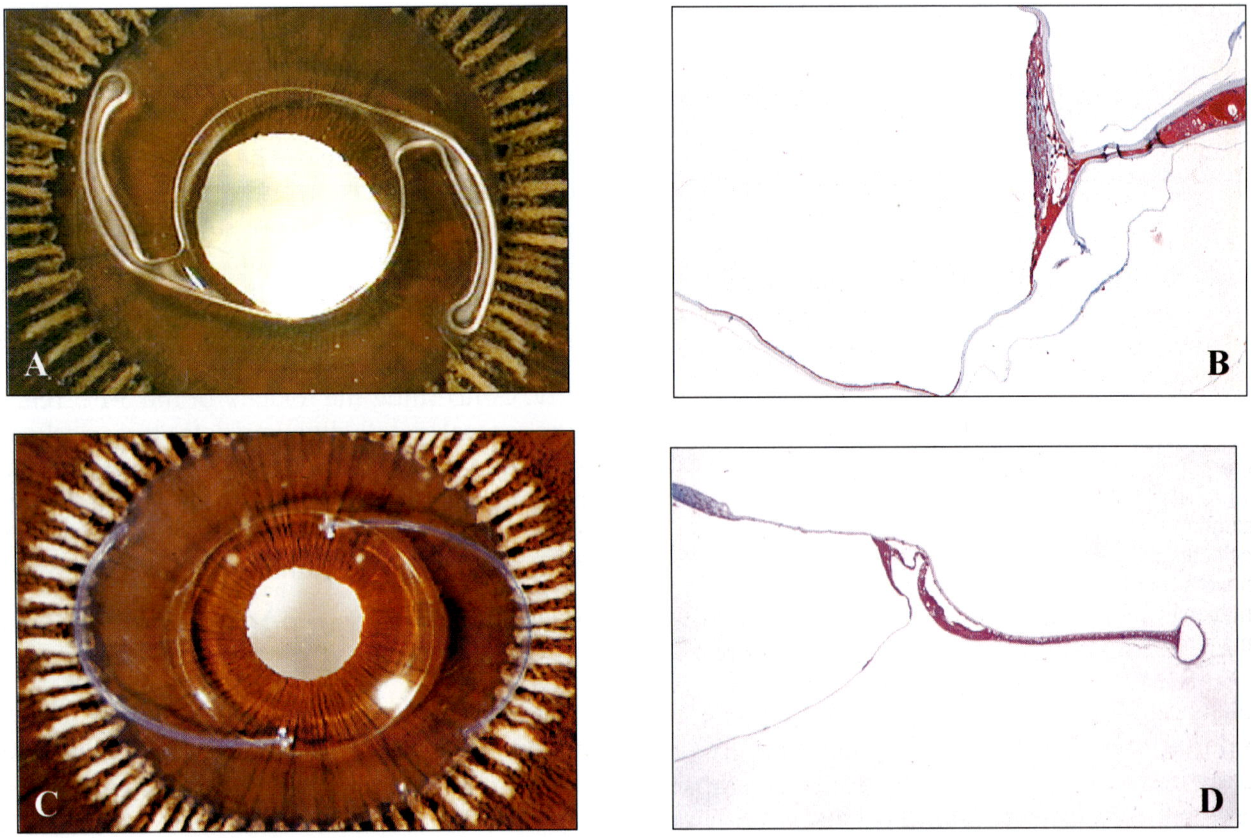

Figs 53.11A to D: Hydrophobic acrylic IOLs had the lowest PCO formation and therefore the Nd:YAG laser posterior capsulotomy rates. The lowest PCO rate was confirmed by gross and histological evaluation: (A) Human eye obtained postmortem, Miyake-Apple posterior photographic technique of a single-piece hydrophobic acrylic optic/haptics (Alcon AcrySof™) PC-IOL showing a symmetric fixation and excellent centration. The surgical technique was excellent and there is virtually no retained/regenerative material (Soemmering's ring). This obviously represents good cortical clean-up, and also suggests good biocompatibility with minimal proliferation, (B) Histological evaluation shows the posterior capsule totally cell-free. The IOL optic is the empty space between the capsules on the left (Masson's trichrome stain, X200), (C) A 3-piece acrylic optic/PMMA haptics (Alcon AcrySof™) showing a good example of excellent cortical clean-up, and also suggesting good biocompatibility, with minimal cellular proliferation, (D) Photomicrograph showing evidence of excellent cortical clean-up. The haptic site is the small round empty space (right) in the equatorial fornix. Note how the regenerative cortical material is blocked at the square/truncated edge of the IOL's optic (Masson's trichrome stain, X100)

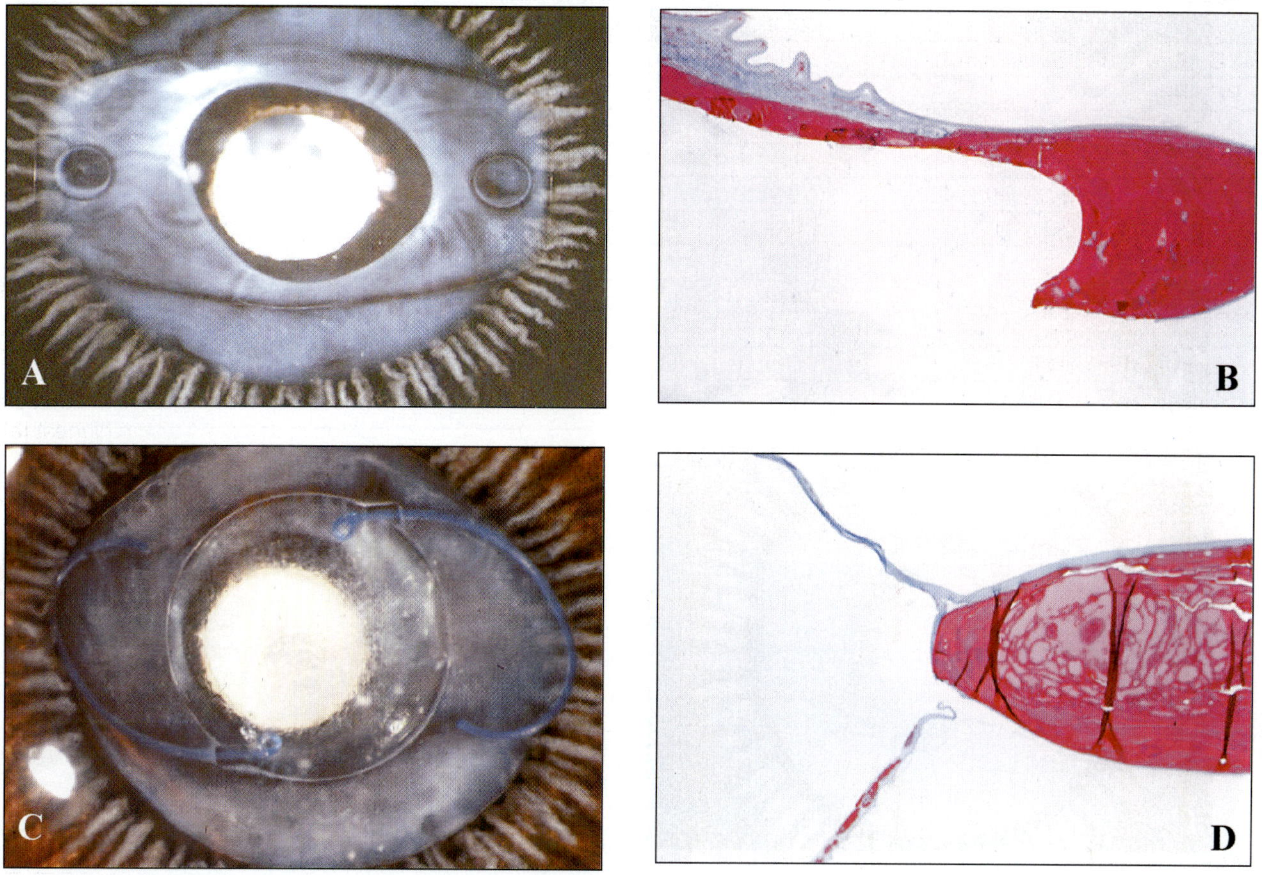

Figs 53.12A to D: The silicone optic IOLs showed less PCO scores: (A) Gross photograph from behind (Miyake-Apple posterior photographic technique) demonstrating a single piece plate-haptic silicone IOL with large positioning holes. There is moderate cell growth/proliferation (Soemmering's ring), but the posterior capsule behind the IOL optic remains clear, (B) Histological evaluation shows how the Soemmering's ring grows above and behind the IOL's optic. Also note the extensive anterior capsule opacification, commonly associated with this IOL design (Masson's trichrome stain, X200), (C) Miyake-Apple posterior view of a 3-piece silicone optic/prolene haptics PC-IOL (Allergan SI 30) with a small amount of Soemmering's ring, and incipient PCO formation under the IOL's optic, (D) Histological evaluation shows the retained/regenerative cortical material (Soemmering's ring) forms a membrane that grows into the visual axis (Masson's trichrome stain, X100)

four lenses with the lowest rates ranging between 3.3 percent and 20.7 percent are modern designs, mostly implanted after 1992 in contrast to the four lenses with the higher rates ranging between 23.3 percent and 33.7 percent. These were all older designs, already in the database prior to 1992. The difference in the Nd: YAG laser rates between the acrylic IOLs and the other IOL types was found to be statistically significant ($P < 0.05$, for all comparisons, chi square test). The Nd: YAG laser rate of all 6 foldable IOLs collectively, 15.3 percent (170/1109), was significantly lower than the rate of the rigid IOLs (Figs 53.11 to 53.13) (32.3%; 1722/5316; $P < 0.05$, chi square test). If one removes the AcrySof™ IOL from the group, the rate noted amongst the other foldable IOLs studied increases to 158/748 (21.1%). In order to evaluate the influence of lens quality vs the influence of the surgical technique on the PCO/Nd: YAG laser posterior capsulotomy rates, it is useful to follow a trend-line over a long-term period. Under optimal conditions, but not possible in this analysis, the information should be viewed considering the age and the duration of each implant. However, the dates of implantation or the time between implantation and death were difficult to determine, due

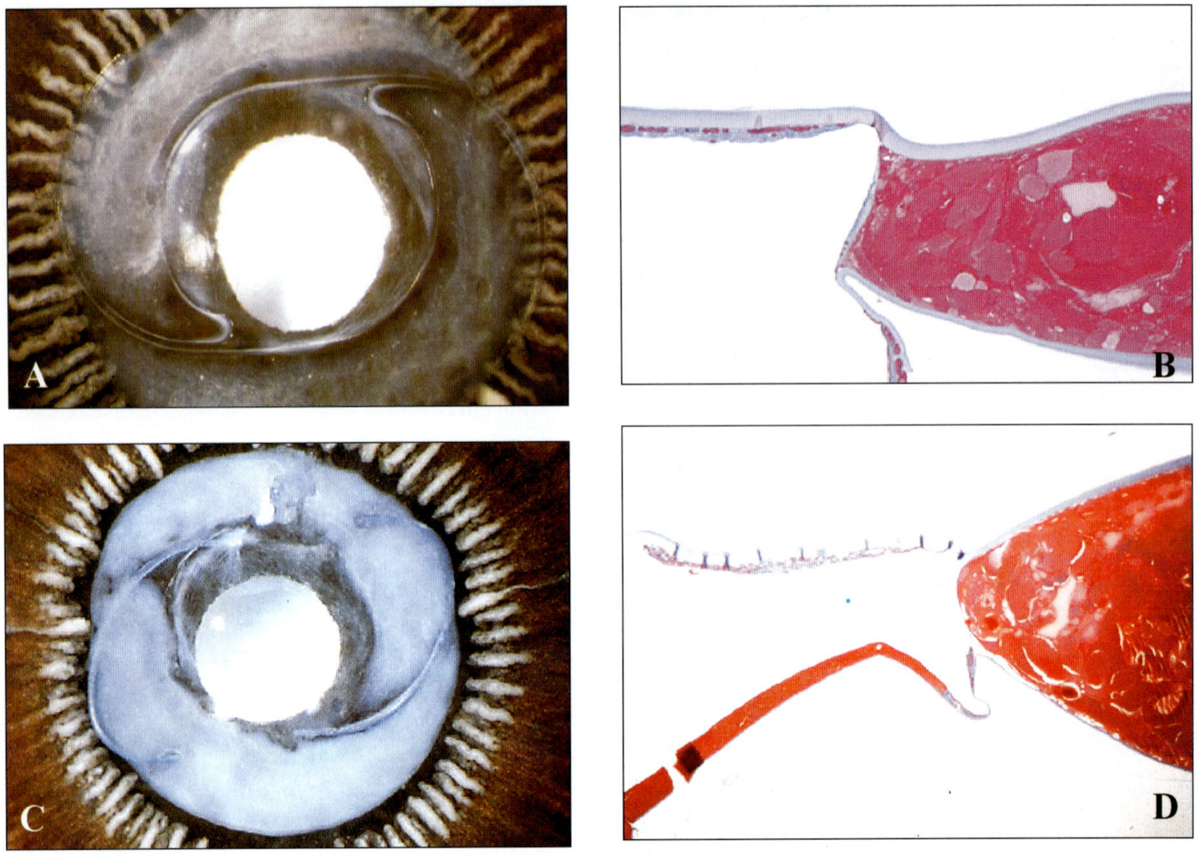

Figs 53.13A to D: A rigid PMMA lenses showed the highest scores, with higher levels of cellular proliferation and PCO formation: (A) Miyake-Apple posterior view of a pseudophakic human eye obtained postmortem, showing a PMMA optic/prolene haptics IOL with moderate Soemmering's ring formation. In this case the barrier effect created by the edge of the IOL optic has retarded a significant growth of cells toward the visual axis, (B) Note the large Soemmering's ring on the right (dark red stain), meaning extensive cellular proliferation (Masson's trichrome stain, X200), (C) This PMMA IOL has extensive Soemmering's ring formation. Note that the central PCO, seen here as a white membrane growing over the posterior surface of the IOL optic, is derived from the Soemmering's ring, (D) Photomicrograph showing the enormous migration of cortical material onto the posterior peripheral surface of the lens optic towards the visual axis (Masson's trichrome stain, X200)

to ethical considerations. These variables are going to factor out over time as larger numbers are obtained and the trend "time line" is extended.

Tracking the trend "time lines" for each lens design will be necessary to help rule out other factors in addition to the duration of each implant in the eye (for example, the quality of surgery) in order to properly assess the differences among the IOLs (Fig. 53.14). Various surgeons' criteria for Nd: YAG laser capsulotomy (e.g., aggressive, conservative) also play a role in the rate. Nevertheless surgeons' criteria, surgical technique, and implant duration will become equalized as the number of accessions and the duration of the study increases.

SUMMARY AND CONCLUSIONS

A major reduction of Nd:YAG laser capsulotomy rates towards single digits is now available because of application of these surgical factors and modern lenses-at least in the industrialized world (Fig. 53.15). This will obviously be of great benefit to patients in achieving improved long-term results and avoidance of Nd:YAG laser capsulotomy complications. Eradication of the Nd:YAG laser procedure will help control what has been the second most expensive cost to the US Medicare System. This evolutionary process is now ongoing, having begun in earnest and volume in approximately 1992 as the major shift towards better

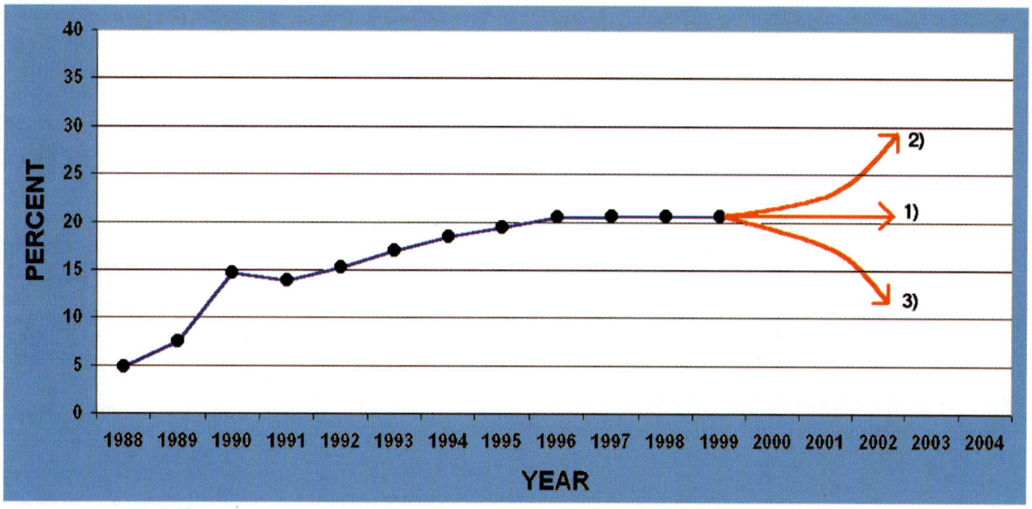

Fig. 53.14: Trend line of a theoretical intraocular lens showing the 3 possible courses with the progression of the analysis in our Center

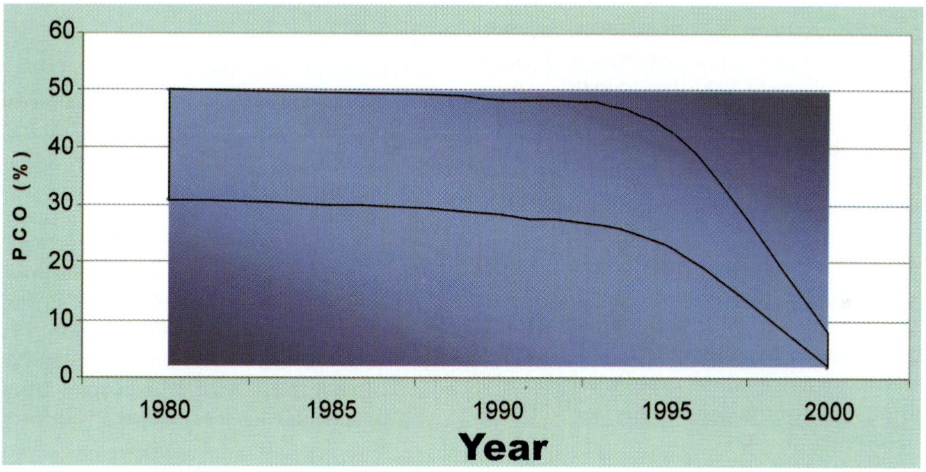

Fig. 53.15: Graph showing the decrease of PCO rates from 30 to 50 percent in the 1980s-early 1990s, to approximately 25 percent in the middle 1990s and probably, as is strongly suggested by our laboratory work, to less than 10 percent in the new millennium

capsular surgery and insertion of foldable IOLs through small incisions occurred.

We believe analyzing human pseudophakic globes obtained postmortem is helpful in understanding how these various lenses are performing in relation to PCO. To date one cannot precisely determine the relative proportion or contribution of IOL design vs surgical techniques to the decrease of Nd:YAG laser rates observed here, but this could be possible with continuing analysis including annual updates and increasing numbers of pseudophakic autopsy eyes. The tools, surgical procedures, skills, and appropriate IOLs are now available to eradicate PCO. Continued motivation to apply the 6 factors noted in this article, the efficacy of which have been further suggested in a recent study, will help diminish this final major complication of cataract-IOL surgery exactly fifty years after Ridley's first encounter with this complication.

REFERENCES

1. Alfaiate M, Leite E, Mira J, Cunha-Vaz JG. Prevalence and surgical complications of pseudoexfoliation syndrome in

Portuguese patients with senile cataract. J Cataract Refract Surg 1996; 22:972-76.
2. Apple D, Lim E, Morgan R, et al. Preparation and study of human eyes obtained postmortem with the Miyake posterior photographic technique. Ophthalmology 1990; 97:810-16.
3. Apple DJ, Auffarth GU, Peng Q, Visessook N. Foldable Intraocular Lenses. Evolution, Clinicopathologic Correlations, Complications. Thorofare, NJ, Slack, Inc., 2000.
4. Apple DJ, Peng Q, Visessook N, Werner L, Pandey SK, Escobar-Gomez M, et al. Eradication of posterior capsule opacification. Documentation of a marked decrease in Nd:YAG laser posterior capsulotomy rates noted in an analysis of 5416 pseudophakic human eyes obtained postmortem. Ophthalmology 2001; 108:505-18.
5. Apple DJ, Peng Q, Visessook N, Werner L, Pandey SK, Escobar-Gomez M, et al. Surgical prevention of posterior capsule opacification. Part I. Progress in eliminating this complication of cataract surgery. J Cataract Refract Surg 2000; 26:180-87.
6. Apple DJ, Ram J, Foster A, Peng Q. Elimination of cataract blindness: A global perspective entering the new millennium. Surv Ophthalmol 2000; 45:S70-S99.
7. Apple DJ, Solomon DK, Tetz, MR, et al. Posterior capsule opacification. Surv Ophthalmol 1992; 37:73-116.
8. Apple DJ. Harold Ridley, MA, MD, FRCS. A golden anniversary celebration and a golden age (editorial). Arch Ophthalmol 1999; 117:827-28.
9. Apple DJ. Intraocular lens biocompatibility (editorial). J Cataract Refract Surg 1992; 18:217-18.
10. Arshinoff S. Classifying capsulorhexis complications (letter). J Cataract Refract Surg 1994; 20:475.
11. Assia E, Apple D, Barden A, et al. An experimental study comparing various anterior capsulectomy techniques. Arch Ophthalmol 1991; 109:642-47.
12. Ayaki M, Ohara K, Ibaraki N, et al. The outgrowth of lens epithelial cells onto the anterior capsule after intraocular lens implantation. Am J Ophthalmol 1993; 115:668-69.
13. Barman SA, Hollick EJ, Boyce JF, et al. Quantification of posterior capsule opacification in digital images after cataract surgery. Inv Ophthalmol Vis Sci 2000; 41:3882-92.
14. Bertelmann E, Kojetinsky C. Posterior capsule opacification and anterior capsule opacification. Curr Opin Ophthalmol 2001; 12:35-40.
15. Bougaran R, Jallet V, Villain F, Colin J. A capsular ring to prevent complications after cataract surgery. ARVO abstract 703. Invest Ophthalmol Vis Sci 1997; 38 (Suppl):144.
16. Brown JD, Pearson PA, Blandford D, et al. Controlled release 5-FU delivery systems: Release studies and HPLC assay. ARVO abstract 3063. Invest Ophthalmol Vis Sci 1991; 32 (Suppl):1293.
17. Cheng CY, Yen MY, Chen SJ, et al. Visual acuity and contrast sensitivity in different types of posterior capsule opacification. J Cataract Refract Surg 2001;27:1055-60.
18. Choung HK, Lee JH. Comparison of the short-term clinical results of silicone and acrylic intraocular lens in patients with diabetes mellitus. Korean J Ophthalmol 2001; 15:15-21.
19. Chung HS, Lim SJ, Kim HB. Effect of mitomycin-C on posterior capsule opacification in rabbit eyes. J Cataract Refract Surg 2000;26:1537-42.
20. Davidson MG, Morgan DK, McGahan MC. Effect of surgical technique on in vitro posterior capsule opacigication. J Cataract Refract Surg 2000;26:1550-54.
21. Davison JA. Capsule contraction syndrome. J Cataract Refract Surg 1993; 19:582-89.
22. Fine IH. Cortical cleaving hydrodissection. J Cataract Refract Surg 1992; 18:508-12.
23. Flach AJ, Dolan BJ. Incidence of postoperative posteior capsular opacification following treatment with diclofenac 0.1% and ketorolac 0.5% ophthalmic solutions: 3-year randomized, double-masked, prospective clinical investigation. Trans Am Ophthalmol Soc 2000;98:101-05.
24. Font RL, Brownstein S. A light and electron microscopic study of anterior subcapsular cataracts. Am J Ophthalmol 1974; 78:972-84.
25. Gayton JL, Apple DJ, Peng Q, Visessook N, Sanders V, Werner L, et al. Interlenticular opacification: Clinicopathological correlation of a complication of posterior chamber piggyback intraocular lenses. J Cataract Refract Surg 2000; 26:330-36.
26. Gayton JL, Sanders VN. Implanting two posterior chamber intraocular lenses in a case of microphthalmos. J Cataract Refract Surg 1993; 19:776-77.
27. Gimbel H, Neuhann T. Development, advantages and methods of the continuous circular capsulorhexis technique. J Cataract Refract Surg 1990; 16:31-37.
28. Gonvers M, Sickenberg M, van Melle G. Change in capsulorhexis size after implantation of three types of intraocular lenses. J Cataract Refract Surg 1997; 23:231-38.
29. Hansen SO, Tetz MR, Solomon KD, et al. Decentration of flexible loop posterior chamber intraocular lenses in a series of 222 postmortem eyes. Ophthalmology 1988; 95:344-49.
30. Hara T, Hara T, Sakanishi K, Yamada Y. Efficacy of equator rings in an experimental rabbit study. Arch Ophthalmol 1995; 113:1060-65.
31. Hara T, Hara T, Yamada Y. Equator ring for maintenance of completely circular contour of the capsular bag equator after cataract removal. Ophthalmic Surg 1991; 22:358-59.
32. Hartman C, Wiedemann P, Gothe K, et al. Prevention of secondary cataract by intracapsular administration of daunomycin. Ophtalmologie 1990; 4:102-06.
33. Hashizoe M, Hara T, Ogura Y, et al. Equator ring efficacy in maintaining capsular bag integrity and transparency after cataract removal in monkey eyes. Graefe's Arch Clin Exp Ophthalmol 1998; 236:375-79.
34. Haus CM, Galand AL. Mitomycin against posterior capsular opacification: an experimental study in rabbits. Br J Ophthalmol 1996; 80:1087-91.

35. Hayashi K, Hayashi H, Nakao F, Hayashi F. Changes in posterior capsule opacification after poly(methyl methacrylate), silicone, and acrylic intraocular lens implantation. J Cataract Refract Surg 2001;27:817-24.
36. Holweger RR, Marefat B. Intraocular pressure change after neodymium:YAG capsulotomy. J Cataract Refract Surg 1997; 23:115-21.
37. Hu CY, Woung LC, Wang MC. Change in the area of laser posterior capsulotomy: 3 months follow-up. J Cataract Refract Surg 2001;27:537-42.
38. Inan UU, Ozturk F, Kaynak S, et al. Prevention of posterior capsule opacification by intraoperative single-dose pharmacologic agents. J Cataract Refract Surg 2001;27:1079-87.
39. Ismail MM, Alio JL, Moreno JMR. Prevention of secondary cataract by antimitotic drugs: Experimental study. Ophthalmic Res 1996; 28:64-69.
40. Javitt JC, Tielsch JM, Canner JK, Kolb MM, Sommer A, Steinberg EP *et al*. National outcomes of cataract extraction. Increased risk of retinal complications associated with Nd:YAG laser capsulotomy. The Cataract Patient Outcomes Research Team. Ophthalmology 1992; 99:1487-97.
41. Koch D, Liu J, Gill P, Parke D. Axial myopia increases the risk of retinal complications after neodymium-YAG laser posterior capsulotomy. Arch Ophthalmol 1989; 107:986-90.
42. Kruger AJ, Schauersberger J, Abela C, et al. Two-year results: Sharp versus rounded optic edges on silicone lenses. J Cataract Refract Surg 2000; 26:566-70.
43. Kucuksumer Y, Bayraktar S, Sahin S, Yilmaz OF. Posterior capsule opacification 3 years after implantation of an AcrySof and a Memory lens in fellow eyes. J Cataract Refract Surg 2000;26:1176-82.
44. Kugelberg U, Zetterstrom C, Lundgren B, et al. After cataract and ocular growth in newborn rabbit eyes implanted with a capsule tension ring. J Cataract Refract Surg 1997; 23:635-40.
45. Legler UFC, Apple DJ, Assia EI, et al. Inhibition of posterior capsule opacification: The effect of colchicine in a sustained drug delivery system. J Cataract Refract Surg 1993; 19:462-70.
46. Linnola RJ, Werner L, Pandey SK, Escobar-Gomez M, Znoiko SL, Apple DJ, et al. Adhesion of fibronectin, vitronectin, laminin and collagen type IV to intraocular lens materials in human autopsy eyes. Part I: histological sections. J Cataract Refract Surg 2000; 26:1792-1806.
47. Linnola RJ, Werner L, Pandey SK, Escobar-Gomez M, Znoiko SL, Apple DJ, et al. Adhesion of fibronectin, vitronectin, laminin and collagen type IV to intraocular lens materials in human autopsy eyes. Part II: explanted IOLs. J Cataract Refract Surg 2000; 26:1807-18.
48. Linnola RJ. Sandwich theory: bioactivity-based explanation for posterior capsule opacification. J Cataract Refract Surg 1997; 23:1539-42.
49. Macky TA, Pandey SK, Werner L, Trivedi RH, Izak A, Apple DJ, et al. Anterior capsule opacification. Int Ophthalmol Clin 2001; 41:17-31.
50. Meacock WR, Spalton DJ, Boyce JF, Jose RM. Effect of optic size on posterior capsule opacification: 5.5 mm versus 6.0 mm AcrySof intraocular lenses. J Cataract Refract Surg 2001;27:1194-98.
51. Meacock WR, Spalton DJ, Holick EJ, et al. The efect of polymethylmethacrylate and acrys of intraocular lenses on the posterior capsule in pateints with a large capsulorhexis. Jpn J Ophthalmol 2001;45:348-54.
52. Menapace R, Findl O, Georgopoulos M, et al. The capsular tension ring: Designs, applications, and techniques. J Cataract Refract Surg 2000; 26:898-912.
53. Miyake K, Miyake C. Intraoperative posterior chamber lens haptic fixation in the human cadaver eye. Ophthalmic Surg 1985; 16:230-36.
54. Miyake K, Ota I, Miyake S, Maekubo K. Correlation between intraocular lens hydrophilicity and anterior capsule opacification and aqueous flare. J Cataract Refract Surg 1996; 22(Supp):764-69.
55. Nagamoto T, Eguchi G. Effect of intraocular lens design on migration of lens epithelial cells onto the posterior capsule. J Cataract Refract Surg 1997; 23:866-72.
56. Nagamoto T, Hara E. Postoperative membranous proliferation from the anterior capsulotomy margin onto the intraocular lens optic. J Cataract Refract Surg 1995; 21:208-11.
57. Nagamoto T, Miyajima HB. A ring to support the capsular bag after continuous curvilinear capsulorhexis. J Cataract Refract Surg 1994; 20:417-20.
58. Nagata T, Minakata A, Watanabe I. Adhesiveness of AcrySof to a collagen film. J Cataract Refract Surg 1998; 24:367-70.
59. Nishi O, Nishi K, Akura J, Nagata T. Effect of round-edged acrylic intraocular lenses on preventing posterior capsule opacification. J Cataract Refract Surg 2001;27:608-13.
60. Nishi O, Nishi K, Fujisawa T, et al. Effects of the cytokines on the proliferation of and collagen synthesis by human cataract lens epithelial cells. Br J Ophthalmol 1996; 80:63-68.
61. Nishi O, Nishi K, Mano C, et al. Inhibition of migrating lens epithelial cells by blocking the adhesion molecule integrin: A preliminary report. J Cataract Refract Surg 1997; 23:860-65.
62. Nishi O, Nishi K, Mano C, et al. The inhibition of lens epithelial cell migration by a discontinuous capsular bend–shaped circular loop or a capsule-bending ring. Ophthalmic Surg Lasers 1998; 29:119-25.
63. Nishi O, Nishi K, Menapace R, Akura J. Capsular bending ring to prevent posterior capsule opacification: 2 year follow-up. J Cataract Refract Surg 2001;27:1359-65
64. Nishi O, Nishi K, Morita T, et al. Effect of intraocular sustained release of indomethacin on postoperative inflammation and posterior capsular opacification. J Cataract Refract Surg 1996; 22:806-10.

65. Nishi O, Nishi K, Ohmoto Y. Synthesis of interleukin-1, interleukin-6, and basic fibroblast growth factor by human cataract lens epithelial cells. J Cataract Refract Surg 1996;22:852-58.
66. Nishi O, Nishi K. Intraocular lens encapsulation by shrinkage of the capsulorhexis opening. J Cataract Refract Surg 1993; 19:544-45.
67. Nishi O, Nishi K. Preventing posterior capsule opacification by creating a discontinuous sharp bend in the capsule. J Cataract Refract Surg 1999; 25:521-26
68. Nishi O. Posterior capsule opacification. Part 1: Experimental investigations. J Cataract Refract Surg 1999; 25:106-17.
69. Nishi O. Removal of lens epithelial cells by ultrasound in endocapsular cataract surgery. Ophthalmic Surg 1987; 18:577-80.
70. Obstbaum SA. The anterior capsulotomy revisited. J Cataract Refract Surg 1998; 24:143-44.
71. Ohmi S, Uenoyama K. Decentration associated with asymmetric capsular shrinkage and intraocular lens design in a rabbit model. J Cataract Refract Surg 1995; 21:293-96
72. Pandey SK, Cochener B, Apple DJ, et al. Intracapsular ring sustained 5-fluorouracil delivery system for prevention of posterior capsule opacification in rabbits: A histological study. J Cataract Refract Surg 2002; 28:139-48.
73. Pandey SK, Wilson ME, Trivedi RH, Izak A, Macky TA, Werner L, et al. Pediatric cataract surgery and intraocular lens implantation: Current techniques, complications and management. Int Ophthalmol Clin 2001; 41:175-96.
74. Peng Q, Apple DJ, Visessook N, et al. Surgical prevention of posterior capsule opacification. Part II. Enhancement of cortical clean-up by focusing on hydrodissection. J Cataract Refract Surg 2000; 26:188-97.
75. Peng Q, Visessook N, Apple DJ, et al. Surgical prevention of posterior capsule opacification. Part III. Intraocular lens optic barrier effect as a second line of defense. J Cataract Refract Surg 2000; 26:198-213.
76. Power WJ, Neylan D, Collum LMT. Daunorubicin as an inhibitor of human lens epithelial cell proliferation in culture. J Cataract Refract Surg 1994; 20:287-90.
77. Rakic JM, Galand A, Vrensen GFJM. Lens epithelial cell proliferation in human posterior capsule opacification. Exp Eye Research 2000;5:489-94.
78. Ram J, Apple DJ, Peng Q, Visessook N, Auffarth GU, Schoderbek RJ, et al. Update on fixation of rigid and foldable posterior chamber intraocular lenses. Part II. Choosing the correct haptic fixation and intraocular lens design to help eradicate posterior capsule opacification. Ophthalmology 1999; 106:891-900.
79. Ram J, Pandey SK, Apple DJ, Werner L, Brar GS, Singh R, et al. Effect of in-the-bag intraocular lens fixation on the prevention of posterior capsule opacification. J Cataract Refract Surg 2001;27:1039-46.
80. Ram J. Kaushik S, Brar GS, Gupta A. Neodymium YAG capsulotomy rates following phacoemulsification with implantation of PMMA, silicone, and Acrylic intraocular lenses. Ophthalmic Surg Lasers 2001;32:375-82.
81. Ravalico Ravalico G, Tognetto D, et al. Capsulorhexis size and posterior capsule opacification. J Cataract Refract Surg 1996;22:98-103.
82. Rootman J, Tisdall J, Gudauskas G, Ostray A. Intraocular penetration of subconjunctivally administered ^{14}C-fluorouracil in rabbits. Arch Ophthalmol 1979; 97:2375-78.
83. Ruiz JM, Medrano M, Alio JL. Inhibition of posterior capsule opacification by 5-Fluorouracil in rabbits. Ophthalmic Res 1990; 22:201-08.
84. Scaramuzza A, Fernando GT, Crayford BB. Posterior capsule opacification and lens epithelial cell layer formation: Hydroview hydrogel versus AcrySof acrylic intraocular lenses. J Cataract Refract Surg 2001;27:1047-54.
85. Schaumberg DA, Dana MR, Christen WG, Glynn RJ. A systematic overview of the incidence of posterior capsular opacification. Ophthalmology 1998; 105:1213-21.
86. Schmidbauer JM, Vargas LG, Peng Q, Escobar-Gomez M, Werner L, Arthur SN, et al. Posterior capsule opacification. Int Ophthalmol Clin 2001;41:109-31.
87. Schmack, Gerstmeyer K. Long-term results of the foldable CeeOn Edge intraocular lens. J Cataract Refract Surg 2000;26:1172-75.
88. Schmidbauer JM, Vargas LG, Apple DJ, et al. Influence of surgery-related factors on the Nd: YAG laser capsulotomy rates of 3-piece silicone IOLs—analysis of 457 pseudophakic human globes obtained postmortem. Klin Montasbl Augenheilkd 2001;218:523-37.
89. Scorolli L, Martini E, Scalinci SZ, et al. Capsule contraction after continuous curvilinear capsulorhexis. J Cataract Refract Surg 1996; 22:1245-46.
90. Shammas HJ. Relaxing the fibrosed capsulorhexis rim to correct induced hyperopia after phacoemulsification. J Cataract Refract Surg 1995; 21:228-29.
91. Solomon KD, VanMeter WS, Pearson PA, et al. Sustained release drug delivery systems in extracapsular cataract surgery. ARVO abstract 1724. Invest Ophthalmol Vis Sci 1990; 31(Suppl):351.
92. Sourdille P, Ducournau Y. Effect of daunomycin on epithelial cells of the crystalline lens. Ophtalmologie 1990; 4:107-08.
93. Spang KM, Rohrbach JM, Weidle EG. Complete occlusion of the anterior capsular opening after intact capsulorhexis: clinicopathologic correlation. Am J Ophthalmol 1999; 127:343-45.
94. Tanaka Y, Ibaraki N, Hongoh M. Histopathological study of rabbit anterior capsule opacification after IOL surgery. Nippon Ganka Gakkai Zasshi 1993; 97:672-77.
95. Tetz MR, Ries MW, Lucas C, et al. Inhibition of posterior capsule opacification by an intraocular–lens–bound sustained drug delivery system: An experimental animal study and literature review. J Cataract Refract Surg 1996; 22:1070-78.

96. Toldos JJM, Roig AA, Benabent EC. Total anterior capsule closure after silicone intraocular lens implantation. J Cataract Refract Surg 1996; 22:269-71.
97. Trivedi RH, Izak A, Werner L, Macky TA, Pandey SK, Apple DJ et al. Interlenticular opacification of piggyback intraocular lenses. Int Ophthalmol Clin 2001; 41:47-62
98. Tsuboi S, Tsujioka M, Kusube T, Kojima S. Effect of continuous circular capsulorhexis and intraocular lens fixation on the blood-aqueous barrier. Arch Ophthalmol 1992; 110:1124-27.
99. Ursell PG, Spalton DJ, Pande MV. Anterior capsule stability in eyes with intraocular lenses made of poly(methyl methacrylate), silicone, and AcrySof. J Cataract Refract Surg 1997; 23:1532-38.
100. Van Horn DL, Sendele DD, Seideman S, Buco PJ. Regenerative capacity of the corneal endothelium in rabbit and cat. Invest Ophthalmol Vis Sci 1977; 16:697-13.
101. Werner L, Apple DJ, Pandey SK, et al. Analysis of elements of interlenticular opacification. Am J Ophthalmol 2002;133:320-26.
102. Werner L, Apple DJ, Pandey SK. Postoperative proliferation of anterior and equatorial lens epithelial cells: A comparison between various foldable IOL designs. In Buratto L, Osher R, Masket S, (Eds): Cataract Surgery in Complicated Cases. Thorofare, NJ, Slack, 2000; pp 399-417.
103. Werner L, Pandey SK, Apple DJ, Escobar-Gomez M, McLendon L, Macky T. Anterior capsule opacification: Correlation of pathological findings with clinical sequelae. Ophthalmology 2001; 108:1675-81.
104. Werner L, Pandey SK, Escobar-Gomez M, et al. Anterior capsule opacification: A histopathological study comparing different IOL styles. Ophthalmology 2000; 107:463-67.
105. Wilson ME, Pandey SK, Werner L, et al. Pediatric cataract surgery: Current techniques, complications and management. In Agarwal A, Agarwal S, Fine H, Sachdeva M, Agarwal A, (Eds): Phacoemulsification, laser cataract surgery and foldable IOLs. Slack Inc., Thorofare, NJ, USA, 2000;369-88.

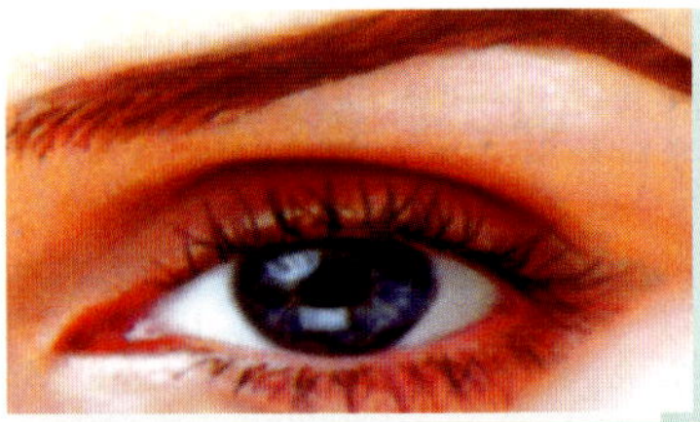

Fifty four

Update on Delayed Postoperative Opacification of Rigid and Foldable Intraocular Lenses

Liliana Werner
Suresh K Pandey
David J Apple
Andrea M Izak (USA)

OVERVIEW

Postoperative opacification of the foldable hydrophilic acrylic lens designs is a major concern among surgeons, and manufacturers. The majority of cases are reported from Asia, Australia, Canada, Europe, Latin America, and South Africa. However, mostly in North America we have noted cases of "snowflake" opacification of the rigid PMMA lenses, a new syndrome of biodegradation of PMMA biomaterial. Our analysis of all 28 cases showed that dense snowflake lesions were clustered in the central part of the lens optic with the peripheral part largely unaffected behind the iris. We classified the cases of snowflake opacification of the PMMA IOLs into four grades according to density and the severity of the lesions. This entity possibly attributed to breakdown of PMMA polymer within the biomaterial. We have termed these lesions "snowflake opacifications" on the basis of morphology. SEMs of the bisected IOL revealed that these lesions were clustered in the anterior 1/3 of the optic substance and the posterior 2/3s remained free.

We have also analyzed 3 major hydrophilic acrylic lenses, explanted due to varying degree of IOL opacification, secondary to different patterns of dystrophic calcification. These designs include the Bausch and Lomb Hydroviewä, Medical Developmental Research- SC60B-OUVä and Ophthalmic Innovations International, Aqua-Senseä. During the past 3 years, we have studied a total of 87 of the aforementioned opacified explanted hydrophilic acrylic designs, which were sent to our laboratory by surgeons worldwide. Clinicopathological studies done at our Center confirmed that the opacification of the Hydroviewä lens appeared to be due to dystrophic calcification on the anterior and posterior lens optic surfaces. This was also confirmed by two different histochemical methods as shown here. In the majority of the SC60B-OUVä lenses, the opacification was also due to precipitation of calcium and was histochemically demonstrated within the substance of the optic biomaterial. Drs Dick and Frohn from Germany attributed the opacification to degeneration of the UV filtration material. Gross microscopic and histochemical examination of the explanted Aqua-Senseä lenses also revealed that opacification was attributed to external and internal precipitation of calcium. Scanning electron microscopic analyses of the external surfaces of Hydroviewa lens designs confirm the presence of cerebriform deposits, as shown in the left top, and left middle photographs. Deposits were present within the optic substance or over its surface of an SC60B-OUV™ and an Aqua-Sense lens, as shown in the middle and right pictures. Spectroscopic analyses of cut sections of the lens optic showed peaks of calcium and phosphate. Together with surgeons, manufacturers, and scientists worldwide, our laboratory is working to explore the etiopathogenesis of the miniepidemic of IOL opacification. In numerous recent publications, we have discussed this complication in detail and cautioned surgeons to be vigilant for timely follow up of patients implanted with these lenses. To prevent the occurrence of lens opacification Bausch and Lomb, Medical Developmental Research and Ophthalmic Innovations International, modified the IOL packaging and/or changed the source of IOL polymers. They now believe the problem is resolved. However, final verification will require further clinical study. In conclusion, possible guidelines for prevention and management of IOL opacification are listed here. The IOL explantation/exchange is currently the only available treatment. Future clinical studies will determine the efficacy of modifications performed on polymers and packaging. Surgeons should remain vigilant in careful follow up of patients implanted with these lenses.

INTRODUCTION

It has been over 50 years since Harold Ridley's first implant and the cataract-IOL procedure has reached an extraordinarily high level of quality and performance. This has no doubt been one of the most satisfying advances of medicine in the 20th Century. Millions of individuals with visual disability or frank blindness from cataracts have and continue to benefit from this procedure. Modern refractive surgery is a first cousin or spin-off of the techniques also preferred by anterior segment surgeons. Continuous high tech innovations now occurring assure that keratorefractive and phakic IOL procedures are and will continue to provide a service to many patients with significant ammetropia.

Since past 3 years, we have extensively studies the opacified explanted rigid PMMA and foldable hydrogel IOL (Pandey SK, Werner L, Apple DJ, Kaskaloglu MM, Izak AM, Cionni RJ. Intraocular Lens Opacification, Second prize in the category Intraocular Lenses at the ASCRS/Alcon Annual Video Festival, Congress of the American Society of Cataract and Refractive Surgeons, Philadelphia, PA, USA, June 2002; Pandey SK, Werner L, Apple DJ, Kaskaloglu MM, Izak AM, Cionni RJ. Intraocular Lens Opacification, Third prize for Scientific Value at the ESCRS/Alcon Annual Video Festival, Congress of the European Society of Cataract and Refractive Surgeons, Nice, France, September 2002; Pandey SK, Werner L, Apple DJ, Kaskaloglu MM, Izak AM, Cionni RJ. Intraocular Lens Opacification, Opacification, Opacification", Best-of-Show video award, Annual Meeting of the American Academy of Ophthalmology, Orlando, Florida, USA, October 2002).

In this write-up we will be discuss striking and often visually disabling opacifications occurring on IOL optics, both on some modern foldable IOLs as well as a PMMA IOL optic degradation occurring with some models a decade or more after implantation (Fig. 54.1). Many of the complications

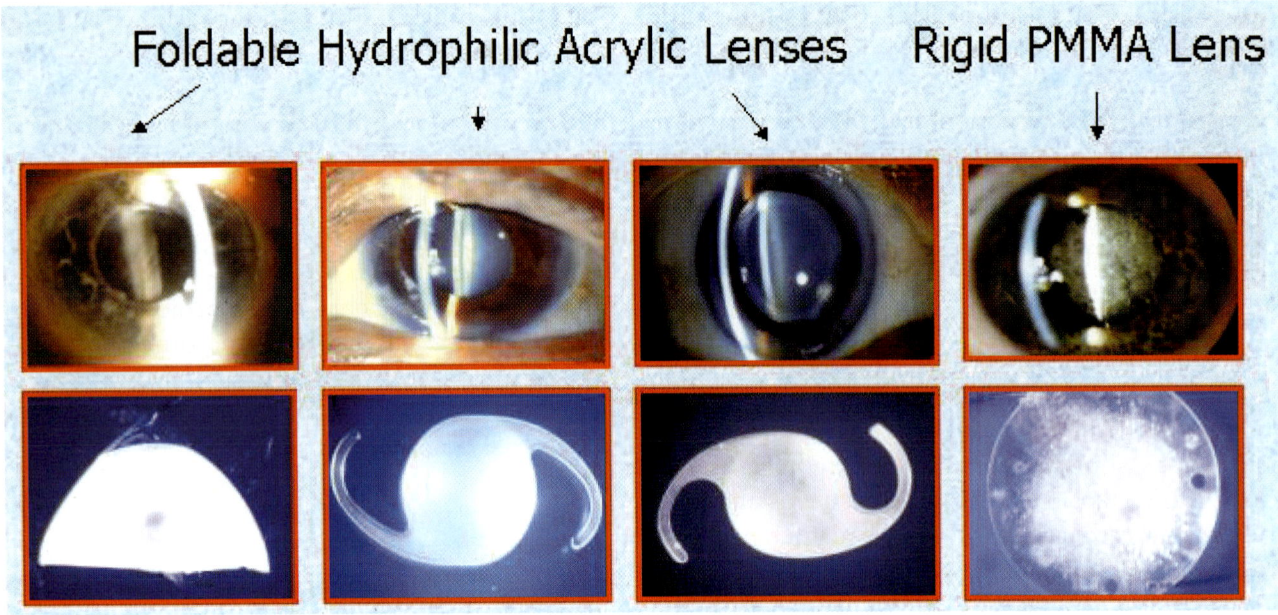

Fig. 54.1: Opacification of rigid and foldable lenses

we will discuss here are totally unexpected and unnecessary vision-threatening and sometimes blinding IOL opacifications—complications that we should not have to concern ourselves within our current advanced stage in the evolution of the cataract-IOL procedure. Some of these are occurring because many surgical procedures today are often performed outside the realm of supervision and oversight of both non-governmental and governmental authorities such as the Food and Drug Administration.

This chapter is divided in 2 sections; in section A, we will address a newly described clinical condition caused by an unexpected late opacification of PMMA, that we termed as "snowflake" opacification or degeneration of polymethyl methacrylate (PMMA) posterior chamber IOL optic biomaterial. In section 2, we will discuss the clinicopathological studies of explanted opacified foldable lenses manufactured from hydrophilic acrylic biomaterial.

SECTION I: DELAYED OPACIFICATION OF PMMA IOL OPTIC BIOMATERIAL: "SNOWFLAKE" OR CRYSTALLINE OPACIFICATION

Over the past 50 years PMMA has been rightly considered a safe, tried and true material for IOL manufacturing with good and high quality control. PMMA biomaterial was used as an optic biomaterial in Sir Harold Ridley's original IOL, manufactured by Rayner Intraocular Lenses Ltd, London, UK, and first implanted in 1949-1950.[1] Although surgeons in the industrialized world and in selected areas in the developing world have largely transitioned to foldable IOL biomaterials, PMMA does remain in widespread use in many regions. Biomaterial studies on PMMA IOL optics were rarely required. Until now, any untoward complications such as PMMA-optic material alteration/breakdown have not been seen with this material and its fabrication.

However, we have recently reported gradual but progressive late postoperative alteration/destruction of PMMA optic biomaterial causing significant decrease in visual acuity, sometimes to a severity that requires IOL explantation (Fig. 54.2). The first clinical case of the type that we observed was a documentation of photographs sent to us by David Davis, MD, of Hayward, CA, in 1993. He noted "crystalline" formations in 7 IOPTEX Research (Azuza, CA) 3-piece PMMA IOLs. Over the past 4 years, 25 cases including 9 explanted IOLs were submitted to Center for Research on Ocular Therapeutics and Biodevices (Fig. 54.2).[2,3]

All of the explanted IOLs were 3-piece posterior chamber (PC)-IOLs with rigid PMMA optical components and blue polypropylene or extruded PMMA haptics. These had been implanted in the

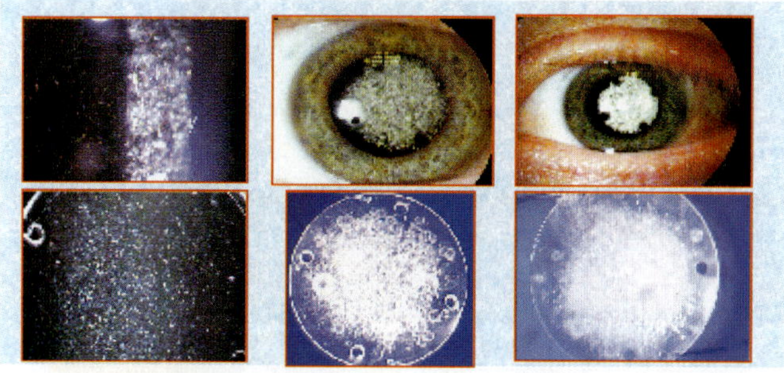

Fig. 54.2: Opacification of rigid and foldable lenses

early 1980s to early 1990s in most cases and the clinical symptoms appeared late postoperatively, ca. 8-15 years after the implantation. The clinical, gross, light and electron microscopic profiles of all the cases showed almost identical findings, differing only in the degree of intensity of the "snowflake" lesions that in turn reflected the severity and probably the duration of the opacification. In the early stages of many of the cases, the lesions were first noted clinically by a routine slit lamp examination, in the absence of visual disturbances. Most examiners described the white-brown opacities within the IOL optics as "crystalline deposits" (Fig. 54.3). They appeared to progress gradually in most cases. Clinically, the slowly progressive opacities of the IOL optics usually start as scattered white-brown spots within the substance of the IOL optic. These usually do not have an impact on the patients' VA. They gradually increase in intensity and number, eventually reaching a point where the VA loss necessitates removal or exchange of the IOL. In addition to visual loss the symptoms included decrease in contrast sensitivity and various visual disturbances and aberrations,

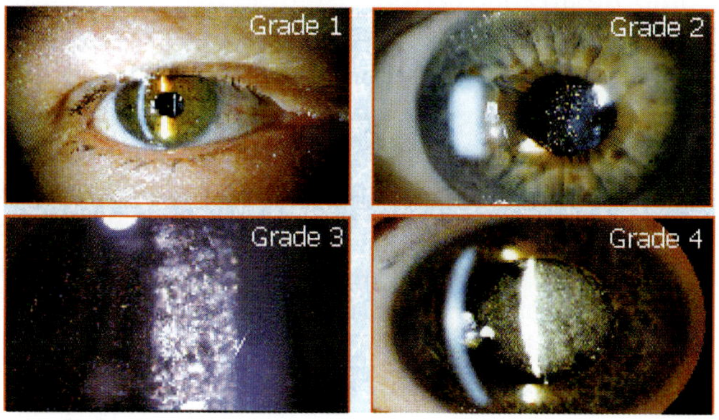

Fig. 54.3: Classification of "snowflake" lesion

including glare. Figure 54.3 presents the classification of snowflake lesions as proposed by Apple and associates.[2,3]

Clinicopathological Study of Explanted Lenses

The opacities of the IOL optics may start as scattered white-brown spots within the substance of the IOL optic and remain stable or slowly progressive. Some may gradually increase in intensity and numbers, eventually reaching a point where a visual acuity loss may necessitate removal or exchange of the IOL. In addition to visual loss the reported symptoms included decrease in contrast sensitivity and various visual disturbances and aberrations, including glare. In early stages there was usually no effect on Snellen visual acuity but a gradual decrease of visual acuity was noted in the late stage of the process. Associated systemic disorders were not described. Metabolic imbalances have not been implicated as pathogenetic factors. Because the lesions invariably appeared years later in a very late postoperative period there is almost certainly no direct connection between the opacities and substances used intraoperatively. In the examinations we performed to identify the nature of the deposits, including energy dispersive spectroscopy (EDS) we did not document any exogenous chemicals apart from elements present in PMMA itself (carbon, oxygen).

High power three-dimensional light microscopy (Fig. 54.4, top left) and SEM (Fig. 54.4 top middle) of the surfaces of bisected IOL optics were the most informative examinations with regard to determining the structure of the opacifications. The term "snowflake" applies best to the clinical and low power microscopic appearance of each lesion (Fig. 54.4, top left). High power examination revealed that the lesions are spherical or stellate, the shape depending on the contour of the surrounding pseudocapsule (Fig. 54.4). The interior of the sphere does not appear to contain fluid.

To date there have not been any clinicopathologic reports on this complication nor any hypotheses regarding its pathogenesis. We suggest that manufacturing variations in some lenses fabricated in the 1980s—early 1990s may be responsible. It is possible that the late change in the PMMA material

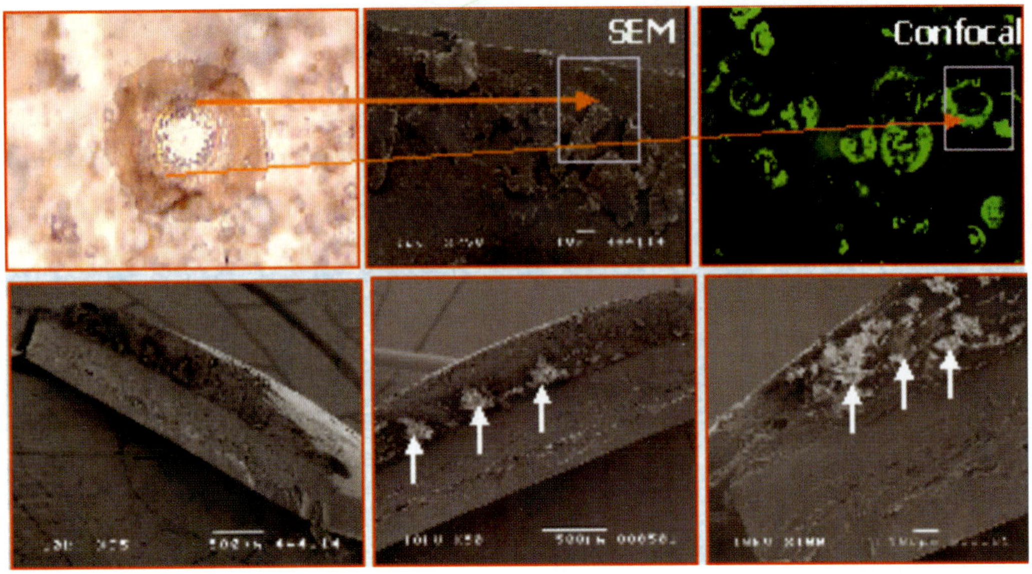

Fig. 54.4: "Snowflake" lesions of PMMA IOL: Microscopic, ultrastructural studies

process is facilitated by long-term ultraviolet (UV, solar) exposure. This is supported by 2 pathologic observations. First, many opacities have been indeed clustered in the central zone of the optic, extending to mid-peripheral portion but often leaving the distal peripheral rim free of the opacities. This observations would support the hypothesis that the slow and sometimes progressive lesion formation noted here might relate to the fact that the IOLs central optic is exposed to ultraviolet radiation over an extended period, whereas the peripheral optic may be protected by the iris. Furthermore, the opacities are present most commonly and intensely within the anterior 1/3 of the optic's substance (Fig. 54.4, bottom). Since the anterior strata of the optic are the first to encounter the ultraviolet light, this might explain why the opacities are seen more frequently in this zone.

Since it is plausible the lesions may be ultraviolet-induced, and it is highly unlikely that non-porous PMMA allows an entrance of aqueous into the optic substance, we postulate that the lesions are "dry" and that the PMMA disruption might be related to a specific manufacturing problem that eaves the optic susceptible to damage.

PMMA is manufactured by polymerization of the MMA monomer. This manufacturing process utilizes many different polymerization techniques, and various components such as UV absorbers and initiators. Therefore various impurity profiles are possible. An initiator substance starts such process. A frequently used initiator is azo-bis-isobutyryl nitrile (AIBN).[4-6] It is possible that UV radiation is a contributing factor, however, the exact pathogenesis can as of now only be hypothesized. Potential causes of a snowflake lesion include (1) insufficient postannealing of the cured PMMA polymer; (2) excessive thermal energy during the curing process leaving voids in the polymer matrix; (3) non-homogeneous dispersement of the UV chromophore and/or thermal initiator into the polymer chain; (4) poor filtration of the pre-cured monomeric components (MMA, UV blocker, thermal initiator). Another possible pathogenic factor could be an inadvertent use of excessive initiator substance during the polymerization process that may facilitate the formation of the snowflake lesions. The N=N bond of the AIBN initiator may be disrupted by gradual UV exposure with a release of nitrogen gas (N_2). Such gas formation can be caused by either heat or UV light exposure. Indeed the normal polymerization process for PMMA synthesis consists in part of a heat-induced N_2 formation as a byproduct. During normal polymerization the N_2 escapes from the mixture. However, with a poor manufacturing process, for example using excessive initiator—more than the fractional amount required—unwanted initiator may be entrapped in the PMMA substance. Slow release of gaseous N_2 within the PMMA substance trigged by long-term UV exposure would explain the formation of the cavitations within the snowflake lesions. The outer "pseudocapsule" might consist of PMMA, whereas the central space contains the N_2 gas admixed with convoluted material also possibly consisting of degenerated PMMA. There is nothing in the molecular structure of the PMMA that in and of itself could be compressed to form such an expansile material that might create the round circular cavitations of the snowflake lesions.

These hypothetical mechanisms have the potential to form micro-heterogeneity within the PMMA polymer that, overtime and potentially with exposure to UV radiation, could result in a lesion within the polymer. Additional experimentation is necessary to determine if any of these proposed mechanisms for the formation of a snowflake lesion are realized.

Awareness of this delayed complication may be warranted in developing countries, where PMMA IOLs are still used in the majority of cases. Virtually all IOLs manufactured today appear to be satisfactory. However, one should always be aware that some early IOLs from American manufacturers, including some described in this report, have been delivered to the developing world over the years, sometimes implanted without regard to expiration dates on the packaging. It would be very unfortunate to see this complication showing up in underprivileged areas where patients have almost no recourse to treat visual loss/blindness of this type.

The emergence of this complication could have represented a true disaster, except for the fact that many of the patients implanted with these IOLs are now deceased. However, there are probably still sufficient number of patients living with varying stages of this complication. This necessitates that today's ophthalmologists to be aware of, to diagnose, and to know when not to explant and/or exchange these lenses. It is important to know the nature of this syndrome in order to spare by now elderly patients and their doctors unwarranted anxiety about the cause of his or her visual problems/loss and also to obviate request for unwarranted diagnostic testing.

SECTION II: OPACIFICATION OF FOLDABLE HYDROPHILIC ACRYLIC LENSES

Introduction

Foldable hydrophilic acrylic intraocular lenses (IOLs), also known as hydrogel lenses are not yet available in the United States but have been marketed by several firms for several years in international markets. Most of the currently available hydrophilic acrylic lenses are manufactured from different copolymers acrylic with water contents raging from 18 to 28 percent, and an incorporated UV absorber.[6,7] They are packaged in a vial containing distilled water or balanced salt solutions, thus being already implanted in the hydrated state and in their final dimensions. Hydration renders these lenses flexible, enabling the surgeons to fold and insert/inject them through small incisions. Many surgeons have adopted the use of hydrophilic acrylic IOLs because of their easier-handling properties and biocompatibility.[8,9] Although hydrophilic surfaces have been shown to lower the inflammatory cytological response to the IOL,[9] some currently available hydrophilic acrylic IOL designs have been associated to reports on late postoperative opacification caused by calcium precipitation.[10-35] Postoperative opacification of the foldable hydrophilic acrylic lens designs is a major concern among surgeons, and manufacturers. The majority of cases are reported from Asia, Australia, Canada, Europe, Latin America, and South Africa.

We describe in this chapter the analyses performed in our laboratory on hydrophilic acrylic lenses of 3 major designs during past 3 years (Fig. 54.5). They were all explanted because of whitish discoloration of the optic component, or of the whole lens, related to different forms and degrees of dystrophic calcification (Werner L, Apple DJ, Pandey SK. "Late postoperative opacification of hydrophilic intraocular lens designs"; presented at the ASCRS Symposium on Cataract, IOL and Refractive Surgery, Best Paper of the Session, San Diego, CA, April 28, 2001; Werner L, Apple DJ,

Pandey SK, Izak AM, et al. Ground glass opalescence of hydrophilic acrylic intraocular lenses"; poster presented at the Annual Meeting of American Academy of Ophthalmology, New Orleans, LA, November 11-14, 2001; Pandey SK, Werner L, Apple D, Kaskaloglu MM, Izak AM, Cionni RJ. Intraocular Lens Opacification, Opacification, Opacification", Second prize in the category Intraocular Lenses at the ASCRS/Alcon Annual Video Festival, Congress of the American Society of Cataract and Refractive Surgeons, Philadelphia, PA, USA).

Bausch and Lomb: Hydroview™ (H60M)

The first group of explanted hydrophilic acrylic lenses analyzed in our Center because of whitish discoloration was represented by the Bausch and Lomb Surgical (Rochester, NY) Hydroview™ IOL (Figs 54.5 and 54.6).[13-18] The optic material of these IOLs is composed of a cross-linked copolymer of 2-hydroxyethyl methacrylate and 6-hydroxyhexyl methacrylate, with a bonded benzotriazole-type UV absorber. The water content of this material is 18 percent and the refractive index is 1.474. The haptics are modified C loops made of blue-colored PMMA, polymerically cross-linked with the optics by means of an interpenetrating polymer network, which provides a one-piece design with a true optic zone of 6.0 mm. This IOL design has been implanted for several years in international markets; over 400,000 have been implanted worldwide. However, although it was cleared for marketing in November 1999 by the United States Food and Drug Administration (FDA), it has not yet been launched for general implantation in this country.

Starting in November 1999, we have received in our Center 25 explanted Hydroview™ lenses for pathological analyses.[13-18] In each case, the lens has been explanted due to the presence of a granularity on its optical surfaces associated with decrease in visual acuity and glare, in the late postoperative period. At the time of explantation, the age of the 25 patients ranged from 54 to 92 years (75.65 ± 8.57). Two patients were in treatment for cardiovascular diseases, 4 were diabetic and the others were otherwise healthy. The lenses were explanted from 4 to 40 months postoperatively (24.42 ± 10.18)

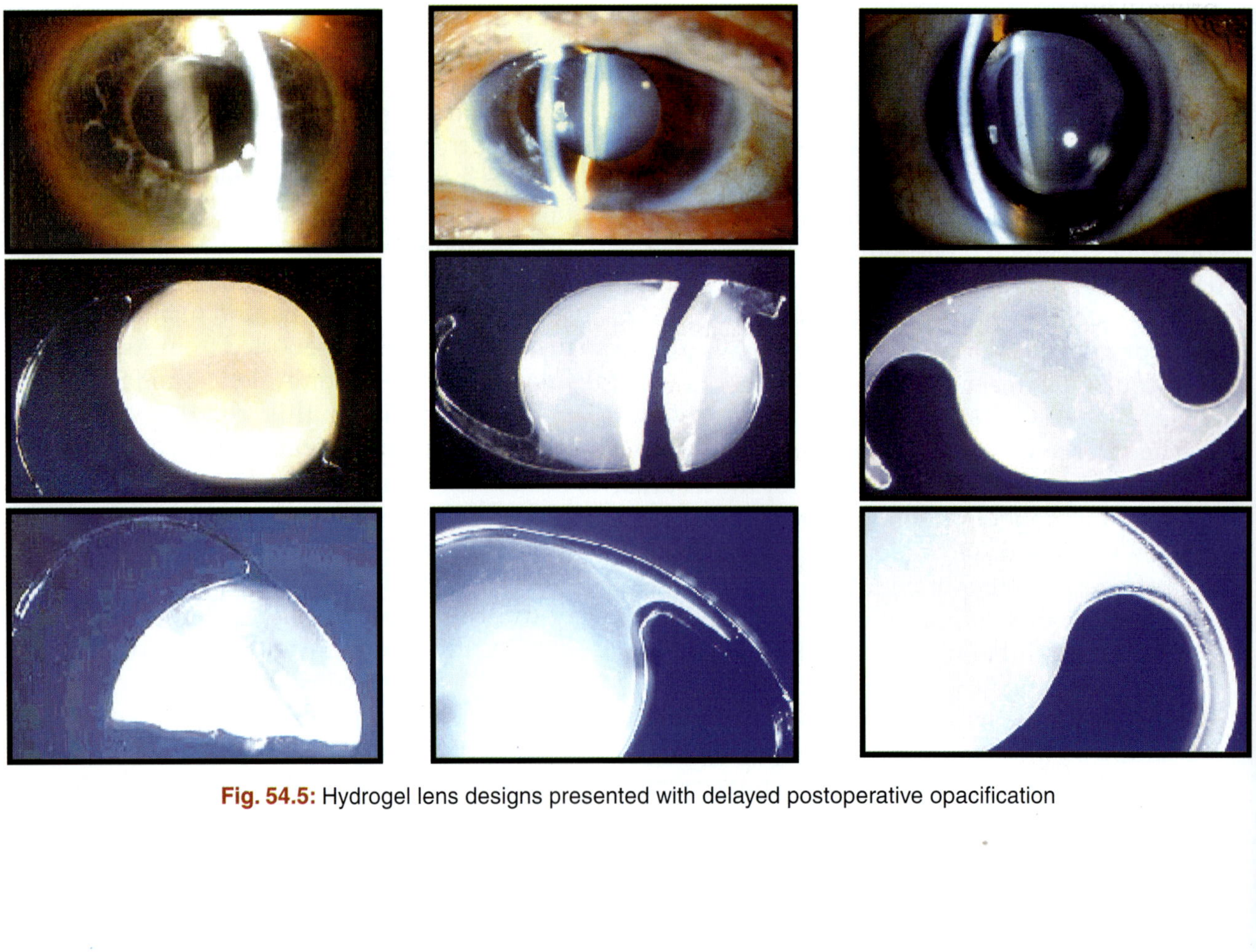

Fig. 54.5: Hydrogel lens designs presented with delayed postoperative opacification

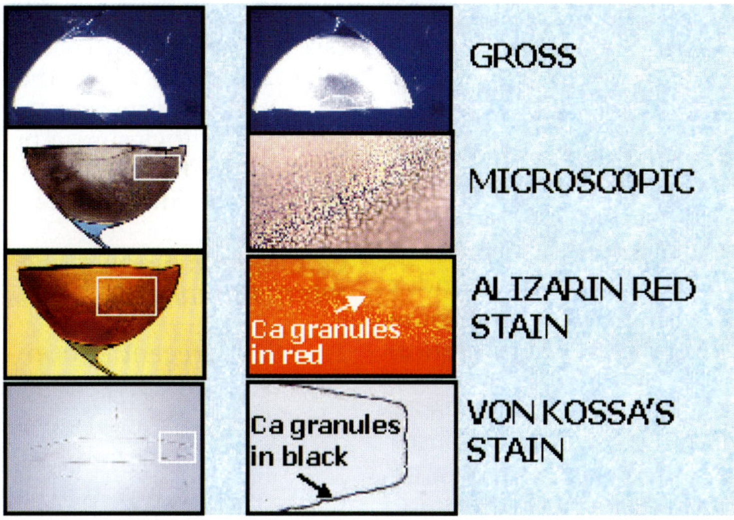

Fig. 54.6: Hydroview™ IOL: microscopic and histochemical evaluation

after the primary procedure due to opacification observed at the level of the optics, associated with decrease in visual acuity (from 20/20 after the primary procedure to hand movements in some cases) and significant glare. In only two cases, the lens was explanted earlier than one year after the primary procedure (4 and 10 months). The surgeons described the findings as a "brown granularity" or "small red corpuscles" present on both external optical surfaces of the lenses (Fig. 54.5, top left). In some cases, the optic of the lenses was almost completely covered by those structures, giving them a "frosty" and very reflective appearance. Nd: YAG laser was performed in many cases in an attempt to clean the optical surfaces, without success.

Medical Developmental Research: SC60B-OUV™

In the second group described here, the hydrophilic IOL to be recently associated with clinically significant postoperative optic opacification is the

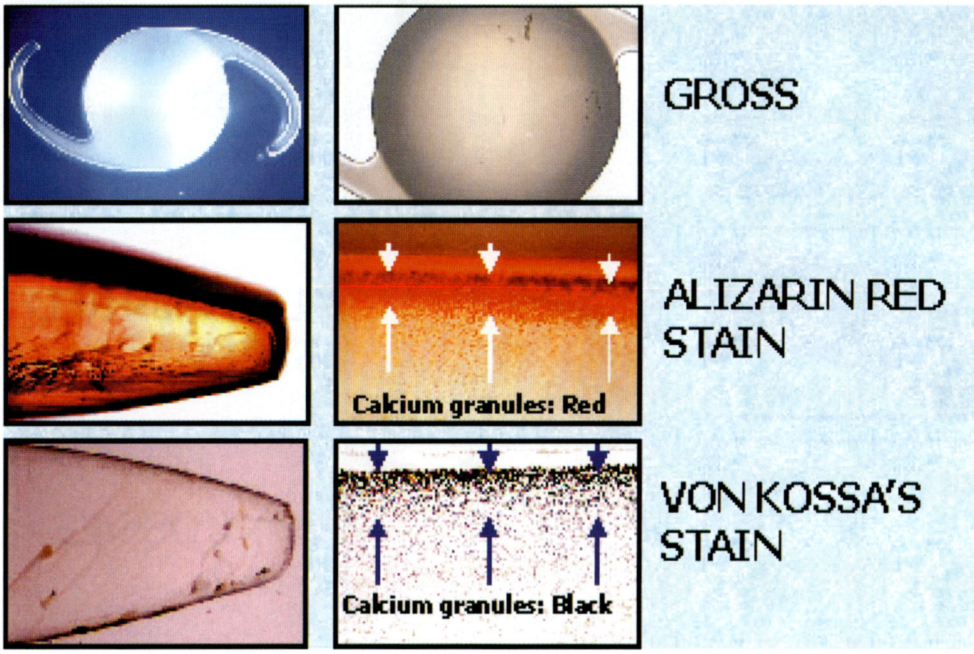

Fig. 54.7: SC60B-OUV™ IOL: Microscopic and histochemical evaluation

SC60B-OUV™ lens (Figs 54.5, middle, and 54.7). The manufacturer and distributor of this design is Medical Developmental Research (MDR Inc., Clearwater, FL). The material used for the manufacture of these IOLs is composed of a cross-linked copolymer of poly 2(hydroxyethyl methacrylate) (HEMA) and methyl methacrylate (MMA), with an incorporated UV absorber. The water content of this material is 28 percent and the refractive index is 1.46. This is a one-piece design, so the haptics are manufactured from the same material as the optical component.

Since 1999 we analyzed 54 explanted SC60B-OUV™ IOLs manufactured by MDR in our Center.[26-29] All of the lenses were explanted because of late postoperative opacification of the optic associated with decreased visual function. At the time of explantation, the ages of the patients ranged from 63 to 82 years (71.00 ± 6.49). Six patients were diabetic, but the majority of the patients did not have any known associated systemic or ocular conditions. The lenses were explanted from 7 to 32 months postoperatively (19.63 ± 7.63). In only two cases, the lens was explanted earlier than one year after the primary procedure (7 and 9 months). In general, the patients returned at around 12 months and later after the surgery complaining of a significant decrease in visual acuity (from 20/20 after the primary procedure to 20/200 in some cases). The clinical characteristics of these lenses were different from the previously described "granularity" covering the optical surfaces of the Hydroview™ design. The clinical appearance of the SC60B-OUV™ lenses was that of a clouding similar to a "nuclear cataract" (Fig. 54.5, middle).

Ophthalmic Innovations International, Inc.: Aqua-Sense™

The third recent group of hydrophilic acrylic designs we analyzed in our Center because of whitish discoloration were explanted Aqua-Sense™ lenses, manufactured by Ophthalmic Innovations International, Inc., (OII), Ontario, CA, USA (Figs 54.5, right, and 54.8).[34,35] This is also a one-piece lens, all manufactured from the same material, a hydrophilic acrylic copolymer with incorporated UV absorber. The material has a refractive index of 1.46 and a water content of 25 percent. Although whitish discoloration was showed with all of the 3 designs, the intensity of the phenomenon with the Aqua-Sense™ is different. The opacity of the lenses available to us for analyses was much more severe than that associated with most cases of the 2 above-mentioned designs.

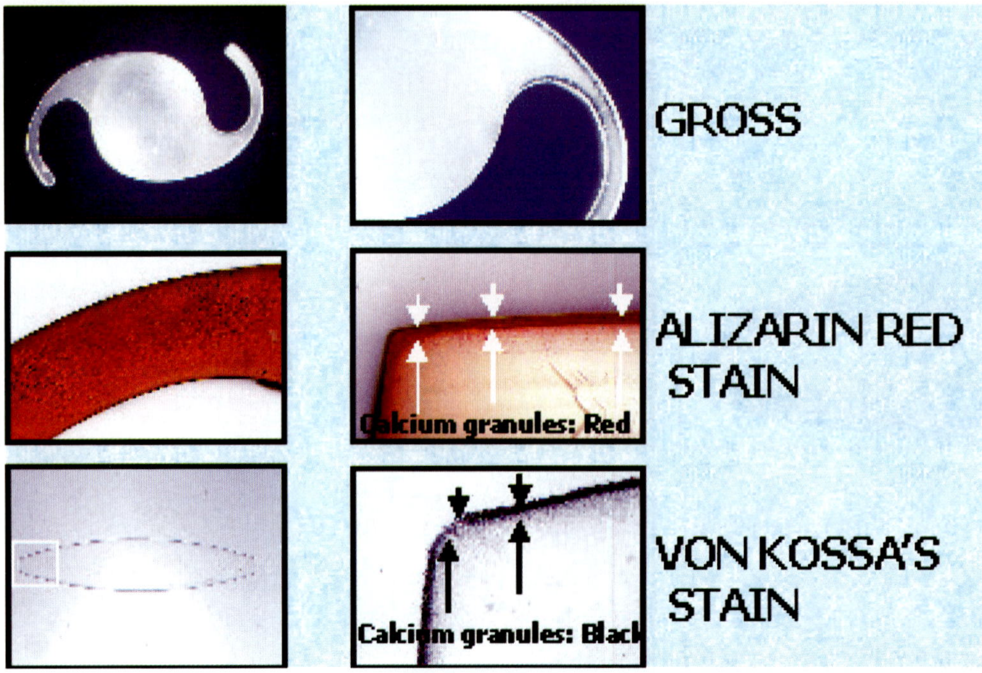

Fig. 54.8: Aqua-senseä IOL: microscopic and histochemical evaluation

Since the beginning of 2001, we received 8 AquaSense™ lenses in our laboratory.[34,35] At the time of explantation, the age of the 8 patients from this group ranged from 25 to 78 years (58.29 ± 16.85). Three patients were diabetic, the others were otherwise healthy. The lenses were explanted from 4 to 14 months postoperatively (10.33 ± 5.51) after the primary surgery. In only one case, the lens was explanted earlier than one year after the primary procedure (4 months). The visual acuity of the patients in general decreased from 20/20 to 20/60 after the primary procedure, with significant associated glare. The clinical appearance of the AquaSense™ lenses was also that of a clouding similar to a "nuclear cataract" (Fig. 54.5, right). As with the two above-mentioned designs, Nd: YAG laser was performed in some cases in an attempt to "clean" the optical surfaces, without success.

Clinicopathological Analyses

The explanted hydrogel IOLs were submitted by several ophthalmic surgeons from various countries (Australia, China, Sweden, Egypt, Germany, South Africa, Turkey, UK, and others) for pathological analysis. Once received in our Center, the IOLs were immediately placed in 4 percent formaldehyde in 0.1 M phosphate buffer, pH 7.4. Care was taken to avoid any manipulation of the IOLs' optics with forceps or other grasping instruments. Some lenses were bisected for explantation, and only one half of them were available to us.

Gross (macroscopic) analysis of the explanted IOLs was performed and gross pictures were taken using a camera (Nikon N905 AF, Nikon Corporation, Tokyo, Japan) fitted to an operating microscope (Leica/Wild MZ-8 Zoom Stereomicroscope, Vashaw Scientific, Inc., Norcross, GA, USA). The unstained lenses were then microscopically evaluated and photographed under a light microscope (Olympus, Optical Co. Ltd., Japan). They were rinsed in distilled water, immersed in a 1 percent alizarin red solution (a special stain for calcium) for 2 minutes, rinsed again in distilled water and reexamined under the light microscope.[35-38]

We then performed full thickness sections through the optic of the explanted lenses. Some of the resultant cylindrical blocks were directly stained with 1 percent alizarin red. The others were dehydrated and embedded in paraffin. Sagittal sections were performed and stained using the von Kossa method for calcium (staining with nitrate solution for 60 minutes; exposure to a 100-watt lamp light; rinsing with distilled water; reaction with sodium thiosulfate solution for 2 minutes; rinsing with distilled water; counterstaining in nuclear fast red solution for 5 minutes). Calcium salts stain in dark brown with this technique.[35-38]

Some lenses in each group were air-dried at room temperature for 7 days, sputter-coated with aluminum and examined under a JEOL JSM 5410LV scanning electron microscope (SEM). The specimens were then further analyzed by Dr. D. G. Dunkelberger (Electron Microscopy Center of the University of South Carolina, Columbia, SC) under a Hitachi 2500 Delta scanning electron microscope equipped with a Kevex X-ray detector with light element capabilities for energy dispersive X-ray analyses (EDS).

Incisional biopsies of conjunctiva and iris were also obtained from one patient during removal and exchange of a Hydroview™ IOL.[18] This was done in order to rule out the presence of dystrophic calcification in those tissues.

Gross and Light Microscopic Analyses

Figures 54.6 to 54.8, summarized the gross, microscopic and histochemical findings in 3 different types of opacified explanted foldable hydrophilic lenses manufactured by the Bausch and Lomb, MDR and OII Inc., respectively. By gross and microscopic evaluations, the presence of granular deposits on the optical surfaces of the Hydroview™ lenses was noted to cause different degrees of IOL haze/opacification, directly proportional to the amount of deposits and the surface of the lenses covered by them. In some cases, both optical surfaces were almost completely covered by a confluent granular layer, whereas in other cases some intervening clear areas were observed. Also, intervening clear areas, probably corresponding to marks caused by forceps during the folding process, were observed in all lenses.

The optical surfaces and the haptics of the SC60B-OUV™ lenses were in general free of deposits. However, there were multiple small structures initially noted to resemble "glistenings" within the central 5-mm of the IOL optical component. These were found to be the cause of each lens opacification. The edges of the optics and the haptics appeared clear in the majority of the cases. However, in one cases, the entire optical component and the haptics were completely opaque (Pandey SK, Werner L, Apple DJ, Kaskaloglu MM, Anand N, Izak AM, et al. "Different patterns of calcium precipitation in the optic and haptics of foldable hydrophilic acrylic lenses"; presented at the ASCRS Symposium on Cataract, IOL and Refractive Surgery, San Diego, CA, April 28, 2001).[29] Light microscopy demonstrated that the opacification was caused by the presence of multiple granular deposits within the optic component of the lenses, sometimes extending to the haptics.

All of the Aqua-Sense™ lenses were completely opacified, presenting a bright whitish discoloration. Multiple, small granular deposits were observed on the external surfaces of the lenses, and also within their substance.

Multiple pits related to Nd: YAG laser treatments were also observed on the posterior surface of some of the IOLs in each group.

Histochemical Stainings

The deposits on the surfaces of the Hydroview™ IOLs stained positive with alizarin red in all cases (Fig. 54.6). No positive staining was observed on the haptics of the IOLs. Sagittal histological sections through the optic of this lens design, stained using von Kossa's method showed a continuous layer of dark brown, irregular granules on the anterior and posterior optical surfaces, and the edges of the lenses (Fig. 54.6). Histochemical evaluations of the conjunctival and iris biopsies obtained from one of the patients were negative.

Alizarin red staining of the surfaces of the SC60B-OUV™ lenses was in general negative. Analysis of the cut sections (sagittal view) of the lens optics revealed multiple granules of variable sizes in a region beneath the external anterior and posterior surfaces of the IOLs. The granules were distributed in a line parallel to the anterior and posterior curvatures of the optics. They stained positive with alizarin red (Fig. 54.7). Sagittal histological sections stained with the von Kossa method also confirmed the presence of multiple dark brown/black granules mostly concentrated in a region immediately beneath the anterior and posterior optical surfaces (Fig. 54.7).

Staining with alizarin red revealed spots of granular deposits on the external surfaces of the Aqua-Sense™ lenses (Fig. 54.8). In some cases, a fine granularity was covering the lenses' external surfaces. Analysis of cut sections (sagittal view) of the lens optic revealed multiple granules of variable sizes in a region beneath the external anterior and posterior surfaces of the IOLs. As with the previous lens design, the granules were distributed in a line parallel to the anterior and posterior curvatures of the optics and they stained positive with alizarin red and the von Kossa method (Fig. 54.8).

Scanning Electron Microscopy

Figure 54.9, summarized the ultrastructural findings in 3 different types of opacified explanted foldable hydrophilic lenses manufactured by the Bausch and Lomb, MDR and OII Inc., respectively. The aspect of the 3 lens designs observed under light microscopy was confirmed by SEM. Analyses of the anterior optical surfaces of some Hydroview™ lenses revealed granular deposits composed of multiple spherical-ovoid globules, scattered in some areas, and confluent in others (Fig. 54.9). SEM analysis of cut sections (sagittal view) of the optic of some SC60B-OUV™ lenses confirmed that the region immediately subjacent to the IOLs' outer surfaces as well as the central area of the optical cut sections were free of deposits. This also revealed the presence of the granules in the intermediate region beneath the anterior and posterior surfaces (Fig. 54.9). With the Aqua-Sense™ lenses, SEM of the anterior surface revealed the presence of small granular deposits (Fig. 54.9). Analyses of cut sections of this lens design demonstrated features similar to those described with the SC60B-OUV™ lens (Fig. 54.9).

Energy Dispersive X-Ray Spectroscopy

With the 3 lens designs, EDS performed precisely on the deposits revealed the presence of calcium

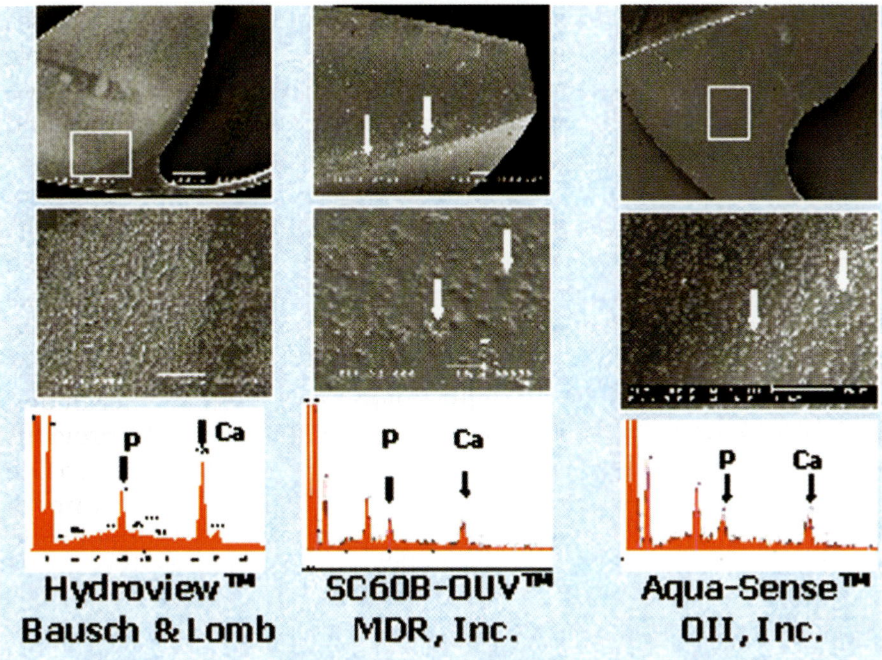

Fig. 54.9: Opacified hydrogel lenses: ultrastructural evaluation

and phosphate peaks (Fig. 54.9). EDS was also performed on areas free of deposits to serve as controls, showing only peaks of carbon and oxygen (Fig. 54.9).

Possible Factors Involved in the Pathological Mechanism

We can divide the phenomenon of crystalline deposition on IOL optics into 2 general time frames: intra or shortly postoperative versus late postoperative (circa 12 months).

Jensen et al[39] in 1994 first described the formation of crystalline deposits on the surface of IOLs during cataract surgery in a series of 11 patients. The deposits would last a long time (at least 6 months) if sequestered by the posterior capsule, and they had a significant effect on the visual acuity (20/40 or worse). The common features in all cases were the use of Healon GVÒ (Pharmacia-Upjohn Ophthalmics, Kalamazoo, MI, USA), a high molecular-weight hyaluronate sodium, and BSS® or BSS Plus® (Alcon Surgical Inc, Forth Worth, TX, USA). The authors hypothesized that the phosphate components used in the viscoelastic preparations to buffer the solution could have reacted with calcium from irrigating solutions or the aqueous humor of the patients, and precipitated. Nevertheless, no analysis of the deposits was performed. Although they were also noted on PMMA IOLs, the severe cases were all associated with silicone lenses, suggesting that silicone is a better substrate for this phenomenon. The same group described later 22 other cases of intraoperative crystallization on IOL surfaces.[39,40] Again, all the severe cases were associated with silicone lenses, but viscoelastics other than Healon GV® have also been used. In these studies, a sample of the material was submitted to scanning electron microscopic analysis and X-ray photoelectron spectroscopy, for elemental identification. The cation of concern was found to be calcium.

Crystalline precipitation on the surface of hydrogel lenses with water content higher than Hydroview™ lenses (Iogel 1103, Alcon Laboratories, Fort Worth, TX, USA) was first described by Amon and Menapace in 1991.[42,43] They evaluated in vivo the surfaces of 200 consecutive IOLs over a 1.5-year postoperative period. In their study, the presence of few, dust-like white precipitates of unknown origin on the surface of 7 percent of the lenses were described. Nevertheless, no comment was made on the time of presentation and the evolution of the deposits.

Bucher et al[44] in 1995 reported a case of dystrophic calcification of the same hydrogel IOL, in an 80-year-old woman with chronic lymphatic leukemia. On the first postoperative day, a brown-white material was observed behind the IOL. During the second postoperative month, the material turned white and changed its shape. Two months after the surgery, granular whitish spots appeared on the anterior surface of the IOL. Their confluence with time formed a band-shaped white layer on the anterior optic surface. White granules also developed in the corneal stroma at the site of a paracentesis, but not at the incision. The lens was explanted due to decreased visual acuity. Special staining and surface analyses revealed the material to contain calcium hydroxyapatite. Intraocular solutions used during the surgery in this case were Ringer's lactate with epinephrine, sodium hyaluronate as viscoelastic and thymoxamine, which is a phosphate-buffered solution used to achieve miosis. Although the patient had chronic lymphatic leukemia, no disturbance of calcium metabolism was detected and the electrolyte levels were normal on several occasions before and after the development of calcification. The authors hypothesized that an oversupply of calcium, from residual lens material, and of phosphates, from the thymoxamine solution, reacted originating the deposits.

All the previous reports concerning crystalline deposit formation on IOL surfaces, mostly in the early postoperative period, seem to be related to calcium-phosphate reaction with formation of calcium salts.[39-44] Indeed, hydroxyapatite is the thermodynamically stable phase of calcium phosphate in biological systems. Calcium and phosphate are present in blood and interstitial fluids at levels that nearly exceed their solubility product. Although the calcium content of the normal aqueous humor is low, about half that of the serum, any cause of a localized increase in calcium or phosphate, such as intraocular inflammation or administration of intraocular drugs rich in these elements might result in dystrophic calcification.[45-47] Some studies reported corneal calcium-phosphate precipitates related to the phosphate buffer concentration in ViscoatÒ (Alcon Laboratories, Fort Worth, TX, USA).[45-46] Viscoat® is a specific formulation of chondroitin sulfate and sodium hyaluronate dissolved in isotonic physiological phosphate-buffered solution.[48] The phosphate buffer concentration was reduced since these reports, in order to prevent the precipitation phenomenon. The crystalline lens itself (or residual cortical material) is a potential source of phosphates. Sources of calcium in cataract surgery scenario could be represented by aqueous humor, intraocular irrigating solutions and also by crystalline lens. Indeed, the concentration of calcium adsorbed to lens proteins is high.

We decided to start the tests by using the alizarin red staining technique. This method is very simple to perform and it is one of the most specific. Demonstration of calcium with this anthraquinone-derivative dye depends on a chelation process with the dye.[36,37] The von Kossa silver test demonstrates the presence of calcium through a metal substitution technique.[38] This method confirmed our findings with alizarin red. Later, scanning electron microscopic (SEM) and energy dispersive X-ray spectroscopic (EDS) analyses revealed the deposits to be composed of calcium and phosphates.

Calcium deposition observed in our cases occurred in the late postoperative period. In the cases of surface deposition, one might speculate that it is similar to the calcium deposition associated with spoilation of soft contact lenses. The term spoilation is used to describe physical and chemical changes in the nature of the hydrophilic soft contact lenses and various deposits that may impair their optical properties and produce discomfort and intolerance. Contact lens spoilage may occur in some cases as early as in 48 hours of wear, but in the majority of cases it occurs after 3-6 months of daily or extended wear. Filmy deposits on the surface of soft contact lenses are in general represented by protein, calcium, lipid and/or bacterial components. Factors that may predispose the formation of calcium deposits on soft contact lenses include dry-eye syndrome, increased levels of calcium and phosphate in the tears and inflammation. In addition to producing a film, calcium can form chalky white granules that may take the shape of barnacles with concentric rings or lamellae. They resemble rock formations and exhibit birefringence under polarized light.[49-54]

Heavy inorganic films often cause damage to the soft contact lens surface, since the material may penetrate into the lens matrix. Thus, after chemical removal of the deposits, pits and other irregularities usually remain.[52-53] In the case of Hydroview™ IOLs, chemical removal of calcium phosphate revealed the presence of few small pits and fissures at SEM, that were found to be artifactual, rather than permanent damage caused by the deposits on the IOLs surfaces (George Green, PhD at Bausch and Lomb, personal communication, February 2000). Yu et al[19,20] and Groh et al[21] in transmission electron analyses of this same lens design, found calcium precipitates within the lens substance, in a region immediately subjacent to the external surfaces.

Chang and associates[10] published the first clinical report on late postoperative opacification of the second group of lenses (SC60B-OUV™ IOL), when they noted a central clouding associated with a decrease in visual acuity. No inflammatory reaction was observed. They speculated whether the IOL opacity could be caused by a process similar to the "glistenings" associated with a hydrophobic acrylic lens, the Alcon AcrySof™.[55-57] We had a similar impression after our initial gross and light microscopic examinations of these lenses. However, the clinical profile noted with the AcrySof™ IOL is different. The occurrence of Alcon AcrySof™-related glistenings has been described as early as 1 week after cataract surgery, and the time frame is highly variable, as opposed to at around 24 months with the SC60B-OUV™ IOLs. Clinical studies on the AcrySof™ IOL have demonstrated that contrast sensitivity has been decreased in some patients, but clinically significant decrease on visual acuity has been rare.[55] In vitro studies have suggested that the occurrence of glistenings in AcrySof™ IOLs may be related to variations in the temperature (êt), with formation of vacuoles within the submersed acrylic polymer when there is a transient increase in temperature above the glass transition temperature, approximately 18.5º C for AcrySof™ (Apple DJ, "Clinicopathological correlation of vacuoles in an acrylic IOL"—Best Paper of the Session–presented at the ASCRS Symposium on Cataract, IOL and Refractive Surgery, April 1998, San Diego, CA, USA). "Glistenings" may then subsequently form from anterior chamber fluid. It has been reported that the IOL packaging, the AcryPak™, and the sterilization technique used with that system may have made the IOL susceptible to the microvacuole formation. In vitro studies have also demonstrated that the temperature at which the IOLs were stored and shipped in the dry state had no influence on the "glistenings" and was thus unrelated to this phenomenon.[56]

In contrast to the findings of what morphologically resembled "glistenings" noted in these clinical and in vitro analyses, light microscopic analyses of the cut sections of the optics (sagittal views) revealed that the structures causing the opacification with the SC60B-OUV™ lenses are not fluid-filled vacuoles, but rather are granules of variable sizes. Frohn A., Dick H.B., and coworkers have evaluated 41 of these lenses by light microscopy, high performance liquid chromatography, sodium dodecyl sulfate polyacrylamide gel electrophoresis, spectrometric analysis, and autoclaving. Neither fatty acids nor proteins could be identified within the IOLs. Spectrometric analysis yielded absorption peaks in the ultraviolet spectral range. According to the same authors, these findings indicate premature aging of the ultraviolet blocking agent within the lenses, the source of the opacification being a change in the IOL material itself. Indeed, the material of these IOLs does contain an incorporated UV absorber which functions to protect the retina from ultraviolet radiation in the 300-400 nm range, protection normally provided by the crystalline lens. We have not yet done studies to verify Frohn's and Dick's findings that unbound UV-absorber monomers or any impurity causes opacification within the IOL optic. Their findings and the calcification process demonstrated by us may be correlated, although our data does not allow us to make definitive conclusions.

There have been reports on brownish discoloration and central haze of silicone lenses, both in the early 1990s, as well as recently (Schulze RR, Apple DJ, "Progressive pigmentation of Staar silicone IOLs: Case report", presented at the ASCRS Symposium on Cataract, IOL and Refractive

Surgery, May 20-24, 2000, Boston, MA, USA).[58-60] This complication has been generally observed in the early postoperative period, e.g. around 6 weeks after cataract surgery and IOL implantation. In general, it is clinically insignificant; IOL explantation has rarely been performed. These reports have suggested that the brown haze was due to light scatter from water vapor that may diffuse into the silicone when immersed in an aqueous medium. This may be caused by some anomaly of the curing process during the manufacture of those lenses or by incomplete extraction of large polymers. UV blocking agents did not seem to be in issue with lens discoloration since the phenomenon was also observed with silicone IOL models not containing these agents. Additional filtration steps in the manufacturing process of silicone lenses seemed to solve the problem. Chromatographic detection and characterization of unbound constituents of the SC60B-OUV™ lenses should be performed to address this issue with this IOL.

Dr Mahmut Kaskaloglu (Turkey) has implanted 361 of these lenses between November 1997 and October 1999. He observed 18 cases of late postoperative opacification of the SC60B-OUV™ lens, 9 of which had associated visual symptoms sufficient to justify explantation and submit for pathological analysis. Of the 18 cases of opacification, 5 patients were diabetic (2 explantations). (Kaskaloglu M, Werner L. "Visual outcomes of the patients with an opacified hydrophilic acrylic IOL"; presented at the ASCRS Symposium on Cataract, IOL and Refractive Surgery, Best Paper of the Session, San Diego, CA, April 29, 2001). [29] To date there is no means to establish a definitive relationship between diabetes and this complication. Again, three separate tests strongly suggested that the granules are at least in part composed of calcium, the alizarin red stain, the von Kossa stain and SEM analyses with EDS. EDS demonstrated the presence of calcium peaks only at the level of the deposits, not in the center of the optic and not in the region immediately subjacent to the surface. Interestingly, although the SC60B-OUV™ design is a single piece lens entirely manufactured from a single acrylic material, the opacifying granules were present only in a specific region of the IOLs' optic. The reasons for this pattern are still unknown to us. It may represent a diffusion-type pattern or absorption of material from aqueous humor.

The Aqua-Sense™ IOL design represents the third group of such cases. Calcium deposition on the external surface of the lens as well as within the substance of the optic and haptic components has been observed with all Aqua-Sense™ lenses analyzed in our Center.[34,35]

Dr. Wynand Troskie (South Africa) has implanted 187 of these lenses between August 1999 and October 2000. Thus far as of the time of this writing, he has observed 23 cases of postoperative opacification of the Aqua-Sense™ lens, 16 of which had associated visual symptoms sufficient to justify explantation and submit the explants for pathological analysis. Of the 23 cases of opacification, 4 patients were diabetic (3 explantations). The Aqua-Sense™ lenses analyzed by us revealed a total opacification occurring to an extent that we have never seen since we began examining IOLs in 1983.

At the time of this writing, the number of reported cases with the Hydroview™ lens is relatively small; 309 of approximately 400,000 lenses implanted worldwide. In 96 cases, the IOL changes were clinically significant, decreasing patient vision enough to result in lens explantation. The clinical reports have not been randomly distributed. Although this IOL model has been implanted in 3,500 centers worldwide, reports have appeared in clusters. The vast majority has come from 31 ophthalmic practices in 11 countries. We have studied cases from several of these centers, including practices in Australia, Canada, and Sweden.

In a February 2001 letter to surgeons who have implanted the Hydroview™ IOL, Bausch and Lomb described their investigation into the phenomenon. Surface chemistry studies identified the lens deposits as a layered mixture of octacalcium phosphate, fatty acids, salts, and small amounts of silicone (Guttman C, "Hydroview calcification resolved". Ophthalmology Times, 2001; 26:No. 4). An in vitro model was then constructed to find out how the material deposited onto the lens. This model, according to the manufacturer, revealed a migration of silicone from a gasket in the lens packaging onto the surface of the IOL. The models also showed that in addition to silicone, fatty acids had to be present to attract calcium ions to the lens surface. A separate retrospective clinical case/control study was also conducted by the manufacturer at the sites where the highest incidences of calcification were reported. A compromised blood-retinal barrier seemed to be associated with the appearance of calcified deposits.

No reports of presumed calcification were received prior to introduction of the SureFold® system. According to Bausch and Lomb studies, part of the components of this packaging contains silicone, which may come off the packaging onto the lens optic. It then appears to be a catalyst for calcium precipitation. Fatty acids and silicone, perhaps in association with a metabolic disease in the affected patient, could result in the calcification.

As of May 2000, MDR had announced 56 cases of late postoperative lens opacification out of over 75,000 SC60B-OUV™ lenses implanted worldwide. They were aware of at least 20 other cases that required explantation because of significant visual loss, in addition to these described here. The manufacturer has withdrawn all SC60B-OUV™ IOLs that have been fabricated from material obtained from their previous polymer supplier and have sent in June of 2000 an informational letter to all lens users. All of these IOLs are now being manufactured from polymer material obtained from a new source.

The manufacturer of the Aqua-Sense™ lens has reported 12 similar cases, besides the cases described here (Mr. Rick Aguilera, President OII, personal communication, Amsterdam, The Netherlands, September 2001). The manufacturer also stated that researchers have found silicone particles on the surface of the lenses. The silicone contaminants appeared to come from some components of the IOL packaging. Those silicone components have been removed and changed to Teflon. Also, the manufacturer stated that they have implemented new manufacturing processes involving proprietary technology to minimize exposure of in-process lenses to chemical agents and remove any residual of these substances during the final stages of manufacture. Residual water-soluble process compounds are now extracted before packaging and sterilization by a process OII named the P.U.R.E™ system (Precision Unresolved-materials Extraction). The Aqua-Sense™ IOL was then re-released in January 2001.

Prevention and Treatment

The opacification described in our reports have an entirely different appearance than classic posterior capsule opacification or anterior lens epithelial cell proliferation.

It is important for the surgeons who implanted lenses from these three groups to recognize this condition. Excessive Nd: YAG laser treatment, in an attempt to clean the optical surfaces of the lenses may jeopardize implantation of a new lens in the capsular bag after explantation of the opacified lens. The adherence of the deposits to the optical surfaces of the lenses seems to be extremely strong and Nd: YAG laser treatment was proven to be ineffective in the cleaning of the lenses' surfaces. The cause of this condition seems to be multifactorial, and until the pathogenic mechanism is not fully clarified, explantation and exchange of the IOL is the only available treatment.

Surgeons usually face two important challenges during explantation of these opacified lenses. Firstly, fibrosis along the capsulorhexis edge and secondly the capsular adhesions around the lens haptics. A few radial incisions may be helpful to increase the rhexis diameter and to remove the capsular flap. It is very important to well visco-dissect the lens from the capsular bag, in order to liberate any adherence to this structure. The lens is removed after being folded inside the eye, bisected, or intact through a larger incision. The status of the capsular bag should then be carefully inspected, which will influence the decision about the site for fixation of the new lens. Methods for the prevention of this condition are also not completely defined to date. Long-term clinical studies will determine the efficacy of modifications performed on IOL polymers and packaging for prevention of lens calcification.

SUMMARY

Each hydrophilic acrylic IOL design available in the market is manufactured from a different copolymer acrylic. To the best of our knowledge, the calcification problem described in this text cannot be generalized to all of the lenses in this category. The incidence of IOL explantation because of calcification remains low, much less than 1 percent in each of the 3 groups described here. The mechanism is not fully understood, but it does not seem to be directed related to substances used during the surgery as it occurred in the late post-operative period. Also, the substances used during the surgery were not the same in all cases. The majority of the patients involved had an associated systemic disease; therefore, the possibility of a patient-related factor, such as a metabolic imbalance cannot be ruled out.

Lot history, component history, process changes, surgical setting and techniques, environmental factors, preexisting patients conditions, and packaging have been examined. It is now important to carefully follow clinical outcomes of these lens designs in order to assure if this phenomenon will disappear following the changes in polymer source or packaging.

ACKNOWLEDGEMENT

The authors would like to thank all the ophthalmic surgeons around the world for submitting the explanted rigid PMMA and hydrogel intraocular lenses for pathological analysis at our Center.

REFERENCES

1. Ridley NHL: Artificial intraocular lenses after cataract extraction. St. Thomas Hospital Reports 1951;7:12-14.
2. Apple DJ, Peng Q, Arthur SN, Werner L, et al. Snowflake degeneration of polymethylmethacrylate (PMMA) posterior chamber intraocular lens optic material: A newly described clinical condition caused by an unexpected late opacification of PMMA. Ophthalmology 2002 (in press).
3. Peng Q, Apple DJ, Arthur SA, et al. "Snowflake" Opacification of polymethylmethacrylate Intraocular Lens Optic Biomaterial: A Newly Described Syndrome. In: Werner L, Apple DJ, (Eds): Complications of Rigid and Foldable Intraocular Lenses. Int Ophthalmol Clin. Lippincott and Wilkins, Philadelphia, PA, USA. 2001;41:91-108.
4. Park JB. Biomaterials—An introduction. New York: Plenum Press, 1979:88-91.
5. Sugaya H. Sakai Y. Polymethylmethacrylate: from polymer to dialyzer. Contributions to Nephrology. 1999;125:1-8.
6. Christ FR, Buchen SY, Deacon J, et al: Biomaterials used for intraocular lenses. In: Wise DL, et al (Eds): Encyclopedic handbook of Biomaterials and Bioengineering. New York: Marcel Dekker Inc., 1995:1277.
7. Chehade M, Elder MJ. Intraocular lens materials and styles: A review. Aust NZ J Ophthalmol 1997;25:255-63.
8. Schauersberger J, Kruger A, Abela C, et al. Course of postoperative inflammation after implantation of 4 types of foldable intraocular lenses. J Cataract Refract Surg 1999; 25:1116-20.
9. Hollick EJ, Spalton DJ, Ursell PG. Surface cytologic features on intraocular lenses: can increased biocompatibility have disadvantages? Arch Ophthalmol 1999;117:872-78
10. Chang BYP, Davey KG, Gupta M, Hutchinson C. Late clouding of an acrylic intraocular lens following routine phacoemulsification. Eye 1999;13:807-08.
11. Murray RI. Two cases of late opacification of the hydroview hydrogel intraocular lens. J Catract Refract Surg 2000;26:1272-73.
12. Fernando GT, Crayford BB. Visually significant calcification of hydrogel intraocular lenses necessitating explantation. Clin Experiment Ophthalmol 2000;28:280-86.
13. Apple DJ, Werner L, Escobar-Gomez M, Pandey SK. Deposits on the optical surfaces of hydroview intraocular lenses (letter). J Cataract Refract Surg 2000;26:796-97.
14. Werner L, Apple DJ, Escobar-Gomez M, et al. Post-operative deposition of calcium on the surfaces of a hydrogel intraocular lens. Ophthalmology 2000;107:2179-85.
15. Izak A, Werner L, Pandey SK, et al. Calcification on the surface of the Bausch and Lomb Hydroview™ intraocular lens. Int Ophthalmol Clin 2001;41:62-78.
16. Apple DJ, Werner L, Pandey SK. Newly recognized complications of posterior chamber intraocular lenses (Editorial). Arch Ophthalmol 2001;119:581-82.
17. Pandey SK, Werner L, Apple DJ, Kaskaloglu M. Hydrophilic acrylic intraocular lens optic and haptics opacification in a diabetic patient: Bilateral case report and clinicopathological correlation. *Ophthalmology* 2002 (in press).
18. Pandey SK, Werner L, Apple DJ, Gravel JP. Calcium precipitation on the optical surfaces of a foldable intraocular lens: A clinicopathological correlation. Arch Ophthalmol 2002;120:391-93.
19. Yu AFK, Shek TWH. Hydroxyapatite formation on implanted hydrogel intraocular lenses. Arch Ophthalmol 2001;107:2179-85.

20. Yu AKF, Kwan KYW, Chan DHY, Fong DYT. Clinical features of 46 eyes with calcified hydrogel intraocular lenses. J Cataract Refract Surg 2001;27:1596-1606.
21. Groh JMM, Schlotzer-Schrehardt U, Rummelt C, et al. Postoperative Kunstlinsen-Eintrubungen bei 12 Hydrogel-Intraokularlinsen (Hydroview). Klin Monatsbl Augenheilkd 2001;218:645-48
22. Shek TW, Wong A, Yau B, Yu Ak. Opacification of artificial intraocular lens: an electron microscopic study. Ultrastruct Pathol 2001;25:281-83.
23. Buchen SY, Cunanan CM, Gwon A et al. Assessing intraocular lens calcification in an animal model. J Cataract Refract Surg 2001;27:1473-84.
24. Frohn A, Dick B, Augustin AJ, Grus FH. Late opacification of the foldable hydrophilic acrylic lens SC60B-OUV. Ophthalmology 2001;108:1999-2004.
25. Mamalis N. Hydrophilic acrylic intraocular lenses (Editorial). J Cataract Refract Surg 2001;27:1339-40.
26. Werner L, Apple DJ, Kaskaloglu M, Pandey SK. Dense Opacification of the optical component of a hydrophilic intraocular lens: A clinicopathological analysis of 9 explanted lenses. J Cataract Refract Surg 2001;27:1485-92.
27. Macky TA, Trivedi RH, Werner L, et al. Degeneration of UV absorber material and calcium deposits within the optic of a hydrophilic IOL lens (manufactured by Medical Developmental Research). In: Werner L, Apple DJ, (Eds). Complications of Aphakic and Refractive Intraocular Lenses. Int Ophthalmol Clin. Lippincott Williams and Wilkins, Philadelphia, PA, USA, 2001; 41:79-90.
28. Apple DJ, Werner L, Pandey SK. Opalescence of hydrophilic acrylic lenses (letter). Eye 2001;15:97-98.
29. Izak AM Werner L, Pandey SK, Apple DJ. Opacification of modern foldable hydrogel intraocular lens designs. Eye. 2002, in press.
30. Sharma TK, Chawdhary S. The opalescence of hydrogel intraocular lens. Eye 2001;15:97-98.
31. Sharma A, Ram J, Gupta A. Late clouding of an acrylic intraocular lens following routine phacoemulsification (letter). Eye 2001; 15:361.
32. Woodruff SA, Khan J, Dhingra N, et al. Late clouding of an acrylic intraocular lens following routine phacoemulsification (letter). Eye 2001; 15:362.
33. Pavlovic S, Magdowski G, Brueckel B, Pavlovic S. Ultrastructural analysis of opacities seen in a hydrophilic acrylic intracular lens. Eye 2001;15:657-59.
34. Werner L, Apple DJ, Izak AM. Discoloration / opacification of modern foldable hydrogel intraocular lens designs. In: Buratto L, Zanini R, Apple DJ, Werner L, (Eds): Phaco 2002, Slack Inc., Thorofare NJ, (in press).
35. Werner L, Izak AM, Apple DJ, Pandey SK, et al. Complete calcification of a hydrogel lens design: Case reports and clinicopathological correlation. Am J Ophthalmol 2002 (submitted).
36. McGee Russell SM. Histochemical methods for calcium. J Histochem Cytochem 1958;6:22-42.
37. Carr LB, Rambo ON, Feichtmeir TV. A method of demonstrating calcium in tissue sections using chloranilic acid. J Histochem Cytochem 1961;9:415-17.
38. Pizzolato P. Histochemical recognition of calcium oxalate. J Histochem Cytochem 1964;12:333-36.
39. Jensen MK, Crandall AS, Mamalis N, Olson RJ. Crystallization on intraocular lens surfaces associated with the use of Healon GV. Arch Ophthalmol 1994;112:1037-42.
40. Olson RJ. New cases of crystalline deposits on intraocular lenses not related to any specific viscoelastic (letter). Arch Ophthalmol 1995; 113:1229.
41. Olson RJ, Caldwell KD, Crandall AS, et al. Intraoperative crystallization on the intraocular lens surface. Am J Ophthalmol 1998; 126:177-84.
42. Amon M, Menapace R. Cellular invasion on hydrogel and polymethyl methacrylate implants: An in vivo study. J Cataract Refract Surg 1991;17:774-79.
43. Amon M, Menapace R. In vivo observation of surface precipitaces of 200 consecutive hydrogel intraocular lenses. Ophthalmologica 1992;204:13-18.
44. Bucher PJM, Buchi ER, Daicker BC. Dystrophic calcification of an implanted hydroxyethylmethacrylate intraocular lens. Arch Ophthalmol 1995; 113:1431-35.
45. Ullman S, Lichtenstein SB, Heerlein K. Corneal opacities secondary to ViscoatÒ. J Cataract Refract Surg 1986;12:489-92.
46. Binder PS, Deg JK, Kohl FS. Calcific band keratopathy after intraocular chondroitin sulfate. Arch Ophthalmol 1987;105: 1243-47.
47. Jensen OA. Ocular calcifications in primary hyperparathyroidism. Histochemical and ultrastructural study of a case. Comparison with ocular calcifications in idiopathic hypercalcemia of infancy and in renal failure. Acta Ophthalmol 1975;53:173-86.
48. Liesegang TJ. Viscoelastics. Int Ophthalmol Clin 1993;33:127-47.
49. Gasset AR, Lobo L, Houde W. Permanent wear of soft contact lenses in aphakic eyes. Am J Ophthalmol 1977; 83:115-20.
50. Winder AF, Ruben M, Sheraidah Ga. Tear calcium levels and contact lens wear. Br J Ophthalmol 1977; 61:539-43.
51. Levy B. Calcium deposits on glyceryl methyl methacrylate and hydroxyethyl methacrylate contact lenses. Am J Optomet Physiol Opt 1984;61:605-07.
52. Bowers RWJ, Tighe BJ. Studies in the ocular compatibility of hydrogels: A review of the clinical manifestations of spoilation. Biomaterial 1987;8:83-88.
53. Bowers RWJ, Tighe BJ. Studies of the ocular compatibility of hydrogels: white spot deposits: chemical composition and geological arrangement of components. Biomaterial 1987;8:172-76.
54. Tripathi RC, Tripathi BJ, Silverman RA, Rao GN. Contact lens deposits and spoilage: Identification and management. Int Ophthalmol Clin 1991;3:91-120.

55. Dhaliwal DK, Mamamlis N, Olson RJ, et al. Visual significance of glistenings seen in the AcrySof intraocular lens. J Cataract Refract Surg 1996;22:452-57.
56. Omar O, Pirayesh A, Mamalis N, Olson RJ. In vitro analysis of AcrySof intraocular lens glistenings in AcryPak and Wagon Wheel Packaging. J Cataract Refract Surg 1998;24:107-13.
57. Anderson C, Koch DD, Green G, et al. Alcon AcrySof™ acrylic intraocular lens. In: Martin RG, Gills JP, Sanders DR, (Eds), Foldable Intraocular Lenses. Thorofare, NJ, Slack, 1993;161-77.
58. Milauskas AT. Silicone intraocular lens implant discoloration in humans (letter). Arch Ophthalmol 1991;109:913.
59. Watt RH. Discoloration of a silicone intraocular lens 6 weeks after surgery (letter). Arch Ophthalmol 1991;109:1494.
60. Koch DD, Heit Le. Discoloration of silicone intraocular lenses (letter). Arch Ophthalmol 1992;110:319-20.

Section Four

Recent Advances and Future Considerations

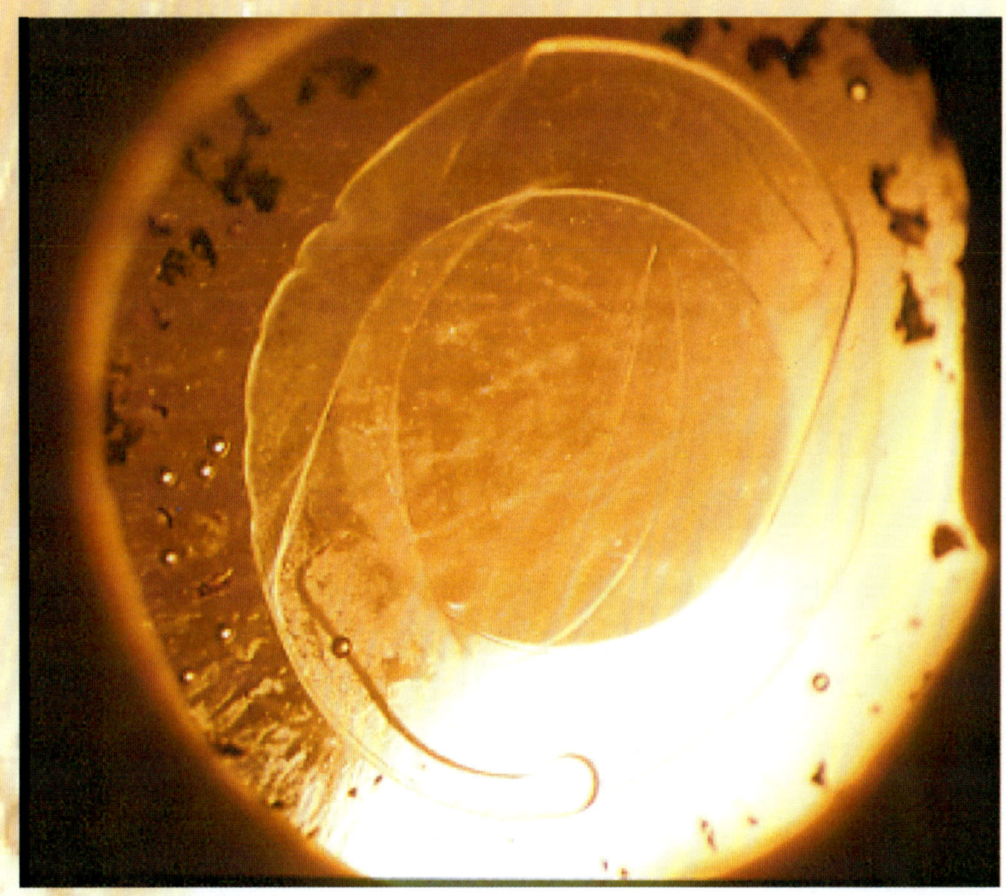

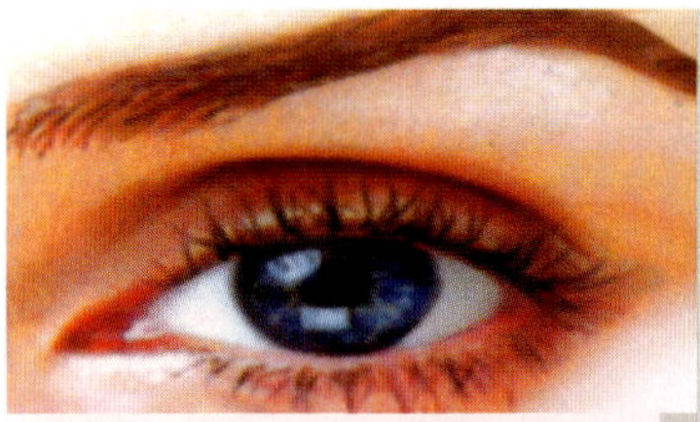

Fifty five

Recent Techniques in Nucleus Delivery in SICS

Arif Adenwala
Ashok Garg (India)

Manual Small Incision Cataract Surgery (MSICS) is a good alternative to expensive technique of phacoemulsification. It can be performed in almost all types of cataract.

This technique has almost all the advantages of phaco surgery. Important steps involved in SICS are:

a. Wound construction: Scleral tunnel is usually preferred.
b. Nucleus Management: This includes:
   - Prolapsing of nucleus in AC.
   - Removal of nucleus out of the wound.
     There are different methods for removal of nucleus out of the wound.
c. Implantation of Intraocular lens.

Nucleus management consists of :

a. Delivery of nucleus into the anterior chamber.
a. Removal of nucleus out of the wound.

DELIVERY OF NUCLEUS INTO THE ANTERIOR CHAMBERS

After construction of good adequate capsulorhxis and hydrodissection, nucleus is prolapsed in the anterior chamber. This is done either by hydrodissection, viscoexpression or with use of Sinskeys hook by rotating the nucleus.

REMOVAL OF NUCLEUS OUT OF THE WOUND[6]

This is very important part of SICS. There are different methods available for it:

1. The Blumenthal technique
3. Use of irrigating vectis
3. Visco-expression
4. Phacofracture
5. Manual phacofracture Cardona's technique
6. Phaco sandwich technique
7. Manual multiple phacofragmentation
8. Prechop manual phacofragmentation
9. Quarter's extraction technique
10. Chopsticks technique
11. Use of claw vectis
12. Plain wire vectis
13. Fish hook technique
14. Phaco-punch technique
15. Hybrid technique
16. Slider pincer technique
17. Double wire Snare splitter technique.

The preliminary step in almost all the methods is prolapse of nucleus in to the anterior chamber:

The Blumenthal Technique[6]

The important feature of nucleus delivery by this technique is hydrodissection of the nucleus followed by its hydrodynamic expression. This technique was indicated by Dr. Michael Blumenthal.

Method Initial step is fixing of Anterior chamber maintainer. It is usually inserted from the temporal side. The tube is attached to BSS bottle which is held 50-60 cm from patient's eye. The height can be adjusted. The next step is to engage the nucleus into the wound. The delivery of nucleus occurs by hydropressure generated by AC Maintainer.

Lens glide is passed below the nucleus and with slight pressure over the scleral lip, the nucleus is removed. Instead of lens glide we can also apply pressure with needle over the scleral lip.

If the AC is shallow you can increase the height of bottle and vice versa.

Advantages[18]

- AC is formed at all the times
- The procedure is not dependent on viscoelastics
- No Sophisticated Instruments are required
- It can be used for all types of Cataract and Capsulotomy.

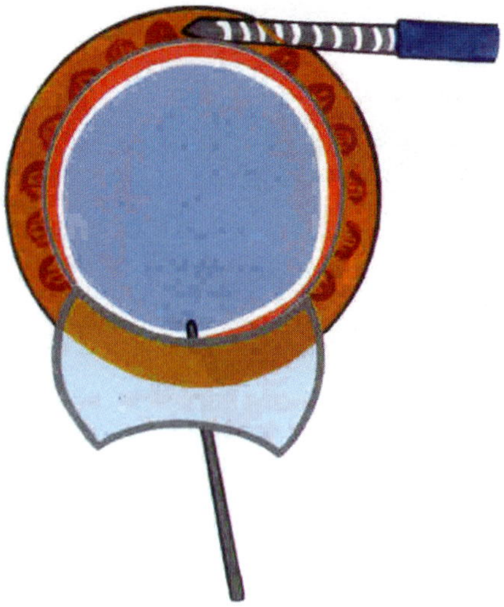

Fig. 55.1: Nuclear Prolapse: Sinskey's hook placed behind the superior pole of nucleus (*Courtesy:* Dr KPS Malik and Dr Ruchi Goel)

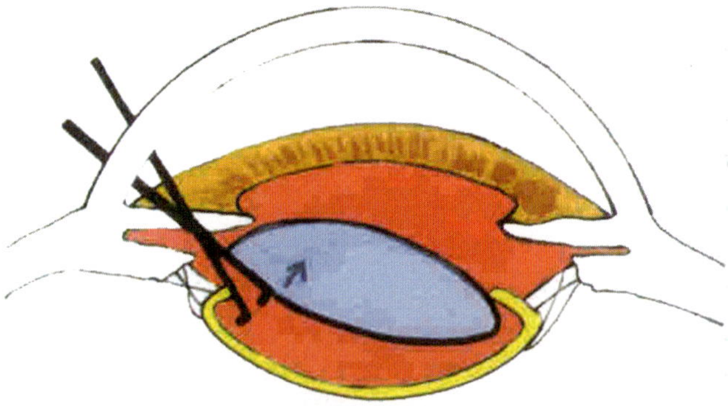

Fig. 55.2: Nuclear prolapse out of the bag: superior pole is lifted up using Sinskey's hook as a crowbar (*Courtesy:* Dr KPS Malik and Dr Ruchi Goel)

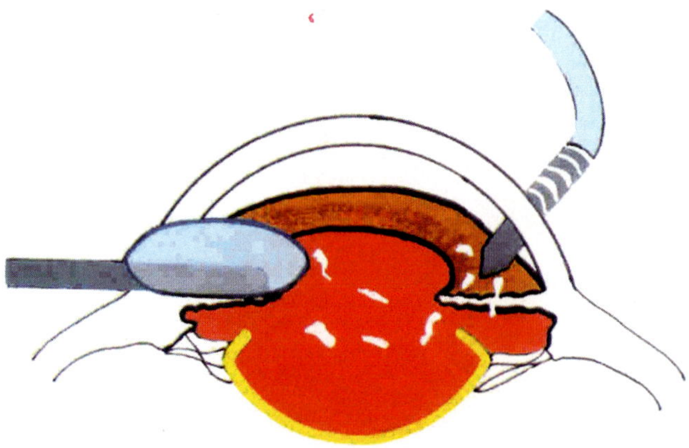

Fig. 55.3: Modified Blumenthal Technique: Nucleus engaged in the section (*Courtesy:* Dr KPS Malik and Dr Ruchi Goel)

Disadvantages[18]

- Failure to manipulate the nucleus in the anterior chamber can cause zonular dialysis
- Keeping the bottle at adequate height is important; otherwise it may lead to frequent changes in the depth of the anterior chamber
- Traumatic delivery can damage the corneal endothelium.

Nucleus Removal using Irrigating Wire Vectis[7]*:* Irrigating Wire Vectis is use to deliver the nucleus either by hydroexpression or by viscoexpression.

Instruments Various sizes of vectis are available. It has two surfaces, viz. anterior concave surface and posterior surface. The anterior end had three 0.3mm openings. The posterior end is attached to syringe or infusion set.

Technique Delivery of nucleus in the anterior chamber. Push the viscoelastic and insinuate the irrigating vectis below the nucleus. Apply counter pressure by holding superior rectus forceps. Now start the irrigation and pull the vectis out of the wound. Give pressure over the scleral lip posteriorly.

Pressure must be built up in the anterior chamber before pulling the nucleus out. Posterior lip depresssion is important part of nucleus delivery.

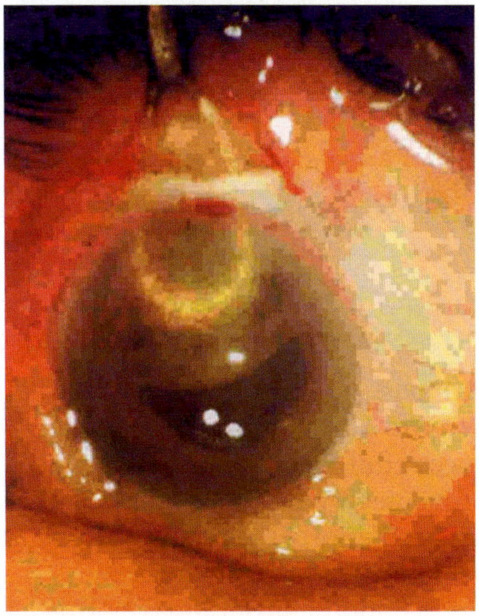

Fig. 55.4: Use of Irrigating Vectis (*Courtesy:* Dr KPS Malik and Dr Ruchi Goel)

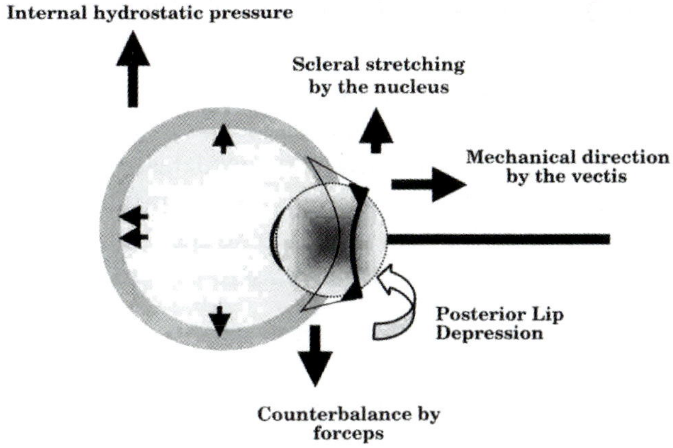

Fig. 55.5: Mechanism of Nucleus Delivery with Irrigating Vectis (*Courtesy:* Dr KPS Malik and Dr Ruchi Goel)

Mechanism of nucleus delivery[7]

It includes:

a. Mechanical pull by irrigating vectis.
b. Internal hydrostatie pressure
c. Scleral stretching by the nucleus
d. Posterior scleral Lip depression.
e. Counter balance force by superior rectus forceps.

Advantages

- Anterior chamber is maintained after the nucleus delivery
- Damage to corneal endothelium is minimal.

Problem Associated

i. *Damage to Iris:* Iris trauma can occur while insinuating the irrigating vectis below the nucleus. This can be prevented by pushing the viscoelastic above and below the nucleus. This pushes the iris posteriorly. Insert the vectis below the nucleus and deliver out the nucleus.
ii. *Posterior Capsular Tears:* It is quite rare with every irrigating vectis.

Visco Expression[6]

This is another technique of removal of nucleus out of the wound. It is a common technique which is used by many surgeons due to its added advantages.

Technique The preliminary step is to prolapse the nucleus out into the anterior chamber. Before this a good hydrodissection and hydrodilineation is very important. Now push viscoelastic into the anterior chamber. While pushing the viscoelastic engage the nucleus into scleral lip and then apply pressure over the posterior scleral lip and deliver the nucleus out. Viscoelastic is continuously pushed while removing the nucleus.

Advantages
- Viscoelastic material acts as a cushion or support to the corneal endothelium and so chances of its damage is minimal.
- Anterior chamber is always maintained.
- Damage to iris tissue is less.
- Incidence of posterior capsule tear is also less.

Disadvantages
- Large quality of viscoelastic is required. This becomes expensive.
- If visocelastic material is not removed completely, there is increase incidence of postoperative uveitis and secondary glaucoma.
- Not suitable for black cataracts.

Phacofracture[3]

This technique was described by Peter Kansas[14,17].

Technique The initial step is to prolapse the nucleus out of the bag. Viscoelastic is pushed both above and below the nucleus in the anterior chamber.

The solid curved vectis is insinuated under the nucleus and the nucleotome is positioned on the anterior surface of nucleus. Both instruments are brought close to each other. This will lead to splitting of the nucleus in to two halves.

Both the halves are seperated and each half is removed with nuclear forceps or by pushing viscoelastic inside the AC.

Modification This technique involves the use of Sinskey hook and wire vectis to sandwich the nucleus and removing it out of the wound.

The anterior chamber should always be deep throughout the surgery.

Advantages
Manual phacofracture is a easy way that eliminates the hazards of the phacomachine with the ability to perform small incision with less expenses.

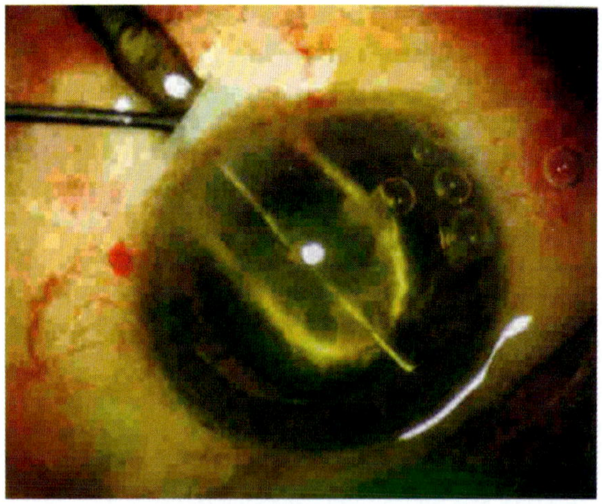

Fig. 55.6: Phacofracture technique using Sinskey Hook and Wire Vectis (*Courtesy:* Dr KPS Malik and Dr Ruchi Goel)

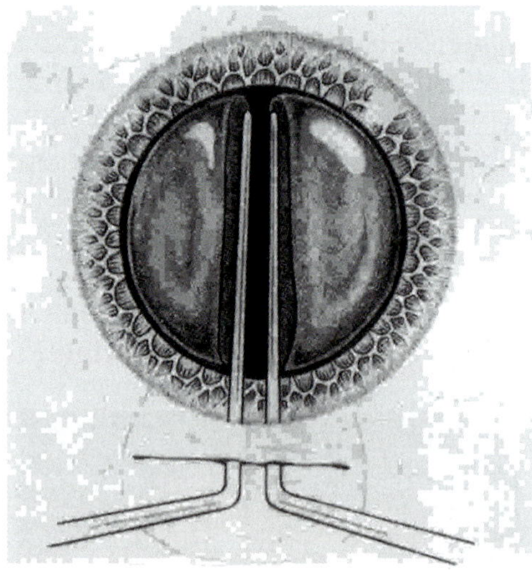

Fig. 55.7: Separation of the nuclear fragments (*Courtesy:* Rozakis Alternative to small incision cataract surgery)

Complications
a. Damage to iris tissue and superior Iridodialysis can occur during fragment extraction. This can be prevented by using lens glide or by pushing the iris posteriorly by pushing viscoelastic.
b. Capsular disruption can occur.
c. Corneal Endothelium damage: This can occur due to passage of 2 instruments in AC and the maneuvering required to sandwich the nucleus and removing it out of the wound.

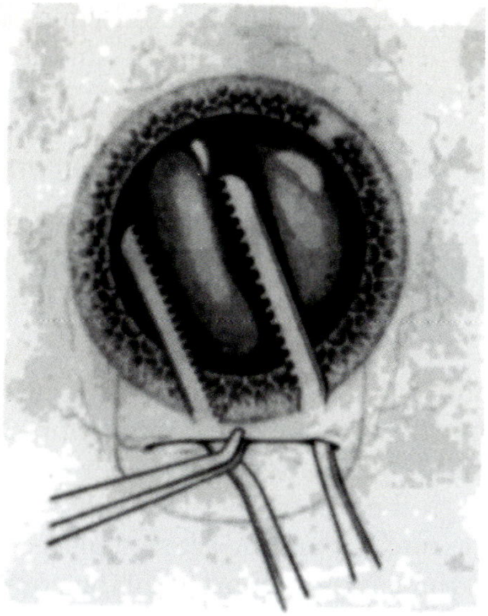

Fig. 55.8: Removal of the nuclear fragment (*Courtesy :* Rozakis Alternative to small incision cataract surgery)

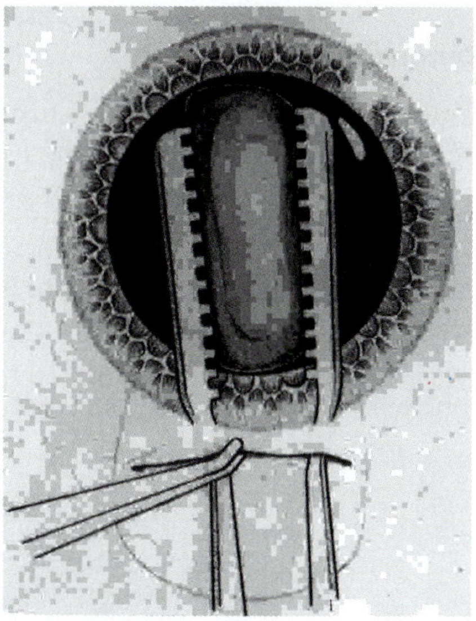

Fig. 55.9: Removal of the last piece of the nucleus (*Courtesy:* Rozakis Alternative to small incision cataract surgery)

The other techniques for phacofracture includes:

A. *Bisector Technique*[6]: This requires the use of bisector. It is type of modification of phacofracture method.

The preliminary step is to insinuate the wire vectis behind the nucleus and the bisector is passed on the anterior surface of the nucleus.

The two instruments are maneuvered toward each other: leading to cleavage of nucleus into two halves. Constant pressure on bisector on vectis splits the nucleus into two halves. Both the halves are seperated and removed by using nucleus holding forceps with vectis or by using viscoelastic material.

B. *Using Trisector*[13]: It is similar technique of phacofracture in which bisector is used thus dividing the nucleus into three pieces.

The trisector consists of 2 longitudinal limits which are sharp in the posterior end. The bisector is passed under the nucleus and pressed toward the nucleus. This divides the nucleus into 3 pieces. Each piece is then removed with serrated forceps.

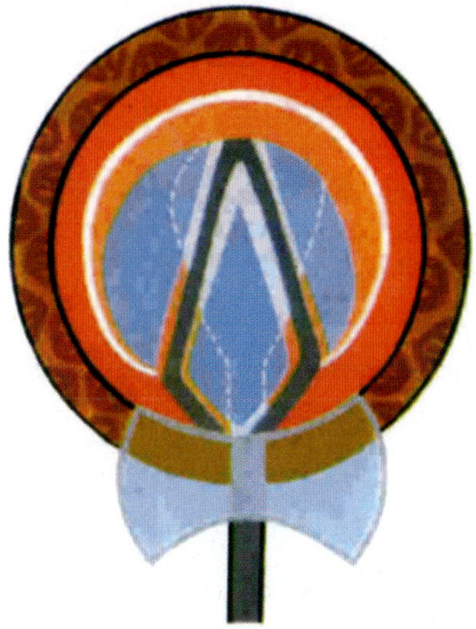

Fig. 55.10: Phacofracture using Trisector (*Courtesy :* Dr KPS Malik and Dr Ruchi Goel)

Advantages

- Safer delivery of nucleus.
- Less dependence on assistant personnel.
- The elimination of phacomachine and
- The cost effectiveness.

C. *Phacosalute and fracture*[6]: The nucleus is prolapsed into the AC. Inject the viscoelastic material. The superior portion of the nucleus is then amputated or pinched off using a capsular forceps and expressed using a irrigating vectis.

Disadvantages:

- Corneal Endothelial damage: Since two instruments are used simultaneously, the chance of endothelial damage is more . This can be prevented by injecting viscoelastic above and below the nucleus.

D. Use of Snare (Wire Loop):- This technique was introduced by Gerard Keener in 1983. He made a snare using 18-19 G blunt tipped needle and 32 G steel wire.

Technique: Nucleus is prolapsed in AC and viscoelastic material is pushed above and below the nucleus. The lens loop / snare is passed below the nucleus. The lens is shifted into vertical position and brought across the nucleus. The loop is constructed by pulling posteriorly on the coil. This leads in the division of nucleus into the halves.

The two halves are then seperated by injecting viscoelastic material. Each halve is the removed with fine toothed forceps.

Advantages

- Fragmentation of the nucleus is safe an non–expensive technique.
- It can be used for hard cataract where phaco is difficult.
- It can also be used in cases of zonular dehisences.
- It is safe, smooth, cost effective and easy to use technique.

Disadvantages

- Difficult in small pupils.
- Difficult in soft nuclei and subluxated lens.
- It can cause some damage to the corneal endothelium

Manual Phacofracture Cardona's Technique

In order to perform the manual bisection of the nucleus according to Cardona's technique, it is important to dislocate the crystalline nucleus in the anterior chamber.

Technique Scleral tunnel of about 5 mm is made. After capsulorhexis and hydroprocedures, nucleus is prolapsed in the anterior chamber.

Through the tunnel incision, vectis is inserted under the nucleus and bisector is placed onto the nucleus. Nucleus is supported by the non-slipping vectis and fragmented into two with the sawing movement of bisector. The nuclear pieces are then removed out of the scleral tunnel wound.

Phaco Sandwich Technique[4,11]

This technique was introduced by Luther L Fry. This procedure require 7.5 mm opening for most of the nuclei and large incision for harder cataract.

Technique Tipping up of the nucleus is very important step. The capsule and iris are hold with iris spatula and the nucleus is nudged toward 6'oclock with hook. The superior pole of nucleus is then caught with spatula and tipped up.

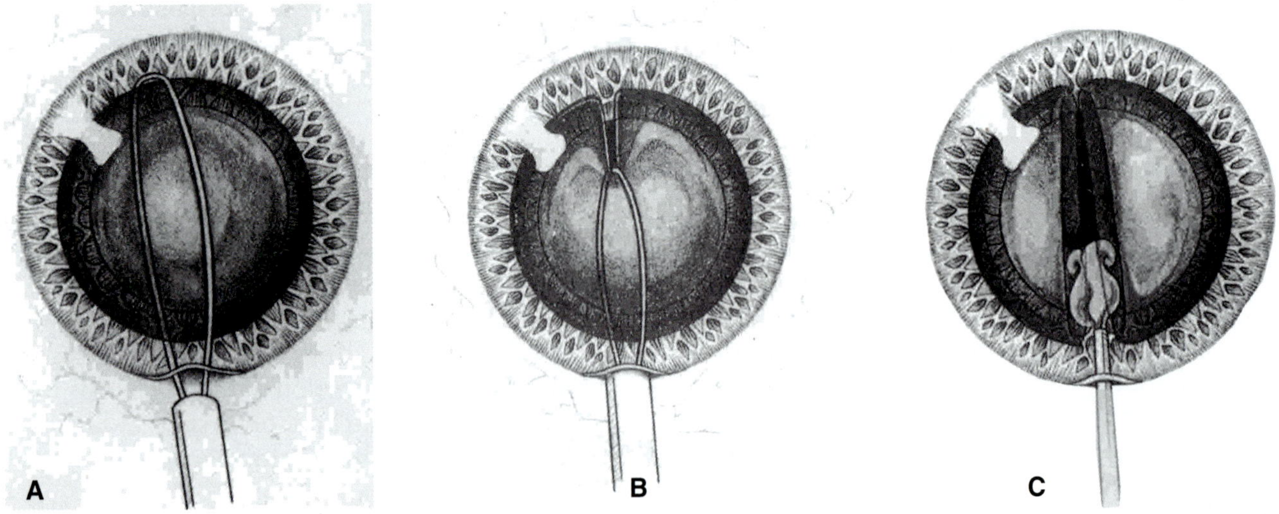

Figs 55.11A to C: Use of Snare
(*Courtesy :* Rozakis Alternative to small incision cataract surgery)

The viscoelastic is placed between superior pole of nucleus and posterior capsule. The iris is pushed posteriorly with viscoelastic and the nucleus is elevated with the spatula. The lens loop is paced beneath the nucleus and spatula is placed on top of nucleus. Both instruments are approximated leading to sandwiching of the nucleus.

Thus with two handed technique the nucleus is removed.

Advantages

- This technique can be used for all pupil sizes and almost all types of nucleus.
- It can be used with large can opener capsulotomy.
- Safe and easy technique which does not require expensive instrumentation.

Disadvantages

- Large amount of viscoelastic material is required.
- Not suitable for very soft cataract.
- Relative contraindication for subluxated cataract.
- Large capsulorrhexis is required.
- Increase chance of damage to the posterior capsule.
- Iridodialysis–Iris may get caught when both the instruments are approximated and removed.

Complications

The most common complication seen in one study done are:

a. Posterior capsular rupture.
b. Loss of vitreous.
c. Transient corneal edema.

Modifications[6] In this technique, the lens loop and spatula is not used. The instruments used are plain wire vectis and viscocannula.

The plain wire vectis is insinuated below the nucleus and viscoselastic is pushed above and below the nucleus. The viscocannula is placed in fornt of the nucleus. The nucleus is sandwich with these instruments and removed. The viscoelastic is injected, while the nucleus is brought out.

Sinskey Hook can also be used instead of cannula.

Manual Multiple Phacofragmentation[6]

It is technique of Manual SICS in which the nucleus is fragmented into multiple pieces and then removed.

Technique

In this procedure special instruments are required.

Instruments

a. *Nucleotome:* It is racquet shaped instrument of length 8mm and width 2mm. It is divided by 3 transverse bars. It is held at 45^0 to long handle.
b. *Spatula:* The shape of spatula should be same as nucleotome.
c. *Manipulators:* Used to collect the nuclear fragments in to center.

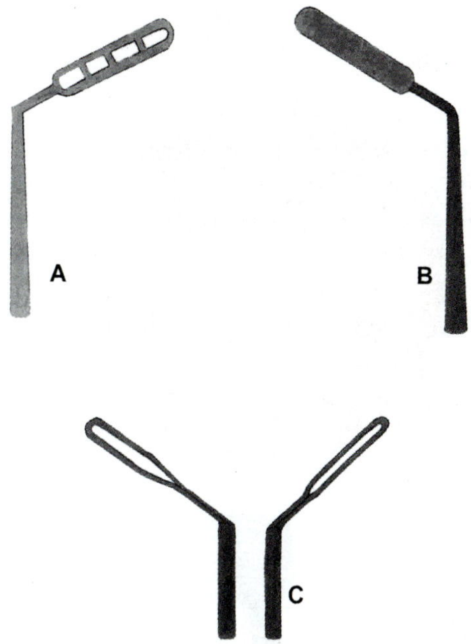

Fig. 55.12: Instruments used for Phaco Fragmentation. **A.** Nucleotome, **B.** Spatula and **C.** Manipulators. (Courtesy*:* Dr KPS Malik and Dr Ruchi Goel.)

Procedure The initial steps remain the same. The spatula is passed below the nucleus present in the anterior chamber and the nucleotome is placed over the nucleus.

Viscoelastic should be sufficient to keep the AC deep. Both the instruments are then brought close to each other. This causes fragmentation of large nucleus into small pieces.

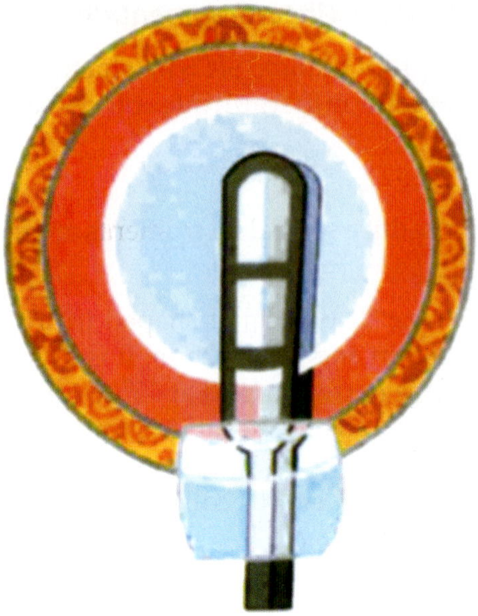

Figs 55.13A and B: Manual Multiphacofragmentation (*Courtesy :* Dr KPS Malik and Dr Ruchi Goel)

The manipulators are used to remove the lens fragments from scleral lip into center of wound. The small pieces are then removed either by using viscoelastic or with the help of nucleus holding forceps.

Advantages

- Hard cataracts can be removed through the small wound by making small nuclear pieces.

Disadvantages

- Damage to corneal endothelium is quite high as two instruments are passed in the anterior chamber.
- Damage to iris tissue is also seen. This is seen both while inserting and removing the instrument.
- Use of special instruments like nucleotome which may not be available everywhere.

Prechop Manual Phacofragementation[12]

In this technique of cataract surgery, the nucleus is manually split into 2 fragments with prechopper forceps and then removed.

Technique After good rhexis and hydroprocedures viscoelastic is injected into the anterior chamber. The sinskey hook is passed through side port to stabilize the nucleus. The prechop forceps is inserted through the wound and passed into center of nucleus core. Opening the forceps will cause splitting of nucleus into 2 pieces. Complete division of nucleus should occur other wise, the steps are repeated. Each piece is prolapsed into anterior chamber and then removed using viscoelastics or serrated with the help of nucleus forceps.

Advantages

- This technique of phacofragmentation is done in the bag and not in anterior chambers and so cause less damage to corneal endothelium.
- Does not require expensive instruments.
- Visual recovery is rapid.

Disadvantages

- Not suitable for hard / black cataracts.
- Also not suitable for subluxated cataract.
- Initial learning curve for nucleus fragmentation is very important.

Quarters Extraction technique for Manual Phacofragmentation[9]

Technique In this procedure the nucleus is manually split and fragments removed. After capsulorhexis, hydrodissection, hydrodelineation and the surface cortex aspiration, the edge of the nucleus is prolapsed into the AC.

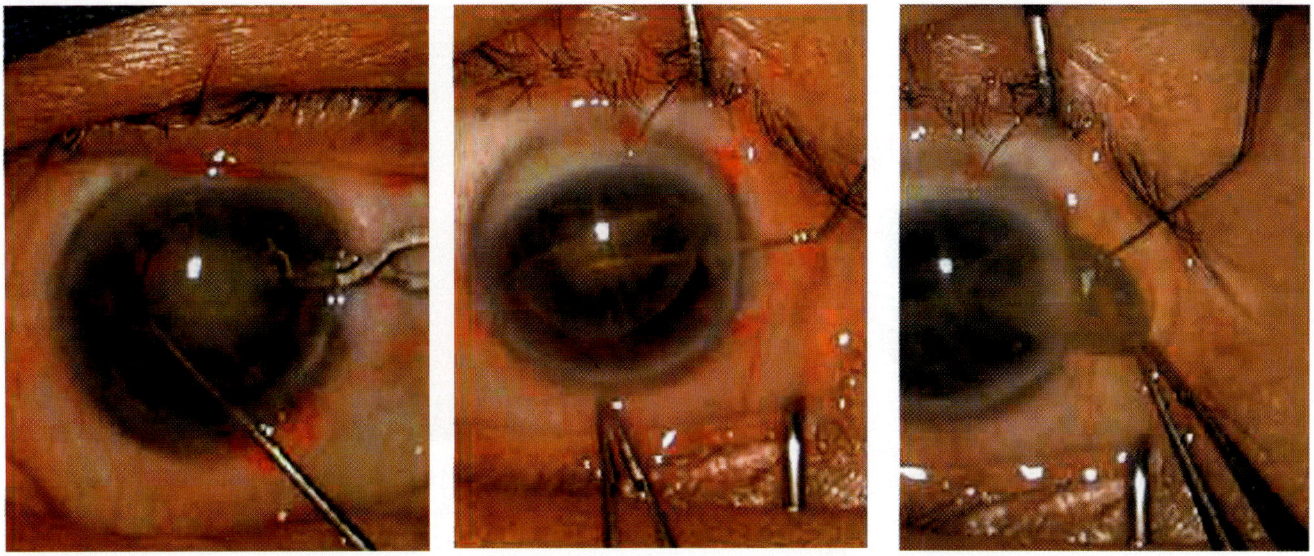

Figs 55.14A to C: Technique of Prechop Manual Phacofragementation (*Courtesy :* Dr. Pipat Kongsap)

The front quarter of the nucleus is cut and removed with nuclear punches. A corner of the remaining three quarter of nucleus is wedged into the wound and rotated out with a claw vectis.

Disadvantages

- This technique is not suitable for very hard/ large nucleus.
- It requires learning curve for fragmentation of the nucleus.

Chop Bisector / Chop Trisector and Chopsticks technique for extraction of the nuclear fragments

It is alternative form of manual phacofragmentation in which chop bisection/chop trisection or chop multisection is done.

Technique The division of the nucleus is carried out by slipping a phacochopper from 6 o'clock to 12 o'clock and applying counter chopper with another manipulator introduced below the nucleus. The extraction of the nuclear fragments is carried out by viscoexpression with the help of vectis or by picking the fragments with the spatula and the chopper. The extraction of nuclear fragments with the Chinese chopsticks technique allows a better adjustment of the final size of the incision to the size of the nuclear fragments.

Use of Claw Vectis[10]

It is simpler one handed technique using a claw vectis. It is a vectis with a claw placed on its tip.

Technique Nucleus is delivered into anterior chamber. Viscoelastic is injected in the anterior chamber. When the nucleus is pulled through the scleral tunnel, it is fixed by the claw and then removed. Viscoelastic is injected while removing the nucleus, so that the corneal endothelium damage is less.

Advantage

- It is better than two handed sandwich technique which may be difficult for many surgeons.

Disadvantage

- Special instruments (claw vectis) are required.
- Damage to iris tissue.

Using of Plain Wire Vectis[6]

Technique The Preliminary step is the delivery of nucleus into the AC. Push viscoelastic above and

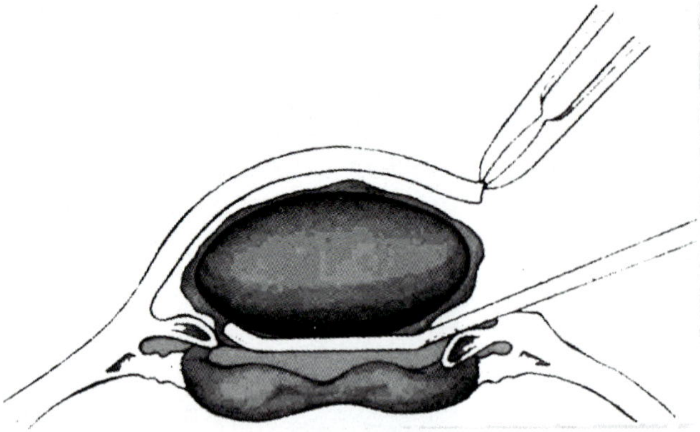

Fig. 55.15: Use of Wire Vectis. (*Courtesy :* Rozakis Alternative to small incision cataract surgery.)

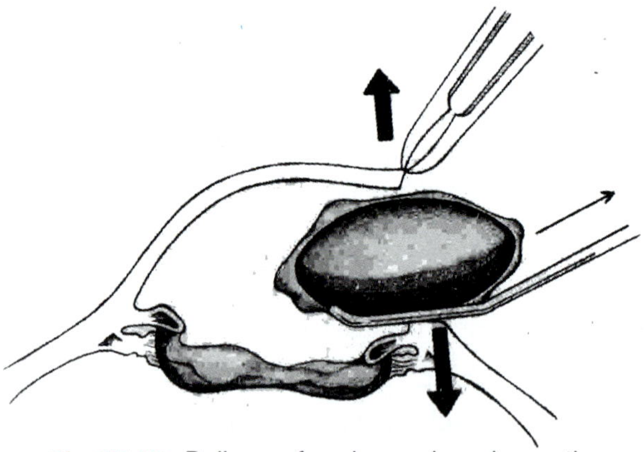

Fig. 55.16: Delivery of nucleus using wire vectis. (*Courtesy :* Rozakis Alternative to small incision cataract surgery.)

below the nucleus. This will prevent the damage of corneal endothelium. Then judge the size of tunnel depending on grade of nucleus.

Pass the wire vectis below the nucleus, so that the nucleus lies in concavity of vectis. Remove the vectis out with simultaneous pressure over the scleral lip posteriorly. The pressure over scleral lip will open the scleral wound and will help in delivery of nucleus.

Advantage

- Use of single instrument and so less chance of damage to surrounding structures.
- Less expensive technique.

Disdvantage

- Increase chance of iridodialysis, common at the 6'O clock position.

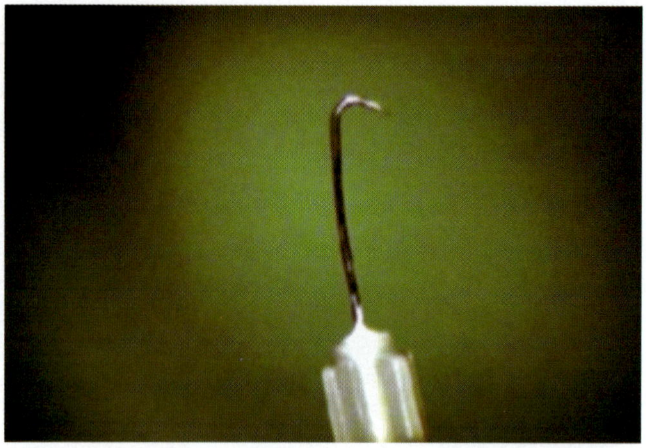

Fig. 55.17: Fish Hook showing the bent top of the 30 G ½ inch needle (*Courtesy :* Dr A Hennig, Nepal.)

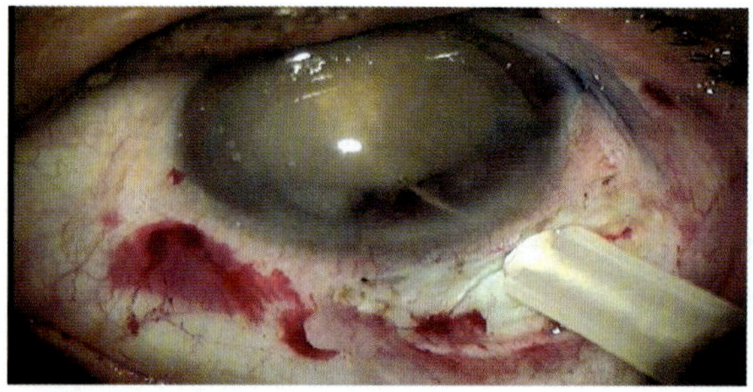

Fig. 55.18A: Insertion of the Hook between Nucleus and posterior capsule (*Courtesy :* Dr A Hennig, Nepal.)

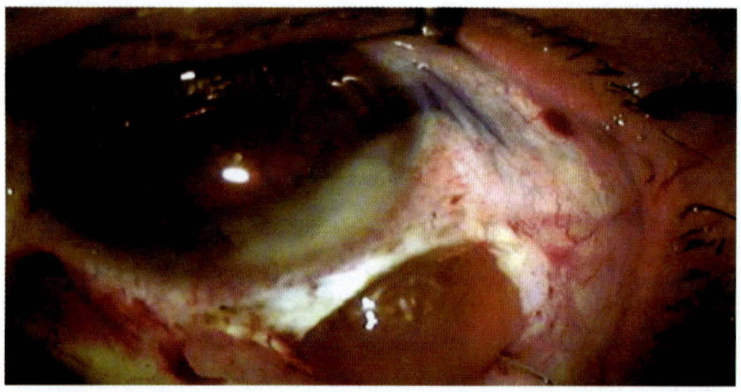

Fig. 55.18B: Hook extraction of the nucleus out of the capsular Bag (*Courtesy :* Dr A Hennig, Nepal.)

- Anterior chamber becomes shallow after delivery of the nucleus.

Fish Hook Technique[8]

In 1997 Dr Albrecht Hennig used a small hook for nucleus extraction instead of anterior chamber maintainer and hydro-expression of the nucleus. It is named as Hennig Technique or Fishhook Technique.

Technique Fish Hook is made of a 30 G ½ inch needle, bending it with fine pliers or a needle older. There are two bends:

1. The tip of the needle which wil insert in the central nucleus.
2. A slight bend between the tip and the plastic mount to assure an easy insertion between the lower part of the nucleus and the posterior capsule.

The hook is mounted on a 1 ml tuberculin syringe and can be reautoclaved.

After completing the rhexis and hydro-procedures, viscoelatic is injected between nuclues and posterior capsule and into the anterior chamber. The bent 30 G needle hook is inserted between nucleus and posterior capsule with the sharp needle tip pointing to the right slide. Then hook is turned and slightly pulled back so that the neelde tip is engaged into the central lower portion of the nucleus.

Without lifting, the nuclues is pulled out of the capsualr bag and through the tunnel. Cortex remains in the anterior chamber, acts as a cushion and thus protects the endothelium from any contact with the nucleus. Once the tip of the hook is correctly inserted into the nucleus, there is no risk to damage any part of the eye.

Advantage

- It is less expensive.
- Sophisticated instruments are not required.
- Easy to learn.
- It can be widely used in case of high volume camps where large numbers of cataract surgery are to be done in short time.

Disadvantage

- Insertion of Fish hook is important. The tip should not touch the corneal endothelium or the Descemet's membrane should not get detached.
- May not be useful in all cases of hard cataract.

Phaco-punch Technique

This technique requires the use of phaco-punch which was designed by Dr. Bidaye.

Instruments It consists of irrigating vectis with a plate in the base and ridge at its distal rim. The three irrigating ports allows viscoexpression, the ridge allow fracture of nucleus and plate help in sandwiching the nucleus between it and scleral corneal lip.

Technique The irrigating phaco-punch is connected to HPMC syringe and is passed below the nucleus. Corneal endothelium is protected by cushion of HPMC. By injecting HPMC pressure is slowly built into the anterior chamber. The increased pressure will push the nucleus out of the wound gape, along the path guide by the punch by depressing the scleral wound with the punch.

The small ridge at distal end prevents the nucleus sliding back into the eye and creates cleavage line for short bite of nucleus. The plate prevents iris prolapse and serves as sandwich plate.

The combined effect removes small bit of the nucleus and converts the round nucleus into bean shaped nucleus. The nucleus is then rotated to align it in vertical direction along its long axis and is removed by injecting viscoelastic material

Hybrid Technique[18]

In the hybrid technique the nucleus is first sculpted with the phacoemulsification. The nucleus is then prolapsed into the anterior chamber and removed by any methods of nucleus delivery.

This technique is mainly useful for beginners who have started learning phacoemulsification. The

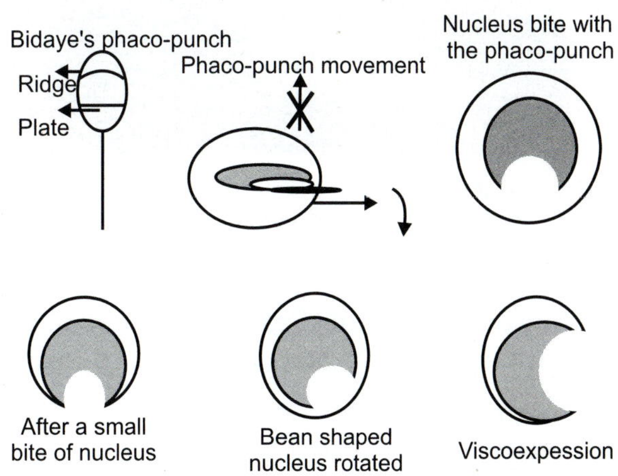

Fig. 55.19: Technique showing the use of Bidayes Phaco Punch (*Courtesy :* Dr Vilas Bidaye)

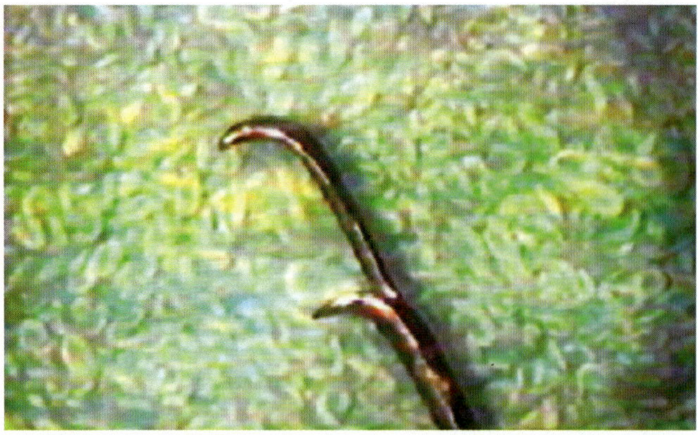

Fig. 55.20: The slider pincer instrument. Note the inner part of the upper slider is sharp while the lowr part is flat to prevent it shipping off the nucleus held

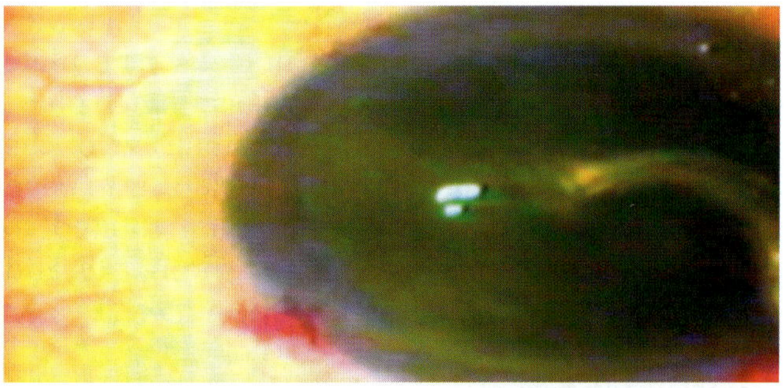

Fig. 55.21: Once the nucleus is in the anterior chamber, the jaws is insetedvia the 3.2 mm incision on the surface of the nucleus

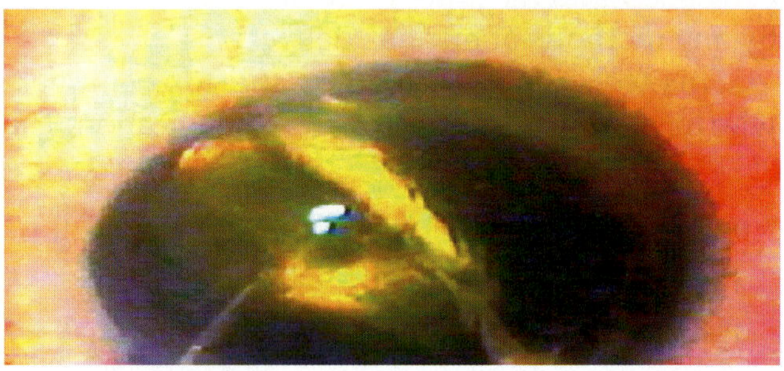

Fig. 55.22: As the slider is approximated it immediately slices through the nucleus. Literlaly with this instrument no resistance is noted even with the hardesh nucleus

technique of phacoemulsification is practiced step by step till the surgeon gain confidence in emulsifying the entire nucleus.

Advantages of nucleus division over phacoemulsification

- It is easier to learn.
- It is not machine dependent.
- It is less expensive.
- The time for removal of nucleus is not time dependent. In phaco the removal of nucleus depends on grade of nucleus.
- High learning curve in phacoemulsification.

Precaution to be taken in nucleus division

a. Initially always attempt the procedures on widely dilated eyes.
b. Approach each care with a mindset that will allow ready conversion to standard extra-capsular cataract extraction, if there is difficulty in prolapsing the nucleus in the AC.
c. Initially the size of incision should be more.
d. While inserting the lens loop beneath the nucleus, it should be directed at an angle toward right edge of nucleus. This will ease in process of learning the loop onto position.
e. Do not fight to extract the nucleus half.

Jaws Slider Pincer Technique

This technique has been developed by Dr Keiki Mehta (India) for small incision, Non-phaco Cataract Surgery. All existing techniques at present are dependent on the lens lying flat with a hard nucleus being sheared off or chopped off with the nucleus lying horizontally flat abutting the posterior capsule. Risk factors involved with these techniques is that the dome of the cornea may be damaged with endothelial cell loss leading to corneal decompensation.

Instrument The jaw slider Pincer forcep is a specially designed instrument to cut even the hardest cataract into the longitudinal slices. It has a tip designed as a beak of a bird and properly rounded to permit its easy entry into the eye. The jaws are made of hardened tungsten steel to prevent any whiplash on handling hard cataracts. The tips of the pincer forceps are designed with the part placed at 12O′ clock being blunt while the 6 O′ clock placement is made curved and sharp to permit easy slicing.

Technique A good capsulorhexis and hydro-dissection is done. Once the lens is made to rotate out. Out of the capsular bag, pincer forcep is introduced via the incision. It is introduced in its closed form, sideways and than gradually opened up to encompass the width of the nucleus. Once it is properly positioned, the jaws are closed which automatically sections the nucleus into two parts. In case of suprahard cataracts, it is necessary to cut the cataract into three or four slices. Always remember to cut the pieces longitudinally as cross cutting makes it more troublesome to remove. With the help of non-apposing curved forceps, the pieces can be easily removed in their entirety.

Advantages

- There is no stress on the incision which does not shear and lead to troublesome irregular astigmatism.
- It prevents the development of extensive endothelial cell loss.
- Simple effective technique which can be done easily with minimal risks.

The Double Wire Snare Splitter Technique

This technique has also been developed by Dr. Keiki Mehta (India) for small incision non-phaco cataract surgery. Many splitting techniques are being used by Ophthalmologists to guillotine the nucleus. Single strands of wire, nylon or polypropylene have been used but the problem is that using a single looped snare does not efficiently work as holding the lens eccentrically leads invariably to the nucleus being irregular cut.

Instrument

A disposable splitter was designed using two strands of wire and a disposable needle. A 20 gauge needle is cut off at the tip and the edges are rounded but maintaining a slight bevel as it permits easier entry into the eye. It is made by using two strands of 28 gauge flexible stainless steel wire threaded through a 20 gauge blunted Disposable needle. Of the two loops of wire, one leg of each is entwined around the other. Thus the two loops are now converted to three strands. Such a dual splitter work simultaneously leaving three fragments of nucleus, each of which is smaller than 4.00 mm (Fig. 55.23).

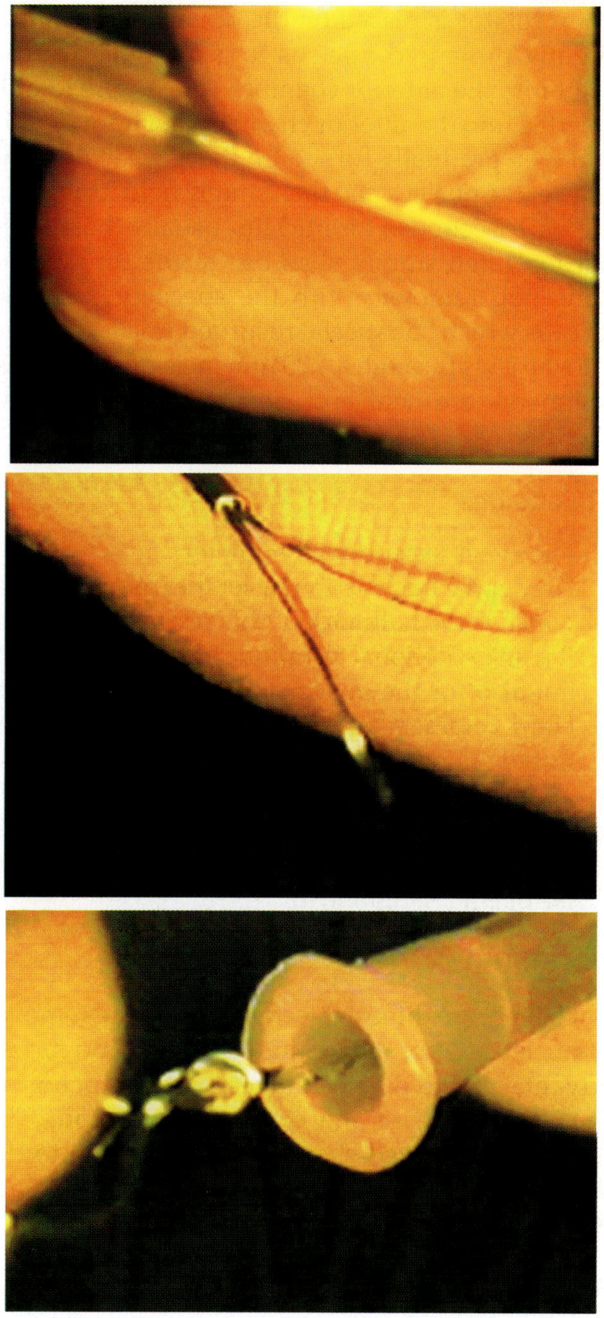

Figs 55.23A to C: Dual splitter: Manner of construction: (A) Standard 20 gauge, 1" length disposable needle selected (B) Loops extended. Note divergence (C) The four wires are knotted together and made into a small loop

Surgical Technique

After excellent workup of Sclero-corneal tunnel incision, wound construction & capsulorrhexis, Viscoelastic is placed in the anterior chamber & a blunt rotator is placed on the opposite pole of the slightly prolapsed nucleus to get it rolls over on itself into the anterior chamber. Now wire loop is inserted into the anterior chamber first horizontally and then gradually turned till they sweep over the edge of the nucleus and then snugly hold it. Following the trisection of the nucleus, usually the middle portion often simply slips out at the time of the wire loop removal. With the specially designed forceps which has special recurved tracks grooved into the jaws through a 4.00 mm incision individual fragments are held and simply removed in the single stroke (Figs 55.24 to 26).

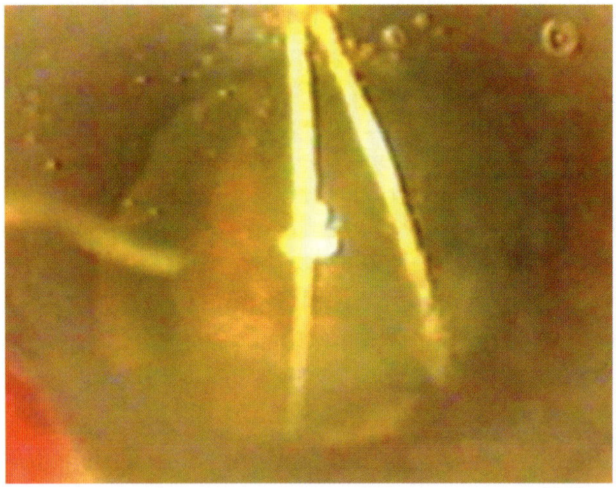

Fig. 55.24: Pull the loops snug to hold the nucleus. Note the spread of the wire loops

Advantages

- The eye is exceptionally quieter.
- Harder the nucleus, the easier the trisector works which is the hallmark of this procedure.
- It is an exceptional technique not only for MSICS but also for the phaco surgeon who often face Hard cataracts usually coupled with compromised endothelium.
- The advantage of splitting the nucleus into three parts permits easier removal of the smaller fragments through small incisions hence less iatrogenic Astigmatism.

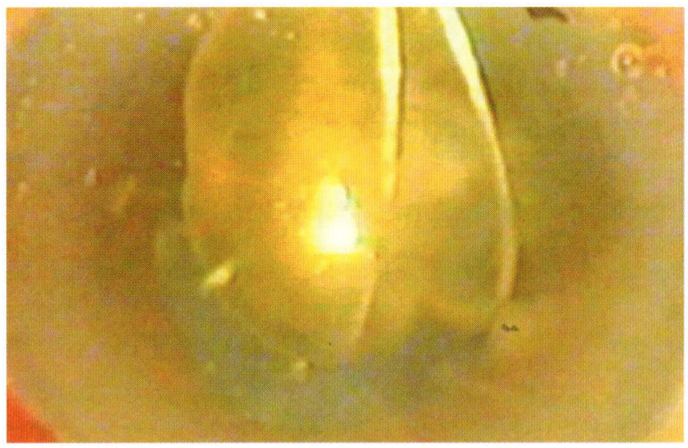

Fig. 55.25: Note how snuggly the nucleus is held. It remains immobile

CONCLUSION

Thus there are different techniques for the removal of nucleus out of the wound. Each method has its advantages and disadvantages, which depends on the experience of the operating surgeon. The technique followed should be comfortable to the doctor and should give good postoperative visual results.

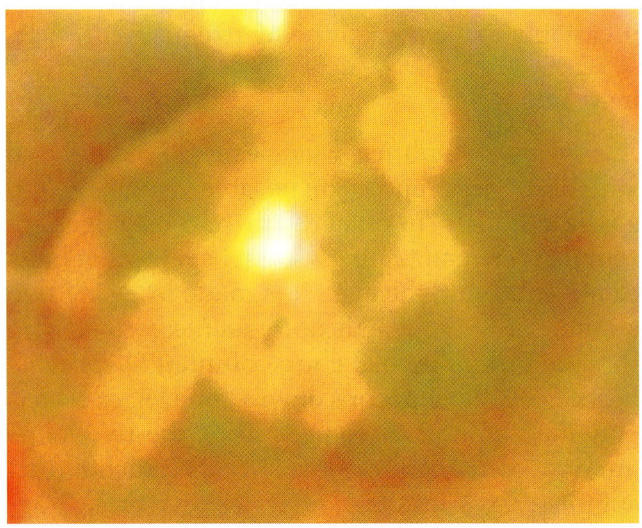

Fig. 55.26: The nucleus is sliced into three parts

REFERENCES

1. Beirouty ZA, Barker NH, Shanmugam NS. Sutureless one-handed small incision cataract surgery by manual nucleosuction: A new technique for cataract extraction. Eur J Implant Ref Surg 1995;7:295-98.
2. Bucher P. Manual Phaco Fragmentation. A small incision cataract operation technique. Basel: University Eye Hospital; 1992.
3. Peter Kansas. Phacofracture. In: Rozakis cataract surgery:Alternative small incision techniques. NJ Slack 1990;45-70.

4. Luther L, Fry. The Phacosandwich Technique. In: Rozakis Cataract Surgery: Alternative Small Incision Techniques. NJ Slack 1990;71-110.
5. Gerald T. Keener Jr. The Nuclear Division Technique for Small Incision Cataract Extraction. In: Rozakis cataract surgery:Alternative small incision techniques NJ Slack 1990;163-191.
6. KPS Malik, Ruchi Goel. Nuclear Management. Manual of Small Incision Cataract Surgery. 39-58.
7. Samas Basak: My Technique of SICS using Irrigating Vectis. Manual of Small Incision Cataract Surgery. 138-145.
8. B P Guliani, OP Ag. Our Technique of SICS, Fish Hook method. Manual of Small Incision Cataract Surgery. 1153-56.
9. Junsuke Akkura, Shuzo Kaneda, M Ishihara, K Matsura. Quarters extraction technique for Manual Phaco Fragmentation. JCRS. 2000;26.
10. Junsuke Akkura, Shuzo Kaneda, Shiro Hatta, Kazuki Matsura. Manual Sutureless Cataract Surgery using Claw Vectis. JCRS 2000;26.
11. Bayramlar H, Cekic O, Totan Y. Manual Tunnel Incision Extra Capsular Cataract Extraction using Sandwich Technique. JCRS 1999;25(3): 312-15.
12. P Kongrap. Pre Chop Manual Phaco Fragmentation; Cataract Surgery without a Phacoemulsification Machine. Asian Journal of Ophthalmology 2002;4(4):7-9.
13. Hepsen IF, Cekic O, Bayramlar H, Totan Y: Small Incision Extra Capsular Cataract Surgery with Phacotrisection. JCRS 2000;26(7);1048-51.
14. Kansas PG. Phacosection.Manual Small Incision Cataract Surgery. Albany : International Ophthalmology Seminar 1994;1-158.
15. Band BF. The Small Incision Phacosection Planned Extracapsular Manual Technique. Highlights Ophthalmology. 1997; 25:15-25.
16. Blumenthal M, Ashkenazi, Assia E, Cahane M. Small Incision Manual Cataract Surgery. Using Selective Hydrodissection.
17. Moustafa Kamal Nassar. Manual Phacofracture, Small Incision Cataract Surgery. Bull Egyptian Ophthalmology Society. 2001; 94(2).
18. Ravi Thomas, A BMS, JK Challa, T George. Methods of Nucleus Extraction. IJO 1993;4(4):202-206.
19. Mr. Vilas Bidaye. Nucleus management in Small Incision Cataract Surgery. Ophthalmology on the Web-Cyber lectures.

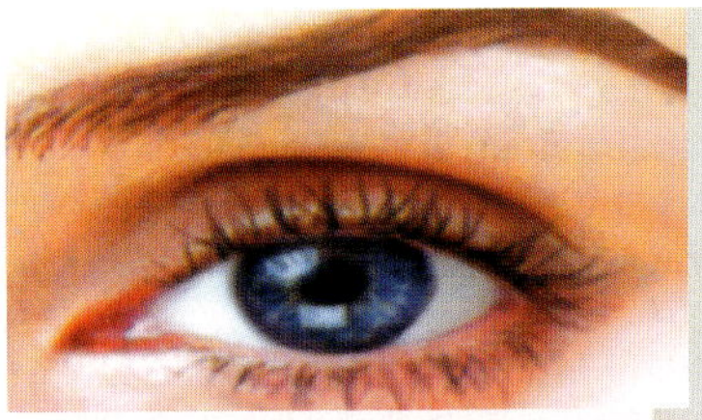

Fifty six

Pediatric Cataract—IOL Surgery: Past, Present and Future

Suresh K Pandey
Edward Wilson
Liliana Werner
David J Apple (USA)
Vidushi Sharma (India)

INTRODUCTION

Several advances for surgical management of childhood cataracts have occurred in the last 2 decades owing to advances in microsurgical techniques, availability of better ophthalmic viscosurgical agents and appropriately sized and styled implants, suitable for small eyes. However, surgeons continue to face the unique challenges posed by children's eyes (Fig. 56.1). This brief write-up is separated in 3 sections (section A, B and C) to summarize the major past, present and future

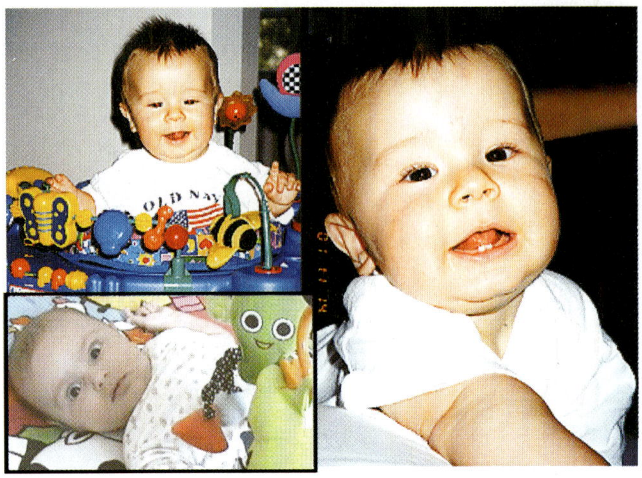

Fig. 56.1: Pediatric cataract IOL surgery: The challenge

advancements in the field of pediatric cataract surgery and intraocular lens implantation. Interested readers can also refer to our recent video on this interesting subject (Wilson ME, Pandey SK, Werner L, Apple DJ. Pediatric cataract surgery: Past, present and future, Third Prize for Special Cases, Annual Video Festival, XXth Congress of the European Society of Cataract and Refractive Surgeons, Nice, France, September 2002).

PEDIATRIC CATARACT—INTRAOCULAR LENS SURGERY: PAST (1951 TO 1989-90S)

It is well-known that Sir Harold Ridley performed the first adult case of intraocular lens implantation in November 1949 on a 46-year-old female (Fig. 56.2).

To the best of our knowledge, Dr Edward Epstein of Johannesburg, South Africa implanted for the first time a Ridley IOL in a child. He operated a 9-year-old child for traumatic cataract in 1951 (Fig. 56.3). In one of his most recent communications, Dr Epstein commented on the fixation and centration of his first pediatric IOL (Fig. 56.4). He metioned *"at first I thought that in those children with the implant remaining central, that irrigation and aspiration had not cleared all the equatorial lens substance which thus favored a Soemmering ring that made a "frame" for the implant. Later it suddenly dawned that the apices of the 4 anterior capsular flaps created by the cruciate discission, pushed by the swelling cortex had become adherent to the posterior surface of the iris... Amazing one did not think that was the way to go, i.e. in-the-bag, when implanting*

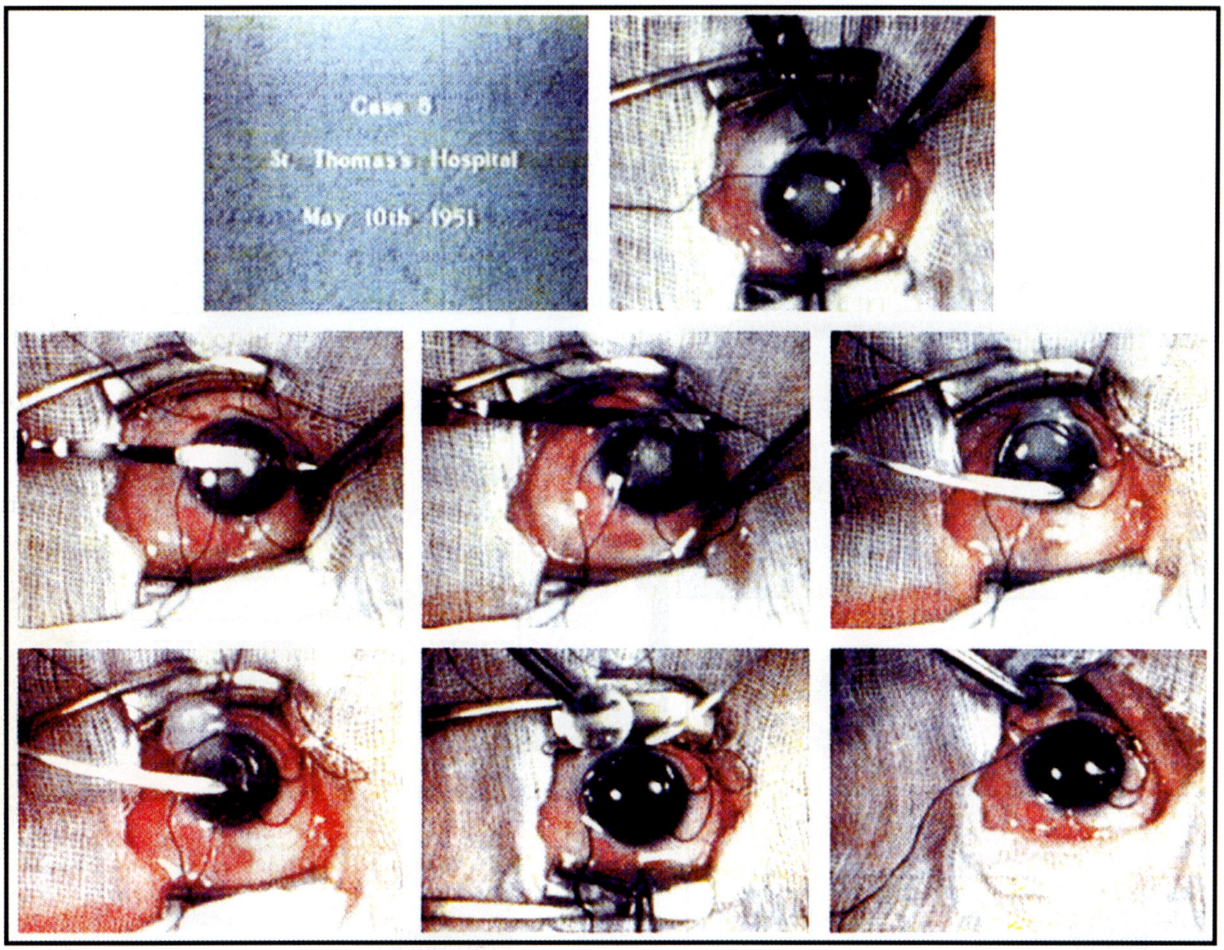

Fig. 56.2: First cataract IOL surgery (Sir Harold Ridley 1949-1950)

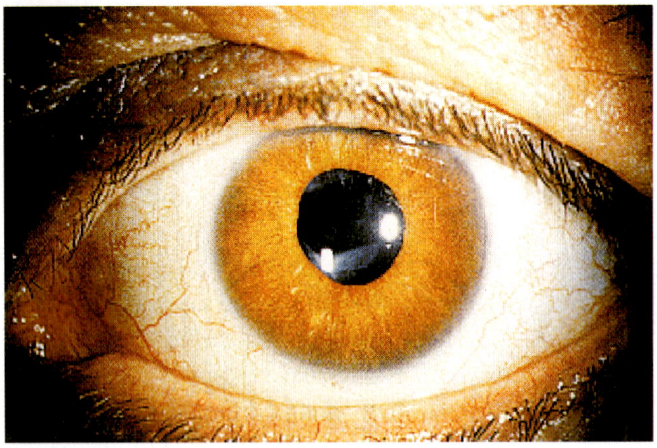

Fig. 56.3: Pediatric cataract IOL surgery: Past (insertion of a Ridley lens in a child) Implantation of Ridley IOL in a 9-year-old child by Dr E Epstein, S Africa (June 26, 1952)

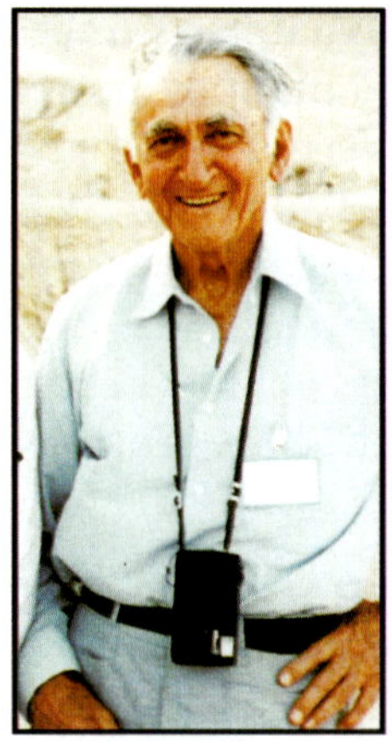

Fig. 56.4: Pediatric cataract—IOL surgery past (Insertion of a Ridley lens in a child)

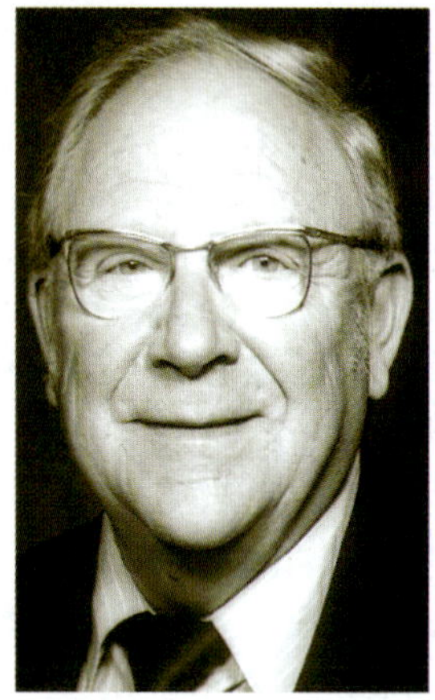

Fig. 56.5: Pediatric cataract—IOL surgery past (Insertion of a Choyce lens in a child)

lenses. But remember in those day microscopes were not used, viscous material not available and the thinnest sutures were 6x0 ropes!!"

Subsequently Dr Peter Choyce from England implanted the Choyce Mark 1 intraocular lenses in the right eye of an eight-year-old child. In a monograph on intraocular lenses and implants published in 1964, Dr Choyce mentioned *"In June, 1957, i.e. only three months after the original injury—a 13 mm (thick haptic) anterior chamber implant was inserted" (Fig. 56.5).*

Some part of the surgical steps of the cataract surgery and implantation of Choyce Mark 1 intraocular lens performed by Dr. Choyce are shown in this Figure 56.6.

Dr Robert Sinskey, Dr David Hiles and others began to implant posterior chamber lenses routinely in the 1980s. Dr Sinskey implanted the very flexible

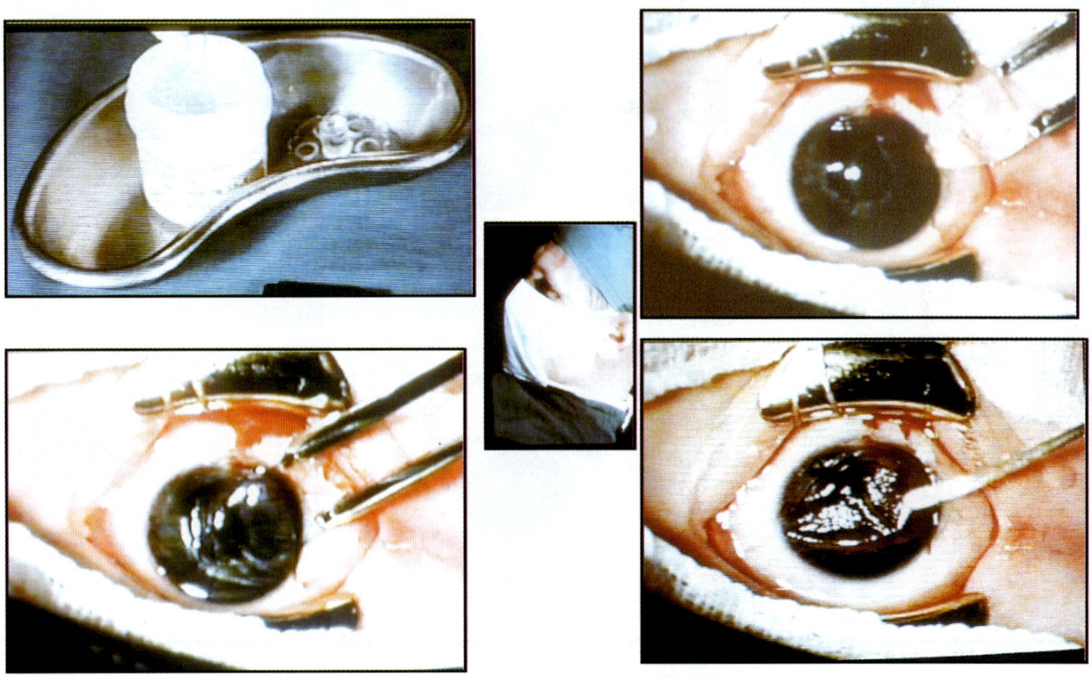

Fig. 56.6: Pediatric cataract—IOL surgery past (Insertion of a Choyce lens in a child)

3-piece Sinskey style posterior chamber intraocular lenses after performing the cataract surgery (Fig. 56.7).

Dr Marshall M Parks, Dr David Taylor and others pioneered the use of primary posterior capsulectomy and anterior vitrectomy for management of pediatric cataracts in the late 70s and early 1980s. This mechanized approach drastically reduced the need for repeated surgeries nearly eliminating secondary membranes. Implantation of intraocular lenses was not common during this period. Therefore, the use of aphakic contact lenses was the preferred method for correction of aphakia in 1980s. Dr Wilson and more than 100 other fellows over the years have learned this technique from Dr Parks (Fig. 56.8).

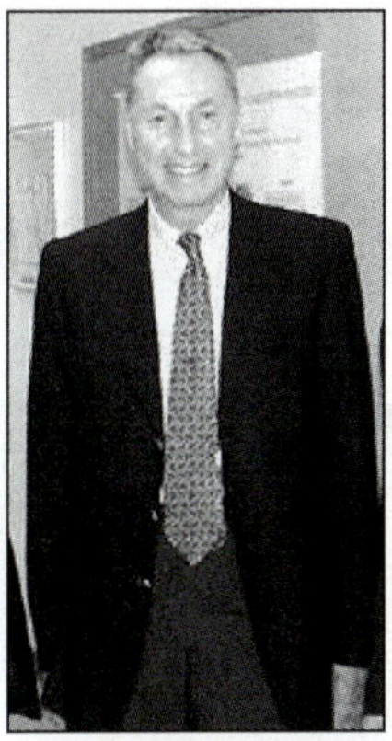

Fig. 56.7: Pediatric cataract—IOL surgery past (Insertion of Sinskey lens in a child)

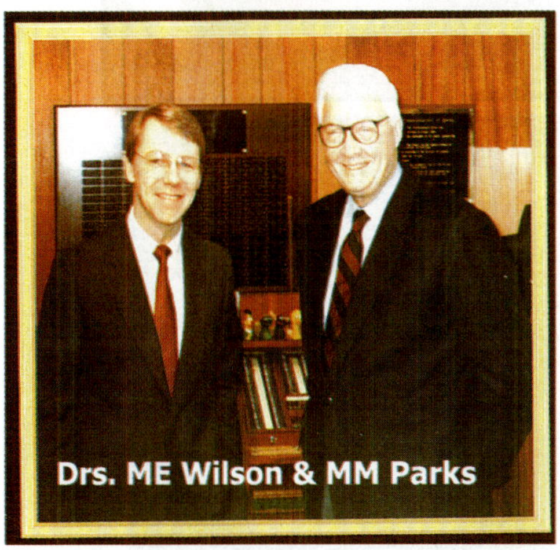

Fig. 56.8: Pediatric cataract—IOL surgery past (Posterior capsule management)

PEDIATRIC CATARACT—INTRAOCULAR LENS SURGERY: PRESENT (1990STO PRESENT)

The last decade witnessed the considerable advances in technology and microsurgical techniques in the field of pediatric cataract surgery and intraocular lens implantation pioneered by several surgeons. During this time implantation of an intraocular lens became common place for correction of aphakia in children beyond their second birthday.

Clinical and research studies done at the Storm Eye Institute and elsewhere helped considerably to select the most suitable technique for capsule management, the selection of appropriate intraocular lens size, design and biomaterial for children and infants (Figs 56.9 to 56.11).

Based on extensive clinical and research work done in this subject at the Storm Eye Institute, our present preferred cataract—IOL surgical technique for infants and children younger than 6 years - anterior capsule can be opened manually, using a vitrector (termed as "Vitrectorhexis") or a bipolar radiofrequency diathermy or by Fugo plasma blade. Aspiration of the lens substance and complete cleaning of the capsular bag; performance of a posterior capsulorhexis using vitrector, which is termed as posterior vitrectorhexis, capsular bag fixation of a single-piece hydrophobic lens through a small incision using the injector. A primary posterior capsulectomy and anterior vitrectomy may be helpful to maintain a long-term clear visual axis, especially in infants and children younger than 6 years of age. For children older than 6 years with relatively less elastic anterior capsule, a manual capsulorhexis, which remains a gold standard, can safely be performed. Additionally, a cortical cleaving hydrodissection can also be used (Fig. 56.12).

Management of the posterior capsule remains a challenge due to very high rate of posterior capsule opacification. Several techniques have been proposed for posterior capsule management on pediatric cataract surgery as shown in this slide. Dr Howard Gimbel from Calgary, Canada proposed a technique of a posterior capsulorhexis with optic capture for maintaining a clear visual axis as shown in this video clip. This procedure is technically

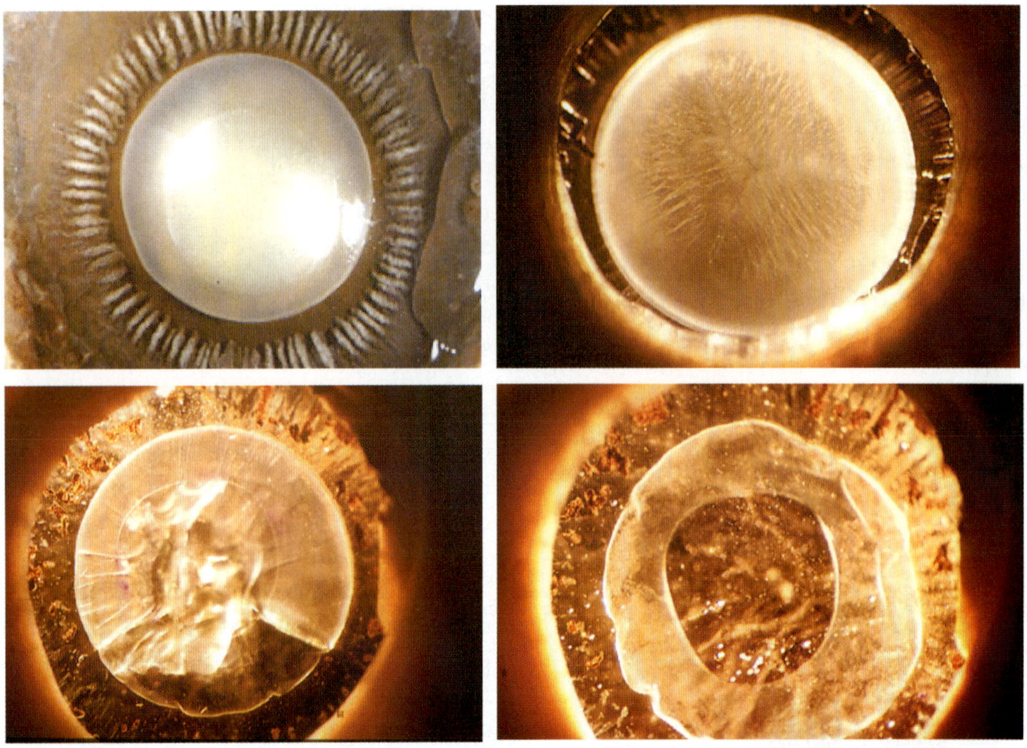

Fig. 56.9: Pediatric cataract—IOL surgery clinical and laboratory research at the Storm Eye Institute

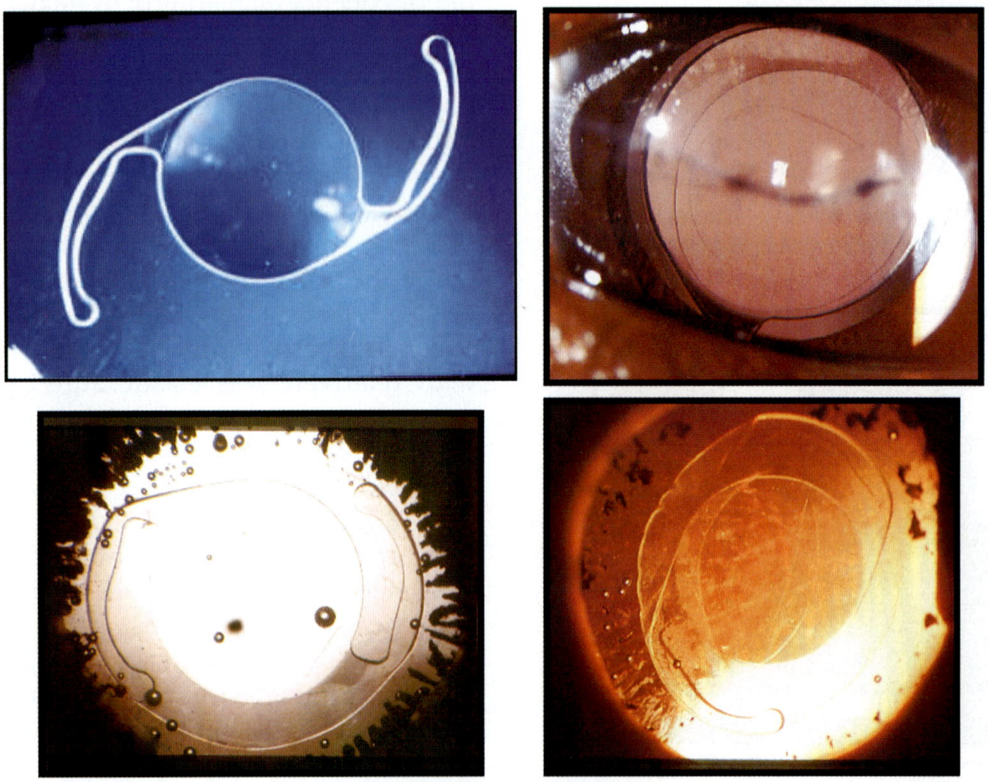

Fig. 56.10: Pediatric cataract—IOL surgery clinical and laboratory research at the Storm Eye Institute

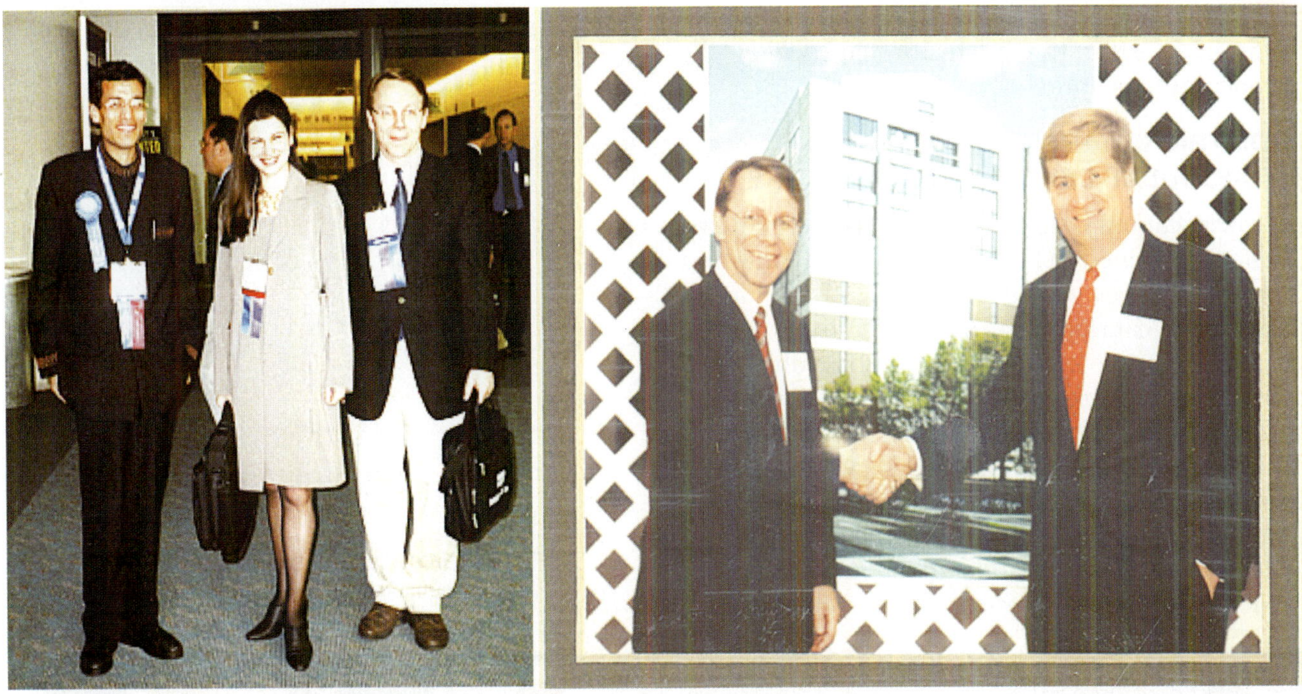

Fig. 56.11: Pediatric Cataract—IOL surgery clinical and laboratory research at the Storm Eye Institute (Storm Eye Institute's Drs Suresh K Pandey, Liliana Werner, M Edward Wilson and David J Apple)

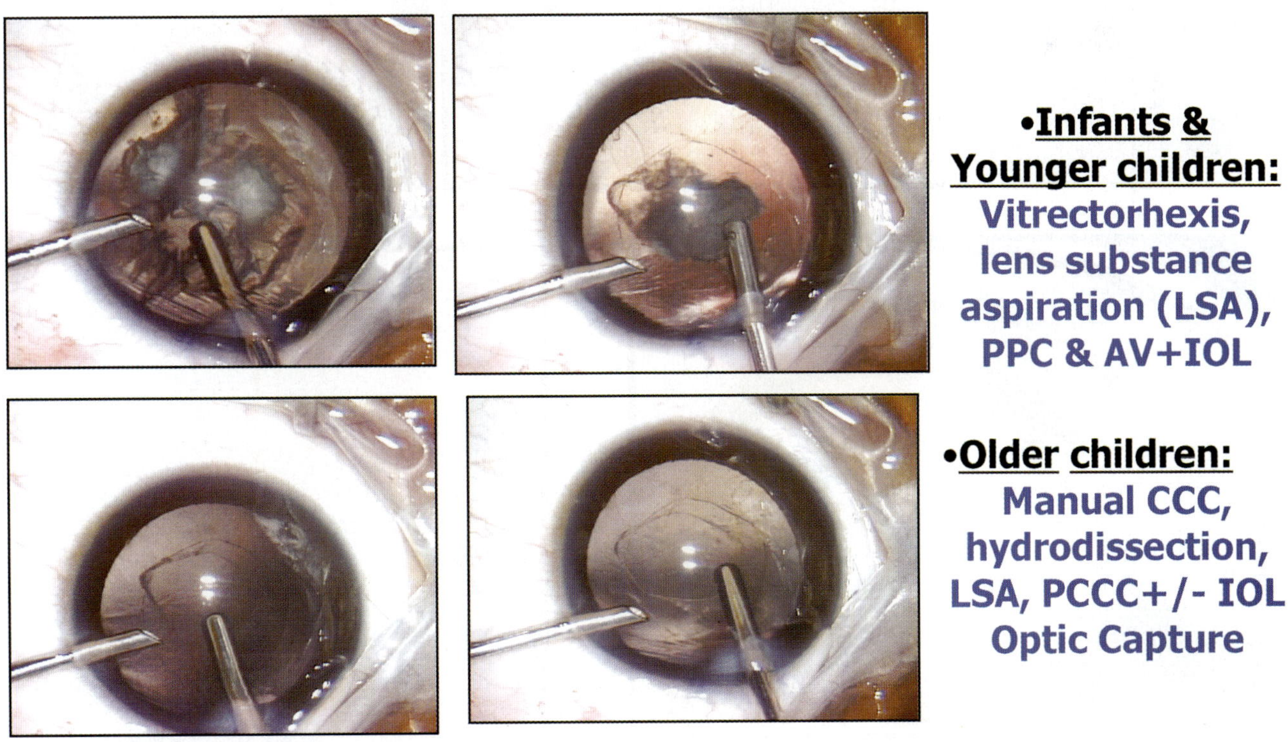

Fig. 56.12: Pediatric cataract—IOL surgery present: Recommendations and guidelines

challenging and opacification of ocular media may occur even after the posterior capture of the intraocular lens optic.

PEDIATRIC CATARACT—INTRAOCULAR LENS SURGERY: FUTURE

Pediatric cataract surgery in the future will be constantly refined to facilitate visual outcome and to reduce the postoperative complications. Pacing with adult cataract surgical procedure, use of intraocular lenses implanted through an ultrasmall incision, as well as implantation of the multifocal and accommodative lenses will increasingly be used for children (Figs 56.13 and 56.14). More research efforts are needed to understand some of the crucial issue such as selection of the intraocular lens power, incidence of postoperative glaucoma and techniques to reduce the posterior capsule opacification.

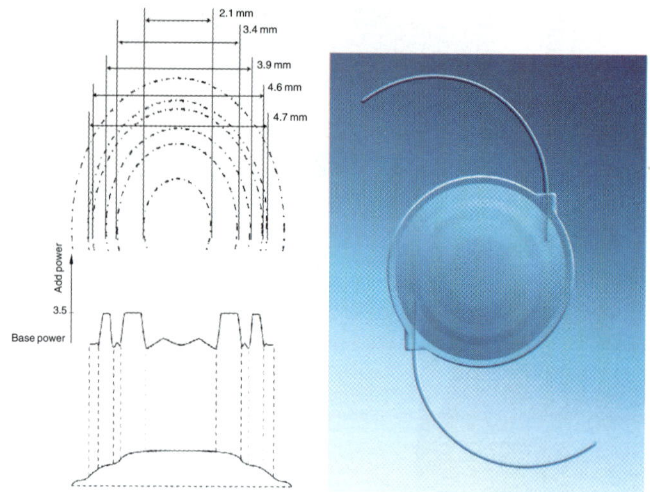

Fig. 56.13: Pediatric cataract—IOL surgery multifocal IOL implantation

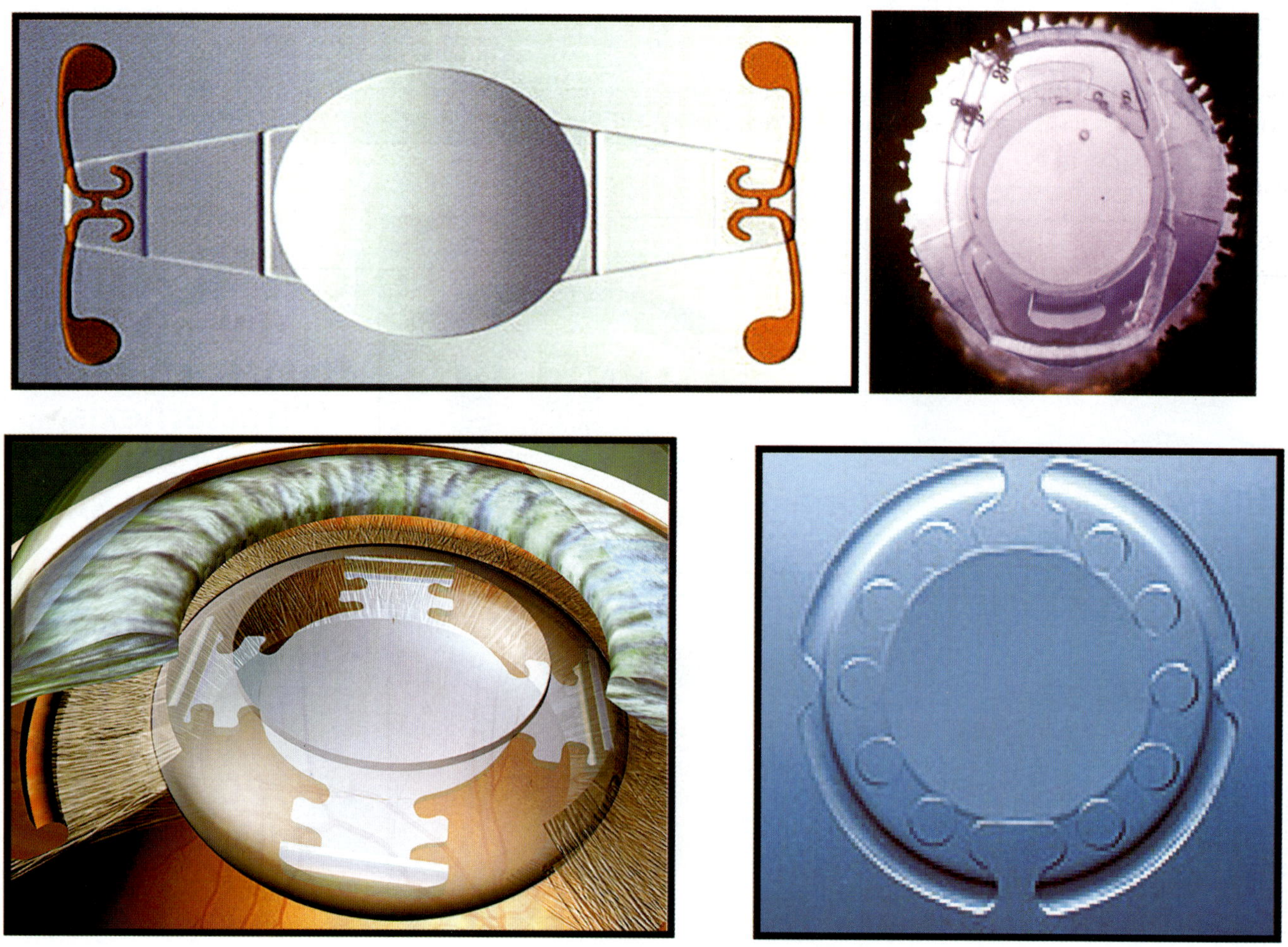

Fig. 56.14: Pediatric cataract—IOL surgery future: Restoration of accommodation

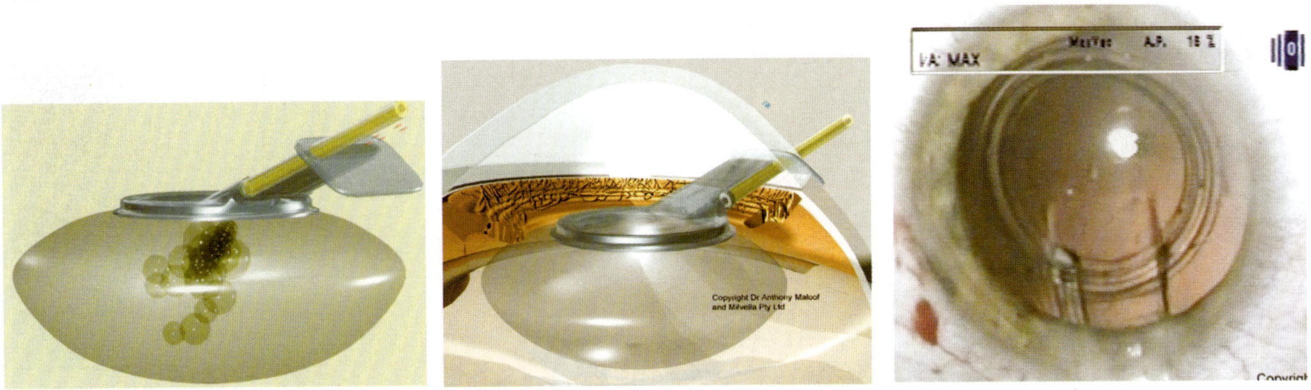

Fig. 56.15: Pediatric cataract—IOL surgery future: Elimination of PCO

Elimination of posterior capsule opacification and restoration of accommodation are 2 major issues that need to be addressed in near future. Solutions are being developed that can potentially eliminate all residual epithelial cells in the pediatric lens capsule. These substances may be delivered via a sealed capsule irrigation device such as one pioneered by Dr Anthony Maloof (Fig. 56.15).

SUMMARY

We attempted to summarize the evolution of pediatric cataract surgery and the intraocular lens in this slide, though it is impossible to mention all the advancements in this field. Most of these advances has been one of the most important achievements in modern ophthalmology. The availability of refined and perfected microsurgical techniques, ophthalmic viscosurgical agents and modern foldable implants represent a major milestone in this evolutionary process. With continued improvements in surgical techniques, availability of multifocal and accommodative lenses the refractive and visual outcomes in pediatric cataract surgery will continue to improve in this century.

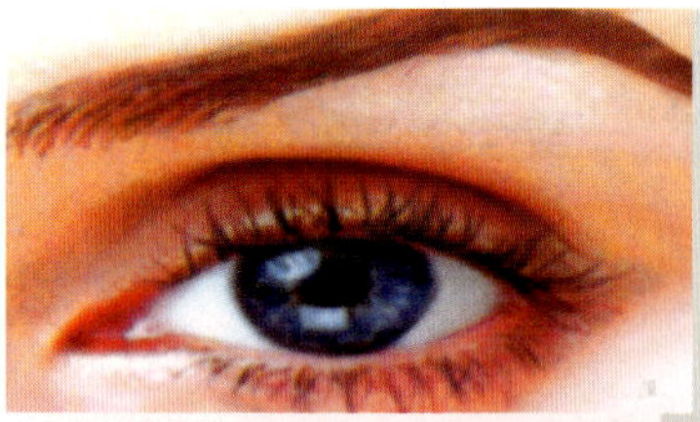

Fifty seven

Suresh K Pandey
Liliana Werner
David J Apple
Andrea M Izak (USA)
Vidushi Sharma
Amar Agarwal
Ashok Garg (India)

Update on Twenty-first Century Cataract—Intraocular Lens Surgery

BACKGROUND

At the beginning of the 21st century, modern cataract-intraocular lens (IOL) surgery has become one of the safest, most successful, and most frequently performed outpatient surgeries in the industrialized world including North America.[1-6] In former times, when anesthesia and fine surgical instrumentation were beyond conception, the cataractous lens was dislocated into the vitreous (couching) (Fig. 57.1). Thanks to considerable advancement in microsurgical techniques modern cataract surgery can be performed using sub-1mm incision and history reaches a full circle with reports of no-anesthesia cataract surgery.[7-9] In this chapter, we attempted to summarize major evolutionary advancements of surgical techniques and IOL designs/biomaterials for cataract surgery. However, it is almost impossible to provide details of each and every evolution.

LARGE INCISION CATARACT SURGERY and IMPLANTATION OF RIGID LENSES

Sir Harold Ridley's cataract extraction and implantation of an IOL marked the beginning of a major change in the practice of ophthalmology (Fig. 57.2). The first operation, done at St. Thomas's

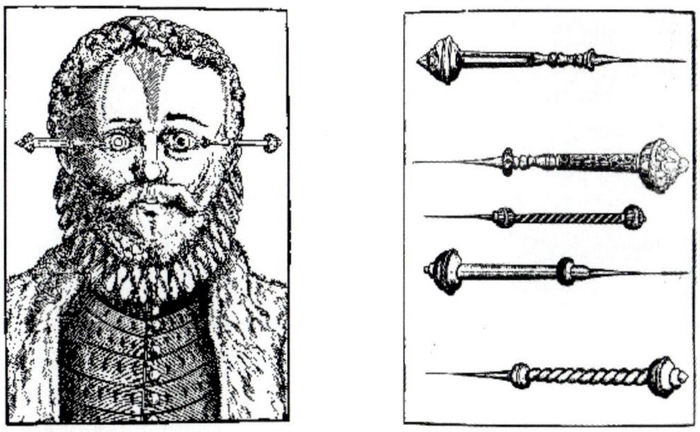

Fig. 57.1: Illustration from a 1966 facsimile of a 1583 German atlas of a renaissance eye surgery showing the ancient technique of couching. Left: Frontal view. Right: An example of ornamental couching needles (From: Bartisch, G: Augendienst, Dresden, Germany, 1583)

Hospital, London, was a two-step procedure. The extracapsular removal of the cataract took place on November 29, 1949. The insertion of the pseudophakos, manufactured by Rayner, Ltd., United Kingdom, occurred as a secondary procedure on February 8, 1950. Ridley selected acrylic as the initial biomaterial based on the experience of ophthalmologists who dealt with World War II injuries involving Perspex plastic[1,2] (Fig. 57.2).

SMALL INCISION CATARACT SURGERY and IMPLANTATION OF FOLDABLE LENSES

Charles D Kelman, MD, believed that cataracts could theoretically be removed through a 2-or 3-mm incision by using vibrational energy to fragment the lens inside the eye. Dr Kelman garnered the idea reportedly after a visit to the dentist, where he found an ultrasonic device being used to help remove plaque and debris from teeth. Phacoemulsification, invented and pioneered by Dr Kelman, has become the most preferred method of cataract surgery in USA and the industrialized world.[4]

Foldable Lenses Manufactured from Hydrophobic and Hydrophilic Acrylic and Silicone Biomaterials

A variety of foldable IOL designs manufactured from hydrophobic or hydrophilic acrylics as well as silicone biomaterials are available to the anterior

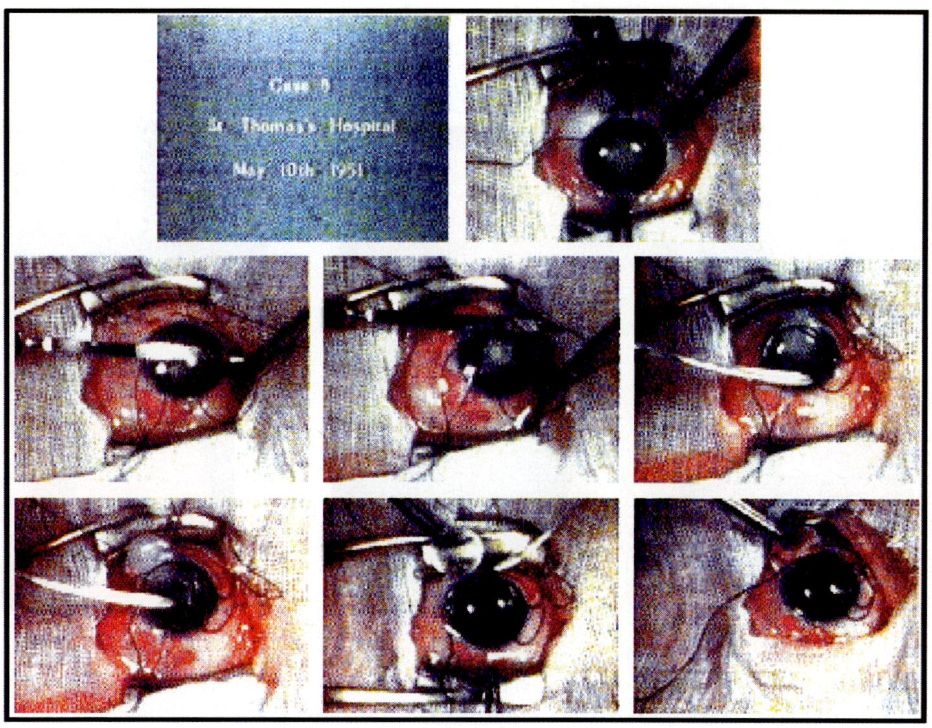

Fig. 57.2: Photographs of Ridley's 8th implant operation, on May 10, 1951. These pictures were taken from the original film. The clips range from the von Graefe incision of approximately 10-11 mm in length (upper left) to the lens removal (lower left) and the IOL insertion (low center and right)

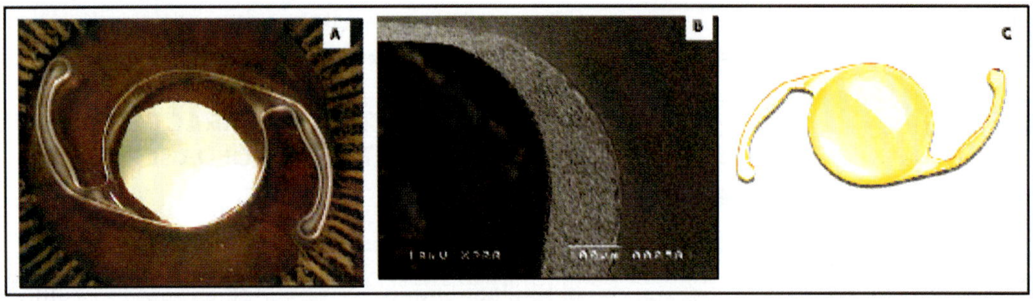

Fig. 57.3A to C: Illustrate characteristics of the single-piece AcrySof™ lens (Alcon Labs., Fort Worth, TX, USA). A: Gross photograph of a human eye obtained postmortem implanted with this lens design, showing optimal centration of the lens and clear capsular bag. B: Scanning electron photomicrograph showing the "velvet" finishing of the lens edge. C: Gross photograph showing the yellow color of the AcrySof™ Natural lens (under investigation)

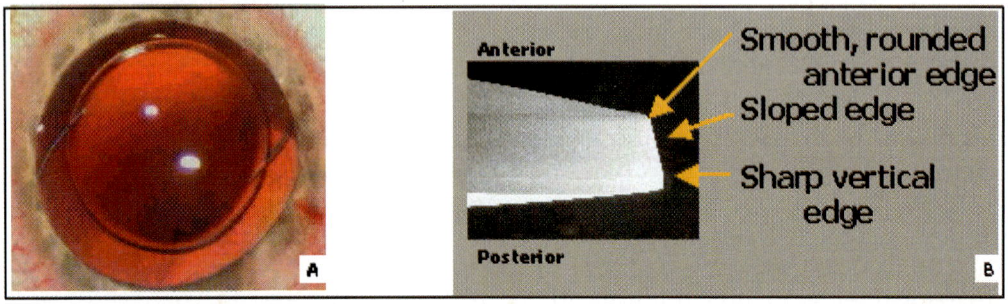

Figs 57.4A and B: present features of the Sensar™ lens with the OptiEdge™ technology (Allergan Inc., Irvine, CA, USA). This design is stated to combine the advantage of truncated optics and at the same time eliminate the drawbacks such as glare, etc. A: Clinical picture of a patient implanted with this lens design (courtesy: Allergan Surgical). B: Scanning electron photomicrograph showing the 3 components of the OptiEdge™

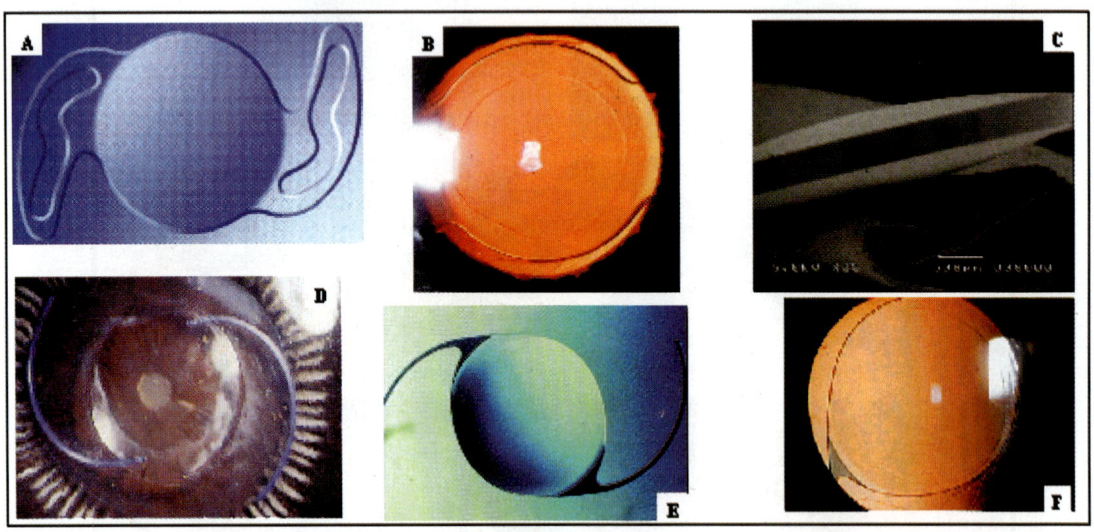

Figs 57.5A to F: Summarize some of the hydrophilic acrylic lenses being used today. A: Gross photograph showing the Rayner Centerflex™ lens. B: Clinical picture of a patient implanted with this lens design (courtesy: Dr. Michael Amon, Vienna, Austria). C: Scanning electron photomicrograph showing the square edge of the Centerflex™ lens. D: Gross photograph of a human eye obtained postmortem implanted with the Ciba Vision MemoryLens™, showing good centration of the lens and clear capsular bag, with the exception of the presence of Soemmering's ring formation limited to one quadrant. E: Gross photograph showing the Bausch and Lomb Hydroview™ lens. F: Clinical picture of a patient implanted with this lens design (courtesy: Dr. Manfred Tetz, Berlin, Germany)

segment surgeon (Figs 57.3 to 57.5).[5,6] Choice of foldable lens design varies from surgeon to surgeon. Foldable lenses with truncated optics manufactured from hydrophobic acrylic lenses are preferred by the surgeons due to reduced incidence of posterior capsule opacification (PCO).

Silicone polymer was the first biomaterial used for foldable lenses (Figs 57.6A to C).

ULTRASMALL INCISION CATARACT SURGERY AND IMPLANTATION OF ROLLABLE LENSES

Bimanual phacoemulsification can now be performed through an ultrasmall (0.9 mm) incision

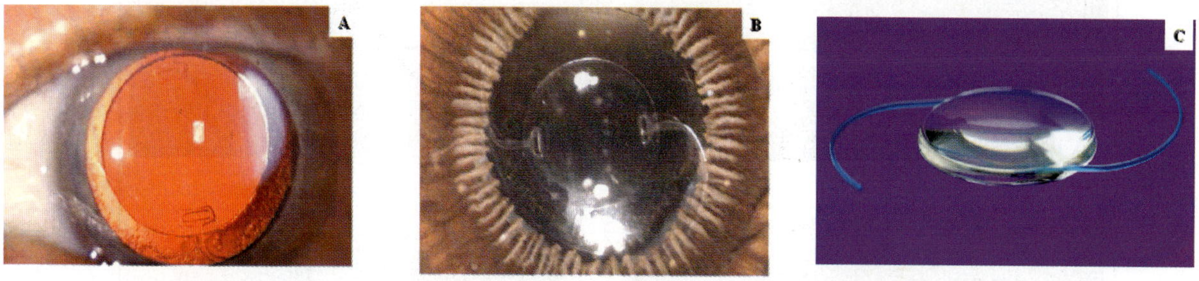

Figs 57.6A to C: Illustrate the newly available silicone lenses. A: Clinical picture of a patient implanted with the CeeOn Edge™ (Pharmacia Inc., Peapack, NJ, USA) lens (Courtesy: Dr KD Solomon, Charleston, SC, USA). B: Gross photograph showing an experimental implantation of the same lens design in a human eye obtained postmortem, prepared according to the Miyake-Apple posterior video-photographic technique. C: Gross photograph showing the ClariFlex™ 3-piece silicone lens with the OptiEdge™ technology (Allergan Inc., Irvine, CA, USA)

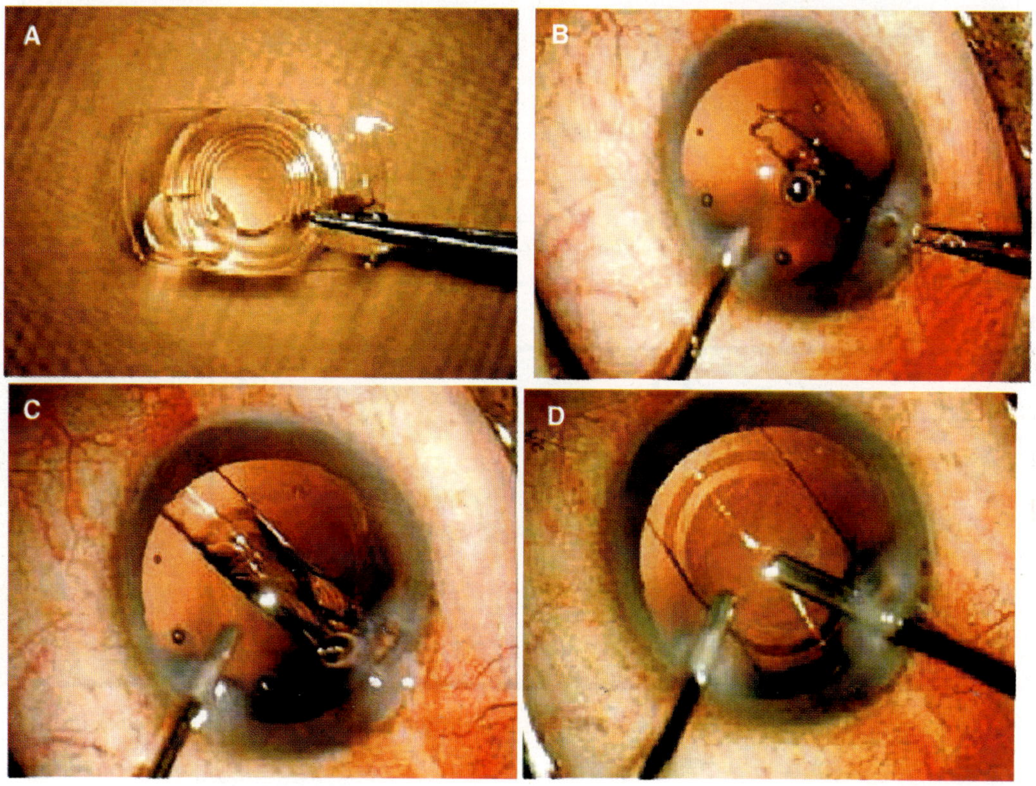

Figs 57.7A to D: Illustrate the Phakonit technique with implantation of the ThinOptX™ rollable IOL (Abingdon, VA, USA). A: Photograph showing the ThinOptX™ rollable IOL. B: The cataract was removed through a 0.9 mm incision using the phakonit technique. The ThinOptX™ IOL was gently rolled between the thumb and index fingers of the surgeon and inserted through a sub-1.5 mm incision. C: The ThinOptX™ IOL is unfolding inside the capsular bag, upon normal body temperature. D: Note the well-centered ThinOptX™ IOL in the capsular bag. Viscoelastic solution is being removed using bimanual irrigation/aspiration probes. AcrySmart™ is another IOL design that can be inserted through ultrasmall incision as shown in Figures 8A-D

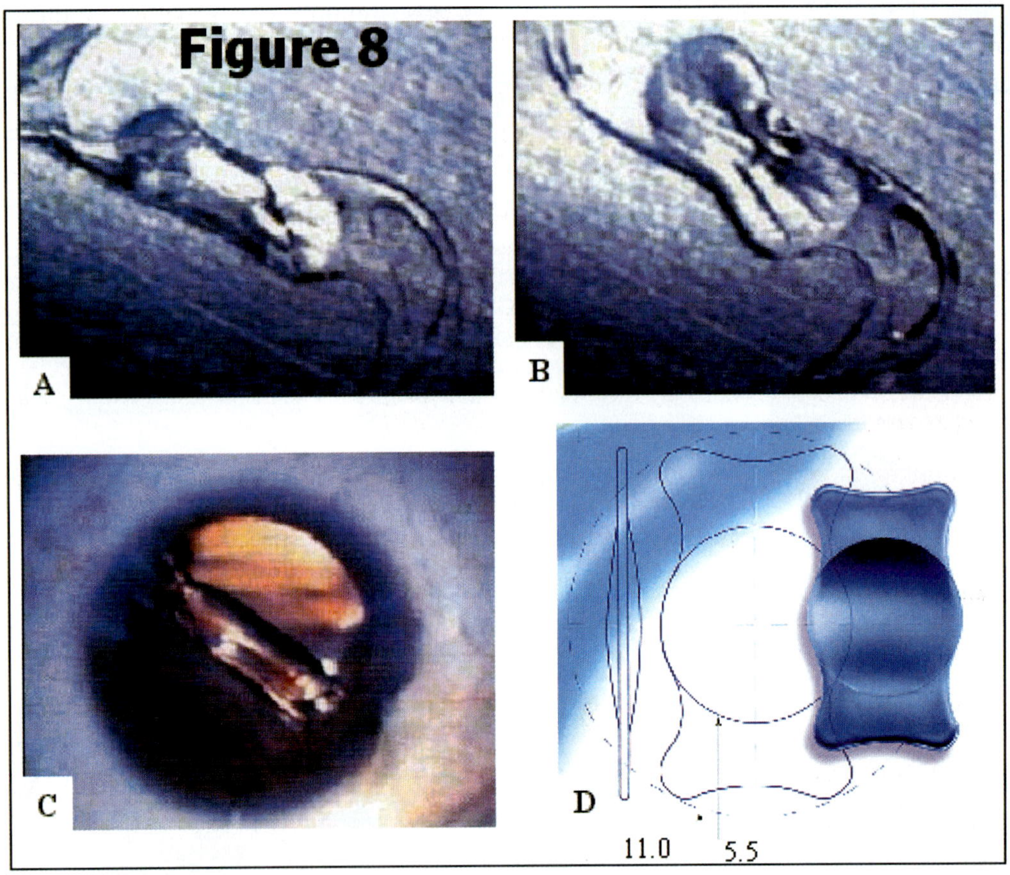

Fig. 57.8A to D: Illustrate the AcrySmart™ IOL design. The pre-folded dehydrated IOL unfolds in balanced salt solution (model H44-IC-1). B: Later stage in the unfolding process. C: The pre-folded dehydrated IOL was inserted in the capsular bag. D: Gross photograph showing the AcrySmart™ model 48 S

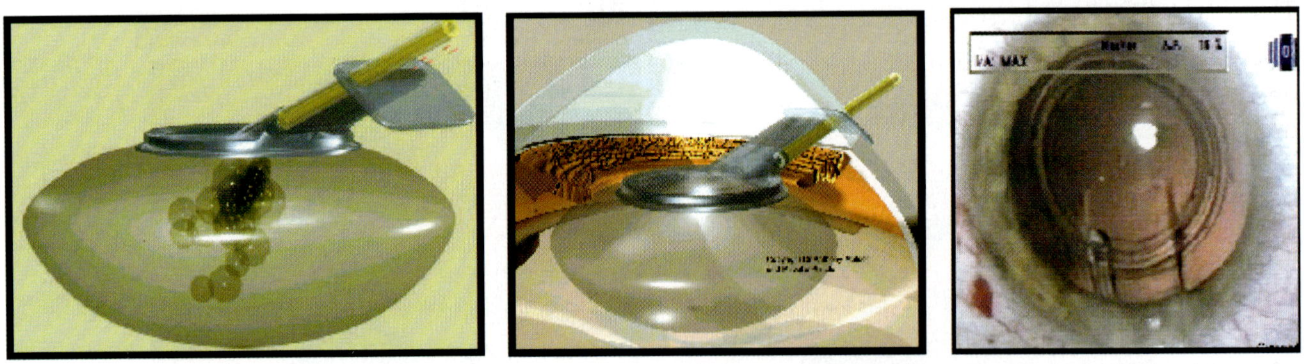

Fig. 57.9: Illustrate the concept of a sealed capsule irrigation device (SCID) or perfect capsule being developed by Dr Anthony Maloof

using the "Phakonit" technique. Pioneered by Dr Amar Agarwal, "Phakonit" had been performed in more than 500 cases without use of topical anesthesia.[7,8] Ongoing research for the development of laser probes, cold phaco, microphaco, and micro-incision cataract surgery (MICS) confirm the interest of leading ophthalmologists and manufacturers in the direction of ultrasmall incisional cataract surgery.

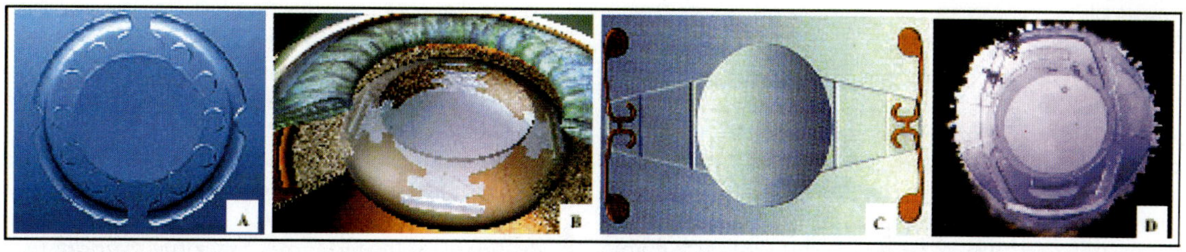

Fig. 57.10A to D: A: Gross photograph showing the Morcher BioComFold™ lens. B: Schematic drawing representing the HumanOptics Accommodative 1 CU lens implanted in the capsular bag of a human eye. C: Schematic drawing representing the C and C CrystaLens™. D: Gross photograph showing an experimental implantation of the Visiogen Inc. (Irvine, CA, USA) intraocular accommodating system in a human eye obtained postmortem, prepared according to the Miyake-Apple posterior video-photographic technique. The capsular bag of the eye was stained with trypan blue, to enhance visualization of the lens. The picture was taken from an anterior view with retroillumination

Table 57.1: Six factors to eradicate PCO

Three surgery-related factors ("capsular" surgery)	*Three IOL-related factors ("Ideal" IOL)*
1. Hydrodissection-enhanced cortical clean-up	1. Biocompatible IOL to reduce stimulation of cellular proliferation
2. In-the-bag fixation	2. Maximal IOL optic-posterior capsule contact, angulated hepatic, "bioadhesive" biomaterial to create a "shrink wrap"
3. Small CCC diameter slightly smaller than that of IOL optic. This places the CCC edge on the anterior surface of the optic and helps sequester the capsular bag. This creates a "shrink wrap" of the capsule around the IOL optic	3. IOL optic geometry square, truncated edge

Section 4

THE FUTURE CHALLENGES

Despite of considerable advancement surgeons need to overcome two important challenges. These include:

A. Eradication of posterior capsule opacification
B. Restoration of accommodation

Eradication of Posterior Capsule Opacification

We have proposed 6 factors to eradicate PCO (Table 57.1).[10] Efforts are in progress to eradicate PCO, a nagging complication of cataract-IOL surgery. Eradication of PCO is critical for success of multifocal and accommodative lenses.

Restoration of Accommodation

Efforts are in progress to restore accommodation after cataract-IOL surgery using accommodative lenses as shown in Figures 57.10A to D.

REFERENCES

1. Apple DJ, Auffarth GU, Peng Q, Visessook N. Foldable intraocular lenses: Evolution, clinicopathologic correlations, complications. Thorofare, NJ, Slack, 2000.
2. Apple DJ, Ram J, Foster A, Peng Q. Elimination of cataract blindness: A global perspective entering the new millennium. Surv Ophthalmol 2000; 45:S1-S160.
3. Pandey SK, Wilson ME, Trivedi RH, Izak A, Macky TA, Werner L, Apple DJ. Pediatric cataract surgery and intraocular lens implantation: Current techniques, complications and management. Int Ophthalmol Clin 2001; 41:175-96.
4. Lineberger EJ, Hardten DR, Shah GK, Lindstrom RL. Phacoemulsification and modern cataract surgery. Surv Ophthalmol 1999; 44:123-47.
5. Werner L, Apple DJ, Schmidbauer JM. New intraocular lenses, new technology. In: Buratto L, Werner L, Zannini M, Apple DJ (Eds): Phacoemulsification Principles and Techniques. Thorofare, Slack, NJ, 2002 (In press).
6. Werner L, Izak AM, Isaacs RT, Pandey SK, Apple DJ. Evolution and pathology of intraocular lens implantation.

In: Yanoff M, Ducker JS (Eds): Ophthalmology. St Louis, Mosby-Yearbook, 2002 (in press).
7. Agarwal A, Agarwal S, Pandey SK, Agarwal A, Bagmar A, Shah SP. Phakonit: Lens removal through 0.9 mm incision. J Cataract Refract Surg 2001; 27:1531.
8. Pandey SK, Werner L, Agarwal A, Agarwal S, Agarwal A, Lal V, Patel N, Hoyos JE, Callahan W, Callahan JS, Callahan JD. Phakonit: Cataract removal through a sub-1mm incision and implantation of ThinOptX® rollable intraocular lens. J Cataract Refract Surg 2002 (in press).
9. Pandey SK, Werner L, Apple DJ, Agarwal A, Agarwal A, Agarwal S. No anesthesia clear corneal phacoemulsification versus topical and topical plus intracameral anesthesia: Randomized clinical trial. J Cataract Refract Surg 2001;27:1643-50.
10. Werner L, Apple DJ, Pandey SK. Postoperative proliferation of anterior and equatorial lens epithelial cells. In: Buratto L, Osher RH, Masket S (Eds): Cataract Surgery in Complicated Cases. Slack Inc., Thorofare, NJ, 2000;399-417.

Index

D

E

F

G

H

I

J

K

L

M

N

Index

R

S

T

U

V

W

Z